Manual of Neonatal Care

Fifth Edition

Manual of Neonatal Care

Fifth Edition

Editors

John P. Cloherty, M.D.
Associate Neonatologist
Children's Hospital, Boston
Associate Clinical Professor
of Pediatrics
Harvard Medical School
Boston, Massachusetts

Eric C. Eichenwald, M.D.
Department of Newborn Medicine
Brigham and Women's Hospital
Assistant Professor of Pediatrics
Harvard Medical School
Boston, Massachusetts

Ann R. Stark, M.D.
Associate Clinical Professor
of Pediatrics
Harvard Medical School
Boston, Massachusetts

LIPPINCOTT WILLIAMS & WILKINS
A **Wolters Kluwer** Company
Philadelphia · Baltimore · New York · London
Buenos Aires · Hong Kong · Sydney · Tokyo

Acquisitions Editor: Timothy Y. Hiscock
Developmental Editor: Kerry B. Barrett
Production Editor: Frank Aversa
Manufacturing Manager: Ben Rivera
Cover Designer: Christine Jenny
Compositor: Print Matters/Compset, Inc.
Printer: RR Donnelley, Crawfordsville

Library of Congress Cataloging-in-Publication Data
Manual of neonatal care / [edited by] John P. Cloherty, Eric C. Eichenwald and Ann R. Stark; Joint Program in Neonatology. —5th ed.
   p. ; cm.
   Includes bibliographical references and index.
   ISBN 0-7817-3599-8 (HC)
   1. Neonatology—Handbooks, manuals, etc.   I. Cloherty, John P.
II. Eichenwald, Eric C.   III. Stark, Ann R.   IV. Joint Program in Neonatology.
   [DNLM: 1. Infant, Newborn, Diseases—Handbooks.   2. Infant Care—
Handbooks.   3. Neonatology—methods—Handbooks.   WS 39 M2945 2003]
   RJ251.M26   2003
   618.92'.01—dc21

                                  2003047702

*We dedicate this edition
to our spouses: Ann, Caryn, and Peter*

*to our children: Maryann, David, Joan, Neil, Danny,
Monica, Tommy, Victoria, Anne, Tim, Zachary,
Taylor, Connor, Laura, and Gregory*

*to our grandchildren: Chrissy, Elizabeth, Daniel,
Sophie, Jack, John, Tom, and Ryan*

*to the many babies and parents
we have cared for, and*

*to the memory of our colleague and friend,
Doug Richardson (1951–2002)*

CONTENTS

CONTRIBUTING AUTHORS

Elisa Abdulhayoglu, M.D.
Associate Chief, Department of Neonatology, Newton-Wellesley Hospital, Newton, Massachusetts, Instructor in Pediatrics, Harvard Medical School, Boston, Massachusetts

Maureen Allen, R.N., B.S.N, I.B.C.L.C.
Lactation Consultant, Neonatal Intensive Care Unit, Brigham and Women's Hospital, Boston, Massachusetts

John Arnold, M.D.
Associate Director, MICU, Medical Director, Respiratory Care, ECMO Program, and Biomedical Engineering, Children's Hospital; Associate Professor of Anesthesia, Harvard Medical School, Boston, Massachusetts

Sanjay Aurora, M.D.
Director, Newborn Medicine, North Shore Medical Center, Salem, Massachusetts

Tara K. Bastek, M.D.
Fellow Newborn Medicine, Division of Newborn Medicine, Children's Hospital, Clinical Fellow in Pediatrics, Harvard Medical School, Boston, Massachusetts

Diana W. Bianchi, M.D.
Chief, Division of Genetics, Department of Pediatrics, Tufts-New England Medical Center, Natalie V. Zucker Professor, Departments of Pediatrics, Obstetrics, and Gynecology, Tufts University School of Medicine, Boston, Massachusetts

Dara D. Brodsky, M.D.
Neonatologist, Children's Hospital, Instructor in Pediatrics, Harvard Medical School, Boston, Massachusetts

Sandra K. Burchett, M.D., M.S.
Clinical Director, Infectious Diseases, Children's Hospital, Assistant Professor of Pediatrics, Harvard Medical School, Boston, Massachusetts

Sule Cataltepe, M.D.
Neonatologist, Brigham and Women's Hospital, Instructor in Pediatrics, Harvard Medical School, Boston, Massachusetts

Kimberlee Chatson, M.D.
Associate Director, Special Care Nursery, Winchester Hospital, Winchester, Massachusetts; Instructor in Pediatrics, Harvard Medical School, Boston, Massachusetts

Helen A. Christou, M.D.
Neonatologist, Children's Hospital; Assistant Professor of Pediatrics, Harvard Medical School, Boston, Massachusetts

John Chuo, M.D.
Fellow in Newborn Medicine, Children's Hospital, Harvard Medical School, Boston, Massachusetts

John P. Cloherty, M.D.
Neonatologist, Children's Hospital; Associate Clinical Professor of Pediatrics, Harvard Medical School, Boston, Massachusetts

William D. Cochran, M.D.
Senior Associate in Medicine, Newborn Intensive Care Unit, Beth Israel Deaconess Medical Center; Associate Clinical Professor of Pediatrics, Emeritus, Harvard Medical School, Boston, Massachusetts

Mehrengise Cooper, M.B.B.S., M.R.C.P.
Fellow in Pediatric Intensive Care, The Hospital for Sick Children, London, United Kingdom

Olivier Danhaive, M.D.
Attending Physician, Department of Neonatology, Bambino Gesù Children's Hospital, Rome, Italy; Former Instructor, Pediatrics, Harvard Medical School, Boston, Massachusetts

Tola Dawodu, Pharm.D.
Clinical Pharmacy Specialist, Brigham and Women's Hospital, Adjunct Instructor Clinical Pharmacy Practice, Massachusetts College of Pharmacy, Boston, Massachusetts

Caryn E. Douma, B.S.N., I.B.C.L.C.
Staff Nurse, Neonatal Intensive Care Unit, Brigham and Women's Hospital, Boston, Massachusetts

Adré J. du Plessis, M.B.Ch.B., M.P.H.
Associate in Neurology, Children's Hospital; Director, Neonatal Neurology Clinical and Research Programs, Associate Professor of Neurology, Harvard Medical School, Boston, Massachusetts

Eric C. Eichenwald, M.D.
Associate Director, Newborn Intensive Care Unit, Brigham and Women's Hospital; Assistant Professor of Pediatrics, Harvard Medical School, Boston, Massachusetts

Deirdre Ellard, M.S., R.D./L.D.N., C.N.S.D.
Neonatal Nutritionist, Brigham and Women's Hospital, Boston, Massachusetts

Marie T. Field, M.S., R.N.
Clinical Education, Pediatrician, Newborn Intensive Care Unit, Brigham and Women's Hospital, Boston, Massachusetts

Allen M. Goorin, M.D.
Associate Professor of Pediatrics, Harvard Medical School, Boston, Massachusetts

James Gray, M.D., M.S.
Associate Neonatologist, Beth Israel Deaconess Medical Center; Instructor in Pediatrics, Harvard Medical School, Boston, Massachusetts

Nicholas G. Guerina, M.D., Ph.D.
Neonatologist, Assistant Professor of Pediatrics, Tufts University-New England Medical Center, Boston, Massachusetts

Munish Gupta, M.D.
Fellow in Newborn Medicine, Children's Hospital, Boston, Massachusetts

Anne R. Hansen, M.D., M.P.H.
Clinical Director of Newborn Intensive Care Unit, Children's Hospital; Assistant Professor of Pediatrics, Harvard Medical School, Boston, Massachusetts

Sandra Harmon, R.N., B.S.
*Staff Nurse, Neonatal Intensive Care Unit, Brigham and Women's Hospital,
Boston, Massachusetts*

Linda J. Heffner, M.D.
*Director of Maternal–Fetal Medicine, Brigham and Women's Hospital; Professor
of Obstetrics, Gynecology and Reproductive Biology, Harvard Medical School,
Boston, Massachusetts*

John T. Herrin, M.B.B.S., F.R.A.C.P.
*Director Dialysis Unit, Division of Nephrology, Children's Hospital; Associate
Clinical Professor, Department of Pediatrics, Harvard Medical School,
Boston, Massachusetts*

Dynio Honrubia, M.D.
*Neonatologist, Cedar-Sinai Medical Center; Assistant Professor of Pediatrics,
U.C.L.A. School of Medicine, Los Angeles, California*

Kathleen M. Howard, R.N., B.S.N., I.B.C.L.C.
*Clinical Research Nurse, Newborn Medicine, Brigham and Women's Hospital,
Boston, Massachusetts*

Kenneth M. Huttner, M.D., Ph.D.
*Neonatologist, Division of Newborn Medicine, Massachusetts General Hospital;
Assistant Professor of Pediatrics, Harvard Medical School, Boston, Massachusetts*

Robert M. Insoft, M.D.
*Medical Director, Neonatal and Pediatric Transport Services, Massachusetts General
Hospital; Assistant Professor of Pediatrics, Harvard Medical School, Boston,
Massachusetts*

Michael R. Jackson, R.R.T.
*Respiratory Care, Neonatal Intensive Care Unit, Brigham and Women's Hospital,
Boston, Massachusetts*

James R. Kasser, M.D.
*Orthopedic Surgeon-in-Chief, Children's Hospital; John E. Hall Professor,
Orthopedic Surgery, Harvard Medical School, Boston, Massachusetts*

Constance H. Keefer, M.D.
*Pediatrician, Instructor in Pediatrics, Harvard Medical School, Brigham and
Women's Hospital, Boston, Massachusetts*

Melanie S. Kim, M.D.
*Associate Residency Director, Department of Pediatrics, Boston Medical Center;
Associate Professor of Pediatrics, Boston University School of Medicine, Boston,
Massachusetts*

Stella Kourembanas, M.D.
*Neonatologist, Brigham and Women's Hospital, Children's Hospital; Associate
Professor of Pediatrics, Harvard Medical School, Boston, Massachusetts*

Jane S. Lee, M.D., M.P.H.
*Neonatologist, Division of Neonatology, Children's Hospital of New York–Presbyterian;
Assistant Professor of Pediatrics, Columbia University College of Physicians and
Surgeons, New York, New York*

Kimberly Gronsman Lee, M.D., M.S., I.B.C.L.C.
Associate Director, Newborn Nursery, Beth Israel Deaconess Medical Center;
Instructor in Pediatrics, Harvard Medical School, Boston, Massachusetts

Aviva Lee-Parritz, M.D.
Medical Director, Labor and Delivery, Brigham and Women's Hospital;
Instructor, Obstetrics, Harvard Medical School, Boston, Massachusetts

Harvey L. Levy, M.D.
Associate Professor of Pediatrics, Harvard Medical School, Boston, Massachusetts

Patricia Wei Lin, M.D.
Neonatologist, Assistant Professor of Pediatrics, Emory University School of
Medicine, Atlanta, Georgia

Nancy A. Louis, M.D.
Neonatologist, Brigham and Women's Hospital, Boston, Massachusetts

Camilia R. Martin, M.D., M.S.
Associate Director, Neonatal Intensive Care Unit, Beth Israel Deaconess Medical
Center; Instructor in Pediatrics, Department of Medicine, Harvard Medical School,
Boston, Massachusetts

Karen R. McAlmon, M.D.
Medical Director, Special Care Nursery, Winchester Hospital, Winchester,
Massachusetts, Instructor in Pediatrics, Newborn Medicine, Harvard Medical School,
Boston, Massachusetts

Ellis Neufeld, M.D.
Director, Clinical Hematology, Director, Boston Center for Genetic Blood Diseases,
Children's Hospital; Associate Professor of Pediatrics, Harvard Medical School,
Boston, Massachusetts

Mark T. Ogino, M.D.
Former Director, NICU, Massachusetts General Hospital, Instructor, Harvard
Medical School, Boston, Massachusetts; Kaiser Permanente Medical Center, NICU,
Honolulu, Hawaii

Irene E. Olsen, Ph.D., R.D.
Postdoctoral Research Fellow, Gastroenterology and Nutrition Division,
Children's Hospital of Philadelphia, Philadelphia, Pennsylvania,

Stephanie Packard, R.N.
Staff Nurse III, Newborn Intensive Care Unit, Children's Hospital, Boston,
Massachusetts

Richard Parad, M.D., M.P.H.
Neonatologist, Brigham and Women's Hospital, Assistant Professor of Pediatrics,
Harvard Medical School, Boston, Massachusetts

Rita Patnode, M.S.N, P.N.P.
Staff Nurse, Brigham and Women's Hospital, Boston, Massachusetts

Corinne Cyr Pryor, R.N.C, B.A., I.B.C.L.C.
Staff Nurse, Brigham and Women's Hospital, Boston, Massachusetts

Karen M. Puopolo, M.D., Ph.D.
Neonatologist, Brigham and Women's Hospital; Instructor in Pediatrics,
Harvard Medical School, Boston, Massachusetts

Steven A. Ringer, M.D., Ph.D.
Chief, Department of Newborn Medicine, Brigham and Women's Hospital, Assistant Professor of Pediatrics, Harvard Medical School, Boston, Massachusetts

Diana Rodriguez-Thompson, M.D., M.P.H.
Maternal Fetal Medicine Specialist, Naval Medical Center Portsmouth, Portsmouth, Virginia

David H. Rowitch, M.D., Ph.D.
Neonatologist, Children's Hospital; Assistant Professor of Pediatrics, Harvard Medical School, Boston, Massachusetts

Sylvia Schechner, M.D., M.P.H.
Harvard Vanguard Medical Associate Neonatologist, Brigham and Women's Hospital, Children's Hospital, Beth Israel Deaconess Medical Center, Assistant Clinical Professor of Pediatrics, Harvard Medical School, Boston, Massachusetts

Mary Deming Scott, M.D.
Associate in Medicine, Children's Hospital; Instructor in Pediatrics, Harvard Medical School, Boston, Massachusetts

Charles F. Simmons Jr., M.D.
Ruth and Harry Roman Chair in Neonatology, Cedar–Sinai Medical Center; Professor of Pediatrics, David Geffen School of Medicine at UCLA, Los Angeles, California

Steven Sloane, M.D.
Medical Director, Blood Bank, Children's Hospital, Assistant Professor of Pathology, Harvard Medical School, Boston, Massachusetts

Evan Y. Snyder, M.D., Ph.D.
Neonatologist, Children's Hospital, Assistant Professor of Pediatrics and Neurology, Harvard Medical School, Boston, Massachusetts,

Janet S. Soul, M.D., C.M. F.R.C.P.C.
Associate Director of Neonatal Neurology Program, Children's Hospital, Boston, Massachusetts, Instructor in Neurology, Harvard Medical School, Boston, Massachusetts

Norman P. Spack, M.D.
Clinical Director, Endocrine Division, Children's Hospital, Assistant Professor of Pediatrics, Harvard Medical School, Boston, Massachusetts

Ann R. Stark, M.D.
Neonatologist, Brigham and Women's Hospital, Associate Clinical Professor of Pediatrics, Harvard Medical School, Boston, Massachusetts

Jane E. Stewart, M.D.
Co-Director, Infant Follow-up Program, Beth Israel Deaconess Medical Center; Instructor in Pediatrics, Harvard Medical School, Boston, Massachusetts

Jeffrey W. Stolz, M.D., M.P.H.
Medical Director, High Risk Infant Follow-up Program, Swedish Medical Center, Seattle, Washington

Yao Sun, M.D., Ph.D.
Neonatologist, Children's Hospital; Instructor in Pediatrics, Harvard Medical School, Boston, Massachusetts

Linda J. Van Marter, M.D.
Neonatologist, Brigham and Women's Hospital, Associate Professor of Pediatrics, Harvard Medical School, Boston, Massachusetts

Louis Vernacchio, M.D., M.Sc.
Pediatrician, Children's Hospital; Instructor in Pediatrics, Harvard Medical School; Adjunct Assistant Professor of Epidemiology, Boston University, Boston, Massachusetts

Stephanie Burns Wechsler, M.D.
Clinical Assistant Professor, Division of Pediatric Cardiology, Departments of Pediatrics and Communicable Diseases, University of Michigan Health System, Ann Arbor, Michigan

Gil Wernovsky, M.D., F.A.C.C., F.A.A.P.
Director, Program Development, Staff Cardiologist, Cardiac Intensive Care Unit, Cardiac Center at the Children's Hospital of Philadelphia; Associate Professor in Pediatrics, University of Pennsylvania School of Medicine, Philadelphia, Pennsylvania

Richard E. Wilker, M.D.
Chief of Neonatology, Newton-Wellesley Hospital, Newton, Massachusetts, Instructor in Pediatrics, Harvard Medical School, Boston, Massachusetts

Louise Wilkins-Haug, M.D., Ph.D.
Director, Center for Fetal Medicine and Prenatal Genetics, Brigham and Women's Hospital; Assistant Professor, Obstetrics, Gynecology, and Reproductive Biology, Harvard Medical School, Boston, Massachusetts

Linda Zaccagnini, R.N.C, M.S., N.N.P.
Neonatal Nurse Practitioner, Beth Israel Deaconess Medical Center, Boston, Massachusetts

John A.F. Zupancic, M.D., Sc.D.
Associate Director, Neonatal Intensive Care Unit, Beth Israel Deaconess Medical Center; Assistant Professor of Pediatrics, Harvard Medical School, Boston, Massachusetts

FOREWORD

Since its inception in 1980, the *Manual of Neonatal Care* has represented an incisive and cogent approach toward the clinical management of critically ill newborns. As our understanding of the pathogenesis of both acquired and constitutional developmental disorders has increased, so has the complexity of our clinical decision-making. Thus, the fifth edition of the *Manual of Neonatal Care* represents our program's state-of-the-art diagnostic and therapeutic guidelines in this rapidly evolving pediatric subspecialty. We are indebted to the faculty and fellows of the Harvard Newborn Medicine Program and especially to the editors—John Cloherty, Ann Stark, and Eric Eichenwald—for their diligent and meticulous efforts in crafting these practice guidelines. Be assured, however, the editors have a keen understanding that the shelf-life of this edition must be monitored closely as the application of new knowledge in mammalian developmental biology and genetics is likely to have its greatest clinical impact in changing the ways in which we diagnose, prevent, and treat newborn diseases.

The logarithmic increase of knowledge in developmental biology will continue to have marked influences on newborn medicine. Developmental biology is concerned with how multicellular structures and processes that characterize the adult animal are generated from the fertilized egg. Recent advances in eukaryotic molecular genetics and experimental embryology have contributed to our understanding of the molecular mechanisms underlying complex differentiative (e.g., cell fates and segmentation) and morphogenic (e.g., limb and organ development) processes.

Indeed, over the past two decades, there has been a dramatic increase in the survival rate of very-low-birth-weight infants; especially those weighing less than 1000 g at birth. In part, this reduction in mortality is due to the application of advanced monitoring and supporting technology, combined with improvements in understanding the basic physiology of the newborn. This reduction in mortality also is due to an increased understanding of developmental systems (e.g., surfactant biosynthesis) and a means either to induce their maturation (e.g., antenatal glucocorticoids) or to correct for their deficiency (e.g., surfactant replacement therapy). However, additional advances in our understanding of developmental systems are required to improve further the outcomes of critically ill newborns.

The expansion in knowledge also has contributed to understanding the ways that cell behavior is controlled during the development of humans and other species. Especially significant has been the realization that there is conservation among animals both in developmental regulatory systems (e.g., control of developmental pathways by complexes of homeotic genes found originally in *Drosophila*, but present in mice and humans) and in the use of proteins that, for example, form the building blocks of the extracellular matrix and of the cytoskeleton—the molecular determinants of cell shape and multicellular organization. Other similarities between these model organisms include tissue responses to injury and wound repair, pathways associated with signal transduction and cell death, and regulation of the cell cycle and gene transcription. Thus, neonatologists can focus justifiably on these regulatory systems and similarities between humans and well-defined model organisms in developing new testable hypotheses that can be used ultimately to formulate novel therapies.

Advances in molecular genetics and genomics further point to new directions in neonatal care. Surprisingly, targeted deletions of genes—for example, *Wnt-1*, *Hox3.1*, *N-myc* (http://tbase.jax.org/) in mice—lead to death at birth or in the newborn period. These observations indicate that these genes function in the adaptation to extrauterine life. Although these results reveal unsuspected functions for several genes, they also emphasize that the developmental function of an increasing number and variety of genes are important for newborn medicine and that neonatologists will play an increasing role in understanding how these genes function. Improvements in genetic mapping techniques, including those for localizing genes associated with complex traits and the variability associated with single nucleotide polymorphisms (SNPs), will facilitate the identification of mutant or modifier genes in a large number of existing mouse mutants with aberrant developmental pathways and in human populations with defined phenotypes. These studies will be critical to understand human developmental abnormalities, such as those associated with neural tube defects and partial trisomies, as well as to understand antecedents of adult diseases, such as diabetes, hypertension, and cancer.

Comparisons between the genomic sequence of model organisms—such as those of roundworms, fruit flies, laboratory rats and mice, and humans—permit the exploration of gene function across several platforms. The advantage of using multiple platforms (organisms) is that simpler organisms often provide clues to gene function that are too expensive or intractable to explore in higher organisms. The accelerated rate at which developmental genes and pathways are being identified suggests that neonatologists would benefit from accessing genome-related databases and using new model systems. Thus, neonatologists with expertise in bioinformatics will help generate new knowledge that can be used to reveal the pathogenesis of newborn diseases.

Finally, high throughput proteomics (e.g., to detect protein-protein interactions); structural biology (e.g., for rational drug design); functional genomics (e.g., for gene expression arrays or promoter assessments); and SNP analysis (e.g., for phenotyping or haplotyping of individual traits, such as the ability to metabolize drugs or the affinity of a dopamine receptor); combined with increased understanding of microbial genomics, promises to revolutionize our approach to clinical medicine and host-pathogen interactions. However, this level of understanding will require a systems-based approach that extends beyond individual cells and molecules to include complex networks in the context of "good old-fashioned" bedside newborn physiology. So enjoy the fifth edition of the *Manual of Neonatal Care*. However, don't get too comfortable with it—the next edition is just over the horizon!

Gary A. Silverman, MD, PhD
Chief, Division of Newborn Medicine
Children's Hospital,
Boston, Massachusetts

1. FETAL ASSESSMENT AND PRENATAL DIAGNOSIS

Louise Wilkins-Haug and Linda J. Heffner

I. **Gestational-age assessment** is important to both the obstetrician and pediatrician, and must be made with a reasonable degree of precision. Elective obstetric interventions such as chorionic villus sampling (CVS) and amniocentesis must be timed appropriately. When premature delivery is inevitable, gestational age is important with regard to prognosis, the management of labor and delivery, and the initial neonatal treatment plan.

   A. **The clinical estimate** of gestational age is usually made based on the first day of the last menstrual period. Accompanied by physical examination, auscultation of fetal heart sounds and maternal perception of fetal movement can also be helpful.

   B. **Ultrasonic estimation** of gestational age. During the first trimester, fetal crown-rump length can be an accurate predictor of gestational age. Crown-rump-length estimation of gestational age is expected to be within 7 days of the true gestational age. During the second and third trimesters, measurements of the biparietal diameter (BPD) and the fetal femur length best estimate gestational age. Strict criteria for measuring the cross-sectional images through the fetal head ensure accuracy. Nonetheless, due to normal biologic variability, the accuracy of gestational age estimated by BPD decreases with increasing gestational age. For measurements made at 14–20 weeks of gestation, the variation is up to 11 days; at 20–28 weeks, up to14 days; and at 29–40 weeks, the variation can be up to 21 days. The length of the calcified fetal femur is often measured and used in validating BPD measurements or used alone in circumstances where BPD cannot be measured (e.g., deeply engaged fetal head) or is inaccurate (e.g., hydrocephalus).

II. **Prenatal diagnosis of fetal disease** continues to improve. The genetic or developmental basis for many disorders is emerging, along with increased test accuracy. Two types of tests are available: screening tests and diagnostic procedures. Screening tests, such as a sample of the mother's blood or an ultrasound, are safe but relatively nonspecific. A positive serum screening test, concerning family history, or a questionable ultrasonic examination may lead patient and physician to consider a diagnostic procedure. Diagnostic procedures, which necessitate obtaining a sample of fetal material, pose a small risk to both mother and fetus but can confirm or rule out the disorder in question.

   A. **Screening by maternal serum analysis** during pregnancy individualizes a woman's risk of carrying a fetus with a neural tube defect (NTD) or an aneuploidy such as trisomy 21 (Down syndrome) or trisomy 18 (Edward syndrome).

      1. **Maternal serum alpha-fetoprotein (MSAFP)** measurement between 15 and 22 weeks' gestation screens for NTDs. MSAFP elevated above 2.5 multiples of the median for gestation age occurs in 70–85% of fetuses with open spina bifida and 95% of fetuses with anencephaly. In half of the women with elevated levels, ultrasonic examination reveals another cause, most commonly an error in gestational age estimate. Ultrasound will often detect an NTD if present.

      2. **MSAFP/triple panel/quad panel:** Low levels of MSAFP are associated with chromosomal abnormalities. Altered levels of human chorionic gonadotropin (hCG), unconjugated estriol (UE3), and inhibin also are associated with fetal chromosomal abnormalities. On average, in a pregnancy with a fetus with trisomy 21, hCG levels are higher than expected and UE3 levels are decreased. A triple-panel screen in combination with maternal age can estimate the risk of trisomy 21 for an individual woman. For women less than 35 years old, 5% will have a positive triple screen, but

1

the majority (98%) will not have a fetus with aneuploidy. However, only about 70% of fetuses with trisomy 21 will have a "positive" maternal serum screen.

3. **First trimester serum screening:** Maternal levels of two analytes, pregnancy associated protein (PAPP-A) and hCG (either free or total) are altered in pregnancies with an aneuploid conception, especially trisomy 21. Like second trimester serum screening, these values can individualize a women's risk of pregnancy complicated by aneuploidy. However, these tests need to be drawn early in pregnancy (optimally at 9–10 weeks) and even if abnormal, detect less than half of the fetuses with trisomy 21.

4. **First trimester nuchal lucency screening:** Ultrasound assessment of the fluid collected at the nape of the fetal neck is a sensitive marker for aneuploidy. With attention to optimization of image and quality control, studies indicate a 70–80% detection of aneuploidy in pregnancies with an enlarged nuchal lucency on ultrasound. In addition, many fetuses with structural abnormalities such as cardiac defects, also will have an enlarged nuchal lucency.

B. In women with a **positive family history of genetic disease,** a positive screening test, or at-risk ultrasound features, diagnostic tests are considered. When a significant malformation or a genetic disease is diagnosed prenatally, the information gives the obstetrician and pediatrician time to educate parents, discuss options, and establish an initial neonatal treatment plan before the infant is delivered. In some cases, treatment may be initiated *in utero* (see Chap. 8).

1. **Chorionic villus sampling (CVS).** Under ultrasonic guidance, a sample of placental tissue is obtained via a catheter placed either transcervically or transabdominally. Performed at or after 10 weeks' gestation, CVS provides the earliest possible detection of a genetically abnormal fetus through analysis of trophoblast cells. Transabdominal CVS can also be used as late as the third trimester when amniotic fluid is not available or fetal blood sampling cannot be performed. Pregnancy loss is approximately 1%, as opposed to 0.5% after second trimester amniocentesis. The possible complications of amniocentesis and CVS are similar. CVS may be associated with an increased risk of fetal limb-reduction defects and oromandibular malformations.

   a. Direct preparations of rapidly dividing cytotrophoblasts can be prepared, making a full karyotype analysis available in 2 days. Although direct preparations minimize maternal cell contamination, most centers also analyze cultured trophoblast cells, which are embryologically closer to the fetus. This procedure takes an additional 8–12 days.

   b. In approximately 2% of CVS samples, both karyotypically normal and abnormal cells are identified. Because CVS-acquired cells reflect placental constitution, in these cases amniocentesis is often performed as a follow-up study to analyze fetal cells. About one-third of CVS mosaicisms are confirmed in the fetus via amniocentesis.

2. **Amniocentesis.** Amniotic fluid is removed from around the fetus via a needle guided by ultrasonic images. The removed amniotic fluid (about 20 mL) is replaced by the fetus within 24 hours. Amniocentesis can technically be performed as early as 10–14 weeks' gestation, although early amniocentesis (< 13 weeks) is associated with a pregnancy loss rate of 1–2%, and an increase incidence of clubfoot. Loss of the pregnancy following an ultrasound-guided second-trimester amniocentesis (16–20 weeks) occurs in 0.5–1.0% cases in most centers, so they are usually performed in the second trimester.

   a. **Amniotic fluid** can be analyzed for a number of compounds, including AFP, acetylcholinesterase (AChE), bilirubin, and pulmonary surfactant. Increased levels of AFP along with the presence of AChE identify NTDs with more than 98% sensitivity when the fluid sample is not contaminated by fetal blood. AFP levels are also elevated when the fetus has abdominal wall defects, congenital nephrosis, or intestinal atresias. In cases of **isoimmune hemolysis,** increased levels of bilirubin in the amniotic fluid reflect erythrocyte destruction. Amniotic fluid bilirubin proportional to the degree of hemolysis is dependent upon gestational age and can be used to predict fetal well-being (Liley curve). Pulmonary surfactant can be measured once or sequentially to assess fetal lung maturity (see Chap. 24).

    b. **Fetal cells** can be extracted from the fluid sample and analyzed for chromosomal and genetic makeup.

        (1) Among second-trimester amniocenteses, 73% of clinically significant karyotype abnormalities relate to one of five chromosomes: 13, 18, 21, X, or Y. These can be rapidly detected using fluorescent *in situ* hybridization, with sensitivities in the 90% range.

        (2) **DNA analysis** is diagnostic for an increasing number of diseases.

            (a) For genetic diseases in which the DNA sequence has not been determined, **indirect DNA studies** use restriction fragment length polymorphism (RFLP) for linkage analysis of affected individuals and family members. Both crossing over between the gene in question and the RFLP probe and the need for multiple informative members from a family limit the number of genetic diagnoses that can be made this way.

            (b) **Direct DNA methodologies** can be used when the gene sequence producing the disease in question is known. Disorders secondary to deletion of DNA (e.g., α-thalassemia, Duchenne and Becker muscular dystrophy, cystic fibrosis, and growth hormone deficiency) can be detected by the altered size of DNA fragments produced following a polymerase chain reaction (PCR). Direct detection of a DNA mutation can also be accomplished by allele-specific oligonucleotide (ASO) analysis. If the PCR-amplified DNA is not altered in size by a deletion or insertion, recognition of a mutated DNA sequence can occur by hybridization with the known mutant allele. ASO analysis allows direct DNA diagnosis of Tay-Sachs disease, alpha- and beta-thalassemia, cystic fibrosis, and phenylketonuria.

        (3) **DNA sequencing** for many genetic disorders has revealed that a multitude of different mutations within a gene can result in the same clinical disease. For example, cystic fibrosis can result from over 1000 different mutations. Thus, for any specific disease, prenatal diagnosis by DNA testing may require both direct and indirect methods.

3. Percutaneous umbilical blood sampling (PUBS) is performed under ultrasonic guidance from the second trimester until term. PUBS can provide diagnostic samples for cytogenetic, hematologic, immunologic, or DNA studies; it can also provide access for treatment *in utero*. An anterior placenta facilitates obtaining a sample close to the cord insertion site at the placenta. Fetal sedation is usually not needed. PUBS has a 1–2% risk of fetal loss along with complications that can lead to a preterm delivery in another 5%.

4. Preimplantation biopsy. Early in gestation (at the eight-cell stage in humans), one or two cells can be removed without known harm to the embryo. In women at risk for X-linked recessive disorders, determination by fluorescent *in situ* hybridization (FISH) of XX-containing embryos can enable transfer of only female embryos through assisted reproduction. Similarly, woman at increased risk of a chromosomally abnormal conception can benefit from pre-implantation biopsy. In women of advanced maternal age or when one member of a couple carries a balanced translocation, only those embryos that screen negative for the chromosome abnormality in question are transferred. Difficulties remain when more cells are needed for molecular diagnoses. An alternative approach is analysis of the second polar body, which contains the same genetic material as the ovum.

5. **Fetal cells in the maternal circulation.** The small number of fetal cells present in the maternal circulation can be separated and analyzed to identify chromosomal abnormalities. However, since there are only about 20 fetal cells in 20 mL of maternal blood, the inability to efficiently identify and separate these fetal cells has prohibited widespread use of this technique. Analysis of free fetal DNA, present at larger quantities in the maternal serum, is being explored as a possible aid in prenatal diagnosis.

III. **Fetal size and growth-rate abnormalities** may have significant implications for perinatal prognosis and care (see Chap. 3). Appropriate fetal assessment is important in establishing a diagnosis and a perinatal treatment plan.

A. **Intrauterine growth restriction (IUGR)** may be due to conditions in the fetal environment (e.g., chronic deficiencies in oxygen or nutrients or both) or to problems intrinsic to the fetus. It is important to identify constitutionally normal fetuses that are affected so that appropriate care can begin as soon as possible. Because their risk of mortality is increased several-fold before and during labor, IUGR fetuses may need preterm intervention for best survival rates. Once delivered, these newborns are at increased risk for immediate complications including hypoglycemia and pulmonary hemorrhage, so they should be delivered at an appropriately equipped facility.

Intrinsic causes of IUGR include chromosomal abnormalities (such as trisomies), congenital malformations, and congenital infections (e.g., cytomegalovirus or rubella). Prenatal diagnosis of malformed or infected fetuses is important so that appropriate interventions can be made. Prior knowledge that a fetus has a malformation (e.g., anencephaly) or chromosomal abnormality (e.g., trisomy 18) that adversely affects life allows the parents to be counseled before birth and may influence the management of labor and delivery.

1. **Definition of IUGR.** There is no universal agreement on the definition of IUGR. Strictly speaking, any fetus that does not reach his or her intrauterine growth potential is included. Historically, fetuses weighing less than the tenth percentile for gestational age or less than two standard deviations below the mean for gestational age have been classified as IUGR. However, many of these fetuses are merely constitutionally small. We consider all fetuses less than the tenth percentile for gestational age as small for gestational age and restrict the use of the term IUGR for those fetuses in whom corroborative evidence is present.

2. **Diagnosis of IUGR.** Clinical diagnostics detect no more than one-half of growth-restricted fetuses; ultrasound is far more sensitive. IUGR may be diagnosed with a single scan when a fetus less than the tenth percentile demonstrates corroborative signs of a compromised intrauterine environment such as oligohydramnios or an elevated head-abdomen ratio, or when the pregnancy is complicated by maternal risk factors such as hypertension. Serial scans documenting absent or poor intrauterine growth regardless of the weight percentile also indicate IUGR. Composite growth profiles derived from a variety of measurements and repeated serially provide the greatest sensitivity and specificity in diagnosing IUGR.

B. **Macrosomia.** Macrosomic fetuses (>4000 g) are at increased risk of shoulder dystocia and traumatic birth injury. Conditions such as maternal diabetes, post-term pregnancy, and maternal obesity are associated with an increased incidence of macrosomia. Unfortunately, efforts to use a variety of measurements and formulas have met with only modest success in predicting the condition.

IV. **Functional maturity of the lungs** is one of the most critical variable in determining neonatal survival in the otherwise normal fetus. A number of tests can be performed on amniotic fluid specifically to determine pulmonary maturity (see Chap. 24).

V. Assessment of fetal well-being. Acute compromise is detected by studies that assess fetal function. Some are used antepartum, while others are used to monitor the fetus during labor.

A. Antepartum tests generally rely on biophysical studies, which require a certain degree of fetal neurophysiologic maturity. The following tests are not used until the third trimester; fetuses may not respond appropriately earlier in gestation.

1. Fetal movement monitoring is the simplest method of fetal assessment. The mother lies quietly for an hour and records each perceived fetal movement. Although she may not perceive all fetal movements that might be noted by ultrasonic observation, she will record enough to provide meaningful data.

Fetuses normally have a sleep-wake cycle, and mothers generally perceive a diurnal variation in fetal activity. Active periods average 30–40 minutes. Periods of inactivity greater than 1 hour are unusual in a healthy fetus and should alert the physician to the possibility of fetal compromise.

2. The nonstress test (NST) is a reliable means of fetal evaluation. It is simple to perform, relatively quick, and noninvasive, with neither discomfort nor risk to mother or fetus.

The NST is based on the principle that fetal activity results in a reflex acceleration in heart rate. The required fetal maturity is typically reached by about 32 weeks of gestation. Absence of these accelerations in a fetus who previously demonstrated them may indicate that hypoxia has sufficiently depressed the central nervous system to inactivate the cardiac reflex.

The test is performed by monitoring fetal heart rate either through a Doppler ultrasound device or through skin-surface electrodes on the maternal abdomen. Uterine activity is simultaneously recorded through a tocodynamometer, palpation by trained test personnel, or the patient's report. The test result may be reactive, nonreactive, or inadequate. The criteria for a reactive test are as follows: (1) heart rate between 120 and 160, (2) normal beat-to-beat variability (5 beats per minute), and (3) two accelerations of at least 15 beats per minute lasting for not less than 15 seconds each within a 20-minute period. A nonreactive test fails to meet the three criteria. If an adequate fetal heart tracing cannot be obtained for any reason, the test is considered inadequate.

Statistics show that a reactive result is reassuring, with the risk of fetal demise within the week following the test at approximately 3 in 1000. A nonreactive test is generally repeated later the same day or is followed by another test of fetal well-being.

3. The contraction stress test (CST) may be used as a backup or confirmatory test when the NST is nonreactive or inadequate.

The CST is based on the idea that uterine contractions can compromise an unhealthy fetus. The pressure generated during contractions can briefly reduce or eliminate perfusion of the intervillous space. A healthy fetoplacental unit has sufficient reserve to tolerate this short reduction in oxygen supply. Under pathologic conditions, however, respiratory reserve may be so compromised that the reduction in oxygen results in fetal hypoxia. Under hypoxic conditions, the fetal heart rate slows in a characteristic way relative to the contraction. Fetal heart rate begins to decelerate 15–30 seconds after onset of the contraction, reaches its nadir after the peak of the contraction, and does not return to baseline until after the contraction ends. This heart-rate pattern is known as a late deceleration because of its relationship to the uterine contraction. Synonyms are type II deceleration or deceleration of uteroplacental insufficiency.

Like the NST, the CST monitors fetal heart rate and uterine contractions. A CST is considered completed if uterine contractions have spontaneously occurred within 30 minutes, lasted 40–60 seconds each, and occurred at a frequency of three within a 10-minute interval. If no spontaneous contractions occur, they can be induced with intravenous oxytocin, in which case the test is called an oxytocin challenge test.

A CST is positive if late decelerations are consistently seen in association with contractions. A CST is negative if at least three contractions of at least 40 seconds each occur within a 10-minute period without associated late decelerations. A CST is suspicious if there are occasional or inconsistent late decelerations. If contractions occur more frequently than every 2 minutes or last longer than 90 seconds, the study is considered a hyperstimulated test and cannot be interpreted. An unsatisfactory test is one in which contractions cannot be stimulated or a satisfactory fetal heart-rate tracing cannot be obtained.

A negative CST is even more reassuring than a reactive NST, with the chance of fetal demise within a week of a negative CST about 0.4 per 1000. If a positive CST follows a nonreactive NST, however, the risk of stillbirth is 88 per 1000, and the risk of neonatal mortality is also 88 per 1000. Statistically, about one-third of patients with a positive CST will require cesarean section for persistent late decelerations in labor.

4. The **biophysical profile** combines an NST with other parameters determined by real-time ultrasonic examination. A score of 0 or 2 is assigned for the absence or presence of each of the following: a reactive NST, adequate amniotic fluid volume, fetal breathing movements, fetal activity, and normal fetal musculoskeletal tone. The total score determines the course of action. Reassuring tests (8–10) are repeated at weekly intervals, while less-reassuring results (4–6) are repeated later the same day. Very low scores (0–2) generally prompt delivery. The likelihood that a fetus will die *in utero* within 1 week of a reassuring test is about the same as that for a negative CST, approximately 0.6–0.7 per 1000.

5. Doppler ultrasonography of **fetal umbilical artery blood flow** is a noninvasive technique to assess downstream (placental) resistance. Poorly functioning placentas with extensive vasospasm or infarction have an increased resistance to flow that is particularly noticeable in fetal diastole. Umbilical artery Doppler flow velocimetry may be used as part of fetal surveillance based on characteristics of the peak systolic frequency shift (S) and the end-diastolic frequency shift (D). The two commonly used indices of flow are the systolic:diastolic ratio (S/D) and the resistance index (S-D/S). Umbilical artery Doppler velocimetry measurements have been shown to improve perinatal outcome only in pregnancies with a presumptive diagnosis of IUGR and should not be used as a screening test in the general obstetric population. Absent or reversed end-diastolic flow is seen in the most extreme cases of IUGR and is associated with a high mortality rate. The use of umbilical artery Doppler velocimetry measurements, in conjunction with other tests of fetal well-being, can reduce the perinatal mortality in IUGR by almost 40%.

B. **Intrapartum assessment of fetal well-being** is important in the management of labor.

1. **Continuous electronic fetal monitoring** is widely used despite the fact that it has not been shown to reduce perinatal mortality or asphyxia relative to auscultation by trained personnel but has increased the incidence of operative delivery. When used, the monitors simultaneously record fetal heart rate and uterine activity for ongoing evaluation.

a. The **fetal heart rate** can be monitored in one of three ways. The noninvasive methods are ultrasonic monitoring and surface-electrode monitoring from the maternal abdomen. The most accurate but invasive method is to place a small electrode into the skin of the fetal presenting part to record the fetal electrocardiogram directly. Placement requires rupture of the fetal membranes. When the electrode is properly placed, it is associated with a very low risk of fetal injury. Approximately 4% of monitored babies develop a mild infection at the electrode site, and most respond to local cleansing.

b. Uterine activity can also be recorded either indirectly or directly. A tocodynamometer can be strapped to the maternal abdomen to record the timing and duration of contractions as well as crude relative intensity. When a more precise evaluation is needed, an intrauterine pressure catheter can be inserted following rupture of the fetal membranes to directly and quantitatively record contraction pressure. Invasive monitoring is associated with an increased incidence of chorioamnionitis and postpartum maternal infection.

c. Parameters of the fetal monitoring record that are evaluated include the following:

   (1) Baseline heart rate is normally between 120 and 160 beats per minute. Baseline bradycardia may result from congenital heart block associated with congenital heart malformation or maternal systemic lupus erythematosus. Tachycardia may result from fetal dysrhythmia, maternal fever, or chorioamnionitis.

   (2) Beat-to-beat variability is recorded from a calculation of each RR interval. The autonomic nervous system of a healthy, awake fetus constantly varies the heart rate from beat to beat by roughly 5–10 beats per minute. Reduced beat-to-beat variability may result from depression of the fetal central nervous system due to hypoxia, fetal sleep, fetal immaturity, or maternal narcotic or sedative use.

   (3) Accelerations of the fetal heart rate are reassuring, as they are during an NST.

   (4) Decelerations of the fetal heart rate may be benign or indicative of fetal distress depending on their characteristic shape and timing in relation to uterine contractions.

   (a) Early, type I, or head-compression decelerations are symmetric in shape and closely mirror uterine contractions in time of onset, duration, and termination. They are benign and usually accompany good beat-to-beat variability. The heart rate may slow to 60–80 beats per minute before returning to baseline. These decelerations are more commonly seen late in labor when the fetal head is compressed within the bony pelvis and vagina, resulting in a parasympathetic effect.

   (b) Late, type II, or uteroplacental insufficiency decelerations indicate fetal distress. Fetal heart rate decelerates 10–30 seconds after the contraction starts and does not return to baseline until after the contraction ends. A fall in the heart rate of only 10–20 beats per minute below baseline (even if still within the range of 120–160) is significant. With increasingly severe hypoxia, (1) beat-to-beat variability will be lost, (2) decelerations will last longer, (3) they will begin sooner following the onset of a contraction, (4) they will take longer to return to baseline, and (5) the rate to which the fetal heart slows will be lower. Repetitive late decelerations demand action. If maternal interventions such as oxygen supplementation fail, then a fetal scalp pH (see V.B.2) should be done to more precisely assess the level of fetal distress.

   (c) Variable, type III, or cord-pattern decelerations vary in their shape and in their timing relative to contractions. They are a cause for concern if they are severe (down to a rate of 60 beats per minute or lasting for 60 seconds or longer, or both), associated with poor beat-to-beat variability, or mixed with late decelerations. This pattern may result from compression of the umbilical cord, and a shift in maternal or fetal position or both will often cause the pattern to resolve.

2. A **fetal scalp blood sample for pH** determination is obtained to confirm or dismiss suspicion of fetal distress. An intrapartum scalp pH above 7.25 is normal. A pH between 7.20 and 7.25 is worrisome. If the pH is between 7.10 and 7.20, the clinical circumstances will dictate appropriate action. Fetuses with a scalp pH below 7.10 should be delivered immediately by the most expedient route.

Suggested Readings

Creasy R.K., Resnik R. (Eds.), *Maternal–fetal medicine: Principles and practice*, 4th ed. Philadelphia: Saunders, 1999.

Hay W.W., Jr, et al. Fetal growth: Its regulation and disorders. *Pediatrics* 1997; 99:585.

2. MATERNAL CONDITIONS THAT AFFECT THE FETUS

Diabetes Mellitus

Aviva Lee-Parritz and John P. Cloherty

I. **Background.** Improved management of diabetes mellitus and advances in obstetrics such as ultrasound and measurement of fetal lung maturity have reduced the incidence of adverse perinatal outcome in infants of diabetes mothers (IDMs). With appropriate management, women with good glycemic control and minimal microvascular disease can expect pregnancy outcomes comparable to the general population. Women with advanced microvascular disease, such as hypertension, nephropathy, and retinopathy, have a 25% risk of preterm delivery as a result of worsening maternal condition or preeclampsia. Pregnancy does not have a significant impact on the progression of diabetes. Women who begin pregnancy with microvascular disease often worsen, but the majority will return to baseline. However, women with ischemic heart disease secondary to diabetes may have up to a 50% mortality risk during pregnancy.

II. **Classification.** Diabetes that antedates the pregnancy is grouped by the White classification, according to the length of disease and presence of vascular complications (see Table 2.1). Gestational diabetes mellitus (GDM) is defined as carbohydrate intolerance of variable severity first diagnosed during pregnancy, and it affects 3% of pregnancies. Risk factors for GDM include advanced maternal age, multifetal gestation, increased body mass index, and strong family history of diabetes. Certain ethnic groups, such as Native Americans, southeast Asians, and African Americans are at increased risk of developing GDM. Approximately 3 to 5% of patients with gestational diabetes actually have underlying type 1 or type 2 diabetes, but pregnancy is the first opportunity for testing. GDM is typically diagnosed during the third trimester of pregnancy and is grouped by diet-controlled (White class A1) or insulin-requiring (White class A2).

III. **Maternal-fetal issues during pregnancy and delivery.** Tight glucose control is paramount during the periconceptional period and throughout pregnancy. The most common complication of IDMs is congenital anomalies. Approximately 6 to 10% of pregnancies complicated with diabetes will demonstrate a structural abnormality directly related to glycemic control in the period of organogenesis. The most common fetal structural defects associated with maternal diabetes are cardiac malformations, neural tube defects, renal agenesis, and skeletal malformations (see VI.F). In addition, maternal hyperglycemia leads to fetal hyperglycemia and fetal hyperinsulinemia, which results in fetal overgrowth. Fetal macrosomia is a risk factor for shoulder dystocia, fetal injury, and need for cesarean delivery (see VI.H).

A. In the first half of pregnancy, **hypoglycemia** is more common than **hyperglycemia** as a result of nausea and vomiting. Hypoglycemia, followed by hyperglycemia from counterregulatory hormones, can complicate diabetic control. Gastroparesis from long-standing diabetes may be a factor as well. There does not appear to be a direct relationship between hypoglycemia alone and adverse perinatal outcome.

B. **Ketoacidosis** is an uncommon complication during pregnancy but carries a 50% risk of fetal death, especially if it occurs before the third trimester. Ketoacidosis can be present in the setting of even mild hyperglycemia (200 mg/dL) and should be excluded in any patient who presents with hyperglycemia or symptoms consistent with ketoacidosis.

C. Throughout pregnancy, **insulin requirements** increase because of placental hormones that antagonize the action of insulin. This is most prominent in

TABLE 2.1. WHITE'S CLASSIFICATION OF MATERNAL DIABETES (REVISED*)

Gestational diabetes (GD):	Diabetes not known to be present before pregnancy
	Abnormal glucose tolerance test in pregnancy
GD diet	Euglycemia maintained by diet alone
GD insulin	Diet alone insufficient; insulin required
Class A:	Chemical diabetes; glucose intolerance before pregnancy; treated by diet alone; rarely seen
	Prediabetes; history of large babies more than 4 kg or unexplained stillbirths after 28 weeks
Class B:	Insulin-dependent; onset after 20 years of age; duration less than 10 years
Class C:	C_1: Onset at 10 to 19 years of age
	C_2: Duration 10 to 19 years
Class D:	D_1: Onset before 10 years of age
	D_2: Duration 20 years
	D_3: Calcification of vessels of the leg (macrovascular disease)
	D_4: Benign retinopathy (microvascular disease)
	D_5: Hypertension (not preeclampsia)
Class F:	Nephropathy with more than 500 mg per day of proteinuria
Class R:	Proliferative retinopathy or vitreous hemorrhage
Class RF:	Criteria for both classes R and F coexist
Class G:	Many reproductive failures
Class H:	Clinical evidence of arteriosclerotic heart disease
Class T:	Prior renal transplantation

Note: All classes below A require insulin. Classes R, F, RF, H, and T have no criteria for age of onset or duration of disease but usually occur in long-term diabetes.
Source: Modified from Hare J. W. Gestational diabetes. In: *Diabetes Complicating Pregnancy: The Joslin Clinic Method.* 1989; New York: Alan R. Liss.

the mid–third trimester and requires intensive blood glucose monitoring and frequent adjustment of insulin dosage.

D. Stillbirth remains an uncommon complication of diabetes is pregnancy. It is most often associated with poor glycemic control, fetal anomalies, severe vasculopathy, and intrauterine growth restriction (IUGR), as well as severe preeclampsia. Shoulder dystocia that cannot be resolved can also result in fetal death.

E. Polyhydramnios is not an uncommon finding in pregnancies complicated by diabetes. It may be due to secondary to osmotic diuresis from fetal hyperglycemia. Careful ultrasound examination is required to rule out structural anomalies, such as tracheal-esophageal fistula as an etiology when polyhydramnios is present.

F. Severe maternal vasculopathy, especially nephropathy and hypertension, is associated with uteroplacental insufficiency, which can result in IUGR, fetal intolerance of labor, and neonatal complications.

IV. Specific management of pregnancy. Management of type 1 or type 2 diabetes during pregnancy begins before conception. Preconception glycemic control has been shown to decrease the risk of congenital anomalies close to the risk of the general population. However, less than 30% of pregnancies are planned. Physicians should discuss pregnancy planning or recommend contraception for all diabetic women of childbearing age until glycemic control is optimized. Tight glucose control requires coordinated care between endocrinologists, maternal-fetal medicine specialists, diabetes nurse educators, and nutritionists.

Most women are screened for GDM between 24 and 28 weeks' gestation by a 50-g, 1-hour glucose challenge. A positive result is equal to or greater than 140 mg/dL, and the diagnosis of GDM is made by two or more elevated values on a 100-g oral glucose tolerance test. Uncontrolled GDM can lead to fetal macrosomia and concomitant risk of fetal injury at delivery. GDM shares many features of type 2 diabetes, and women diagnosed with GDM have a 50% lifetime risk of developing overt type 2 diabetes.

A. Diabetic control. Strict control is achieved with nutritional modification and insulin therapy, with the goals of fasting glucose concentration less than 95 mg/dL and postprandial values less than 140 mg/dL for 1 hour and 120 mg/dL for 2 hours. Recent data has suggested that oral hypoglycemic agents may be used in the setting of GDM, but are untested in pre-gestational diabetes.

B. First trimester testing
1. **Measurement of glycosylated hemoglobin** in the first trimester can give a risk assessment for congenital anomalies by reflecting ambient glucose concentrations during the period of organogenesis.
2. **Accurate dating of the pregnancy** is performed by ultrasound.
3. **Ophthalmologic exam** is mandatory, as retinopathy may progress as a result of the rapid normalization of glucose concentration in the first trimester. Women with retinopathy need periodic examinations throughout pregnancy and are candidates for laser photocoagulation as indicated.
4. **Renal function** is assessed by 24-hour urine collection for protein excretion and creatinine clearance. Patients with recent diagnosis of diabetes can have screening of renal function with urine microalbumin, followed by a 24-hour collection if abnormal.
5. **Evaluate thyroid function**

C. Second trimester testing
1. **Maternal serum screening** for neural tube defects and Down syndrome screening is performed between 15 and 19 weeks' gestation.
2. All patients undergo a thorough **ultrasound survey** for structural anomalies, including fetal echocardiography.
3. Women older than 35 years of age or with other risk factors for fetal aneuploidy are offered **chorionic villus sampling** or **amniocentesis** for karyotyping.

D. Third trimester testing
1. **Ultrasound examinations** are performed periodically through the third trimester for fetal growth measurement.
2. **Weekly fetal surveillance** using nonstress testing or biophysical profiles are implemented between 28 and 32 weeks' gestation, depending on glycemic control and other complications (see Chap. 1).
3. **Delivery is planned** for 39 to 40 weeks, unless other pregnancy complications dictate earlier delivery. Elective delivery after 39 weeks does not require fetal lung maturity testing. Nonemergent delivery before 39 weeks requires documentation of fetal lung maturity testing using the lecithin-sphingomyelin (L/S) ratio >3.5:1, positive Amniostat (phosphatidyglycerol present), saturated phosphatidylcholine (SPC) >1000 µg/dL or mature FLM (fetal lung maturity) (see Table 2.2 and Fig. 2.1). Emergent delivery should be carried out without fetal lung maturity testing.
4. **Risk of preterm labor** is not increased in patients with diabetes, although risk of iatrogenic preterm delivery is increased for patients with microvascular disease as a result of IUGR, fetal distress, and maternal hyper-

TABLE 2.2.   LECITHIN-SPHINGOMYELIN RATIO, SATURATED PHOSPHATIDYLCHOLINE LEVEL, AND RESPIRATORY DISTRESS SYNDROME IN INFANTS OF DIABETIC MOTHERS AT THE BOSTON HOSPITAL FOR WOMEN 1977–1980

SPC level (μg/dL)	L/S ratio			Mild, moderate, or severe RDS/total
	<2.0 : 1.0	2.0–3.4 : 1	≥3.5 : 1.0	
Not done	0/1	0/12	0/13	0/26 (0%)
≤500	6/6	1/9	1/2	8/17 (47%)
501–1000	0/2	3/20	1/15	4/37 (11%)
>1000	0/0	2/22	0/142	2/164 (1.2%)
Total (RDS)	6/9 (67%)	6/63 (10%)	2/172 (1.2%)	14/244 (5.7%)

L/S = lecithin/sphingomyelin; RDS = respiratory distress syndrome; SPC = saturated phosphatidylcholine.

tension. Antenatal corticosteroids for induction of fetal lung maturity should be employed for the usual obstetric indications. Corticosteroids can cause temporary hyperglycemia; therefore, patients often need to be managed with continuous intravenous insulin infusions until the effect of the steroids wear off.

E. Delivery
1. **Route of delivery** is determined by ultrasound estimated fetal weight, maternal and fetal condition, and previous obstetric history. The ultrasound estimated weight at which an elective cesarean delivery would be recommended is controversial.
2. **Blood glucose concentration** is tightly controlled during labor and delivery. If an induction of labor is planned, patients are instructed to take one-half of their usual intermediate-acting insulin on the morning of induction. During spontaneous or induced labor, blood glucose concentration is measured every 1 to 2 hours. Blood glucose concentration higher than 120 to 140 mg/dL is treated with an infusion of intravenous short acting insulin. Intravenous insulin is very short acting, allowing for quick response to changes in glucose concentration. Active labor may also be associated with hypoglycemia, because the contracting uterus uses circulating metabolic fuels.
3. **Continuous fetal monitoring** is mandatory during labor. Cesarean delivery is performed for obstetric indications. The risk of cesarean section for obstetric complications is approximately 50%.
4. **Patients with advanced microvascular disease** are at increased risk of cesarean delivery because of the increased incidence of IUGR, preeclampsia, and nonreassuring fetal status. A history of retinopathy that has been treated in the past is not necessarily an indication for cesarean delivery. Patients with active proliferative retinopathy that is unstable or active hemorrhage may benefit from elective cesarean delivery.
5. **Postpartum period patients** are at increased risk of hypoglycemia, especially in the postoperative setting with minimal oral intake. Patients with type 1 diabetes may also experience a "honeymoon" period immediately after delivery, with greatly reduced insulin requirements that can last up to several days. Insulin is adjusted to approximate the prepregnancy dose. For women with type 2 diabetes, the use of oral hypoglycemic agents

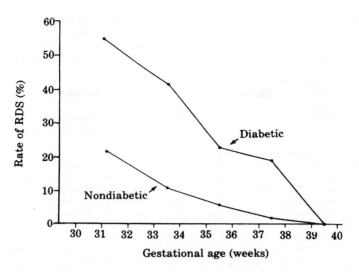

FIG. 2.1. Rate of respiratory distress syndrome (RDS) versus gestational age in nondiabetic and diabetic pregnancies at the Boston Hospital for Women from 1958 to 1968. (Reprinted with permission from Robert M. Association between maternal diabetes and the respiratory distress syndrome in the newborn. *N Engl J Med* 1976;294:357.)

during breastfeeding remains controversial, and insulin management may need to be continued.

V. Evaluation of the infant

    A. The evaluation of the infant begins **before the actual delivery**. If pulmonary maturity is not certain, amniotic fluid can be obtained by aspiration of the amniotic sac before it is opened at cesarean section. Fluid may be evaluated by gram stain, culture, shake test, L/S ratio, FLM testing, or saturated phosphatidylcholine (SPC) content (see IV.D and Chap. 24).

    B. After the baby is born, assessment is made on the basis of Apgar scores to determine the need for any resuscitative efforts (see Chap. 4). The infant should be dried and placed under a warmer. The airway is bulb suctioned for mucus, but the stomach is not aspirated, because of the risk of reflex bradycardia and apnea from pharyngeal stimulation in the first 5 minutes of life. A screening physical examination for the presence of major congenital anomalies should be performed and the placenta examined. A glucose level and pH may be determined on cord blood.

    C. In the nursery, **supportive care** should be given while a continuous evaluation of the infant is made. This includes providing warmth, suction, and oxygen as needed, while checking vital signs (e.g., heart and respiratory rates, temperature, perfusion, color, and blood pressure). Cyanosis should make one consider cardiac disease, respiratory distress syndrome (RDS), transient tachypnea of the newborn, or polycythemia. An examination should be repeated for possible anomalies because of the 6 to 9% incidence of major congenital anomalies in IDMs. Special attention should be paid to the brain, heart, kidneys, and skeletal system. Reports indicate that IDMs have a 47% risk of significant hypoglycemia, 22% risk of hypocalcemia, 19% risk of hyperbilirubinemia, and a 34% risk of polycythemia; therefore, the following studies are performed:

        1. Blood glucose levels are checked at 1, 2, 3, 6, 12, 24, 26, and 48 hours. Glucose is measured with Chemstrip B-G (Bio-Dynamics, BMC, Indianapolis, Indiana). Readings less than 40 mg/dL should be checked rapidly by a clinical laboratory or by Ames eyetone instrument (Ames Company, Division of Miles Laboratories, Inc., Elkhart, Indiana). The infant is fed orally or given intravenous (IV) glucose by 1 hour of age (see VI. and Chap. 29).

2. **Hematocrit levels** are checked at 1 and 24 hours (see Chap. 26).

3. **Calcium levels** are checked if the baby appears jittery or is sick for any reason (see VI.C and Chap. 29).

4. **Bilirubin levels** are checked if the baby appears jaundiced.

5. Every effort is made to involve the parents in infant care as soon as possible.

VI. Specific problems frequently observed in IDMs

A. **Respiratory distress.** With changes in pregnancy management resulting in longer gestations and more vaginal deliveries, the incidence of RDS in IDMs has fallen from 28% during 1950–1960 to 4% in 1990, with the major difference in the incidence of RDS between diabetics and nondiabetics in infants born before 37 weeks' gestation. Most of the deaths from RDS also are in infants less than 35 weeks' gestation who were delivered by cesarean section because of fetal distress or maternal indications.

Delayed lung maturity in IDMs may occur because hyperinsulinemia blocks cortisol induction of lung maturation. Causes of respiratory distress besides RDS are cardiac or pulmonary anomalies (4%), hypertrophic cardiomyopathy, transient tachypnea of the newborn, and polycythemia. Pneumonia, pneumothorax, and diaphragmatic hernia also should be considered. The following studies should be done in infants with respiratory distress:

1. **Chest X ray** to evaluate aeration, presence of infiltrates, cardiac size and position, and the presence of pneumothorax or anomalies.

2. **Blood gases** to evaluate gas exchange and the presence of right-to-left shunts.

3. Electrocardiogram, blood pressure measurements, and an echocardiogram if **hypertrophic cardiomyopathy** or **a cardiac anomaly** is thought to be present.

4. **Blood cultures, with spinal-fluid examination and culture** if the infant's condition allows and infection is a possibility. (See Chap. 24 for the differential diagnosis and management of respiratory disorders.)

B. **Hypoglycemia.** Hypoglycemia is defined as a blood glucose level less than 40 mg/dL in any infant, regardless of gestational age and whether symptomatic or not. Previously, we used a level of less than 30 mg/dL as the definition of hypoglycemia (see Chap. 29).

1. With less than 30 mg/dL as the definition, the **incidence of hypoglycemia** in IDMs is 30 to 40%. The onset is frequently within 1 to 2 hours of age and is most common in macrosomic infants.

2. The **pathogenesis of neonatal hypoglycemia in IDMs** is explained by Pederson's maternal hyperglycemia–fetal hyperinsulinism hypothesis. The correlation between fetal macrosomia, elevated HbA_1 in maternal and cord blood, and neonatal hypoglycemia, as well as between elevated cord blood C-peptide or immunoreactive insulin levels and hypoglycemia, suggests that control of maternal blood sugar in the last trimester may decrease the incidence of neonatal hypoglycemia in IDMs. Mothers should not receive large doses of glucose before or at delivery because this may stimulate an insulin response in the hyperinsulinemic offspring. We attempt to keep maternal glucose level at delivery at approximately 120 mg/dL. Hypoglycemia in small-for-gestational-age (SGA) infants born to mothers with vascular disease may be due to inadequate glycogen stores; it may also present later (e.g., at 12 to 24 hours of age). Other factors that may cause hypoglycemia in IDMs are decreased catecholamine and glucagon secretion as well as inadequate substrate mobilization (dimin-

ished hepatic glucose production and decreased oxygenation of fatty acids).

3. **Symptomatic, hypoglycemic IDMs** usually are quiet and lethargic rather than jittery. Symptoms such as apnea, tachypnea, respiratory distress, hypotonia, shock, cyanosis, and seizures may occur. If symptoms are present, the infant is probably at greater risk for sequelae than if asymptomatic. The significance of asymptomatic hypoglycemia is unclear, but conservative management to maintain the blood sugar level in the normal range (>40 mg/dL) appears to be indicated.

4. **Diagnosis.** Our neonatal protocol was explained in V.C.1. The blood glucose level is measured more often if the infant is symptomatic, if the infant has had a low level, and to see the response to therapy.

5. **Therapy**
   a. **Asymptomatic infants with normal blood glucose levels:**
      (1) In our nursery, we begin **feeding "well" IDMs** by bottle or gavage with dextrose 10% (5 mL/kg body weight) at or before 1 hour of age. Infants weighing less than 2 kg should have parenteral dextrose starting in the first hour of life. Larger infants can be fed hourly for three or four feedings until the blood sugar determinations are stable; infants should be switched to formula feeding (20 cal/oz) if the feedings are 2 hours apart or more. This schedule prevents some of the insulin release associated with oral feeding of pure glucose. The feedings can then be given every 2 hours and later every 3 hours as the interval between feedings increases, the volume is increased.
      (2) If by 2 hours of age the blood glucose level is less than 40 mg/dL despite feeding, or if feedings are not tolerated, as indicated by large volumes retained in the stomach, **parenteral treatment** is indicated.
   b. **Symptomatic infants, infants with a low blood glucose level after enteral feeding, sick infants, or infants less than 2 kg in weight:**
      (1) The basic treatment element is **IV glucose administration** through reliable access.
      (2) Administration of IV glucose is usually by **peripheral IV catheter.** Peripheral lines may be difficult to place in obese IDMs, and sudden interruption of the infusion may cause a reactive hypoglycemia in these hyperinsulinemic infants. Rarely, in emergency situations with symptomatic babies, we have used umbilical venous catheters in the inferior vena cava until a stable peripheral line is placed.
      (3) Specific treatment is determined by the baby's condition. If the infant is in **severe distress** (e.g., seizure or respiratory compromise), 0.5 to 1.0 g of glucose per kg of body weight is given by an IV push of 2 to 4 mL/kg 25% dextrose in water (D/W) at a rate of 1 mL/min/kg. For example, a 4-kg infant would receive 8 to 16 mL of 25% D/W over 2 to 4 minutes. This is followed by a continuous infusion at a rate of 4 to 8 mg of glucose per kg of body weight per minute. The concentration of dextrose in the IV fluid will depend on the total daily fluid requirement. For example, on day 1, the usual fluid intake is 65 mL/kg, or 0.045 mL/kg/min. Therefore, 10% D/W would provide 4.5 mg of glucose per kg per minute, and 15% D/W would provide 6.75 mg of glucose per kg per minute. In other words, 10% D/W at a standard IV fluid maintenance rate usually supplies sufficient glucose to raise the blood glucose level above 40 mg/dL. The concentration of dextrose and the infusion rates, however, are increased as necessary to maintain the blood glucose level in the normal range (see Fig. 29.1).

      The **usual method** in an infant not in severe distress is to give 200 mg of glucose per kg of body weight (2 mL/kg 10% dextrose) over 2 to

3 minutes. This is followed by a maintenance drip of 6 to 8 mg of glucose per kg per minute (10% dextrose at 80 to 120 mL/kg/day) (see Chap. 29).

(4) **If the infant is asymptomatic** but has a blood glucose level in the hypoglycemic range, an initial push of concentrated sugar should not be given in order to avoid a hyperinsulinemic response. Rather, an initial infusion of 5 to 10 mL of 10% D/W at 1 mL/min is followed by continuous infusion at 4 to 8 mg/kg per minute. Blood glucose levels must be carefully monitored at frequent intervals after beginning IV glucose infusions, both to be certain of adequate treatment of the hypoglycemia and to avoid hyperglycemia and the risk of osmotic diuresis and dehydration.

(5) Parenteral sugar should never be abruptly discontinued, because of the risk of a **reactive hypoglycemia.** As oral feeding progresses, the rate of the infusion can be decreased gradually, and the concentration of glucose infused reduced by using 5% D/W. It is vital to measure blood glucose levels during tapering of the IV infusion.

(6) **In difficult cases,** hydrocortisone (5 mg/kg per day intramuscularly (IM) in two divided doses) has occasionally been helpful. In our experience, other drugs (epinephrine, diazoxide, or growth hormone) have not been necessary in the treatment of the hypoglycemia of IDMs.

(7) In a hypoglycemic infant, **if difficulty is experienced in achieving vascular access,** we administer crystalline glucagon IM or subcutaneously (300 mg/kg to a maximum dose of 1.0 mg), which causes a rapid rise in blood glucose levels in large IDMs who have good glycogen stores; the response is not reliable in smaller infants of maternal classes D, E, F, and others. The rise in blood glucose may last 2 to 3 hours and is useful until parenteral glucose can be started. This method is rarely used.

(8) The hypoglycemia of most IDMs usually responds to the above treatment and resolves by 24 hours. **Persistent hypoglycemia** is usually due to a continued hyperinsulinemic state and may be manifested by glucose use of more than 8 mg of glucose per kg per minute (see Fig. 29.1). Efforts should be made to decrease islet cell stimulation (e.g., keeping blood glucose adequate but not high, moving a high umbilical artery line to a low line, etc.).

(9) **If the hypoglycemia lasts more than 7 days,** consider other etiologies (see Chap. 29).

C. **Hypocalcemia** (see Chap. 29, Hypocalcemia, Hypercalcemia, and Hypermagnesemia) is found in 22% of IDMs and is not related to hypoglycemia. Hypocalcemia in IDMs may be caused by a delay in the usual postnatal rise of parathyroid hormone or vitamin D antagonism at the intestinal level from elevated cortisol and hyperphosphatemia that is due to tissue catabolism. There is no evidence of elevated serum calcitonin concentrations in these infants in the absence of prematurity or asphyxia. Other causes of hypocalcemia, such as asphyxia and prematurity, may be seen in IDMs. The nadir in calcium levels occurs between 24 and 72 hours, and 20 to 50% of IDMs will become hypocalcemic as defined by a total serum calcium level less than 7 mg/dL.

Hypocalcemia in "well" IDMs usually resolves without treatment, and we do not routinely measure serum calcium levels in asymptomatic IDMs. Infants who are sick for any reason—prematurity, asphyxia, infection, respiratory distress—or IDMs with symptoms of lethargy, jitteriness, or seizures that do not respond to glucose should have their serum calcium levels measured. If an infant has symptoms that coexist with a low calcium level, has an illness that will delay onset of calcium regulation, or is unable to feed, treatment with calcium may be necessary (see Chap. 29). Hypomagnesemia should be considered in hypocalcemia in IDMs because the hypocalcemia may not respond until the hypomagnesemia is treated.

D. Polycythemia (see Chap. 26, Polycythemia) is common in IDMs. In infants who are small for gestational age, polycythemia may be related to placental insufficiency, causing fetal hypoxia and increased erythropoietin. In IDMs it may be due to reduced oxygen delivery secondary to elevated HbA_1 in both maternal and fetal serum. If fetal distress occurred, there may be a shift of blood from the placenta to the fetus.

E. Jaundice. Hyperbilirubinemia (bilirubin >15 mg/dL) is seen with increased frequency in IDMs. Bilirubin levels higher than 16 mg/dL were seen in 19% of IDMs at the Brigham and Women's Hospital. Bilirubin production is increased in IDMs as compared with infants of nondiabetic mothers. Insulin causes increased erythropoietin. When measurement of carboxyhemoglobin production is used as an indicator of increased heme turnover, IDMs are found to have increased production as compared with controls. There may be decreased erythrocyte life span because of less deformable cell membranes, possibly related to glycosylation of the erythrocyte cell membrane. This mild hemolysis is compensated for but may cause increased bilirubin production. Other factors that may account for jaundice are prematurity, impairment of the hepatic conjugation of bilirubin, and an increased enterohepatic circulation of bilirubin as a result of poor feeding. Infants born to well-controlled diabetic mothers have fewer problems with hyperbilirubinemia. The increasing gestational age of IDMs at delivery has contributed to the decreased incidence of hyperbilirubinemia. Hyperbilirubinemia in IDMs is diagnosed and treated as in any other infant (see Chap. 18).

F. Congenital anomalies are found more frequently in IDMs than in infants of nondiabetic mothers.

   1. Incidence. As mortality from other causes such as prematurity, stillbirth, asphyxia, and RDS falls, malformations become the major cause of perinatal mortality in IDMs. Infants of diabetic fathers show the same incidence of anomalies as the normal population; consequently, the maternal environment may be the important factor. Most studies show a 6 to 9% incidence of major anomalies in IDMs, compared with a usual major anomaly rate for the general population of 2% (see Chap. 8). The types of anomalies seen in IDMs involve the central nervous system (anencephaly, meningocele syndrome, holoprosencephaly); cardiac, vertebral, skeletal, and renal systems; situs inversus; and caudal regression syndrome (sacral agenesis). The central nervous system and cardiac anomalies make up two-thirds of the malformations seen in IDMs. Although there is a general increase in the anomaly rate in IDMs, no anomaly is specific for IDMs, although half of all cases of caudal regression syndrome are seen in IDMs.

   2. There have been several studies correlating poor metabolic control of diabetes in early pregnancy with **malformations in the IDM**. Among more recent studies, one performed by the Joslin Clinic again showed a relationship between elevated HbA_1 in the first trimester and major anomalies in IDMs. The data are consistent with the hypothesis that poor metabolic control of maternal diabetes in the first trimester is associated with an increased risk for major congenital malformations.

G. Poor feeding is a major problem in IDMs, occurring in 37% of a series of 150 IDMs at the Brigham and Women's Hospital. Sometimes poor feeding is related to prematurity, respiratory distress, or other problems; however, it is often present in the absence of other problems. In our most recent experience (unpublished), it was found in 17% of class B to D IDMs and in 31% of class F IDMs. Infants born to class F mothers are often preterm. There was no difference in the incidence of poor feeding in large-for-gestational-age infants versus appropriate-for-gestational-age infants, and there was no relation to polyhydramnios. Poor feeding is a major reason for prolonged hospital stays and parent-infant separation.

H. Macrosomia, defined as a birth weight higher than the ninetieth percentile or more than 4000 g, may be associated with an increased incidence of primary cesarean section or obstetric trauma, such as fractured clavicle, Erb's palsy, or phrenic nerve palsy as a result of shoulder dystocia. The incidence of macrosomia was 28% at the Brigham and Women's Hospital from 1983 to 1984. An association was found between third-trimester elevated maternal blood sugar and macrosomia. There also was an association between hyperinsulinemia in IDMs and macrosomia, and between macrosomia and hypoglycemia. Macrosomia is not usually seen in infants born to class F mothers.

 I. Myocardial dysfunction. Transient hypertrophic subaortic stenosis resulting from ventricular septal hypertrophy in IDMs has been reported. Infants may present with heart failure, poor cardiac output, and cardiomegaly. The cardiomyopathy may complicate the management of other illnesses such as RDS. The diagnosis is made by echocardiography, which shows hypertrophy of the ventricular septum, the right anterior ventricular wall, and the left posterior ventricular wall in the absence of chamber dilation. Cardiac output decreases with increasing septal thickness. Most symptoms resolve by 2 weeks of age, and septal hypertrophy resolves by 4 months. Most infants will respond to supportive care. Inotropic drugs are contraindicated unless myocardial dysfunction is seen on echocardiography; propranolol is the most useful agent. The differential diagnosis of myocardial dysfunction that is due to diabetic cardiomyopathy of the newborn includes (1) postasphyxial cardiomyopathy, (2) myocarditis, (3) endocardial fibroelastosis, (4) glycogen storage disease of the heart, and (5) aberrant left coronary artery coming off the pulmonary artery (see Chap. 25). There is some evidence that good diabetic control during pregnancy may reduce the incidence and severity of hypertrophic cardiomyopathy (see Chap. 25 and VI.C).

 J. Renal vein thrombosis. Renal vein thrombosis may occur in utero or postpartum. Intrauterine and postnatal diagnosis may be made by ultrasonographic examination. Postnatal presentation may include hematuria, flank mass, hypertension, or embolic phenomena. Most renal vein thrombosis can be managed conservatively, allowing preservation of renal tissue (see Chaps. 26, 31, and 33).

 K. Other thrombosis (see Chap. 26, Major Arterial and Venous Thrombosis Management)

 L. Small left colon syndrome presents as generalized abdominal distension because of inability to pass meconium. Meconium is obtained by passage of a rectal catheter. An enema performed with meglumine diatrizoate (Gastrografin) will make the diagnosis and often results in evacuation of the colon. The infant should be well hydrated before Gastrografin is used. The infant may have some problems with passage of stool in the first week of life, but this usually resolves after treatment with half-normal saline enemas (5 mL/kg) and glycerine suppositories. Other causes of intestinal obstruction should be considered (see Chap. 33).

 M. Genetics. The parents of IDMs are often concerned about the eventual development of diabetes in their children. There are conflicting data on the incidence of insulin-dependent diabetes in IDMs. In the general population, a person has a less than 1% chance of becoming a type I diabetic. The offspring of one parent with type 1 diabetes has a 5 to 10% risk of developing the disease. If both parents have type 1 diabetes, the risk is about 20%. In type 2 diabetes, the average person has a 12 to 18% chance of developing the disease. If one parent has it, the risk to offspring is 30%; if both parents have it, the risk is 50–60%.

 N. Perinatal survival. Despite all problems, a diabetic woman has a 95% chance of having a healthy child if she is willing to participate in a program of pregnancy management and surveillance at an appropriate perinatal center. In a series of 215 IDMs at the Brigham and Women's Hospital from 1983 to 1984, the total perinatal mortality, from 23 weeks of gestation to 28 days postpartum, was 28 per 1000. There was one intrauterine demise of a singleton near term.

Suggested Readings

American College of Obstetricians and Gynecologists. ACOG Practice Bulletin No. 30, *Obstet Gynecol* 2001;89:525.

American Diabetes Association. Gestational diabetes mellitus. *Diabetes Care Supplement* 25(Suppl. 1): 2002;S94–96.

Buchanan T.A., et al: Insulin sensitivity and B-cell responsiveness to glucose during late pregnancy in lean and moderately obese women with normal glucose tolerance or mild gestational diabetes. *Am J Obstet Gynecol* 1990;162:1008.

Cloherty J.P. Neonatal management. In: Brown F. (Ed.), *Diabetes Complicating Pregnancy: The Joslin Clinic Method,* 2nd ed. New York: Wiley, 1995, 169–186.

Kitzmiller J.L., et al. Preconception care of diabetes: Glycemic control prevents congenital anomalies. *JAMA* 1991;265:731.

Landon M.B. Diabetes in pregnancy. *Clin Perinatol* 1993;20:507.

Landon M.B., et al. Fetal surveillance in pregnancies complicated by insulin-dependent diabetes mellitus. *Am J Obstet Gynecol* 1992;167:617.

Langer O., et al. Shoulder dystocia: Should the fetus weighing >4000 grams be delivered by cesarean section? *Am J Obstet Gynecol* 1991;165:831–837.

Reece E.A., et al. Infant of the diabetic mother. *Semin Perinatol* 1994;18:459.

Thyroid Disorders*

Camilia R. Martin

I. **Thyroid metabolism in pregnancy.** Multiple changes occur in maternal thyroid physiology during pregnancy.
   A. **Increased uptake and clearance of iodine.** Increased renal glomerular filtration rate, a by-product of an enhanced hemodynamic state during pregnancy (increased cardiac output, increased stroke volume, increased heart rate, and decreased systemic vascular resistance), and increased placental transfer of iodide and iodothyronines promote accelerated iodine turnover.
   B. **Thyroid gland volume** may enlarge in regions deficient in iodine, yet remains stable in iodine-sufficient areas (e.g., the United States).
   C. **Increased thyroxine-binding globulin (TBG) levels.** Elevated estrogen levels lead to an increase in TBG levels. Estrogen stimulates TBG hepatic synthesis. In addition, estrogen promotes sialylation of the protein, which, in turn, increases the half-life and reduces hepatic clearance. Elevated TBG levels are evident very early in gestation and plateau midway through the pregnancy.
   D. **Increased total T_4 and T_3 levels.** An increase in TBG results in an increase in total T_4 and T_3 levels. Free hormone concentrations, however, remain relatively unchanged. There may be a slight increase in free T_4 and T_3 early in pregnancy and then a decline to low-normal levels late in pregnancy. Throughout these changes, levels should remain within normal reference ranges and the woman should remain euthyroid.

* This is a revision of a chapter by Mary D. Scott in the 4th Edition.

   E. **Human chorionic gonadotropin (hCG) has thyrotropin (TSH)-like activity** because of its structural similarity. There is a linear relationship between the rise in hCG and the rise in free T_4 levels and the fall in TSH levels. Once again, the rise of free T_4 levels to toxic ranges would be unusual.
   F. There is minimal difference in the **hypothalamic–pituitary–thyroid (HPT) axis response** to thyrotropin-releasing hormone (TRH) between nonpregnant and pregnant women. First-trimester TSH response is more blunted (when free T_4 levels are the highest) compared with the second trimester; however, the TSH response is not flat, as seen in hyperthyroidism.
   G. The **negative feedback control mechanisms of the HPT axis** remain intact.
   H. **Transplacental passage.** Iodide and TRH readily cross the placenta. Transplacental passage of T_4, T_3, and rT_3 occur in limited but critical amounts. Maternal thyroid hormones are important for fetal development in the first trimester before establishment of the fetal HPT axis. Late transfer of maternal thyroid hormones is not as important to the fetus but may be neuroprotective for a fetus with congenital hypothyroidism. Maternal thyroid-stimulating immunoglobulins (TSI) and TSH-binding inhibitory immunoglobulins (TBII) also cross the placenta and can cause transient hyper- or hypothyroidism in the newborn. The placenta is impermeable to TSH.
II. **Maternal hypothyroidism.** The incidence of maternal hypothyroidism is 3/1000.
   A. **Common causes** of hypothyroidism include autoimmune (Hashimoto's) and previous treatment for hyperthyroidism that included radioiodine ablation or thyroidectomy. Less common causes include thyroiditis, external radiation, drug-induced hypothyroidism, and congenital hypothyroidism.
   B. **Recognizing the typical symptoms** of hypothyroidism during pregnancy may be difficult because of the hypermetabolic state that normally occurs.
   C. **Unrecognized or untreated maternal hypothyroidism** may result in an increased frequency of maternal and neonatal complications. Maternal complications include first-trimester miscarriages, preeclampsia, placental abruption, preterm delivery, and postpartum hemorrhage. Neonatal complications include intrauterine growth restriction (IUGR) and poor neurodevelopmental outcome. Treatment includes L-thyroxine replacement with the goal of maintaining TSH levels in the normal range. Thyroid function tests should be monitored every 4 weeks until this goal is achieved.
   D. **Women with a prenatal diagnosis of hypothyroidism** who are appropriately treated typically deliver normal infants. Pregnant women who have primary hypothyroidism should have thyroid function tests as soon as pregnancy is confirmed and again at 6 weeks' gestation, 16 to 20 weeks' gestation, and 28 to 32 weeks' gestation. The thyroxine dose may need to be increased during pregnancy to keep TSH in the normal range and should be adjusted to normalize TSH as rapidly as possible.
   E. **There is limited transfer of L-thyroxine into breast milk.** There is no contraindication to taking thyroxine while breastfeeding.
   F. **In women who make TBII**, placental transfer of the immunoglobulins may cause fetal hypothyroidism (VI.E.2.a.). TBII and TSI screening in the last trimester may aid in determining the risk to the fetus for altered thyroid physiology.
III. **Maternal hyperthyroidism.** Graves' disease complicates 1/1000–2000 pregnancies.
   A. **Untreated** maternal hyperthyroidism carries a significant risk to the mother and fetus. Potential maternal risks include miscarriage, pregnancy-induced hypertension, preterm delivery, congestive heart failure, thyroid storm, and placental abruption. Risks to the fetus include hyperthyroidism and IUGR.
   B. **Treatment and obstetric monitoring.** Once maternal hyperthyroidism is diagnosed, prompt treatment should be established. Antithyroid drugs, including propylthiouracil (PTU) and methimazole (MMI), are the treatments of choice. There is some preference for PTU because of the reduced passage across the placenta and limited excretion into breast milk. In addition, small case series

have suggested an association between MMI and aplasia cutis congenita, a focal scalp lesion. However, this has not been consistently proven in larger studies. Beta-adrenergic blocking agents may be added to aid in controlling hypermetabolic symptoms. However, long-term use should be avoided because of potential neonatal morbidities. Iodides are generally contraindicated because of secondary neonatal goiter and hypothyroidism. However, brief exposure to control hyperthyroid symptoms or to prepare for surgery seems to be well tolerated. Radioactive iodine is contraindicated, especially after the twelfth week of gestation when the fetal thyroid develops iodine concentration abilities. Pregnant women with Graves' disease should have regular monitoring of thyroid function and fetal well-being. The goal of treatment is to maintain free thyroxine levels in the upper third of the normal range.

   C. Thyroid function in neonates. All fetuses of pregnant women with Graves' disease should be monitored for intrauterine hyperthyroidism. Transplacental passage of TSI and TBII does occur that may be significant enough to alter neonatal thyroid function. However, neonatal hyperthyroidism occurs in only 1 to 5% of infants born to mothers with Graves' disease. Fetal thyroid dysfunction is related to the duration of thyrotoxicosis in pregnancy, dosage levels of maternal antithyroid drugs, and maternal antibody levels at delivery. Measurements of TSI and TBII levels in the last trimester may be helpful in determining the risk of neonatal thyrotoxicosis. TSI values greater than 300% or TBII values greater than 30% of control values can be predictive of neonatal thyrotoxicosis. If values are elevated, neonates should be closely monitored for the development of thyrotoxicosis in the first 2 weeks of life.

   D. Maternal medications, complications, and breastfeeding
   1. **Antithyroid** drugs cross the placenta, are associated with fetal goiters (see IV.A), and are excreted into breast milk. As stated, transplacental passage of PTU and excretion into breast milk are less than for MMI. Excretion into breast milk is limited and it is considered safe to breastfeed while receiving either PTU or MMI. Complications in breastfeeding newborns are rare with maternal doses less than 450 mg per day of PTU and less than 20 mg per day of MMI. Within these ranges, the infant does not require more than routine thyroid function testing if somatic and mental development are normal.
   2. **Propranolol** can cause impaired responses to hypoxia, bradycardia, and hypoglycemia in the fetus. There is limited transfer of propranolol into breast milk. It is considered safe to breastfeed while taking Propranolol. However, studies are lacking regarding long-term exposure.

IV. Fetal and neonatal goiter
   A. PTU-induced fetal goiter can be seen, although the occurrence does not always correlate with level of maternal dosing. Transient neonatal hypothyroidism also may be evident. After delivery, neonates eliminate PTU in 2 to 4 weeks, with normal thyroid function tests by 4 to 6 weeks (Table 2.3). Newborns with PTU-induced goiter should be treated with thyroxine for about 1 month. Enlarging fetal goiters in PTU-treated pregnant women may be due to either TSI-induced hyperthyroidism or PTU-induced hypothyroidism. Fetal blood sampling is diagnostic (see Chap. 1, II.B.3). Third-trimester goitrous fetal hypothyroidism has been successfully treated with weekly intraamniotic injections of 250 to 500 mg of L-thyroxine.
   B. Other forms of goiter. Neonatal goiter may be seen in inherited hypothyroidism or after maternal ingestion of iodine. The differential diagnosis includes hemangiomas or lymphangiomas. Iodine-induced goiter resolves over 2 to 3 months, with resolution accelerated by thyroxine treatment. T_4, T_3, and TSH determinations should be obtained from the infant before treatment to exclude permanent defects in T_4 synthesis.

V. Neonatal hyperthyroidism. Neonatal hyperthyroidism is uncommon, accounting for approximately 1% of hyperthyroidism seen during childhood. Most often infants are born to mothers with Graves' disease. A rare, autosome-dominant,

TABLE 2.3. NORMAL THYROID FUNCTION PARAMETERS IN INFANTS AGED 2 TO 6 WEEKS*

Serum constituent	Concentration
T_4	84–210 nmol/L (6.5–16.3 µg/dL)
T_3	1.5–4.6 nmol/L (100–300 ng/dL)
Free T_4[†]	12–28 pmol/L (0.9–2.2 ng/dL)
TSH	1.7–9.1 mU/L (1.7–9.1 U/mL)
TBG	160–750 nmol/L (1.0–4.5 mg/dL)
Thyroglobulin[‡]	15–375 pmol/L (10–250 ng/mL)

T_3 = triiodothyronine; T_4 = thyroxine; TBG = thyroxine-binding globulin; TSH = thyroid-stimulating hormone.
*Data from Nichols Institute reference values unless indicated otherwise.
†Measured by direct dialysis.
‡Thyroglobulin from Vulsma et al., *N Engl J Med* 1989;321:13.
Source: From Fisher D. A. Management of congenital hypothyroidism. *J Clin Endocrinol Metab* 1991;72:525.

nonimmune cause of neonatal hyperthyroidism is characterized by an activating mutation of the TSH receptor. This condition results in permanent hyperthyroidism and may require thyroid gland ablation. *Autoimmune, transient* neonatal hyperthyroidism will be discussed.

A. **Incidence.** Of infants born to mothers with Graves' disease, 1 to 5% will go on to develop hyperthyroidism.

B. **Pathogenesis**

1. **Altered thyroid function** results from transplacental passage of TSI and TBII. Because both stimulating and blocking antibodies are made and cross the placenta. Infants may initially present with hypothyroidism or have a delay in the development of thyrotoxicosis. Initial hypothyroidism may also be present as a result of the transplacental passage of PTU or MMI.

2. **Neonatal hyperthyroidism** usually occurs with active maternal disease. However, hyperthyroidism may also occur with inactive maternal disease because of the continued presence of thyroid autoantibodies.

3. Measurements of maternal TSI and TBII levels may be predictive for the likelihood of **neonatal thyrotoxicosis**. Maternal TSI activity greater than 300% or TBII levels greater than 30% of control values are likely to result in thyrotoxicosis. Symptoms may persist for 2 to 4 months.

C. **Clinical findings.** Thyrotoxic newborns may present within 24 hours to 6 weeks of life. Usual clinical manifestations include microcephaly, low birth weight, prematurity, irritability, fever, tachycardia, heart failure, goiter, vomiting, diarrhea, hepatosplenomegaly, failure to thrive despite hyperphagia, flushing, hypertension, exophthalmos, and craniosynostosis. Arrhythmias and cardiac failure may be fatal. Measurements of TSI, TBII, T_4, free T_4, and TSH can be diagnostic.

D. **Treatment.**

1. **In severe cases PTU** (5 to 10 mg/kg/day in three divided doses) or **MMI** (0.5 to 1.0 mg/kg/day in three divided doses) may be used. If there is no response in 36 to 48 hours, the drug dose is increased by 50%.

2. An **iodine preparation** such as Lugol's (or strong iodine) solution containing 4.5 to 5.5 g of elemental iodine and 9.5 to 10.5 g of potassium iodide per dL is given in a dose of 1 drop three times a day. If there is no response in 48 hours, the dose is increased by 25% per day until control is obtained. Iopanoic acid (Telepaque) or sodium ipodate (Oragrafin) at 600 mg/m²/day

may be preferable to iodine solutions. Sodium ipodate decreases serum T_3 by 50% within 24 hours and appears to be safe and effective in newborns.

3. Approximately 2 mg/kg/day of **propranolol** (range 1 to 3.5 mg/kg/day) in three divided doses is used to control tachycardia and congestive heart failure.

4. Additional therapy may include **prednisone** at 1 to 2 mg/kg/day.

5. **Supportive care** maintains adequate oxygenation, positive fluid balance, sufficient caloric intake and growth, and temperature regulation.

6. **Treatment may be required for 4 to 12 weeks.** Once control is gained, the infant can be discharged with close follow-up. Iodine solutions are given for only 10 to 14 days. Infants are weaned off propranolol as indicated by heart rate, and then the dose of PTU is tapered as allowed by T_4 level and clinical situation.

E. **Prognosis.** Most newborns have rapid improvement and are able to withdraw treatment over several months. Rarely, the disease persists for more than 6 months. Mortality can be as high as 15%. Long-term morbidities include retarded growth, craniosynostosis, hyperactivity, and intellectual and developmental impairment.

VI. **Congenital hypothyroidism (CH)**

A. **Thyroid embryogenesis** occurs during the first trimester. By 10 to 12 weeks, the fetal thyroid gland demonstrates the ability to concentrate iodide and synthesize iodothyronines. TRH, somatostatin, and TSH are also detectable by this age. However, activity of the HPT axis is low, and circulating TSH and T_4 levels are minimal until about 18 to 20 weeks. After 20 weeks, there is a progressive increase in TSH and free T_4 levels. There is also an increase in the T_4:TSH ratio, suggesting maturation of the negative feedback control of the HPT axis. T_3 levels also progressively increase, although later, after approximately 30 weeks of gestation.

B. **Neonatal physiology.** At birth there is a sharp increase in TSH as a result of neonatal cooling. This surge peaks at 30 minutes and declines over the next few days. The increased TSH results in a concomitant sharp rise in T_4 and T_3 levels, peaking at 36 to 48 hours of life, and then steadily declining to adult values over 4 to 5 weeks. Preterm infants demonstrate similar changes in thyroid hormone levels as full-term newborns. However, quantitatively the response is blunted because of axis immaturity, resulting in overall lower levels of total T_4, free T_4, and T_3. Thyroid hormone levels are related to gestational age and birth weight (Table 2.4). Hypothyroxinemia of prematurity is discussed further in section VI.E.2.c.

C. **Screening.** Newborn screening for CH is routine in developed countries. Most North American programs use a spot T_4 measurement and TSH confirmation of low T_4 values.

1. **Screening and early discharge.** With many neonates discharged on day 1 of life, obtaining early TSH measurements has increased the false-positive rate for CH screening. Because T_4 is also elevated on days 1 and 2 of life, mild cases of CH may be missed if T_4 is within the low-normal range. If the infant is tested before 24 hours of age, he or she should be retested 24 to 48 hours after discharge.

2. **Prematurity and low birth weight.** Total T_4 levels are related to gestational age and birth weight. A majority of preterm, low-birth-weight infants may have T_4 levels in the hypothyroid range. In addition, truly hypothyroid, low-birth-weight infants may demonstrate a delayed rise in TSH 2.5 to 7 weeks after birth (see section VI.E.1.d). These factors make the diagnosis of hypothyroidism more challenging in this group. As a result, it is recommended to repeat state newborn screening specimens at 2, 6, and 10 weeks of life for all newborns less than 1500 g.

3. If **signs of hypothyroidism** appear (prolonged jaundice, delayed stooling, hypothermia, poor tone, mottled skin, poor feeding), screening should be repeated even if the original screen was normal. Screening programs miss some cases of CH as a result of early discharge, laboratory error, improper

TABLE 2.4.   REFERENCE RANGES FOR SERUM FREE T$_4$ AND THYROTROPIN IN PREMATURE AND TERM INFANTS DURING THE FIRST WEEK OF LIFE

Age Groups	Age (wk)	Weight, g (SD)	Free T$_4$ ng/dL (mean)	Thyrotropin (mU/L)
Premature infants*	25–27	772 (233)	0.6–2.2 (1.4)	0.2–30.3
	28–30	1260 (238)	0.6–3.4 (2.0)	0.2–20.6
	31–33	1786 (255)	1.0–3.8 (2.4)	0.7–27.9
	34–36	2125 (376)	1.2–4.4 (2.8)	1.2–21.6
Term infants†	37–42	>2500	2.0–5.3 (3.8)	1.0–39

SD = standard deviation.
*Adams L.M., Emery J.R., Clark S.J. Reference ranges for newer thyroid function test in premature infants. *J Pediatr* 1995;126:122.
†Nelson J.C., Clark S.J., Borut D.L., Tomei R.T., Carleton E.I. Age-related change in serum free thyroxine during childhood and adolescence. *J Pediatr* 1993;123:899–905.
Source: Fisher D.A. Thyroid function in premature infants: The hypothyroxinemia of prematurity. *Clin Perinatol* 1998;25:999–1014.

or no specimen collection, hospital transfers, sick neonates, prematurity, low birth weight, and home deliveries.
  D. **CH is seen more frequently** in infants with Down syndrome, trisomy 18, neural tube defects, congenital heart disease, metabolic disorders, familial autoimmune thyroid disorders, and Pierre Robin syndrome.
  E. **Etiologies of CH**
   1. **Permanent conditions.** The overall incidence of conditions leading to permanent hypothyroidism is 1 in 3500 to 4000 live births.
      a. **Thyroid dysgenesis** (aplasia, hypoplasia, ectopic thyroid) is the most common cause of permanent CH with an incidence of 1 in 4000 births (approximately 80% of cases). Thyroid dysgenesis is least common in black (1:32,000) and most common in Hispanic infants (1:2000). It is usually sporadic, but may be familial if the cause is cytotoxic antibodies crossing the placenta in pregnant women with autoimmune thyroid disease. The female-to-male ratio is 2:1. Infants have no goiter, low T$_4$ and free thyroxine (T$_4$), low triiodothyronine (T$_3$), elevated thyroid-stimulating hormone (TSH), normal thyroxin-binding globulin (TBG), no or ectopic radioactive iodine uptake (RAIU), and an increased response to thyrotropin-releasing hormone (TRH) at 30 minutes.
      b. **Thyroid hormone synthetic defects** (autosomal recessive) have an incidence of 1 in 30,000 (approximately 10% of permanent CH cases). Synthetic defects may be anywhere along the synthetic pathway, including abnormalities in trapping, organification, deiodination, storage, or release. **Pendred's syndrome** is an organification defect coupled with sensorineural deafness. Check for family history of deafness or goiter or for consanguinity. RAIU scans are typically normal, and a gland is present on ultrasound. Thyroglobulin may be low; T$_3$, T$_4$, and free T$_4$ are low; TSH is high; TBG is normal; and there is an increased response to TRH at 30 minutes. A goiter is usually present.
      c. **Hypothalamic-pituitary hypothyroidism.** The incidence is 1 in 100,000. T$_4$, free T$_4$, and T$_3$ are low, with low-to-normal TSH, normal TBG, and a low or delayed response to TRH infusion. Infants with suspected hypothalamic or pan-hypopituitarism also may have hypoglycemia and microphallus. Cortisol and growth hormone measurements should be obtained and a magnetic resonance imaging scan done to visualize the hypothalamus and pituitary. Goiter is not present.

      d. Hypothyroxinemia with delayed TSH elevation. The incidence is 1 in 100,000 of all newborns, but 1/300 in very-low-birth-weight infants. On initial screening, TSH is normal, with low T_4, low free T_4, low T_3, and normal TBG. On subsequent testing 2.5 to 7 weeks later, TSH levels are found to be elevated with a pattern typical of primary hypothyroidism. Etiology remains unclear, with possibilities including an abnormality of the pituitary-thyroid feedback mechanism or a type of acquired hypothyroidism.

  2. Transient conditions are seen frequently in sick or preterm neonates.

      a. Thyroid-blocking antibodies. Transient hypothyroidism that is due to thyroid-blocking antibodies has an incidence of 1 in 50,000. This is seen in maternal autoimmune thyroid disease. Antibodies freely cross the placenta and are secreted in breast milk. Antibodies may inhibit TSH binding to receptors TSH-binding inhibitory immunoglobulins (TBII), inhibit TSH-mediated thyroid cell growth thyroid growth inhibitory immunoglobulin (TGII), or block the effects of TSH on cell function. Antibodies with blocking or stimulating properties may be found in the same pregnant woman and may have different or subsequent effects on the fetus, exerting their influence for as long as 9 months after birth. Hypothyroidism may persist for that length of time. T_4, free T_4, and T_3 are low, TSH is increased, TBG is normal, and antibodies are present in both mother and infant. TRH test shows an increased TSH response. RAIU may be absent, but a gland will be present on ultrasound.

      b. Iodine exposure. Sick and preterm infants are at risk for transient hypothyroxinemia because of the exposure to iodine-containing disinfectant solutions. Exposed infants may demonstrate depressed free T_4 levels and elevated TSH and urinary iodine levels. Use of iodine-containing disinfectant solutions should be avoided or minimized in preterm, low-birth-weight newborns.

      c. Transient hypothyroxinemia of prematurity. Transient hypothyroxinemia of prematurity is a poorly understood disorder, affecting as many as 85% of preterm infants. Typically, total T_4 levels are low, but free T_4, T_3, and TSH values are normal. Most values normalize within a few months. Previously, this transient phenomenon was attributed to a normal adaptive response of an immature hypothalamic-pituitary axis or to sick euthyroid syndrome and was considered clinically insignificant. However, more recently, hypothyroxinemia during the neonatal period in the preterm infant has been linked with significant postneonatal morbidities. Decreased total thyroxine levels are associated with intraventricular hemorrhage, white matter damage, cerebral palsy, poor neurodevelopment, and death. Treatment considerations are discussed under section VI.G.2–3.

F. Diagnosis. Infants with abnormal newborn state screen thyroid-function results ($T_4 < 6$, TSH > 20) should have the tests repeated by venipuncture (Fig. 2.2). In addition to TSH and total T_4 levels, free T_4, T_3 resin uptake, TBG, and thyroglobulin levels should be considered to aid in diagnosis. Bone age evaluation (e.g., knee, foot) may show delay in epiphyseal maturation. RAIU with I-123 may be helpful in differentiating aplasia from synthetic defects. Absent uptake may also be seen in TSH receptor defects and iodide-trapping defects. TSH receptor blockade by maternal TSH receptor–blocking antibodies (TBA in figure) in maternal autoimmune thyroid disease may also cause absent RAIU. Thyroglobulin levels will be low in agenesis or thyroxine synthetic defects and elevated in thyroid dysgenesis, depending on the quantity of thyroid tissue and degree of TSH stimulation. TRH testing (7 mg/kg given intravenously; TSH release measured at 30 minutes and 1 to 2 hours) will show a subnormal response in pituitary CH (<10 mU/mL) and a delayed response in hypothalamic CH.

G. Treatment and monitoring of CH

  1. Preterm and term infants with low T_4 and elevated TSH must be treated as primary hypothyroidism. All infants with an uncertain diagnosis or

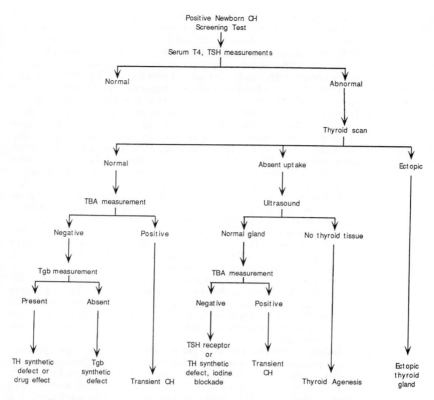

FIG. 2.2. Possible initial approaches to a newborn infant with presumptive positive test results for congenital hypothyroidism (CH) from a screening laboratory. All such infants require measurements of serum thyroxine (T_4) and thyroid-stimulating hormone (TSH) concentrations. Those infants with low T_4 and elevated TSH concentrations can be further screened by a thyroid scan using technetium or radioiodine 123. Finding an ectopic gland provides a definitive diagnosis. Infants with absent uptake or a normally appearing thyroid gland by scan can be evaluated further by ultrasound scanning and measurements of TBA and serum thyroglobulin (Tgb) concentrations. Infants with TBA-induced transient CH may have a normal scan if their CH is partially compensated. This initial evaluation should be accomplished within 2 to 5 days. (From Fisher D.A. Management of congenital hypothyroidism. *J Clin Endocrinol Metab* 1991;72: 525.)

suspected transient disease should have a brief trial off medication between 3 and 4 years of age to determine whether they have transient disease or if permanent thyroxine replacement is necessary.

2. **Treatment with L-thyroxine** should be initiated at 10 to 15 µg/kg/day, using the highest dose for infants with the lowest T_4, highest TSH values, and most delayed bone ages. A term infant receiving 50 µg/day will have normal T_4 and TSH levels within 2 weeks. Keeping T_4 in the upper half of the normal range (10 to 16 µg/dL) should keep TSH levels below 20 mU/mL in a majority of infants, but as many as 20% of infants with CH will continue to have abnormal T_4-to-TSH feedback for the first decade of life. Thyroxine doses should be adjusted at 6-week intervals for the first 6 months of life and at 2-month intervals during the next 12 months to

keep T_4 in the 10 to 16 µg/dL range and TSH below 5 mU/L. Thyroxine must be crushed and fed directly to the infant. It cannot be made into a liquid or added to breast milk or formula in a bottle. Soy-based formulas and ferrous sulfate interfere significantly with L-thyroxine absorption. Soy-based formula and/or ferrous sulfate should be administered at least 2 hours apart from the L -thyroxine dose.

3. The question of whether **T$_4$ supplementation in preterm infants (<30 weeks' gestation) with low T$_4$ and *normal* TSH levels** might improve outcome remains controversial. Recent studies have suggested that supplementation in extremely preterm infants may demonstrate long-term benefit. However, present opinion, including the New England Hypothyroid Collaborative and the Cochrane Neonatal Collaborative Review, is that there is no clear benefit to routine T_4 supplementation in these infants. Larger clinical trials, especially among the most vulnerable preterm infants born at less than 28 weeks' gestation, are needed.

H. **Prognosis.** Prompt, early thyroxine replacement, close monitoring, and maintenance of T_4 levels in the upper half of reference range has significantly improved neurodevelopment, even in the most severe cases of congenital hypothyroidism. Although mental retardation can be avoided with early treatment, subtle neurocognitive deficits may persist, including poor visuospatial abilities, attention, and memory skills.

Acknowledgment
I thank Drs. Marvin L. Mitchell, P. Reed Larsen, and Catherine M. Gordon for their review of the chapter.

Suggested Readings
Azizi F., et al. Thyroid function and intellectual development of infants nursed by mothers taking methimazole. *J Clin Endocrinol Metab* 2000;85:3233–3238.

Berghout A., Wiersinga W. Thyroid size and thyroid function during pregnancy: An analysis. *Eur J Endocrinol* 1998;138:536–542.

Briet J.M., et al. Neonatal thyroxine supplementation in very preterm children: Developmental outcome evaluated at early school age. *Pediatrics* 2001;107:712–718.

Buckingham B. The hyperthyroid fetus and infant. *NeoReviews* 2000;1:e103–e109.

Burrow G.N., Fisher D.A., Larsen P.R. Maternal and fetal thyroid function. *N Engl J Med* 1994;331:1072–1078.

Den Ouden A.L., et al. The relation between neonatal thyroxine levels and neurodevelopmental outcome at age 5 and 9 years in a national cohort of very preterm and/or very low birth weight infants. *Pediatr Res* 1996;39:142–145.

Dubuis J.M., et al. Outcome of severe congenital hypothyroidism: Closing the developmental gap with early high dose levothyroxine treatment. *J Clin Endocrinol Metab* 1996;81:222–227.

Fantz C.R., et al. Thyroid function during pregnancy. *Clin Chem* 1999;45:2250–2258.

Fisher D.A. Hypothyroidism. *Pediatr Rev* 1994;15:227–232.

Fisher D.A. Thyroid function in premature infants: The hypothyroxinemia of prematurity. *Clin Perinatol* 1998;25:999–1014, viii.

Haddow J.E., et al. Maternal thyroid deficiency during pregnancy and subsequent neuropsychological development of the child. *N Engl J Med* 1999;341:549–555.

Kaplan M.M. Monitoring thyroxine treatment during pregnancy. *Thyroid* 1992;2: 147–152.

Leviton A., et al. Hypothyroxinemia of prematurity and the risk of cerebral white matter damage. *J Pediatr* 1999;134:706–711.

Lucas A., Morley R., Fewtrell M.S. Low triiodothyronine concentration in preterm infants and subsequent intelligence quotient (IQ) at 8 year follow up. *BMJ* 1996;312:1132–1133; discussion 1133–1134.

Mandel S.J., Cooper, D.S. The use of antithyroid drugs in pregnancy and lactation. *J Clin Endocrinol Metab* 2001;86:2354–2359.

Meijer W.J., et al. Transient hypothyroxinaemia associated with developmental delay in very preterm infants. *Arch Dis Child* 1992;67:944–947.

Mestman J.H. Hyperthyroidism in pregnancy. *Endocrinol Metab Clin North Am* 1998;27:127–149.

Mitchell M.L. Potential pitfalls in screening programs for congenital hypothyroidism. *NeoReviews* 2000;1:e110–e115.

Montoro M.N. Management of hypothyroidism during pregnancy. *Clin Obstet Gynecol* 1997;40:65–80.

Parravicini E., et al. Iodine, thyroid function, and very low birth weight infants. *Pediatrics* 1996;98:730–734.

Paul D.A., et al. Low serum thyroxine on initial newborn screening is associated with intraventricular hemorrhage and death in very low birth weight infants. *Pediatrics* 1998;101:903–907.

Rapaport R., Rose S.R., Freemark M. Hypothyroxinemia in the preterm infant: The benefits and risks of thyroxine treatment. *J Pediatr* 2001;139:182–188.

Reuss M.L., et al. The relation of transient hypothyroxinemia in preterm infants to neurologic development at two years of age. *N Engl J Med* 1996;334:821–827.

Reuss M.L., et al. Correlates of low thyroxine values at newborn screening among infants born before 32 weeks' gestation. *Early Hum Dev* 1997;47:223–233.

Reuss M.L., et al. Thyroxine values from newborn screening of 919 infants born before 29 weeks' gestation. *Am J Public Health* 1997;87:1693–1697.

Rovet J.F., Ehrlich R. Psychoeducational outcome in children with early-treated congenital hypothyroidism. *Pediatrics* 2000;105:515–522.

Smit B.J., et al. Neurologic development of the newborn and young child in relation to maternal thyroid function. *Acta Paediatr* 2000;89:291–295.

Toft A.D. Thyroxine therapy. *N Engl J Med* 1994;331:174–180.

van Wassenaer A.G., et al. Effects of thyroxine supplementation on neurologic development in infants born at less than 30 weeks' gestation. *N Engl J Med* 1997;336:21–26.

Wing D.A., et al. A comparison of propylthiouracil versus methimazole in the treatment of hyperthyroidism in pregnancy. *Am J Obstet Gynecol* 1994;170:90–95.

Preeclampsia and Related Conditions

Diana Rodriguez-Thompson

I. **Terminology of preeclampsia and related conditions**
   A. **Chronic hypertension.** Hypertension preceding pregnancy or before 20 weeks gestation.
   B. **Chronic hypertension with superimposed preeclampsia.** Worsening hypertension with new onset proteinuria, hyperuricemia, or thrombocytopenia in latter half of pregnancy in a woman with chronic hypertension.
   C. **Pregnancy-induced hypertension.** Hypertension without proteinuria.
   D. **Preeclampsia.** Hypertension with proteinuria.
   E. **Eclampsia.** Preeclampsia with seizure activity.

II. **Incidence and epidemiology.** Hypertensive disorders are a major cause of maternal morbidity and mortality, accounting for 15 to 20% of maternal deaths worldwide. In the United States, hypertensive disorders are the second leading cause of maternal mortality. Preeclampsia complicates 6% of pregnancies beyond 20 weeks' gestation; severe preeclampsia, less than 1%. Eclampsia itself is much less frequent, occurring in 0.1% of pregnancies. Several risk factors have been identified (Table 2.5).

   More recently the genetic thrombophilias (factor V Leiden mutation, prothrombin gene mutation, methylenetetrahydrofolate reductase mutation) have been associated with severe preeclampsia.

III. Many **etiologies** have been proposed: (1) an increased ratio of thromboxane to prostacyclin, which may lead to vasoconstriction, hypertension, and end-organ changes; (2) abnormal trophoblast invasion; (3) cardiovascular maladaptation; (3) increased circulating lipid peroxides, which may inhibit endogenous nitric oxide, a vasodilator, leading to vasoconstriction and hypertension; (4) endothelial-cell injury, with causative agent not yet identified; and (5) vasculitis that is

TABLE 2.5. RISK FACTORS FOR HYPERTENSIVE DISORDERS

Risk factor	Risk ratio
Nulliparity	3
Age > 40	3
African-American race	1.5
Family history of PIH	5
Chronic HTN	10
Chronic renal disease	20
Antiphospholipid antibody syndrome	10
Diabetes	2
Twin gestation	4

Angiotensinogen gene T235
    Homozygous
    Heterozygous
	
	20
	4

HTN = hypertension; PIH = pregnancy-induced hypertension.
Source: ACOG. Hypertension in pregnancy. Technical Bulletin # 219, January 1996.

due to circulating immune complexes, although supporting evidence for the last is inconsistent.

IV. **Diagnosis.** The classic triad defining preeclampsia is hypertension, proteinuria, and edema. The clinical spectrum of preeclampsia ranges from mild to severe. Most patients have mild disease that develops late in the third trimester.

A. **Criteria for the diagnosis of mild preeclampsia**

 1. **Hypertension** defined as a sustained blood pressure elevation of 140 mm Hg systolic or 90 mm Hg diastolic. Measurements should be taken in the sitting position, and proper cuff size should be ensured.
 2. **Proteinuria** defined as at least 300 mg of protein in a 24-hour period.
 3. **Nondependent edema** (e.g., periorbital, hands) is sometimes listed, but it is common and not as useful.

B. **Criteria for the diagnosis of severe preeclampsia**

 1. **Blood pressure** greater than 160 mm Hg systolic or 110 mm Hg diastolic with the diagnostic readings taken twice at least 6 hours apart.
 2. **Proteinuria** greater than 5 g per 24-hour collection.
 3. **Symptoms suggestive of end-organ damage.** Visual disturbances such as scotomata, diplopia or blindness, persistent severe headache, and epigastric pain.
 4. **Pulmonary edema.**
 5. **Oliguria** defined as less than 500 mL of urine per 24-hour collection.
 6. **Microangiopathic hemolysis.**
 7. **Thrombocytopenia.**
 8. **Hepatocellular dysfunction.** Elevated transaminases.
 9. **Intrauterine growth restriction (IUGR) or oligohydramnios.**

C. **HELLP syndrome** (hemolysis, elevated liver enzymes, and low platelets) represents advanced preeclampsia associated with disseminated intravascular coagulation (DIC) and reflects systemic end-organ damage. HELLP syndrome often appears without hypertension or proteinuria.

V. Complications of preeclampsia result in a **maternal mortality rate** of 3 per 100,000 live births in the United States. Maternal morbidity may include central nervous system complications (e.g., strokes, seizures, intracerebral hemorrhage, and blindness), DIC, hepatic failure or rupture, pulmonary edema, and abruptio placentae leading to maternal hemorrhage and/or acute renal failure. Fetal mortality markedly increases with rising maternal diastolic blood pressure and proteinuria. Diastolic blood pressures greater than 95 mm Hg are associated with a threefold rise in the fetal death rate. Fetal morbidity may include IUGR, fetal acidemia, and complications from prematurity.

VI. **Considerations in management**

A. **The definitive treatment for preeclampsia is delivery.** However, the severity of disease, ripeness of maternal cervix, gestational age at diagnosis, and pulmonary maturity of the fetus influence obstetric management. Delivery is usually indicated if there is nonreassuring fetal testing in a viable fetus, regardless of gestational age or fetal pulmonary maturity.

B. **Delivery should be considered** for all term patients with any degree of preeclampsia. Patients with very mild disease and an unfavorable cervix can be closely monitored in order to await a more favorable cervix; however, prolongation of pregnancy beyond 40 weeks is not recommended.

C. For patients with **preterm gestation and mild preeclampsia,** their pregnancies may continue with close observation as outlined in section VII until the development of severe preeclampsia, nonreassuring fetal testing, or fetal maturity.

D. **Consideration for delivery should be made in all patients with severe preeclampsia.** Conservative therapy of severe preeclampsia early in gestation has been suggested, with one study showing that in pregnancies between 28 and 32 weeks, conservative management resulted in a mean prolongation of pregnancy of 2 weeks. However, conservative management of severe preeclampsia may be associated with serious sequelae, such as acute renal failure, DIC, HELLP syndrome, abruptio placentae, eclampsia, and intrauterine fetal death. Patients should be counseled that prolongation of pregnancy in the setting of severe preeclampsia is for fetal benefit only, and conservative management should only be undertaken in centers where there is rapid availability of immediate obstetrical and neonatal care.

E. **Conservative management entails antihypertensive therapy and frequent maternal and fetal surveillance.** It should only be undertaken in carefully selected patients after an initial period of observation of 24 to 48 hours to ensure stability of the pregnant woman. Women with uncontrolled hypertension, thrombocytopenia, hepatocellular dysfunction, pulmonary edema, compromised renal function, or persistent headache or visual changes are not candidates for conservative management of severe preeclampsia remote from term.

F. **Although a trial of labor induction is not contraindicated in patients with severe preeclampsia, the success rate is low** in patients with severe preeclampsia remote from term with an unfavorable cervix (approximately 15% of patients in our center).

VII. **Clinical management of mild preeclampsia**
  A. **Antepartum management.** Conservative management of mild preeclampsia generally includes hospitalization with bed rest and close maternal and fetal observation. Outpatient management is an option for carefully selected patients. Compliant patients may be monitored at home; however, a period of initial observation to serially assess maternal and fetal status is recommended.
    1. **Fetal evaluation**
      a. An initial **ultrasound** should be performed at the time of diagnosis to rule out IUGR and/or oligohydramnios. A **nonstress test** or **biophysical profile** should also be performed.
      b. **Betamethasone** to accelerate fetal maturity should be administered if less than 34 weeks of gestation and no maternal contraindications exist.
      c. If the fetus is appropriately grown with reassuring fetal testing, **testing should be repeated weekly**.
      d. If the estimated fetal weight is < 10th percentile or there is oligohydramnios (amniotic fluid index ≤ 5), then **testing should be performed at least twice weekly** after consideration of delivery.
      e. Any **change in maternal status** should prompt evaluation of fetal status.
      f. **Fetal indications for delivery** include severe fetal growth restriction, nonreassuring fetal testing, and oligohydramnios.
    2. **Maternal evaluation**
      a. Women should be **evaluated for signs and symptoms** of preeclampsia and severe preeclampsia.
      b. **Laboratory evaluation** includes hematocrit, platelet count, quantification of protein excretion in the urine, serum creatinine, transaminase, and uric acid level in addition to albumin, lactate dehydrogenase, prothrombin time/partial thromboplastin time, and fibrinogen.
      c. **If criteria for mild preeclampsia is met,** laboratory studies should be performed at frequent intervals. At Brigham and Women's Hospital, women with mild preeclampsia have laboratory testing twice weekly.
      d. **Maternal indications for delivery** include gestational age greater than or equal to 38 weeks, thrombocytopenia (<100,000), progressive deterioration in hepatic or renal function, abruptio placentae, and persistent severe headaches, visual changes, or epigastric pain.
      e. **Antihypertensive agents** are not given to the mother because they have not been shown to improve outcome in cases of mild preeclampsia.
      f. **When early delivery is indicated,** it is our practice to induce labor. Cesarean delivery should be performed in cases of suspected fetal distress, when further fetal evaluation is not possible, or when a rapidly deteriorating maternal condition mandates expeditious delivery (e.g., HELLP with decreasing platelet counts, abruption).

B. Intrapartum management of preeclampsia

1. **Magnesium sulfate** (6 g intravenous [IV] load followed by 2 g/h infusion), used to prevent seizures, is started when the decision to proceed with delivery is made and continued for at least 24 hours postpartum or until symptoms are resolving in the mother. Unless contraindicated, magnesium sulfate has been shown to be the agent of choice for seizure prophylaxis. In patients with a contraindication to magnesium sulfate (e.g., myasthenia gravis, hypocalcemia), other antiseizure agents such as Dilantin may be used. Magnesium sulfate is renally cleared, thus urine output should be carefully monitored. Signs and symptoms of maternal toxicity include loss of deep tendon reflexes, somnolence, respiratory depression, cardiac arrhythmia, and, in extreme cases, cardiovascular collapse.

2. **Careful monitoring of fluid balance** is critical because preeclampsia is associated with capillary leaking, decreased intravascular volume, pulmonary edema, and oliguria.

3. **Severe hypertension** may be controlled with agents including hydralazine, labetalol, nifedipine, or nitroglycerin. We avoid sodium nitroprusside before delivery because of potential fetal cyanide toxicity. It is important to avoid large or abrupt reductions in blood pressure because decreased intravascular volume and poor uteroplacental perfusion can lead to acute changes suggestive of fetal compromise.

4. **Continuous electronic fetal monitoring** is recommended given the risk of fetal compromise. Patterns that suggest fetal compromise include persistent tachycardia, decreased short- and long-term variability, and recurrent late decelerations not responsive to standard resuscitative measures. Reduced fetal heart rate variability may also result from maternal administration of magnesium sulfate.

5. Patients may be safely administered **epidural anesthesia** in the absence of thrombocytopenia or DIC. Consideration should be given for early epidural catheter placement when the platelet count is reasonable and there is concern that it is decreasing. Any anesthesia should be carefully administered by properly trained personnel experienced in the care of women with preeclampsia given the hemodynamic changes associated with the condition. Adequate preload should be ensured to minimize the risk of hypotension.

6. **Invasive central monitoring** of the mother is rarely needed, even in the setting of severe preeclampsia.

C. Postpartum management. The mother's condition may worsen immediately after delivery. Signs and symptoms usually begin to resolve within 24 to 48 hours postpartum, however, and completely resolve within 1 to 2 weeks. Because postpartum eclamptic seizures generally occur within the first 48 hours and usually within the first 24 hours after delivery, magnesium sulfate is continued for at least 24 hours. Close monitoring of fluid balance is continued. Maternal diuresis is a sign that the disease process is resolving.

VIII. Management of eclampsia

A. About half of **eclamptic seizures** occur before delivery. Twenty percent occur during delivery, and another 30% occur in the postpartum period. There is no clear constellation of symptoms that will accurately predict those patients who will have an eclamptic seizure.

B. **Basic principles of maternal resuscitation** should be followed in the initial management of an eclamptic seizure: airway protection, oxygen, left lateral displacement to prevent uterine compression of vena cava, intravenous access, and blood pressure control.

C. Magnesium sulfate should be initiated for **prevention of recurrent seizures**. If untreated, 10% of women with eclamptic seizures will have a recurrent seizure.

D. A **transient fetal bradycardia** is usually seen during the seizure followed by a **transient fetal tachycardia** with loss of variability. It may take as long as

20 to 30 minutes for the fetal heart rate tracing to return to baseline. The fetus should be resuscitated in utero.

E. **Eclampsia is an indication for delivery but not necessarily an indication for cesarean delivery.** No intervention should be initiated until maternal stability is ensured and the seizure is over. Because of the risk of DIC, coagulation parameters should be assessed and appropriate blood products should be set up if necessary.

F. A **neurologic exam** should be performed once the patient recovers from the seizure. If the seizure is atypical or any neurologic deficit persists, **brain imaging** is indicated.

IX. **Recurrence risk.** Patients who have a history of preeclampsia are at increased risk for hypertensive disease in a subsequent pregnancy. Recurrence risk is as high as 40% in women with preeclampsia before 30 weeks of gestation in contrast to 10% or less in women with mild preeclampsia near term. Severe disease and eclampsia are also associated with recurrence. Racial differences exist, with black women having higher recurrence rates. The recurrence rate for HELLP syndrome is about 5%. The presence of a thrombophilia also confers an increase risk.

X. **Risk of chronic hypertension.** Preeclampsia may be linked to the development of chronic hypertension later in the mother's life. Women with recurrent preeclampsia, women with early-onset preeclampsia, and multiparas with a diagnosis of preeclampsia (even if not recurrent) are at an increased risk.

XI. **New treatments**

A. Because preeclampsia is associated with an increased thromboxane-prostacyclin ratio, **selective use of low-dose aspirin** has been evaluated. However, no clear benefit has been shown. The use of low-dose aspirin has been evaluated both in women considered low risk and high risk (insulin-dependent diabetes mellitus, chronic hypertension, multiple gestations, history of preeclampsia), and no benefit was shown in either group. In fact, within the low-risk population, there were more abruptions in the patients receiving low-dose aspirin compared with those receiving placebo. Although there may be a subgroup of patients that may benefit from low-dose aspirin, current data do not support its use.

B. Although earlier studies suggested that **antenatal calcium supplementation** may reduce the incidence of hypertensive disorders of pregnancy, a large National Institutes of Health–sponsored placebo-controlled trial did not show any benefit when given to healthy nulliparous women. Calcium supplementation did not decrease the incidence, severity, or timing of preeclampsia. Mean systolic and diastolic blood pressures were no different between the two groups. The question of whether calcium supplementation can benefit select high-risk groups has not been adequately addressed. There are no known apparent maternal, fetal, or neonatal side effects from calcium supplementation.

C. More recently, **a randomized controlled trial comparing supplementation with both vitamin C and E to placebo** in women with a history of preeclampsia or abnormal uterine artery Doppler revealed a significant reduction in the incidence of preeclampsia.

D. The efficacy of **heparin therapy** for the prevention of preeclampsia in women with a genetic thrombophilia is unknown.

XII. **Implications for the newborn**

A. Infants born to mothers with moderate or severe preeclampsia may show evidence of intrauterine growth restriction **(IUGR)** (see Chaps. 1 and 3) and are frequently delivered prematurely. They may tolerate labor poorly and require resuscitation.

B. **Medications used ante- or intrapartum** may affect the fetus.

1. **Short-term sequelae of hypermagnesemia,** such as hypotonia and respiratory depression, are sometimes seen (see Chap. 29). Long-term maternal administration of magnesium sulfate has rarely been associated with neonatal parathyroid abnormalities and other abnormalities of calcium homeostasis.

2. **Antihypertensive medications,** including calcium-channel blockers, may have fetal effects. Antihypertensive medications and magnesium sulfate generally are not contraindications to breastfeeding.
3. **Low-dose aspirin therapy** does not appear to increase the incidence of intracranial hemorrhage, asymptomatic bruising, bleeding from circumcision sites, or persistent pulmonary hypertension.
4. About one-third of infants born to mothers with preeclampsia have **decreased platelet counts at birth,** but the counts generally increase rapidly to normal levels. About 40 to 50% of newborns have neutropenia that generally resolves before 3 days of age. These infants may be at increased risk of neonatal infection.

Suggested Readings

American College of Obstetricians and Gynecologists. Technical Bulletin 219: Hypertension in Pregnancy. January 1996.

Caritis S., et al., National Institute of Child Health and Human Development Network of Maternal–Fetal Medicine Units. Low-dose aspirin to prevent preeclampsia in women at high risk. *N Engl J Med* 1998;338:701–705.

Chappeli L.C., et al. Effect of antioxidants on the occurrence of pre-eclampsia in women at increased risk: A randomized trial. *Lancet* 1999;354:810–816.

Cunningham F.G., et al. Hypertensive disorders in pregnancy. In: MacDonald, PC et al. (Eds.), *William's Obstetrics,* 19th ed. 1993; Norwalk, CT: Appleton & Lange, 763–817.

Levine R.J., et al. Trial of calcium to prevent preeclampsia. *N Engl J Med* 1997; 337:69–76.

Sibai B.M., et al. Maternal and perinatal outcome of conservative management of severe preeclampsia in midtrimester. *Am J Obstet Gynecol* 1985;152:32–37.

Sibai B.M., et al. Aggressive versus expectant management of severe preeclampsia at 28 to 32 weeks gestation: A randomized controlled trial. *Am J Obstet Gynecol* 1994;171:818–822.

3. ASSESSMENT OF THE NEWBORN

History and Physical Examination of the Newborn

William D. Cochran and Kimberly G. Lee

I. **History.** The family, maternal, pregnancy, and perinatal history should be reviewed (Table 3.1).

II. **Routine physical examination of the neonate.** Although no statistics are available, the first routine examination probably reveals more abnormalities than any other routine examination done.

A. **General examination.** At the initial examination, attention should be directed to determine (1) whether any congenital anomalies are present, (2) whether the infant has made a successful transition from fetal life to air breathing, (3) to what extent gestation, labor, delivery, analgesics, or anesthetics have affected the neonate, and (4) whether he or she has any sign of infection or metabolic disease.

1. The baby should be naked. Naked newborns are easily chilled, so they should not be kept uncovered for a long time unless they are in or under a warming device. A general appraisal of a naked newborn allows one to assess quickly whether any major anomalies are present, whether jaundice or meconium staining is present, and whether the infant is having trouble making the adjustment to breathing air. At least half of all infants will exhibit jaundice, although usually only at its peak on the third or fourth day of life. Visible jaundice usually means the bilirubin level is at least 5 mg/dL.

2. It is usually wise to examine infants in the order listed because they will be quieter at the beginning, when you most need their cooperation. If the infant being examined is fretful, offer the baby a pacifier or nipple.

B. **Cardiorespiratory system**

1. **Color.** Skin color is probably the single most important index of cardiorespiratory function. Good color in caucasian infants means an overall reddish pink hue, except for possible cyanosis of the hands, feet, and occasionally the lips (acrocyanosis). The mucous membranes of dark-skinned infants are more reliable indicators of cyanosis than skin. Infants of diabetic mothers and premature infants are pinker than average, and postmature infants are paler.

2. **Respiratory rate** is usually 40–60 breaths per minute. All infants are **periodic** rather than regular breathers, and premature infants are more so than term infants. Thus, babies may breathe at a fairly regular rate for a minute or so and then have a short period of no breathing (usually 5–10 seconds). **Apnea,** often defined as periods of no breathing during which an infant's color changes from normal to grades of cyanosis, is not normal, whereas periodic breathing is. Apnea is thus an abnormal prolongation of periodic breathing (see Chap. 24, Apnea).

3. In a warm infant there should be no expiratory grunting and little or no flaring of the nostrils. When crying, infants (especially premature infants) exhibit mild chest retraction; if unaccompanied by grunting, such retraction may be considered normal.

4. When an infant is pink and breathing without retractions or grunting at a rate of less than 60 breaths per minute, the respiratory system is usually intact. Significant respiratory disease in the absence of tachypnea is rare unless the infant also has severe central nervous system (CNS) depression. Rales, decreased heart or breath sounds, or asymmetry of breath sounds are occasionally found in an asymptomatic infant and may

TABLE 3.1.   IMPORTANT ASPECTS OF MATERNAL AND PERINATAL HISTORY

FAMILY HISTORY
   Inherited diseases (e.g., metabolic disorders, hemophilia, cystic fibrosis, polycystic kidneys, history of perinatal deaths)

MATERNAL HISTORY
   Age
   Blood type
   Transfusions
   Blood group sensitizations
   Chronic maternal illness
   Diabetes
   Hypertension
   Renal disease
   Cardiac disease
   Bleeding disorders
   Sexually transmitted diseases, including herpes and HIV/AIDS
   Infertility IVF (*in vitro* fertilization)
   Recent infections or exposures

PREVIOUS PREGNANCIES: PROBLEMS AND OUTCOMES
   Abortions
   Fetal demise
   Neonatal deaths
   Prematurity
   Postmaturity
   Malformations
   Respiratory distress syndrome
   Jaundice
   Apnea

DRUG HISTORY
   Medications
   Drug abuse
   Alcohol
   Tobacco

CURRENT PREGNANCY
   Probable gestational age
   Quickening (normally 16–18 weeks)
   Fetal heart heard with fetoscope (normally 18–20 weeks)

(continues)

TABLE 3.1.   (continued)

Results of any fetal testing (e.g., amniocentesis, ultrasound examination, estriols, fetal monitoring, tests of fetal lung maturity, and prenatal infection screening [hepatitis, group B streptococci, syphilis, etc.])

Preeclampsia

Bleeding

Trauma

Infection

Surgery

Polyhydramnios

Oligohydramnios

Glucocorticoids

Labor suppressant

Antibiotics

LABOR AND DELIVERY (PERINATAL)

Presentation

Onset of labor

Rupture of membranes

Duration of labor

Fever

Fetal monitoring

Amniotic fluid (blood, meconium, volume)

Analgesic

Anesthesia

Maternal oxygenation and perfusion

Method of delivery

Initial delivery room assessment (shock, asphyxia, trauma, anomalies, temperature, infection)

Apgar scores

Resuscitation

Placental examination

---

reveal occult disease that is confirmed by chest X ray (e.g., dextrocardia, pneumothorax, pneumomediastinum).

5. The **heart** should be examined. The examiner should observe precordial activity, rate, rhythm, the quality of the heart sounds, and the presence or absence of murmurs.

   a. It should be determined whether the heart is on the right or left side. This is done by auscultation and by palpation.

   b. The **heart rate** is normally 120–160 beats per minute. It varies with changes in the infant's activity, increasing when he or she is crying, active, or breathing rather rapidly, and decreasing when the baby is quiet and breathing slowly. To some, this physiologic slowing provides an important indicator that there is no significant cardiac stress. An occasional term or postmature infant may, at rest, have a heart rate well below 100. In a normal infant, the heart rate will increase if the baby is stimulated.

   c. **Murmurs** mean less in the newborn period than at any other time. Infants can have extremely serious heart anomalies without any murmurs. On the other hand, a closing ductus arteriosus may cause a murmur that is only transient, but at the time is very loud and worrisome. Gallop sounds may be an ominous finding, while the presence of a split S2 may be reassuring.

   d. If there is any question after auscultation and observation that the heart is abnormally placed, abnormally large, or overactive, a **chest X ray** is the best means of further assessment. Distant heart sounds, especially if accompanied by respiratory symptoms, are often secondary to pneumothorax or pneumomediastinum.

   e. The **femoral pulses** should be felt, although often they are weak in the first day or two. If there is doubt about the femoral pulses by time of discharge, the blood pressure in the upper and lower extremities should be checked. In infants with coarctation, pulses and pressures may be normal in the first few days of life while the ductus is still open (see Chap. 25).

C. **Abdomen.** The abdominal examination of a newborn differs from that of older infants in that observation can again be used to greater advantage.

   1. The anterior abdominal organs (e.g., liver, spleen, bowel) can often be seen through the abdominal wall, especially in thin or premature infants. The edge of the liver is occasionally seen, and intestinal patterning is easily visible. Asymmetry due to congenital anomalies or masses often is first appreciated by observation.

   2. When palpating the abdomen, start with gentle pressure or stroking, moving from lower to upper quadrants to reveal the edges of the liver or spleen. Try to appreciate mushiness when palpating over the intestine compared with the firmer feel over the liver or other organs or masses. The normal newborn liver extends 2.0–2.5 cm below the costal margin. The spleen is usually not palpable. Remember there may be situs inversus.

   3. After the abdomen has been gently palpated, **deep palpation** is possible, not only because of the lack of developed musculature but also because there is no food and little air in the intestine. Abnormal, absent, or misplaced kidneys and other deep masses should be felt for. Only during the first day or two of life is it possible for the kidneys to be routinely palpated with relative ease and reliability (see Chap. 31).

D. **Genitalia and rectum**

   1. **Male**

      a. Males almost invariably have marked **phimosis.**

      b. The **scrotum** is often quite large, since it is an embryonic analogue of the female labia and therefore has responded to maternal hormones.

      c. **Hydroceles** are not uncommon, but unless they are communicating types, they will disappear in time without being the forerunner of an inguinal hernia.

      d. The **testes** should be palpated, with the epididymis and vas identified. The testis is best found by running a finger from the internal ring down on either side of the upper shaft of the penis, thus pushing and trapping the testes in the scrotum. Each testis should be the same size, and they should not appear blue (a sign of torsion) through the scrotal skin.

      e. If present, the degree of **hypospadias** should be noted.

      f. The length and width of the penis should be measured. Length under 2.5 cm is abnormal and requires evaluation (see Chap. 30). Torsion of the penis is seen in 1.5% of normal males.

2. Female
   a. Female genitalia at term are most noticeable for their enlarged **labia majora.**
   b. Occasionally, a **mucosal tag** from the wall of the vagina is noted.
   c. A **discharge** from the vagina, usually creamy white in color, is commonly found and, on occasion, replaced after the second day by pseudomenses.
   d. The **labia** should always be spread, and cysts of the vaginal wall, imperforate hymen, or other less common anomalies should be sought.
3. The **anus** and **rectum** should be checked carefully for patency, position, and size (normal diameter is 10 mm). Occasionally, large fistulas are mistaken for a normal anus, but if one checks carefully, it will be noted that a fistula will be either anterior or posterior to the usual location of a normal anus.

E. Skin (see Chap. 34). The epidermis of a newborn (especially a premature infant) is thin; therefore, the oxygenated capillary blood makes it very pink. Common abnormalities include tiny **milia** (plugged sweat glands) on the nose, unusually brown-pigmented nevi scattered around any body part, and what are referred to as **mongolian spots.** Mongolian spots are bluish, often large areas most commonly seen on the back, buttocks, or thighs that fade slightly over the first year of life.

   Erythema toxicum may be noted occasionally at birth, although it is more common in the next day or two. These papular lesions with an erythematous base are found more on the trunk than the extremities and fade without treatment by 1 week of age.

   Look for **jaundice.**

F. Palpable **lymph nodes** are found in about one-third of normal neonates. They are usually under 12 mm in diameter and are often found in the inguinal, cervical, and occasionally the axillary area.

G. Extremities, spine, and joints (see Chap. 28)
   1. Extremities. Anomalies of the digits (too few, too many, syndactyly, or abnormal placement), club feet, and hip dislocation are the common problems. Because of fetal positioning, many infants have forefoot adduction, tibial bowing, or even tibial torsion. Forefoot adduction, if correctable with stretching, will often correct itself in weeks and is no cause for concern. Mild degrees of tibial bowing or torsion are also normal. Decreased motion of an arm should make one consider **Erb's palsy** or a **fracture** of a clavicle or other bone (see Chap. 20).
   2. To check for **hip dislocation** (if present, remember that the head of the femur will most often have been displaced superiorly and posteriorly), place the infant's legs in the frogleg position. With the third finger on the greater trochanter and the thumb and index finger holding the knee, attempt to relocate the femoral head in the acetabulum by pushing upward away from the mattress with the third finger and toward the mattress and laterally with the thumb at the knee. If there has been a dislocation, a distinct upward movement of the femoral head will be felt as it relocates in the acetabulum. Hip "clicks," due to movement of the ligamentum teres in the acetabulum, are much more common than dislocated hips (hip "clunks") and are not a cause for concern. It has been shown that not all dislocated hips are present at birth, hence the recent designation "developmental dysplasia of the hip."
   3. Back. The infant should be turned over and held face down on your hand. The back, especially the lower lumbar and sacral areas, should be examined. Special care should be taken to look for pilonidal sinus tracts and small soft midline swellings that might indicate a small meningocele or other anomaly (see Chap. 27).

H. Head, neck, and mouth
   1. Head
      a. The average full-term **head circumference** is 33–38 cm.

    b. The infant's **scalp** should be inspected for cuts or bruises due to forceps application or fetal monitor leads. Check laterally for erosions from the bony spines of the maternal pelvis, which may be difficult to see under hair. Scalp aplasia may also be present.

    c. **Caput succedaneum** (edema of the scalp from labor pressure) should be checked to see if there are underlying early cephalohematomas; **cephalohematomas** usually do not become full-blown until the third or fourth day.

    d. **Mobility of the suture lines** will rule out **craniosynostosis.** Mobility is checked by putting each thumb on opposite sides of the suture and then pushing in alternately while feeling for motion. The skull should be observed for **deformational plagiocephaly.**

    e. The degree of **molding of the skull bones** themselves should be noted, and it may be considerable. Usually, such molding will subside within 5 days.

    f. Occasional infants have **craniotabes,** a soft ping-pong ball effect of the skull bones (usually the parietal bones). It is most common in postmature or dysmature infants. If present, craniotabes is usually only an incidental finding that disappears in a matter of weeks, even if marked at birth.

    g. **Fontanelles.** As long as the head circumference is within normal limits and there is motion of the suture lines, one need pay little attention to the size (large or small) of the fontanelles. Very large fontanelles reflect a delay in bone ossification and may be associated with hypothyroidism (see Chap. 2, Thyroid Disorders), trisomy syndromes, intrauterine malnutrition, hypophosphatasia, rickets, and osteogenesis imperfecta. Normal tension is that in which the fontanelle softens when the infant is raised to the sitting position.

    h. **Ears.** Note size, shape, position, and presence of auditory canals as well as preauricular sinus, pits or skin tags.

  2. The **neck** should be checked for range of motion, goiter, and thyroglossal or branchial-arch sinus tracts. Occasionally, marked asymmetry is noted with a deep concavity on one side. Although the uninitiated might interpret this as possible agenesis of a muscle or muscle group, it is most commonly due to persistent fetal posture with the head tilted to one side **(asynclitism).** This is most easily confirmed by noting that the mandibular gum line is not parallel to the maxillary line, further evidence of unequal pressure on the jaw as a result of the head's being held tilted *in utero* over time (see Chap. 28).

  3. The **mouth** should be checked to ensure that there are neither hard nor soft palatal clefts, no gum clefts, and no deciduous teeth present. Rarely, cysts appear on the gum or under the tongue. **Epstein's pearls** (small white inclusion cysts clustered about the midline at the juncture of the hard and soft palate) are normal.

I. Neurologic examination. Much has been written about neonatal neurologic examinations, but more will have to be learned before the examination becomes an accurate evaluation—especially one with prognostic significance—when done at birth. A carefully performed, detailed examination will reveal more than a superficial one. Many senior physicians can recall an infant with hydranencephaly or a similar gross internal neurologic lesion that was completely missed by careful neurologic examination only to be found later by ultrasound of the head or even simple transillumination.

  1. Probably the most reliable information that can be obtained quickly is gained while handling the infant during the preceding parts of the examination. With experience, the examiner is able to carry out at least two examinations concurrently, that is, the examination of organ and physiologic systems and a simultaneous neurologic evaluation. Symmetry of movement and posturing, body tone, and response to being handled and disturbed (i.e., crying appropriately and quieting appropriately) can all be evaluated while other body parts are being tested.

2. The amount of crying should be carefully noted as well as the pitch. When the infant is crying, seventh nerve weaknesses should be sought (the affected side of the mouth does not pull down). **Erb's palsy,** if present, will usually be revealed by lack of motion of the shoulder and arm; the arm will lie beside the body in repose rather than being normally flexed with fist near mouth. Jitteriness that is present but disappears in the prone position is usually benign (see Chap. 27, Neonatal Seizures). Persistent crying should make one search for the cause of pain (e.g., fracture).

3. The essentials of a neurologic examination (beyond that acquired while carrying out other components of the physical examination) may be covered by doing the following:

   a. Put your index fingers in the infant's palms to obtain the Palmer grasp. Then hold the infant's fingers between your thumb and forefinger and pull him or her to a sitting position. Note the degrees of head lag and head control; remember a crying infant often throws the head back in anger. The infant should be held in a sitting position and the trunk moved forward and back enough to test head control again. Then let the trunk and head slowly fall back.

   b. To test the Moro reflex, pull your fingers quickly from his or her grasp just before the head touches the mattress, allowing the infant to fall onto the back. Usually the Moro reflex will result, although a "complete" Moro is demonstrable in only about 20% of cases.

   c. Touching the upper lip laterally will cause most infants to turn toward the touch and open their mouths; the hungrier and more vigorous the infant, the more intense is the rooting response. Placing a nipple in the mouth will initiate a sucking response.

4. **Stepping (and placing)** can be elicited by holding the infant upright with the feet on the mattress and then leaning the baby forward. This forward motion often sets off a slow alternate stepping action. However, a normal infant frequently will not perform the reflex.

5. The complete **behavioral examination** is more dependent on infant–examiner interaction. Much depends on the infant's relative wakefulness, whether the baby has just been fed or not, and to a degree, on the analgesia and anesthesia used during delivery. Eye opening is elicited when the infant is sucking or being held vertically. Some infants will appear alert and listen when they are spoken to in a pleasant voice. Almost all infants enjoy being cuddled. If some of these behavioral responses cannot be elicited, they may indicate either temporary or permanent problems. The more detailed behavioral examination also involves habituation to repeated stimuli of various sorts (noxious and otherwise) that will not be discussed here.

J. **Head circumference and length.** These measurements are usually last in the examination. The head circumference of a term (38- to 40-week) infant of normal weight (2.7–3.6 kg, or 6–8 lb) is usually 33–38 cm (13–15 in.). Crown-foot length is 48–53 cm (19–21 in.).

K. **Eye examination.** The eyes should be examined for the presence of scleral hemorrhages, icterus, conjunctival exudate, iris coloring, and pupillary size, equality, extraocular muscle movement, and centering. The red reflex should be obtained, and cataracts sought. Glaucoma is manifest by a large cloudy cornea. The normal cornea in a neonate measures less than 10.5 mm in horizontal diameter. In the first 2 days of life, puffy eyelids sometimes make examination of the eyes impossible. If so, it should be noted so that the eyes will be examined upon follow-up.

III. **Discharge examination.** At discharge, the infant should be reexamined with the following points considered:

A. **Heart.** Development of murmur, cyanosis, failure, femoral pulses.

B. **CNS.** Fullness of fontanelles, sutures, activity.

C. **Abdomen.** Any masses previously missed, stools, urine output.
D. **Skin.** Jaundice, pyoderma.
E. **Cord.** Infection.
F. **Infection.** Signs of sepsis.
G. **Feeding.** Spitting, vomiting, distension, degree of weight loss (or gain), dehydration.
H. **Parental competence.** To provide adequate care.
I. **Follow-up.** Arrangements made with infant's primary physician.

Suggested Readings
Bamji M., et al. Palpable lymph nodes in healthy newborns and infants. *Pediatrics* 78:573, 1986.

Ben-Ari J., et al. Characteristics of the male genitalia in the newborn. *J Urol* 135:521, 1985.

Brazelton T. B. *Neurobehavioral Assessment Scale.* Philadelphia: Lippincott, 1973.

El-Haddao M., et al. The anus in the newborn. *Pediatrics* 76:927, 1985.

Faix R. G. Fontanelle size in black and white term newborn infants. *J Pediatr* 100:304, 1982.

Nelson L. B. *Pediatric Ophthalmology.* Philadelphia: Saunders, 1984.

Scanlon J. W. *A System of Newborn Physical Examination.* Baltimore: University Park Press, 1979.

IDENTIFYING THE HIGH-RISK NEWBORN AND EVALUATING GESTATIONAL AGE, PREMATURITY, POSTMATURITY, LARGE-FOR-GESTATIONAL-AGE, AND SMALL-FOR-GESTATIONAL-AGE INFANTS

Kimberly G. Lee and John P. Cloherty

I. **High-risk newborns** are associated with certain conditions; when one or more of these are present, nursery staff should be aware and prepared for possible difficulties. The cord blood and placenta should be saved after delivery in all cases of high-risk delivery, including cases that involve transfer from the birth hospital. An elusive diagnosis such as toxoplasmosis may be made based on placental pathology. The following factors are associated with high-risk newborns:

A. **Maternal conditions**   **Associated risk for fetus or neonate**
  1. **Age at delivery**
    a. Over 40 years   Chromosomal abnormalities, macrosomia, intrauterine growth restriction (IUGR), blood loss (abruption, previa)
    b. Under 16 years   IUGR, prematurity, child abuse/neglect (mother herself may be abused)

  2. **Personal factors**
    a. Poverty   Prematurity, infection, IUGR
    b. Smoking   IUGR, increased perinatal mortality
    c. Drug, alcohol abuse   IUGR, fetal alcohol syndrome, withdrawal syndrome, sudden infant death syndrome, child abuse/neglect

d. Poor diet	Mild IUGR to fetal demise in severe malnutrition
e. Trauma (acute, chronic)	Fetal demise, prematurity
3. Medical history	
a. Diabetes mellitus	Congenital anomalies, stillbirth, respiratory distress syndrome (RDS), hypoglycemia, macrosomia/birth injury
b. Thyroid disease	Goiter, hypothyroidism, hyperthyroidism
c. Renal disease	IUGR, stillbirth, prematurity
d. Urinary tract infection	Prematurity, sepsis
e. Heart, lung disease	IUGR, stillbirth, prematurity
f. Hypertension (chronic or preeclampsia)	IUGR, stillbirth, asphyxia, prematurity
g. Anemia	IUGR, stillbirth, asphyxia, prematurity, hydrops
h. Isoimmunization (red cell antigens)	Stillbirth, anemia, jaundice, hydrops
i. Isoimmunization (platelets)	Stillbirth, bleeding
j. Thrombocytopenia	Stillbirth, bleeding
4. Obstetric history	
a. Past history of infant with prematurity, jaundice, RDS, or anomalies	Same with current pregnancy
b. Maternal medications	See specific medication insert and see Appendix C
c. Bleeding in early pregnancy	Stillbirth, prematurity
d. Hyperthermia	Fetal demise, fetal anomalies
e. Bleeding in third trimester	Stillbirth, anemia
f. Premature rupture of membranes, fever, infection	Infection/sepsis
g. TORCH infections	(See Chap. 23, Infections)
B. Fetal conditions	**Associated risk for fetus or neonate**
1. Multiple gestation	Prematurity, twin–twin transfusion syndrome, IUGR, asphyxia, birth trauma
2. Intrauterine growth restriction (IUGR)	Fetal demise, congenital anomalies, asphyxia, hypoglycemia, polycythemia
3. Macrosomia	Congenital anomalies, birth trauma, hypoglycemia
4. Abnormal fetal position	Congenital anomalies, birth trauma, hemorrhage
5. Abnormality of fetal heart rate or rhythm	Hydrops, asphyxia, congestive heart failure, heart block
6. Decreased activity	Fetal demise, asphyxia
7. Polyhydramnios	Anencephaly, other central nervous system (CNS) disorders, neuromuscular disorders, problems with swallowing (e.g., agnathia, esophageal atresia), chylothorax, diaphragmatic hernia, omphalocele, gastroschisis, trisomy, tumors, hydrops, isoimmunization, anemia, cardiac failure, intrauterine infection, inability to concentrate urine, maternal diabetes

8. Oligohydramnios	IUGR, placental insufficiency, postmaturity, fetal demise, intrapartum distress, renal agenesis, pulmonary hypoplasia, deformations
C. Conditions of labor and delivery	**Associated risk for fetus or neonate**
1. Premature labor	Respiratory distress syndrome (RDS), other issues of prematurity further elaborated in subsequent chapters
2. Labor occurring 2 weeks or more after term	Stillbirth, asphyxia, meconium aspiration (see **VI**)
3. Maternal fever	Infection/sepsis
4. Maternal hypotension	Stillbirth, asphyxia
5. Rapid labor	Birth trauma, intracranial hemorrhage (ICH)
6. Long labor	Stillbirth, asphyxia, birth trauma
7. Abnormal presentation	Birth trauma, asphyxia
8. Uterine tetany	Asphyxia
9. Meconium-stained amniotic fluid	Stillbirth, asphyxia, meconium-aspiration syndrome, persistent pulmonary hypertension
10. Prolapsed cord	Asphyxia, ICH
11. Cesarean section	RDS, retained fetal lung fluid/transient tachypnea, blood loss
12. Obstetric analgesia and anesthesia	Respiratory depression, hypotension, hypothermia
13. Placental anomalies	
a. Small placenta	IUGR
b. Large placenta	Hydrops, maternal diabetes
c. Torn placenta	Blood loss
d. Vasa praevia	Blood loss
D. Immediate neonatal conditions	**Associated risk for fetus or neonate**
1. Prematurity	RDS, other sequelae of prematurity
2. Low 5-minute Apgar score	Prolonged transition (especially respiratory)
3. Low 15-minute Apgar score	Cardiac failure, renal failure, severe neurologic damage
4. Pallor or shock	Blood loss
5. Foul smell of amniotic fluid or membranes	Infection
6. Small for gestational age	(see **IV**)
7. Postmaturity	(see **VI**)

II. **Gestational age estimation and birth weight classification**
   A. Attempts should be made to classify neonates by gestational age, as this is more meaningful than birth weight.
      1. Assessment based on **obstetric information** is covered in Chap. 1, Assessment and Prenatal Diagnosis, I. Note that gestational age estimates by first-trimester ultrasound are accurate within 4 days.
      2. To confirm or supplement obstetric dating, the modified Dubowitz (Ballard) examination for newborns (Fig. 3.1) may be useful in gestational age estimation. There are limitations to this method, especially with use of the neuromuscular component in sick newborns.
      3. **Infant classification by gestational (postmenstrual) age**
         a. **Preterm.** Less than 37 completed weeks (259 days).
         b. **Term.** 37 to 41 6/7 weeks (260–294 days).
         c. **Postterm.** 42 weeks (295 days) or more.
   B. Although there is no universal agreement on birth weight subclassifications, the commonly accepted definitions are as follows:
      1. **Normal birth weight (NBW).** 2500–3999 g.

Neuromuscular Maturity

	-1	0	1	2	3	4	5
Posture							
Square Window (wrist)	>90°	90°	60°	45°	30°	0°	
Arm Recoil		180°	140°-180°	110°-140°	90°-110°	<90°	
Popliteal Angle	180°	160°	140°	120°	100°	90°	<90°
Scarf Sign							
Heel to Ear							

Physical Maturity

Skin	sticky friable transparent	gelatinous red, translucent	smooth pink, visible veins	superficial peeling &/or rash, few veins	cracking pale areas rare veins	parchment deep cracking no vessels	leathery cracked wrinkled	
Lanugo	none	sparse	abundant	thinning	bald areas	mostly bald		
Plantar Surface	heel-toe 40-50mm: -1 <40mm: -2	>50mm no crease	faint red marks	anterior transverse crease only	creases ant. 2/3	creases over entire sole		
Breast	imperceptible	barely perceptible	flat areola no bud	stippled areola 1-2mm bud	raised areola 3-4mm bud	full areola 5-10mm bud		
Eye/Ear	lids fused loosely:-1 tightly:-2	lids open pinna flat stays folded	sl. curved pinna; soft; slow recoil	well-curved pinna; soft but ready recoil	formed & firm instant recoil	thick cartilage ear stiff		
Genitals male	scrotum flat, smooth	scrotum empty faint rugae	testes in upper canal rare rugae	testes descending few rugae	testes down good rugae	testes pendulous deep rugae		
Genitals female	clitoris prominent labia flat	prominent clitoris small labia minora	prominent clitoris enlarging minora	majora & minora equally prominent	majora large minora small	majora cover clitoris & minora		

Maturity Rating

score	weeks
-10	20
-5	22
0	24
5	26
10	28
15	30
20	32
25	34
30	36
35	38
40	40
45	42
50	44

Expanded NBS includes extremely premature infants and has been refined to improve accuracy in more mature infants.

FIG. 3.1. New Ballard score. (From J. L. Ballard, et al. New Ballard Score, expanded to include extremely premature infants. *J. Pediatr* 1991;119:417.)

   2. **Low birth weight (LBW).** Less than 2500 g. Note that, while most LBW infants are preterm, some are term but SGA. LBW infants can be further subclassified as follows:
      a. **Very low birth weight (VLBW).** Less than 1500 g.
      b. **Extremely low birth weight (ELBW).** Less than 1000 g.
III. **Prematurity.** A **preterm neonate** is one whose birth occurs through the end of the last day of the thirty-seventh week (259th day; i.e., 36 6/7 weeks) following onset of the last menstrual period.
   A. **Incidence.** Approximately 12% of all U.S. births are premature, and about 2% are less than 32 weeks' gestation. In some population segments, demographics play a major role in the incidence of prematurity.
   B. **Etiology** is unknown in most cases. Premature and/or LBW delivery is associated with the following conditions:
      1. **Low socioeconomic status** (SES), whether measured by family income, educational level, residency, social class, or occupation
      2. **African-American women's** rate of very premature (<32 weeks' gestation) delivery is almost three times that of Caucasian women, and their

rate of moderately premature (32–36 weeks) delivery is about one and a half times that of Caucasian women. Disparities persist even when SES is taken into account.

3. **Women under age 16 or over 35** are more likely to deliver LBW infants; the association with age is more significant in Caucasians than in African-Americans.

4. **Maternal activity** requiring long periods of standing or substantial amounts of physical stress may be associated with IUGR and prematurity. This is not significant in mothers from higher-SES groups, possibly because they are less likely to continue working in such jobs once they encounter pregnancy complications.

5. **Acute or chronic maternal illness** is associated with early delivery, whether spontaneous or, not infrequently, induced.

6. **Multiple-gestation births** frequently occur prematurely (57% of twins and 93% of triplets in 2000). Birth-weight–specific mortality is no higher in multiples than in singletons; thus their higher rate of neonatal mortality is primarily due to prematurity.

7. **Prior poor birth outcome** is the single strongest predictor of poor birth outcome. A preterm first birth is the best predictor of a preterm second birth.

8. **Obstetric factors** such as uterine malformations, uterine trauma, placenta previa, abruptio placentae, hypertensive disorders, preterm cervical shortening or "incompetence," previous cervical surgery, premature rupture of membranes, and amnionitis also contribute to prematurity.

9. **Fetal conditions** such as nonreassuring testing (see Chap. 1, Fetal Assessment and Prenatal Diagnosis), IUGR, or severe hydrops may require preterm delivery.

10. **Inadvertent early delivery** because of incorrect estimation of gestational age is now rare.

C. **Problems of prematurity**, which are related to difficulty in extrauterine adaptation due to immaturity of organ systems, are noted here but discussed in greater detail in other chapters.

1. **Respiratory**. Premature infants may experience:
   a. **Perinatal depression** in the delivery room due to poor adaptation to air breathing (see Chap.4, Resuscitation)
   b. **RDS** due to surfactant deficiency (see Chap. 24, Respiratory Disorders)
   c. **Apnea** due to immaturity in mechanisms controlling breathing (see Chap. 24).
   d. **Chronic lung disease,** variously described/classified as bronchopulmonary dysplasia, Wilson-Mikity disease, and chronic pulmonary insufficiency of prematurity (see Chap. 24)

2. **Neurologic**. Premature infants have a higher risk for neurologic problems including:
   a. Perinatal depression
   b. Intracranial hemorrhage (see Chap. 27, Neurology)
   c. Periventricular white-matter disease (see Chap. 27)

3. **Cardiovascular**. Premature infants may present with cardiovascular problems including:
   a. Hypotension.This may be due to
      (1) Hypovolemia,
      (2) Cardiac dysfunction, and/or
      (3) Vasodilation due to sepsis
   b. Patent ductus arteriosus is common and may lead to congestive heart failure (see Chap. 25, Cardiac Disorders).

4. **Hematologic**
   a. Anemia (see Chap. 26, Hematologic Problems)
   b. Hyperbilirubinemia (see Chap. 18, Neonatal Hyperbilirubinemia)

5. **Nutritional** Premature infants require specific attention to the content, amount, and route of feeding (see Chap. 10, Nutrition).

6. **Gastrointestinal.** Prematurity is the single greatest risk factor for necrotizing enterocolitis; formula feeding is also a significant risk factor; breast milk is protective (see Chap. 32, Necrotizing Enterocolitis).

7. **Metabolic** problems, especially in glucose and calcium metabolism, are more common in premature infants (see Chap. 29, Metabolic Problems).

8. **Renal.** Immature kidneys are characterized by low glomerular filtration rate and an inability to handle water, solute, and acid loads; fluid and electrolyte management can be difficult (see Chaps. 9, Fluid and Electrolyte Management, 31, Renal Conditions).

9. **Temperature regulation.** Premature infants are especially susceptible to hypothermia and hyperthermia (see Chap. 12, Temperature Control).

10. **Immunologic.** Because of deficiencies in both humoral and cellular response, premature infants are at greater risk for infection than are term infants.

11. **Ophthalmologic.** Retinopathy of prematurity may develop in the immature retina in infants < 32 weeks or < 1500 g birth weight (see Chap. 35, Auditory and Ophthalmologic Problems).

D. **Management of the premature infant**
   1. **Immediate postnatal management**
      a. **Delivery** in an appropriately equipped and staffed hospital is most important. Risks to the very premature or sick preterm infant are greatly increased by delays in initiating necessary specialized care.
      b. **Resuscitation and stabilization** require the immediate availability of qualified personnel and equipment. Anticipation and prevention are always preferred over reaction to problems already present. Adequate oxygen delivery and maintenance of proper temperature are immediate postnatal goals (see Chap. 4, Resuscitation).
   2. **Neonatal management**
      a. **Thermal regulation** should be directed toward achieving a neutral thermal zone, that is, the environmental temperature at which oxygen consumption is minimal yet sufficient to maintain body temperature. For the small preterm infant, this will require either an overhead radiant warmer (with the advantages of infant accessibility and rapid temperature response) or a closed incubator (with the advantages of diminished insensible water loss) (see Chap. 12, Temperature Control).
      b. **Oxygen therapy and assisted ventilation** (see Chap. 24, Respiratory Disorders)
      c. **Patent ductus arteriosus** in premature infants with birth weight >1000 g usually requires only conservative management: adequate oxygenation, fluid restriction, and possibly intermittent diuresis. In smaller infants, a prostaglandin antagonist such as indomethacin may be necessary. In the most symptomatic infants or those for whom indomethacin fails to close the ductus, surgical ligation may become necessary (see Chap. 25, Cardiac Disorders).
      d. **Fluid and electrolyte therapy** must account for potentially high insensible water loss while maintaining proper hydration and normal glucose and plasma electrolyte concentrations (see Chap. 9, Fluid and Electrolyte Management).
      e. **Nutrition,** which may be limited by the inability of many preterm infants to suck and swallow effectively or to tolerate enteral feedings, may require gavage feeding or parenteral nutrition. Mother's milk is the optimal primary source of enteral nutrition (see Chap. 10, Nutrition).
      f. **Hyperbilirubinemia,** which is inevitable in the smallest infants, can usually be managed effectively by careful monitoring of bilirubin levels and judicious use of phototherapy. In the most severe cases, exchange transfusion may be necessary (see Chap. 18, Neonatal Hyperbilirubinemia).
      g. **Infection** is always possible after preterm delivery. Broad-spectrum antibiotics should be begun when suspicion is strong. Consider anti-

staphylococcal antibiotics for VLBW infants who have undergone multiple procedures or have remained for long periods in the hospital and are at increased risk of nosocomial infection (see Chap. 23, Infections).

h. **Immunization.** Hepatitis B (HBV), diphtheria, pertussis, and tetanus (DPT), polio, multivalent pneumococcal, and hemophilus influenzae type B (HIB) vaccines are given in full doses to premature infants based on their chronologic age (i.e., weeks after birth), not postconceptional age.

(1) If the infant is hospitalized at the appropriate chronologic age (usually at 2, 4, and 6 months), acellular **DPT**, multivalent pneumococcal, and HIB vaccine are given. Pertussis vaccine is contraindicated in infants with possible or documented evolving neurologic disorders; these infants must receive pediatric DT, not adult DT vaccine. Infants with stable neurologic conditions may receive acellular DPT.

(2) Oral polio vaccine should not be given. Administer inactivated polio vaccine (IPV).

(3) Preterm infants whose mothers test positive for hepatitis B surface antigen (HBsAg-positive) should receive hepatitis B immune globulin within 12 hours of birth with the appropriate dose of HBV vaccine given concurrently at a different site, or as soon as possible thereafter, and always within the first month of life (see Chap. 23, Viral Infections in the Newborn).

The optimal timing for HBV vaccination in preterm infants with birthweight less than 2 kg whose mothers are HBsAg-negative is not clear. However, some studies have reported seroconversion rates in VLBW infants in whom vaccination was initiated shortly postpartum to be lower than in preterm infants vaccinated later or in term infants vaccinated shortly postpartum. The first vaccination in preterm infants with birthweight less than 2 kg and HBsAg-negative mothers should thus be delayed until just before hospital discharge if the infant weighs 2 kg or more, or until approximately 2 months, when other immunizations are given.

(4) Preterm infants with chronic respiratory disease should receive influenza immunization at 6 months if they are not hospitalized. To protect hospitalized infants with respiratory or other chronic conditions who are younger than 6 months, family and other caretakers should be immunized against influenza.

(5) Respiratory syncytial virus (RSV) prophylaxis (intramuscular immune globulin; Palivizumab) should be considered during RSV season for infants who meet any of the following criteria:

(a) born at less than 32 weeks' gestation;

(b) born between 32 and 35 weeks with

(i) plans for day care during RSV season;

(ii) smoker(s) in the household

(iii) other young children in the household

(c) chronic lung disease.

(6) Immunizations should be given at least 48 hours prior to discharge so that any febrile response will occur in the hospital.

E. **Survival of premature infants.** Figure 3.2 shows the survival rates by birthweight category of 118,448 VLBW infants admitted to the 362 NICUs participating in the Vermont Oxford Network over a 9-year period from 1991–1999. Mortality was highest (around 50%) in the smallest group of babies (501–750 g) and lowest (<10%) in the heaviest group (1000–1500 g). Similarly, in a series of 20,488 infants admitted to Canadian NICU Network facilities from 1996–1997, Lee, et al. noted that survival rates increased markedly with increasing GA between 22 and 26 weeks.

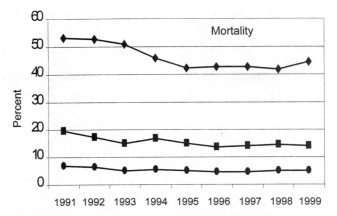

FIG. 3.2 Mortality for infants 501–1500 g, 1991 to 1999, by birth weight category at all 362 network hospitals (501–750 g: diamond markers; 751–1000 g: square markers; 1001–1500 g: circle markers). (From Horbar J. D. et al. Trends in mortality and morbidity for very low birth weight infants, 1991–1999. *Pediatr* 2002;110:143–151.)

    F. Long-term problems of prematurity. Premature infants are vulnerable to a wide spectrum of morbidity. The risk of morbidity, like that of mortality, declines markedly with increasing gestational age (GA). Although severe impairment occurs in a small population, the prevalence of lesser morbidities is less clearly defined, although large controlled multicenter trials are now providing a more comprehensive picture both of these sequelae and of the effects of intervention.

      1. Developmental disability.

        a. Major handicaps (cerebral palsy, mental retardation).

        b. Sensory impairments (hearing loss, visual impairment) (see Chap. 35, Auditory and Ophthalmologic Problems).

        c. Minimal cerebral dysfunction (language disorders, learning disability, hyperactivity, attention deficits, behavior disorders).

      2. Retinopathy of prematurity (see Chap. 35, Auditory and Ophthalmologic Problems).

      3. Chronic lung disease (see Chap. 24, Respiratory Disorders).

      4. Poor growth (see Chap. 10, Nutrition).

      5. Increased rates of postneonatal illness and rehospitalization

      6. Increased frequency of congenital anomalies

  IV. Infants who are SGA (see Chap. 1, Assessment and Prenatal Diagnosis)

    A. Definition. There is no uniform definition of SGA, although most reports define it as two standard deviations below the mean for gestational age or as below the tenth percentile. For practical purposes, infants with birth weights less than the third percentile for gestational age are at the greatest risk of perinatal morbidity and mortality. Further, babies who are constitutionally SGA are at lower risk compared to those who have experienced intrauterine growth restriction (IUGR) due to some pathologic process. Numerous "normal birth curves" have been defined using studies of large infant populations (see Fig. 3.3); it should be noted that over the past 30 years birth weight has increased in the general population.

    B. Etiology. Approximately one-third of LBW infants are SGA. There is an association of the following factors with SGA infants:

      1. Maternal factors.

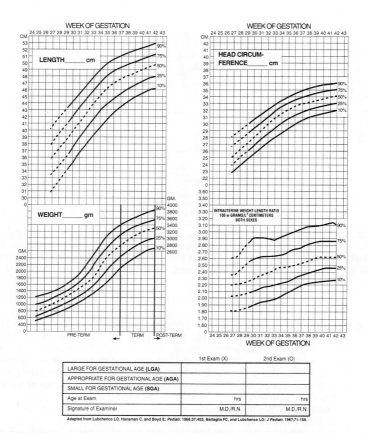

FIG. 3.3. Sample of a form used to classify newborns based on maturity and intrauterine growth. (Reproduced with permission from a form developed by Kay J. L., Seton Medical Center, Austin, TX, with Mead Johnson & Co., Evansville, IN.)

a. Genetic size
b. Demographics
    (1) Age (extremes of reproductive life)
    (2) Race
    (3) Socioeconomic status
c. Underweight before pregnancy (e.g., malnutrition)
d. Chronic disease
e. Factors interfering with placental flow and oxygenation
    (1) Heart disease
    (2) Renal disease
    (3) Hypertension (chronic or preeclampsia)
    (4) Tobacco use
    (5) Cocaine use
    (6) Sickle-cell anemia and other hemoglobinopathies
    (7) Pulmonary disease
    (8) Collagen-vascular disease
    (9) Diabetes (e.g., classes D, E, F, and R) (see Chap. 2, Diabetes Mellitus)
   (10) Postmaturity

(11) Multiple gestation/placentation
(12) Uterine anomalies
(13) Thrombotic disease
(14) High-altitude environment
f. Parity (nulliparity, grand multiparity)
g. Malnutrition
h. Exposure to teratogens such as alcohol, drugs, and radiation

2. **Placental factors**
   a. Malformations (e.g., vascular malformations, velamentous cord insertion)
   b. Chorioangioma
   c. Infarction
   d. Abruption
   e. Previa
   f. Abnormal trophoblast invasion

3. **Fetal factors**
   a. **Constitutional**—the majority of SGA infants: normal, "genetically small"
   b. **Chromosomal abnormality**—under 5% of SGA infants; more likely in the presence of malformation
   c. **Malformations,** especially abnormalities of CNS and skeletal system
   d. **Congenital infection,** especially rubella and cytomegalovirus (see Chap. 23, Infections).
   e. **Multiple gestation**

C. **Management of intrauterine growth restriction**
   1. **Pregnancy** (see Chap. 1, Assessment and Prenatal Diagnosis)
      a. Determination of the cause should be attempted when IUGR is detected. The investigation includes a search for relevant factors (listed in IV.B) and includes thorough ultrasonic examination.
      b. An attempt should be made to assess fetal well-being. Antepartum fetal monitoring, including nonstress testing, oxytocin challenge testing, a biophysical profile, and serial ultrasonic examinations, is generally used (see Chap. 1, Assessment and Prenatal Diagnosis). Doppler evaluation of placental flow may be used to evaluate uteroplacental insufficiency.
      c. Treatment (e.g., for hypertension) should be initiated when available.
      d. Determination of fetal pulmonary maturity should be considered if early delivery is contemplated (see Chaps. 1, Fetal Assessment and Prenatal Diagnosis; 24, Respiratory Disorders).
   2. **Delivery.** Early delivery is necessary if the risk of remaining *in utero* is considered greater for the fetus than the risk of prematurity.
      a. Generally, indications for delivery are arrest of fetal growth, fetal distress, and pulmonary maturity near term, especially in a mother with hypertension.
      b. Acceleration of pulmonary maturity with glucocorticoids administered to the mother should be considered if amniotic fluid analyses suggest pulmonary immaturity, or delivery is anticipated remote from term.
      c. If there is poor placental blood flow, the fetus may not tolerate labor and may require cesarean delivery.
      d. As noted in IV. A., very IUGR infants are at risk for perinatal problems and often require specialized care in the first few days of life. Thus, if possible, delivery should occur at a center with a special care nursery. The delivery team should be prepared to manage fetal distress, perinatal depression, meconium aspiration, hypoxia, hypoglycemia, and heat loss.
   3. **In the nursery**
      a. If not yet known, the cause of IUGR should be investigated; in many cases the etiology will remain unclear.
         (1) Newborn examination.The infant should be evaluated for signs of any of the previously listed causes of poor fetal growth, especially chromosomal abnormalities, malformations, and congenital infection.

(a) Infants who had growth restriction due to factors active during the phase of cellular hypertrophy in the last part of pregnancy (e.g., preeclampsia) will have a relatively normal head circumference, some reduction in length, but a more profound reduction in weight (see Figs. 3.4, 3.5). This is thought to be due to the redistribution of fetal blood flow preferentially to vital organs (e.g., brain), hence the term "head-sparing IUGR." Use of the ponderal index (birth weight in grams $\times$ 100 / [length in centimeters]^3) or the weight-length ratio will quantify weight loss. These infants may have little subcutaneous tissue, peeling loose skin, a wasted appearance, and meconium staining. The usual physical markers of gestational age (e.g., vernix, breast buds) may not be reliable due to the "head-sparing" redistribution of perfusion.

(b) Infants whose growth restriction began in early pregnancy, during the phase of early fetal cellular hyperplasia, will have proportionally small head circumference, length, and weight. These infants are sometimes referred to as "symmetrically IUGR" and their ponderal index may be normal. As compared with infants whose IUGR began in late pregnancy, symmetrically IUGR infants are more likely to have significant intrinsic fetal problems (e.g., chromosomal defects, malformations, and congenital infection).

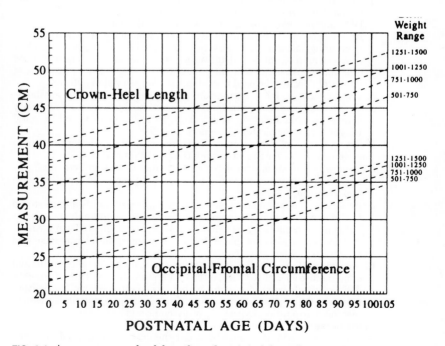

FIG. 3.4. Average crown–heel length and occipital-frontal circumference (centimeters) versus postnatal age (days) for infants with birth-weight ranges 501–750 g, 751–1000 g, 1001–1250 g, and 1251–1500 g. (From Wright K. et al. New postnatal growth grids for very low birth weight infants. *Pediatrics* 1993;91:922.)

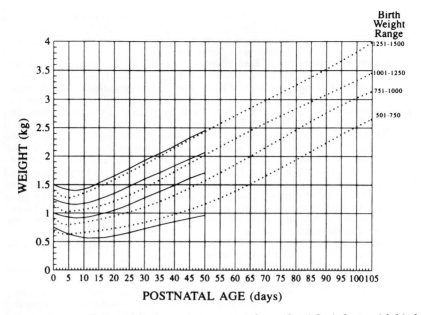

FIG. 3.5. Average daily weight (grams) vs. postnatal age (days) for infants with birth weight ranges 501–701 g, 751–1000 g, 1001–1250 g, and 1250–1500 g (dotted lines), plotted with the curves of Dancis et al. for infants with birth weights 750, 1000, 1250, and 1500 g (solid lines).

(2) **Pathologic examination of the placenta** for infarction or congenital infection may be helpful.

(3) Generally, **serologic screening** for congenital infection is not indicated unless history or examination suggests infection as a possible cause.

b. Potential complications related to IUGR

(1) **Congenital anomalies**

(2) **Perinatal depression**

(3) **Meconium aspiration**

(4) **Pulmonary hemorrhage**

(5) **Persistent pulmonary hypertension**

(6) **Hypothermia**

(7) **Hypoglycemia**

(8) **Hypocalcemia**

(9) **Acute tubular necrosis/renal insufficiency**

(10) **Polycythemia**

(11) **Thrombocytopenia**

(12) **Neutropenia**

c. **Specific management considerations**

(1) SGA infants in general require **more calories per kilogram** than AGA infants for "catch-up" growth; term SGA infants will often regulate their intake accordingly.

(2) **Blood glucose level** should be monitored every 2–4 hours until in the normal range and stable.

(3) **Serum calcium levels** may be significantly depressed in preterm SGA infants and/or those who have experienced hypoperfusion.

(4) The **serum sodium concentration** may also be low (see Chap. 9, Fluid and Electrolyte Management).

D. **Long-term problems of SGA infants.** As noted in IV.A., the majority of SGA infants have not experienced IUGR and are at low risk. However, it is difficult to determine specific effects of IUGR because of the multifactorial etiologies involved. Further, not all studies control well for parental height and socioeconomic status, and there are often overlapping effects from prematurity and asphyxia. The comparison groups vary as well: while SGA infants have a lower risk of neonatal death compared with premature AGA infants of the same birth weight, they have a higher perinatal mortality rate than AGA infants of the same gestational age. They also have a greater risk of morbidity at 1 year of age. In general, SGA infants are at higher risk for poor postnatal growth. Those who are preterm and/or from poor socioeconomic environments may also be at increased risk for adverse cognitive outcomes. Finally, some adults who were SGA at birth appear to have a higher risk of coronary heart disease and related health problems, including hypertension, non-insulin-dependent diabetes, and stroke.

E. **Management of subsequent pregnancies** is important because IUGR commonly recurs. Specific recommendations include:
1. The mother should be cared for by personnel experienced with high-risk pregnancies.
2. The health of mother and fetus should be assessed throughout pregnancy by ultrasound and nonstress tests (see Chap. 1, Assessment and Prenatal Diagnosis).
3. Early delivery should be considered if fetal growth is poor.

V. **Infants who are large for gestational age (LGA)** (see Chap. 1, Fetal Assessment and Prenatal Diagnosis)

A. **Definition.** The newborn's birth weight is two standard deviations above the mean or above the ninetieth percentile (see Fig. 3.3).

B. **Etiology**
1. Constitutionally large infants (large parents)
2. Infants of diabetic mothers (e.g., classes A, B, and C)
3. Some postterm infants
4. Beckwith-Wiedemann and other syndromes

C. **Management**
1. The baby should be evaluated for problems listed in V.B.
2. Look for possible evidence of birth trauma, including brachial plexus injury and perinatal depression (see Chaps. 20, Birth Trauma; 27, Neurology).
3. The infant should be allowed to feed early, and the blood sugar level should be monitored. Some LGA infants may have hyperinsulinism and hence be prone to hypoglycemia (especially infants of diabetic mothers, infants with Beckwith-Wiedemann syndrome, or infants with erythroblastosis [see Chaps. 2, Diabetes Mellitus, and 29, Hypoglycemia and Hyperglycemia]).
4. Consider the possibility of polycythemia (see Chap. 26, Hematologic Problems).

VI. **Postterm infants**

A. **Definition.** The newborn's gestation exceeds 42 completed weeks. Between 3% and 12% of pregnancies reach this point.

B. **Etiology.** The cause of prolonged pregnancy is unknown in the majority of cases. The following are known associations:
1. **Anencephaly**. An intact fetal pituitary-adrenal axis is involved in the initiation of labor.
2. **Trisomies 16 and 18**
3. **Seckel's syndrome** (bird-headed dwarfism)
4. **Erroneous estimation of gestational age**

C. Syndrome of postmaturity. These infants usually have normal length and head circumference. If they have postmaturity syndrome, however, they will have lost weight. SGA infants also may have these signs and symptoms, and postmature infants may also be SGA. Postmature infants may be classified as follows:

1. Stage 1
  a. Dry, cracked, peeling, loose, and wrinkled skin
  b. Malnourished appearance
  c. Decreased subcutaneous tissue
  d. Skin "too big" for baby
  e. Open-eyed and alert baby

2. Stage 2
  a. All features of stage 1
  b. Meconium staining
  c. Perinatal depression (in some cases)

3. Stage 3
  a. The findings in stages 1 and 2
  b. Meconium staining of cord and nails
  c. A higher risk of fetal, intrapartum, or neonatal death

D. Management

1. Prepartum management
  a. Careful estimation of true gestational age, including ultrasound data.
  b. Antepartum assessments by cervical examination and monitoring of fetal well-being (see Chap. 1, Fetal Assessment and Prenatal Diagnosis) should be initiated between 41 and 42 weeks on at least a weekly basis. If fetal testing is not reassuring, delivery is usually indicated. In most instances, a patient is a candidate for induction of labor if the pregnancy is at greater than 41 weeks of gestation and the condition of the cervix is favorable.

2. Intrapartum management involves use of fetal monitoring and preparation for possible perinatal depression and meconium aspiration.

3. Postpartum management
  a. Evaluation for complications related to postmaturity. The following conditions occur more frequently in postmature infants:
    (1) Congenital anomalies
    (2) Perinatal depression
    (3) Meconium aspiration
    (4) Persistent pulmonary hypertension
    (5) Hypoglycemia
    (6) Hypocalcemia
    (7) Polycythemia
  b. Attention to proper nutritional support.

Suggested Readings

American Academy of Pediatrics and American College of Obstetricians and Gynecologists. *Guidelines for perinatal care*, 4th edition. Evanston, Ill.,: American Academy of Pediatrics and American College of Obstetricians and Gynecologists, 1997.

American Academy of Pediatrics Committee on Infectious Diseases. Policy statement: recommendations for the prevention of pneumococcal infections, including the use of pneumococcal conjugate vaccine (Prevnar), pneumococcal polysaccharide vaccine, and antibiotic prophylaxis. *Pediatrics* 2000;106:362.

Barker D.J. Early growth and cardiovascular disease. *Arch Dis Child* 1999;80:305.

Dancis J., et al. A grid for recording the weight of premature infants. *J Pediatr* 1948;33:570–572.

Horbar J.D., Badger G.J., Carpenter J.H., et al. Trends in mortality and morbidity for very low birth weight infants, 1991–1999. *Pediatrics* 2002;110:143–151.

Lee S., et al. Variations in practice and outcomes in the Canadian NICU Network: 1996–97. *Pediatrics* 2000;106:1070.

McCormick M., et al. Early educational intervention for very low birth weight infants: results from the Infant Health and Development Program. *Pediatrics* 1993;123:527.

National Center for Health Statistics. Births: final data for 2000. National Vital Statistics Reports 50(5):15,16. Hyattsville, Md.: U.S. Dept of Health and Human Services, February 12, 2002.

Report of Committee on Infectious Disease: The Red Book. Evanston, Ill.: American Academy of Pediatrics, 2000.

Vohr B.R., et al., Neurodevelopmental and functional outcomes of extremely low birth weight infants in the National Institute of Child Health and Human Development Neonatal Research Network, 1993–1994. *Pediatrics* 2000;105:1216.

4. RESUSCITATION IN THE DELIVERY ROOM

Steven A. Ringer

I. **General principles.** A person skilled in basic neonatal resuscitation should be present at every delivery. Delivery of all high-risk infants should be attended by skilled personnel whose sole responsibility is the newborn.

The highest standard of care requires the following: (1) knowledge of perinatal physiology and principles of resuscitation; (2) mastery of the technical skills required; and (3) a clear understanding of the roles of other team members, which allows accurate anticipation of each person's reactions in a specific instance. Certification of each caregiver by the Newborn Resuscitation Program of the American Academy of Pediatrics/American Heart Association (NRP) ensures that each employs a consistent approach to resuscitations.

A. **Perinatal physiology.** Resuscitation efforts at delivery are designed to help the newborn make the respiratory and circulatory transitions that must be accomplished rapidly and effectively: The lungs expand, clear fetal lung fluid, and establish effective air exchange, and the right-to-left circulatory shunts terminate. The critical period for these physiologic changes is during the first several breaths, which result in lung expansion and elevation of the partial pressure of oxygen (PO_2) in both the alveoli and the arterial circulations. Elevation of the PO_2 from the fetal level of approximately 25 mm Hg to values of 50–70 mm Hg is associated with (1) decrease in pulmonary vascular resistance, (2) decrease in right-to-left shunting via the ductus arteriosus, (3) increase in venous return to the left atrium, (4) rise in left atrial pressure, and (5) cessation of right-to-left shunt through the foramen ovale. The end result is conversion from fetal to transitional to neonatal circulation pattern. Adequate systemic arterial oxygenation results from perfusion of well-expanded and well-ventilated lungs and adequate circulation.

Conditions at delivery may compromise the fetus's ability to make the necessary transitions. Alterations in tissue perfusion and oxygenation ultimately result in depression of cardiac function, but human fetuses initially respond to hypoxia by becoming apneic. Even a relatively brief period of oxygen deprivation may result in this **primary apnea**. Rapid recovery from this state is generally accomplished with appropriate stimulation and oxygen exposure. If the period of hypoxia continues, the fetus will irregularly gasp and lapse into **secondary apnea**. This state may occur remote from birth or in the peripartum period. Infants born during this period require resuscitation with assisted ventilation and oxygen (see III.B).

B. **Goals of resuscitation** are directed toward the following:
1. **Minimizing immediate heat loss** by drying and providing warmth, thereby decreasing oxygen consumption by the neonate.
2. **Establishing normal respiration and lung expansion** by clearing the upper airway and using positive-pressure ventilation if necessary.
3. **Increasing arterial PO_2** by providing adequate alveolar ventilation. The **routine** use of added oxygen is not warranted, but this therapy may be necessary in some situations.
4. **Supporting adequate cardiac output.**

II. **Preparation.** Anticipation is key in ensuring that adequate preparations have been made for a neonate likely to require resuscitation at birth. It is estimated that as many as 10% of neonates require some assistance at birth for normal transition.

A. **Perinatal conditions associated with high-risk deliveries.** Ideally, the obstetrician should notify the pediatrician well in advance of the actual birth. The pediatrician may then review the obstetric history and events leading to the high-risk delivery and prepare for the specific problems that may be anticipated. If time permits, the problems should be discussed with the parent(s). The following antepartum and intrapartum events warrant the presence of a resuscitation team at delivery.

1. **Evidence of nonreassuring fetal status**
   a. Serious heart-rate abnormalities, for example, sustained bradycardia
   b. Scalp pH of 7.20 or less
   c. Nonreassuring heart-rate pattern (see Chap. 1, Fetal Assessment and Prenatal Diagnosis)
2. **Evidence of fetal disease or potentially serious conditions (see Chap. 3)**
   a. Meconium staining in amniotic fluid and other evidence of possible fetal compromise (see Chap. 24, Respiratory Disorders)
   b. Prematurity (<36 weeks), postmaturity (>42 weeks), anticipated low birth weight (<2.0 kg), or high birth weight (>4.5 kg)
   c. Major congenital anomalies diagnosed prenatally
   d. Hydrops fetalis
   e. Multiple gestation (see Chap. 7, Multiple Births)
   f. Cord prolapse
   g. Abruptio placentae
3. **Labor and delivery conditions**
   a. Significant vaginal bleeding
   b. Abnormal fetal presentation
   c. Prolonged, unusual, or difficult labor

B. The following conditions do not require a pediatric team to be present, but personnel should be available for assessment and triage.
1. **Neonatal conditions**
   a. Unexpected congenital anomalies
   b. Respiratory distress
   c. Unanticipated neonatal depression, for example, Apgar score of less than 6 at 5 minutes
2. **Maternal conditions**
   a. Signs of maternal infection
      (1) Maternal fever
      (2) Membranes ruptured for more than 24 hours
      (3) Foul-smelling amniotic fluid
      (4) History of sexually transmitted disease
   b. Maternal illness or other conditions
      (1) Diabetes mellitus
      (2) Rh or other isoimmunization without evidence of hydrops fetalis
      (3) Chronic hypertension or pregnancy-induced hypertension
      (4) Renal, endocrine, pulmonary, or cardiac disease
      (5) Alcohol or other substance abuse

C. **Necessary equipment** must be present and operating properly. Each delivery room should be equipped with the following:
1. **Radiant warmer** with procedure table or bed. The warmer must be turned on and checked before delivery. Additional heat lamps for warming a very low-birth-weight (VLBW) infant should be available.
2. **Oxygen source (100%)** with adjustable flowmeter and adequate length of tubing. A humidifier and heater may be desirable. While not available currently in many delivery rooms, pulse oximetry and a system for providing an air–oxygen mixture of adjustable content may become standard equipment in the future.
3. Flow-through **anesthesia bag** with adjustable pop-off valve or self-inflating bag with reservoir. The bag must be appropriately sized for neonates (generally about 750 mL) and capable of delivering 100% oxygen.
4. **Face mask(s)** of appropriate size for the anticipated infant.
5. **A bulb syringe** for suctioning.
6. **Stethoscope** with infant- or premature-sized head.
7. **Equipped emergency box.**

    a. Laryngoscope with no. 0 and no. 1 blades
    b. Extra batteries
    c. Uniform diameter endotracheal tubes (2.5-, 3.0-, and 3.5-mm internal diameters), two of each
    d. Drugs, including epinephrine (1:10,000), sodium bicarbonate (0.50 mEq/mL), naloxone, albumin 5%, and NaCl 0.9%
    e. Umbilical catheterization tray with 3.5 and 5F catheters
    f. Syringes (1.0, 3.0, 5.0, 10.0, and 20.0 mL), needles (18–25 gauge), T-connectors, and stopcocks
  8. Transport incubator with battery-operated heat source and portable oxygen supply should be available if delivery room is not close to the nursery.
  9. The utility of equipment for continuous monitoring of cardiopulmonary status in the delivery room is hampered by difficulty in effectively applying monitor leads.

D. Preparation of equipment. Upon arrival in the delivery room, check that the transport incubator is plugged in and warm, and has a full oxygen tank. The specialist should introduce himself or herself to the obstetrician and anesthesiologist, the mother (if she is awake), and the father (if he is present). While the history or an update is obtained, the following should be done:

  1. Ensure that the radiant warmer is on, and that dry, warm blankets are available.
  2. Turn on the oxygen source and adjust the flow to 5–8 L/min.
  3. Test the anesthesia bag for pop-off control and adequate flow. Be sure the proper-sized mask is present.
  4. Make sure the laryngoscope light is bright and has an appropriate blade (no. 1 for full-term neonates, no. 0 for premature neonates).
  5. Set out an appropriate endotracheal tube for the expected birth weight (3.5 mm for full-term infants, 3.0 mm for premature infants >1250 g, and 2.5 mm for smaller infants). The NRP recommends a 4.0-mm tube for larger babies, but this is rarely necessary. For all babies, the tube should be 13 cm long. An intubation stylet may be used, if the tip is kept at least 0.5 cm from the distal end of the endotracheal tube.
  6. If the clinical situation suggests that extensive resuscitation may be needed, the following actions may be required:
    a. Set up an umbilical catheterization tray for venous catheterization.
    b. Draw up sodium bicarbonate (0.5 mEq/mL) solution, 1:10,000 epinephrine, and isotonic saline for catheter flush solution.
    c. Check that other potentially necessary drugs are present and ready for administration.

E. Universal precautions. Exposure to blood or other body fluids is inevitable in the delivery room. Universal precautions must be practiced by wearing caps, goggles or glasses, gloves, and impervious gowns until the cord is cut and the newborn is dried and wrapped.

III. During delivery, the team should be aware of the type and duration of anesthesia, extent of maternal bleeding, and newly recognized problems such as meconium in the amniotic fluid or nuchal cord.

A. Immediately following delivery, begin a process of evaluation, decision, and action (resuscitation).

  1. Place the newborn on the warming table.
  2. Dry the infant completely and discard the wet linens, including those upon which the infant is lying. Make sure the infant is warm. Extremely small infants may require extra warming with rubber gloves filled with warm water or additional warming lamps (see Chap. 6, Care of the Extremely Low-Birth-Weight Infant).
  3. Place the infant with head in midline position, with slight neck extension.
  4. Suction the mouth, oropharynx, and nares thoroughly with a suction bulb. Deep pharyngeal stimulation with a suction catheter may cause arrhythmias that are probably of vagal origin, and should be avoided. A suc-

TABLE 4.1. APGAR SCORING SYSTEM

Sign	Score		
	0	1	2
Heart rate	Absent	Under 100 beats per minute	Over 100 beats per minute
Respiratory effort	Absent	Slow (irregular)	Good crying
Muscle tone	Limp	Some flexion of extremities	Active motion
Reflex irritability	No response	Grimace	Cough or sneeze
Color	Blue, pale	Pink body, blue extremities	All pink

Source: From Apgar V. A proposal for a new method of evaluation of the newborn infant. *Anesth Analg* 1953;32:260.

tion bulb should be used instead. If meconium-stained amniotic fluid is present and the infant is not vigorous, suction the oropharynx and trachea as quickly as possible (see **IV.A** and Chap. 24, Meconium Aspiration).
B. **Sequence of intervention.**While Apgar scores (Table 4.1) are assigned at 1 and 5 minutes, resuscitative efforts should begin during the initial neonatal stabilization period. The NRP recommends that at the time of birth, the baby should be assessed by posing five questions: (1) is the baby or amniotic fluid clear of meconium?; (2) is the baby crying or breathing?; (3) does the baby have good muscle tone?; (4) is the baby centrally pink?; (5) is it a term gestation? If the answer to any of these questions is "no," the intial steps of resuscitation should commence.

First, assess whether the infant is **breathing spontaneously.** Next, assess whether the **heart rate is greater than 100 beats per minute (bpm).** Finally, evaluate whether the infant's overall color is pink (acrocyanosis is normal). If any of these three characteristics is abnormal, take immediate steps to correct the deficiency, and reevaluate every 15–30 seconds until all characteristics are present and stable. In this way, adequate support will be given while overly vigorous interventions are avoided when newborns are making adequate progress on their own. This approach will help avoid complications such as laryngospasm and cardiac arrhythmias from excessive suctioning or pneumothorax from injudicious bagging. Some interventions are required in specific circumstances.

1. **Infant breathes spontaneously, heart rate is greater than 100 bpm, and color is becoming pink (Apgar score of 8–10).** This situation is found in over 90% of all term newborns, with a median time to first breath of about 10 seconds. Following (or during) warming, drying, positioning, and oropharyngeal suctioning, the infant should be assessed. If respirations, heart rate, and color are normal, the infant should be wrapped and returned to the parents.

   Some newborns do not immediately establish spontaneous respiration but will rapidly respond to tactile stimulation, including vigorous flicking of the soles of the feet or rubbing the back (e.g., cases of **primary apnea**). More vigorous or other techniques of stimulation have no therapeutic value and are potentially harmful. If breathing does not start after **two** attempts at tactile stimulation, the baby may well be in **secondary apnea,** and respiratory support should be initiated. It is better to overdiagnose secondary apnea in this situation than to continue attempts at stimulation that are not successful.

2. **Infant breathes spontaneously, heart rate is greater than 100 bpm, but the overall color remains cyanotic (Apgar score of 5–7).** This situation

is not uncommon and may follow primary apnea. The newborn should be given blow-by oxygen (100%) at a rate of 5 L/min by mask or by tubing held about 1 cm from the face. If color improves, oxygen should be gradually withdrawn while color is reassessed. If cyanosis recurs, the oxygen source should be moved closer to the infant. There is evidence that resuscitaion with room air alone may be as effective as providing additional oxygen. Current recommendations,however, still include the use of supplemental oxygen. In either case, unregulated continuous positive airway pressure by face mask has no role in resuscitation.

3. **The infant is apneic despite tactile stimulation or has a heart rate of less than 100 bpm despite apparent respiratory effort (Apgar score of 3–4).** This represents **secondary apnea** and requires treatment with bag-and-mask ventilation. A bag of approximately 750 mL volume should be connected to oxygen (100%) at a rate of 5–8 L/min and to a mask of appropriate size. The mask should cover the chin and nose but leave eyes uncovered. After positioning the newborn's head in the midline with slight extension, the initial breath should be delivered at a peak pressure that is adequate to produce appropriate chest rise, which may be as high as 30–40 cm H_2O. This will establish functional residual capacity, and subsequent inflations will be effective at lower inspiratory pressures.

   The inspiratory pressures for subsequent breaths should again be chosen to result in adequate chest rise. In infants with normal lungs, this inspiratory pressure is usually no more than 15–20 cm H_2O. In infants with known or suspected disease causing decreased pulmonary compliance, continued inspiratory pressures of 20–40 cm H_2O may be required. A rate of 40–60 breaths per minute should be used, and the infant should be reassessed in 15–30 seconds. Aiming for a rate closer to 40 bpm is often helpful in ensuring adequate breaths. Support should be continued until respirations are spontaneous, and the heart rate is greater than 100 bpm.

   Such moderately depressed infants will be acidotic but generally able to correct this respiratory acidosis spontaneously after respiration is established. This process may take up to several hours, but unless the pH remains less than 7.25, acidosis does not need further treatment.

4. **The infant is apneic, and the heart rate is below 100 bpm despite 30 seconds of assisted ventilation (Apgar score of 0–2).** If the heart rate is greater than 60, positive-pressure ventilation should be continued, and the heart rate rechecked in 30 seconds. It is appropriate to carefully assess the effectiveness of support during this time period using the following steps.

   a. **Adequacy of ventilation** is most important, and should be assessed by observing chest-wall motion at the cephalad portions of the thorax and listening for equal breath sounds laterally over the right and left hemithoraces at the midaxillary lines. The infant should be ventilated at 40–60 breaths per minute using the minimum pressure that will move the chest and produce audible breath sounds. Infants with respiratory distress syndrome, pulmonary hypoplasia, or ascites may require higher pressures.

      By current recommendations, be certain that 100% oxygen is being delivered and that the mask has a good seal with the face. Recheck head position and clear the airway again. Continue bag-and-mask ventilation and reassess in 15–30 seconds. The most important measure of ventilation adequacy is infant response. If, despite good air entry, the heart rate fails to increase and color remains poor, intubation may be considered (see Chap. 36). Air leak (e.g., pneumothorax) should be ruled out.

   b. **Intubation is absolutely indicated** only when a diaphragmatic hernia or similar anomaly is suspected or known to exist. It may be warranted when bag-and-mask ventilation is ineffective, when an endotracheal tube is needed for emergency administration of drugs, or when the infant requires transportation for more than a short distance after stabilization. Even in these situations, effective ventilation with a bag and mask may be done for long periods, and it is preferred over repeated unsuccessful attempts at intubation or attempts by unsupervised personnel unfamiliar with the procedure.

Intubation should be accomplished rapidly (limiting each attempt to 20 seconds with intervening bag-and-mask ventilation) by a skilled person. If inadequate ventilation was the sole cause of the bradycardia, intubation should result in an increase in heart rate to over 100 bpm, and a rapid improvement in color. Intubation skills can be readily learned and maintained through practice utilizing one of several commercially available models or through humane use of ketamine-anesthetized kittens.

The key to successful intubation is to correctly position the infant and laryngoscope and to know the anatomic landmarks. If the baby's chin, sternum, and umbilicus are all lined up in a single plane, and if, after insertion into the infant's mouth, the laryngoscope handle and blade are aligned in that plane and held at about a 60 degree angle to the baby's chest, only one of four anatomic landmarks will be visible to the intubator: from cephalad to caudad these include the posterior tongue, the vallecula and epiglottis, the larynx (trachea and vocal cords), or the esophagus. The successful intubator will view the laryngoscope tip and a landmark, and should then know whether the landmark being observed is cephalad or caudad to the larynx. The intubator can adjust the position of the blade by several millimeters and locate the vocal cords. The endotracheal tube can then be inserted under direct visualization.

c. **Circulation.** If, after intubation and 30 seconds of ventilation with 100% oxygen, the heart rate remains below 60 bpm, cardiac massage should be instituted. The best technique is to stand at the foot of the infant and place both thumbs at the junction of the middle and lower thirds of the sternum, with the fingers wrapped around and supporting the back. Alternatively, one can stand at the side of the infant and compress the lower third of the infant's sternum with the index and third fingers of one hand. In either method, compress the sternum about one-third the diameter of the chest at a rate of 90 times per minute in a ratio of three compressions for each breath. Positive pressure ventilation should be continued at a rate of 30 breaths per minute, interspersed in the period following every third compression. Determine effectiveness of compressions by palpating the femoral, brachial, or umbilical cord pulse.

After 30 seconds, suspend both ventilation and compression for 6 seconds as heart rate is assessed. If the rate is greater than 60 bpm, chest compression should be discontinued and ventilation continued until respiration is spontaneous. If no improvement is noted, compression and ventilation should be continued for successive periods of 30 seconds interposed with 6-second periods of assessment.

Infants requiring ventilatory and circulatory support are markedly depressed and require immediate, vigorous resuscitation (Fig. 4.1). Resuscitation may require at least three trained people working together.

d. **Medication.** If, despite adequate ventilation with 100% oxygen and chest compressions, a heart rate of more than 60 bpm has not been achieved by 1–2 minutes after delivery, **or if the initial heart rate is zero,** medications such as chronotropic and inotropic agents should be given to support the myocardium, correct acidosis, and ensure adequate fluid status. (See Table 4.2 for drugs, indications, and dosages.) Medications provide substrate and stimulation for the heart so that it can support circulation of oxygen and nutrients to the brain. For rapid calculations, use 1, 2, or 3 kg as the estimate of birth weight.

(1) The most accessible intravenous route for neonatal administration of medications is catheterization of the umbilical vein (see Chap. 36,

Baby limp and blue; heart rate <100

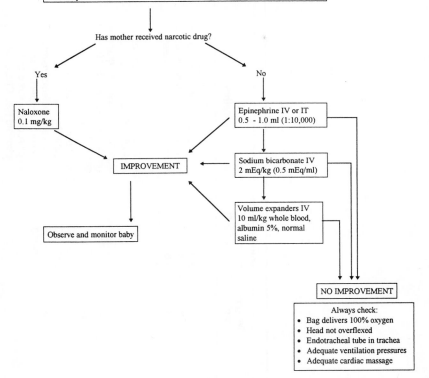

- Perform initial stabilization (dry, warm position)
- Suction oropharynx, nasopharynx
- Stimulate, give bag-and-mask ventilation (40-60 breaths per minute)
- Heart rate < 60; < 80, not increasing: begin cardiac massage (120 bpm)
- Bag and mask inadequate → intubate
- No improvement in 1 minute or heart rate = 0, place intravenous or umbilical line

Has mother received narcotic drug?

Yes

No

Naloxone
0.1 mg/kg

Epinephrine IV or IT
0.5 - 1.0 ml (1:10,000)

IMPROVEMENT

Sodium bicarbonate IV
2 mEq/kg (0.5 mEq/ml)

Volume expanders IV
10 ml/kg whole blood,
albumin 5%, normal
saline

Observe and monitor baby

NO IMPROVEMENT

Always check:
- Bag delivers 100% oxygen
- Head not overflexed
- Endotracheal tube in trachea
- Adequate ventilation pressures
- Adequate cardiac massage

FIG. 4.1. Flow sheet for resuscitation of the newborn. (Modified from Perinatal Continuing Education Program, University of Virginia. Courtesy of J. Kattwinkel.)

Common Neonatal Procedures), which can be done rapidly and aseptically. Although the saline-filled catheter can be advanced into the inferior vena cava (i.e., 8–10 cm), in 60–70% of neonates the catheter may become wedged in an undesirable or dangerous location (e.g., hepatic, portal, or pulmonary vein). Therefore, insertion of the catheter approximately 2–3 cm past the abdominal wall (4–5 cm total in a term neonate), just to the point of easy blood return, is safest prior to injection of drugs. In this position, the catheter tip will be in or just below the ductus venosus; it is important to flush all medications through the catheter because there is no flow through the vessel after cord separation.

(2) **Drug therapy** as an adjunct to oxygen is to support the myocardium and correct acidosis. Continuing bradycardia is an indication for **epinephrine** administration, once effective ventilation has been

TABLE 4.2. NEONATAL RESUSCITATION

Drug/Therapy	Dose/kg	Weight (kg)	Volume (mL) IV	Volume (mL) IT	Method	Indication
Epinephrine 1:10,000 0.1 mg/mL	0.01–0.03 mg/kg IV IT dose is 2–3 × IV	1 2 3 4	0.2 0.4 0.6 0.8	0.5 1.0 1.5 2.0	Give IV push or IT diluted with 1–2 mL of normal saline; do not give into an artery; *do not mix* with bicarbonate; repeat in 5 min PRN	Asystole or severe bradycardia
Sodium bicarbonate 0.5 mEq/ml	2 mEq/kg IV	1 2 3 4	4 8 12 16		Give IV over 2 minutes; do not mix with epinephrine, calcium, or phosphate; assure adequate ventilation; repeat in 5–10 min PRN	Metabolic acidosis
Naloxone (Narcan) 0.4 mg/mL	0.1–0.2 mg/kg	1 2 3 4	0.25–0.5 0.50–1.0 0.75–1.5 1.0–2.0		Give IV push, IM, SQ, or IT; repeat PRN 3 times if no response; *if maternal narcotic addiction is suspected do not give*; do not mix with bicarbonate (see Chap. 19)	Narcotic depression

Volume expanders				Hypotension due to intravascular volume loss (see Chap. 17)
Normal saline	10 ml/kg			
5% Albumin		1	10 mL	
Plasma		2	20 mL	Give IV over 5–10 min
Whole blood		3	30 mL	Slower in premature infants
		4	40 mL	

Dopamine — Begin at 5 µg/kg/min IV (may increase up to 20 µg/kg/min)

$$\frac{6 \times \text{wt (kg)} \times \text{desired dose (µg/kg/min)}}{\text{desired fluid rate (ml/h)}} = \text{mg of dopamine per 100 mL of solution; give as continuous infusion with pump}$$

Hypotension due to poor cardiac output (see Chap. 17)

Cardioversion/defibrillation (see Chap. 25) — 1 to 4 Joules/kg increase 50% each time — Ventricular fibrillation, ventricular tachycardia

ET tube (see Chap. 36)

Weight	Internal diameter (mm)	Distance of tip of ET tube
<1000 g	2.5 uncuffed	7 cm
1000–2000 g	3.0 uncuffed	8 cm
2000–4000 g	3.5 uncuffed	9 cm
>4000 g	3.5–4.0 uncuffed	10 cm

(for nasal intubation add 2 cm)

Laryngoscope blades (see Chap. 36)

<2000 g	0 (straight)
>2000 g	1 (straight)

IM = intramuscular; IT = intratracheal; IV = intravenous; SQ = subcutaneous.

established. Epinephrine is a powerful adrenergic agonist, and works in both adults and neonates by inducing an intense vasoconstriction and improved coronary (and cerebral) artery perfusion. The recommended dose is extrapolated from the apparently efficacious dose in adults, and is based on both measured responses and empiric experience. The dose of 0.1–0.3 mL/kg (up to 1.0 mL) of a 1:10,000 epinephrine solution should ideally be given through the umbilical venous catheter and flushed into the central circulation. This dose may be repeated every 3–5 minutes if necessary, and there is no apparent benefit to higher doses.

When access to central circulation is difficult or delayed, epinephrine may be delivered via an endotracheal tube for transpulmonary absorption. Studies in asphyxiated animals have demonstrated the rapid absorption and action of endotracheally administered epinephrine, leading to increased heart rate and arterial blood pressure even in the presence of severe acidosis. Case reports support the same effect in newborns, although larger experiences and controlled studies are lacking. Nevertheless, it appears that intratracheal administration of 0.1–0.3 mL/kg of 1:10,000 epinephrine is more rapid and safer than intracardiac administration. In emergent situations, use estimated volumes of 0.5 mL of solution in small infants and 1.0 mL in larger infants. More effective delivery may be accomplished by diluting the epinephrine with an equal volume of normal saline.

If two doses of epinephrine do not produce improvement, additional doses may be given, but one should consider other causes for continuing depression. Documented or suspected acidosis should be treated with 2 mEq of bicarbonate per kilogram body weight. The **bicarbonate** should be given as **4 mL/kg of 0.5 mEq/mL of sodium bicarbonate** administered over 2–4 minutes through the umbilical vein.

Because there are potential risks as well as benefits for all medications (see Table 4.2), drug administration through the umbilical vein should be reserved for those newborns in whom bradycardia persists despite adequate oxygen delivery and ventilation. If an adequate airway has been established, adequate ventilation achieved, and the heart rate exceeds 100 bpm, the infant should be moved to the neonatal intensive care unit (NICU), where physical examination, determination of vital signs, and test results such as chest radiographic appearance will more clearly identify needs for specific interventions.

(3) Volume expansion. If oxygenation and blood pH are satisfactory, but blood pressure is still low and peripheral perfusion poor, volume expansion may be indicated through the use of normal saline, 5% albumin, packed red blood cells, or whole blood (see IV.B and Chap. 17, Shock). Additional indications for volume expansion include evidence of acute bleeding or poor response to resuscitative efforts. Volume expansion should be carried out cautiously in newborns in whom hypotension may be caused by asphyxial myocardial damage rather than hypovolemia. It is important to use the appropriate gestational age– and birth weight–related blood-pressure norms to determine volume status (see Chap. 26, Hematologic Problems).

(4) Reversal of narcotic depression. If the mother has received narcotic analgesia within a few hours of delivery, the newborn may manifest respiratory depression due to transplacental passage. The depression usually presents as apnea, bradycardia, and cyanosis that easily correct with bag-and-mask ventilation but recur upon cessation of support. These infants should be treated with naloxone

(0.4 mg/mL), in a dose of 0.25 mL/kg (e.g., 0.1 mg/ kg). Naloxone should not be used if the mother is a chronic user of narcotics. Respiratory support should be maintained until spontaneous respirations occur.

IV. **Special situations**

   A. **Meconium aspiration** (see Chap. 24, Respiratory Disorders).

   1. In the presence of any meconium staining of the amniotic fluid, the obstetrician should suction the mouth and pharynx with a bulb syringe or suction catheter after delivery of the head and before breathing begins.

   2. The newborn should immediately be assessed to determine whether it is vigorous, as defined by strong respiratory effort, good muscle tone, and a heart rate greater than 100 bpm. Infants who are vigorous should be treated as normal, despite the presence of meconium-stained fluid. Infants who are not clearly vigorous should be rapidly intubated and their trachea suctioned for meconium, preferably before the first breath. In many cases, even if the infant has gasped, some meconium may still be removed with direct tracheal suction. Suctioning is accomplished via adapters that allow connection of the endotracheal tube to the suction catheter. The resuscitator should avoid suction techniques that could allow self-contamination with blood or vaginal contents.

   3. For infants at risk of meconium aspiration syndrome who show initial respiratory distress, care should be taken at all times in the delivery room and NICU to provide adequate oxygen and prevent even transient hypoxemia.

   B. **Shock.** Some newborns present with pallor and shock in the delivery room (see Chaps. 17, Shock; 26, Hematologic Problems). Shock may result from significant intrapartum blood loss due to placental separation, fetal-maternal hemorrhage, avulsion of the umbilical cord from the placenta, vasa or placenta previa, incision through an anterior placenta at cesarean section, twin–twin transfusion, or rupture of an abdominal viscus (liver or spleen) during a difficult delivery. It may also result from vasodilation or loss of vascular tone due to septicemia or hypoxemia and acidosis. These newborns will be pale, tachycardic (over 180 bpm), tachypneic, and hypotensive with poor capillary filling and weak pulses.

   After starting respiratory support, immediate transfusion with O-negative packed red blood cells and 5% albumin may be necessary if acute blood loss is the underlying cause. A volume of 20 mL/kg can be given through an umbilical venous catheter. If clinical improvement is not seen, causes of further blood loss should be sought, and more vigorous blood and colloid replacement should be continued. It is important to remember that the hematocrit may be normal immediately after delivery if the blood loss was acute during the intrapartum period.

   Except in cases of massive acute blood loss, the emergent use of blood replacement is not necessary and acute stabilization can be achieved with colloid solutions. Normal saline is the primary choice of replacement fluid. This allows time to obtain proper products from the blood bank, if blood replacement is subsequently needed.

   Except in the most extreme emergency situation where no other therapeutic option exists, the use of autologous blood from the placenta is not recommended.

   C. **Air leak.** If an infant fails to respond to resuscitation despite apparently effective ventilation, chest compressions, and medications, consider the possibility of air-leak syndromes. Pneumothoraces (uni- or bilateral) and pneumopericardium should be ruled out by transillumination or diagnostic thoracentesis (see Chap. 24, Respiratory Disorders).

   D. **Prematurity.** Premature infants require additional special care in the delivery room, including precautions to prevent heat loss because of thinner skin and an increased surface-area-to-body-weight ratio. Apnea due to respiratory insufficiency is more likely at lower gestational ages, and support should be provided. Surfactant-deficient lungs are poorly compliant, and higher venti-latory pressures may be needed for the first and subsequent breaths. De-pending on the reason for premature birth, perinatal infection is more likely in premature infants, which increases their risk of perinatal depression.

V. **Apgar scores.** Evaluation and decisions regarding resuscitation measures should be guided by assessment of respiration, heart rate, and color. Apgar scores are conventionally assigned after birth and recorded in the newborn's chart. The Apgar score consists of the total points assigned to five objective signs in the newborn. Each sign is evaluated and given a score of 0, 1, or 2. Total scores at 1 and 5 minutes after birth are usually noted. If the 5-minute score is 6 or less, the score is then noted at successive 5-minute intervals until it is greater than 6 (see Table 4.1). A score of 10 indicates an infant in perfect condi-tion; this is quite unusual because most babies have some degree of acro-cyanosis. The scoring, if done properly, yields the following information:

A. **One-minute Apgar score.** This score generally correlates with umbilical cord blood pH and is an index of intrapartum depression. It does not corre-late with outcome. Babies with a score of 0–4 have been shown to have a sig-nificantly lower pH, higher partial pressure of carbon dioxide ($PaCO_2$), and lower buffer base than those with Apgar scores greater than 7. In the VLBW infant a low Apgar may not indicate severe depression. As many as 50% of infants with gestational ages of 25–26 weeks and Apgar scores of 0–3 have a cord pH of greater than 7.25. Therefore, a VLBW infant with a low Apgar score cannot be assumed to be severely depressed. Nonetheless, such infants should be resuscitated actively and will usually respond more promptly and to less invasive measures than newborns whose low Apgar scores reflect acidemia.

B. **Apgar scores beyond 1 minute** are reflective of the infant's changing condi-tion and the adequacy of resuscitative efforts. Persistence of low Apgar scores indicates need for further therapeutic efforts and usually the severity of the baby's underlying problem. In assessing the adequacy of resuscitation, the most common problem is inadequate pulmonary inflation and ventilation. It is important to verify a good seal with the mask, correct placement of the en-dotracheal tube, and adequate peak inspiratory pressure applied to the bag if the Apgar score fails to improve as resuscitation proceeds.

The more prolonged the period of severe depression (i.e., Apgar score 3), the more likely is an abnormal long-term neurologic outcome. Nevertheless, many newborns with prolonged depression (>15 minutes) are normal in follow-up. Moreover, most infants with long-term motor abnormalities such as cerebral palsy have not had periods of neonatal depression after birth (see Chap. 27, Perinatal Asphyxia). Apgar scores were designed to monitor neonatal transi-tion and the effectiveness of resuscitation, and their utility remains essen-tially limited to this important role.

VI. **Evolving practices.** The practice of neonatal resuscitation continues to evolve with the availablity of new devices and enhanced understanding of the best ap-proach to resuscitation.

A. **Laryngeal mask airways.** Masks that fit over the laryngeal inlet have been developed and are effective for ventilating newborn infants. Ease of inser-tion and the ability to maintain a stable airway with these devices without the need for skill at intubation may make these a preferred method of air-way support in many instances. These airways have been most widely stud-ied in full-term infants, but there have been case reports of their utility in ventilating even small premature infants for extended periods of time. How-ever, these masks have not been evaluated in small, preterm infants, and relative effectiveness for the suctioning of meconium has not been reported.

B. **The Neopuff Infant Resuscitator** (Fisher & Paykel, Inc.). This is a manually triggered, pressure-limited, and manually cycled device that is pneumatically powered by a flowmeter. This device offers greater control over manual venti-lation by delivering breaths of reproducible size (peak and end-expiratory pressures) and a simplified method to control breath rate. One important use for this device is to transport preterm infants requiring supported ventilation, when the use of a powered mechanical ventilator is not possible.

C. **Room-air resuscitation.** The NRP continues to recommend the use of 100% oxygen in the conduct of neonatal resuscitation, but there is some evidence that room air resuscitation is equally effective and potentially safer. Animal studies have shown that neither hyperbaric nor normobaric oxygen is more efficient in the resuscitation of newborn rabbits, and that high oxygen levels may result in increases mortality and worse neurologic outcome among survivors. In studies of human infants, the groups treated with oxygen and room air had equal times until the normalization of heart rate after birth, and similar Apgar scores at 1 and 5 minutes. Blood gases normalized at the same rate in both groups, except for higher carbon dioxide tensions in the oxygen-treated group. The time until first cry was prolonged in the oxygen-treated group, and neonatal mortality was similar in both groups. As better understanding is developed regarding the normal changes in oxygen saturation at birth, it seems likely that respiratory support with 100% oxygen will be replaced by regulated blended oxygen, or room air.

Suggested Readings

Burchfield D.J. Medication use in neonatal resuscitation. *Clin Perinat* 1999;26:683.

Ostrea E.M., Odell G.B. The influence of bicarbonate administration on blood pH in a "closed system": clinical implications. *J Pediatr* 1972;80:671.

Perlman J.M., Rissewr R. Cardiopulmonary resuscitation in the delivery room. *Arch Pediatr Adolesc Med* 1995;149:20.

Saugstad O.D., Rootwelt T., Aalen O. Resuscitation of asphyxiated newborn infants with room air or oxygen: an international controlled trial. *Pediatrics* 1998;102:e1.

Saugstad O.D. Resuscitation of newborn infants with room air or oxygen. *Semin Neonatol* 2001;6:233.

Textbook of Neonatal Resuscitation, 4th ed. Kattwinkel J (Ed.). Dallas: American Academy of Pediatrics and American Heart Association, 2000.

5. NURSERY CARE OF THE WELL NEWBORN

Constance H. Keefer

I. **The guiding philosophy for nursery care of the well newborn**
   A. Nursery care should be **family-focused and infant-centered,** respecting the event as a major family turning point. Particular attention should be paid to **allow contact between mother and infant** and to avoid their separation from each other. We encourage **pediatric exams and nursing procedures** to be done interactively **in the parents' presence**. Pediatric and nursing assessments should include behavioral as well as physical aspects of the infant. Avoidance-reduction of infant's experience of pain has been reinforced by JCAHO (Joint Commission on Accreditation of Healthcare Organizations) standards. We give 1 to 3 cc sucrose per minute p.o. before procedures such as heel stick, injection, and venipuncture. A developmental model for maternal postpartum care can be applied to guide relational care that supports parental competence in caring for the infant. Nurse assignment to mother-infant pairs encourages rooming-in and seamlessness of care. Seamlessness is also addressed by ensuring appropriate pediatric and obstetric posthospital follow-up before discharge from the hospital.
   B. Take advantage of the **opportunities for preventative public health** available during the postpartum in-hospital stay. These include:
      1. Counseling parents about proper use of **car seats**, avoidance of **air bags** for young children, and their own use of **seat belts**.
      2. Requesting parents to provide a **smoke-free environment** for the infant and providing information for smoking cessation services, which are more available since the litigation-required payments by the tobacco companies.
      3. Support for **breastfeeding initiation** throughout the hospital stay, especially for first-time mothers (see Chap. 11).
      4. Screen mothers for risk of **postpartum depression** and other mental-health problems.
   C. In these few days in the hospital, the newborn should be evaluated.
      1. **Rule out any:**
         a. **Malformation.**
         b. **Infectious disease.**
         c. **Genetic problems.**
         d. **Metabolic problems.**
         e. **Neurologic problems.**
         f. **Inappropriate jaundice.**
      2. The pediatrician should be certain that the baby is making a **good transition from fetal to neonatal life,** especially in the areas of:
         a. **Respiration.**
         b. **Cardiac function.**
         c. **Feeding.**
         d. **Urination.**
         e. **Stooling.**
      3. The **paternal/maternal/infant interaction and the dynamics of the family** should be evaluated to assess the ability of the family to care for the new infant.
II. **Initial period**
   A. **Protective gloves** should be worn when one is handling newborns who have not been bathed and when in contact with an infant's blood, saliva, meconium, or stool.

B. The **newborn's temperature** should be stabilized with warming lights or an incubator, or skin-to-skin contact with the mother; initial skin care should be deferred until temperature is stable. Temperature regulation will be more difficult in preterm and small-for-gestational-age infants.

C. On admission to the nursery, **repeat the initial physical examination** (see Chap. 3, History and Physical Examination of the Newborn), looking for the following:
   1. **Respiratory distress** (see Chap. 24).
   2. **Poor color,** including pallor, plethora, cyanosis, and jaundice (see Chaps. 18, 25, 26).
   3. **Malformation.**
   4. **Signs of infection** (see Chap. 23).
   5. **Jitteriness.** If present, consider hypoglycemia/hypocalcemia or hypomagnesemia (see Chap. 29), drug withdrawal (see Chap. 19), and central nervous system injury or disease (see Chap. 27).
   6. **Hypo- or hyperthermia.**

D. **Classify weight** as appropriate, small, or large for gestational age (AGA, SGA, and LGA, respectively; see Chap. 3).
   1. If the infant is **SGA,** check for possible causes and complications (see Chap. 3, Identifying the High-Risk Newborn).
   2. If the infant is **LGA, check for hypoglycemia.** (see Chap. 29).

E. **Skin care.** Examine skin for signs of trauma, infection, malformation, or lesions (see Chaps. 3, 23, 34).
   1. Use **cotton cloth with tap water and nonmedicated soap** to remove blood and meconium. Do not remove the vernix caseosa. Afterward, skin can be cleaned as needed with nonmedicated soap and water.
   2. If the nursery is having problems with *Staphylococcus aureus* **infections,** a hexachlorophene soap can be used until the epidemic has passed. Remember, hexachlorophene can be absorbed through intact skin and is potentially toxic to neonates. Leave on skin 5 minutes and rinse well.
   3. **Skin abrasions** should be carefully cleaned with soap and water. Topical antibiotics may be reasonable to use in infants who will have short hospital stays. Use of topical antibiotics for routine skin care in infants who have prolonged hospitalizations has been associated with the emergence of multiple antibiotic-resistant organisms. Such medications should only be used for specific indications.

F. **Cord care.** We use a plastic cord clamp (double-grip umbilical cord clamp, Hollister, Inc., Libertyville, Illinois), which is removed 24 hours after birth. There are several methods of cord care, and no single method has proved superior. We do not use alcohol or any topical medication. We fold the diaper down to expose the cord to air.

G. **Eye care.** Erythromycin ointment is applied in the delivery room within 1 hour of life to prevent gonococcal ophthalmia. Silver nitrate drops 1% are effective and will kill erythromycin-resistant gonococci if that is a consideration (see Chap. 23).

H. **Vitamin K** (1.0 mg vitamin K_1 oxide, phytonadione) is administered within 2 hours of life to prevent hemorrhagic disease. The association of vitamin K administration to newborns with increased cancer rates in childhood, found in several small studies, was not substantiated in a National Institute of Child Health and Human Development (NICHD) case-control study of the Collaborative Perinatal Project (see Chap. 26).

III. **Subsequent period**
   A. **Measure weight daily.**
   B. **Record time and amount for stools and urine, as well as pulse, respiration rate, and axillary temperature, at least every 8 hours.** Pulse and respiration should be recorded every 4 hours for infants with any risk factors for infection, pulmonary or cardiac disease.
   C. **Feeding.** The first feedings are at the breast within an hour of delivery. Bottle-fed infants are fed by one hour of life (see Chaps. 10, 11).

1. **Breastfeeding** is preferred, unless contraindications exist (see Chap. 11).
2. If **formula** is used, the first feed should be within 1 hour of birth and the baby fed every 3 to 4 hours after that. The first few feeds should be limited to 1 oz.

D. **Infant sleep position** should be on the side for the first few days of life. After that, the supine position is the one recommended by the American Academy of Pediatrics. The infant should sleep on a firm infant mattress with only a thin covering between the infant and the mattress.

1. **Certain infants** with craniofacial anomalies (e.g., Pierre-Robin), gastroesophageal reflux, or preterm infants while they are experiencing respiratory disease **should not sleep in a supine position.** Preterm infants who have recovered from respiratory disease should sleep in the supine position.
2. We recommend that parents allow the infant, when awake, some periods of time each time in the **prone position.** This may help to decrease the apparently dramatic increase seen in craniofacial clinics of occipital deformational plagiocephaly. In addition, the prone position in the awake infant allows for use of neck and shoulder muscles.

E. **Family-focused care,** practiced in our nurseries, includes maternal and infant care provided by the same nurse. The infant is kept in the mother's room as much as possible, consistent with the health of the infant and parental ability to care for him or her.

IV. **Nursery assessment** should include a review of maternal records. We review prenatal ultrasound findings, rubella immunity, hepatitis B antigen, tuberculosis, gonorrhea, chlamydia, and syphilis testing. Reasons for incomplete prenatal care are explored, as is history of previous pregnancy losses and medical and social history, including history of postpartum depression (see Chap. 3).

V. **Interventions**

A. **Circumcision**

1. The following policy for **nonritual circumcision** exists in our nurseries:
   a. There is **no absolute medical indication** for routine neonatal circumcision.
   b. **Pros and cons of circumcision** should be discussed with parents before the birth.
   c. Infants who have potential **problems that may make lifelong penile hygiene difficult** should probably have a circumcision.
   d. In certain infants, **circumcision should not be performed routinely:**
      (1) Infants with **chordee or hypospadias** because foreskin may be used in later repair.
      (2) Infants with **ambiguous genitalia.**
      (3) Infants with **bleeding disorders** (see Chap. 26).
   e. Circumcision should be performed only on **infants who are stable and healthy** and should be done by **well-trained personnel.** When done before the initial full pediatric examination, the genitalia should be confirmed as normal. It is not necessary to restrict oral intake for a period before the circumcision. We do not delay discharge awaiting first postcircumcision void.

2. **Complications**
   a. If circumcision is performed, **analgesia** should be provided. Swaddling, sucrose by mouth, and acetaminophen administration may reduce the stress response but are not sufficient for the operative pain and can not be recommended as the sole method of analgesia. Although local anesthesia and EMLA cream provides some anesthesia benefit, both ring blocks and dorsal penile blocks have proved more effective.
   b. **Risks of surgery.** There is a 0.2 to 0.6% complication rate. Risks include the following:
      (1) **Hemorrhage.**
      (2) **Infection.**

(3) Surgical trauma (partial amputation, denudation).
(4) Late complications—meatal stenosis and ulceration.
3. The **uncircumcised penis** is easy to keep clean. The foreskin usually does not fully retract for several years and should not be forced. Gentle washing of the genital area while bathing is sufficient for normal hygiene. Later, when the foreskin is fully retractable, boys should be taught the importance of washing underneath the foreskin on a regular basis.
B. **Hepatitis B immunization** for prophylaxis is offered to all newborns (see Chap. 23).
C. **Indications for social service consultation** include incomplete prenatal care, maternal substance abuse, and maternal medical diagnoses such as depression, other psychiatric diagnosis, and mental retardation. Other indicators for consultation include inadequate housing or support and young maternal age.
D. **Pain management** includes offering 23% sucrose solution, 5 to 10 cc, 5 minutes before injections, heel sticks, and other painful procedures.
VI. **Screening**
  A. **Cord blood**
  1. Cord blood is **saved for 2 weeks**.
  2. **Blood type and Coombs' test** on infants born to Rh-negative mothers, mothers with a positive finding on antibody screening, mothers whose previous infant had a Coombs positive hemolytic anemia, and type O mothers if the infant is to be discharged before the age of 24 hours (see Chap. 18).
  3. Blood type and Coombs' test if **jaundice** is noted within 24 hours after birth.
  4. **Later screening for intrauterine infection** if indicated. Note cord blood should not be used for syphilis testing because of a high false-positive rate (see Chap. 23).
  B. **Metabolic disease screening.** In Massachusetts, screening for phenyl-ketonuria, maple syrup urine disease, galactosemia, homocystinuria, hypo-thyroidism, biotinidase deficiency, hemoglobinopathies, congenital adrenal hyperplasia, medium chain acetyl Co-A dehydrogenase deficiency (MCAD) and toxoplasmosis is mandated (see Chaps. 2, 23, 29). Our routine is to obtain a specimen between 24 and 72 hours of life, as close to 48 hours as possible. Screening for cystic fibrosis is being offered in Massachusetts.
  1. Infants who are transferred to other institutions, admitted to the neonatal intensive care unit (NICU), or discharged before 24 hours are the **most likely to miss the screening**.
    a. Infants **discharged before the age of 24 hours** should have a specimen collected while in the hospital and a follow-up sample obtained between days 3 and 7.
    b. We obtain a **blood sample from sick infants** before transfer from our institution and remind the receiving institution to get another sample. Sick or preterm infants should have a specimen drawn at 48 to 72 hours of age and a second specimen at 2 weeks of age or at discharge, whichever is earlier. If the birth weight is less than1500 g, obtain specimens at 2, 4, 6, and 10 weeks of age, or until the baby weighs 1500 g. Specimen should be obtained before blood transfusion and repeated 3 to 7 days post-transfusions.
  2. **Newborn screening for galactosemia.** If serum galactose level is used as the marker, the test will miss infants with galactosemia who are fed lactose-free formulas from birth.
  C. **Developmental dysplasia of the hip.** This is one of the most commonly missed diagnoses in the normal newborn nursery (see Chaps. 3, 28).
  D. **Hearing screening** is mandated for all newborns before discharge in our state (see Chap. 35).
VII. **Administrative policies in effect in our nurseries:**
  A. **Visitors to mother and infant**

1. **Father or significant other** may visit anytime, and healthy siblings of any age, adults, and other children older than age 12 may visit during visiting hours.
2. During **unusual viral epidemics,** visiting may need to be curtailed.

B. **Readmission to the regular nursery** is restricted to infants younger than 2 weeks who have been diagnosed with hyperbilirubinemia requiring phototherapy.

C. **A healthy infant may be a visitor** to a readmitted mother if the mother is able to care for the infant or has a responsible adult to care for the infant on a 24-hour basis.

D. Security
   1. Infants are given **two identical ankle bands** at birth that match the number on a wrist band given to the mother.
   2. Fathers or a designated other are given an **identification sticker for a photographic identification** (e.g., driver's license) **or identification band** for access to the hospital after visiting hours and for taking the infant from the nursery.
   3. **All staff are required to wear a picture identification card.** Parents are instructed to allow the infant to be taken only by someone with appropriate picture identification.
   4. **All stairwell exits and internal elevators** from the nursery, NICU, and labor and delivery floors are by access ID only.

VIII. **Parental education** includes instruction by the primary nurse on feeding and infant care, distribution of booklets and pamphlets on care of the healthy newborn, and the availability of hospital television with continuous maternal and child health teaching programs.

IX. **Discharge plan**

A. The **discharge examination is covered in Chapter 3,** History and Physical Examination of the Newborn. The physician or primary nurse should answer parents' questions and **review the following issues:** observation for possible jaundice, skin infection, and subtle signs of infant illness (e.g., fever, fussiness, lethargy, change in feeding behavior); adequacy of intake in breastfed infants (e.g., minimum of eight nursings, six wet diapers, and two stools each 24 hours); use of car seat, seat belts. and smoke detectors; lowering of hot-water temperature; and forbidding smoking in the home.

B. **Pediatric follow-up appointment** should be made before discharge.
   1. **Two-week visits are routine** for healthy infants leaving after 48 hours.
   2. **High-risk infants** need a follow-up visit for weight check or other examination before 2 weeks.
   3. **Breastfed infants,** especially if small, preterm, or firstborn, should be monitored closely for signs of dehydration until the milk comes in and weight stabilizes. These infants are usually seen 2 to 3 days after discharge.

C. **Discharge of low-risk infants before 24 hours** with home visitation at 3 days by a nurse has been demonstrated to be safe. It should be done only when the mother, the pediatrician, and the obstetrician are comfortable with the plan. Decisions should be based on medical rather than financial grounds. We use the following guidelines from the *Guidelines for Perinatal Care:*

Each mother-neonate dyad should be evaluated individually to determine the optimal time of discharge. Institutions should develop guidelines through their professional staff in collaboration with appropriate community agencies, including third-party payers, to establish hospital stay programs for mothers and their healthy term newborns. State and local public health agencies also should be involved in the oversight of existing hospital stay programs for quality assurance and monitoring.

The following **minimum criteria** should be met before a newborn is discharged from the hospital after an **uncomplicated pregnancy, labor, and delivery prior to 24 hours after birth.**

1. Delivery was **vaginal.**
2. The neonate is **38 to 42 weeks of gestation,** and birth weight is **appropriate for gestational age.**
3. The neonate's vital signs are documented to be normal and **stable for the 12 hours before discharge.**
4. The neonate has **urinated and passed at least one stool.**
5. The neonate has **completed at least two successful feedings,** and documentation has been made that the neonate is able to coordinate sucking, swallowing, and breathing while feeding.
6. Physical examination reveals **no abnormalities** that require continued hospitalization.
7. There is no evidence of excessive bleeding at the circumcision site for at least 2 hours.
8. There is **no evidence of significant jaundice** in the first 24 hours of life (noninvasive means of detecting jaundice may be useful) (see Chap. 18).
9. The mother's (or preferably, both **parents') knowledge, ability, and confidence to provide adequate care** for the neonate are documented by the fact that the following training and information has been received:
   a. Condition of the neonate.
   b. The breastfeeding mother-neonate dyad should be assessed by trained staff regarding nursing position, latch-on, adequacy of swallowing, and woman's knowledge of urine and stool frequency.
   c. Umbilical cord, skin, and newborn genital care as well as temperature assessment and measurement with a thermometer should be reviewed.
   d. The mother should be able to recognize signs of illness and common newborn problems, particularly jaundice.
   e. Instruction in proper newborn safety (e.g., proper use of a car seat and positioning for sleeping) should be provided.

D. **Discharge of all infants** should include the following steps:
   1. Family members or other **support persons,** including health-care providers such as the family pediatrician or his or her designees, who are familiar with newborn care and are knowledgeable about lactation and the recognition of jaundice and dehydration, are available to the mother and the neonate for the first few days after discharge.
   2. Instructions to follow in the event of a complication or **emergency.**
   3. **Laboratory data** are available and have been reviewed, including:
      a. Maternal syphilis, hepatitis B virus surface antigen (HbsAg), and HIV status.
      b. Umbilical cord or newborn blood type and direct Coombs' test are preformed when the mother is Rh negative, type O, has abnormal antibodies, and has had a previously jaundiced child.
   4. **Screening tests** have been performed in accordance with state requirements. If a test was performed **before 24 hours of milk feeding,** a system for **repeating the test in 3 to 7 days** must be in place in accordance with local or state policy.
   5. Initial **hepatitis B** vaccine has been administered or an appointment scheduled for its administration and the importance of maintaining newborn immunizations stressed.
   6. A physician-directed source of continuing medical care for both the mother and the neonate has been identified. For newborns discharged before 24 hours after delivery, an appointment has been made for the neonate to be examined within 48 hours of discharge. The follow-up visit can take place in a home or clinic setting, as long as the personnel examining the neonate are competent in newborn assessment and the results of the follow-up visit are reported to the neonate's physician or designees on the day of the visit.
   7. **Family, environment, and social risk factors** have been assessed. When risk factors are present, the discharge should be delayed until they are

resolved or a plan to safeguard the newborn is in place. Such factors may include, but are not limited to:

    a. Untreated parental substance use or positive urine toxicology test results in the mother or the newborn.

    b. History of child abuse or neglect.

    c. Mental illness in a parent who is in the home.

    d. Lack of social support, particularly for single, first-time mothers.

    e. No fixed home.

    f. History of untreated domestic violence, particularly during this pregnancy.

    g. Adolescent mother, particularly if other risk factors are present.

8. All newborns having a **shortened hospital stay** should be **examined by experienced health-care providers within 48 hours of discharge.** If it cannot be assure that this examination will take place, discharge should be deferred until a mechanism for follow-up evaluation is identified. The follow-up visit is designed to fulfill the following functions:

    a. Assess the newborn's general health, hydration, and degree of jaundice and identify any new problems.

    b. Review feeding pattern and technique, including observation of breast-feeding for adequacy of position, latch-on, and swallowing.

    c. Assess historical evidence of adequate stool and urine patterns.

    d. Assess quality of mother-neonate interaction and details of newborn behavior.

    e. Reinforce maternal or family education in neonatal care, particularly regarding feeding and sleep position.

    f. Review results of laboratory tests performed at discharge.

    g. Perform screening tests in accordance with state regulations and other tests that are clinically indicated.

    h. Identify a plan for health-care maintenance, including a method for obtaining emergency services, preventive care and immunizations, periodic evaluations and physical examinations, and necessary screening."

9. Maternal contact telephone number is documented in the chart.

E. Copies of initial and discharge summaries are given to parents or sent to the physician or clinic rendering follow-up care. These should include all test results, social service referrals, and plans for any special follow-up care. Early discharge has been associated with problems such as hyperbilirubinemia, kernicterus, sepsis, feeding problems resulting in severe weight loss, missed metabolic diseases, and late diagnosis of congenital heart disease.

F. Infants should be taken home early in an appropriate infant car seat that is correctly installed in the car. Massachusetts has a program for teaching parents how to install the car seat and how to safely secure the infant in the seat. Infants weighing less than 1500 g or born at less than 37 weeks' gestation are tested for apnea in the car seat. Those who fail are offered/sold an infant car bed for use for the first 3 months and then retested.

Suggested Readings

American Academy of Pediatrics/American College of Obstetricians and Gynecologists. *Guidelines for Perinatal Care,* 5th ed. Elk Grove Village, IL, 2002.

American Academy of Pediatrics. Controversies concerning vitamin K and the newborn. *Pediatrics* 1993;91:1001.

American Academy of Pediatrics. Family shopping guide to car seats. AAP Safe Ride Program, 141 Northwest Point Blvd., P.O. Box 927, Elk Grove Village, IL 60009–0927.

American Academy of Pediatrics. Newborn screening fact sheet. *Pediatrics* 1996; 98:473.

American Academy of Pediatrics. Newborn screening for sickle disease and other hemoglobinopathies. *Pediatrics* 1989;84:813.

American Academy of Pediatrics. Newborns: Care of the uncircumcised penis. *Pediatrics* 1987;80:765.

American Academy of Pediatrics. *Report of the Committee on Infectious Diseases.* 2000; Elk Grove, IL: American Academy of Pediatrics.

American Academy of Pediatrics. Task Force on Circumcision. Circumcision policy statement. *Pediatrics* 1999;103:686–693.

American Academy of Pediatrics. Task Force on Infant Sleep Positioning and Sudden Infant Death Syndrome. Changing concepts of sudden infant death syndrome: Implications for infant sleep environment and sleep position. *Pediatrics* 2000;105:650–696.

Charles S., Prystowsky B. Early discharge, in the end: maternal abuse, child neglect and physician harassment. *Pediatrics* 1995;96:746.

Elders J.M. Reducing the risk of sudden infant death syndrome. *JAMA* 1994;272:1646.

Gray J.E., et al. Failure to screen newborns for inborn disorders: Lessons from current experience. *Early Hum Dev* 1997;48:279.

Herzog L. Urinary tract infections and circumcision: A case-control study. *Am J Dis Child* 1989;143:348.

Klebanoff M.A., et al. The risk of childhood cancer after neonatal exposure to vitamin K. *N Engl J Med* 1993;329:905.

Massachusetts Department of Public Health. *Newborn Screening Program Specimen Collection Protocol* March 1994; Boston: Massachusetts Department of Public Health, Regional Newborn Screening Program.

Norr K.F., et al. Early discharge with home follow-up: Impacts on low-income mothers and infants. *J Obstet Gynecol Neonatal Nurs* 1988;17:133.

Phillips C.R. *Family-Centered Maternity/Newborn Care: A Basic Text.* 1991; St. Louis: Mosby-Year Book.

Sotolongo J.R., et al. Penile denudation injuries after circumcision. *J Urol* 1985;133:102.

Stein M.T. The hospital discharge examination: Getting to know the individual child. In: Dixon, S and Stein, MT (Eds.), *Encounters with Children: Pediatric Behavior and Development.* 1992; St. Louis: Mosby-Year Book.

Williams L.R., Cooper M.K. Nurse-managed postpartum home care. *J Obstet Gynecol Neonatal Nurs* 1993;21:25.

6. CARE OF THE EXTREMELY LOW-BIRTH-WEIGHT INFANT

Steven A. Ringer

I. **Introduction.** Extremely low-birth-weight infants (ELBW, birth weight less than 1000 g) are a unique subclass of patients in the Newborn Intensive Care Unit (NICU). Because these infants are so physiologically immature, they are extremely sensitive to small changes in respiratory management, control of blood pressure, fluid administration, nutrition, and virtually all other aspects of care. The optimal way to care for these infants ultimately will be established by ongoing research. However, the most effective care based on currently available evidence is best ensured through the implementation of standardized protocols for the care of the ELBW infant within individual NICUs. Our approach is outlined in Table 6.1. Uniformity of approach within an institution and a commitment to provide and evaluate care in a collaborative manner may be the most important aspects of such protocols.

II. **Prenatal considerations.** If possible, extremely premature infants should be delivered in a facility with a high-risk obstetrical service and a level III NICU. The safety of maternal transport must be weighed against the risks of infant transport (see Chap. 13, Neonatal Transport). Prenatal administration of glucocorticoids to the mother reduces the risk of respiratory distress syndrome (RDS) and the other sequelae of prematurity.

A. **Neonatology consultation.** If delivery of an extremely premature infant is threatened, a neonatologist should consult with the mother, with both parents and the obstetrician present if possible. The consultation should address the following:

1. **Survival.** To most parents, the impending delivery of an extremely premature infant is frightening, and their initial concern is the chance for infant survival. In our consultations, we use survival data from our experience based on the best obstetrical estimate of gestational age. Most published data on survival is based on birth weight because it can be determined with greater accuracy than gestational age. However, birth weight is not available until after birth, it does not account for the impact of intrauterine growth restriction, and gestational maturity is a more important factor in determining survival and outcome. One recent study reported that the survival rate for infants at less than 23 weeks' gestational age was zero and at 23, 24, and 25 weeks the rates were 15, 55, and 79%, respectively. Published data are helpful in counseling, but the importance of local, single institution results should not be underestimated, especially in antenatal counseling. The best obstetrical estimate of gestational age may vary between institutions, and local practices and capabilities may significantly affect both mortality and morbidity in ELBW infants. For this reason, a general assessment of the gestational age at which an infant has any hope of survival should be agreed upon by all caregivers within an institution. If only birth weight-stratified data are available, gestational age estimates for appropriate for gestational age (AGA) fetuses can be roughly converted as follows: 600 g = 24 weeks; 750 g = 25 weeks; 850 g = 26 weeks; 1000 g = 27 weeks.

In discussions with parents, we advocate attempting resuscitation of all newborns who are potentially viable. Realistically, the lower gestational age limit is between 23⅓ and 23⅔ weeks. The addition of medical problems other than prematurity may result in extremely low survival even at higher gestational ages. Parents are counseled that delivery room resuscitation has a high (but not absolute) chance of success, unless the infant appears more immature than the estimated gestational age would suggest, or weighs less than 500 g. We stress that the moments following

TABLE 6.1. ELEMENTS OF A PROTOCOL FOR STANDARDIZING CARE OF THE ELBW INFANT

1. Prenatal consultation
Parental education
Determining parental wishes when viability is questionable
Defining limits of parental choice; need for caregiver-parent teamwork

2. Delivery room care
Define limits of resuscitative efforts
Respiratory support
Low tidal volume ventilation strategy
Prevention of heat and water loss
Early surfactant therapy

3. Ventilation strategy
Low tidal volume, short inspiratory time
Avoid hyperoxia and hypocapnia
Surfactant therapy as indicated
Define indications for high-frequency ventilation

4. Fluids
Early use of incubators to limit fluid and heat losses
Judicious use of fluid bolus therapy for hypotension
Careful monitoring of fluid and electrolyte status
Use of double-lumen umbilical venous catheters for fluid support

5. Nutrition
Initiation of parenteral nutrition shortly after birth
Early initiation of trophic feeding with maternal milk
Advancement of feeding density to provide adequate calories for healing and growth

6. Cardiovascular support
Maintenance of blood pressure within standard range
Use of dopamine for support as indicated
Corticosteroids for unresponsive hypotension

7. Patent ductus arteriosus (PDA)
Avoidance of excess fluid administration
Early medical therapy when PDA suspected
Surgical ligation after failed medical therapy

8. Infection control
Scrupulous handwashing, use of bedside alcohol gels
Limiting blood drawing, skin punctures
Protocol for CVL care, acceptable dwell time
Minimal entry into central venous lines (CVLs), no use of fluids prepared in NICU

delivery are a poor time to make reliable decisions about viability or long-term outcome. Parents should also know that the initiation of support in no way mandates that it be continued if it is later determined to be futile, or very likely to result in a poor long-term outcome. We assure parents that initial resuscitation is always followed by frequent reassessment in the NICU. Intensive support may be withdrawn if the degree of immaturity results in no response to therapy, or if a catastrophic and irreversible complication occurs. Parents are counseled that the period of highest vulnerability may last several weeks in infants of lowest gestational ages. If parents disagree with our recommended approach to resuscitation and care, we first attempt to resolve differences directly. If an impasse continues, we seek consultation from the institutional Ethics service.

2. **Morbidity.** We try to inform parents as fully as possible about short- and long-term prognosis. Before delivery, particular attention is paid to the problems that might appear at birth or shortly thereafter. We explain the risk of respiratory distress syndrome (RDS) and the potential need for ventilatory support. In our NICU, all infants of 24 weeks' gestation require some ventilatory support; at 25 to 26 weeks, this proportion drops to 80 to 90%; at 27 to 28 weeks, about 50 to 60% of infants require ventilatory support. We also inform parents of the likelihood of infection at birth as well as our plan to screen for it and begin prophylactic antibiotic therapy while final culture results are pending.

3. **Potential morbidity.** We avoid giving parents lists of potential sequelae because they may be too overwhelmed to process extensive information during the period surrounding premature birth. However, we do discuss problems that are either likely to occur in many ELBW infants or will be specifically screened for during hospitalization. These include apnea of prematurity, intraventricular hemorrhage (IVH), nosocomial sepsis (or evaluations for possible sepsis), and feeding difficulties, as well as long-term sensory disabilities. We specifically discuss retinopathy of prematurity and subsequent visual deficits, and the need for hearing screening and potential for hearing loss.

4. **Parents' desires.** In most instances parents are the best surrogate decision makers for their child. During the consultation, the neonatologist should try to understand parental wishes about resuscitative efforts and subsequent support especially when chances for infant survival are slim. We encourage parents to voice their understanding of the planned approach and their expectations for their soon-to-be born child, and we reassure them that the strength of their wishes does help guide caregivers in determining whether and how long to continue resuscitation attempts. It is important to clarify for parents their role in decision making as well as the limitations of that role. We believe that there should be a uniform approach to parental demands for attempting or withholding resuscitation at very low gestational ages. The best practice is for caregivers to formulate decisions in concert with parents, after providing them with clear, realistic, and factual information about the possibilities for success of therapy and its long-term outcome.

III. **Delivery room care.** The pediatric team should include an experienced pediatrician or neonatologist, particularly when the fetus is less than 26 weeks' gestational age. The approach to resuscitation is similar to that in more mature infants (see Chap. 4, Resuscitation in the Delivery Room). Special attention should be paid to the following:

A. **Warmth and drying.** The ELBW neonate is at particular risk for rapid cooling. The infant should be placed under a preheated warmer and quickly dried. Wet toweling should be expeditiously removed. Additional warming lights should be placed near the radiant warmer.

B. **Respiratory support.** Most ELBW infants require ventilatory support because of pulmonary immaturity and limited respiratory muscle strength. If the neonate cries vigorously, we administer blow-by oxygen as required and observe the infant for signs of distress. Many of these infants require bag-and-mask ventilation for apnea or ineffective respiratory drive. The resolution of bradycardia is the best indicator of adequate response to resuscitation. If the infant's lungs are deficient in surfactant, high inflating pressures may be necessary for the initial breaths, but the peak pressure should be rapidly lowered to minimize lung injury. Because these infants generally require continued respiratory support and benefit from early application of end-expiratory pressure, we generally perform endotracheal intubation and ventilation shortly after birth. After initial lung inflation, the use of a Neopuff Infant Resuscitator (Fisher and Paykell) is preferred over hand-bagging because it ensures uniform breaths and regulated inflation pressures. The goal is to use the lowest tidal volumes possible while still adequately ventilating the infant. Initiation of exogenous surfactant therapy before the first breath has not been proven to be more beneficial than administration after initial stabilization of the infant. Exogenous surfactant may be safely administered in the delivery room once correct endotracheal tube position has been confirmed clinically.

The pediatrician should assess the response to resuscitation and gauge the need for further interventions. If the infant fails to respond, the team should recheck that all support measures are being effectively administered. Support for apnea or poor respiratory effort must include intermittent inflating breaths or regulated nasal continuous positive airway pressure (CPAP). Face-mask CPAP alone is not adequate support for an apneic baby, and failure to respond to this limited intervention does not mean that the infant is too immature to be resuscitated. If no positive response to resuscitation occurs after a reasonable length of time, we consider withdrawing support.

C. **Care after resuscitation.** Immediately after resuscitation the infant should be wrapped in warmed towels and placed in a prewarmed transport incubator for transfer to the NICU. We always show the baby to the parents in the delivery room (while in the transport incubator) because this is important for the beginning of parent–infant interaction. In the NICU, the infant is moved to a radiant warmer where a complete assessment is done and treatment initiated. The infant's temperature should be rechecked at this time and closely monitored. As soon as possible, the infant should be moved to an incubator for continued care. In addition to reducing insensible fluid losses and thereby simplifying fluid therapy, the use of incubators aids in reducing unnecessary stimulation and noise experienced by the baby. Newer convertible beds that easily change between radiant warmer and incubator (Giraffe Bed, Ohmeda Medical) are the ideal bed type, and can be used starting right from birth.

IV. **Care in the intensive care unit.** Careful attention to detail and frequent monitoring are the basic components of care of the ELBW infant, because critical changes can occur rapidly. Large fluid losses, balances between fluid intake and blood glucose levels, delicate pulmonary status, and the immaturity and increased sensitivity of several organ systems all require close monitoring. Monitoring itself, however, may pose increased risks because of small blood volumes, tiny-caliber vessels, and limited skin integrity. Issues in routine care that require special attention in ELBW infants include the following:

A. **Survival.** The first 24 to 48 hours are the most critical for survival. Infants who require significant respiratory, cardiovascular, and/or fluid support are assessed continuously, and their chances for survival are estimated. If caregivers and the parents determine that death is imminent, continued treatment is futile, or treatment is likely to result in survival of a neurologically devastated infant, we recommend the withdrawal of ventilator support and redirection of care to comfort measures only.

B. **Respiratory support.** Most ELBW infants require initial respiratory support.

1. **Conventional ventilation.** We generally use conventional ventilation and prefer synchronized intermittent mandatory ventilation (SIMV) (see Chap. 24, Mechanical Ventilation). The lowest possible tidal volume to provide adequate ventilation and oxygenation and a short inspiratory time should be used. Special effort should be made to avoid hyperoxia by setting the limits of oxygen saturation at lower than have been used in the past. A recent report suggested that limits of 85% to 93% and staff training programs designed to reduce the number of hypoxia-hyperoxia fluctuations might reduce the incidence of retinopathy of prematurity. It is hypothesized that limiting hyperoxia may also reduce the incidence or severity of chronic lung disease. It is important as well to avoid hypocapnia, although the potential benefit of permissive hypercapnia as a ventilatory strategy remains a subject of debate.

2. **Surfactant therapy** (see Chap. 24, Respiratory Distress Syndrome/Hyaline Membrane Disease). We administer surfactant to infants with RDS who are ventilated with a mean airway pressure of at least 7 cm H_2O and an inspired oxygen concentration (FiO_2) of 0.30 or higher in the first 2 hours after birth. We give the first dose as soon as possible after birth, preferably within the first hour.

3. **High-frequency oscillatory ventilation (HFOV)** is used in infants who fail to improve after surfactant administration, and require conventional ventilation at high peak inspiratory pressures. For infants with air leak, especially pulmonary interstitial emphysema (see Chap. 24, Pulmonary Air Leak), high-frequency jet ventilation may be the preferred mode of ventilation.

4. **Vitamin A Supplementation.** All infants with birth weight of 1000 g and less should receive 5000 IU of Vitamin A intramuscularly 3 times a week for the first 4 weeks. This therapy has been shown to slightly reduce the incidence of chronic lung disease.

C. **Fluids and electrolytes** (see Chaps. 9 and 31). Fluid requirements increase tremendously as gestational age decreases below 28 weeks, due to both an increased surface area–body weight ratio and immaturity of the skin. Renal immaturity may result in large losses of fluid and electrolytes that must be replaced. Early use of incubators significantly reduces insensible fluid losses and therefore the total administered volume necessary to maintain fluid balance.

1. **Route of administration.** Whenever possible, an umbilical arterial line and a double-lumen umbilical venous line are placed shortly after birth. Arterial lines are maintained for 7 to 10 days and then replaced by peripheral arterial lines if needed. Umbilical venous lines may be used for as long as 7 to 14 days, and are often replaced by percutaneously inserted central venous catheters (PICC) when the UVC is removed.

2. **Rate of administration.** Table 6.2 presents initial rates of fluid administration for different gestational ages and birth weights. We monitor weight, blood pressure, urine output, and serum electrolyte levels frequently. Fluid rate is adjusted to avoid dehydration or hypernatremia. We generally measure electrolytes before the age of 12 hours (6 hours for infants <800 g), and repeat as often as every 6 hours until the levels are stable. By the second day, many infants have a marked diuresis and natriuresis and require continued frequent assessment and adjustment of fluids and electrolytes. Insensible water loss diminishes as the skin thickens and dries over the first few days of life.

3. **Fluid composition.** Initial intravenous (IV) fluids should consist of dextrose solution in a concentration sufficient to maintain serum glucose levels higher than 45 to 50 mg/dL. Immature infants often do not tolerate

TABLE 6.2.   FLUID ADMINISTRATION RATES FOR THE FIRST 2 DAYS OF LIFE FOR INFANTS ON RADIANT WARMERS*

Birth Weight (g)	Gestational Age (weeks)	Fluid Rate (mL/kg per day)	Frequency of Electrolyte Testing
500–600	23	140–200	q6h
601–800	24	120–130	q8h
801–1000	25–26	90–110	q12h

*Rates may be 25–30% lower if incubator or shield is used. Urine output and serum electrolytes should be closely monitored.

dextrose concentrations higher than 10% at high fluid rates, so we generally use dextrose 7.5% or 5% solutions. Usually, a glucose administration rate of 4 to 10 mg/kg per minute is sufficient. If hyperglycemia results, we lower dextrose concentrations, but avoid hypoosmolar solutions (dextrose <5%). If hyperglycemia persists at levels above 180 mg/dL with glycosuria, we begin an insulin infusion at a dose of 0.05 to 0.1 unit/kg per hour and adjust as required (see Chap. 29).

ELBW infants begin losing protein and develop negative nitrogen balance soon after birth. To avoid this, we start parenteral nutrition immediately upon admission to the NICU, using a premixed solution of amino acids and trace elements in dextrose 5%. Multivitamin solutions are not included in this initial parenteral nutrition because of shelf-life issues, but are added within 24 hours after delivery. No electrolytes are added to the initial solution other than the small amount of potassium phosphate needed to buffer the amino acids. The solution is designed so that the administration of 60 mL/kg per day (the maximum infusion rate used) provides 1.5 g of protein/kg per day. Additional fluid needs are met by the solutions described above. Customized parenteral nutrition, including lipid infusion, is begun as soon as it is available, generally within the first day.

4. **Skin care.** Immaturity of skin and susceptibility to damage requires close attention to maintenance of skin integrity (see Chap. 34). Topical emollients or petroleum-based products are not used except under extreme situations, but semipermeable coverings (Tegaderm and Vigilon) are used over areas of skin breakdown.

D. **Cardiovascular support**
   1. **Blood pressure.** There is disagreement over acceptable values for blood pressure in extremely premature infants, and some suggestion that cerebral perfusion may be adversely affected at levels below 30 mm Hg. In the absence of data demonstrating an impact on long-term neurologic outcome, we accept mean blood pressures of 26 to 28 mm Hg for infants 24 to 26 weeks' gestational age if the infant appears well perfused and has a stable heart rate. Early hypotension is more commonly due to altered vasoreactivity than hypovolemia, so therapy with fluid administration is limited to 10 to 20 mL/kg, after which pressor support, initially with dopamine, is begun. Stress dose hydrocortisone (1 mg/kg every 12 hours for two doses) may be useful in infants with hypotension refractory to this strategy (see Chap. 17).
   2. **Patent ductus arteriosus (PDA).** The incidence of symptomatic PDA is as high as 70% in infants with a birth weight lower than 1000 g. The initial presentation occurs most commonly between 24 and 72 hours after birth and may be evident with increasing need for ventilatory support or an increase in oxygen requirement. A murmur may be absent or difficult to hear, and the physical signs of increased pulses or an active precordium may be difficult to discern. Indomethacin therapy (see Chap. 25) should be initiated when clinical criteria alone are present, or after a suspected PDA is confirmed by echocardiography. Prophylactic treatment with indomethacin has been demonstrated to reduce the incidence and severity of PDA. However, because it has not yet been demonstrated to result in a change in long-term neurologic outcome, it has not become routine therapy. Persistent or recurrent PDA is confirmed by echocardiography and treated with indomethacin. Recurrence after a second treatment course is generally an indication for surgical ligation.

E. **Blood transfusions.** These are often necessary in small infants because of large obligatory phlebotomy losses. Infants who weigh less than 1000 g at birth and are moderately or severely ill may receive as many as eight or nine transfusions in the first few weeks of life. Donor exposure can be limited by reducing laboratory testing to the minimum necessary level, employing strict uniform criteria for transfusion, and by identifying a specific unit of blood for each patient likely to need several transfusions (see Chap. 26). Each such unit can be split to provide as many as eight transfusions for a single patient over a period of 21 days with only a single donor exposure. Erythropoietin therapy in conjunction with adequate iron therapy will result in accelerated erythropoiesis, but it has not been shown to reduce the need for transfusion. It is not routinely used in these patients.

F. **Infection and infection control** (see Chap. 23). Premature birth in general is associated with an increased incidence of early-onset sepsis, with an incidence of 1.5 % of infants less than 1500 g birth weight. Group B streptococcus (GBS) remains an important pathogen, but gram-negative organisms now account for a majority of early-onset sepsis in infants less than 1500 g. We almost always screen for infection immediately after birth, and treat with prophylactic antibiotics (ampicillin and gentamicin) pending culture results. Extremely low-birth-weight (ELBW) infants are also particularly susceptible to nosocomial infections (occurring at >72 hours after birth). About one-third of infants less than 1000 g at birth will have at least one episode of late-onset sepsis, although wide variations in its incidence between centers is observed. Almost half of late-onset infections are due to coagulase-negative staphylococcus, 18% to gram-negative organisms, and 12% due to fungi. Mortality is higher among infants who develop these late-onset infections, primarily in those with gram-negative organisms. Risk factors for late-onset infection include longer duration of mechanical ventilation, umbilical and central venous lines, and parenteral nutrition support.

Comparison of practices among institutions with different rates of nosocomial infection has led to a number of recommendations that we have employed to potentially reduce the incidence within our NICUs. Foremost among these is meticulous attention to handwashing. We have added the use of alcohol-based gels, available at every bedside, and a strict policy for use before patient contact. In-line suctioning is used in respiratory circuits to minimize disruption, and every effort is made to minimize the duration of mechanical ventilation. We only use hyperalimentation solutions that have been prepared under laminar flow, and never alter them after preparation. The early introduction of feedings, preferably with human milk, minimizes the need for central lines and provides the benefits of milk-borne immune factors. Laboratory testing is kept to a minimum, and tests clustered whenever possible, to reduce the number of skin punctures and to reduce patient handling. These practices are part of a standardized protocol for skin care for all neonates born at less than 1000 g. Finally, the establishment of a uniform NICU culture that encompasses pride in care and cooperation has fostered an environment of blameless questioning between practitioners.

G. **Nutritional support**
   1. **Initial management.** In all infants who weigh less than 1200 g at birth, parenteral nutrition is begun shortly after birth using a standard solution administered at a rate of 60 mL/kg per day (see IV. C. above), resulting in protein administration of 1.5 g/kg per day. On subsequent days, customized parenteral solutions are formulated to increase the protein administration rate by 1 g/kg per day up to a maximum of 3.5 g/kg per day. Parenteral lipids are begun on day 2 and advanced each day to a maximum of 3 g/kg per day. Enteral feeding is not attempted until the patient is clinically stable, and not receiving indomethacin or pressor therapy.
   2. The safe initiation of enteral feeds often begins with small trophic feedings of breast milk (10 mL/kg per day). These may be started even in the presence of an umbilical arterial line. Feedings of 20 calories per 30 mL breast milk or formula are then slowly advanced (10 to 20 mL/kg per day) while monitoring for signs of feeding intolerance such as abdominal distention, vomiting (which is rare), and increased gastric residuals. It is important but often difficult to differentiate the characteristically poor gastrointestinal motility of ELBW infants from signs of a more serious

gastrointestinal disorder such as necrotizing enterocolitis (see Chap. 32). At least two-thirds of our ELBW infants have episodes of feeding intolerance that result in interruption of feeds. Once successful tolerance of feedings is established at 90 to 100 mL/kg per day, caloric density is advanced to 24 cal /30 mL, and then the volume is advanced (see Chap. 10). This eliminates a drop in caloric intake as parenteral nutrition is weaned while feedings advance. Once tolerance of full feedings of 24 cal/30 mL is established, the density of feedings may be advanced by 2 cal/30 mL per day up to a maximum of 30 to 32 cal/30 mL. Protein powder is added to a total protein content of 4 g/kg per day, as this promotes improved somatic and head growth over the first several weeks of life. Many extremely small infants benefit from restriction of total fluids to 130 to 140 mL/kg per day. This minimizes problems with fluid excess while still providing adequate caloric intake.

Suggested Readings

El-Metwally D., Vohr B., Tucker R.B. Survival and neonatal morbidity at the limits of viability in the mid 1990s: 22 to 25 weeks. *J Pediatr* 2000;137(5):616–622.

Horbar J.D., Rogowski J., Plsek P., et al. Collaborative quality improvement for neonatal intensive care. *Pediatrics* 2001;107:14–22.

Stoll B.J., Hansen N., Fanaroff A.A., et al. Late-onset sepsis in very low birth weight neonates: The experience of the NICHD Neonatal Research Network. *Pediatrics* 2002;110:285–291.

Wood N.S., et al. for the EPICure Study Group. Neurologic and developmental disability after extremely preterm birth *N Engl J Med* 2000;343:378–384.

7. MULTIPLE BIRTHS

Olivier Danhaive

I. **Classification**
   A. **Zygosity.** Monozygous (MZ) twins develop from a single fertilized egg and are identical. Dizygous (DZ) twins derive from two fertilized eggs and are fraternal. Naturally occurring higher-order pregnancies are usually multizygous, although they can be monozygous, or, rarely, a combination.
   B. **Placentation.** Twins have either one single placenta (monochorionic), frequently with shared vasculature, or two separate (dichorionic) placentas with no shared vasculature. Dichorionic placentas may fuse and appear single, but are usually divided by a clearly identifiable ridge. The amniotic sac may be single (monoamniotic) or separated (diamniotic) (See Fig. 7.1).

II. **Epidemiology**
   A. **Natural incidence.** The rate of twin pregnancies in the United States in 1980 (before the era of assisted reproduction) was approximately 11 per 1000 pregnancies. Triplet and higher-order multiple pregnancies occurred in 0.4 per 1000 pregnancies. The rate of MZ twinning is relatively constant (3.5 per 1000). However, the rate of DZ pregnancy is influenced by several factors, such as ethnicity (greater in African-Americans and lower in Asians than in whites and Hispanics), greater maternal age (twinning peaks at 35 years and then declines) and greater parity. In the United States, approximately two-thirds of twins are DZ.
   B. **Influence of assisted reproduction.** Ovulation-inducing drugs (e.g., clomiphene, gonadotropins), assisted reproduction techniques (e.g., *in vitro* fertilization, gamete intrafallopian transfer), and increased maternal age have contributed to a substantial increase in multiple births in Western societies. From 1980 to 1999, the rate of twin births increased from 18.9 to 28.9 per 1000 live births (53% increase), and the rate of higher-order multiple births increased more than fourfold to 1.7 per 1000 live births.

III. **Etiology**
   A. **MZ pregnancies** result from the splitting of a single egg during the first 10 days of development. This is thought to be due to a teratogenic event that leads to separation of embryonic cells but leaves intact the already formed cavities. In the first 3 days after ovulation, such an event leads to complete separation of the embryos and their placental tissues, resulting in **diamniotic-dichorionic placentation.** If splitting occurs on days 4–8, at the time of implantation, the placenta stays fused but two amniotic sacs develop (**diamniotic-monochorionic placentation**). From day 9 to days 12–15, when the amniotic cavity forms, the two separate embryos develop in a single sac (**monoamniotic-monochorionic twins**). Thereafter, once the embryonic axis is established, splitting results either in conjoined twins or a single individual with malformations involving symmetry or complex midline defects.
   B. **DZ or multizygous pregnancies** result from multiple ovulation. The greater incidence of DZ twinning in certain ethnic groups and with greater maternal age or multiparity is likely due to higher levels of gonadotropins (FSH and LH). Occasional familial predisposition suggests that genetic factors play a role in some cases. Assisted reproductive techniques such as ovarian stimulation and multiple embryo transfer increase the risk of multizygous pregnancies. However, 1 in 10–15 multiple pregnancies that follow infertility treatment is MZ.

IV. **Obstetrical management**
   A. **Diagnosis of zygosity.** Detecting and identifying MZ twins is important because specific risk factors are associated with monochorionic and monoamniotic placentation.

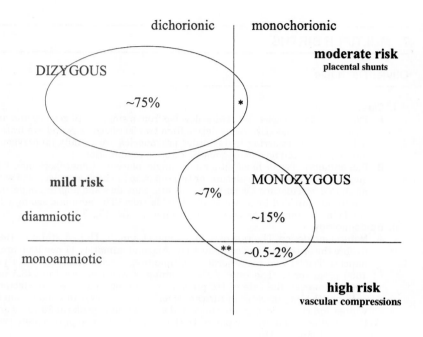

* false positive: fused placentas
** false positive: ruptured septum

FIG. 7.1. Distribution of zygocity according to the type of placentation. (With permission from Bernischke K. Multiple pregnancy. In: Polin R. A., Fox W. W. (Eds.). *Fetal and Neonatal Physiology,* 2nd ed. Philadelphia: Saunders, 1998;115–123.)

1. **Ultrasonography** can detect multiple gestational sacs at 5 weeks and cardiac activity from more than one fetus at 6 weeks. From 10 to 14 weeks, fused dichorionic placentas may often be distinguished from true monochorionic ones by the presence of an internal dividing membrane or a ridge at the placental surface (lambda sign). In the former, the dividing septum appears thicker and includes two amnions and two chorionic layers; in the latter, it consists only of two thin amnions. The absence of a dividing septum suggests monoamniotic twins, but may also be due to septal disruption. Both conditions have a poor prognosis.
2. **Genetic techniques** can be used to determine zygosity in same-sex twins. DNA obtained by chorionic villus sampling or amniocentesis can be compared by restriction fragment length polymorphism analysis. Unlike-sex twins are always DZ.
B. **Management**
   1. **Assisted reproduction.** Spontaneous abortion and preterm birth are strongly correlated to the number of fetuses. Thus, techniques that limit the number of reimplanted eggs or transferred embryos, or selective reduction of higher-order multiples may improve the likelihood of successful outcome.
   2. **Maternal complications.** Multifetal pregnancies have an increased risk of complications. These include preterm labor, premature rupture of the

membranes, hypertension (2.5 times greater than singleon pregnancies), preeclampsia and hemolysis, elevated liver enzymes, low platelet count (HELLP) syndrome, acute liver fatty necrosis, glucose intolerance, anemia, and urinary-tract infections. Postpartum complications, such as infection or hemorrhage, also occur more frequently.

V. Fetal and neonatal complications

A. Prematurity and low birth weight. The average duration of gestation is shorter in multifetal pregnancies, and shortens more as the number of fetuses increases. The mean gestational age at birth is 36, 32, and 31 weeks, respectively, for twins, triplets, and quadruplets. Approximately 10% of triplets deliver before 28 weeks' gestation. In developed countries, the incidence of preterm birth in twins was 53 percent in 1997, compared to 9–10% in singletons. Although most of this increased incidence is due to mild prematurity, multifetal pregnancy increases the risk of severe prematurity and very low birth weight (VLBW). The likelihood of a birth weight less than 1500 g is 8 and 33 times greater in twins and triplets or higher-order multiples, respectively, compared to singletons. In two multicenter surveys, multiples occurred in 21–24% of births less than 1500 g and 30% less than 1000 g. The risk of delivering a VLBW infant is higher in women who conceived spontaneously after a long period of infertility or who had infertility treatment.

1. Causes of preterm deliveries in multiples include preterm labor in half, preterm rupture of the membranes in one-fourth, and delivery for maternal and fetal indications, such as preeclampsia, fetal distress, growth restriction or single fetal demise, in one-fourth.

2. Whether twins reach maturity earlier than singletons is uncertain. At gestational ages greater than 31 weeks, results of lung maturity tests such as the Fetal Lung Maturity test (FLM II) are higher in twins than singletons; however, results do not correlate with a lower incidence of respiratory distress syndrome. Thus, these tests may overestimate lung maturity in twins.

B. Growth restriction and weight discordance. Fetal growth is independent of the number of fetuses until approximately 30 weeks' gestation, after which growth of multiples gradually falls off compared to singletons (Fig. 7.2). The mechanism is likely uterine crowding and limitation of placental perfusion. Growth restriction is more likely to affect monochorionic than dichorionic twins, affecting one fetus in 52% and 36% and both twins in 17% and 7%, respectively.

1. **Moderate discordant growth.** The second twin is more likely to have growth restriction, suggesting that implantation may be a determining factor. If the weight discordance is <20% and both fetuses follow their respective growth curves, it is usually safe for the pregnancy to continue under close monitoring.

2. **Severe discordance in growth** (>30%) that occurs before 30 weeks' gestation may reflect chronic fetal distress and is associated with an increased rate of intrauterine demise, perinatal death, and preterm birth before 32 weeks. Severe growth restriction or discordant growth may be due to other conditions, such as congenital anomalies, fetal infection, twin–twin transfusion syndrome, or placental dysfunction.

C. Malformations. Malformations occur in approximately 6% of twin pregnancies, or 3% of individual twins. The risk in MZ twins is approximately 2.5-fold greater than DZ twins or singletons. Structural defects specific to MZ twins are (1) early malformations that share a common origin with the twinning process and (2) vascular disruption syndromes. Twin pregnancies should be evaluated for fetal anomalies by fetal ultrasonography or more invasive procedures if indicated.

1. **Chromosomal anomalies, isolated malformations, and single-gene defects.** The likelihood of finding an anomaly in at least one of DZ twins is slightly greater than twice that of a singleton fetus. The risk of a mendelian or chromosomal abnormality is independent for each fetus. The risk is due in part to increased maternal age, a predisposing factor

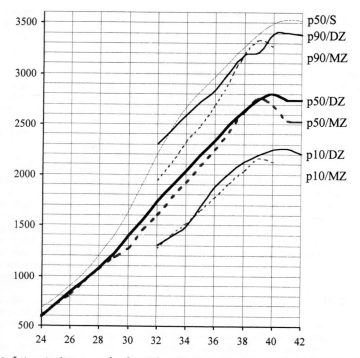

FIG. 7.2. Intrauterine growth chart for dizygotic and monozygotic twins. (From Naeye R., Bernischke K., Hagstrom J., Marcus C.C. Intrauterine growth of twins as estimated from liveborn birth-weight data. *Pediatrics* 1966;37:409. American Academy of Pediatrics, 1966.)

for both DZ twinning and chromosomal anomalies. The risk of mendelian and chromosomal abnormalities in MZ twins is equivalent to a singleton.

2. **Early structural defects** are more frequent in MZ twins, and may share a common etiology with the embryonic splitting process. These include caudal malformations (sirenomelia, sacrococcygeal teratoma), urological malformations (cloacal or bladder exstrophy), the VATER spectrum (vertebral anomalies, anal atresia, tracheoesophageal fistula, renal agenesis, cardiac defects), neural tube defects (anencephaly, encephalocoele, or holoprosencephaly), and defects of laterality (situs inversus, polysplenia, or asplenia). Anomalies are concordant (both fetuses equally affected) only in a minority of cases, even in MZ twins. Thus, the presence of an anomaly in only one twin does not indicate they are DZ. Whether embryo manipulations lead to birth defects is uncertain. In a large study, the risk of a major birth defect was greater in infants conceived with assisted reproduction methods (odds ratio 2.0), compared with natural conception. However, smaller studies in the past failed to show a difference.

3. **Conjoined twins** are rare (incidence: 1/14,000–1/80,000) and result from embryonic splitting after 2 weeks. Three-quarters are joined at the chest and/or abdomen. Thoracopagus twins lie face-to-face and are joined at the thoracic and abdominal level. The hearts are joined with complex anatomy of the great vessels in 75%, segments of the gastrointestinal tract are shared in 50%, and the biliary tree is common in 25%. A subset of thoraco-

pagus twins is xyphopagus twins, who are joined through the anterior abdominal wall, sharing a common peritoneal cavity but usually with separate organs. The other variants have pelvic (ischiopagus), sacral, or cranial fusion (craniopagus). Prenatal (40%) and perinatal mortality (35%) of conjoined twins are high. Extensive assessment of fetal anatomy should be performed to determine management options.

4. **Vascular disruption sequences** may occur early or late in gestation.

   a. Large arterial anastomoses between the two embryos may occur early in development and lead to unequal arterial perfusion, in which one embryo receives only low-pressure blood flow through the umbilical artery and preferentially perfuses its lower extremities. This results in **acardia**, a rare condition (1 in 35,000) characterized by profound malformations ranging from complete amorphism to severe upper-body abnormalities, such as anencephaly, holoprosencephaly, rudimentary facial features and limbs, and absent thoracic or abdominal organs. The other twin is usually well formed. The incidence of spontaneous abortion and prematurity is 20% and 60%, respectively, in acardiac twin pregnancies. Perinatal mortality in the donor twin is 40%.

   b. Vascular disruption syndromes that occur later in gestation may result in exchange of tissue between twins through placental anastomoses. This often occurs after the demise of one fetus. Resulting malformations include aplasia cutis, limb interruption, intestinal atresia, gastroschisis, anorchia or gonadal dysgenesis, hemifacial microsomia, Goldenhaar syndrome (facio-auriculo-vertebral), or Poland sequence. Cranial abnormalities include porencephalic cysts, hydranencephaly, microcephaly, and hydrocephalus.

5. **Deformations,** such as clubfoot, are more frequent in multiple pregnancies. They result from crowding of the uterine environment.

D. **Placental vascular anomalies**

1. **Twin-to-twin transfusion syndrome (TTS)** complicates 10–15% of monochorionic twin pregnancies, although this may underestimate early-onset cases that lead to silent fetal loss. The diagnosis is usually made between 17 and 26 weeks' gestation, although the process begins as early as 13 weeks.

   a. Vascular communications occur in essentially all monochorionic placentas but are exceptional in dichorionic ones. There are two categories: (1) superficial arterial-to-arterial and venous-to-venous anastomoses that are potentially bidirectional, and (2) deep interfetal artery-to-vein communications located in the placental cotyledons that are supplied by one fetus and drained by the other.

   b. TTS results when intertwin arteriovenous shunts are improperly compensated by the superficial network of anastomoses. One fetus (the donor) slowly pumps blood into the other's circulation. This may result in progressive anemia, hypovolemia, growth restriction, brain ischemic lesions, renal insufficiency, oligohydramnios ("stuck twin"), lung hypoplasia, limb deformation, and ultimately fetal demise in the donor. Plethora, heart failure, cerebral emboli, thrombosis, disseminated intravascular coagulation, renal failure, hydrops, and polyhydramnios may occur in the recipient. The mortality rate of severe untreated TTS is 60–90%. This is due in part to preterm birth, which occurs frequently as a consequence of polyhydramnios.

   c. Neonatal criteria of TTS are mostly nonspecific. The diagnosis is suggested by a difference between twins of 15% in hematocrit or 20% in birth weight.

   d. Resuscitation may be necessary at birth, including ventilatory and cardiac support, rapid vascular access for glucose supply and volume expanders, or partial exchange transfusion. Postnatal evaluation, including cranial ultrasonography, should be performed to detect prenatally acquired lesions.

2. **Velamentous cord insertion and vasa previa** occur 6–9 times more often in twins than singletons, and even more often in higher-order gestations. They probably result from placental crowding and abnormal blastocyst nidation. All types of placentation can be affected. The result is that the umbilical vessels are unprotected by Wharton jelly and are more prone to compression or disruption, leading to acute fetal distress or hemorrhage.

3. **Cord blood-flow interruption.** Overall perinatal mortality in monoamniotic twins is more than 20%. The high rate of intrauterine death of one or both twins results from frequent cord accidents (e.g., entanglement, compression). The period of highest risk is 26–32 weeks. Management includes daily assessments of fetal well-being, and delivery when the lungs are mature.

E. **Intrauterine death**

1. The death of one fetus in multiple pregnancies is a common event during the first trimester (>20%) and is often not recognized. Possible causes include abnormal nidation, chromosomal abnormalities, and fetal malformations. The diagnosis is sometimes made at birth, when the placenta appears double or contains a "fetus papyraceus." In other cases, it presents as a "vanishing twin," seen in early ultrasound examinations, then subsequently absent. The prognosis for the second twin is usually excellent.

2. The death of one twin is less common in the second and the third trimesters, occurring in ~9% of multiple pregnancies. The risk is 4–6 times greater in monochorionic pregnancies, and even more in monoamniotic ones. In monochorionic pregnancies, the death of one twin jeopardizes the second. Preterm labor occurs in many cases. Multicystic encephalopathy is a severe complication in the surviving twin after death of the co-twin, and is probably related to hypotension or thromboembolic events. In one series, mortality was 4% for the second twin, and neurological complications occurred in 12% of the survivors.

VI. **Outcomes**

A. **Mortality**

1. **Fetal mortality.** The death of at least one fetus will occur in ~9% of twin pregnancies between 10 and 24 weeks of gestation. Fetal loss before 24 weeks is greater in monochorionic than dichorionic twins (12.2 vs. 1.8%).

2. **Intrapartum mortality** is 4–11 times higher in twins than in singletons, and worsens in higher-order multiples. The second twin is at greater risk, being more prone to malpresentation (35–40% of the second-presenting vs. 15–20% of the first-presenting twin are nonvertex), cord compression, asphyxia, perinatal depression, and longer exposure to anesthesia.

3. **Neonatal mortality** remains strongly related to prematurity and low birth weight.

4. **Mortality** during the first year is almost three times higher in twins than singletons. This is due to prematurity and congenital anomalies.

B. **Long-term morbidity**

1. **Cerebral palsy (CP)** and other neurological handicaps affect more twins and multiples than singletons. Twins account for 5–10% of all cases of CP in the United States. The prevalence of CP in twins is 7.4%, compared to 1% in singletons. This is related to the increased risk of prematurity and low birth weight in multiple births. In addition, other factors such as TTS and demise of one twin (associated with 20% risk of CP in the surviving co-twin) play a role.

2. **Consequences of prematurity and growth restriction** affect many multiples. These are discussed elsewhere. (See appropriate chapters.)

C. **Economic impact.** Hospital stays for mothers and babies are typically longer for multiple gestations. In a study performed at our institution in the early 1990s, average hospital charges were estimated to be 3 and 6 times higher for twins and triplets, respectively, compared to singletons; the total family charges were 4 and 11 times higher, respectively. In that study, 35% of twins and 75% of triplets resulted from assisted reproduction techniques, emphasizing the contribution of fertility treatment to overall costs.

Suggested Readings

Bejar R., Vigliocco G., Gramajo H. et al. Resnik, R. Antenatal origin of neurologic damage in newborn infants II. Multiple gestations. *Am J Obstet Gynecol* 1990;162:1230–6.

Callahan T.L., Hall J.E., Ettner S.L., et al. The economic impact of multiple-gestation pregnancies and the contribution of assisted reproduction techniques to their incidence. *N Engl J Med* 1994;331:244–9.

Gardner M.O., Goldenberg R.L., Cliver S.P., et al. The origins and outcome of preterm twin pregnancies. *Obstet Gynecol* 1995;85:553–7.

Joseph K.S., Allen A.C., Dodds L., et al. Causes and consequences of recent increases in preterm birth among twins. *Obstet Gynecol* 2001;98:57–64.

Lemons J.A., Bauer C.R., Oh W., et al., for the NICHD Neonatal Research Network. Very Low Birth Weight Outcomes of the National Institute of Health and Human Development Neonatal Research Network, january 1995 through december 1996. *Pediatrics* 2001;107:e1.

Schieve L.A., Meikle S.F., Ferre C., et al. Low and very low birth weight in infants conceived with use of assisted reproductive technology. *N Engl J Med* 2002; 346:731–7.

Sebire N.J., Snijders R.J.M., Hughes K., et al. The hidden mortality of monochoroinic twin pregnancies. *Br J Obstet Gynecol* 1997;104:1203–7.

Tommiska V., Heinonen K., Ikonen S., et al. A national short-term follow-up study of extremely low birth weight infants born in Finland in 1996–1997. *Pediatrics* 2001;107:e2.

Williams K., Hennessy E., Alberman E. Cerebral palsy: effects of twinning, birth weight and gestational age. *Arch Dis Child* 1996;75:F178–82.

8. GENETIC ISSUES PRESENTING IN THE NURSERY

Diana W. Bianchi

I. **Introduction.** Although as many as 40% of pediatric hospital admissions have a genetic basis, it is usually the infant with major malformations or an inborn error of metabolism who presents in the nursery setting. **Major malformations** are defined as anomalies that are prenatal in origin and have cosmetic, medical, or surgical significance. The birth of an infant with major malformations, whether diagnosed antenatally or not, evokes an emotional parental response. The medical staff must ensure that the affected infant has an expedient but thorough evaluation so appropriate diagnostic procedures and therapy may proceed.

II. **Incidence.** Major malformations occur in 2 to 3% of live births and have surpassed prematurity as the leading cause of neonatal death. The incidence of congenital anomalies is doubled above the general population for an individual twin.

III. **Etiology.** The etiologies of congenital anomalies are shown in Table 8.1. Note that the cause is unknown in the majority of cases. Only about 10% are associated with a chromosomal abnormality.

IV. **Approach to the infant**

    A. History

        1. Prenatal. The obstetric chart should be reviewed for the presence or absence of the following:

            a. History of possible teratogenic exposure, including chronic maternal illness, for example, diabetes, phenylketonuria, Graves' disease, myasthenia gravis, myotonic dystrophy, or systemic lupus erythematosus (Table 8.2).

            b. Specific exposure to drugs or alcohol during pregnancy (Table 8.2).

            c. Abnormal uterine shape.

            d. Infections during pregnancy.

            e. Multiple gestation.

            f. Fetal growth pattern (e.g., relationship of uterine size to gestational age)

            g. Results of antenatal ultrasonographic examinations (were anomalies, polyhydramnios, or oligohydramnios diagnosed? Was there an increased nuchal translucency measurement in the first trimester?)

            h. Results of maternal serum screening (see Chap. 1, Fetal Assessment and Prenatal Diagnosis). A **low alpha-fetoprotein** (AFP) level may be seen in the presence of trisomy 18 or 21. A **high AFP** level may indicate a multiple gestation, impending fetal demise, open neural tube defect, abdominal wall defect, congenital nephrosis, epidermolysis bullosa, or Turner syndrome. A high human chorionic gonadotropin (hCG) level is also associated with trisomy 21.

            i. Quality and frequency of fetal movements.

        2. Family history. The parents and, if possible, the grandparents should be asked the following:

            a. Have there been any prior affected infants in the family?

            b. Is there a history of infertility, multiple miscarriages, neonatal death, or newborns with other malformations?

            c. What is the ethnic background of both mother and father?

            d. Is there a history of consanguinity?

        3. Perinatal events.

            a. Fetal position *in utero*.

            b. Significant events during labor and type of delivery.

            c. Length of umbilical cord (e.g., a positive association exists between fetal motor activity and cord length).

            d. Placental appearance.

        4. Neonatal course.

TABLE 8.1. ETIOLOGY OF CONGENITAL ANOMALIES: BRIGHAM AND WOMEN'S HOSPITAL MALFORMATIONS SURVEILLANCE DATA FROM 69,227 NEWBORNS

	Number	Percent
Single gene (mendelian inheritance)	48	4.1
Chromosome abnormality	157	10.1
Familial	225	14.4
Multifactorial	356	22.8
Teratogens	49	4.1
Uterine factors	39	2.5
Twinning	6	0.4
Unknown	669	43.1
Total	1549	100

Source: From Nelson K., Holmes L. B. *N Engl J Med* 1989;320:19.

B. **Physical examination.** A complete physical examination is essential to making an accurate diagnosis. Often, however, the critically ill neonate is partially hidden by monitoring equipment. Beware of making a diagnosis when (1) the midface is obscured by adhesive tape securing endotracheal and nasogastric tubes, (2) the extremities cannot be visualized because there are peripheral intravenous (IV) lines in place, or (3) the infant is hydropic.
   1. **Anthropometrics.** Specific physical parameters that should be measured include length, head circumference, outer and inner canthal distance, palpebral fissure length, interpupillary distance, ear length, philtrum length, internipple distance, chest circumference, upper-lower segment ratio, and hand and foot length. Normal standards exist for all these measurements in infants of 27 to 41 weeks' gestation.
   2. Aspects of the physical examination to be emphasized include a thorough inspection of the skin, the position of the hair whorls, head shape and facial characteristics, and dermatoglyphics, and a description of the extremities. The dermatoglyphic pattern of low-arch dermal ridges is particularly useful in the bedside diagnosis of trisomy 18 (Table 8.3).
   3. Examine both parents, if possible.
C. **Laboratory and other studies**
   1. **Placental pathology,** if possible.
   2. **Chromosome studies.** Skin and peripheral blood are the most available sources of cells for chromosome analysis. Generally, 1 mL of peripheral blood is collected in a green-top tube (sodium heparin being the anticoagulant). The sample should be kept at room temperature. For chromosomal analysis, it does not matter if the infant has received transfusions, because blood for neonates is generally irradiated. Irradiation prevents cell division, therefore the dividing cells in the karyotype originate from the newborn. Results of chromosome analysis are usually available within 48 hours. Although 0.6% of newborns have abnormal chromosomes, only a third of these have serious malformations. (See Table 8.3 for a summary of physical findings in the three major live-born autosomal trisomies.) For all newborns with **conotruncal heart malformations** (e.g., interrupted aortic arch, truncus arteriosis, tetralogy of Fallot), particularly in the setting of additional malformations such as cleft palate or single kidney, fluorescence *in situ* hybridization (FISH) studies should be performed, with

TABLE 8.2. KNOWN HUMAN TERATOGENS

DRUGS	MATERNAL CONDITIONS
Aminopterin/amethopterin	Alcoholism
Androgenic hormones	Graves' disease
Busulfan	Insulin-dependent diabetes mellitus
Chlorobiphenyls	Maternal phenylketonuria
Cocaine	Myasthenia gravis
Cyclophosphamide	Myotonic dystrophy
Diethylstilbestrol	Systemic lupus erythematosus
Iodide	
Isotretinoin (13-*cis*-retinoic acid)	INTRAUTERINE INFECTIONS
Lithium	Cytomegalovirus
Phenytoin	Herpes simplex
Propylthiouracil	Rubella
Tetracycline	Syphilis
Trimethadione	Toxoplasmosis
Valproic acid	Varicella
Warfarin	Venezuelan equine encephalitis virus
HEAVY METALS	OTHER EXPOSURES
Lead	Gasoline fumes
Mercury	Heat
	Hypoxia
	Maternal smoking
RADIATION	
Cancer therapy	

specific emphasis on using probes that recognize long-arm deletions of chromosome 22. The FISH test is the diagnostic test of choice for DiGeorge syndrome. Similarly, for newborns with severe unexplained hypotonia and oral feeding difficulties, consider a diagnosis of Prader-Willi syndrome. The FISH test diagnoses long-arm deletions of chromosome 15. Other disorders that present in the newborn period that may be diagnosed by FISH are listed in Table 8.4. Clinical applications of FISH include: rapid screening for aneuploidy, identification of microdeletion syndromes, and cancer cytogenetics. FISH studies are not automatically performed when a chromosome analysis is ordered; the particular probe for the condition being sought must be specified.

3. **DNA-based diagnosis and/or banking.** An increasing number of diseases presenting in the nursery result from single-gene mutations. Many are potentially lethal. The relevant disorders are listed in Table 8.5. Obtaining blood or skin fibroblasts for DNA studies may facilitate genetic counseling and prenatal diagnosis in future pregnancies. Note that if an infant

TABLE 8.3. PHYSICAL FINDINGS IN THE THREE MAJOR LIVE-BORN
AUTOSOMAL TRISOMIES

	Trisomy 13	Trisomy 18	Trisomy 21
Birth weight:	Normal range	Growth retarded	Normal range
Skin:	Scalp defects		
CNS:	Major malformations Holoprosencephaly Neural tube defects	Microcephaly	
Facies:	Abnormal midface	Micrognathia	Upslanting eyes
	Microphthalmia		Flattened facies
	Cleft lip/palate		Epicanthal folds
			Prominent tongue
			Small ears
Heart:	VSD, PDA, ASD	VSD, ASD, PDA	AV canal
	Dextrocardia		VSD, PDA
Abdomen:	Polycystic kidneys	Omphalocele	
Extremities:	Polydactyly	Camptodactyly	Brachydactyly
		Overlapping fingers	Simian crease in 45%
		Abnormal dermato-glyphics	Fifth finger clinodactyly
		Nail hypoplasia	Wide space between first and second toe
Neurologic:		Hypertonic	Muscular hypotonia
			Weak Moro reflex

VSD = ventricular septal defect; ASD = atrial septal defect; PDA = patent ductus arteriosus;
AV = atrioventricular.

TABLE 8.4. FISH TESTS COMMONLY ORDERED IN THE NEWBORN SETTING

Condition	Chromosome Location	Symptoms
DiGeorge syndrome	22q11	Congenital heart disease, cleft palate, other malformations, hypocalcemia
Miller-Dieker syndrome	17p13	Lissencephaly
Prader-Willi syndrome	15q11–13	Hypotonia, feeding problems
Steroid sulfatase deficiency (X-linked ichthyosis)	Xp22	Skin rash, low maternal estriol
Williams syndrome	7q11	Hypercalcemia, aortic stenosis

TABLE 8.5. DNA MUTATIONS PRESENTING AS SERIOUS NEONATAL ILLNESS

Hemophilia

Ornithine transcarbamylase deficiency

Autosomal dominant polycystic kidney disease

Alpha-1-antitrypsin deficiency

Chronic granulomatous disease

21-OH deficiency (congenital adrenal hyperplasia)

Cystic fibrosis

Phenylketonuria

Myotonic dystrophy

Osteogenesis imperfecta

Spinal muscular atrophy

has been transfused, the donor white blood cells will contribute DNA to the sample. Therefore, in infants who have received transfusions, a fibroblast culture obtained from a skin biopsy is preferable. DNA mutation analysis for infants suspected to have cystic fibrosis is recommended for premature infants, who cannot have a sweat test. DNA studies are also useful in the determination of twin zygosity and paternity.

4. **Radiographic studies** are important in the overall assessment.
   a. **Ultrasonographic examinations** can detect cranial malformations, congenital heart disease, and liver and renal anomalies.
   b. **Radiographs** can define bony malformations or skeletal dysplasias.
   c. Magnetic resonance imaging may be helpful in defining brain and abdominal anatomy.
5. **Ophthalmologic examination** is indicated if there is suspicion of congenital infection, or there are central nervous system (CNS) or craniofacial anomalies.
6. **Determination of toxoplasmosis, rubella, cytomegalovirus, herpes simplex, and "other," which may include parvovirus, syphillis, and immunedeficiency virus (TORCH)** titers is only indicated if the physical findings are suggestive of congenital infection (see Chap. 23, Infections).
7. **Measurement of urinary organic acids** is useful to diagnose metabolic disease in the dysmorphic newborn with metabolic acidosis (see Chap. 29, Inborn Errors of Metabolism).
8. Serum cholesterol level (if low) may diagnose Smith-Lemli-Opitz syndrome.

V. **Diagnosis.** After all results are known, a diagnosis may be possible. In many cases it is not possible to make a diagnosis in the nursery. Because of major changes in facial features over the first year after birth, as well as failure to achieve certain developmental milestones, certain diagnoses may become apparent later. Careful follow-up is vital.

VI. **Counseling.** If a diagnosis is made, genetic counseling should be offered to discuss prognosis and potential therapy. A future counseling session should be scheduled to provide a recurrence risk and give information about the possibility of prenatal diagnosis.

VII. **Perinatal death of an infant with malformations**
   A. Have a complete **autopsy** performed, including radiographs and photographs.
   B. Obtain a sterile **skin biopsy specimen** for tissue culture. Cultured fibroblasts may serve as a source of chromosomes, enzymes, or DNA (see Chap.

29, Inborn Errors of Metabolism). The umbilical cord or placenta can serve as an alternate source of fetal cells for study.

C. Arrange a follow-up meeting with the family to summarize the results of studies.

Suggested Readings

Baraitser M., et al. *A Colour Atlas of Clinical Genetics.* London: Wolfe Medical Publications, 1983.

Biggio J.R. Jr., Wenstrom K. D. Biochemical screening for fetal aneuploidy. *Infert Reprod Clin N Amer* 2001;12:713.

Briggs G.G., et al. *Drugs in pregnancy and lactation* (6th Ed.). Philadelphia: Lippincott Williams & Wilkins, 2001.

Goldmuntz E., et al. Microdeletions of chromosomal region 22q11 in patients with congenital conotruncal cardiac defects. *J Med Genet* 1993;30:807.

Jones K. L. *Smith's Recognizable Patterns of Human Malformation*, 5th Ed. Philadelphia: Saunders, 1997.

Malcolm S. Microdeletion and microduplication syndromes. *Prenat Diagn* 1996; 16:1213.

McKusick V. *Mendelian Inheritance in Man*, 12th Ed. Baltimore: Johns Hopkins University Press, 1998.

Merlob P., et al. Arthropometric measurements of the newborn infant (27 to 41 gestational weeks). *Birth Defects* 1984;20:1.

Parad R.B. Buccal DNA mutation analysis for diagnosis of cystic fibrosis in newborns and infants inaccessible to sweat chloride measurement. *Pediatrics* 1998;101:851.

Taybi H., et al. *Radiology of Syndromes and Metabolic Disorders*, 4th Ed. St. Louis: Mosby-Year Book Inc., 1996.

9. FLUID AND ELECTROLYTE MANAGEMENT

Patricia W. Lin and Charles F. Simmons Jr.

Dramatic changes in body composition and skin, renal, and neuroendocrine function accompany the transition to extrauterine life. The skin regulates fluid and electrolyte balance in newborns. Developmental immaturity in extremely premature neonates contributes substantially to possible mortality and morbidity.

I. **Principles of water and electrolyte metabolism.** Fluid and electrolyte therapy must be individualized, and an infant's requirements can be determined only after careful assessment of clinical and laboratory status.

   A. **Compartmentation of total-body water (TBW).** TBW is divided into **intracellular fluid (ICF)** and **extracellular fluid (ECF)** (Fig. 9.1). ECF is composed of intravascular and interstitial fluid, and is readily assessed when evaluating fluid and electrolyte therapy. The goals of therapy are (1) to maintain an appropriate ECF volume, which is determined primarily by total-body sodium (Na), and (2) to maintain appropriate ICF and ECF osmolality, determined by the amount of TBW relative to solutes.

   B. **Perinatal changes in TBW.** In term infants, a physiologic diuresis of TBW and ECF occurs within 3 to 5 days after birth. This results in a weight loss of 5 to 10%. The diuresis may be desirable in preterm infants because excessive parenteral fluid and Na administration may increase risk of chronic lung disease (CLD), patent ductus arteriosis, and other diseases. At lower gestational ages, ECF accounts for a greater proportion of birth weight (see Fig. 9.1). Therefore, very-low-birth-weight (VLBW) infants must lose a greater percentage of birth weight (5 to 15%) during the first week of life to maintain ECF proportions equivalent to those of term infants.

   C. **Renal and hormonal maturation.** Renal function matures with increasing gestational age. Consequently, urinary water and electrolyte losses can vary greatly. Premature infants often manifest immature Na and water homeostasis. Contributing factors include (1) decreased glomerular filtration rate (GFR), (2) reduced maximal proximal and distal tubule Na reabsorption, (3) diminished renal capacity for concentration and dilution of urine, and (4) decreased bicarbonate reabsorption and potassium (K) and hydrogen ion secretion. Profoundly immature renal function often leads to water and electrolyte imbalance in extremely premature newborns (see Chaps. 6, 31).

   D. **Extrarenal sources of water and electrolyte loss.** Insensible water loss in VLBW infants can exceed 150 mL/kg per day because of radiant warmers, phototherapy, loss of skin integrity, or extreme prematurity (Table 9.1). Losses of other fluids such as cerebrospinal fluid (ventriculostomy drainage or repeated lumbar punctures), stool (diarrhea or ostomy drainage), and nasogastric tube or thoracostomy tube drainage should be quantitated, characterized, and replaced if significant.

II. **Assessment of fluid and electrolyte status**

   A. **History.** Newborn fluid and electrolyte status partially reflects maternal hydration and drug administration. Excessive use of oxytocin, diuretics, and hypotonic intravenous (IV) fluid can lead to maternal and fetal hyponatremia.

   B. **Physical examination**

      1. **Body weight.** Acute changes in TBW cause weight changes. Therefore, infants should be weighed at least daily. The distribution of water in body compartments reflects both total-body solute distribution and vascular permeability characteristics. Thus, acute changes in body weight may not reflect changes in intravascular volume. For example, neuromuscular paralysis or peritonitis can lead to weight gain and interstitial edema but decreased intravascular volume.

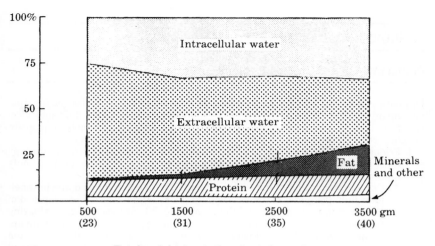

Fetal weight (gestational age in weeks)

FIG. 9.1. Body composition in relation to fetal weight and gestational age. (From Dweck H. S. *Clin Perinatol* 1975;2:183; data from Widdowson E. M. Growth and composition of the fetus and newborn. In Assali N. S. (Ed.). *Biology of Gestation,* Vol. 2. New York: Academic Press, 1968.)

2. **Skin.** ECF volume abnormalities can lead to altered skin turgor, altered anterior fontanelle tension, variations in mucous membranes, and edema. These findings are not sensitive indicators of fluid or electrolyte balance.
3. **Cardiovascular.** Tachycardia can result from ECF excess (e.g., heart failure) or hypovolemia. **Delayed capillary refill time** can signify reduced cardiac output, and **hepatomegaly** can suggest an increased ECF volume. **Blood pressure changes** occur late in the sequence of responses to reduced cardiac output.
C. **Laboratory evaluation**
  1. **Serum electrolytes and plasma osmolarity** reflect the composition and tonicity of ECF.
  2. **Urine electrolytes and specific gravity** can reflect renal capacity to concentrate or dilute urine and reabsorb or excrete Na. If the patient's hydration and ECF tonicity are normal, urine electrolytes do not correlate well with replacement needs. **Diuretic therapy** causes wide diurnal varia-

TABLE 9.1. INSENSIBLE WATER LOSS (IWL)*

Birth weight (g)	IWL (mL/kg/day)
750–1000	82
1001–1250	56
1251–1500	46
>1501	26

*Values represent mean IWL for infants in incubators during the first week of life. IWL is increased by phototherapy (up to 40%), radiant warmers (up to 50%), and fever. IWL is decreased by the use of humidified gas with respirators and heat shields in incubators [4,5,10,18].

tion in urine electrolyte composition and increased Na, K, calcium (Ca), and chloride (Cl) excretion.

3. **Urine output** falls with ECF depletion (dehydration), often to less than 1 mL/kg per hour. In neonates with immature renal function, urine output may not decrease despite ECF volume depletion.

4. **Fractional excretion of Na (FE-Na)** reflects the balance between glomerular filtration and tubular reabsorption of Na. FE-Na is determined after measuring Na and creatinine (Cr) concentrations in both urine and plasma:

$$\% \text{ filtered Na excreted} = \frac{\text{excreted Na}}{\text{filtered Na}} \times 100$$

$$= \frac{\text{urine Na} \times \text{plasma Cr}}{\text{urine Cr} \times \text{plasma Na}} \times 100$$

Newborns with FE-Na values less than 1% manifest oliguria due to prerenal factors reducing renal blood flow, such as hypovolemia or poor cardiac output. Values higher than 2.5% occur with acute renal failure (ARF) and in infants receiving diuretics. FE-Na is frequently higher than 2.5% in infants less than 32 weeks' gestation, irrespective of fluid and electrolyte status: FE-Na is less helpful in the evaluation of oliguria in these infants. Diuretic use in any infant will make the measurement meaningless.

5. **Blood urea nitrogen (BUN) and serum Cr** values provide indirect information about ECF volume and GFR. Values in the early postnatal period reflect placental clearance.

6. **Arterial pH, carbon dioxide tension (PCO_2), and Na bicarbonate** determinations can provide indirect evidence of intravascular volume depletion because poor tissue perfusion leads to high-anion-gap metabolic acidosis (lactic acidosis).

III. **Management of fluids and electrolytes.** The goal of early management is to allow initial ECF loss over the first 5 to 6 days as reflected by weight loss, while maintaining normal tonicity and intravascular volume as reflected by blood pressure, heart rate, urine output, serum electrolyte levels, and pH. Subsequent fluid management should maintain water and electrolyte balance, including requirements for body growth.

A. **The term infant.** Body weight decreases by 3 to 5% over the first 5 to 6 days. Subsequently, fluids should be adjusted so that changes in body weight are consistent with caloric intake. Clinical status should be monitored for maldistribution of water (e.g., edema). Na supplementation is not usually required in the first 24 hours unless ECF expansion is necessary. Small-for-gestational-age term infants may require early Na supplementation to maintain adequate ECF volume.

B. **The premature infant.** Allow a 5 to 15% weight loss over the first 5 to 6 days. Table 9.2 summarizes initial fluid therapy. Then, adjust fluids to maintain stable weight until an anabolic state is achieved and growth occurs. Frequently assess response to fluid and electrolyte therapy during the first 2 days of life. **Physical examination, urine output and specific gravity, and serum electrolyte determinations may initially be required as frequently as every 6 to 8 hours in infants less than 1000 g** (see VIII.A).

Water loss through skin and urine may exceed 200 mL/kg per day, which can represent up to **one-third of TBW.** IV Na supplementation is not required for the first 24 hours unless ECF volume loss exceeds 5% of body weight per day (see Chap. 6). If ECF volume expansion is necessary, **normal saline (NS) is preferred over 5% albumin solutions** in order to reduce risk of CLD.

TABLE 9.2. INITIAL FLUID THERAPY*

Birth weight (kg)	Dextrose (g/100 mL)	Fluid rate (mL/kg/d)		
		<24 h	24–48 h	>48 h
<1.0	5–10	100–150†	120–150	140–190
1.0–1.5	10	80–100	100–120	120–160
>1.5	10	60–80	80–120	120–160

*Infants in humidified incubators. Infants under radiant warmers usually require higher initial fluid rates.
†VLBW infants frequently require even higher initial rates of fluid administration, and frequent reassessment of serum electrolytes, urine output, and body weight.

IV. **Approach to disorders of Na and water balance.** Abnormalities can be grouped into disorders of **tonicity** or **ECF volume.** The conceptual approach to disorders of tonicity (e.g., hyponatremia) depends on whether the newborn exhibits normal ECF (euvolemia), ECF depletion (dehydration), or ECF excess (edema).
   A. **Isonatremic disorders**
      1. **Dehydration**
         a. **Predisposing factors** frequently involve equivalent losses of Na and water (via thoracostomy, nasogastric, or ventriculostomy drainage) or third-space losses that accompany peritonitis, gastroschisis, or omphalocele. Renal Na and water losses in the VLBW infant can lead to hypovolemia despite normal body tonicity.
         b. **Diagnosis.** Dehydration is usually manifested by weight loss, decreased urine output, and increased urine-specific gravity. However, infants fewer than 32 weeks' gestation may not demonstrate oliguria in response to hypovolemia. Poor skin turgor, tachycardia, hypotension, metabolic acidosis, and increasing BUN may coexist. A low FE-Na (<1%) is usually only seen in infants beyond 32 weeks' gestational age (see II.C.4).
         c. **Therapy. Administer Na and water** to first correct deficits and then adjust to equal maintenance needs plus ongoing losses. Acute isonatremic dehydration may require IV infusion of 10 mL/kg of NS if acute weight loss exceeds 10% of body weight with signs of poor cardiac output.
      2. **Edema**
         a. **Predisposing factors** include excessive isotonic fluid administration, heart failure, sepsis, and neuromuscular paralysis.
         b. **Diagnosis.** Clinical signs include periorbital and extremity edema, increased weight, and hepatomegaly.
         c. **Therapy** includes **Na restriction** (to decrease total-body Na) and water restriction (depending on electrolyte response).
   B. **Hyponatremic disorders** (Table 9.3). Consider **factitious hyponatremia** due to hyperlipidemia or **hyperosmolar hyponatremia** due to osmotic agents. True hyposmolar hyponatremia can then be evaluated.
      1. **Hyponatremia due to ECF volume depletion**
         a. **Predisposing factors** include diuretic use, osmotic diuresis (glycosuria), VLBW with renal water and Na wasting, adrenal or renal tubular salt-losing disorders, gastrointestinal losses (vomiting, diarrhea), and third-space losses of ECF (skin sloughing, early necrotizing enterocolitis [NEC]).
         b. **Diagnosis.** Decreased weight, poor skin turgor, tachycardia, rising blood urea nitrogen (BUN), and metabolic acidosis are frequently observed. If

TABLE 9.3. HYPONATREMIC DISORDERS

Clinical diagnosis	Etiology	Therapy
Factitious hyponatremia	Hyperlipidemia	
Hypertonic hyponatremia	Mannitol	
	Hyperglycemia	
ECF volume normal	SIADH	Restrict water intake
	Pain	
	Opiates	
	Excess intravenous fluids	
ECF volume deficit	Diuretics	Increase Na intake
	Late-onset hyponatremia of prematurity	
	Congenital adrenal hyperplasia	
	Severe glomerulotubular imbalance (immaturity)	
	Renal tubular acidosis	
	Gastrointestinal losses	
	Necrotizing enterocolitis (third-space loss)	
ECF volume excess	Heart failure	Restrict water intake
	Neuromuscular blockade (e.g., pancuronium)	
	Sepsis	

renal function is mature, the newborn may develop decreased urine output, increased urine-specific gravity, and a low FE-Na.

    c. Therapy. If possible, reduce ongoing Na loss. Administer Na and water to replace deficits and then adjust to match maintenance needs plus ongoing losses.

  2. Hyponatremia with normal ECF volume

    a. Predisposing factors include excess fluid administration and the syndrome of inappropriate antidiuretic hormone secretion (SIADH). Factors that cause SIADH include pain, opiate administration, intraventricular hemorrhage (IVH), asphyxia, meningitis, pneumothorax, and positive-pressure ventilation.

    b. Diagnosis of SIADH. Weight gain usually develops without edema. Excessive fluid administration without SIADH results in low urine-specific gravity and high urine output. In contrast, SIADH leads to **decreased urine output** and **increased urine osmolarity.** Urinary Na excretion in infants with SIADH varies widely and reflects Na intake. The diagnosis of SIADH presumes no volume-related stimulus to antidiuretic hormone (ADH) release, such as reduced cardiac output or abnormal renal, adrenal, or thyroid function.

    c. Therapy. Water restriction is therapeutic unless (1) serum Na concentration is less than approximately 120 mEq/L or (2) neurologic signs such as obtundation or seizure activity develop. In these instances, **furosemide** 1 mg/kg IV q6h can be initiated while replacing urinary Na excretion with **hypertonic NaCl (3%) (1 to 3 mL/kg initial dose).** This strategy leads to loss of free water with no net change in total-body Na. Fluid restriction alone can be utilized once serum Na concentration exceeds 120 mEq/L and neurologic signs abate.

  3. Hyponatremia due to ECF volume excess

    a. Predisposing factors include sepsis with decreased cardiac output, late NEC, heart failure, abnormal lymphatic drainage, and neuromuscular paralysis. Weight increase with edema is observed. Decreasing urine output, increasing BUN and urine-specific gravity, and a low FE-Na are often present in infants with mature renal function.

    b. Diagnosis. Weight increase with edema is observed. Decreasing urine output, increasing BUN and urine-specific gravity, and a low FE-Na are often present in infants with mature renal function.

    c. Therapy. Treat the underlying disorder and **restrict water** to alleviate hypotonicity. Na restriction and improving cardiac output may be beneficial.

C. Hypernatremic disorders

  1. Hypernatremia with normal or deficient ECF volume

    a. Predisposing factors include increased renal and insensible water loss in VLBW infants. Skin sloughing can accelerate water loss. ADH deficiency secondary to IVH can occasionally exacerbate renal water loss.

    b. Diagnosis. Weight loss, tachycardia and hypotension, metabolic acidosis, decreasing urine output and increasing urine-specific gravity may occur. Urine may be dilute if the newborn exhibits central or nephrogenic diabetes insipidus.

    c. Therapy. Increase **free water administration** to reduce serum Na no faster than 1 mEq/kg per hour. If signs of ECF depletion or excess develop, adjust Na intake. **Hypernatremia does not necessarily imply excess total-body Na.** For example, **hypernatremia in the VLBW infant in the first 24 hours of life is almost always due to free-water deficits** (see VIII.A.1).

  2. Hypernatremia with ECF volume excess

    a. Predisposing factors include excessive isotonic or hypertonic fluid administration, especially in the face of reduced cardiac output.

    b. Diagnosis. Weight gain associated with edema is observed. The infant may exhibit normal heart rate, blood pressure, and urine output and specific gravity, but an elevated FE-Na.

    c. Therapy. Restrict Na administration.

V. Oliguria exists if urine flow is less than 1 mL/kg per hour. Although delayed micturition in a healthy infant is not of concern until 24 hours after birth, urine output in a critically ill infant should be assessed by 8 to 12 hours of life, using urethral catheterization if indicated. Diminished urine output may reflect abnormal prerenal, renal parenchymal, or postrenal factors (Table 9.4). The most common causes of neonatal acute renal failure are asphyxia, sepsis, and severe respiratory illness. It is important to exclude other potentially treatable etiologies. (See Chap. 31.) Oliguria in VLBW infants may be normal in the first 24 hours of life (see VIII.A.1).

A. History and physical examination. Screen the maternal and infant history for maternal diabetes (renal vein thrombosis), birth asphyxia (acute tubular necrosis), and oligohydramnios (Potter's syndrome). Force of the infant's urinary stream (posterior urethral valves), rate and nature of fluid administration and urine output, and nephrotoxic drug use (aminoglycosides, indomethacin, furosemide) should be evaluated. **Physical examination** should determine blood pressure and ECF volume status; evidence of cardiac disease, abdominal masses, or ascites; and the presence of any congenital anomalies associated with renal abnormalities (e.g., Potter's syndrome, epispadias).

TABLE 9.4. ETIOLOGIES OF OLIGURIA

Prerenal	Renal parenchymal	Postrenal
Decreased inotropy	Acute tubular necrosis Ischemia (hypoxia, hypo- volemia)	Posterior urethral valves
Decreased preload	Disseminated intravascular coagulation Renal artery or vein thrombosis	Neuropathic bladder
Increased peripheral resistance	Nephrotoxin Congenital malformation Polycystic disease Agenesis Dysplasia	Prune-belly syndrome Uric acid nephropathy

B. **Diagnosis**
   1. **Initial laboratory examination** should include urinalysis, BUN, Cr, and FE-Na determinations. These aid in diagnosis and provide baseline values for further management.
   2. **Fluid challenge,** consisting of a total of 20 mL/kg of normal saline, is administered as two infusions at 10 mL/kg per hour if no suspicion of structural heart disease or heart failure exists. Decreased cardiac output not responsive to ECF expansion may require the institution of inotropic/chronotropic pressor agents. Dopamine at a dose of 1 to 5 µg/kg per minute may increase renal blood flow and a dose of 2 to 15 µg/kg per minute may increase total cardiac output. These effects may augment GFR and urine output. (See Chap. 17.)
   3. **If no response to fluid challenge occurs,** one may induce diuresis with **furosemide** 2 mg/kg IV.
   4. Patients who are unresponsive to increased cardiac output and diuresis should be evaluated with an **abdominal ultrasound** to define renal, urethral, and bladder anatomy. IV pyelography, renal scanning, angiography, or cystourethrography may be required (see Chap. 31).
C. **Management. Prerenal** oliguria should respond to increased cardiac output. **Postrenal** obstruction requires urologic consultation, with possible urinary diversion and surgical correction. If parenchymal **ARF** is suspected, minimize excessive ECF expansion and electrolyte abnormalities. If possible, eliminate reversible causes of declining GFR, such as nephrotoxic drug use.
   1. **Monitor** daily weight, input and output, and BUN, Cr, and serum electrolytes.
   2. **Fluid restriction.** Replace insensible fluid loss plus urine output. **Withhold K supplementation** unless hypokalemia develops. Replace urinary Na losses unless edema develops.
   3. **Adjust dosage and frequency of drugs** eliminated by renal excretion. Monitor serum drug concentrations to guide drug-dosing intervals.
   4. **Peritoneal or hemodialysis** may be indicated in patients whose GFR progressively declines causing complications related to ECF volume or electrolyte abnormalities (see Chap. 31).
VI. **Metabolic acid–base disorders**
A. **Normal acid–base physiology.** Metabolic acidosis results from excessive loss of buffer or from an increase of volatile or nonvolatile acid in the extracellular space. Normal sources of acid production include the metabolism of amino acids containing sulfur and phosphate, as well as hydrogen ion re-

leased from bone mineralization. Intravascular buffers include bicarbonate, phosphate, and intracellular hemoglobin. Maintenance of normal pH depends on excretion of volatile acid (e.g., carbonic acid) from the lungs, skeletal exchange of cations for hydrogen, and renal regeneration and reclamation of bicarbonate. Kidneys contribute to maintenance of acid–base balance by reabsorbing the filtered load of bicarbonate, secreting hydrogen ions as titratable acidity (e.g., H_2PO_4), and excreting ammonium ions.

B. Metabolic acidosis (see Chap. 29, Inborn Errors of Metabolism)

    1. Anion gap. Metabolic acidosis can result from accumulation of acid or loss of buffering equivalents. Anion gap determination will suggest mechanism. Na, Cl, and bicarbonate are the primary ions of the extracellular space and exist in approximately electroneutral balance. The **anion gap,** calculated as the difference between the Na concentration and sum of the Cl and bicarbonate concentrations, reflects the unaccounted-for anion composition of the ECF. An increased anion gap indicates an accumulation of organic acid whereas a normal anion gap indicates a loss of buffer equivalents. Normal values for the neonatal anion gap are 5 to 15 mEq/L and vary directly with serum albumin concentration.

    2. Metabolic acidosis associated with an increased anion gap (>15 mEq/L). Disorders (Table 9.5) include renal failure, inborn errors of metabolism, lactic acidosis, late metabolic acidosis, and toxin exposure. Lactic acidosis results from diminished tissue perfusion and resultant anaerobic metabolism in infants with asphyxia or severe cardiorespiratory disease. Late metabolic acidosis typically occurs during the second or third week of life in premature infants who ingest high casein-containing formulas. Metabolism of sulfur-containing amino acids in casein and increased hydrogen ion release due to the rapid mineralization of bone cause an increased acid load. Subsequently, inadequate hydrogen ion excretion by the premature kidney results in acidosis.

    3. Metabolic acidosis associated with a normal anion gap (<15 mEq/L) results from buffer loss through the renal or gastrointestinal systems (see Table 9.5). Premature infants less than 32 weeks' gestation frequently manifest a proximal or distal renal tubular acidosis (RTA). Urine pH persistently higher than 7.0 in an infant with metabolic acidosis suggests a distal RTA. Urinary pH less than 5.0 documents normal distal-tubule hydrogen ion secretion but proximal tubular bicarbonate resorption could

TABLE 9.5. METABOLIC ACIDOSIS

Increased anion gap (>15 mEq/L)	Normal anion gap (<15 mEq/L)
Acute renal failure	Renal bicarbonate loss
Inborn errors of metabolism	Renal tubular acidosis
Lactic acidosis	Acetazolamide
Late metabolic acidosis	Renal dysplasia
Toxins (e.g., benzyl alcohol)	Gastrointestinal bicarbonate loss
	Diarrhea
	Cholestyramine
	Small-bowel drainage
	Dilutional acidosis
	Hyperalimentation acidosis

still be inadequate (proximal RTA). IV Na bicarbonate infusion in infants with proximal RTA will result in a urinary pH higher than 7.0 prior to attaining a normal serum bicarbonate concentration (22 to 24 mEq/L).

4. **Therapy.** Whenever possible, **treat the underlying cause.** Lactic acidosis due to low cardiac output or to decreased peripheral oxygen delivery should be treated with specific measures. The use of a low-casein formula may alleviate late metabolic acidosis. Treat normal-anion-gap metabolic acidosis by decreasing the rate of bicarbonate loss (e.g., decreased small-bowel drainage) or providing buffer equivalents. **IV Na bicarbonate or Na acetate** (which is compatible with Ca salts) is most commonly used to treat arterial pH less than 7.25. Oral buffer supplements can include Bicitra or Na citrate (1 to 3mE/kg per day). Estimate bicarbonate deficit from the following formula:

$$\text{Deficit} = 0.4 \times \text{body weight} \times (\text{desired bicarbonate} - \text{actual bicarbonate})$$

The premature infant's acid–base status can change rapidly, and frequent monitoring is warranted. The infant's ability to tolerate an increased Na load and to metabolize acetate is an important variable that influences acid–base status during treatment.

C. **Metabolic alkalosis.** The etiology of metabolic alkalosis can be clarified by determining urinary Cl concentration. Alkalosis accompanied by ECF depletion is associated with decreased urinary Cl, whereas states of mineralocorticoid excess are usually associated with increased urinary Cl (Table 9.6). Treat the underlying disorder.

VII. **Disorders of K balance.** K is the fundamental intracellular cation. Serum K concentrations do not necessarily reflect total-body K because extracellular and intracellular K distribution also depends on the pH of body compartments. **An increase of 0.1 pH unit in serum results in approximately a 0.6 mEq/L fall in serum K concentration due to an intracellular shift of K ions.** Total-body K is regulated by balancing K intake (normally 1 to 2 mEq/kg per day) and excretion through urine and the gastrointestinal tract.

A. **Hypokalemia** can lead to arrhythmias, ileus, renal concentrating defects, and obtundation in the newborn.

1. **Predisposing factors** include nasogastric or ileostomy drainage, chronic diuretic use, and renal tubular defects.

2. **Diagnosis.** Obtain serum and urine electrolytes, pH, and an ECG to detect possible conduction defects (prolonged QT interval and U waves).

3. **Therapy.** Reduce renal or gastrointestinal losses of K. Gradually increase K intake as needed.

TABLE 9.6. METABOLIC ALKALOSIS

Low urinary Cl (<10 mEq/L)	High urinary Cl (>20 mEq/L)
Diuretic therapy (late)	Barter's syndrome with mineralocorticoid excess
Acute correction of chronically compensated respiratory acidosis	Alkali administration
Nasogastric suction	Massive blood product transfusion
Vomiting	Diuretic therapy (early)
Secretory diarrhea	Hypokalemia

B. Hyperkalemia. The normal serum K level in a nonhemolyzed blood specimen at normal pH is 3.5 to 5.5 mEq/L; symptomatic hyperkalemia may begin at a serum K level higher than 6 mEq/L.

1. **Predisposing factors.** Hyperkalemia can occur unexpectedly in any patient but should be **anticipated** and **screened** for in the following scenarios:

   a. Increased K release secondary to tissue destruction, trauma, cephalhematoma, hypothermia, bleeding, intravascular or extravascular hemolysis, asphyxia/ischemia, and IVH.

   b. Decreased K clearance due to renal failure, oliguria, hyponatremia, and congenital adrenal hyperplasia.

   c. Miscellaneous associations including dehydration, birth weight lower than 1500 g (see VIII.A.2), blood transfusion, inadvertent excess (KCl) administration, CLD with KCl supplementation, and exchange transfusion.

   d. Up to 50% of VLBW infants born before 25 weeks' gestation manifest serum K levels higher than 6 mEq/L in the first 48 hours of life (see VIII.A.2). **The most common cause of sudden unexpected hyperkalemia in the neonatal intensive care unit (NICU) is medication error.**

2. **Diagnosis.** Obtain serum and urine electrolytes, serum pH, and Ca concentrations. The hyperkalemic infant may be asymptomatic or may present with a spectrum of signs including bradyarrhythmias or tachyarrhythmias, cardiovascular instability or collapse. The ECG findings progress with increasing serum K from peaked T waves (increased rate of repolarization), flattened P waves and increasing PR interval (suppression of atrial conductivity), to QRS widening and slurring (conduction delay in ventricular conduction tissue as well as in the myocardium itself), and finally supraventricular/ventricular tachycardia, bradycardia, or ventricular fibrillation. The ECG findings may be the first indication of hyperkalemia (see Chap. 25).

   Once hyperkalemia is diagnosed, **remove all sources of exogenous K (change all IV solutions and analyze for K content, check all feedings for K content), rehydrate the patient if necessary, and eliminate arrhythmia-promoting factors.** The pharmacologic therapy of neonatal hyperkalemia consists of three components:

   a. **Goal 1: Stabilization of conducting tissues.** This can be accomplished by Na or Ca ion administration. **Ca gluconate (10%) given carefully at 1 to 2 mL/kg IV (over 0.5 to 1 hour)** may be the most useful in the NICU. Treatment with hypertonic NaCl solution is not done routinely. However, if the patient is both hyperkalemic and hyponatremic, NS infusion may be beneficial. Use of antiarrhythmic agents such as lidocaine and bretylium should be considered for refractory ventricular tachycardia. (See Chap. 25.)

   b. **Goal 2: Dilution and intracellular shifting of K.** Increased serum K in the setting of dehydration should respond to fluid resuscitation. Alkalemia will promote intracellular K-for-hydrogen-ion exchange. **Na bicarbonate 1 to 2 mEq/kg per hour IV** may be used, although the resultant pH change may not be sufficient to markedly shift K ions. Na treatment as described in 1 may be effective. **In order to reduce risk of IVH, avoid rapid Na bicarbonate administration, especially in infants born before 34 weeks' gestation and younger than 3 days.** Respiratory alkalosis may be produced in an intubated infant by hyperventilation, although the risk of hypocarbia-diminishing cerebral perfusion may make this option more suited to emergency situations. Theoretically, every 0.1 pH unit increase leads to a decrease of 0.6 mEq/L in serum K.

   Insulin enhances intracellular K uptake by direct stimulation of the membrane-bound Na-K ATPase. Insulin infusion with concomitant glucose administration to maintain normal blood glucose concentration is relatively safe as long as serum or blood glucose levels are frequently monitored. **This therapy may begin with a bolus of insulin and glucose (0.05 unit/kg of human regular insulin with 2 mL/kg of dextrose 10% in water [D10W]) followed by continuous infusion of D10W at 2 to 4 mL/kg per hour and human regular insulin (10 units/ 100 mL) at 1 mL/kg per hour.** To minimize the effect of binding to IV tubing, insulin diluted in D10W may be flushed through the tubing. Adjustments in infusion rate of either glucose or insulin in response to hyperglycemia or hypoglycemia may be simplified if the two solutions are prepared individually (see Chap. 29).

Beta-2-adrenergic stimulation enhances K uptake, probably via stimulation of the Na-K ATPase. The immaturity of the beta-receptor response in preterm infants may contribute to nonoliguric hyperkalemia in these patients (see VIII.A.2). To date, beta stimulation is not primary therapy for hyperkalemia in the pediatric population. However, if cardiac dysfunction and hypotension are present, use of dopamine or other adrenergic agents could, through beta-2 stimulation, lower serum K.

   c. Goal 3: Enhanced K excretion. Diuretic therapy (e.g., **furosemide 1 mg/kg IV**) may increase K excretion by increasing flow and Na delivery to the distal tubules. In the clinical setting of inadequate urine output and reversible renal disease (e.g., indomethacin-induced oliguria), **peritoneal dialysis** and **double volume exchange transfusion** are potentially lifesaving options. Peritoneal dialysis can be succcessful in infants weighing less than 1000 g and should be considered if the patient's clinical status and etiology of hyperkalemia suggest a reasonable chance for good long-term outcome. **Use fresh whole blood (<24 hours old) or deglycerolized red blood cells reconstituted with fresh-frozen plasma for double volume exchange transfusion.** Aged, banked blood may have K levels as high as 10 to 12 mEq/L; aged, washed packed red blood cells will have low K levels (see Chap. 26).

Enhanced K excretion using cation exchange resins such as Na or Ca polystyrene sulfonate has been studied primarily in adults. The resins can be administered orally per gavage (PG) or rectally. A study involving uremic and control rats demonstrated that Na polystyrene sulfonate (Kayexelate) administered by rectum with sorbitol was toxic to the colon, but rectal administration after suspension in distilled water produced only mild mucosal erythema in 10% of animals. Another possible complication of resins is bowel obstruction secondary to bezoar or plug formation.

The reported experience with resin use in neonates covers those born at 25 to 40 weeks' gestation. **PG administration of Kayexelate is not recommended in preterm infants because they are prone to hypomotility and are at risk for NEC. Rectal administration of Kayexelate (1 g/kg at 0.5 g/mL of NS) with a minimum retention time of 30 minutes should be effective in lowering serum K levels by approximately 1 mEq/L. The enema should be inserted 1–3 cm using a thin Silastic feeding tube.** Published evidence supports the efficacy of this treatment in infants. Kayexelate prepared in water or NS (eliminating sorbitol as a solubilizing agent) and delivered rectally should be a therapeutic agent with an acceptable risk-benefit ratio.

The clinical condition, ECG, and actual serum K level all affect the choice of therapy for hyperkalemia. Figure 9.2 contains guidelines for treatment of hyperkalemia.

VIII. Common clinical situations
   A. VLBW infant
      1. VLBW infants undergo three phases of fluid and electrolyte homeostasis: prediuretic (first day of life), diuretic (second to third day of life), and postdiuretic (fourth to fifth day of life). Marked diuresis and natriuresis can occur

Remove all sources of exogenous potassium.

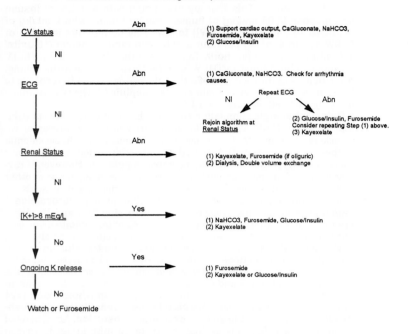

In general, if [K+] acceptable for 6 hours cease therapy but continue monitoring.

Drug doses:

CaGluconate	1-2ml/kg IV	
NaHCO3	1-2 mEq/kg IV	
Furosemide	1 mg/kg IV	
Glucose/Insulin	Bolus:	D10W 2ml/kg
		Humulin 0.05 U/kg
	Infusion:	D10W 2-4 ml/kg/hr
		Humulin, 10 U/100 ml D10W or 5% Albumin, 1 ml/kg/hr
Kayexelate	1 gm/kg PR, used cautiously in the setting of an immature ischemic GI tract	

FIG. 9.2. Treatment of hyperkalemia (CV = cardiovascular; Nl = normal; Abn = abnormal). For a given algorithm outcome proceed by administering the entire set of treatments labeled (1). If unsuccessful in lowering [K+] or improving clinical condition, proceed to the next set of treatments, e.g., (2) then (3).

during the diuretic phase leading to **hypernatremia** and the need for frequent serum electrolyte determinations (q6 to 8h) and increased rates of parenteral fluid administration. Increased free water loss through skin and dopamine-associated natriuresis (due to increased GFR) can further complicate management. Hypernatremia often occurs despite a total body Na deficit. Lack of a brisk diuretic phase has been associated with increased CLD incidence.

In addition, **impaired glucose tolerance** can lead to hyperglycemia, requiring reduced rates of parenteral glucose infusion (see Chap. 29, Hypoglycemia and Hyperglycemia). This combination frequently leads to administration of reduced dextrose concentrations (below 5%) in parenteral solutions. Avoid the infusion of parenteral solutions containing less than

200 mOsmol/L (i.e., D3W), to minimize local osmotic hemolysis and thus reduce renal K load.

2. **VLBW infants often develop a nonoliguric hyperkalemia** in the first few days of life. This is caused by a relatively low glomerular filtration rate (GFR) combined with an intracellular to extracellular K shift due to decreased Na, K ATPase activity. Postnatal glucocorticoid use may further inhibit Na, K ATPase activity. Insulin infusion to treat hyperkalemia may be necessary but elevates the risk of iatrogenic hypoglycemia. Treatment with Kayexelate (see VII.B.2.c) can occasionally be beneficial in infants born before 32 weeks' gestation despite the obligate Na load and potential irritation of bowel mucosa by rectal administration. Na restriction can reduce the risk of CLD.

3. **Late-onset hyponatremia of prematurity** often occurs 6 to 8 weeks postnatally in the growing premature infant. Failure of the immature renal tubules to reabsorb filtered Na in a rapidly growing infant often causes this condition. Other contributing factors include the low Na content in breastmilk and diuretic therapy for CLD. Infants at risk should be monitored with periodic electrolytes measurements and if affected, treated with simple Na supplementation (start with 2 mEq/kg per day).

B. **Severe Chronic Lung Disease (CLD)** (see Chap. 24, Chronic Lung Disease). CLD requiring **diuretic** therapy often leads to **hypokalemic, hypochloremic metabolic alkalosis.** Affected infants frequently have a chronic respiratory acidosis with partial metabolic compensation. Subsequently, vigorous diuresis can lead to total-body K and ECF volume depletion, causing a superimposed metabolic alkalosis. If the alkalosis is severe, alkalemia (pH >7.45) can supervene and result in central hypoventilation. If possible, gradually reduce urinary Na and K loss by reducing the diuretic dose, and/or increase K intake by administration of KCl (starting at 1 mEq/kg per day). Rarely, administration of ammonium chloride (0.5 mEq/kg) is required to treat the metabolic alkalosis. Long-term use of loop diuretics such as furosemide promotes excessive urinary Ca losses and nephrocalcinosis. Urinary Ca losses may be reduced through concomitant thiazide diuretic therapy (see Chap. 24).

Suggested Readings

Anand S. K. Acute renal failure in the neonate. *Pediatr Clin North Am* 1982;29:791.

Baumgart S, et al. Water and electrolyte metabolism of the micropremie. *Clin Perinatol* 2000;27(1):131.

Bell E. F., et al. Effect of fluid administration on the development of symptomatic patent ductus arteriosus and congestive heart failure in premature infants. *N Engl J Med* 1980;302:598.

Bell E. F., et al. Heat balance in premature infants: Comparative effects of convectively heated incubator and radiant warmer, with or without plastic heat shield. *J Pediatr* 1980;96:460.

Bell E. F., et al. The effects of thermal environment on heat balance and insensible water loss in low-birth-weight infants. *J Pediatr* 1980;96:452.

Brown E. R., et al. Bronchopulmonary dysplasia: Possible relationship to pulmonary edema. *J Pediatr* 1978;92:982.

Celsi G, et al. Sensitive periods for glucocorticoids' regulation of Na+,K(+)-ATPase mRNA in the developing lung and kidney. *Pediatr Res* 1993;33(1):5.

Cheek D. B., et al. Further observations on the corrected bromide space of the neonate and investigation of water and electrolyte status in infants born of diabetic mothers. *Pediatrics* 1961;28:861.

Costarino A. T., Jr., et al. Sodium restriction versus daily maintenance replacement in very low birth weight premature neonates: A randomized, blind therapeutic trial. *J Pediatr* 1992;120:99.

Fanaroff A. A., et al. Insensible water loss in low birth weight infants. *Pediatrics* 1972;50:236.

Fink C. W., et al. The corrected bromide space (extracellar volume) in the newborn. *Pediatrics* 1960;26:397.

Fisher D. A., et al. Control of water balance in the newborn. *Am J Dis Child* 1963;106:137.

Gruskay J., et al. Nonoliguric hyperkalemia in the premature infant weighing less than 1000 grams. *J Pediatr* 1988;113:381.

Leake R. D. Perinatal nephrobiology: A developmental perspective. *Clin Perinatol* 1977;4:321.

Lorenz J. M., et al. Water balance in very low-birth-weight infants: Relationship to water and sodium intake and effect on outcome. *J Pediatr* 1982;101:423.

Lorenz J. M., et al. Phases of fluid and electrolyte homeostasis in the extremely low birth weight infant. *Pediatrics* 1995;96(3 Pt 1):484.

Norman M. E., et al. A prospective study of acute renal failure in the newborn infant. *Pediatrics* 1979;63:475.

Okken A., et al. Insensible water loss and metabolic rate in low birth weight newborn infants. *Pediatr Res* 1979;13:1072.

Rahman N., et al. Renal failure in the perinatal period. *Clin Perinatol* 1981;8:241.

Shaffer S. G., et al. Hyperkalemia in very low birth weight infants. *J Pediatr* 1992;121:275.

Skorecki K. L., et al. Body fluid homeostasis in man. A contemporary overview. *Am J Med* 1981;70:77.

Stefano J. L., et al. Nitrogen balance in extremely low birth weight infants with nonoliguric hyperkalemia. *J Pediatr* 1993;123:632.

Stevenson J. G. Fluid administration in the association of patent ductus arteriosus complicating respiratory distress syndrome. *J Pediatr* 1977;90:257.

Wu P. Y. K., et al. Insensible water loss in pre-term infants: Changes with postnatal development and non-ionizing radiant energy. *Pediatrics* 1974;54:704.

10. NUTRITION

Deirdre Ellard, Irene E. Olsen, and Yao Sun

Following birth, term infants rapidly adapt from a relatively constant intrauterine supply of nutrients to intermittent feedings of milk. Preterm infants, however, are at increased risk of potential nutritional compromise. These infants are born with limited nutrient reserves, immature pathways for absorption and metabolism, and increased nutrient demands. In addition, medical and surgical conditions commonly associated with prematurity frequently alter nutrient requirements and complicate adequate nutrient delivery. As mortality rates for these high-risk newborns continue to improve, optimizing nutritional care, beginning in the immediate postnatal period, has become an important topic of clinical research. Current investigations suggest that earlier, more aggressive nutrition intervention is desirable.

I. **Growth**
   A. Fetal body composition changes throughout gestation, with accretion of most nutrients occurring primarily in the late second and throughout the third trimester. Term infants will normally have sufficient glycogen and fat stores to meet energy requirements during the relative starvation of the first days of life. In contrast, preterm infants will rapidly deplete their limited nutrient reserves, becoming both hypoglycemic and catabolic unless appropriate nutritional therapy is provided. In practice, it is generally assumed that the severity of nutrient insufficiency is inversely related to gestational age at birth and birth weight.
   B. Postnatal growth varies from intrauterine growth in that it begins with a period of weight loss, primarily through the loss of extracellular fluid. The typical loss of 5 to 10% of birth weight for a full-term infant may increase to as much as 15% of birth weight in infants born preterm. The nadir in weight loss usually occurs by 4 to 6 days of life, with birth weight being regained by 14 to 21 days of life in most preterm infants. Currently, there is no widely accepted measure of neonatal growth that captures both the weight loss and subsequent gain characteristic of this period. Our goals are to limit the degree and duration of initial weight loss in preterm infants and to facilitate regain of birth weight within 7 to 14 days of life.
   C. After achieving birth weight, intrauterine growth and nutrient accretion rate data are widely accepted as reference standards for assessing growth and nutrient requirements. We use goals of: 10 to 20 g/kg per day weight gain (15 to 20 g/kg per day for infants ≤1500 g), ~1 cm/week in length, and 0.5 to 1.0 cm/week in head circumference. Although these goals are not initially attainable in most preterm infants, replicating growth of the fetus at the same gestational age remains an appropriate goal as recommended by the American Academy of Pediatrics.
   D. Along with monitoring rates of growth, serial measurements of weight, head circumference, and length plotted on growth curves provide valuable information in the nutritional assessment of the preterm infant. Available intrauterine growth curves are criticized for limited sample sizes, lack of racial diversity, and being out-of-date. However, until more contemporary curves are available, we use the Lubchenco intrauterine growth curves (1966) (Fig. 10.1) because these are based on a reasonably sized sample, provide curves to monitor weight, length and head circumference, and are easy to use and interpret.
      A number of other growth curves are also available, but we do not recommend their use in the neonatal intensive care unit (NICU). Postnatal growth curves follow the same infants over time (i.e. longitudinal growth curves), and

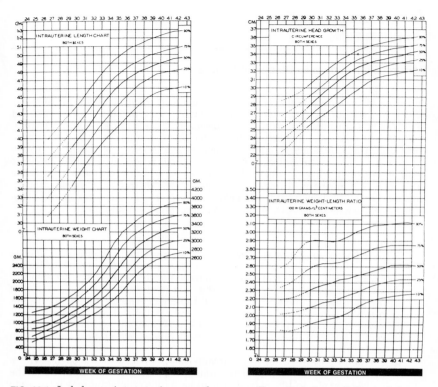

FIG. 10.1. Lubchenco intrauterine growth curves. (From Lubchenco L.O. et al. Intrauterine growth in length and head circumference as estimated from live births at gestational ages from 26 to 42 weeks. *Pediatrics* 1966;37:403.)

are available from a number of single-NICU studies and more recently from the National Institute for Child Health and Human Development (NICHD) multi-center study (2000). The problem with these curves, however, is that they show *actual*, not ideal growth. Although these curves provide interesting information by allowing comparison of the growth of infants in one NICU to those in another, they do not indicate if either group of infants is growing adequately. Intrauterine growth remains the gold standard for comparison.

E. When an infant is full-term-corrected gestational age, the monitoring of growth should take place on the 2000 Centers for Disease Control (CDC) United States Growth Charts (formerly, the National Center for Health Statistics, NCHS, growth curves). Alternative growths curves, based on a sample of low-birth-weight infants (1501 to 2500 g at birth) and very-low-birth-weight infants (<1500 g at birth), are also available for this age group. However, these curves are subject to the same criticisms as the postnatal growth curves. We do not recommend their use in former preterm infants, because these infants should still be striving to grow at the rate of their average peers.

II. Nutrient Recommendations

A. Sources for nutrient recommendations for preterm infants include the American Academy of Pediatrics Committee on Nutrition (AAP-CON), the European Society of Paediatric Gastroenterology and Nutrition Committee on Nutrition (ESPGAN-CON), and the consensus recommendations published by Tsang and colleagues (Table 10.1). These recommendations are based on: (1) intrauterine accretion rate data, (2) the nutrient content of human milk, (3) the assumed decreased nutrient stores and higher nutritional needs in preterm infants, and (4) the available data on biochemical measures reflecting adequate intake. However, due to the limitations of the currently available data, the goals for nutrient intake for preterm infants are considered to be recommendations only.

B. **Fluid** (see Chap. 9, Fluid and Electrolyte Management). The initial step in nutritional support is to determine an infant's fluid requirement, which is dependent on gestational age, postnatal age, and environmental conditions. Generally, baseline fluid needs are inversely related to gestational age at birth and birth weight. During the first week of life, very-low-birth-weight (VLBW) infants are known to experience increased water loss because of the immaturity of their skin, which has a higher water content and increased permeability, and the immaturity of their renal function with a decreased ability to concentrate urine. Environmental factors, such as radiant warmers, phototherapy, and low humidity, also increase insensible losses and raise fluid requirements. Conversely, restriction of fluid intake may be necessary to assist with the prevention and/or treatment of patent ductus arteriosus, renal insufficiency, and chronic lung disease. Fluid requirements in the first weeks of life are, therefore, continually reassessed, as the transition is made from fetal to neonatal life, and at least daily afterward.

C. **Energy**. Estimates suggest that preterm infants in a thermoneutral environment require approximately 40 to 60 kcal/kg per day for maintenance of body weight, assuming adequate protein is provided. Additional calories are needed for growth, with the smallest neonates tending to demonstrate the greatest need, as their rate of growth is highest (Table 10.2). In practice, we generally strive for energy intakes of 120 to 160 kcal/kg per day. Lesser intakes (90 to 120 kcal/kg per day) may sustain intrauterine growth rates, if energy expenditure is minimal or if parenteral nutrition is used.

III. **Parenteral Nutrition (PN)**

A. **Nutrient Goals.** Historically, the initiation of nutrition support was withheld for the first weeks of life. This practice has changed as research suggests that earlier nutrition intervention is desirable. Our initial goal for PN is to provide sufficient calories and amino acids to prevent negative energy and nitrogen balance. Goals thereafter include the promotion of appropriate weight gain and growth, while awaiting the attainment of adequate enteral intake.

B. **Indications for Initiating PN**
   1. Infants with a birth weight $\leq$ 1500 g. For those infants weighing >1000 g, this is often done in conjunction with slowly advancing enteral nutrition.
   2. Infants with a birth weight of 1501 to 1800 g for whom significant enteral intake is not expected for > 3 days.
   3. Infants with a birth weight >1800 g for whom significant enteral intake is not expected for > 5 days.

C. **Peripheral versus Central PN**
   1. Parenteral solutions may be infused via peripheral veins or a central vein, usually the superior or inferior vena cava. The AAP recommends that peripheral solutions maintain an osmolarity between 300 and 900 mOsm/L. Because of this limitation, peripheral solutions often cannot adequately support growth in extremely low-birth-weight infants. Central PN allows for the use of more hypertonic solutions but also incurs greater risks, particularly catheter-related sepsis.
   2. We consider central PN to be warranted under the following conditions:
      a. Nutritional needs exceed the capabilities of peripheral PN.
      b. An extended period (e.g., >7 days) of inability to take enteral feedings, such as in infants with necrotizing enterocolitis and in some postoperative infants.
      c. Imminent lack of peripheral venous access.

TABLE 10.1. COMPARISON OF ENTERAL INTAKE RECOMMENDATIONS OF THE PREMATURE INFANT PER KILOGRAM PER DAY*

Nutrient	Unit	Tsang et al. [3]	AAP-CON[1]†	ESPGAN-CON [2]†	24 kcal/oz Similac Special Care Advance w/Iron	24 kcal/oz Enfamil Premature LIPIL w/Iron	Mature‖ Human Milk	Mature Human Milk plus (4 packets Enfamil LIPIL HMF/dL)	Mature Human Milk plus (4 packets Similac Advance HMF/dL)
Protein	g/kg/day		3.5–4.0	2.7–3.7	3.3	3.6	1.6	3.3	3.1
Infants < 1000 g	g/kg/day	3.6–3.8							
Infants > 1000 g	g/kg/day	3.0–3.6							
Carbohydrate	g/kg/day		10.8–15.6	8.4–16.8	12.9	13.2	10.7	11	13.4
Fat	g/kg/day		5.4–7.2	4.3–8.4	6.6	6.1	5.9	7.5	6.3
Vitamin A	IU/kg/day	700–1500	90–270	324–540	1522	1500	338	1778	1331
Vitamin D	IU/day	150–400§‡	500§/day	800–1600/day§	183	288	3.1	231	197
Vitamin E	IU/kg/day	6–12	>1.3	0.72–12	4.9	7.6	0.6	7.5	5.8
Vitamin K	µg/kg/day	8–10	4.8	4.8–18.0	15	9.6	0.3	6.9	14
Ascorbate (vit C)	mg/kg/day	18–24	42	8.4–48.0	45	24	6.1	24	46.4
Thiamine	µg/kg/day	180–240	>48	24–300	304	240	32	259.5	408
Riboflavin	µg/kg/day	250–360	>72	72–720	755	360	52	382	725
Pyridoxine	µg/kg/day	150–210	>42	42–300	304	180	30.6	204	371
Niacin	mg/kg/day	3.6–4.8	>0.3	1–6	6	4.8	0.2	4.7	6
Pantothenate	mg/kg/day	1.2–1.7	>0.36	>0.36	2.3	1.44	0.27	1.3	2.7
Biotin	µg/kg/day	3.6–6.0	>1.8	>1.8	45	4.8	0.6	4.7	42.7
Folate	µg/kg/day	25–50	39.6	>72	45	48	7.1	44.9	44

Nutrient	Units								
Vitamin B$_{12}$	μg/kg/day	0.3	>0.18	>0.18	0.67	0.3	0.07	0.3	1.1
Sodium	mEq/kg/day	2–3	2.5–3.5	1.2–2.8	2.3	3	1.2	2.2	2.2
Potassium	mEq/kg/day	2–3	2–3	2.8–4.6	4	3	2	3.1	4.6
Chloride	mEq/kg/day	2–3		1.9–3.0	2.8	3	1.8	2.3	3.5
Calcium	mg/kg/day	120–230	210	84–168	219	198	42	179.7	230
Phosphorus	mg/kg/day	60–140	110	60–104	122	100	21	96.3	129
Magnesium	mg/kg/day	7.9–15.0		7.2–14.4	14.6	10.8	5.2	6.6	16.4
Iron	mg/kg/day	2	2–3	1.8	2.2	2.2	0.04	2.2	0.6
Zinc	μg/kg/day	1000	>600	660–1320	1830	1800	184	1263	1800
Copper	μg/kg/day	120–150	108	108–144	304	144	38	103.8	312
Selenium	μg/kg/day	1.3–3.0			2.2	3.4	2.2	2.2	3.0
Chromium	μg/kg/day	0.1–0.5							
Manganese	μg/kg/day	7.5	>6	1.8–9.0	14.6	7.6	1	16	12.6
Molybdenum	μg/kg/day	0.3							
Iodine	μg/kg/day	30–60	6	12–54	7	30	16	16	16
Taurine	mg/kg/day	4.5–9.0				7.2			
Carnitine	mg/kg/day	2.9		>1.4		2.9			
Inositol	mg/kg/day	32–81			7.3	52.8	22.5		28.1
Choline	mg/kg/day	14.4–28.0			12.2	24	14.3		17.1

HMF = human milk fortifier.

*Recommendations and calculated intakes of formulas and human milk are based on 150 mL/kg/d.

†Recommendations per 100 calories were converted to 120 cal/kg/day values for comparison.

‡Aim for 400 IU/d.

§Total recommended vitamin D is IU/day.

||Denotes milk of mothers of preterm infants post the first 21 days of lactation.

TABLE 10.2. ENERGY UTILIZATION OF INFANTS

	Kcal/kg/day		
	Preterm	0–6 Months	6–12 Months
Basal	55	55	55
Activity	15	17	20
SDA	8	7	7
Stool loss	12	11	13
Subtotal	90	90	95
Growth*	40–85	20–40	5–15
Total	130–175	110–130	100–110

*5 kcal/g weight gain.
Source: From Reichman B., et al. Partition of energy metabolism and energy cost of growth in the very-low-brith-weight infant. Pediatrics 1982;69:446.

D. **Carbohydrate.** Dextrose (D-glucose) is the carbohydrate source in intravenous solutions.
   1. The caloric value of dextrose is 3.4 kcal/g.
   2. Because dextrose contributes to the osmolarity of a solution, it is generally recommended that the concentration administered via peripheral veins be limited to $\leq$ 12.5% dextrose. We also limit concentrations delivered via umbilical arterial catheters to $\leq$ 12.5% dextrose but will use up to 25% dextrose for central venous infusions. In unusual circumstances, higher concentrations have been used, if the fluid volume must be severely restricted.
   3. Dextrose infusions are typically referred to in terms of the milligrams of glucose per kilogram per minute (mg/kg/min) delivered, which expresses the total glucose load and accounts for infusion rate, dextrose concentration, and patient weight (Fig. 10-2).
   4. The initial glucose requirement for term infants is defined as the amount that is necessary to avoid hypoglycemia. In general, this may be achieved with initial infusion rates of approximately 4 mg/kg/min.
   5. Preterm infants usually require higher rates of glucose, as they have a higher brain-to-body weight ratio and higher total energy needs. Initial infusion rates of 4 to 8 mg/kg/min are generally required to maintain euglycemia.
   6. Initial rates may be advanced, as tolerated, by 1 to 2 mg/kg/min daily to a maximum of 11 to 14 mg/kg/min. This may be accomplished by increasing dextrose concentration, by increasing infusion rate, or by a combination of both. Infusion rates above 11 to 14 mg/kg/min may exceed the infant's oxidative capacity and are generally not recommended, as this may cause the excess glucose to be converted to fat, particularly in the liver. This conversion may also increase oxygen consumption, energy expenditure, and CO_2 production.
   7. The quantity of dextrose that an infant can tolerate will vary with gestational and postnatal age. Signs of glucose intolerance include hyperglycemia and secondary glucosuria with osmotic diuresis.
E. **Protein.** Crystalline amino acid solutions provide the nitrogen source in PN.
   1. The caloric value of amino acids is 4 kcal/g.

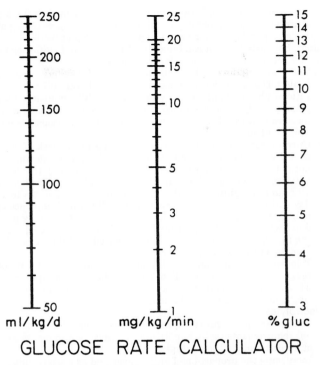

GLUCOSE RATE CALCULATOR

Use a straight edge to determine the volume required per 24 hours.

FIG. 10.2. Interconversion of glucose infusion units. (From Klaus M. H., Faranoff A. A. (Eds.). *Care of the High-Risk Neonate*, 2nd ed. Philadelphia: Saunders, 1979, 430.)

2. At present, two pediatric amino acid formulations are commercially available in the United States: Aminosyn-PF, Abbott Laboratories, and TrophAmine, B. Braun. In theory, these products are better adapted to the needs of newborns than are standard adult formulations, as they have been modified for improved tolerance and contain conditionally essential amino acids. However, the optimal amino acid composition for neonatal PN has not yet been defined, and there are no products currently available that are specifically designed for preterm infants.

3. It has been demonstrated that VLBW infants who do not receive amino acids in the first days of life catabolize body protein at a rate of at least 1 g/kg per day. Studies investigating the use of early amino acids have consistently shown a reversal of this catabolism without adverse metabolic consequences. Current data therefore support the infusion of amino acids in a dose of at least 1 g/kg per day beginning in the first 24 hours of life.

4. We provide all infants with a birth weight < 1250 g with 1.5 g/kg per day beginning immediately after birth. Infants with a birth weight between 1250 and 1500 g are initiated on 1.5 g/kg per day within the first 24 to 48 hours of life. Infants > 1500 g are only initiated on 1.5 g/kg per day if indicated; depending on their size, clinical condition, and estimated time to achieve significant enteral volumes.

   5. Infusion rates are generally advanced by approximately 1 g/kg per day to a target of 3.5 g/kg per day for all infants weighing ≤ 1500 g at birth and 3.0 g/kg per day for neonates weighing > 1500 g at birth.

F. Lipid. Soybean oil, or a combination of soybean and safflower oil, provides the fat source for intravenous fat emulsions.

   1. The caloric value of 20% lipid emulsions is 2 kcal/mL (approximately 10 kcal/g). The use of 20% emulsions is preferred over 10% because the higher ratio of phospholipids to triglyceride in the 10% emulsion interferes with plasma triglyceride clearance. Twenty percent emulsions also provide a more concentrated source of calories. For these reasons, we only use 20% lipid emulsions.

   2. Current data suggest that preterm infants are at risk of essential fatty acid (EFA) deficiency within 72 hours of life, if an exogenous fat source is not delivered. This deficiency state can be avoided by the administration of 0.5 to 1.0 g/kg per day of lipid emulsion. Therefore, in our institutions, all infants weighing < 1000 g at birth are initiated on 0.5 to 1.0 g/kg per day within the first 24 to 48 hours of life. This rate is advanced by approximately 0.5 g/kg per day, as tolerated, to a target of 3.0 g/kg per day. All infants weighing > 1000 g at birth are initiated on 1.0 g/kg per day within the first 24 to 48 hours of life and advanced by 1.0 g/kg per day, as tolerated, to a target of 3.0 g/kg per day.

   3. Tolerance also correlates with hourly infusion rate, and no benefit to a rest period has been identified. We, therefore, infuse lipid emulsions over 24 hours for optimal clearance. However, due to sepsis risk factors, syringes are changed every 12 hours.

G. Electrolytes

   1. Sodium and potassium concentrations are adjusted daily based on individual requirements (see Chap 9). Maintenance requirements are estimated at approximately 2 to 4 mEq/kg.

   2. Increasing the proportion of anions provided as acetate aids in the treatment of metabolic acidosis in VLBW infants.

H. Vitamins. The current vitamin formulation (MVI Pediatric, NeoSan Pharmaceuticals) does not maintain blood levels of all vitamins within an acceptable range for preterm infants. However, there are no products currently available that are specifically designed for preterm infants. Table 10.3 provides guidelines for the use of the available formulations for term and preterm infants. We typically add 1.5 mL MVI Pediatric/100 mL PN administered at a rate of 150 mL/kg. For those infants receiving < 150 mL/kg, the American Society of Clinical Nutrition and AAP guidelines of 40% of the currently available single dose vial per kg (not to exceed 5 mL per day) may need to be considered. Vitamin A is the most difficult to provide in adequate amounts to the VLBW infant without providing excess amounts of the other vitamins, as it is subject to losses via photodegradation and absorption to plastic tubing and solution-containing bags. B vitamins may also be affected by photodegradation. This is of particular concern with long-term PN use and for this reason PN-containing plastic bags and tubing should be shielded from light.

I. Minerals. The amount of calcium and phosphorus that can be administered via IV is limited by the precipitation of calcium phosphate. Unfortunately, the variables that determine calcium and phosphate compatibility in PN are complex and what constitutes maximal safe concentrations is controversial. We adhere to the following guidelines:

   1. Calcium. Our standard, **peripheral PN solution** contains 30 mg/dL (1.5 mEq/dL) of elemental calcium.

   2. Phosphorus. 1.0 mEq/dL of potassium phosphate is also routinely added to our standard, **peripheral PN.** This provides approximately 21 mg/dL of phosphate (0.68 mM/dL of phosphate).

   3. These standard mineral concentrations provide only about one-third of daily intrauterine accretion rates for calcium and phosphorus. Therefore,

TABLE 10.3. SUGGESTED INTAKES OF PARENTERAL VITAMINS IN INFANTS

Vitamin	Estimated Needs		40% of a Single-dose Vial MVI Pediatric (NeoSan) per Kilogram of Body Weight	1.5 mL MVI Pediatric per 100 mL PN Administered at a Rate of 150 mL/kg/day[†]
	Term Infants (dose/day)	Preterm Infants (dose/ kg/day)*		
LIPID SOLUBLE				
A (μg)[‡]	700	500	280	315
D (IU)[‡]	400	160	160	180
E (IU)[‡]	7	2.8	2.8	3.2
K (μg)	200	80	80	90
WATER SOLUBLE				
Thiamine (mg)	1.2	0.35	0.48	0.54
Riboflavin (mg)	1.4	0.15	0.56	0.63
Niacin (mg)	17	6.8	6.8	7.65
Pantothenate (mg)	5	2.0	2.0	2.25
Pyridoxine (mg)	1.0	0.18	0.4	0.45
Biotin (μg)	20	6.0	8.0	9.0
Vitamin B_{12} (μg)	1.0	0.3	0.4	0.45
Vitamin C (mg)	80	25	32	36
Folate (μg)	140	56	56	63

*Maximum not to exceed term dose.
†Assumes 150 mL/kg is the average PN administration rate.
‡700 μg retinol equivalent = 2300 IU; 7 mg alpha-tocopherol = 7 IU; 10 μg vitamin D = 400 IU.
Source: From Greene H. L., et al. Guidelines for the use of vitamins, trace elements, calcium, magnesium, and phosphorus in infants and children receiving total parenteral nutrition. *Am J Clin Nutr* 1988;48:1324.

preterm infants receiving prolonged PN are at increased risk for metabolic bone disease (see Chap. 29).

4. Increasing the mineral content of these solutions may diminish metabolic bone complications. However, this also increases the risk of precipitation and administration requires central venous access. Our standard, **central PN solution** contains 50 mg/dL of elemental calcium and 2.0 mEq/dL potassium phosphate with a goal calcium to phosphorus ratio of approximately 1.3:1 to 1.7:1 by weight (1.1:1 to 1.3:1 molar).

5. We do not use 3-in-1 PN solutions (dextrose, amino acid, and lipid mixed in single bag) for the following reasons:

    a. The pH of lipid emulsions is more basic and increases the pH of the total solution, which decreases the solubility of calcium and phosphorus and limits the amount of these minerals in the solution.

    b. If the calcium and phosphorus in a 3-in-1 solution did precipitate, it would be difficult to detect, as the solution is already cloudy.

    c. 3-in-1 solutions require either a larger-micron filter or no filter, which may pose a greater sepsis risk.

J. Trace elements

  1. We currently add 0.2 mL/dL of NeoTrace and 1.5 µg/dL of selenium beginning in the first days of PN. However, when PN is supplementing enteral nutrition or limited to < 2 weeks, only zinc may be needed.

  2. As copper and manganese are excreted in bile, we routinely reduce or omit these trace elements if impaired biliary excretion and/or cholestatic liver disease is present.

K. General PN procedures

  1. If possible, the continuity of a central line should not be broken for blood drawing or blood transfusion because of the risk of infection.

  2. Most medications are not given in PN solutions. If necessary, the PN catheter may be flushed with saline solution and a medication then infused in a compatible IV solution. Refer to the table in Appendix A for our guidelines for PN/IL and medication compatibility.

  3. Heparin is added to all central lines at a concentration of 0.5 unit/mL of solution.

L. Metabolic monitoring for infants receiving PN. All infants receiving PN are monitored according to the schedule indicated in Table 10.4.

M. Potential complications associated with PN

  1. Cholestasis (see Chap. 18) may be seen and is more often transient than progressive. Experimentally, even short-term PN can reduce bile flow and bile salt formation.

    a. Risk factors include:

      (1) Prematurity

      (2) Duration of PN administration

      (3) Duration of fasting (lack of enteral feeding also produces bile inspissation and cholestasis)

TABLE 10.4. SCHEDULE FOR METABOLIC MONITORING OF INFANTS RECEIVING PARENTERAL NUTRITION

Measurement	Frequency of Measurement
BLOOD	
Glucose, electrolytes, including total carbon dioxide or pH	Daily for 2–3 days, then twice weekly
Blood urea nitrogen, creatinine, calcium, phosphorus, magnesium, total protein, albumin, transaminases, (ALT, AST), bilirubin, alkaline phosphatase, triglycerides, hematocrit	Weekly or every other week
URINE	
Specific gravity, reducing substances, total volume	Daily

      (4) Infection

      (5) Narcotic administration

   b. Recommended management

      (1) Attempt enteral feeding. Even minimal enteral feedings may stimulate bile secretion.

      (2) Avoid overfeeding.

      (3) Provision of a mixed fuel source may be helpful.

  2. Metabolic bone disease (see Chap. 29). The use of earlier enteral feedings and central PN, with higher calcium and phosphorus ratios, has reduced the incidence of metabolic bone disease. However, this continues to be seen with the prolonged use of PN in place of enteral nutrition.

  3. Metabolic abnormalities. Azotemia, hyperammonemia, and hyperchloremic metabolic acidosis have become uncommon since introduction of the current crystalline amino acid solutions. These complications may occur, however, with amino acid intakes exceeding 4 g/kg per day.

  4. Metabolic abnormalities related to lipid emulsions

   a. Hyperlipidemia/hypertriglyceridemia. The incidence is inversely related to gestational age at birth and postnatal age. A short-term decrease in the lipid infusion rate usually is sufficient to normalize serum lipid levels. We typically aim to maintain serum triglyceride levels below 200 mg/dL.

   b. Indirect Hyperbilirubinemia. Since free fatty acids can theoretically displace bilirubin from albumin-binding sites, the use of lipid emulsions during periods of neonatal hyperbilirubinemia has been questioned. Recent research however suggests that infusion of lipid at rates up to 3 g/kg per day is unlikely to displace bilirubin. However, during periods of extreme hyperbilirubinemia (e.g., requiring exchange transfusion), rates < 3 g/kg per day should be provided.

   c. Sepsis has been associated with decreased lipoprotein lipase activity and impaired triglyceride clearance. Therefore, during a sepsis episode, it may be necessary to temporarily limit the lipid infusion to approximately 2.0 g/kg per day if the triglyceride level is > 150 mg/dL.

   d. The potential adverse effects of lipid emulsions on pulmonary function, the risk of chronic lung disease, and impaired immune function remain subjects of debate. Because of the concern about toxic products of lipid peroxidation, lipid emulsions should also be protected from both ambient and phototherapy lights.

N. Current controversies

  1. Carnitine facilitates the transport of long-chain fatty acids into the mitochondria for oxidation. However, this nutrient is not routinely added to PN solutions. Preterm infants who receive prolonged, unsupplemented PN are at risk of carnitine deficiency due to their limited reserves and inadequate rates of carnitine synthesis. For those infants who are able to tolerate enteral nutrition, we assume their needs are met by the use of human milk and/or carnitine-containing infant formula. However, for infants requiring prolonged (e.g., > 4 weeks) PN, we will routinely supplement carnitine at an initial dose of approximately 10 mg/kg per day until enteral nutrition can be established.

  2. Cysteine is not a component of current crystalline amino acid solutions, as it is unstable over time and will form a precipitate. Cysteine is ordinarily synthesized from methionine and provides a substrate for taurine. However, this may be considered an essential amino acid for preterm infants due to low activity of the enzyme hepatic cystathionase, which converts methionine to cysteine. Supplementation with L-cysteine hydrochloride lowers the pH of the PN solution and may necessitate the use of additional acetate to prevent acidosis. However, the lower pH also enhances the solubility of calcium and phosphorus and allows for improved mineral intake. We routinely supplement cysteine at a rate of approximately 40 mg/g protein.

3. **Glutamine** is an important fuel for intestinal epithelial cells and lymphocytes, however, due to its instability, it is presently not a component of crystalline amino acid solutions. Its use as an additive to PN solutions is currently under review.

4. **Insulin** is not routinely added to PN. Its use must be weighed against the risk of wide swings in blood glucose levels, as well as the concerns surrounding the overall effects of the increased uptake of glucose. When hyperglycemia is severe or persistent, an insulin infusion may be useful. We initiate an infusion of regular insulin at a rate of 0.05 unit/kg per hour, with the dose titrated to maintain blood glucose concentrations of 100 to 200 mg/dL. A convenient initial solution is 10 units of insulin per 100 mL of fluid (0.1 unit/mL). The IV tubing should first be thoroughly flushed with the solution (see Chap. 29).

5. **Vitamin A** is important for normal growth and differentiation of epithelial tissue, particularly the development and maintenance of pulmonary epithelial tissue. Extremely-low-birth-weight (ELBW) infants are known to have low vitamin A stores at birth, minimal enteral intake for the first several weeks after birth, poor enteral absorption of vitamin A, and unreliable parenteral delivery. Studies have suggested that vitamin A supplementation can reduce the risk of chronic lung disease. At present, we supplement infants weighing < 1000 g at birth with 5000 IU vitamin A intramuscularly three times per week for the first 4 weeks of life, beginning in the first 72 hours of life (see Chap. 24).

IV. Enteral Nutrition

A. Early enteral feeding

1. The structural and functional integrity of the gastrointestinal (GI) tract is dependent upon the provision of enteral nutrition. Withholding enteral feeding after birth places the infant at risk for all the complications associated with luminal starvation, including mucosal thinning, flattening of the villi, and bacterial translocation. **Trophic feedings** (also referred to as "gut priming" or "minimal enteral feedings") may be described as feedings that are delivered in very small volumes (≤ 10 mL/kg per day) for the purpose of induction of gut maturation rather than nutrient delivery.

2. **Benefits associated with trophic feedings include:**
   a. Improved levels of gut hormones.
   b. Less feeding intolerance.
   c. Earlier progression to full enteral feedings.
   d. Improved weight gain.
   e. Improved calcium and phosphorus retention.
   f. Fewer days on parenteral nutrition.

3. **We adhere to the following guidelines for the use of trophic feedings:**
   a. Begin as soon after birth as possible, ideally by day of life 2 to 3.
   b. Use full-strength human milk or full-strength 20 kcal/oz preterm formula at a volume of ≤ 10 mL/kg per day. We administer trophic feedings every 4, 6, or 8 hours.
   c. We do not use trophic feedings in infants with severe hemodynamic instability, suspected or confirmed NEC, evidence of ileus, or clinical signs of intestinal pathology. We also do not feed infants who are undergoing treatment with indomethacin for patent ductus arteriosus.
   d. Controlled trials of feeding with umbilical arterial catheters (UACs) in place have not shown an increased incidence of NEC. We do not consider the presence of a UAC to be a contraindication to trophic feeding. However, the clinical condition accompanying the prolonged use a UAC may serve as a contraindication.

B. Preterm Infants

1. **Fortified human milk.** Human milk provides the gold standard for feeding term infants, and although there is no such gold standard for preterm infants, we consider the use of fortified human milk to be the most nutritionally optimal diet for preterm infants.

a. Preterm human milk contains higher amounts of protein, sodium, chloride, and magnesium than term milk (see Table 10.1). However, the levels of these nutrients remain below preterm recommendations, the differences only persist for the first 21 days of lactation, and composition is known to vary.

b. For these reasons, we routinely supplement human milk for preterm infants with human milk fortifier (HMF). The addition of HMF to human milk (Table 10.1) increases energy, protein, vitamin, and mineral contents to levels more appropriate for preterm infants.

c. Infants born weighing < 1500 g are supplemented with HMF once they are tolerating 100 mL/kg of human milk. Infants > 1500 g are supplemented once they achieve full volume feedings.

d. Because the addition of HMF has resulted in hypercalcemia in the past, we may monitor calcium and phosphorus levels. Hypercalcemia has been less of a problem with the newer HMF formulations.

e. When human milk is fed via continuous infusion, incomplete delivery of nutrients may occur, in particular, the nonhomogenized fat and nutrients in the HMF may cling to the tubing. Small, frequent bolus feedings may result in improved nutrient delivery and absorption compared with continuous feedings.

f. Our protocols for the collection and storage of human milk are outlined in Chap. 11.

2. Preterm formulas (see Tables 10.1 and 10.6) are designed to meet the nutritional and physiologic needs of preterm infants and have some common features:

a. Whey-predominant, taurine-supplemented protein source, which is better tolerated and produces a more normal plasma amino acid profile than casein-predominant protein.

b. Carbohydrate mixtures of 40 to 50% lactose and 50 to 60% glucose polymers to compensate for preterm infants' relative lactase deficiency.

c. Fat mixtures containing approximately 50% medium-chain triglycerides, to compensate for limited pancreatic lipase secretion and small bile acid pools, as well as 50% long-chain triglycerides to provide a source of EFAs.

d. Higher concentrations of protein, vitamins, minerals, and electrolytes to meet the increased needs associated with rapid growth, decreased intestinal absorption, and limited fluid tolerance.

3. Feeding advancement. When attempting to determine how best to advance a preterm infant to full enteral nutrition, there is very limited data to support any one method as optimal. The following guidelines reflect our current practice:

a. We use full-strength, 20 kcal/oz human milk or preterm formula and advance feeding volume according to the guidelines in Table 10.5 for any infant being fed by tube feedings.

b. For those infants with a birth weight < 1500 g, caloric density is advanced from 20 to 24 kcal/oz at 100 mL/kg of volume. As previously discussed, in the case of human milk–fed infants, this is accomplished through the addition of HMF. This volume is then maintained for approximately 24 hours before the advancement schedule is resumed. For those > 1500 g, caloric density is advanced after achieving full volume feedings.

c. As enteral volumes are increased, the rate of any IV fluid is reduced accordingly so that the total daily fluid volume remains the same. Enteral nutrients are taken into account when administering any supplemental PN.

C. Term Infants

1. Human milk is considered the preferred feeding choice for term infants.

2. Term formulas. The AAP provides specific guidelines for the composition of infant formulas so that term infant formulas approximate human milk in general composition. Table 10.6 describes the composition of commonly available formulas, many of which are derived from modified cow's milk.

TABLE 10.5. TUBE FEEDING GUIDELINES*,†,‡,§

Birth Weight (g)	Initial Rate (mL/kg/day)	Volume Increase (mL/kg/day)
<800	10	10–20
800–1000	10–20	10–20
1001–1250	20	20–30
1251–1500	30	30
1501–1800	30–40	30–40
1801–2500	40	40–50
>2500	50	50

*This table does not apply to infants capable of PO feeding.
†The above guidelines must always be individualized based on the infant's clinical status/severity of illness.
‡Consider advancing feeding volume more rapidly than the above guidelines once tolerance of ≥100 mL/kg/day is established, but do not exceed increments of 30 mL/kg/day in most infants weighing less than 1500 g.
§The recommended volume goal for feedings is 140–160 mL/kg/day.

D. Specialized formulas have been designed for a variety of congenital and neonatal disorders, including milk protein allergy, malabsorption syndromes, and several inborn errors of metabolism. Indications for the most commonly used of these specialized formulas are briefly reviewed in Table 10.7, while composition is outlined in Table 10.6. However, it is important to note that **these formulas were not designed to meet the special nutritional needs of preterm infants.** Preterm infants fed these formulas require vigilant nutritional assessment and monitoring for protein, mineral, and multivitamin supplementation.

E. Caloric-enhanced feedings. Many ill and preterm infants require increased energy/nutrient intakes in order to achieve optimal rates of growth.

1. In general, we first increase caloric density by concentrating feedings to 24 kcal/oz; if needed, MCT oil and/or Polycose are added in increments of 2 kcal/oz.
2. We also supplement protein intake with Promod for all VLBW infants in order to increase the protein content to approximately 4.0 g/kg per day.
3. These supplements are further described in Table 10.8.
4. Growth patterns of infants receiving these supplements are monitored closely and the nutritional care plan is adjusted accordingly.

F. Feeding method. These should be individualized based on gestational age, clinical condition, and feeding tolerance.

1. **Nasogastric/orogastric feedings.** We utilize nasogastric tube feedings more frequently, as orogastric tubes tend to be more difficult to secure.
   a. **Candidates**
      (1) Infants <34 weeks' gestation, as most do not yet have the ability to coordinate suck-swallow-breathe patterns.
      (2) Infants with impaired suck/swallow coordination due to conditions such as encephalopathy, hypotonia and maxillofacial abnormalities.
   b. **Bolus versus continuous.** Studies may be found in support of either method and, in practice, both are utilized. We tend to initiate with bolus feedings every 3 to 4 hours. If difficulties with feeding tolerance occur, we will lengthen the amount of time over which a feeding is given (e.g., feed over a 2-hour period based on a 4-hour feeding interval).

2. Transpyloric feedings
  a. Candidates. There are only a few indications for transpyloric feedings.
  (1) Infants intolerant to nasogastric/orogastric feedings.
  (2) Infants at increased risk for aspiration.
  (3) Severe gastric retention or regurgitation.
  (4) Anatomic abnormalities of the GI tract such as microgastria.
  b. Other considerations
  (1) Transpyloric feedings should be delivered continuously, as the small intestine does not have the same capacity for expansion as does the stomach.
  (2) There is an increased risk for fat malabsorption, as lingual and gastric lipase secretions are bypassed.
  (3) These tubes are routinely placed under guided fluoroscopy.
3. Transition to breast/bottle feedings is a gradual process. Infants who are approximately 34 weeks' gestation who have coordinated suck-swallow-breathe patterns and respiratory rates <60 per minute are appropriate candidates for introducing breast/bottle feedings.
4. Gastrostomy feedings
  a. Candidates
  (1) Infants whose transition to breast/bottle feedings is expected to be prolonged (e.g., > 2 months).
  (2) Infants with neurological impairment and/or those who are unable to take sufficient volumes via breast/bottle feeding to maintain adequate growth/hydration status.
G. Iron. The AAP recommends that preterm infants receive a source of iron, provided at 2 to 4 mg/kg per day, by the time they are 2 months of age or have doubled their birth weight. We administer iron supplementation according to the guidelines outlined in Table 10.9. Iron supplementation is recommended until the infant is 2 years of age.
  1. Vitamin E is an important antioxidant that acts to prevent fatty acid peroxidation in the cell membrane. The recommendation for preterm infants is 6 to 12 IU vitamin E/kg per day, with the upper limit being desirable. Preterm infants are not initiated on iron supplements until they are tolerating full enteral volumes of 24 kcal/oz feedings, which provides vitamin E at the low to mid-range of the recommendations. An additional vitamin E supplement would be required to meet the upper end of the recommendation.
H. Current controversies
  1. Glutamine. As with parenteral glutamine supplementation, there are presently no recommendations for enteral glutamine supplementation in preterm infants.
  2. Long-chain polyunsaturated fatty acids (LCPUFAs). The inclusion of LCPUFAs, specifically docosahexaenoic acid (DHA) and arachidonic acid (ARA), in infant formulas has been the subject of much debate in recent years. These LCPUFAs are derivatives of the essential fatty acids, linoleic acid and α-linolenic acid, and they are important in cognitive development and visual acuity. Human milk contains these LCPUFAs but, until recently, standard infant formula did not. Controlled trials investigating the effects of LCPUFA-supplemented formula on cognitive development in preterm infants have been inconclusive. The effects on visual acuity have more consistently suggested an advantage. Furthermore, no adverse effects were noted.
V. Special Considerations
  A. Gastro-esophageal reflux (GER). Episodes of gastroesophageal reflux, as monitored by esophageal pH probes, are common in both preterm and full-term infants. The majority of infants, however, do not exhibit clinical compromise from GER.
  1. Introduction of enteral feeds. Emesis can be associated during the introduction and advancement of enteral feeds in preterm infants. These epi-

TABLE 10.6. HUMAN MILK AND FORMULA COMPOSITION

Formula (distributor)	kcal/30 mL	Protein (gm/dL)	Fat (gm/dL)	Carbo-hydrate* (gm/dL)	Minerals (mg/dL)			Electro-lytes (mEq/dL)			Vitamins (IU/dL)			Folate (μg/dL)	Osmolality (mOsmo/Kg H_2O)	Renal Solute Load (mOsmol/L)‡
					Ca	P	Fe‡	Na⁺	K†	C‡	A	D	E			
Breast milk (composition varies)	20	1.1	3.9	7.2	28	14	0.03	0.8	1.3	1.2	233	2.2	0.31	5	290–300	93
Standard cow's milk–based formulas																
Similac 20 (Ross)	20	1.4	3.7	7.3	53	28	1.2	0.7	1.8	1.2	203	41	1.0	10	300	93.6
Enfamil 20 (Mead Johnson)	20	1.5	3.6	7.3	53	36	1.22	0.8	1.8	1.2	200	41	1.35	10.8	300	132
Enfamil 24 (Mead Johnson)	24	1.7	4.3	8.8	63	43	1.46	1.0	2.3	1.4	240	49	1.62	13	360	158
Milk Protein, lactose free																
Lactofree (Mead Johnson)	20	1.4	3.6	7.4	55	37	1.2	0.9	1.9	1.3	200	41	1.35	10.8	200	132
Similac Advance lactose free (Ross)	20	1.4	3.6	7.2	57	38	1.2	0.9	1.9	1.2	203	41	2.0	10.1	200	97.6
Soy Formulas																
Isomil (Ross)	20	1.7	3.7	7.0	71	51	1.2	1.3	1.9	1.2	203	41	1.0	10.1	200	110
Prosobee (Mead Johnson)	20	1.7	3.6	7.2	71	56	1.2	1.0	2.1	1.5	200	41	1.35	10.8	200	161
Preterm formulas																
Similac Special Care (Ross)	20	1.8	3.7	7.2	122	68	1.2	1.3	2.2	1.5	845	101	2.7	25	235	124

Formula															
Similac Special Care (Ross)	24	2.2	4.4	8.6	146	81	1.5	1.5	2.7	1.9	1014	122	3.3	30	280	149
Enfamil Premature (Mead Johnson)	20	2	3.5	7.5	112	56	1.22	1.13	1.8	1.6	850	183	4.3	24	260	175
Enfamil Premature (Mead Johnson)	24	2.4	4.1	9	134	67	1.46	1.4	2.1	1.9	1010	220	5.1	28	310	210
Transitional formulas															
Similac NeoSure (Ross)	22	1.9	4.1	7.7	78	46	1.3	1.1	2.7	1.6	342	52	2.7	18.7	250	131
EnfaCare (Mead Johnson)	22	2.1	3.9	7.9	89	49	1.3	1.1	2.0	1.6	330	59	3	19.2	230	181
Specialized formulas															
Pregestimil (Mead Johnson)	20	1.9	3.8	6.9	78	51	1.3	1.4	1.9	1.6	260	34	2.6	10.8	280	174
Alimentum (Ross)	20	1.9	3.7	6.9	71	51	1.2	1.3	2.0	1.5	203	30	2.0	10	370	123
Neocate (SHS)	20	2.1	3	7.8	83	62	1.2	1.1	2.6	1.5	272	57.8	0.7	6.8	342	
Nutramigen (Mead Johnson)	20	1.9	3.4	7.5	64	43	1.2	1.4	1.9	1.6	200	34	1.35	10.8	320	173
Portagen (Mead Johnson)	20	2.4	3.2	7.8	64	47	1.3	1.6	2.2	1.6	530	53	2.1	10.6	230	200
Similac PM 60/40 (Ross)	20	1.5	3.8	6.9	38	19	0.5	0.7	1.5	1.1	203	41	1.7	10	280	92.2

CA = calcium; P = phosphorus; Fe = iron; Na$^+$ = sodium; K$^+$ = potassium; Cl = chloride

*See text for types of carbohydrates used in formula.

†In instances where high and low Fe formulations are available, the iron fortified value appears.

‡Estimated renal solute load = [Protein (g) $\times$ 4] + [Na(mEq) + K(mEq) + Cl (mEq)].

TABLE 10.7. INDICATIONS FOR USE OF INFANT FORMULAS

Clinical Condition	Suggested Formula	Rationale
Allergy to cow's milk protein or soy protein	Pregestimil, Nutramigen, Alimentum, Neocate	Protein hydrolysate due to protein sensitivity
Bronchopulmonary dysplasia	High-energy, nutrient-dense	Increased energy requirement, fluid restriction
Biliary atresia	Pregestimil	Impaired intraluminal digestion and absorption of long-chain fats
Chylothorax (persistent)	Portagen, Pregestimil	Decrease lymphatic absorption of fats
Congestive heart failure	High-energy formula	Lower fluid and sodium intake; increased energy requirement
Cystic fibrosis	Pregestimil or standard formula with pancreatic enzyme supplementation	Impaired intraluminal digestion and absorption of long-chain fats
Diarrhea		
Chronic nonspecific	Standard formula	Appropriate distribution of calories
	Lactose free	If malabsorbing lactose
Intractable	Pregestimil	Impaired digestion of intact protein, long-chain fats, and disaccharides
Galactosemia	Lactose free	Lactose free
Gastroesophageal reflux	Standard formula, Enfamil AR	Thicken with 1–3 tsp of cereal per ounce; small, frequent feedings

Condition	Formula	Reason
GI bleeding (due to cow's milk protein intolerance)	Soy formula or other cow's milk-free formula	Milk protein intolerance
Hepatic insufficiency	Portagen, Pregestimil	Impaired intraluminal digestion and absorption of long-chain fats
Hypoparathyroidism, late-onset hypocalcemia	PM 60/40	Low phosphate content
Lactose intolerance	Lactose free	Impaired digestion or utilization of lactose
Lymphatic anomalies	Portagen	Impaired absorption of long-chain fats
Necrotizing enterocolitis	Preterm Formula or Pregestimil (when feeding is resumed)	Impaired digestion
Renal insufficiency	PM 60/40	Low phosphate content, low renal solute load

Source: Modified from Gryboski J., Walker W. A. *Gastrointestinal Problems in the Infant*, 2nd Ed. Philadelphia: Saunders, 1983.

TABLE 10.8. ORAL DIETARY SUPPLEMENTS AVAILABLE FOR USE IN INFANTS

Nutrient	Product	Source	Energy Content
Fat	MCT oil (Mead Johnson)	Medium-chain triglycerides	8.3 kcal/g 7.7 kcal/mL
	Microlipid (Mead Johnson)	Long-chain triglycerides	4.4 kcal/mL
	Corn oil	Long-chain triglycerides	9 kcal/gm 8.4 kcal/mL
Carbohydrate	Polycose (Ross)	Glucose polymers	3.8 kcal/gm 8 kcal/tsp (powder) 2 kcal/mL (liquid)
Protein	Promod (Ross)	Whey concentrate	4.2 kcal/g 5.5 kcal/tsp

MCT = medium-chain triglyceride.

sodes are most commonly related to intestinal dysmotility secondary to prematurity, and will respond to modifications of the feeding regimen.

  a. Temporary reductions in the feeding volume, removal of nutritional additives, lengthening the duration of the feeding (sometimes to the point of using continuous feeding), and temporary cessation of enteral feeds are all possible strategies depending upon the clinical course of the infant.

  b. Rarely, specialized formulas are used when all other feeding modifications have been tried without improvement. In general, these formulas should only be used for short periods of time with close nutritional monitoring.

  c. Infants who have repeated episodes of symptomatic emesis that prevent achievement of full volume enteral feeds may require evaluation for anatomic problems such as malrotation or Hirschsprung's disease. In general, radiographic studies are not undertaken unless feeding problems have persisted for 2 or more weeks, or unless bilious emesis occurs.

2. **Established feeds.** Preterm infants on full-volume enteral feeds will have occasional episodes of symptomatic emesis. If these episodes do not compromise the respiratory status or growth of the infant, no intervention is required other than continued close monitoring of the infant. If symptomatic emesis is associated with respiratory compromise, repeated apnea, or growth restriction, therapeutic maneuvers are indicated.

  a. **Positioning.** Re-position the infant to elevate the head and upper body, in either a prone or right side down position.

  b. **Feeding intervals.** Shortening the interval between feeds to give a smaller volume during each feed may sometimes improve signs of GER. Infants fed by gavage may have the duration of the feed increased.

  c. **Metoclopramide.** Infants who remain clinically compromised from GER after positioning and feeding interval changes can have a therapeutic trial of metoclopramide, at a dose of 0.03 to 0.1 mg/kg po/pg q8 hours. The metoclopramide should be discontinued after 1 week if there is no improvement in clinical status.

  d. **Thickened feeds.** Infants who are nipple feeding may benefit from feeds thickened with rice cereal, starting at 1/2 teaspoon per ounce of feed, if clinically compromised by GER.

  e. Full-term infants may benefit from therapeutic trials of **anti-reflux positioning** and/or **thickened feeds.**

TABLE 10.9. IRON SUPPLEMENTATION GUIDELINES IN THE PREMATURE INFANT*

	Birth Weight				Notes
	<1000 g	1000–1500 g	1500–1800 g	>1800 g	
Total dose	4 mg/kg/day	3–4 mg/kg/day	2–3 mg/kg/day	2 mg/kg/day	—
Formula					
Low iron	Supplement with elemental iron 4 mg/kg/day	Supplement with elemental iron 3–4 mg/kg/day	Supplement with elemental iron 2–3 mg/kg/day	Supplement with elemental iron 2 mg/kg/day	—
Iron fortified	Supplement with elemental iron 2 mg/kg/day	Additional elemental iron 1–2 mg/kg/day	Additional 1 mg/kg/day as needed	No additional supplementation	—
Human milk (HM) only	Elemental iron 4 mg/kg/day (see Notes)	Elemental iron 3–4 mg/kg/day (see Notes)	Elemental iron 2 mg/kg/day (see Notes)	Elemental iron 2 mg/kg/day	Infants under 1800 g should be on 24 cal/oz HM (with human milk fortifier) before iron supplementation is begun
Combination (formula plus HM)					
Low iron	Supplement with elemental iron 4 mg/kg/day	Supplement with elemental iron 3–4 g/kg/day	Supplement with elemental iron 2–3 mg/kg/day	Supplement with elemental iron 2 mg/kg/day	—
Iron fortified	Calculate for total iron dose of 4 mg/kg/day	Calculate for total dose of 3–4 mg/kg/day	Additional 1 mg/kg/day as needed	No additional supplementation	—

*Early initiation of iron supplementation in the premature infant reduces the risk of later iron deficiency and its sequelae. These guidelines are based on an intake of 150 mL/kg/day of 24 cal/oz. The clinician must consider iron content in formula or human milk fortifier when determining additional iron supplementation. Low-iron and iron-fortified formulas provide 0.3 and 2.2 mg/kg/day, respectively.

3. **Apnea.** Studies using pH probes have not shown an association between GER and apnea episodes. Treatment with promotility agents should not be used for uncomplicated apnea of prematurity.

B. **Necrotizing enterocolitis (NEC) (See Chapter 32, Necrotizing Enterocolitis).** Nutritional support of the patient with NEC focuses around providing complete parenteral nutrition during the acute phase of the disease, followed by gradual introduction of feeds after the patient has stabilized and the gut has been allowed to heal.

1. **Parenteral nutrition.** For at least 2 weeks after the initial diagnosis of NEC, the patient is kept NPO and receives total parenteral nutrition. The goals for PN were delineated previously in section III.

2. **Initiation of feeds.** If the patient is clinically stable after a minimum 2 weeks of bowel rest, feeds are introduced at approximately 10 mL/kg per day, preferably with human milk, although a standard formula appropriate for the gestational age of the patient may also be used (i.e., preterm formula for the typical NICU infant). More specialized formulas containing elemental proteins are rarely indicated.

3. **Feeding advancement.** If trophic feedings (10 mL/kg per day) are tolerated for 24 to 48 hours, gradual advancement of feeding volume is continued at approximately 10 mL/kg every 12 to 24 hours for the next 2 to 3 days. If this advancement is tolerated, further advancement proceeds according to the guidelines in Table 10.5. Supplemental PN is continued until enteral feeds are providing ≥75% of goal volume.

4. **Feeding intolerance.** Signs of feeding intolerance include large gastric residuals, emesis, abdominal distension, and increased numbers of apnea episodes. Reduction of feeding volume or cessation of feeding is usually indicated. If these clinical signs prevent attainment of full-volume enteral feeds despite several attempts to advance feeds, radiographic contrast studies may be indicated to rule out intestinal strictures. This type of evaluation would typically take place after 1 to 2 weeks of attempting to achieve full-volume enteral feeds.

5. **Enterostomies.** If one or more enterostomies are created as a result of surgical therapy for NEC, it may be difficult to achieve full nutritional intake by enteral feeds. Depending on the length and function of the upper intestinal tract, increasing feeding volume or nutritional density may result in problems with malabsorption, dumping syndrome, and poor growth.

a. **Re-feeding.** Output from the proximal intestinal enterostomy can be re-fed into the distal portion(s) of the intestine through the mucous fistula(s). This may improve the absorption of both fluid and nutrients.

b. **PN support.** If growth targets cannot be achieved using enteral feeds, continued use of supplemental PN may be indicated depending on the patient's overall status and liver function. Enteral feeding should be continued at the highest rate and nutritional density tolerated, and supplemental PN should be given to achieve the nutritional goals outlined in section III.

C. **Chronic Lung Disease.** Preterm infants who have chronic lung disease (CLD) have increased caloric requirements due to their increased metabolic expenditure, and at the same time have a lower tolerance for excess fluid intake.

1. **Fluid restriction.** Total fluid intake is typically restricted from the usual 150 mL/kg per day to 140 mL/kg per day. In cases of severe CLD, further restriction to 130 and, rarely, 120 mL/kg per day may be required. Careful monitoring is required when fluid restrictions are implemented to ensure adequate caloric and micronutrient intake. Growth parameters must also be monitored so that continued growth is not compromised.

2. **Caloric density.** Infants with CLD will commonly require up to 30 kcal/oz feeds in order to achieve the desired growth targets. In fluid-restricted infants with severe CLD, the maximum density of 32 kcal/oz is used on an infrequent basis.

VI. Nutritional Considerations in Discharge Planning. Recent data describing post-natal growth in the United States suggest that a significant number of VLBW and ELBW infants continue to have catch-up growth requirements at the time of discharge from the hospital.

A. Human milk. The use of human milk and efforts to transition to full breast-feeding in former preterm infants who continue to require enhanced caloric density feedings poses a unique challenge. We plan individualized care in order to support the transition to full breastfeeding while continuing to allow for optimal rates of growth. Usually this is accomplished by a combination of a specified number of nursing sessions per day, supplemented by feedings of calorically enhanced breast milk. Growth rate data obtained in the hospital are forwarded to infant follow-up clinics and the private pediatrician for all VLBW and ELBW infants.

B. Formula choices

    1. Transitional formulas. Preterm infants fed nutrient-enriched postdischarge formulas grow better than infants fed standard term formulas. The AAP suggests these nutrient-enriched formulas may be used to a postnatal age of 9 months. We consider all preterm infants to be appropriate candidates for the use of transitional formulas, either as an additive to human milk or as a sole formula choice, once they are ≥2000 g and 35 weeks' corrected.

    2. Term formulas may also be utilized; however, careful attention must be paid to ensure adequate caloric and micronutrient intake.

C. Vitamin supplementation. We presently adhere to the following vitamin supplementation guidelines:

    1. Preterm infants who are >2000 g and 35 weeks' corrected gestational age, and human milk-fed, are supplemented with 1 mL of pediatric MVI and 0.6 mg/kg zinc daily for their remaining period of hospitalization.

    2. Human-milk-fed infants are discharged on 1 mL QD of pediatric MUI in accordance with the AAP recommendation for 200 IU per day vitamin D until they are weaned to at least 500 mL per day of vitamin D-fortified formula or milk.

    3. Iron supplementation is provided as previously described.

Suggested Readings

American Academy of Pediatrics, Committee on Nutrition (AAP-CON). *Pediatric Nutrition Handbook.* Elk Grove Village, Ill.: American Academy of Pediatrics, 1998.

European Society of Paediatric Gastroenterology and Nutrition, Committee on Nutrition of the Preterm Infant (ESP-AN-CON). *Nutrition and Feeding of Preterm Infants.* Oxford: Blackwell Scientific, 1987.

Tsang R. C., et al. (Eds.). *Nutritional Needs of the Premature Infant: Scientific Basis and Practical Guidelines.* Baltimore: Williams & Wilkins, 1993.

11. BREASTFEEDING

Kathleen M. Howard and Maureen Allen

I. **Introduction.** Breastfeeding is a learned art that requires education and support to be successful. Its health and socioeconomic benefits are well documented. The American Academy of Pediatrics (AAP) encourages the promotion of breastfeeding as the preferred source of nutrition for at least the first year after birth. The health-care team is in a unique position to promote and support breastfeeding, especially during the first 2 to 3 weeks postpartum when most difficulties occur.

II. **Physiology of lactation. Hormonal influences** during pregnancy prepare the breast for lactation. Colostrum is secreted as early as the second trimester due to placental **lactogen.** After delivery, the release of **prolactin** stimulates milk production. Breastfeeding is the most effective stimulant for continued prolactin production. Tactile stimulation of the nerve endings in the areola and nipple result in **oxytocin** release from the pituitary gland that causes myoepithelial breast cells to contract and eject milk. Milk ejection, or the **letdown reflex,** is a neuroendocrine reflex that is negatively affected by maternal stress or pain. **Environmental influences** including pain, stress, separation from the infant, and maternal illness can all negatively affect lactogenesis and result in delayed or decreased milk production.

A. **Benefits of breastfeeding**

1. **Decreased incidence and severity of infection** due to the presence in milk of secretory antibodies, leukocytes, and carbohydrates active against viruses, bacteria, and parasites.

2. **Improved function of immune system** and effectiveness of response to immunizations.

3. **Improved nutrition and growth** due to properties that make human milk more easily digestible. The pattern of growth is different for breastfed than formula-fed infants. Breast-fed infants are less likely to develop obesity as adults.

4. **Decreased incidence of chronic diseases,** including type 1 and 2 diabetes, celiac disease, inflammatory bowel disease, childhood cancer, and allergic disease, including asthma.

5. **Potential effects on cognitive development.** Long-chain polyunsaturated fatty acids present in human milk are important for brain growth and development.

6. **Maternal health and psychosocial benefits** include assistance in expulsion of the placenta, minimizing maternal blood loss, and facilitating more rapid uterine involution. Health benefits appear to be cumulative over a mother's lifetime, and may reduce the risk of breast and ovarian cancer. Breastfeeding increases maternal self-confidence and may enhance maternal–infant bonding.

7. **Socioeconomic benefits** include the cost saving of not buying formula and of reduced illness in the breastfed infant.

III. **Potential contraindications to breastfeeding.** There are few contraindications to breastfeeding or the use of expressed breastmilk.

A. Mothers with the following conditions should be advised **not** to breastfeed.

1. **HIV infection** is a contraindication to breastfeeding in developed countries, due to the risk of transmission via the milk. In developing countries, the mortality risks associated with not breastfeeding must be weighed against the risk of transmission of HIV.

2. **Cytomegalovirus (CMV)** may be shed intermittently in human milk. Infants born to CMV-seronegative women who seroconvert during lactation and premature infants with low concentrations of transplacentally acquired maternal antibodies to CMV can develop symptomatic disease and should

not be breastfed or receive expressed milk. Pasteurization of milk appears to inactivate CMV; freezing milk at $-20°C$ ($-4°F$) decreases viral titers but does not reliably eliminate CMV. Disease transmission is uncommon in term infants, most likely because of passively transferred maternal antibodies.

3. **Human T-Cell lymphotropic virus type I,** a retrovirus associated with development of malignant neoplasms and neurologic disorders in adults, appears to be transmitted through breastfeeding. Women who are HTLV-I seropositive should not breastfeed.

4. **Human T-Cell lymphotropic virus type II,** a retrovirus, may also be transmitted through breastfeeding, although the rate and timing are uncertain. Seropositive women should not breastfeed.

5. **Herpes simplex virus type I** has been isolated from human milk in the absence of vesicular lesions or drainage from the breast or concurrent positive cultures from the maternal cervix, vagina, or throat. Women with herpetic lesions on their breasts should refrain from breastfeeding; active lesions elsewhere should be covered.

6. **Infants with galactosemia** cannot breastfeed because they cannot metabolize lactose, a sugar present in human milk.

7. **Drugs of abuse** such as amphetamines, cocaine, heroin, marijuana, and phencyclidine are hazardous to the nursing infant.

B. Conditions in which breastfeeding may be considered.

1. **Hepatitis B** surface antigen (HbsAg) has been detected in milk from HbsAg-positive women. Infants born to known HbsAg-positive women should receive Hepatitis B Immune Globulin (HBIG) and hepatitis B virus vaccine to eliminate the risk of transmission through breastfeeding.

2. **Hepatitis C** transmission through human milk has not been shown. Thus, the risk of infection is no greater for breastfed than bottle-fed infants. Transmission may occur if the mother has cracked or bleeding nipples.

3. **Rubella** virus has been isolated from human milk, but the presence of the virus in milk has not been associated with significant disease in infants. Women with rubella or who have just been immunized with rubella live-attenuated virus vaccine may breastfeed.

4. **Varicella** vaccine may be considered for a susceptible breastfeeding mother if the risk of exposure to natural varicella-zoster virus is high. It is not known whether varicella vaccine virus is secreted in human milk or whether the virus would infect a breastfeeding infant.

5. **Infants with phenylketonuria** can breastfeed with special clinical management.

6. **Tobacco and alcohol** are not absolutely contraindicated in breastfeeding. Alcohol is present in breastmilk, and intake should be limited, or the milk discarded. Nicotine appears in milk of mothers who smoke and may decrease their milk supply. However, the benefits of human milk outweigh the risks of nicotine exposure.

IV. **Prenatal education.** Breastfeeding support and education should begin during the prenatal period. This should include a history of previous breastfeeding experience and any breast surgery or disease. A nipple assessment should be made to identify anatomic deviations that may interfere with breastfeeding success. Women should be encouraged to attend prenatal breastfeeding classes and informed of community resources available to assist with breastfeeding. Breastfeeding promotion should be viewed as health education, as important as discussions of infant car seat safety and immunizations.

V. **Breastfeeding the healthy term infant**

A. **Guidelines for the initial postpartum period**

1. Infants should nurse as soon as possible after delivery, preferably during the initial alert phase, and subsequently should nurse on demand (on average 8 to 12 times per 24 hours) in response to early feeding cues (i.e., rooting, hands to face and mouth). Rooming-in facilitates demand feeding.

2. Infants should nurse on the first breast until satisfied and come off spontaneously before offering the second side. This ensures they receive the high-fat hindmilk component of the feeding.
3. Pacifiers and supplemental feedings should be avoided during the first 2 weeks unless medically indicated while the milk supply is being established.
4. A deep latch is essential to milk transfer at the breast. The infant's gums should be as far back on the areola as possible (0.5 to 1.0 cm) for efficient and comfortable nursing.
5. Signs of adequate milk transfer include a minimum of 15 to 20 minutes of rhythmic sucking with audible swallowing, breast softening, milk in the infant's mouth, satiation, and six to eight wet diapers and at least two soft yellow stools per day. If milk transfer is inadequate, supplementation (usually by bottle) may be required. This should ideally be done with expressed breastmilk.
6. Follow-up is recommended 1 to 2 days following discharge.

B. **Common problems in the postpartum period**

1. **Sore nipples** are almost always due to shallow latch (the infant sucking on the tip of the nipple rather than farther back on the areola). Correct positioning should be demonstrated for the mother. Interventions include nursing first on the least sore side, bathing nipples in breastmilk and allowing them to air-dry after nursing or pumping, and avoiding the use of drying agents such as soaps or lotions on the nipples. Purified lanolin, applied sparingly 3 or 4 times per day with the mother's milk, may hasten healing. It does not need to be washed off before feeding.. Hydrogel dressings or breast shells worn between feedings may be helpful. When nipple damage is severe, the mother should uses a breastpump and the infant fed expressed milk while the nipples heal. Nipple shields can be used to protect sore nipples.
2. **Engorgement** may present at 2 to 5 days postpartum as bilateral generalized breast swelling. The breasts become hard and do not always soften with feeding. Infants often have difficulty latching on. The mother may have a low-grade fever and usually experiences discomfort. If untreated, engorgement can lead to decreasing milk supply and plugged ducts. Frequent breastfeeding is the best prevention and treatment for engorgement. Full breasts should be emptied frequently (every 2 to 3 hours). The use of heat and massage may facilitate milk removal. If breasts are engorged, it may be helpful to hand express or pump for a few minutes to soften the areola and evert the nipple before nursing. Applying ice packs to breasts for 5 to 10 minutes before and after feeding and/or pumping decreases edema and promotes milk flow. Engorgement usually resolves within 24 hours with treatment.
3. **Plugged ducts** present as isolated, tender lumps in an otherwise well mother. Heat and massage applied to the area before and during breastfeeding may facilitate drainage. Positioning the infant's jaw toward the plugged duct may help release the plug during feeding. Prevention includes frequent milk removal and avoiding potential interference with removal, such as underwire bras or constrictive clothing. If untreated, plugged ducts can lead to mastitis.
4. **Mastitis** usually presents after the initial postpartum period as an erythematous, painful, hardened area in the breast. Mothers are usually febrile and have flulike symptoms. Mothers with mastitis should continue breastfeeding and contact their physician who will prescribe the appropriate antibiotic. Most antibiotics are compatible with breastfeeding.
5. **Topical or intraductal candidiasis** can occur. Symptoms include itching, burning, and shooting pain in the breast that is not associated with feeding. A fine, pinpoint-raised red shiny rash may occur on the nipple and areola. Susceptibility is increased in mothers with cracked nipples and

those who received antibiotics during pregnancy or after delivery. Prevention includes keeping the nipples as dry as possible between feeds, and changing pads that absorb leaking milk frequently. Treatment includes a topical antifungal agent. Infections that do not respond to topical therapy are considered intraductal and require systemic treatment. The infant of an affected mother should be treated with an oral antifungal agent, even if there are no symptoms. Breastfeeding can continue if both mother and infant are treated. Breast milk that is pumped while the mother is infected should be discarded.

VI. Special situations.

A. Hyperbilirubinemia is not a contraindication to breastfeeding. Frequent breastfeeding should be encouraged to enhance gut motility and bilirubin excretion. (See Chap. 18, Neonatal Hyperbilirubinemia.)

B. Hypoglycemia can usually be prevented in term infants with early, frequent breastfeeding.

C. Near-term infants (35 to 37 weeks) may not be developmentally able to breastfeed consistently like term infants. They may require supplementation for 2 to 3 weeks until their feeding abilities mature. Weighing the infant before and after feeding may help determine appropriate volumes and frequency of supplementation. Mothers should pump after feedings to help initiate and maintain an adequate supply; this milk can be used for supplementation while the baby matures.

D. Cesarean delivery and anesthesia should not cause a delay in breastfeeding once the mother is alert enough to hold the infant safely. However, maternal anesthesia may reduce the infant's level of alertness and ability to feed. Also, maternal intravenous fluid may lead to edema of breast tissue and make it more difficult for the infant to latch on. Because pain may inhibit the letdown reflex, analgesics should not be discouraged.

E. Multiple births. These infants are able to breastfeed because the supply of milk increases to meet the demand.

F. Birth defects. Infants with birth defects can often benefit from breastfeeding but may need special management.

1. Ankyloglossia (tongue tie). Severe ankyloglossia may interfere with nursing, although indications for and timing of frenectomy are controversial.

2. Craniofacial anomalies. Infants with cleft lip/palate may have difficulty latching on to the breast. Assistance with positioning and devices may help achieve a complete seal.

3. Cardiac defects. Infants with cardiac defects who become stressed or fatigued during nursing may require more frequent feedings for shorter durations. An upright position may improve comfort with feeding.

4. Developmental and neurological problems. Poor muscle tone, weak suckling, and sleepiness may interfere with nursing. These infants often require supplementation.

VII. Premature and hospitalized infants.
Mothers of premature infants should be encouraged to provide breast milk for their infants because of the nutritional and other health advantages over formula feedings. (See Chap. 10, Nutrition.)

A. Initiating and maintaining lactation. Mothers must pump in order to establish and maintain an adequate supply of milk. An adequate milk volume is defined as 18 to 20 oz of milk over a 24-hour period at 2 weeks postpartum.

1. Pumping should begin as soon after delivery as possible, preferably within 6 hours.

2. Mothers should pump frequently, at least 8 to 12 times per 24 hours. Simultaneous pumping of both breasts is most efficient. Pumping should last 10 to 15 minutes during the first few days. Once the breasts fill with milk, pumping should continue for 1 to 2 minutes after milk flow stops to empty the breasts and remove the high fat hindmilk.

3. Mothers should use the best available pump, preferably a hospital-grade electric breastpump (e.g., Medela Classic) with a double collection kit.

Vacuum should be sufficient to just draw the nipple into the tunnel and to make milk flow. Increased vacuum will not yield more milk, but may lead to nipple damage.

B. Delay or decrease in milk production. Onset of lactation may be delayed for up to a week in women with complications of pregnancy such as hemorrhage, hypertension, infection, preterm labor, and cesarean delivery. Stress and fatigue can also cause the milk supply to fluctuate.

1. Mothers should be reassured that milk volume will eventually increase if they continue to pump diligently.
2. Kangaroo care (skin-to-skin holding) may help increase milk supply.
3. Herbs (fenugreek, blessed thistle) and medications (metoclopromide, domperidone) have been used as galactagogues with varying results. These medications are not approved in the United States for this indication.

C. Storage of breast milk. (See Table 11.1)

1. Expressed breast milk should be stored in small sterile containers. Glass or hard plastic is preferred to plastic bags for storage in the hospital. The container should be labeled with the infant's name, medical record number, date and time pumped, and any maternal medication. A new container should be used for each pumping session.
2. Fresh milk should be refrigerated after it is expressed until it is frozen or used. Frozen milk should not be allowed to thaw during transport.
3. Expressed breastmilk should be warmed or thawed in a warm water bath. Microwave heating of breast milk is not recommended. Milk that has been warmed and not used should be discarded.

D. Early feedings at the breast

1. **Expectations.** Premature infants can be put to breast as soon as they are extubated and stable. These sessions should be regarded as "getting acquainted." Although nearly all nutrition will come from gavage feedings, these sessions allow the mother to become comfortable holding the baby and provide the breast as the baby's first oral experience. They also motivate many mothers to continue pumping.
   a. Expectations should be based on gestational and developmental ability. In general, infants do not breastfeed consistently well until they reach 38 to 40 weeks postmenstrual age.
   b. An early feeding typically lasts only a few minutes. Following that, a gavage feeding should be given.
   c. If the baby cannot coordinate oral feeding well, the mother can pump before putting the baby to breast.
   d. Mothers should put their babies to breast with each visit as tolerated.

TABLE 11.1. RECOMMENDATIONS FOR STORAGE OF BREAST MILK FOR AN INFANT IN THE NICU

Room temperature	1 h
Refrigerator (<4° C <39° F)	Store fresh milk up to 48 h
Thawed frozen milk	Store in refrigerator up to 24 h
Milk with additives	Store in refrigerator up to 24 h
Freezer compartment (<−20° C <−4° F)	Store up to 3 months
Deep freezer (<−20° C <−4° F)	Store up to 3 months

2. **Nipple shields.** Silicone nipple shields may help premature infants to achieve and maintain latch and increase the volume of milk intake. The need should be assessed on an individual basis. Nipple shields should be considered only after infants have developed the ability to coordinate sucking, swallowing, and breathing. Milk supply and infant growth should be monitored closely.

3. **Supplementation.** Premature infants often require supplementation of nursing and continued fortification of breast milk because of increased nutritional requirements. Supplementation with nasogastric tube feeding is preferred in the hospital. After discharge, supplementation is usually provided by bottle (preferably slow flow), although other methods, such as cupfeeding, fingerfeeding, spoonfeeding, and supplemental nutrition system at the breast, are sometimes used.

4. **Test weights.** Weighing the infant before and after feeding may help to plan the volume and frequency of supplementation required and validate the mother's assessment of the sufficiency of nursing.

E. **Discharge planning.** Few premature infants are discharged from the NICU exclusively breastfeeding because discharge often occurs before breastfeeding behaviors are developmentally mature. The discharge feeding plan should consider the infant's gestational age at birth, postmenstrual age at discharge, the mother's breastfeeding goals and milk supply, and observations of the baby at breast during hospitalization. Parents should be comfortable and confident in the plan.

1. The pediatrician should provide close follow-up until supplementation is no longer needed. The pediatrician should see the infant within a day or two of discharge to assess the weight and revise the breastfeeding plan if indicated. A visiting nurse, if available, should see the mother and baby the day after discharge to assess breastfeeding and check the weight.

2. The mother should continue to pump to maintain her milk supply until the baby is breastfeeding well and no longer needs supplements.

VIII. **Medications.** Medications taken by a lactating mother often can appear in her milk. In general, if medication is safe to administer to an infant, it is safe to give to a lactating woman. (See Appendix B.)

A. The amount of drug transferred to the infant through breast milk depends on a number of factors, including maternal dose, frequency and duration of administration, absorption, and distribution characteristics of the drug. The concentration of drug in the infant is usually less than a therapeutic dose.

B. The potential effect on the infant of a medication taken by the mother is influenced by the infant's maturity, postnatal age, clinical issues, and pattern of breastfeeding.

C. Physicians caring for breastfed infants should be aware of potential interactions of drugs that the mother and infant are receiving.

D. When appropriate medications are prescribed for a lactating woman, the benefits of breastfeeding should be weighed against the infant's risk of exposure to the drug. In most cases, the benefits far exceed the risks.

Professional Resources

Hale T.W. *Medications and Mothers' Milk.* Amarillo, Tex.: Pharmasoft Publishing, 2000.

Lawrence R.A., Lawrence R.M. *Breastfeeding: A Guide for the Medical Profession.* St. Louis, Mo.: Mosby, 1999.

Mohrbacher N., Stock J. *The Breastfeeding Answer Book.* Schaumburg, Ill.: La Leche League International, 2002.

Riordan J., Auerbach K.G. (Eds.). *Breastfeeding and Human Lactation.* Boston: Jones and Bartlett, 1998.

Parent Resources

Meek J.Y. (Ed.). *American Academy of Pediatrics New Mother's Guide to Breastfeeding*. New York, Bantam Books, 2002.

Cox S. *Breastfeeding: I Can Do That*. Tasmania, Australia: TasLaC, 1997.

Huggins K. *The Nursing Mother's Companion*. Boston: The Harvard Common Press, 1999.

La Leche League International. *The Womanly Art of Breastfeeding*. Schaumburg, Ill.: La Leche League International, 1999.

Internet Resources

International Lactation Consultants Association (www.Ilca.org)

La Leche League International (www.Lalecheleague.org)

Texas Tech University School of Medicine—Breastfeeding pharmacology (www. neonatal.ttuhsc.edu/lact/)

Academy of Breastfeeding Medicine (www. Bfmed.org)

12. TEMPERATURE CONTROL

Kimberlee Chatson

I. **Heat production.** Thermoregulation in adults is achieved by both metabolic and muscular activity (e.g., shivering). During pregnancy, maternal mechanisms maintain intrauterine temperature. After birth, newborns must adapt to their relatively cold environment by the metabolic production of heat because they are not able to generate an adequate shivering response.

Term newborns have a source for thermogenesis in brown fat, which is highly vascularized and innervated by sympathetic neurons. When these infants face cold stress, norepinephrine levels increase and act in the brown-fat tissue to stimulate lipolysis. Most of the free fatty acids (FFAs) are reesterified or oxidized; both reactions produce heat. Hypoxia or beta-adrenergic blockade decreases this response.

II. **Temperature maintenance**

A. **Premature infants** have special problems in temperature maintenance that put them at a disadvantage compared to term infants. These include:

1. A higher ratio of skin surface area to weight.
2. Decreased subcutaneous fat, with less insulative capacity.
3. Less-developed stores of brown fat.
4. The inability to take in enough calories to provide nutrients for thermogenesis and growth.
5. Limitation of oxygen consumption in some preterm infants because of pulmonary problems.

B. **Cold stress.** Premature infants subjected to acute hypothermia respond with peripheral vasoconstriction, causing anaerobic metabolism and metabolic acidosis, which can cause pulmonary vessel constriction, leading to further hypoxemia, anaerobic metabolism, and acidosis. Hypoxemia further compromises the infant's response to cold. Premature infants are therefore at great risk for hypothermia and its sequelae (i.e., hypoglycemia, metabolic acidosis, increased oxygen consumption). The more common problem facing premature infants is caloric loss from unrecognized chronic cold stress, resulting in excess oxygen consumption and inability to gain weight.

C. **Neonatal cold injury** occurs in low-birth-weight infants (LBWs) and term infants with central nervous system (CNS) disorders. It occurs more often in home deliveries, emergency deliveries, and settings where inadequate attention is paid to the thermal environment and heat loss. These infants may have a bright red color because of the failure of oxyhemoglobin to dissociate at low temperature. There may be central pallor or cyanosis. The skin may show edema and sclerema. Core temperature is often below 32.2°C (90°F). Signs may include the following: (1) hypotension, (2) bradycardia, (3) slow, shallow, irregular respiration, (4) decreased activity, (5) poor sucking reflex, (6) decreased response to stimulus, (7) decreased reflexes, and (8) abdominal distention or vomiting. Metabolic acidosis, hypoglycemia, hyperkalemia, azotemia, and oliguria are present. Sometimes there is generalized bleeding, including pulmonary hemorrhage. It is uncertain whether warming should be rapid or slow. Setting the abdominal skin temperature to 1°C higher than the core temperature in a radiant warmer will produce slow rewarming and setting it to 36.5°C will result in slow rewarming. If the infant is hypotensive, normal saline (10 to 20 mL/kg) should be given; sodium bicarbonate is used to correct metabolic acidosis. Infection, bleeding, or injury should be evaluated and treated.

D. **Hyperthermia,** defined as an elevated core body temperature, may be caused by a relatively hot environment, infection, dehydration, CNS dysfunction, or medications. Placing newborns in sunlight to control bilirubin is hazardous and may be associated with significant hyperthermia.

TABLE 12.1. NEUTRAL THERMAL ENVIRONMENTAL TEMPERATURES

Age and weight	Temperature*	
	At start (°C)	Range (°C)
0–6 hours		
Under 1200 g	35.0	34.0–35.4
1200–1500 g	34.1	33.9–34.4
1501–2500 g	33.4	32.8–33.8
Over 2500 g (and >36 weeks' gestation)	32.9	32.0–33.8
6–12 h		
Under 1200 g	35.0	34.0–35.4
1200–1500 g	34.0	33.5–34.4
1501–2500 g	33.1	32.2–33.8
Over 2500 g (and >36 weeks' gestation)	32.8	31.4–33.8
12–24 h		
Under 1200 g	34.0	34.0–35.4
1200–1500 g	33.8	33.3–34.3
1501–2500 g	32.8	31.8–33.8
Over 2500 g (and >36 weeks' gestation)	32.4	31.0–33.7
24–36 h		
Under 1200 g	34.0	34.0–35.0
1200–1500 g	33.6	33.1–34.2
1501–2500 g	32.6	31.6–33.6
Over 2500 g (and >36 weeks' gestation)	32.1	30.7–33.5
36–48 h		
Under 1200 g	34.0	34.0–35.0
1200–1500 g	33.5	33.0–34.1
1501–2500 g	32.5	31.4–33.5
Over 2500 g (and >36 weeks' gestation)	31.9	30.5–33.3
48–72 h		
Under 1200 g	34.0	34.0–35.0
1200–1500 g	33.5	33.0–34.0
1501–2500 g	32.3	31.2–33.4
Over 2500 g (and >36 weeks' gestation)	31.7	30.1–33.2

(continues)

TABLE 12.1. *(continued)*

Age and weight	Temperature*	
	At start (°C)	Range (°C)
72–96 h		
Under 1200 g	34.0	34.0–35.0
1200–1500 g	33.5	33.0–34.0
1501–2500 g	32.2	31.1–33.2
Over 2500 g (and >36 weeks' gestation)	31.3	29.8–32.8
4–12 days		
Under 1500 g	33.5	33.0–34.0
1501–2500 g	32.1	31.0–33.2
Over 2500 g (and >36 weeks' gestation)		
4–5 days	31.0	29.5–32.6
5–6 days	30.9	29.4–32.3
6–8 days	30.6	29.0–32.2
8–10 days	30.3	29.0–31.8
10–12 days	30.1	29.0–31.4
12–14 days		
Under 1500 g	33.5	32.6–34.0
1501–2500 g	32.1	31.0–33.2
Over 2500 g (and >36 weeks' gestation)	29.8	29.0–30.8
2–3 weeks		
Under 1500 g	33.1	32.2–34.0
1501–2500 g	31.7	30.5–33.0
3–4 weeks		
Under 1500 g	32.6	31.6–33.6
1501–2500 g	31.4	30.0–32.7
4–5 weeks		
Under 1500 g	32.0	31.2–33.0
1501–2500 g	30.9	29.5–35.2
5–6 weeks		
Under 1500 g	31.4	30.6–32.3
1501–2500 g	30.4	29.0–31.8

*In their version of this table, Scopes and Ahmed (*Arch Dis Child* 1966;47:417–419) had the walls of the incubator 1–2° C warmer than ambient air temperatures. Generally speaking, the smaller infants in each weight group will require a temperature in the higher portion of the temperature range. Within each time range, the younger infants require the higher temperatures. Source: Klaus M., Fanaroff A. The physical environment, in *Care of the High Risk Neonate,* 5th ed. Philadelphia: Saunders, 2001.

If environmental temperature is the cause of hyperthermia, the trunk and extremities are the same temperature and the infant appears vasodilated. In contrast, infants with sepsis are often vasoconstricted and the extremities are 2 to 3°C colder than the trunk.

III. Mechanisms of heat loss

    A. Radiation. Heat dissipates from the infant to a colder object in the environment.

    B. Convection. Heat is lost from the skin to moving air. The amount lost depends on air speed and temperature.

    C. Evaporation. The amount of loss depends primarily on air velocity and relative humidity. Wet infants in the delivery room are especially susceptible to evaporative heat loss.

    D. Conduction. This is a minor mechanism of heat loss that occurs from the infant to the surface on which he or she lies.

IV. Neutral thermal environments minimize heat loss. Thermoneutral conditions exist when heat production (measured by oxygen consumption) is minimum and core temperature is within the normal range (see Table 12.1).

V. Management to prevent heat loss

    A. Healthy infant

        1. Newborns should be dried and wrapped in a warmed blanket after delivery.

        2. Examination in the delivery room should be done with the infant under a radiant warmer. A skin probe with servocontrol to keep skin temperature at 36.5°C (97.7°F) should be used for prolonged examinations.

        3. A cap is very useful in preventing significant heat loss through the scalp.

        4. If the temperature is stable, the infant can be placed in a crib with blankets.

    B. Sick infant

        1. The infant should be dried.

        2. A heated incubator should be used for transport.

        3. A radiant warmer should be used during procedures.

        4. Sick or premature infants require a thermoneutral environment to minimize energy expenditure; the incubator should be kept at an appropriate temperature (see Table 12.1) if a skin probe cannot be used because of the potential damage to skin in small premature infants.

        5. Servocontrolled open warmer beds may be used for very sick infants when access is important. The use of a tent made of plastic wrap is effective in preventing both convection heat loss and insensible water loss (see Chap. 9, Fluid and Electrolyte Management).

        6. Double-walled incubators limit radiant heat loss.

        7. Premature infants in relatively stable condition can be dressed in clothes and caps and covered with a blanket. We try to do this as soon as possible even if the infant is on a ventilator. Heart rate and respiration should be continuously monitored because the clothing may limit observation.

VI. Hazards of temperature control methods

    A. Hyperthermia. A servocontrolled warmer can generate excess heat, causing severe hyperthermia if the probe becomes detached from the infant's skin. Temperature alarms are subject to mechanical failure.

    B. Undetected infections. Servocontrol of temperature may mask the hypothermia or hyperthermia associated with infection. A record of both environmental and core temperatures, along with observation for other signs of sepsis, will help detect this problem.

    C. Volume depletion. Radiant warmers can cause increased insensible water loss. Body weight and input and output should be closely monitored in infants cared for on radiant warmers.

Suggested Readings

Klaus M. A., Martin R. J., Fanaroff A. A. (Eds.). The physical environment. In *Care of the High Risk Neonate*, 5th Ed. Philadelphia, Saunders, 2001.

Sinclair, J. C. Servo-control for maintaining abdominal skin termperature at 36°C in low-birth-weight infants. *Cochrane Database Syst Rev* 2002;(1):CD001074.

13. NEONATAL TRANSPORT

Robert M. Insoft

I. **Indications**
   A. Interhospital transport should be considered if the medical resources or personnel needed for a high-risk infant are not available at the hospital currently providing care. Ideally, the pregnant mother should be transferred before delivery to a high-risk perinatal center capable of caring for both her and her newborn when a problem is known or arises in early labor. If a high-risk newborn is delivered at a hospital without advanced services, a medical team should be available that is capable of performing the initial stabilization.
   B. Transfer to the regional neonatal tertiary center should be expedited following initial stabilization. Medical personnel from the referring center should contact their affiliated Neonatal Intensive Care Unit (NICU) transport service to arrange transfer and agree upon a treatment plan to optimize patient care prior to the transport team's arrival at the referring center.
   C. **Criteria for neonatal transfer** depend on the capability of the hospital. Conditions that require transfer to a center that provides neonatal intensive care include:
      1. Prematurity and/or birth weight <1500 g.
      2. Gestational age < 32 weeks.
      3. Respiratory distress requiring ventilatory support (CPAP, ventilation).
      4. Seizures.
      5. Congenital anomalies and/or inborn errors of metabolism.
      6. Congenital heart disease or cardiac arrhythmias requiring cardiac services.
      7. Severe hypoxic-ischemic injury.
      8. Other conditions requiring neonatology consultation and consideration of transfer.
         a. Severe hyperbilirubinemia possibly requiring exchange transfusion.
         b. Infant of diabetic mothers.
         c. Severe intrauterine growth restriction.
         d. Birth weight between 1500 and 2000 g and gestational age between 32 and 36 weeks.
         e. Procedures unavailable at referring hospital.
II. **Organization of Transport Services**
   A. All hospitals with established maternity services should have **agreements** with regional perinatal centers outlining criteria for perinatal consultations and neonatal transfer.
   B. The regional NICU transport team should have an appointed **Medical Director.** Neonatologists should monitor the protocols and procedures carried out by the team.
   C. **Transport teams** consist of a combination of at least two or three trained personnel. Advanced practice nurses, neonatal nurse practitioners, respiratory therapists, and physicians may be team members. Senior resident and subspecialty fellows provide the physician component for many teams. Skills of team members must be assessed and arrangements made for advice and supervision. Each transport should be supervised by a medical control officer, who may be the attending neonatologist.
   D. **Modes of transport** include ambulance, helicopter, or fixed-wing aircraft depending on distance, acuity, and geography. Some hospitals own, maintain, and insure ambulances or helicopters. Other hospitals contract with commercial ambulance or rotor-wing services that can accommodate a transport incubator and appropriate equipment.
   E. **Equipment.** The team should be self-sufficient in terms of equipment, medications, and other supplies. Packs especially designed for neonatal transport are

TABLE 13.1. TRANSPORT TEAM EQUIPMENT

Transport incubator equipped with monitors for heart rate, vascular pressures, oxygen saturation, temperature

Suction device

Infusion pumps

Gel-filled mattress

Adaptors to plug into both hospital and vehicle power

Airway equipment

Anesthesia bag with manometer

Laryngoscopes with no. 0 and no. 1 blades

Magill forceps

Instrument tray for chest tubes and vascular catheters

Stethoscope

Tanks of oxygen and compressed air oxygen, compressed air, heat, light, and a source of electrical power

The carrier must be ready to depart within 30 min

---

commercially available. These packs or other containers should be stocked by members of the transport team. The weight of the stocked packs should be documented for air transport. (see Tables 13.1, 13.2, and 13.3).

   F. **Legal issues.** The transport process may raise legal issues, which vary from state to state. We periodically review all routine procedures and documentation forms with hospital legal counsel and provide the team with access to legal advice by phone when problems occur.

   G. **Malpractice insurance coverage** is required for all team members. The tertiary hospital should decide whether transport is considered an off-site or extended on-site activity because this can affect the necessary coverage.

   H. **Carrier regulations** vary from state to state and may conflict with transport goals. For example, some states require that an ambulance stop at the scene of an unattended accident until a second ambulance arrives. If this is an issue, it should be reviewed with the medical director of the commercial carrier.

III. Referring Hospital Responsibilities

   A. **Documentation.** A complete transfer note should be available at time of transfer. Initial transport consent should be obtained by the referring hospital staff and documented in the patient's medical record. Any risk to the patient for communicable diseases must be disclosed to the tertiary center. We recommend that a senior pediatric clinician remain in attendance until the patient leaves the referring hospital with the transport team.

   B. If the patient is known prior to transfer to require a specialized medical and/or surgical service (e.g., surfactant, nitric oxide, surgery, extracorporeal membrane oxygenation [ECMO]), the referring hospital and transport team staff should ensure that the service is available at the referral center. If it is not, alternative tertiary centers should be considered for that patient.

   C. The speed of the transfer should never take precedence over ensuring the correct level of transport staff and accepting facilities for a critically ill neonatal patient.

IV. Transport Team Responsibilities

   A. The referral center should provide a team of skilled personnel and appropriate equipment.

TABLE 13.2. SUPPLIES USED BY TRANSPORT TEAMS

Airways	Kelly clamp
Alcohol swabs	Lubricating ointment
Armboards	Monitor leads and transducers
Batteries	Needles: 18, 20, 26 gauge
Benzoin	Oxygen tubing
Betadine swabs	Replogle nasogastric tube
Blood culture bottles	Scalpel blades, no. 11
Blood pressure cuff	Sterile gown
Butterfly needles: 23 and 25 gauge	Stopcocks
Chest tubes: 10 and 12F, and connectors	Stylus
Chemstrip	Suction catheters: 6, 8, and 10F and traps
Clipboard with transport data	Suture material (silk 3-0, 4-0, on curved needle)
forms, permission forms, progress notes, and booklet for parents	
Culture tubes	Syringes: 1, 3, 10, 50 mL
Endotracheal tubes: 2.5, 3.0, 3.5, 4.0 mm	Tape
Face mask, term and premature	T-connectors
Feeding tubes: 5 and 8F	Thermometer
Gauze pads	Tubes for blood specimens
Gloves, sterile and exam	Umbilical catheters: 3.5 and 5F (double lumen)
Heimlich valves	Urine collection bags
Intravenous tubing	Xeroform gauze
Intravenous catheters: 22 and 24 gauge	

B. The medical control officer or attending neonatologist should discuss the patient's condition and potential therapies with team members prior to departure. Recommendations should focus on respiratory, cardiovascular, and metabolic stabilization. Interventions concerning airway management and vascular access should be specific. All recommendations should be documented.

C. The team should obtain consent for transfer as well as any other anticipated procedures upon arrival to the NICU.

D. Team members should introduce themselves clearly and politely to the referring hospital staff and family members. Appropriate photo identification should be worn.

E. Transfer of patient information (sign out) should be clear and there should be agreement on when the transport team assumes responsibility for management.

F. The team should work collegially with the referring hospital staff and be objective in their assessment and stabilization. The referring staff should be included in as much of the care as appropriate.

TABLE 13.3. MEDICATIONS USED ON TRANSPORT

Albumin 5%	Gentamicin
Ampicillin	Heparin
Atropine	Isoproterenol
Calcium	Lidocaine
Calcium gluconate	Midazolan
Dexamethasone	Morphine
Dextrose 50% in water	Naloxone
Dextrose 10% in water	Normal saline
Diphenylhydantoin	Pancuronium
Digoxin	Phenobarbital
Dobutamine	Potassium chloride
Dopamine	Prostaglandin E_1 (on ice)
Epinephrine	Sodium bicarbonate
Erythromycin eye ointment	Sterile water
Fentanyl	Vitamin K_1

G. The referring and primary physicians should be identified and their names documented.

H. The parents should have time to see their newborn before the team leaves the referring hospital. We take instant photos for the parents to keep.

I. The team's policy regarding parents traveling with their newborn on transport should be reviewed with the family. We allow one parent to travel by ambulance as long as all team members agree that the family member will not interfere with medical care. The team should have policies regarding the presence of parents during air transport.

J. The team should call back the referring hospital staff after the transport is complete with pertinent follow-up while respecting the confidentiality of the patient and family.

K. Outreach education should be provided to referring hospital staff in the form of transport conferences, in-service presentations, and case reviews.

V. **Medical management prior to transport**

A. The tertiary center should mobilize their transport team as soon as possible. While the transport team is en route, the responsible neonatologist should discuss additional treatment strategies with the referring hospital staff.

B. The referring staff should stabilize the patient in conjunction with recommendations from the transport medical control officer or neonatologist. While awaiting the transport team, the referring staff should:

1. Maintain airway, oxygenation, and thermal stability.
2. Normalize circulatory deficits.
3. Maintain adequate blood glucose concentration.
4. Secure umbilical venous access, if appropriate.
5. Secure umbilical arterial access, if appropriate.
6. Obtain appropriate cultures and give first doses of antibiotics.
7. Insert a nasogastric tube and decompress the stomach.
8. Have a recent chest X ray and other applicable studies available.
9. Obtain initial transport consent from parents.

10. Maximize the parents' ability to be near their newborn.
11. Obtain copies of obstetrical and neonatal charts for the transport team.

VI. **Returning to the NICU.** If the patient has been stabilized, most return trips are uneventful. Continuous direct observation of the infant is one of the most important forms of monitoring. During the transport, the benefit of handling the patient and taking vital signs must be weighed against the possibility of an accidental extubation or thermal loss incurred by opening the transport incubator. We prepare in advance all medications and intravenous. fluids that may be needed during the transport. Many teams routinely use wireless telephones or direct radios to maintain contact with the NICU and seek advice for unexpected events.

VII. **Arrival at the NICU**
   A. The team should give the NICU caregivers a complete sign-out and copies of charts, consents, and X rays.
   B. A team member should telephone the parents to tell them their child has arrived safely.
   C. All transport medications should be immediately restocked and all equipment checked and secured for subsequent calls.
   D. A team member should telephone the referring and primary physicians to inform them of the patient's status and who will be providing further communication.
   E. Quality assurance documentation used to monitor transport activities should be done immediately and the team's medical director notified of any issues that require follow-up.

VIII. **Special medical conditions and therapies**
   A. Most infants with **congenital diaphragmatic hernia** require immediate intubation and mechanical ventilation. Placement of a nasogastric tube prevents gaseous distention of herniated viscera during respiratory support.
   B. When **cyanotic congenital heart disease** is a possible diagnosis, prostaglandin E_1 (PGE_1) must be available during transport. Ideally, treatment should be initiated at the referring hospital and administered through a central venous catheter, such as an umbilical venous catheter. Apnea, hypothermia, and hypotension are common side effects of PGE_1. Endotracheal intubation is usually warranted for transport of an infant requiring PGE_1 infusion.
   C. **Anemia** may result from a variety of conditions, including fetal-maternal hemorrhage, abruption, hydrops fetalis, and twin-to-twin transfusion. Acute blood loss may not be reflected in a hematocrit drop for several hours but may be suggested by the history and clinical presentation. In such cases, cross-matching of blood should begin at the referring hospital while the transport team is en route. Infants in urgent need of a transfusion can be given non-cross-matched type O-negative packed cells until matched blood is available.
   D. **Abdominal wall defects:** Both gastroschisis and omphalocele are treated by placing a nasogastric tube and immediately wrapping exposed abdominal contents with warm, sterile, saline-soaked (noncling) gauze. We use an outer wrapping with a plastic bag or plastic wrap to decrease heat and insensible water losses.
   E. **Tracheoesophageal fistula and esophageal atresia.** A Replogle-type (sump) tube should be placed gently in the esophageal pouch to minimize the risk of aspiration. Positive-pressure ventilation should be avoided if possible in order to avoid overdistention of the GI tract.
   F. **Neural tube defects** should be wrapped in warm, sterile, saline-soaked noncling gauze and plastic wrap for protection and to minimize heat and fluid loss, as well as to prevent contamination with stool.
   G. Premature infants with respiratory distress syndrome (RDS) and newborns with other disorders may require **surfactant administration.** We have adopted our NICU-based protocols for surfactant administration on transport. The transport team should consult the medical control physician prior to surfactant administration, and the consultation should be documented. After

TABLE 13.4. FiO₂ REQUIRED TO MAINTAIN A CONSTANT PaO₂ AT INCREASING ALTITUDE

Sea Level	F_iO_2 at Altitude (ft) of									
	2000	4000	6000	8000	10,000	12,000	14,000	16,000	18,000	20,000
0.21	0.23	0.24	0.27	0.29	0.31	0.34	0.37	0.41	0.45	0.49
0.30	0.32	0.35	0.38	0.41	0.45	0.49	0.53	0.59	0.64	0.71
0.40	0.43	0.47	0.51	0.55	0.60	0.65	0.71	0.78	0.85	0.94
0.50	0.54	0.58	0.63	0.69	0.75	0.81	0.89	0.98		
0.60	0.65	0.70	0.76	0.83	0.99	0.98				
0.70	0.76	0.82	0.89	0.96						
0.80	0.86	0.94								
0.90	0.97									
1.00										

Key: FiO₂ = fractional concentration of inspired oxygen; PaO₂ = arterial oxygen tension.

administration, we wait at least 30 minutes prior to moving the newborn to the transport incubator. This provides time for direct observation and initial ventilatory changes, thus minimizing the risk of morbidity such as a plugged endotracheal tube or a pneumothorax from acute changes in compliance.

IX. **Air transports**

   A. **Changes in barometric pressure.** Barometric pressure decreases as altitude increases, leading to a decrease in oxygen tension. This is important even in aircraft with pressurized cabins because pressure is usually maintained at a level equal to 8000 to 10,000 feet above sea level. To correct for this, FiO_2 must be increased to result in an adequate PaO_2. Oxygen saturation should be continuously monitored and FiO_2 adjusted as needed.. If oxygen saturation monitoring is unavailable, PaO_2 can be estimated using the alveolar gas equation. Values of FiO_2 needed to maintain a constant PaO_2 at any altitude are shown in Table 13.4.

   B. **Gas expansion.** As barometric pressure decreases with increasing altitude, gases trapped in closed spaces will expand. Even a small pneumothorax or the normal gaseous distention of the gastrointestinal (GI) tract may result in clinical deterioration and should be drained or vented with a nasogastric tube before an air transport.

X. **Nitric oxide**

   A. Inhaled nitric oxide (iNO) reduces the need for ECMO in critically ill term or near-term infants with pulmonary hypertension and hypoxemic respiratory failure. In some cases (e.g., anticipated prolonged transport time or rapid deterioration of the patient), it may be appropriate to begin Ino treatment on transport. In patients already receiving Ino, treatment should be continued if transfer to an ECMO center is required.

   B. Protocols should be developed by each transport team for the use of iNO. The protocol should be acceptable to all associated ambulance and aircraft vendors and referral hospital staff.

   C. A certified neonatal respiratory therapist or other appropriately trained team member should be responsible for the administration of iNO on transport, including management of the needed equipment. Initiation of iNO at the referring hospital or during the transport should be done with the supervision of the responsible transport medical control physician or neonatologist.

   D. Prior to initiating iNO therapy on transport, we document the presence of pulmonary hypertension by echocardiogram or a difference in preductal and postductal oxygen saturation (See Persistent Pulmonary Hypertension of the Newborn, Chap. 24). Nitric oxide should not be used for newborns who have or are highly suspected to have certain congenital heart disease.

Suggested Readings

American Academy of Pediatrics. *Guidelines for Air and Ground Transport of Neonatal and Pediatric Patients.* Elk Grove Village, Ill.: American Academy of Pediatrics, 1999.

Krug S.E. Principles and Philosophy of Transport Stabilization. In McCloskey K., Orr R. (Eds.). *Pediatric Transport Medicine.* St. Louis: Mosby, 1995, 132–142.

Insoft R.M. Neonatal Transport. In Finberg L., Kleinman R. (Eds.). *Saunders Manual of Pediatric Practice.* Philadelphia: Harcourt, 2002.

Insoft R.M. The Use of Inhaled Nitric Oxide in Neonatal Transport. In Jaimovich D.G., Vidyasagar D. (Eds.). *The Handbook of Pediatric and Neonatal Transport Medicine.* Philadelphia: Hanley and Belfus, 2002.

14. DEVELOPMENTALLY SUPPORTIVE CARE

Marie T. Field and Sandra L. Harmon

I. **Introduction.** Current research suggests that children born very prematurely suffer significantly higher incidences of long-term morbidity relative to cognitive and behavioral performance (1–4). Our challenge, as neonatal caregivers, is to cultivate interventions and an environment that optimize the care rendered to this fragile and still developing population. Developmentally supportive care (DSC) is an effective means of meeting this challenge. The pioneering work of Als and others (5–7) has provided a greater understanding of preterm infant brain development, preterm infant behavior, and the importance of individualized DSC. The belief is that employing the principles of DSC in a neonatal intensive care unit (NICU) environment will lead to improved neurodevelopmental outcomes in the preterm infant population (8).

II. **Neurobehavioral assessment.** Neurobehavioral assessment begins with an appreciation of an individual infant's level of organized functioning and threshold to stimulation and stress. Accurate identification of stress responses and self-regulating behaviors presented by a preterm infant are essential to formulating and modifying neurodevelopmentally supportive plans of care.

   A. **Stress responses.** Autonomic, motoric, state organizational behavior, and attentional/interactive signs of stress combine to provide a baseline profile of an infant's overall response to stimulation. Autonomic signs of stress include changes in color, heart rate, and respiratory patterns, as well as visceral changes, such as gagging, hiccupping, vomiting, and stooling. Motoric signs of stress include facial grimacing, gaping mouth, twitching, hyperextension of limbs, finger splaying, back arching, flailing, and generalized hypotonia. State alterations suggesting stress include rapid state transitions, diffuse sleep states, irritability, and lethargy. Changes in attention or the interactional availability of preterm infants, exhibited by covering eyes/face, gaze aversion, frowning, and hyperalert or panicked facial presentation, represent signs of stress.

   B. **Self-regulating behavior.** Preterm infants elicit a number of self-consoling behaviors that facilitate their coping responses to stress. Self-regulating behaviors include hand or feet bracing, sucking, hands to face, flexed positioning, cooing, and grasping of linens or their own body parts, such as thumbs.

III. **Developmentally supportive extrauterine environment.** Preterm exposure to an extrauterine environment during a time of rapid brain growth may adversely affect neurodevelopmental outcomes of preterm infants (8). The goal of DSC is to soften the gap between a mother's womb and the high-technology environment of a NICU. Neonatal caregivers can potentially minimize negative outcomes by providing preterm infants with a modified extrauterine environment designed to support neurologic and sensory development. In addition to the neurological and sensory supports, a developmentally supportive extrauterine environment must be designed to nurture parents and foster positive family growth and development.

   A. **Structuring the physical environment.** Noise reduction, soft lighting, limited bedside activity, and soothing visual surroundings are essential to a DSC physical environment. Preterm infants should be placed in an incubator as soon as medically possible. The incubator should be covered with a thick, dark-colored blanket to further reduce light and muffle environmental noise. Staff, family members, and visitors should be reminded to refrain from activities that disrupt the confines of the incubator (bumping into the incubator, placing items on top of incubator) or create unnecessary noise around the incubator (slamming doors, drawers, and trash can lids; loud voices; ringing telephones; unanswered alarms; loud music). When babies come out of their incubators for care or to be held, the environment around the baby must become as soft and as soothing as possible.

B. **Promoting the social environment.** Parents and other family members should be shown measures that will facilitate infant self-regulating behaviors, such as swaddling, suckling at breast, nonnutritive sucking on a pacifier, containment by holding the baby close in a flexed position against the body or during kangaroo care (skin-to-skin contact between parent and infant) visits. Provisions for comfortable family visits, such as the availability of rocking chairs and recliners at the bedside or private family areas, promote positive family development. Families should be encouraged to personalize their infant's bed space by providing items from home, such as family photos, quilts, soft infant blankets, clothes, and toys.

IV. **Developmentally supportive direct infant care practices.** Care plans must be designed to meet both the medical and developmental needs of the preterm infant. This can be accomplished through a coordinated, primary-team effort designed to cluster care and interventions around the infant's state of alertness, sleep cycles, and family visits. The goal is to maximize rest, minimize stress, and optimize healing and growth.

A. **Positioning.** Positioning of preterm infants should focus on comfort and self-regulatory competency. The use of "nesting materials," such as sheepskin and soft blanket rolls, as well as swaddling assists the infant in maintaining flexed posturing. Hands-on containment after a procedure assists the infant in transitioning to a restful sleep state. Positioning of preterm infants should focus on comfort and self-regulatory competency.

B. **Feeding.** Preterm infants can begin to breastfeed at as early as 28 weeks' gestation but are not generally mature enough to bottlefeed until 33 weeks or more. Infants should be swaddled and/or cuddled securely in a flexed, upright position for bottle feeding. Nipple choice should consider size and shape and rate of flow relative to the level of competence of each infant. The feeding environment should be relaxed and quiet with low lighting.

V. **Comfort and pain-relieving measures.** Preterm infants must endure many uncomfortable/painful procedures necessary to meet their medical needs. Freedom from pain is a basic right of *all* patients. Research suggests that providing continuous infusion of morphine to preterm infants requiring ventilatory support may decrease the incidence of poor neurological outcomes (9). Nonpharmacological interventions include swaddling, pacifiers, and administration of sucrose by nipple if the infant can suck and swallow (see Chap. 27).

VI. **Discharge planning.** Parents must be educated that brain development in preterm infants occurs at a slower rate than in babies born at term (3) and that a preterm infant cannot, therefore, be expected to behave as a term infant would. DSC must be continued at home as the preterm's central nervous system remains immature for several months past discharge from the NICU (10) (see Chap. 16).

VII. **Infant follow-up and early-intervention programs.** Research suggests that infants born prematurely are at high risk for long-term cognitive and developmental delay (4). Close follow-up is paramount to maximizing developmental outcome. At Brigham and Women's Hospital, all infants born at less than 32 weeks' gestation, as well as those with complex medical issues, are referred to state-run early-intervention programs. In addition, any infant born at less than 1500 g or having risk factors for long-term morbidity meets the criteria for the Infant Follow-up Program.

References

1. Huppi P., et al. Quantitative magnetic resonance imaging of brain development in premature and mature newborns. *Ann Neurol* 1998;43:224.
2. Huppi P., et al. Microstructural development of human newborn cerebral white matter assessed *in vivo* by diffusion tensor magnetic resonance imaging. *Pediatr Res* 1998;44:584.

3. Huppi P., et al. Structural and neurobehavioral delay in postnatal brain development of preterm infants. *Pediatr Res* 1996;39:895.
4. Peterson B., et al. Regional brain volume abnormalities and long-term cognitive outcome in preterm infants. *JAMA* 2000;284:1939.
5. Als H., et al. Individualized developmental care for the very low birth weight preterm infant. *JAMA* 1994;272:853.
6. McGrath J. Developmental physiology of the neurological system. *Central Lines* 2000;16:1.
7. Vandenberg K. Basic principles of developmental caregiving. *Neonatal Network* 1997;16:69.
8. Buehler D., et al. Effectiveness of individualized developmental care for low-risk preterm infants: Electrophysiologic evidence. *Pediatrics* 1995;96:923.
9. Anand K.J.S., et al. Analgesia and sedation in preterm neonates who require ventilatory support. *Arch Pediatr Adolesc Med* 1999;153:331.
10. Vandenberg K. What to tell parents about the developmental needs of their baby at discharge. *Neonatal Network* 1999;18:57.

15. FOLLOW-UP CARE OF VERY-LOW-BIRTH-WEIGHT INFANTS*

Jane E. Stewart

I. **Introduction.** The number of surviving very-low-birth-weight (VLBW) infants (birth weight < 1500 g) has increased from 1.21% to 1.43% live births from 1985 to 2000. Although this represents a small percentage of total births, approximately 58,000 VLBW infants were born in 2000, and an estimated 75% to 84% survived. These infants are at risk for sequelae of prematurity, including medical and developmental problems. Survival rates have also increased to 40% to 55% for extremely low-birth-weight (ELBW) infants (birth weight < 1000 g). ELBW infants are at the highest risk of long-term morbidity. VLBW infants have unique follow-up needs and often require utilization of special medical and educational resources.

II. **Medical issues**

A. **Respiratory problems and infections.** (see Chap. 24). Approximately 23% of VLBW infants and 35 to 46% of ELBW infants develop bronchopulmonary dysplasia (BPD). Infants with BPD have twice the risk of normal birth weight (NBW) infants of developing reactive airway disease, particularly in the setting of viral respiratory infections. They often require supplemental oxygen at home, as well as bronchodilator or diuretic therapy. Infants with severe BPD may require tracheostomy and long-term ventilator support. These infants are also at increased risk of feeding problems, gastroesophageal reflux, poor weight gain, and delays in achieving early developmental milestones.

1. **Hospitalizations.** VLBW infants are 4 times more likely to be rehospitalized during the first year than NBW infants, most often for complications of respiratory infections. Up to 60% are rehospitalized at least once by the time they reach school age. The increased risk of hospitalization persists into early school age; 7% of VLBW children are hospitalized in a year, compared with 2% of NBW children.

2. **Respiratory syncytial virus** (RSV) is the most important cause of bronchiolitis and pneumonia in premature infants, especially in those with BPD. VLBW infants should receive palivizumab (Synagis) monoclonal antibody to prevent illness with RSV. The American Academy of Pediatrics recommends treatment during RSV season for at least the first year of life in infants born ≤ 28 weeks' gestation and for at least the first 6 months of life for those born between 28 and 32 weeks' gestation. Other preventive strategies that should be recommended to families include good handwashing for all those in close contact with infants, avoidance of exposure to others with respiratory infections (especially young children during the winter season), and avoidance of cigarette smoke.

3. **Air travel.** In general, air travel is not recommended for infants with BPD because of the increased risk of exposure to infection and because of the lowered cabin pressure resulting in lower oxygen concentration in the cabin air. If flying cannot be avoided, infants with $PaO_2 \leq 80$ mm Hg, should be given supplemental oxygen while en route.

B. **Immunizations.** VLBW infants should receive their routine pediatric immunizations on the same schedule as term infants with the exception of hepatitis B vaccine, which should not be administered until an infant is 2 kg or 2 months of age (unless exposed). Although studies evaluating the long-term immune response to routine immunizations have shown that antibody titers are lower in preterm infants, most achieve titers in the therapeutic range.

Influenza vaccine is also recommended for VLBW infants when they are older than 6 months. Until then, care providers in close contact with the infant should consider receiving the vaccine.

*This is a revision of a chapter by Marie C. McCormick and Jane E. Stewart in the 4th edition.

C. Growth. Many VLBW infants have feeding and growth problems for multiple reasons. Infants with severe BPD have increased caloric needs for appropriate weight gain. Many also develop oral motor problems and have oral aversion because of negative oral stimulation during their early life.

1. **Monitoring.** Growth should be followed carefully on standardized growth curves. The child's age should be corrected for prematurity (corrected age) for at least the first 2 years of life.

2. **Caloric supplementation.** Supplemental caloric density is usually required to optimize growth. Specialized premature infant formulas with increased protein, calcium, and phosphate (either added to breast milk or used alone) should be considered in infants with borderline growth for the first 6 to 12 months of life. Growth in ELBW infants is typically close to or below the fifth percentile. A growth pattern is usually considered healthy if it runs parallel to the normal curve.

3. **Evaluation.** Infants whose growth curve plateaus or falls off the normal curve should be evaluated by a dietician to assess caloric intake. Referral to a gastroenterologist should be considered to rule out gastrointestinal pathology such as severe gastroesophageal reflux disease (GERD) or to an endocrinologist for possible growth hormone deficiency. Infants with oral aversion should be referred to an oral motor specialist (occupational or speech therapist) experienced in the management of infants with oral motor sensory problems.

4. **Gastrostomy.** G-tube placement is necessary in a small subset of patients with severe feeding problems. Long-term problems may persist, and children usually require specialized feeding and oral motor therapy to wean eventually from G-tube feedings.

D. Anemia. VLBW infants are at risk for iron deficiency anemia and should receive supplemental iron for the first 12 to 15 months of life.

E. Rickets. VLBW infants who have had nutritional deficits in calcium, phosphorous, or vitamin D intake are at risk for rickets. Infants at highest risk are those who received prolonged parenteral nutrition, furosemide therapy, or have fat malabsorption resulting in decreased vitamin D absorption. Infants with rickets diagnosed in the NICU may need continued supplementation of calcium, phosphorous, and vitamin D during the first year of life. Supplemental vitamin D (400 IU/day) should also be provided to all infants discharged home on breast milk.

F. Sensory problems

1. **Ophthalmologic follow-up** (see Chap. 35).

Infants with severe retinopathy of prematurity (ROP) and retinal detachment are at risk of significant vision loss or blindness. The incidence of blindness is 2 to 9% in ELBW infants, who have the highest risk of severe ROP.

a. Preterm infants with no ROP or with mild or moderately severe ROP that has regressed remain at increased risk of ophthalmologic problems. These include refractive error (myopia is most common), strabismus (both esotropia and exotropia), amblyopia, and glaucoma.

b. All VLBW infants should have follow-up with an ophthalmologist who is experienced with problems related to prematurity. This should occur by 8 months of age and then as recommended by the ophthalmologist, but usually by 3 years of age at the latest.

2. **Hearing follow-up.** Hearing loss occurs in 2% to 11% of VLBW infants. Prematurity increases the risk of both sensorineural and conductive hearing loss. All VLBW infants should be screened in the neonatal period and again at 1 year of age. They should be screened before 1 year if there are parental concerns or if the infant has additional risk factors for hearing loss. VLBW infants also appear to be at increased risk for central auditory processing problems.

G. Dental problems. VLBW infants have an increased incidence of enamel hypoplasia and discoloration. Long-term oral intubation in the neonatal period may result in palate and alveolar ridge deformation affecting tooth development. We recommend referral to a pediatric dentist in the first 18 months of life. Supplemental fluoride should be given.

III. **Neurodevelopmental outcomes.** Infants with intracranial hemorrhage, especially parenchymal hemorrhage, or periventricular white matter injury are at increased risk of neuromotor and cognitive delay. Infants with white matter injury are also at risk of visuomotor problems and visual field deficits. Poor outcome is most likely in ELBW infants with serious neonatal complications, such as BPD, brain injury (intraparenchymal echodensity, periventricular leukomalacia, porencephalic cyst, grade 3 or 4 intraventricular hemorrhage), and severe ROP (threshold or stage 4 or 5 in one or both eyes). In a large study, 88% of infants with these complications had poor neurosensory outcomes (cerebral palsy, cognitive delay, severe hearing loss, or bilateral blindness) at 18 months' corrected age.

A. **Neuromotor problems.** The incidence of cerebral palsy is 7 to 12% in VLBW and 11 to 15% in ELBW infants. The most common type of cerebral palsy is spastic diplegia. This correlates with injury to the corticospinal tracts in the periventricular white matter.

   1. **Management.** Diagnosis should be made early in infants at risk. A neurologist and orthopedic specialist should evaluate infants with CP. They should be referred promptly for appropriate early intervention services such as physical and occupational therapy. Some infants will benefit from orthotics or other adaptive equipment. Those with severe spasticity may benefit from treatment with botulinum-A toxin (Botox) injections. Treatment with baclofen (oral or via an intrathecal catheter with a subcutaneous pump) may be helpful for severe spasticity. Older children may require surgical procedures.

B. **Cognitive delay.** Progress should be assessed with some form of intelligence or development quotient (DQ) on an established scale, such as the Bayley Scales of Infant Development. VLBW infants tend to average somewhat lower than NBW infants on such scales, but many still fall within the normal range.

   1. Scores lower than 68 to 70 (below two standard deviations) are reported in 5 to 20% in VLBW and 14 to 40% in ELBW infants. Most studies reflect children tested at less than 2 years of age. The proportion of those severely affected is similar in older children. However, the rate of school failure or school problems is as high as 50%, with rates of 20% even among children with average IQ scores. Learning disabilities, especially related to visuospatial and visuomotor abilities, written output, and verbal functioning, are more common in ELBW infants (without neurologic problems) tested at 8 to 11 years of age, compared to term infants matched for sociodemographic status. Some type of special education assistance is required by >50% of ELBW infants, compared to <15% of healthy term controls. Measures of self-esteem in teenage children who were born ELBW do not differ from control infants.

   2. **Management.** VLBW infants should be referred to early intervention programs at the time of discharge from the NICU. This allows early identification of children with delays and appropriate referral for therapy from educational specialists and speech therapists. Children with severe language delays may benefit from referral to special communication programs that utilize adaptive technology to enhance language and communication.

C. **Emotional and behavioral health**

   1. **Sleep problems.** Parents frequently report sleep difficulties in VLBW infants. The etiology is multifactorial, with medical and behavioral components. Parents often benefit from utilizing books on sleep training. In more severe cases, referral to a sleep specialist may be helpful.

   2. **Behavior problems.** Behavior problems related to hyperactivity and/or attention deficit are more common in VLBW children. Additional risk factors include stress within the family, maternal depression, and smoking. Behavior problems can contribute to school difficulties. In relation to both

school problems and other health issues, VLBW children are seen as less socially competent than NBW children.

a. Behavior problems are detected using scales developed to elicit parental and teacher concerns. These standardized scales are available for children > 2 years old.

b. Management depends on the nature of the problem and the degree of functional disruption. Some problems may be managed with special educational programs. Others may need referral for psychotherapy services and/or medication.

IV. **Developmental follow-up.** Follow-up programs help to optimize health outcomes for NICU graduates. They also provide feedback for improvement of medical care in the NICU. A number of activities can be included.

A. **Management of sequelae associated with prematurity.** This is especially important with the increased survival of ELBW infants.

B. **Consultative assessment and referral.** NICU graduates require surveillance for the emergence of a variety of problems that may require referral to and coordination of multiple preventive and rehabilitative services.

C. **Monitoring outcomes.** Information on health problems and use of services by NICU graduates is integral to the assessment of the effect of services on outcomes and for counseling of parents regarding an individual child's future.

V. **Program structure**

A. NICUs differ in the population requiring follow-up care and the availability and quality of community resources. Criteria used by most programs are a combination of birth weight (or gestational age) and specific complications. The criteria must be explicit and well understood by all members of the NICU team. Mechanisms should be developed for identifying and referring appropriate children. We target all NICU graduates with a birth weight of <1500 g.

B. The timing of visits depends on the infant's needs and community resources. Some programs recommend a first visit within a few weeks of discharge to assess the transition to home. If not dictated by acute problems, future visits are scheduled to assess progress in key activities. In the absence of acute-care needs, we assess patients routinely at 6-month intervals.

C. Because the focus of follow-up care is enhancement of individual and family function, personnel must include individuals with expertise in multiple areas. These include clinical skill in the management of sequelae of prematurity; the ability to perform neurologic and cognitive diagnostic assessment; familiarity with general pediatric problems presenting in premature infants; the ability to manage children with complex medical, motor, and cognitive problems; and knowledge of the availability of and access to community programs.

D. Methods used to measure a child's progress depend on the need for direct assessment by health professionals and the availability and quality of primary-care and early-intervention services.

1. A variety of indirect approaches exist for children with few problems and access to adequate community resources. These provide information needed by NICU programs and operate at minimal inconvenience to parents.

2. For direct assessment, a multidisciplinary team is needed. Staff team members and consultants should include a pediatrician (developmental specialist or neonatologist), neonatology fellows or pediatric residents (for training), pediatric neurologist, physical therapist, psychologist, occupational therapist, dietician, speech and language specialist, and social worker.

3. Both transient and long-term motor problems in infants require assessment and treatment by physical therapists. These services are usually provided at home through local programs. Infants with sensorineural handicaps require coordination of appropriate clinical services and developmental programs. For older children, consultation with the schools and participation in an educational plan are important.

Suggested Readings

Doyle L.W., Betharas F.R., Ford G. W., et al. Survival, cranial ultrasound and cerebral palsy in very low birth weight infants: 1980 versus 1990s. *J Paediatr Child Health* 2000;36:7–12.

Escobar G. J., Littenberg B., Pettiti D. B. Outcome among very low birth weight infants: a meta-analysis. *Arch Dis Child* 1991;66:204–211.

Hack M., Wilson-Costello D., Friedman H., et al. Neurodevelopment and predictors of outcomes of children with birth weights of less than 1000g. *Arch Pediatr Adolesc Med* 2000;154:725–731.

McCormick M. C., Stewart M. C., Cohen R., et al. Follow-up of NICU graduates: Why, what, and by whom. *J Intensive Care Med* 1995;10:213–225.

Lorenz J.M., Wooliever D. E., Jetton J.R., et al. A quantitative review of mortality and developmental disability in extremely premature newborns. *Arch Pediatr Adolesc Med* 1998;152:425–435.

McCormick M.C., Workman-Daniels K., Brooks-Gunn J. The behavioral and emotional well-being of school-age children with different birth weights. *Pediatrics* 1996;97:18–25.

McCormick M.C., McCarton C., Tonascia J., et al. Early educational intervention for very low birth weight infants: results from the Infant Health and Development Program. *J Pediatr* 1993;123:527–533.

Schmidt B., Asztalos E. V., Roberts R.S., et al. Impact of bronchopulmonary dysplasia, brain injury, and severe retinopathy of prematurity on the outcome of extremely low-birth-weight infants at 18 months. *JAMA* 2003;289:112–1129.

Vohr B., Wright L.L., Dusick A. M., et al. Neurodevelopmental outcomes of extremely low birth weight infants in the National Institute of Child Health and Human Development Neonatal Research Network, 1993–1994. *Pediatrics* 2000;105: 1216–1226.

16. DISCHARGE PLANNING*

Linda Zaccagnini

The survival rate for low-birth-weight (less than 2500 g), moderately low-birth-weight (1500 to 2500 g), very-low-birth-weight (less than 1500 g), and extremely low-birth-weight (less than 1000 g) infants has increased in the past three decades. The infant who weighs less than 750 g has a greater than 30% chance of survival, while survival rates for the infant weighing more than 1000 g are 90% (see Table 3.2 in Chap. 3). Greater survival rates for preterm infants have created a population with unique long-term health-care needs. Changes in the health-care system in the United States are encouraging earlier discharge and more out-of-hospital care.

Effective discharge planning ensures continuity of care from hospital to home. The plan must provide for individualized family and infant needs and prepare family members and health-care providers for infant-care requirements.

I. **Features of a good discharge plan**
   A. Individualized to meet infant and family needs and resources.
   B. Begins early.
   C. Includes clearly identified goals.
   D. Decreases fragmentation and duplication of services.
   E. Decreases delays in accessing care and progressing through the provider system.
   F. Anticipates potential delays in development and directs care toward prevention and early intervention.
   G. Is community-based.
   H. Increases quality of care.

II. **System assessment.** Assign a primary team upon admission to assist the family in developing trusting relationships with staff. This enhances communication and minimizes the number of staff with whom the family will need to interact. It is important to know how your facility functions, who assumes responsibility for various components of discharge planning, and how communication is carried out. Early planning will expedite discharge. Delays in discharge can be costly, and readmissions can be traumatic to the infant and the family.
   A. A **primary physician** or **nurse practitioner** is assigned to the infant at admission. That person is responsible for daily management of issues. In teaching institutions where staff rotate monthly, families may need to adjust to many different primary providers. It is helpful for an assigned primary attending physician or practitioner to follow up infants with complex cases throughout their stay and provide continuity.
   B. **Primary and associate nurses** follow the family through the NICU stay, co-ordinating and implementing the care plan developed by the team.
   C. **Social workers** support the family in crisis and assist in locating available resources.
   D. **Discharge planners** vary from institution to institution. They may be specialized advance practice nurses, clinical specialists, primary nurses, social workers, or a combination of players.
   E. **Respiratory, physical, and occupational therapists** can teach families skills and can transfer care to community resources.
   F. **Payer resources.** HMOs and third-party payers may have case managers or resource personnel to assist and approve coordination of services. Preferred providers may be contractually required to be used. Case managers can clarify coverage issues or advise on availability.

---

*This is a revision of a chapter in the 4th edition originally written by Kimberly Cox and Linda Zaccagnini.

III. Family assessment may begin prior to admission. Ongoing communication between professionals and the family will allow providers to develop a multidisciplinary, individualized care plan that includes discharge planning. Involving the family in developing the plan optimizes its success by individualizing the plan and adding to the parents' feeling of control. The transition to home can go smoothly, even in the most complex cases, with early planning, ongoing teaching, and attention to the family's needs and resources.

A. Family dynamics. Include the following issues when assessing the family's readiness for discharge:

1. Willingness to assume responsibility for care.
2. Previous or present experiences with infant care and medical procedures.
3. The actual as well as perceived complexity of the skills required to care for the infant.
4. Family structure.
5. Financial concerns.
6. Home setting.
7. Coping skills.
8. Supports.
9. Medical and psychological history (ongoing illness may impact caretaking needs).
10. Cultural beliefs (bonding, roles, and available supports).
11. Language barriers (may require an interpreter).

B. Home environment. Structural components of the home may need alteration. Confirm electrical, water, heating, and cooling resources.

C. Stress and coping. In the NICU, discuss what it will be like to have the infant at home. Consider who will be involved for the extended duration and for available support. Referral to a parent group or specialized support group may be helpful. Explore the availability of community services for counseling and social needs. The following are common issues:

1. **Grief.** Parents need to cope with the loss of their "perfect" infant. The four psychological effects of a high-risk pregnancy are denial, blame and guilt, feelings of failure, and ambivalence.
2. **Abandonment and isolation.** Much attention and support are available while the infant is hospitalized. After discharge, parents may feel alone and abandoned.
3. **Siblings** may delay reacting until the new baby comes home and then respond with regressive or acting-out behaviors.
4. **Parenting disorders.** When the child is well, parents may be so overburdened with the memories of severe illness that they never treat the infant as a healthy child.
5. **Privacy.** Infants requiring complex care at home may require "blocks" of nursing or ancillary care at home; these disrupt space and privacy. An array of "strangers" in the home adds stress to the family.

D. Financial resources. Complete a financial assessment early. Early delivery or complex care can alter the family's plans for work and child care. Loss of work, income changes, cost of copayments, and inability to make career moves because of insurance coverage all impact the family's financial stability.

IV. Infant's readiness for discharge

A. Healthy, growing, preterm infants are considered ready for discharge when they meet the following criteria:

1. Ability to maintain temperature in an open crib.
2. Ability to take all feedings by bottle or breast without respiratory compromise.
3. No apnea or bradycardia for 5 days (see Chap. 24).
4. Steady weight gain.

B. Infants with specialized needs require a complex, flexible, ongoing discharge and teaching plan. Discharge specifics may not be identified until just prior to discharge. It is important to consider the relative fragility and stability of various systems and the complexity of interventions. Include assessment of behavioral and developmental issues, and evaluate parental recognition and response.

C. **Discharge screening.** Complete routine screening tests and immunizations according to individual institutional guidelines (Fig. 16.1).

1. **Hearing screening** (see Chap. 35 and Fig. 16.1).

2. **Eye exams** (see Chap. 35 and Fig. 16.1).

3. Perform **cranial ultrasound** (see Chap. 27 and Fig. 16.1) screening for intra-ventricular hemorrhage and periventricular leukomalacia for all infants who

   a. weigh less than 1500 g or under 32 weeks gestational age.

   b. are under 34 weeks gestational age if mechanically ventilated.

   Perform **head ultrasound** at

   day of life 1 to 3 if results alter clinical management,

   day of life 7 to 10, then

   day of life 21 to 28.

4. **Immunizations.** Administer according to American Academy of Pediatrics guidelines based on chronological, not postconceptional, age (see Chap. 3).

V. **Follow-up care** for the infant with special needs may involve many different services and providers to meet all of the child's needs.

A. **Primary care** is usually provided through a pediatrician, family practitioner, or nurse practitioner. Ongoing communication between NICU staff and the primary-care provider begins long before discharge. This maintains continuity and improves the infant's chances of receiving appropriate medical care after discharge.

B. **Specialty services** may be required.

C. **Infant follow-up programs** affiliated with many Level III nurseries offer multidisciplinary services including developmental assessments, hearing and visual screening, physical therapy assessments, and referrals to community-based providers and support groups (see Chap. 15).

D. **Early intervention programs** are community-based and offer multidisciplinary services for children from birth to age 3. Children deemed at biological, environmental, or emotional risk are eligible. Programs are partially federally funded and are offered free or on a sliding scale. They provide multidisciplinary services including physical therapy, early childhood education, social services, and parental support groups. Services may be home-based or center-based. Make referrals early in the child's hospital stay, as some centers have long waiting lists.

VI. **Preparing the home for the infant's discharge**

A. **Home-care services** are becoming more widely available; however, their ability to provide specialized pediatric or neonatal services is variable. Assess individual programs separately before making a referral.

B. **Skilled nursing care**

1. **Public health nurses** may do home visits before discharge to assess the family's readiness and the home situation. They may also do well-baby and basic health-care teaching.

2. **Visiting nurse associations** provide home visits for reinforcement of teaching, health and psychosocial assessments, and short-term treatments or nursing care. They usually charge service fees.

3. **Home health-care agencies** provide skilled nursing care, home health aids, physical and/or occupational therapy, and medical equipment and supplies. Fees for service and insurance coverage are highly variable.

C. **Respite care.** Many parents do not realize how emotionally and physically draining it can be to care for a child with complex medical needs. The usual support people, such as relatives, friends, and babysitters, may be uncomfortable or be unable to deal with the added responsibility. Explore resources for respite care before discharge.

D. **Notify emergency care providers** including community hospital emergency wards and local emergency medical technicians (EMT) or fire responders of the child's presence, medical needs, and likely problems. This will assure appropriate emergency response.

Newborn State Screening for Metabolic Disease (see Chap. 29)

Criteria
- All infants admitted to the NICU

Initial
- Day 3 or D/C date (whichever comes first)

Follow-up
- Day 14 or D/C date (whichever comes first)
- Week 6 (if birth weight < 1500 g)
- Week 10 (if birth weight < 1500 g)

Head Ultrasound (see Chap. 27)

Criteria
- All infants with gestational age <32 weeks (an ultrasound would be done at any gestational age at any time if thought to be clinically indicated)

Initial
- Day 7–10 (in the case of critically ill infants, when results of an earlier ultrasound may alter clinical management, an ultrasound should be performed at the discretion of the clinician)

Follow-up (minimum if no abnormalities noted)
- If no hemorrhage or germinal matrix hemorrhage
  - If < 28 weeks: week 4 *and* at 36 weeks corrected age (or discharge if <36 weeks)
  - If < $28^{0/7}$–$31^{6/7}$ weeks: week 4 *or* 36 weeks corrected age (or discharge if <36 weeks)
- If intraventricular (grade 2+) or intraparenchymal hemorrhage: follow-up at least weekly until stable (more frequently if unstable post-hemorrhagic hydrocephalus and clinically indicated)

Ophthalmologic Examination (see Chap. 35)

Criteria
- All infants with birth weight <1500 g or gestational age <32 weeks

Initial
- If <27 weeks: week 6
- If 27–28 weeks: week 5
- If 29–30 weeks: week 4
- If 31–$31^{6/7}$ weeks: week 3

Note:
- If the infant is transferred to another nursery prior to 4 weeks of age, recommend exam at the receiving hospital
- If the infant is discharged home prior to 4 weeks of age, examine prior to discharge

Follow-up (based on initial exam findings)
- Immature retina zone 1 or zone 2, or low-grade ROP: follow-up every 2 weeks
- Immature retina zone 3: follow-up in 4–10 weeks
- Prethreshold ROP: follow-up weekly
- Regressing ROP: follow-up every 1–10 weeks depending on zone

Audiology Screening (see Chap. 35)

Criteria
- All infants to be discharged home from NICU

Timing
- Examine at 34 weeks gestation or greater

(continues)

FIG. 16.1. Guidelines for routine screening, testing, treatment, and follow-up, Neonatal Intensive Care Unit, Beth Israel Deaconess Medical Center.

FIG. 16.1. *(continued)*

Car Seat Testing

Criteria
- All infants to be discharged from NICU *and* born at less than 37 weeks or with other conditions that may compromise respiratory status

Timing
- Examine prior to discharge home

Hepatitis B Vaccination (see Chap. 3)

Criteria
- All infants to be discharged home from NICU or at 2 months of age

Initial
- If weight ≥2000 g: vaccinate prior to discharge home or at 2 months
- If weight <2000 g: vaccinate at 2 months of age

Follow-up (dose #2)
- Vaccinate 1 month after initial vaccine dose

Occupational Therapy Consultation

Criteria
- All infants meeting one of the following conditions:
  - Birth at or below 28 weeks' gestation
  - Birth weight < 1000 g
  - Neurological insults including IVH, PVL, seizure disorder
  - Genetic syndromes that affect quality of movement or state regulation
  - Symptoms associated with Neonatal Abstinence Syndrome
  - Orthopedic or musculo–skeletal impairments
  - Born to parents with physical disabilities
  - Brachial plexus palsy (Erb's or Klumpke's palsy)
  - Critically ill term infants

Social Security

Criteria
- All infants meeting one of the following conditions:
  - Birth weight < 1200 g
  - Birth weight 1200–2000 g and at least 4 weeks small for gestational age (refer to growth curve)
  - Any infant with serious handicapping conditions

Timing
- Application completed during first week of life

Follow-up
- Parent notifies SSI office of baby's discharge via form letter.

Infant Follow-up Program (IFUP)

Criteria
- All infants meeting one of the following conditions:
  - Birth weight < 1000 g
  - Birth weight 1000–1499 g with one of the following:
    - Maternal age < 20
    - IVH (Grades 2–4)
    - PVL
    - Surgical NEC
    - ROP
    - Psychosocial concerns

Timing
- Referral completed prior to discharge

(continues)

Neonatal Neurology Program
Criteria
- All infants meeting one of the following conditions:
  - Neurologic disorders (e.g., stroke, intracranial hemorrhage, and neonatal seizures)
  - Neuromuscular disorders
  - Birth weight <1500 g with IVH (Grades 2–4) or PVL (referral to IFUP also)

Timing
- Referral completed prior to discharge

Early Intervention Program (EIP)
Criteria
- Infant meeting *four* or more of the following criteria:
  - BW < 1200 g
  - GA < 32 weeks
  - NICU admission > 5 days
  - Apgar < 5 at 5 min
  - IUGR or SGA (refer to growth curves)
  - Hospital stay > 25 days
  - Chronic feeding difficulties
  - Insecure attachment
  - Suspected central nervous system abnormality
  - Maternal age <17 *or* 3 or more births at maternal age < 20
  - Maternal education < 10 years
  - Parental chronic illness or disability affecting caregiving
  - Lack of family supports
  - Inadequate food, shelter, and clothing
  - Open or confirmed protective service investigation ("51-A")
  - Substance abuse in the home
  - Domestic violence in the home

Timing
- Referral complete prior to discharge

FIG. 16.1. *(continued)*

E. **Local utility companies** (telephone, electricity, fuel) should be notified in writing of the child's presence in the home so they will assign priority resumption of services if there is an interruption.

F. **Supplies and equipment**
   1. Order **supplies and equipment** well before discharge to ensure availability. Have caregivers care for their child using the home monitors and oxygen equipment in the NICU. This increases their skill and confidence.
   2. **Medications and special formulas** or dietary supplements should also be ordered early and delivered to the home. Many preparations are not readily available in the community.
   3. It is helpful to locate a **home health agency** that can be contracted to coordinate equipment delivery and repair, reorder and deliver medical supplies and medications, and arrange for home-care providers. It enables the family to deal with only one person for all of their home-care needs.

VII. **Preparing the family for discharge**
   A. **Simplify care** by thoroughly reviewing the infant's care regimen. Alter medication schedules to fit the family's schedule. Eliminate unnecessary medications. Formulas and additives can be changed to less-expensive or more easily obtained products, such as substituting corn oil for medium-chain triglyceride

(MCT) oil. Get the infant used to the daily schedule that will be followed at home.

B. Begin **teaching** early to allow the caregivers adequate time to process information, practice skills, and formulate questions. Make teaching protocols detailed and thorough. Include written information for the family to take home to use as reference (see Figs. 16.2 and 16.3). Standardize information

BETH ISRAEL DEACONESS MEDICAL CENTER
A member of CAREGROUP
Boston, MA 02215

NEONATAL INTENSIVE CARE UNIT
DISCHARGE INSTRUCTION SHEET

Baby's Caregivers:
Attending Neonatologist at Discharge: ______________
Primary Nurse & Team: ______________
Social Worker: ______________

PARENT INFORMATION

	Reviewed	N/A	RN Signature	Date
NICU parent packet	☐		________	___/___/___
WIC form	☐	☐	________	___/___/___
Immunization booklet	☐	☐	________	___/___/___
Synagis information sheet	☐	☐	________	___/___/___
Hepatitis B information sheet	☐	☐	________	___/___/___
Other ________	☐	☐	________	___/___/___

PREPARATION FOR DISCHARGE

	Reviewed	RN Signature	Date
Feeding: breast milk or formula	☐	________	___/___/___
Bowel and bladder pattern	☐	________	___/___/___
Bulb syringe use	☐	________	___/___/___
Bathing, skin care, cord care	☐	________	___/___/___
Temperature taking	☐	________	___/___/___
Circumcision care (if applicable)	☐	________	___/___/___
CPR instruction	☐	________	___/___/___
When to call your baby's doctor	☐	________	___/___/___
Car seat instruction	☐	________	___/___/___
Car seat screening	☐	________	___/___/___
Protection from infection	☐	________	___/___/___
Other ________	☐	________	___/___/___

DATE OF DISCHARGE: ___/___/___

Discharge Measurements:		RN Signature	Date
Weight	______ gms (___ lbs ___ oz)	________	___/___/___
Length	______ cm (___ in)	________	___/___/___
Head Circumference	______ cm (___ in)	________	___/___/___

STATE NEWBORN SCREENING: Most recent test: ___/___/___

NEWBORN HEARING SCREEN: ☐Pass ☐Refer (see follow-up care)

ADDITIONAL NOTES:

BABY'S FOLLOW UP CARE

Primary Pediatric Provider: ☐N/A
Name: ______________
Telephone: ______________
Appt. Date: ___/___/___ Time: ________

Early Intervention: ☐N/A
Center Name/Town: ______________
Telephone: ______________
Initial Contact: ___/___/___ Date Confirmed: ___/___/___

Visiting Nurse: ☐N/A
Center Name/Town: ______________
Telephone: ______________
Date Contacted: ___/___/___ ☐ referral faxed

Infant Follow-up Program: (617) 667-1330 ☐N/A
(<1500g-see criteria on referral sheet)
Date Contacted: ___/___/___ ☐ referral faxed

Neonatal Neurology Program: (617) 355-6388 ☐N/A
Children's Hospital
(see criteria on referral sheet)
Date Contacted: ___/___/___

Lactation Consultant: ☐N/A
Name: ______________
Telephone: ______________

Ophthalmologist: ☐N/A
Name: ______________
Telephone: ______________
Date: ___/___/___ Time: ________
☐ Recommended Follow-up at 8 months

Follow-up Hearing Screen: ☐N/A
Date: ___/___/___ Time: ________
Location:
☐ Children's Hospital - Fegan 11 (617) 355-6461
☐ Children's Hospital - Lexington (781) 672-2000
☐ HVMA - Kenmore (617) 421-8888
☐ Other: ________ ( ) ___-____

Other:

Medication/Feeding Additives	Reason	Amount to give	When to give	How to give
☐ Check medroom for stored breastmilk				

This information has been reviewed with me, and my questions have been answered. I authorize the NICU staff to provide necessary information from my child's medical record to the above named providers/services.

________________ Parent Signature ☐ Copy given to parent ________________ RN Signature ___/___/___ Date

MC0104 Revised 5/00 White - Medical Record Yellow - Parent

***Note:** This is a general guideline, and it does not represent a professional standard of care governing providers' obligations to patients. Care is revised to meet individual patient needs.*

FIG. 16.2. Newborn discharge instruction sheet.

PARENT RESOURCES

At Beth Israel Deaconess Medical Center
- Neonatal Intensive Care Unit .... (617) 667–4042
- NICU Transitional Care Unit (TCU) .... (617) 667–4062
- Social Work Office .... (617) 667–3421
- Birth Certificate Office .... (617) 667–4167
- Learning Center .... (617) 667–9100

Community Resources
- **NICU: Parent Support, Inc.** If you would like to talk to a parent who has gone through a NICU experience, call ... (617) 964-8778/(800) 964-6428
- **Poison Control Center** .... (617) 232-2120/(800) 682-9211
- **Children's Hospital (Boston) Emergency Room** .... (617) 355-6611
- **Parental Stress Line** .... (800) 632–8188
- **Battered Women's Hotline** *(24 hour)* .... (617) 661–7203
- **Statewide Alcohol and Drug Hotline** .... (800) 327–5050
- **Mother of Twins Association** .... (781) 646–TWIN
- **Triplets, Moms and More** .... (781) 449–3261

Breastfeeding
- La Leche League of Mass .... (617) 469–9423
- Women, Infants and Children (WIC) Office ... (617) 624-6100/(800) 682–9211
- Massachusetts Lactation Consultant Association .... (617) 662–7910
- Boston Association for Childbirth Education and Nursing Mother's Council .... (617) 244–5102
- BI-Deaconess Learning Center—Lactation Consultation and Support Group .... (617) 667–9100

WHEN TO CALL YOUR BABY'S DOCTOR

Any sudden changes in baby's usual patterns of behavior:
- increased sleepiness
- increased irritability
- feeding poorly

Any of the following:
- breathing difficulties
- blueness around lips, mouth, or eyes
- fever (by rectal temperature) over 100° or 99.6° under the arm or low temperature under 97° (rectal)
- vomiting or diarrhea
- dry diapers for more than 12 hours
- no bowel movement for more than 4 days
- black or bright red color seen in stool

PROTECTING YOUR BABY FROM INFECTION

Your baby's immune system is still quite immature. This makes him/her especially vulnerable to colds and other communicable diseases. To protect your baby from infections we advise that you
- avoid taking your baby to crowded indoor places
- avoid contact with anyone who has a cold, flu, or other active infection
- do not allow anyone to smoke around baby
- encourage anyone who comes into close contact with your baby to wash their hands

SAFETY

It is a Massachusetts state law that all children 12 years old and under must be fastened in a properly adjusted car seat or safety belt. It is recommended that children under 40 pounds always ride in car seats.

BACK TO SLEEP

The Academy of Pediatrics has recommended that infants be placed on their backs to sleep to prevent SIDS. Avoid sleeping on stomach, sleeping on a soft surface, overheating, and exposure to secondary smoke. "Tummy Time" should be provided during awake and supervised periods.

FIG. 16.3. Additional discharge instruction sheet.

to ensure that every family member receives the same essential information. Address well-baby care, developmental issues, and necessary medical information. Include several family members in the learning process so that the parents can get needed support.

   C. Provide transitional programs for parents. Schedule blocks of hands-on care or have the parents room in with the infant in the NICU. This maximizes parental confidence and competence and helps strengthen the parent–infant bond.

   D. Retrotransfer to a Level II nursery in the community. This may allow the family to spend more time with the infant, and facilitate learning in a less acute environment.

   E. It is vital to **include the family** in formulating all plans and, whenever possible, choosing care providers.

VIII. Communication with community providers is essential for a smooth transiton home. Identification of the primary-care provider early allows for ongoing updates in complex situations. Utilizing the primary-care providers network along with insurance guidelines will avoid confusion for an already anxious family. A verbal conversation prior to discharge promptly followed up with the faxed dictated summary (Fig 16.4) and copies of in-house studies will allow for optimal communication. A dictated summary may need to be also faxed to follow-up programs as deemed appropriate.

IX. Alternatives to home discharge may be temporary or permanent. Integrating the child into the home may be difficult because of medical needs or family dynamics. Decisions regarding alternative placement may be painful for the family. Alternatives vary widely from community to community.

   A. Specialized foster care places the special-needs infant in a home setting with specially trained caregivers. The ultimate goal is to place the infant back with the family.

   B. Pediatric rehabilitation hospitals can be used for the high-risk infant who requires ongoing but less-acute hospital care.

   C. Pediatric nursing homes provide extended care at a skilled level.

   D. Hospice care may be institutional or home-based. It focuses on maximizing the quality of life when cure is no longer possible.

X. Financial concerns

   A. Neonatal intensive care, especially for very-low-birth-weight infants, ranks among the most costly of all hospital admissions. Health insurance may not cover 100% of costs.

   B. Home care benefits are often limited. Prior authorization is almost universally required. Services may be restricted to a particular provider or to a finite period.

   C. Alternative funding

      1. Social Security. Several states have programs that waive parental income criteria and provide Medicaid benefits to infants and children or to those whose hospitalization may be extended if home-care services are not provided.

      2. State government financial assistance. The maternal and child health agencies in most state governments will provide some financial assistance for follow-up of certain infants whose families meet state-established financial criteria. Services vary from state to state but may include physical therapy services, equipment, and diagnostic and treatment services.

      3. Private charities such as the Easter Seal Society and the March of Dimes Birth Defects Foundation have local chapters that provide specialized services on an ability-to-pay or free basis.

      4. Public health departments may offer immunizations and well-child clinics at no cost or very low cost.

      5. Women, Infants and Children Program (WIC) is federally funded and provides nutrition education and supplemental formula to financially eligible pregnant women and to children up to 5 years of age who are assessed as being at risk.

NICU Discharge/Interim Summary Dictation Guideline

Department of Neonatology
Beth Israel Deaconess Medical Center

Begin dictation when you hear the tone.
1. Name of dictator (spell name).
2. Name of attending (spell name).
3. Patient's name (spell name). Use _only_ *"Boy"* or *"Girl"* for first name.
4. Service ("Neonatology").
5. Patient unit number.
6. Date of birth and sex of patient.
7. Date of admission.
8. Date of discharge. *Use the best estimate. A date _must_ be entered.* If interim summary, state "interim date."
9. History.
   • If interim summary, specify dates covered and author/date of prior summary.
   • Include reason for admission, birth weight, gestational age.
   • Maternal history—including prenatal labs, pregnancy, labor, and birth history.
10. Physical examination on admission.
    • Include weight head circumference, and length—note percentile.
11. Summary of hospital course by systems (concise). Include pertinent lab results.
    a. *Respiratory*—Initial impression. Surfactant given? Maximum level of support. Days on ventilation, CPAP, supplemental oxygen. If apnea, report how patient was treated, when treatment ended, and condition resolved (levels if still on therapy).
    b. Cardiovascular—Diagnoses/therapies in summary form. Echo/ECG results.
    c. *Fluids, Electrolytes, Nutrition*—Brief feeding history. Include recent weight, length and head circumference.
    d. *GI*—Pertinent diagnoses and treatment. Maximum bilirubin and therapy used.
    e. *Hematology*—Patient blood type, brief transfusion summary, recent Hct.
    f. *Infectious Disease*—Cultures, antibiotic courses.
    g. *Neurology*—Describe ultrasound findings.
    h. *Sensory*—
       i. *Audiology*—"Hearing screening was performed with automated auditory brainstem responses." Results. [If baby didn't pass or testing not performed, indicated date/location of follow-up test or recommend test prior to discharge].
       ii. *Ophthalmologic findings:*
    • **Not Examined:** Patient is due for a first exam on _____.
    • **Immature:** Eyes examined most recently on _____ revealing immaturity of the retinal vessels but no ROP as of yet. A follow-up examination should be scheduled for the week of _____.
    • **ROP:** Eyes examined most recently on _____, revealing ROP _____.
      A follow-up examination by a pediatric ophthalmologist should be scheduled for _____.
    • **Mature:** Eyes were examined most recently on _____, revealing mature retinal vessels. A follow-up exam is recommended in 6 months.
    i. *Psychosocial*—BIDMC Social Work involved with family. The contact social worker is [name], and she can be reached at 667-4700. Follow-up will be provided by [name of agency/social worker and telephone number]. [If applicable, "A 51-A has been filed."]

(continues)

FIG. 16.4. NICU Discharge/Interim Summary Dictation Guideline.

FIG. 16.4. *(continued)*

12. Condition at discharge.
13. Discharge disposition (e.g., home, [Level II], [Level III], chronic care]).
14. Name of primary pediatrician (spell name). Phone #: _____ Fax #: _____.
15. Care/recommendations (quick summary for those assuming care of the infant).
    a. Feeds at discharge.
    b. Medications.
    c. State newborn screening status.
    d. Immunizations received.
    e. Immunizations recommended (Dictate verbatim).
        i. "Synagis RSV prophylaxis should be considered from October through April for infants who meet any of the following three criteria: (1) born at <32 wks; (2) born between 32 and 35 wks with plans for daycare during RSV season, with a smoker in the household, or with preschool sibs; or (3) with chronic lung disease."
        ii. "Influenza immunization should be considered annually in the fall for preterm infants with chronic lung disease once they reach 6 months of age. Before this age, the family and other caregivers should be considered for immunization against influenza to protect the infant."
    f. Follow-up appointments scheduled/recommended.
16. Discharge Diagnoses List. [Be complete; this is used by medical records coders].

D. Social services or continuing-care departments are invaluable in determining existing coverage and in accessing alternative sources of financial support.

Suggested Readings

American Academy of Pediatrics, Task force on Infant Positioning and SIDS Positioning and SIDS. Changing concepts of sudden infant death syndrome: Implications for infant sleep environment and sleep position. *Pediatrics.* 2000;105:650–656.

Damato E. Discharge planning from the neonatal intensive care unit. *J Perinatal Neonatal Nurs* 1991;5(1):43.

Hulseman M. L., Lee N. The neonatal ICU graduate: Part I. Common problems. *Am Fam Physician* 1992;45(3):1301.

Hulseman M. L., Lee N. The neonatal ICU graduate: Part II. Fundamentals of outpatient care. *Am Fam Physician* 1992;45(4):1696.

Hutt H. L. Home care. In: Kenner C., Brueggemeyer A., Gunderson L. P. (Eds.). *Comprehensive Neonatal Nursing.* Philadelphia: Saunders, 1991.

Kenner C., Bagwell G. Assessment and management of the transition to home. In: Kenner C., Brueggemeyer A., Gunderson L. P. (Eds.). *Comprehensive Neonatal Nursing.* Philadelphia: Saunders, 1991.

Leonard C. High-risk infant follow-up programs. In: Ballard R. (Ed.). *Pediatric Care of the ICN Graduate.* Philadelphia: Saunders, 1988.

17. SHOCK

Stella Kourembanas

I. **Background.** Shock is an acute, complex state of circulatory dysfunction resulting in insufficient oxygen and nutrient delivery to satisfy tissue requirements. Systemic hypotension is the key presenting sign of uncompensated shock that eventually progresses to metabolic acidosis. However, the lowest acceptable normal blood pressure is not well established in newborns, particularly preterm infants. As a result, the blood pressure that triggers a decision to treat infants who do not have acidosis is somewhat arbitrary. One study reported continuous arterial blood pressure measurements in 103 neonates between 23 and 43 weeks' gestation. Based on these data, the statistically defined lower limit of mean arterial pressure during the first postnatal day roughly equals the gestational age of the infant. However, by the third day, >90% of preterm infants <26 weeks' gestation have a mean arterial blood pressure >30 mm Hg.

II. **Causes of Shock.** In the immediate postnatal period, abnormal regulation of peripheral vascular resistance is a frequent cause of hypotension, especially in preterm infants. Hypovolemia is another common cause.

  A. **Hypovolemia.** Hypovolemia should always be considered as an underlying cause of shock in the newborn. A decrease in blood volume can result from loss of whole blood, plasma, or extravascular fluid (see Chap. 26).

  1. Placental hemorrhage, as in abruptio placentae or placenta previa.

  2. Fetal-to-maternal hemorrhage (diagnosed by the Kleihauer-Betke test of the mother's blood for fetal erythrocytes).

  3. Twin-to-twin transfusion (see Chap. 7).

  4. Intracranial hemorrhage (see Chap. 27).

  5. Intraabdominal bleeding from liver laceration caused by gastrointestinal surgery or traumatic breech delivery. Necrotizing enterocolitis or other causes of peritonitis can cause plasma loss.

  6. Massive pulmonary hemorrhage (see Chap. 24).

  7. Disseminated intravascular coagulation (DIC) or other severe coagulopathies.

  8. Plasma loss into the extravascular compartment, as seen with low oncotic pressure states or capillary leak syndrome (e.g., sepsis).

  9. Excessive extracellular fluid losses, as seen with volume depletion from insensible water loss or inappropriate diuresis, commonly seen in extremely low-birth-weight infants.

  B. **Distributive causes.** Abnormalities of circulatory distribution can cause inadequate tissue perfusion. This may result from increased venous capacitance, vasomotor paralysis from pharmacologic agents, or shunting past capillary beds. Etiologies of maldistribution include the following:

  1. **Sepsis.** The precise mechanisms underlying circulatory dysfunction in septic shock are not clear. Multiple factors can interact to alter blood flow: (1) direct depressive effect of microbial products, including endotoxin on the cardiovascular system and/or (2) release of other vasoactive agents, including nitric oxide, serotonin, prostaglandins, histamine, and endorphins resulting in peripheral vasodilation and relative hypovolemia.

  2. **Drugs** that decrease vascular tone include muscle relaxants and anesthetic. Vancomycin has been reported to cause acute circulatory failure in newborn infants.

  C. **Cardiogenic shock.** Although an infant's myocardium normally exhibits good contractility, various perinatal insults, congenital abnormalities, or arrhythmias can result in heart failure.

  1. Intrapartum asphyxia can cause poor contractility and papillary muscle dysfunction with tricuspid regurgitation, resulting in low cardiac output.

2. Myocardial dysfunction can occur secondary to infectious agents (bacterial or viral) or metabolic abnormalities such as hypoglycemia. Cardiomyopathy can be seen in infants of diabetic mothers (IDMs) with or without hypoglycemia (see Chap. 2).

3. Obstruction to blood flow resulting in decreased cardiac output can be seen with many congenital heart defects (see Chap. 25).

   a. **Inflow obstructions**
      (1) Total anomalous pulmonary venous return.
      (2) Cor triatriatum.
      (3) Tricuspid atresia.
      (4) Mitral atresia.
      (5) Acquired inflow obstructions can occur from intravascular air or thrombotic embolus, or from increased intrathoracic pressure caused by high airway pressures, pneumothorax, pneumomediastinum, or pneumopericardium.

   b. **Outflow obstructions**
      (1) Pulmonary stenosis or atresia.
      (2) Aortic stenosis or atresia.
      (3) Hypertrophic subaortic stenosis seen in IDMs with compromised left ventricular outflow, particularly when cardiotonic agents are used.
      (4) Coarctation of the aorta or interrupted aortic arch.
      (5) Arrhythmias, if prolonged. Supraventricular arrhythmias such as paroxysmal atrial tachycardia are most common.

III. **Pathophysiology of circulatory failure**

   A. Abnormal peripheral vasoregulation results in **systemic hypotension** that is often observed in preterm infants in the immediate postnatal period. This is primarily due to immature neurovascular pathways as well as proinflammatory cascades that lead to vasodilation.

   B. **Hypovolemic shock.** In the compensated phase, central venous pressure (CVP) and urine output are decreased, and tachycardia and increased systemic vascular resistance are present. In very premature infants, acute hypotension with bradycardia can occur without preceding tachycardia.

   C. **Distributive shock** presents initially with a hyperdynamic state of tachycardia, normal blood pressure and urine output, and bounding pulses. The arteriovenous oxygen saturation difference, when measured, is narrow. Eventually, cardiogenic shock ensues.

   D. In **cardiogenic shock,** compensatory mechanisms can have deleterious effects. Increased vascular resistance maintains adequate blood supply to vital organs but increases left ventricular afterload and cardiac work. Decreased renal perfusion from low cardiac output results in sodium and water retention, causing increased central blood volume, increased left ventricular pressure and volume, and therefore pulmonary edema, with hypoxia and acidosis further compromising cardiac function. Tachycardia, hypotension, oliguria, and acidosis dominate the presentation of cardiogenic shock.

IV. **Clinical presentation.** In addition to hypotension and tachycardia (except in very premature infants; see III.B), shock is manifested principally by (1) pallor and poor skin perfusion, (2) cool extremities, (3) central nervous system signs, and (4) decreased urine output. Organ dysfunction occurs because of inadequate blood flow and oxygenation, and cellular metabolism becomes predominantly anaerobic, producing lactic and pyruvic acid. Hence, metabolic acidosis often indicates inadequate circulation. In preterm infants, the associated decrease in brain blood flow and oxygen supply during severe hypotension predisposes to intraventricular hemorrhage and periventricular leukomalacia with long-term neurodevelopmental abnormalities. Abnormalities are seen in many organ systems:

   A. **Brain.** Lethargy.

   B. **Heart.** Decreased cardiac output and increased pulmonary blood volume.

   C. **Lungs.** Release of vasoactive substances, pulmonary edema, and decreased compliance.

D. Gastrointestinal tract. Mucosal dysfunction, diarrhea, sepsis, hemorrhage, and perforation.

E. Kidneys. Reduced glomerular filtration rate (GFR) and urinary output, loss of renal tubular epithelium, uremia, electrolyte abnormalities.

V. Treatment always begins by ensuring a patent airway, assessing ventilation, and providing supplemental oxygen. Heart rate, blood pressure, and oxygenation should be monitored continuously. An infusion of 10 to 20 mL/kg isotonic saline solution will help establish etiology. If hypovolemia exists, the saline infusion will be therapeutic, at least temporarily, until the underlying cause is corrected. Albumin solutions should not be given.

A. Measurement of central venous pressure (CVP) may help management, especially in term or near-term infants. CVP is measured using a catheter with its tip in the right atrium or in the intrathoracic superior vena cava. The catheter can be placed through the umbilical vein or percutaneously through the external or internal jugular or subclavian vein. In many infants, maintaining CVP at 5 to 8 mm Hg with volume infusions is associated with improved cardiac output. If CVP exceeds 5 to 8 mm Hg, additional volume will usually not be helpful. CVP is influenced by noncardiac factors such as ventilator pressures and by cardiac factors such as tricuspid valve function. Both types of factors may affect the interpretation and usefulness of CVP measurements.

B. Correction of negative inotropic factors such as hypoxia, acidosis, hypoglycemia, and other metabolic derangements will improve cardiac output. Sodium bicarbonate infusion at a dose of 1 to 2 mEq/kg is indicated for metabolic acidosis with pH below 7.20 if there is adequate ventilation (PCO_2 less than 44 to 50 mm Hg). More sodium bicarbonate can be infused if the pH remains low. In addition, hypocalcemia frequently occurs in infants with circulatory failure, especially if they have received large amounts of volume resuscitation; this must be corrected. In this setting, calcium frequently produces a positive inotropic response. Calcium gluconate 10% (1 mL/kg) can be infused slowly on an empirical basis or after measurement of the ionized calcium level. (see Chap. 29).

C. Positive inotropic agents should be used to increase cardiac output.

1. Sympathomimetic amines are commonly used in infants. The advantages include rapidity of onset, ability to control dosage, and ultrashort half-life.

a. Dopamine is a naturally occurring catecholamine. Exogenous dopamine activates receptors in a dose-dependent fashion. At low doses (0.5 to 2 µg/kg/min), dopamine stimulates peripheral dopamine receptors (DA_1 and DA_2) and increases renal, mesenteric, and coronary blood flow with little effect on cardiac output. In intermediate doses (2 to 6 µg/kg/min), dopamine has positive inotropic and chronotropic effects (beta-1 and beta-2). At high doses (6 to 10 µg/kg/minute), dopamine stimulates alpha-1 and alpha-2 adrenergic receptors and serotonin receptors, resulting in vasoconstriction and increased peripheral vascular resistance. High-dose dopamine also increases venous return. In preterm infants, dopamine may stimulate the alpha receptors at lower doses. The increase in myocardial contractility depends in part on myocardial norepinephrine stores. Dopamine has been used at high infusion rates (>25 µg/kg/min) to normalize blood pressure in preterm newborns without detrimental vasoconstrictive effects, probably due to the decreased cardiovascular sensitivity to sympathomimetic agents that is prevalent in these infants.

b. Dobutamine is a synthetic catecholamine with relatively cardioselective inotropic effects. In doses of 5 to 15 µg/kg per minute, dobutamine increases cardiac output (alpha-1 receptors) with little effect on heart rate. Dobutamine can decrease systemic vascular resistance (beta-receptors). Dobutamine is often used with dopamine to improve cardiac output in cases of decreased mycardial function as its inotropic effects, unlike those of dopamine, are independent of norepinephrine stores. However, because hypotension is a result of decreased systemic vascular resistance in the majority of nonasphyxiated newborns, dopamine remains the first line of pressor therapy.

c. **Epinephrine** increases myocardial contractility and peripheral vascular resistance (beta- and alpha-receptors). It is not a first-line drug in newborns; however, it may be effective in patients who do not respond to dopamine and dobutamine. Epinephrine may be helpful in conditions such as sepsis when low perfusion is due to peripheral vasodilatation. The starting dose is 0.05 to 0.1 µg/kg per minute and can be increased rapidly as needed while dopamine infusion rates are decreased. Epinephrine is an effective adjunct therapy to dopamine because cardiac norepinephrine stores are readily depleted with prolonged and higher rate dopamine infusions.

2. **Other agents**

a. **Corticosteroids** may be useful in extremely premature infants with hypotension refractory to volume expansion and vasopressors, but this usage has not been adequately tested in clinical trials. Hydrocortisone stabilizes blood pressure through multiple mechanisms. It induces the expression of the cardiovascular adrenergic receptors that are down-regulated by prolonged use of sympathomimetic agents and also inhibits catecholamine metabolism. Moreover, some extremely preterm infants have adrenal insufficiency, especially in the setting of prolonged illness. After hydrocortisone administration, there is a rapid increase in intracellular calcium availability, resulting in enhanced responsiveness to adrenergic agents. The blood pressure response is evident as early as 2 hours after hydrocortisone treatment. For refractory hypotension, we use hydrocortisone in a dose of 1 mg/kg. If efficacy is noted, we repeat the dose every 12 hours for 2 to 3 days, especially if low serum cortisol levels are documented prior to hydrocortisone treatment. High-dose steroids have been used in sepsis, but their efficacy remains controversial, perhaps because administration is initiated late in the clinical course after the cascade of inflammatory mediators has begun.

Suggested Readings

Nuntnarumit P., Yang W., Bada-Ellzey H.S. Blood pressure measurements in the newborn. *Clin Perinatal* 1999;26:981–996.

Seri I., Tan R., Evans J. Cardiovascular effects of hydrocortisone in preterm infants with pressor-resistant hypotension. *Pediatrics* 2001;107:1070–1074.

18. NEONATAL HYPERBILIRUBINEMIA

Camilia R. Martin and John P. Cloherty

I. **Background.** The normal adult serum bilirubin level is less than 1 mg/dL. Adults appear jaundiced when the serum bilirubin level is greater than 2 mg/dL, and newborns appear jaundiced when it is greater than 7 mg/dL. Between 25 and 50% of all term newborns and a higher percentage of premature infants develop clinical jaundice. Also, 6.1% of well term newborns have a maximal serum bilirubin level over 12.9 mg/dL. A serum bilirubin level over 15 mg/dL is found in 3% of normal term babies. **Physical exam is not a reliable measure of the serum bilirubins.**

A. **Source of bilirubin.** Bilirubin is derived from the breakdown of heme-containing proteins in the reticuloendothelial system. The normal newborn produces 6 to 10 mg of bilirubin per kilogram per day, as opposed to the production of 3 to 4 mg/kg per day in the adult.

1. The major heme-containing protein is **red blood cell (RBC) hemoglobin.** Hemoglobin released from senescent RBCs in the reticuloendothelial system is the source of 75% of all bilirubin production. One gram of hemoglobin produces 34 mg of bilirubin. Accelerated release of hemoglobin from RBCs is the cause of hyperbilirubinemia in isoimmunization (e.g., Rh and ABO incompatibility), erythrocyte biochemical abnormalities (e.g., glucose-6-phosphate dehydrogenase(G6PD) and pyruvate kinase deficiencies), abnormal erythrocyte morphology (e.g., hereditary spherocytosis), sequestered blood (e.g., bruising and cephalohematoma), and polycythemia.

2. The other 25% of bilirubin is called **early labeled bilirubin.** It is derived from hemoglobin released by ineffective erythropoiesis in the bone marrow, from other heme-containing proteins in tissues (e.g., myoglobin, cytochromes, catalase, and peroxidase), and from free heme.

B. **Bilirubin metabolism.** The heme ring from heme-containing proteins is oxidized in reticuloendothelial cells to **biliverdin** by the microsomal enzyme heme oxygenase. This reaction releases **carbon monoxide (CO)** (excreted from the lung) and **iron** (reutilized). Biliverdin is then reduced to bilirubin by the enzyme **biliverdin reductase.** Catabolism of 1 mol of hemoglobin produces 1 mol each of CO and bilirubin. Increased bilirubin production, as measured by CO excretion rates, accounts for the higher bilirubin levels seen in Asian, Native American, and Greek infants.

1. **Transport.** Bilirubin is nonpolar and insoluble in water and is transported to liver cells bound to serum **albumin.** Bilirubin bound to albumin does not usually enter the central nervous system and is thought to be nontoxic. Displacement of bilirubin from albumin by drugs, such as the sulfonamides, or by free fatty acids (FFA) at high molar ratios of FFA:albumin, may increase bilirubin toxicity (Table 18.1).

2. **Uptake.** Nonpolar, fat-soluble bilirubin (dissociated from albumin) crosses the hepatocyte plasma membrane and is bound mainly to cytoplasmic **ligandin** (Y protein) for transport to the smooth endoplasmic reticulum. Phenobarbital increases the concentration of ligandin.

3. **Conjugation.** Unconjugated (indirect) bilirubin (UCB) is converted to water-soluble conjugated (direct) bilirubin (CB) in the smooth endoplasmic reticulum by **uridine diphosphate glucuronyl transferase (UDPG-T).** This enzyme is inducible by phenobarbital and catalyzes the formation of bilirubin monoglucuronide. The monoglucuronide may be further conjugated to bilirubin diglucuronide. Both mono- and diglucuronide forms of CB are able to be excreted into the bile canaliculi against a concentration gradient.

Inherited deficiencies and polymorphisms of the conjugating enzyme gene can cause severe hyperbilirubinemia in neonates. **Bilirubin uridine**

TABLE 18.1. DRUGS THAT CAUSE SIGNIFICANT DISPLACEMENT OF BILIRUBIN FROM ALBUMIN *IN VITRO*

Sulfonamides

Moxalactam

Fusidic acid

Radiographic contrast media for cholangiography (sodium iodipamide, sodium ipodate, iopanoic acid, meglumine ioglycamate)

Aspirin

Apazone

Tolbutamide

Rapid infusions of albumin preservatives (sodium caprylate and N-acetyltryptophan)

Rapid infusions of ampicillin

Long-chain free fatty acids (FFA) at high molar ratios of FFA:albumin

Source: From Roth P., Polin R. A. Controversial topics in kernicterus. *Clin Perinatol* 1988;15:970.

5′-diphosphate-glucuronyltransferase gene (UGT1A1) polymorphisms have been described which diminish the expression of the UDPG-T enzyme. The **TATA box mutation** is the most common mutation found and is implicated in Gilbert's syndrome in the Western population. Instead of the usual six (TA) repeats in the promotor region, there is an extra two-base pair (TA) repeat resulting in seven (TA) repeats ([TA]7TAA). The estimated allele frequency among whites is 0.33 to 0.40 and among Asians it is less frequent at 0.15. Alone, this mutation may not result in significant neonatal hyperbilirubinemia; however, with other risk factors for hyperbilirubinemia present (G6PD deficiency, ABO incompatibility, hereditary spherocytosis, breast milk jaundice), the presence of this mutation may confer a significant risk for neonatal hyperbilirubinemia. The **211G→A (G71R)** mutation has been found with increased frequency among the Japanese population and the presence of this mutation alone (homozygote or heterozygote) can result in reduced enzyme activity and neonatal hyperbilirubinemia. This mutation is also the most common mutation in Japanese patients with Gilbert's syndrome. The G71R mutation has not been found in the white population. Other mutations have been described, such as **1456T→G** and the **CAT box mutation** (CCAAT→ GTGCT), however, less is known about these mutations and further investigation is needed to determine their role in the development of nonphysiologic hyperbilirubinemia in the newborn. The population differences in allele frequencies may account for some of the racial and ethnic variation seen in the development of jaundice.

4. **Excretion.** CB in the biliary tree enters the gastrointestinal (GI) tract and is then eliminated from the body in the stool, which contains large amounts of bilirubin. CB is not normally resorbed from the bowel unless it is converted back to UCB by the intestinal enzyme **beta-glucuronidase.** Resorption of bilirubin from the GI tract and delivery back to the liver for reconjugation is called **enterohepatic circulation.** Intestinal bacteria can prevent enterohepatic circulation of bilirubin by converting CB to **urobilinoids,** which are not substrates for beta-glucuronidase. Pathologic con-

ditions leading to increased enterohepatic circulation include decreased enteral intake, intestinal atresias, meconium ileus, and Hirschsprung's disease.

5. **Fetal bilirubin metabolism.** Most UCB formed by the fetus is cleared by the placenta into the maternal circulation. Formation of CB is limited in the fetus because of decreased fetal hepatic blood flow, decreased hepatic ligandin, and decreased UDPG-T activity. The small amount of CB excreted into the fetal gut is usually hydrolyzed by beta-glucuronidase and resorbed. Bilirubin is normally found in amniotic fluid by 12 weeks' gestation and is usually gone by 37 weeks' gestation. Increased amniotic fluid bilirubin is found in hemolytic disease of the newborn and in fetal intestinal obstruction below the bile ducts.

II. **Physiologic hyperbilirubinemia.** The serum UCB level of most newborn infants rises to over 2 mg/dL in the first week of life. This level usually rises in full-term infants to a peak of 6 to 8 mg/dL by 3 days of age and then falls. A rise to 12 mg/dL is in the physiologic range. In premature infants, the peak may be 10 to 12 mg/dL on the fifth day of life, possibly rising over 15 mg/dL without any specific abnormality of bilirubin metabolism. Levels under 2 mg/dL may not be seen until 1 month of age in both full-term and premature infants. This "normal jaundice" is attributed to the following mechanisms:

A. **Increased bilirubin production** due to
   1. Increased RBC volume per kilogram and decreased RBC survival (90-day versus 120-day) in infants compared with adults.
   2. Increased ineffective erythropoiesis and increased turnover of nonhemoglobin heme proteins.
B. Increased enterohepatic circulation caused by high levels of intestinal beta-glucuronidase, preponderance of bilirubin monoglucuronide rather than diglucuronide, decreased intestinal bacteria, and decreased gut motility with poor evacuation of bilirubin-laden meconium.
C. **Defective uptake** of bilirubin from plasma caused by decreased ligandin and binding of ligandin by other anions.
D. **Defective conjugation** due to decreased UDPG-T activity.
E. **Decreased hepatic excretion** of bilirubin.

III. **Nonphysiologic hyperbilirubinemia** (Fig. 18.1 and Table 18.2). Nonphysiologic jaundice may not be easy to distinguish from physiologic jaundice. The following situations suggest nonphysiologic hyperbilirubinemia and require investigation:

A. **General conditions**
   1. Onset of jaundice before 24 hours of age.
   2. Any elevation of serum bilirubin that requires phototherapy (see Fig. 18.2 and VI.D).
   3. A rise in serum bilirubin levels of over 0.5 mg/dL/hour.
   4. Signs of underlying illness in any infant (vomiting, lethargy, poor feeding, excessive weight loss, apnea, tachypnea, or temperature instability).
   5. Jaundice persisting after 8 days in a term infant or after 14 days in a premature infant.
B. **History**
   1. A family history of jaundice, anemia, splenectomy, or early gallbladder disease suggests hereditary hemolytic anemia (e.g., spherocytosis, G6PD deficiency).
   2. A family history of liver disease may suggest galactosemia, alpha-1-antitrypsin deficiency, tyrosinosis, hypermethioninemia, Gilbert's disease, Crigler-Najjar syndrome types I and II, or cystic fibrosis.
   3. Ethnic or geographic origin associated with hyperbilirubinemia (East Asian, Greek, and American Indian) (see I.B.3 for potential genetic influences).
   4. A sibling with jaundice or anemia may suggest blood group incompatibility, breast-milk jaundice, or Lucey-Driscoll syndrome.

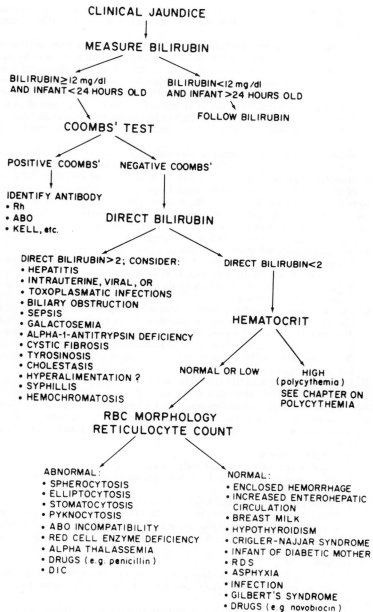

FIG. 18.1. Diagnosis of the etiology of hyperbilirubinemia. Rh = rhesus factor; RBC = red blood cell; DIC = disseminated intravascular coagulation; RDS = respiratory distress syndrome.

5. Maternal illness during pregnancy may suggest congenital viral or toxo-plasmosis infection. Infants of diabetic mothers tend to develop hyper-bilirubinemia (see Chap. 2).

6. Maternal drugs may interfere with bilirubin binding to albumin, making bilirubin toxic at relatively low levels (sulfonamides) or may cause he-molysis in a G6PD-deficient infant (sulfonamides, nitrofurantoin, anti-malarials).

7. The labor and delivery history may show trauma associated with extra-vascular bleeding and hemolysis. Oxytocin use may be associated with neonatal hyperbilirubinemia, although this is controversial. Asphyxiated infants may have elevated bilirubin levels caused either by inability of the liver to process bilirubin or by intracranial hemorrhage. Delayed cord clamping may be associated with neonatal polycythemia and increased bilirubin load.

8. The infant's history may show delayed or infrequent stooling, which can be caused by poor caloric intake or intestinal obstruction and lead to increased enterohepatic circulation of bilirubin. Poor caloric intake may also decrease bilirubin uptake by the liver. Vomiting can be due to sepsis, pyloric stenosis, or galactosemia.

9. **Breastfeeding.** A distinction has been made between breast-milk jaun-dice, in which jaundice is thought to be due to the breast milk itself, and breastfeeding jaundice, in which low caloric intake may be responsible.

   a. **Breast-milk jaundice** is of late onset and has an incidence in term infants of 2 to 4%. By day 4, instead of the usual fall in the serum bilirubin level, the bilirubin level continues to rise and may reach 20 to 30 mg/dL by 14 days of age. If breastfeeding is continued, the levels will stay ele-vated and then fall slowly at 2 weeks of age, returning to normal by 4 to 12 weeks of age. If breastfeeding is stopped, the bilirubin level will fall rapidly in 48 hours. If nursing is then resumed, the bilirubin may rise 2 to 4 mg/dL but usually will not reach the previous high level. These infants show good weight gain, have normal liver function test results, and show no evidence of hemolysis. Mothers with infants who have breast-milk jaundice syndrome have a recurrence rate of 70% in future pregnancies (see I.B.3 for potential genetic influences). The mechanism of true breast-milk jaundice is unknown but is thought to be due to an unidentified factor (or factors) in breast milk interfering with bilirubin metabolism. Additionally, compared with formula-fed infants, breastfed infants are more likely to have increased enterohep-atic circulation because they ingest the beta-glucuronidase present in breast milk, are slower to be colonized with intestinal bacteria that convert CB to urobilinoids, and excrete less stool. There are reports of kernicterus in otherwise healthy, breastfed, term newborns.

   b. **Breastfeeding jaundice.** Infants who are breastfed have higher biliru-bin levels after day 3 of life compared to formula-fed infants. The dif-ferences in the levels of bilirubin are usually not clinically significant. The incidence of peak bilirubin levels >12 mg/dL in breastfed term infants is 12 to 13%. The main factor thought to be responsible for breast-feeding jaundice is a decreased intake of milk that leads to increased enterohepatic circulation.

C. **The physical examination.** Jaundice is detected by blanching the skin with finger pressure to observe the color of the skin and subcutaneous tissues. Jaundice progresses in a cephalocaudal direction. The highest bilirubin lev-els are associated with jaundice below the knees and in the hands. However, visual inspection is not a reliable indicator of serum bilirubin levels.

   Jaundiced infants should be examined for the following physical findings:

   1. **Prematurity.**

   2. **Small size for gestational age (SGA),** which may be associated with poly-cythemia and in utero infections.

TABLE 18.2. CAUSES OF NEONATAL HYPERBILIRUBINEMIA

Overproduction	Undersecretion	Mixed	Uncertain mechanism
Fetomaternal blood group incompatibity (e.g., Rh, ABO)	**Metabolic and endocrine conditions**	Sepsis	Chinese, Japanese, Korean, and American Indian infants (see polymorphism discussion, section I.B.3)
Hereditary spherocytosis, eliptocytosis, somatocytosis	Galactosemia	Intrauterine infections	
Nonspherocytic hemolytic anemias	Familial nonhemolytic jaundice types 1 and 2 (Crigler-Najjar syndrome)	Toxoplasmosis	
G6PD deficiency and drugs	Gilbert's disease	Rubella	
Pyruvate-kinase deficiency	Hypothyroidism	CID	
Other red-cell enzyme deficiencies	Tyrosinosis	Herpes simplex	
Alpha thalassemia	Hypermethioninemia	Syphilis	Breast-milk jaundice
Delta-beta thalassemia	Drugs and hormones	Hepatitis	
Acquired hemolysis due to vitamin K, nitrofurantoin, sulfonamides, antimalarials, penicillin, oxytocin, bupivacaine, or infection	Novobiocin	Respiratory distress syndrome	
	Pregnanediol	Asphyxia	
	Lucy-Driscoll syndrome	Infant of diabetic mother	
	Infants of diabetic mothers	Severe erythroblastosis fetalis	
Extravascular Blood	Prematurity		
Petechiae	Hypopituitarism and anencephaly		
Hematomas	**Obstructive Disorders**		
Pulmonary, cerebral or occult hemorrhage	Biliary atresia*		
Polycythemia	Dubin-Johnson and Rotor's syndrome*		
Fetomaternal or fetofetal transfusion	Choledochal cyst*		
Delayed clamping of the umbilical cord	Cystic fibrosis (inspissated bile)*		
	Tumor* or band* (extrinsic obstruction)		

Increased enteropathic circulation
Pyloric stenosis*
Intestinal atresia or stenosis including annular pancreas
Hirschsprung's disease
Meconium ileus and/or meconium plug syndrome
Fasting or hypoperistalsis from other causes
Drug-induced paralytic ileus (hexamethonium)
Swallowed blood

Alpha-1-antitrypsin deficiency*
Parenteral nutrition

G6PD = glucose-6-phosphate dehydrogenase; CID = cytomegalovirus inclusion disease, as in TORCH (toxoplasmosis, other, rubella, cytomegalovirus, herpes simplex).
*Jaundice may not be seen in the neonatal period.
Source: Modified from Odell G. B., Poland R. L., Nostrea E. Jr., Neonatal Hyperbilirubinemia. In Klaus M. H., Fanaroff A. (Eds.). *Care of the High Risk Neonate.* Philadelphia: Saunders, 1973; Chap. 11.

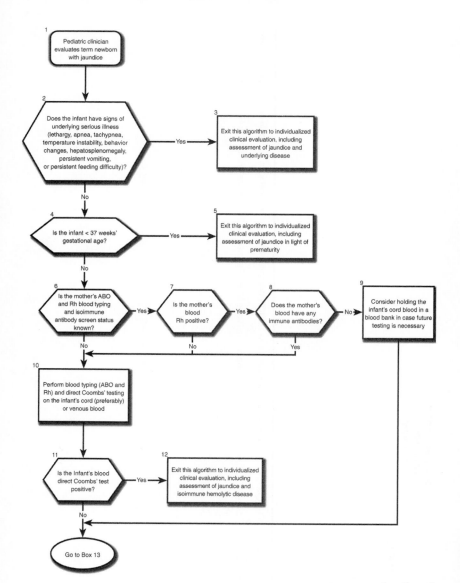

(continues)

FIG. 18.2. Algorithm: Management of hyperbilirubinemia in the healthy term infant. From AAP. Practice parameter: Management of hyperbilirubinemia in the healthy term newborn. *Pediatrics* 1994; 94:558. This practice guideline was being revised by the AAP in 2003. The new guideline was not yet available.

3. **Microcephaly,** which may be associated with *in-utero* infections.
4. **Extravascular blood:** bruising, cephalohematoma, or other enclosed hemorrhage.
5. **Pallor** associated with hemolytic anemia or extravascular blood loss.
6. **Petechiae** associated with congenital infection, sepsis, or erythroblastosis.

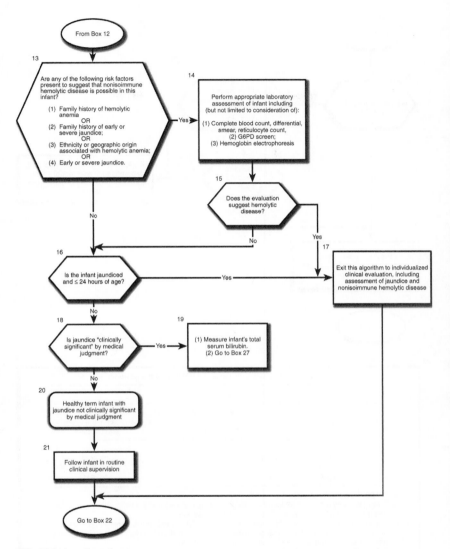

FIG. 18.2. *(continued)*

7. **Hepatosplenomegaly** associated with hemolytic anemia, congenital infection, or liver disease.
8. **Omphalitis.**
9. **Chorioretinitis** associated with congenital infection.
10. Evidence of **hypothyroidism** (see Chap. 2).

D. **Prediction of nonphysiologic hyperbilirubinemia**
   1. A **screening total serum bilirubin (TSB)** collected predischarge from the newborn nursery and plotted on a "hour-specific bilirubin nomogram" (see Fig. 18.3) has been shown to be helpful in identifying infants at high risk of developing nonphysiologic hyperbilirubinemia.

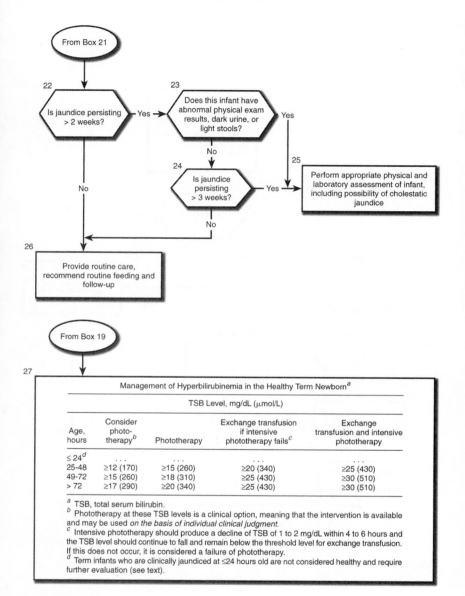

FIG. 18.2. *(continued)*

2. In infants > 30 weeks' gestation, **transcutaneous bilirubin (TcB)** using multiple wavelength analysis (versus two-wavelength method) can reliably estimate serum bilirubin levels independent of skin pigmentation, gestational age, postnatal age, and weight of infant. Similar to TSB, TcB can be used as a screening tool to identify infants at high risk for severe hyperbilirubinemia by plotting obtained values on a hour-specific bilirubin nomogram. Despite advancements in transcutaneous technology, ex-

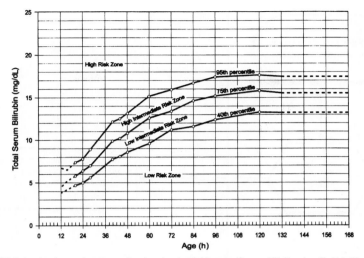

Risk designation of term and near-term well newborns based on their hour-specific serum bilirubin values. The high-risk zone is designated by the 95th percentile track. The intermediate-risk zone is subdivided to upper- and lower-risk zones by the 75th percentile track. The low-risk zone has been electively and statistically defined by the 40th percentile track. (Dotted extensions are based on <300 TSB values/epoch). This study is based on heel stick venous bilirubins and lower bilirubins.

FIG. 18.3. Hour-specific bilirubin nomogram. Reprinted with permission from Bhutani VK, et al. Predictive ability of a predischarge hour-specific serum bilirubin for subsequent significant hyperbilirubinemia in healthy term and near-term newborns. *Pediatrics* 1999; 103:6–14.

trapolation to serum bilirubin levels from TcB should continue to be done with caution. TcB values of > 13 mg/dL should be correlated with TSB values. Likewise, TcB values of 75th percentile or greater on a hour-specific nomogram should be given serious consideration. TcB as a screening tool has the potential to reduce the number of invasive blood tests performed in newborns and reduce related health-care costs.

3. Due to the production of carbon monoxide during bilirubin metabolism (see I.B), **end-tidal carbon monoxide (ETCOc)** has been hypothesized as a potential screening tool. In a recent study, ETCOc was not shown to improve the sensitivity or specificity of predicting nonphysiologic hyperbilirubinemia over TSB or TcB alone. However, it may offer insight to the underlying pathologic process contributing to the hyperbilirubinemia (hemolysis versus conjugation defects).

E. **Clinical tests** (Figs. 18.1, 18.2, and 18.4). The following tests are indicated in the presence of nonphysiologic jaundice:

1. **Total serum bilirubin.**

2. **Blood type, Rh, and direct Coombs' test of the infant** to test for isoimmune hemolytic disease. Infants of women who are Rh-negative should have a blood type, Rh, and Coombs' test performed at birth. Routine blood typing and Coombs' testing of all infants born to O-positive mothers to determine whether there is risk for ABO incompatibility is probably unnecessary. Such testing is reserved for infants with clinically significant jaundice, those in whom follow-up is difficult, or those whose skin pigmentation is such that jaundice may not be easily recognized. Blood typing and Coombs' testing should be considered for infants who are to be discharged early, especially if the mother is Type O (see Chap. 5).

3. **Blood type, Rh, and antibody screen of the mother** should have been done during pregnancy and the antibody screen repeated at delivery.

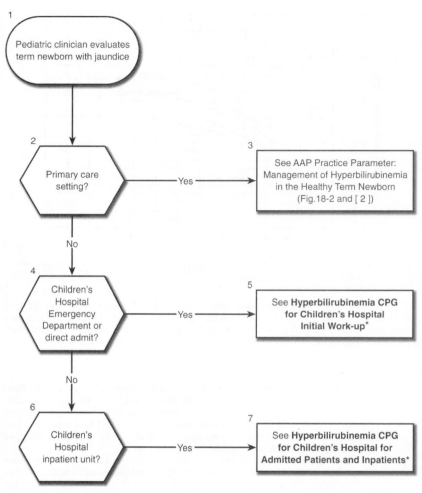

FIG. 18.4A. Children's Hospital hyperbilirubinemia clinical practice guide (CPG) for evaluation of infants with jaundice who have been discharged from the birth hospital.

4. **Peripheral smear for RBC morphology and reticulocyte count** to detect causes of Coombs'-negative hemolytic disease (e.g., spherocytosis).
5. **Hematocrit** will detect polycythemia or suggest blood loss from occult hemorrhage.
6. Identification of **antibody on infant's RBCs** (if result of direct Coombs' test is positive).
7. **Direct bilirubin** determination is necessary when jaundice persists beyond the first 2 weeks of life or whenever there are signs of cholestasis (light-colored stools and bilirubin in urine).
8. In prolonged jaundice, tests for liver disease, congenital infection, sepsis, metabolic defects, or hypothyroidism are indicated. Total parenteral nutrition is a well-recognized cause of prolonged direct hyperbilirubinemia.

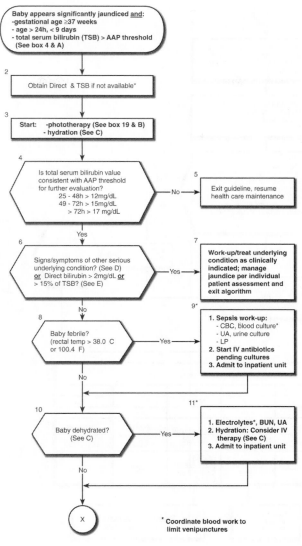

FIG. 18.4B. Hyperbilirubinemia CPG Children's Hospital initial workup.

9. **A G6PD screen** may be helpful, especially in male infants of African, Asian, Southern European, and Mediterranean or Middle Eastern descent. The incidence of G6PD among African-Americans is 11 to 13%, comprising the most affected subpopulation in America. Previously, term black infants with G6PD deficiency were not thought to be at significant risk for hyperbilirubinemia. However, recent literature suggests otherwise. Not all infants with G6PD deficiency will manifest neonatal hyperbilirubinemia. A combination of genetic and environmental risk factors will determine

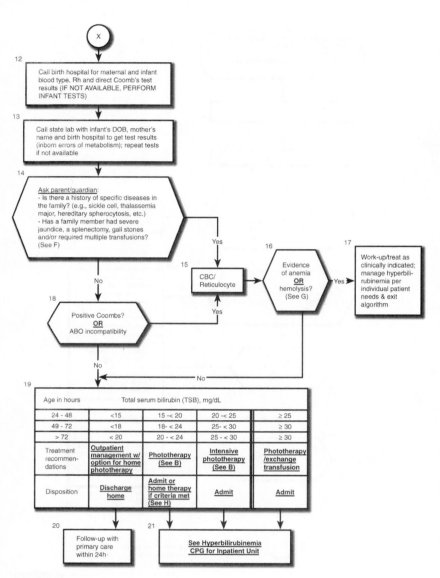

FIG. 18.4B. *(continued)*

the individual risk (see I.B.3 for potential genetic influences). Screening the parents for G6PD deficiency is also helpful in making the diagnosis. Infants who had G6PD deficiency and were discharged early have been reported with severe hyperbilirubinemia and significant sequelae.

IV. Diagnosis of neonatal hyperbilirubinemia (see Table 18.2 and Fig. 18.1).

V. Bilirubin toxicity. This area remains highly controversial. The problem is that bilirubin levels that are toxic to one infant may not be toxic to another, or even to the same infant in different clinical circumstances. Currently, major debate

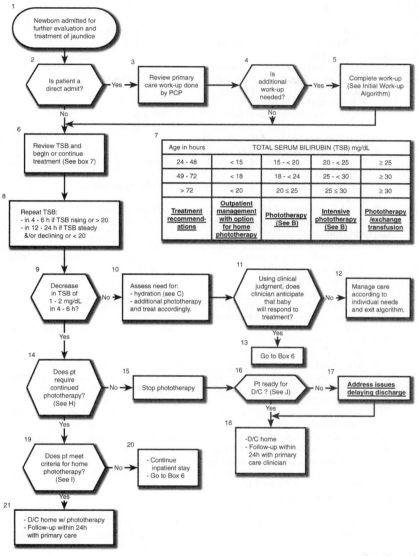

(continues)

FIG. 18.4C. Hyperbilirubinemia CPG Children's Hospital, Boston, for admitted patients or inpatients.

surrounds the toxicity of bilirubin in otherwise healthy full-term infants and in premature, low-birth-weight infants.

Bilirubin levels refer to total bilirubin. Direct bilirubin is not subtracted from the total unless it constitutes more than 50% of total bilirubin.

A. Bilirubin entry into the brain occurs as free (unbound) bilirubin or as bilirubin bound to albumin in the presence of a disrupted blood–brain barrier. It is estimated that 8.5 mg of bilirubin will bind tightly to 1 g of albumin

Annotations for Hyperbilirubinemia CPG (Fig. 18-4A and B)

A. Exclusion Statement
1. If infant is less than 24 hours old, exit this algorithm to individualized clinical evaluation, including assessment of jaundice and nonisoimmune hemolytic disease.
2. Patients with jaundice limited to the head and neck and not deemed to be clinically significant may be excluded from the CPG.

B. Phototherapy
1. Initiate phototherapy (preferably with blanket) as soon as feasible; shield eyes if not using blanket.
2. Light source recommendations:
   - Fiber optic (425–475 nm).
   - Overhead banks/spots (425–475/550–600 nm).
3. Continuous; interruptions for breastfeeding may be considered.
4. To achieve intensive phototherapy:
   - Maximal surface area must be exposed.
   - Requires two or more lights (any combination of overheads, spots, bili blankets).
5. Maximal intensity for overheads: as close to baby as possible without hyperthermia or burn.
6. Overhead banks of phototherapy are associated with increased insensible fluid loss, and this loss should be considered when calculating intake needs.

C. Hydration
1. *Definition of dehydration (any one of the following):* no urine within 4–6 hours, tachycardia, decreased skin turgor, sunken eyes, sunken fontanelle, delayed cap refill, serum Na > 145, HCO_3 < 17.
2. Management:
   - Oral hydration preferred.
   - Breast milk preferred; otherwise, use formula. Supplementation with dextrose water or sterile water is not indicated.
   - IV hydration if maintenance deficit cannot be provided by oral route.

D. Signs and Symptoms of Serious Underlying Condition
1. *Sepsis / Galactosemia:* vomiting, lethargy, poor feeding, excessive weight loss, hepatosplenomegaly, apnea, temperature instability, tachypnea.
2. *Cholestatic Jaundice:* dark urine, positive bilirubin in urine, light-colored stools, persistent jaundice > 3 weeks.

E. Direct Bilirubin Results
A direct bilirubin level of 2.0 mg/dL or a level that is ≥ 15% of the TSB indicates cholestasis, which is a sign of hepatic or biliary-tract malfunction. Work-up and treat underlying condition as clinically indicated.

F. Family History—Ethnic or Geographic Origin
1. Black infants at risk for hemoglobinopathies S,C.
2. Southeast Asians or Mediterranean origin at risk for G6PD deficiency or other hemoglobinopathies.

G. Anemia/Hemolysis
Normal blood values for hemoglobin (Hgb) in newborns range from 13.7 to 20.1 g/dL with a mean of 16.8 g/dL based on studies of cord blood levels in term newborns. An elevated reticulocyte count of >6% accompanied by a Hgb of <13 g/dL is suggestive of hemolysis.

H. Response to Phototherapy [2]

Bili	Age	Action
<18	—	Wean to single phototherapy
≤12	—	Discharge home
≤14	49–72h	Discontinue phototherapy, discharge home*
≤15	>72h	Discontinue phototherapy, discharge home*

*Check rebound TSB 12–24 hours after discharge.

(continues)

I. Home Phototherapy
1. Parents must agree.
2. Community pediatrician must agree.
3. Insurance approval.
4. Treatment and monitoring must be readily accessible.

J. Discharge Criteria
1. Infant feeds normally and family has access to lactation consultation if breastfeeding.
2. Parents have received education as to normal infant well-being, including feeding, voiding, stooling, sleep patterns and position, signs of acute illness, and infant safety.
3. Follow-up appointments have been scheduled with primary pediatrician and appropriate home health services, and parents agree to such care.
4. Hearing screening test should be scheduled as part of follow-up after discharge for infants who reached TSB levels exceeding indication for exchange transfusion.

(molar ratio of 1), although this binding capacity is less in small and sick prematures. Free fatty acids and certain drugs (see Table 18.1) interfere with bilirubin binding to albumin, while acidosis affects bilirubin solubility and its deposition into brain tissue. Factors that disrupt the blood–brain barrier include hyperosmolarity, anoxia, and hypercarbia, and the barrier itself may be more permeable in premature infants.

B. Kernicterus is a pathologic diagnosis and refers to **yellow staining** of the brain by bilirubin together with evidence of **neuronal injury.** Grossly, bilirubin staining is most commonly seen in the basal ganglia, various cranial nerve nuclei, other brain stem nuclei, cerebellar nuclei, hippocampus, and anterior horn cells of the spinal cord. Microscopically, there is necrosis, neuronal loss, and gliosis.

C. Acute bilirubin encephalopathy is classically seen in term infants dying of Rh hemolytic disease with high (>20 mg/dL) bilirubin levels who have kernicterus on autopsy. The clinical presentation of acute bilirubin encephalopathy can be divided into three phases:
1. Hypotonia, lethargy, high-pitched cry, and poor suck.
2. Hypertonia of extensor muscles (with opisthotonus, rigidity, oculogyric crisis, and retrocollis), fever, and seizures. Many infants die in this phase. All infants who survive this phase develop chronic bilirubin encephalopathy.
3. Hypotonia replaces hypertonia after about 1 week of age.

D. Chronic bilirubin encephalopathy is marked by athetosis, partial or complete sensorineural deafness, limitation of upward gaze, dental dysplasia, and mild intellectual deficits.

E. Bilirubin toxicity and hemolytic disease. There is general agreement that in Rh hemolytic disease there is a direct association between marked elevations of bilirubin and signs of bilirubin encephalopathy with kernicterus at autopsy. Studies and clinical experience have shown that in full-term infants with hemolytic disease, if the total bilirubin level is kept under 20 mg/dL, bilirubin encephalopathy is unlikely to occur. Theoretically, this should apply to other causes of isoimmune hemolytic disease, such as ABO incompatibility, and to hereditary hemolytic processes such as hereditary spherocytosis, pyruvate kinase deficiency, or glucose-6-phosphate dehydrogenase (G6PD) deficiency.

F. Bilirubin toxicity and the healthy full-term infant. In contrast to infants with hemolytic disease, there is little evidence showing adverse neurologic outcome in healthy term neonates with bilirubin levels below 25 to 30 mg/dL. A large prospective cohort study failed to demonstrate a clinically significant association between bilirubin levels above 20 mg/dL and neurologic abnormality, long-term hearing loss, or intelligence quotient (IQ) deficits. However, an increase in minor motor abnormalities of unclear significance was detected in those with serum bilirubin levels over 20 mg/dL. Hyperbilirubinemia in term infants has been associated with abnormalities in brain-stem audiometric-evoked responses (BAER), cry characteristics, and neurobehavioral measures. However, these changes disappear when bilirubin levels fall and there are no measurable long-term sequelae. Kernicterus has been reported in jaundiced healthy, full-term, breastfed infants. **All predictive values for bilirubin toxicity are based on heel stick values.**

G. **Bilirubin toxicity and the low-birth-weight infant.** Initial early studies of babies of 1250 to 2500 g and 28 to 36 weeks' gestational age showed no relationship between neurologic damage and bilirubin levels over 18 to 20 mg/dL. Later studies, however, began to report "kernicterus" at autopsy or neurodevelopmental abnormalities at follow-up in premature infants under 1250 g who had bilirubin levels previously thought to be safe (e.g., under 10 to 20 mg/dL). Because kernicterus in preterm infants is now considered uncommon, hindsight suggests that this so-called "low bilirubin kernicterus" was largely due to factors other than bilirubin alone. For example, unrecognized intracranial hemorrhage, inadvertent exposure to drugs that displace bilirubin from albumin, or the use of solutions (e.g., benzyl alcohol) that can alter the blood–brain barrier may have accounted for developmental handicaps or kernicterus in infants with low levels of serum bilirubin. In addition, premature infants are more likely to suffer from anoxia, hypercarbia, and sepsis, which also open the blood–brain barrier and lead to enhanced bilirubin deposition in neural tissue. Finally, the pathologic changes seen in postmortem preterm infant brains has been more consistent with nonspecific damage than with true kernicterus. Thus, bilirubin toxicity in low-birth-weight infants may not be a function of bilirubin levels per se but of their overall clinical status.

VI. **Management of unconjugated hyperbilirubinemia.** Given the uncertainty of determining what levels of bilirubin are toxic, these are general clinical guidelines only and should be modified in any sick infant with acidosis, hypercapnia, hypoxemia, asphyxia, sepsis, hypoalbuminemia (<2.5 mg/dL), or signs of bilirubin encephalopathy.

A. **General principles.** Management of unconjugated hyperbilirubinemia is clearly tied to the etiology. Early identification of known causes of nonphysiologic hyperbilirubinemia (see III. B, C, and D) should prompt close observation for development of jaundice, appropriate laboratory investigation, and timely intervention. Any medication (see Table 18.1) or clinical factor that may interfere with bilirubin metabolism, bilirubin binding to albumin, or the integrity of the blood–brain barrier should be discontinued or corrected. Infants who are receiving inadequate feedings, or who have decreased urine and stool output, need increased feedings both in volume and in calories to reduce the enterohepatic circulation of bilirubin. Infants with hypothyroidism need adequate replacement of thyroid hormone. If levels of bilirubin are so high that the infant is at risk for kernicterus, bilirubin may be removed mechanically by exchange transfusion, its excretion increased by alternative pathways using phototherapy, or its normal metabolism increased by drugs such as phenobarbital.

B. **Infants with hemolytic disease**
1. In Rh disease we start intensive phototherapy immediately. An exchange transfusion is performed if the bilirubin level is predicted to reach 20 mg/dL (see Fig. 18.5, A and B).
2. In ABO hemolytic disease we start phototherapy if the bilirubin level exceeds 10 mg/dL at 12 hours, 12 mg/dL at 18 hours, 14 mg/dL at 24 hours, or 15 mg/dL at any time. If the bilirubin reaches 20 mg/dL, an exchange transfusion is done.
3. In hemolytic disease of other causes we treat as if it were Rh disease (Tables 18.3, 18.4, 18.5).

C. **Healthy term infants** (Fig. 18.2). The American Academy of Pediatrics (AAP) has published a set of practice parameters for the treatment of unconjugated hyperbilirubinemia in healthy, full-term neonates.

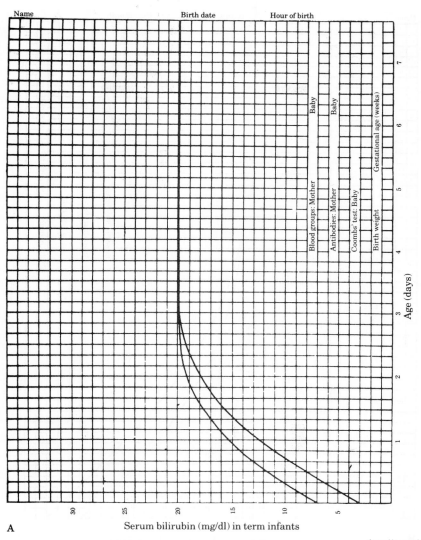

A   Serum bilirubin (mg/dl) in term infants

(continues)

FIG. 18.5. Serum bilirubin levels plotted against age in term infants (**A**) and premature infants (**B**) with erythroblastosis.

1. We have begun to use TcB (see IIID) measurements and the hour-specific bilirubin nomogram to identify infants at risk for significant hyperbilirubinemia.
2. Serum bilirubin levels are not routinely screened on our healthy term infants unless jaundice occurs in the first 2 days of life or other risk factors are present. Most of our term infants are sent home by 24 to 48 hours of age; therefore, parents should be informed about neonatal jaundice prior to discharge from the hospital. **Arrangements should be made for follow up in 1 or 2 days. This is especially true if the infant is under 38 weeks**

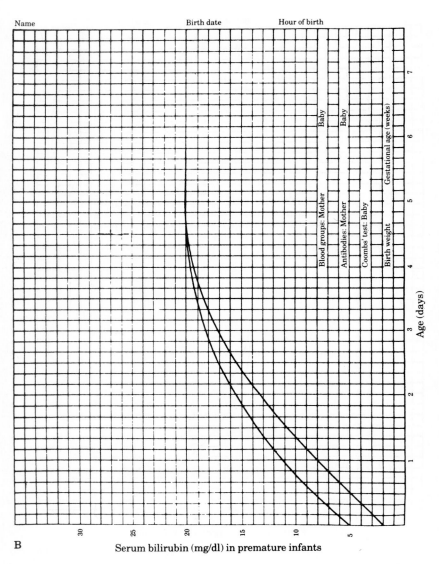

B

Serum bilirubin (mg/dl) in premature infants

FIG. 18.5. *(continued)*

gestation, is the first child, is breast feeding, or has any other risk factors for hyperbilirubinemia.

3. In healthy term infants who are jaundiced, we follow the guidelines published by the AAP (Fig. 18.2) and have a local clinical practice guideline based on these recommendations (Fig. 18.4). For example, if the bilirubin level of a 2½-day-old infant is 25 to 30 mg/dL, intensive phototherapy will be started as preparations are made to perform an exchange transfusion. If a repeat bilirubin determination 4 to 6 hours later shows the bilirubin remaining above 25 mg/dL, an exchange transfusion will be performed.

TABLE 18.3. COMMON ANTIGENS OTHER THAN RH IMPLICATED IN HEMOLYTIC DISEASES OF THE NEWBORN

Antigen	Alternative Symbol or Name	Blood Group System
Do^a		Dombrock
Fy^a		Duffy
Jk^a		Kidd
Jk^b		Kidd
K	K:1	Kell
Lu^a	Lu:1	Lutheran
M		MNSs
N		MNSs
S		MNSs
s		MNSs

However, if total serum bilirubin declines to under 25 mg/dL, exchange transfusion will be held as intensive phototherapy continues.

4. In healthy term **breastfed infants** with hyperbilirubinemia, preventive measures are the best approach and include encouragement of frequent nursing (at least every 3 hours) and, if necessary, supplementation with formula (not dextrose water) (see III.B.9).

TABLE 18.4. OTHER ANTIGENS INVOLVED IN HEMOLYTIC DISEASES OF THE NEWBORN

Antigen	Alternative Symbol or Name	Blood Group System
Co^a		Colton
Di^b		Diego
Ge		Gerbich
Hy	Holley	
Jr		
Js^b	Matthews, K:7	Kell
k	Cellano, K:2	Kell
Kp^b	Rautenberg, K:4	Kell
Lan	Langereis	
Lu^b		Lutheran
LW	Landsteinder-Weiner	
$P,P1,P^k$	Tj^a	P
U		MNSs
Yt^a		Cartwright

TABLE 18.5. INFREQUENT ANTIGENS IMPLICATED IN HEMOLYTIC DISEASES OF THE NEWBORN

Antigen	Alternative Symbol or Name	Blood Group System
Be^a	Berrens	Rh
Bi	Biles	
By	Batty	
C^w	Rh:8	Rh
C^x	Rh:9	Rh
Di*^{a}		Diego
Evans		Rh
E^w	Rh:11	Rh
Far	See Kam	
Ga	Gambino	
Go^a	Gonzales	Rh
Good		
Heibel		
Hil	Hill	MNSs Mi sub+
Ht^a	Hunt	
Hut	Hutchinson	MNSs Mi sub
Js^a	Sutter	Kell
Kam (Far)	Kamhuber	
Kp^a	Penney	Kell
Mit	Mitchell	
Mt^a	Martin	MNSs#
Mull	Lu:9	Lutheran
Mur	Murrell	MNSs Mi sub
Rd	Radin	
Re^a	Reid	
R^N	Rh:32	Rh
Vw(Gr)	Verweyst (Graydon)	MNSs Mi sub
Wi^a	Wright	
Zd		

This may not be a complete list. Any antigen that the father has and the mother does not have and that induces an IgG response in the mother may cause sensitization.

5. Guidelines for phototherapy and exchange transfusion are identical for breastfed and formula-fed infants. However, in **breastfed infants,** a decision is often made whether or not to discontinue breastfeeding. In a randomized controlled trial of breastfed infants with bilirubin levels of at least 17 mg/dL, 3% of those who switched to formula and received phototherapy reached bilirubin levels above 20 mg/dL compared with 14% of those who continued nursing while they were receiving phototherapy. In infants not receiving phototherapy, 19% of those who switched to formula reached bilirubin levels over 20 mg/dL compared with 24% of those who simply continued nursing. No infant in any group had a bilirubin over 23 mg/dL, and none required exchange transfusion. However, discontinuing breastfeeding entirely may not be necessary. In a later prospective trial, breastfed infants who continued to breastfeed and were supplemented with formula had a comparable response to treatment to infants who stopped breastfeeding and fed formula alone.

In general, **our current practice** is that if the bilirubin reaches a level that would require phototherapy and is predicted to exceed 20 mg/dL, we will start phototherapy, and discontinue breastfeeding for 48 hours and supplement with formula. The mother requires much support through this process and is encouraged to pump her breasts until breastfeeding can be resumed.

6. Failure of bilirubin levels to fall after the interruption of breastfeeding may indicate other causes of prolonged indirect hyperbilirubinemia, such as hemolytic disease, hypothyroidism, and familial nonhemolytic jaundice (Crigler-Najjar syndrome).

D. **Premature infants.** There are no consensus guidelines for phototherapy and exchange transfusion in low-birth-weight infants. The following statement from the Guidelines for Perinatal Care from the American Academy of Pediatrics and the American Academy of Obstetricians and Gynecologists emphasize our current lack of knowledge in this area:

"Some pediatricians use guidelines that recommend aggressive treatment of jaundice in low-birth-weight neonates, initiating phototherapy early and performing exchange transfusions in certain neonates with very low bilirubin levels (<10 mg/dL). However, this approach will not prevent kernicterus consistently. Some pediatricians prefer to adopt a less-aggressive therapeutic stance and allow serum bilirubin concentrations in low-birth-weight neonates to approach 15 to 20 mg/dL (257 to 342 mmol/L), before considering exchange transfusions. At present, both of these approaches to treatment should be considered reasonable. In either case, the finding of low bilirubin kernicterus at autopsy in certain low-birth-weight neonates cannot necessarily be interpreted as a therapeutic failure or equivalent to bilirubin encephalopathy. Like retinopathy of prematurity, kernicterus is a condition that cannot be prevented in certain neonates, given the current state of knowledge. Although there is some evidence of an association between hyperbilirubinemia and neurodevelopmental handicap less severe than classic bilirubin encephalopathy, a cause-and-effect relationship has not been established. Furthermore, there is no information presently available to suggest that treating mild jaundice will prevent such handicaps."

Our current practice for treating jaundiced premature infants is as follows:

1. **Infants <1000 g.** Phototherapy is started within 24 hours, and exchange transfusion is performed at levels of 10 to 12 mg/dL.

2. **Infants 1000 to 1500 g.** Phototherapy at bilirubin levels of 7 to 9 mg/dL and exchange transfusion at levels of 12 to 15 mg/dL.

3. **Infants 1500 to 2000 g.** Phototherapy at bilirubin levels of 10 to 12 mg/dL and exchange transfusion at levels of 15 to 18 mg/dL.

4. **Infants 2000 to 2500 g.** Phototherapy at bilirubin levels of 13 to 15 mg/dL and exchange transfusion at levels of 18 to 20 mg/dL.

VII. **Phototherapy.** Although bilirubin absorbs visible light with wavelengths of about 400 to 500 nm, the most effective lights for phototherapy are those with high-energy output near the maximum adsorption peak of bilirubin (450 to 460 nm). Special blue lamps with a peak output at 425 to 475 nm are the most efficient for phototherapy. Cool white lamps with a principal peak at 550 to 600 nm and a range of 380 to 700 nm are usually adequate for treatment. Fiberoptic phototherapy (phototherapy blankets) have been shown to reduce bilirubin levels although less effectively for term infants; likely due to the limited skin exposure it can offer.

A. **Photochemical reactions.** When bilirubin absorbs light, three types of photochemical reactions occur.

   1. **Photoisomerization** occurs in the extravascular space of the skin. The natural isomer of unconjugated bilirubin (4Z,15Z) is instantaneously converted to a less-toxic polar isomer (4Z,15E) that diffuses into the blood and is excreted into the bile without conjugation. However, excretion is slow, and the photoisomer is readily converted back to unconjugated bilirubin, which is resorbed from the gut if the baby is not having stools. After about 12 hours of phototherapy, the photoisomers make up about 20% of total bilirubin. Standard tests do not distinguish between naturally occurring bilirubin and the photoisomer, so bilirubin levels may not change much even though the phototherapy has made the bilirubin present less toxic. Photoisomerization occurs at low-dose phototherapy (6 μW/cm² per nanometer) with no significant benefit from doubling the irradiance.

   2. **Structural isomerization** is the intramolecular cyclization of bilirubin to **lumirubin.** Lumirubin makes up 2 to 6% of serum concentration of bilirubin during phototherapy and is rapidly excreted in the bile and urine without conjugation. Unlike photoisomerization, the conversion of bilirubin to lumirubin is irreversible, and it cannot be reabsorbed. It is the most important pathway for the lowering of serum bilirubin levels and is strongly related to the dose of phototherapy used in the range of 6 to 12 μW/cm² per nanometer.

   3. The slow process of **photo-oxidation** converts bilirubin to small polar products that are excreted in the urine. It is the least important reaction for lowering bilirubin levels.

B. **Indications for phototherapy**

   1. Phototherapy should be used when the level of bilirubin may be hazardous to the infant if it were to increase, even though it has not reached levels requiring exchange transfusion (see VI).

   2. Prophylactic phototherapy may be indicated in special circumstances, such as extremely low-birth-weight infants or severely bruised infants. In hemolytic disease of the newborn, phototherapy is started immediately while the rise in the serum bilirubin level is plotted (see Fig. 18.5) and during the wait for exchange transfusion.

   3. Phototherapy is usually contraindicated in infants with direct hyperbilirubinemia caused by liver disease or obstructive jaundice because indirect bilirubin levels are not usually high in these conditions and because phototherapy may lead to the **"bronze baby" syndrome.** If both direct and indirect bilirubin are high, exchange transfusion is probably safer than phototherapy because it is not known whether the bronze pigment is toxic.

C. **Technique of phototherapy**

   1. We have found that **light banks** with alternating special blue (narrow-spectrum) and daylight fluorescent lights are effective and do not make the baby appear cyanotic. The irradiance can be measured at the skin by a radiometer and should exceed 5 μW per cm² at 425 to 475 nm. There is not much benefit in exceeding 9 μW/cm² per nanometer. Bulbs should be changed at intervals specified by the manufacturer. Our practice is to change all the bulbs every 3 months because this approximates the correct number of hours of use in our unit.

   2. For infants under radiant warmers, we lay infants on fiberoptic blankets and/or use **spot phototherapy** overhead with quartz halide white light having output in the blue spectrum.

3. **Fiberoptic blankets** with light output in the blue-green spectrum have proved very useful in our unit, not only for single phototherapy but also for delivering **"double phototherapy"** in which the infant lies on a fiberoptic blanket with conventional phototherapy overhead.

4. Infants under phototherapy lights are kept naked except for eye patches and a face mask used as a diaper to ensure light exposure to the greatest skin surface area. The infants are turned every 2 hours. Care should be taken to ensure that the eye patches do not occlude the nares, as asphyxia and apnea can result.

5. If an incubator is used, there should be a 5- to 8-cm space between it and the lamp cover to prevent overheating.

6. The infants' temperature should be carefully monitored and servo-controlled.

7. Infants should be weighed daily (small infants are weighed twice each day). Between 10 and 20% extra fluid over the usual requirements is given to compensate for the increased insensible water loss in infants in open cribs or warmers who are receiving phototherapy. Infants also have increased fluid losses caused by increased stooling (see Chap. 9).

8. Skin color is not a guide to hyperbilirubinemia in infants undergoing phototherapy; consequently, bilirubin level should be monitored at least every 12 to 24 hours.

9. Once a satisfactory decline in bilirubin levels has occurred (e.g., exchange transfusion has been averted), we allow infants to be removed from phototherapy for feedings and brief parental visits.

10. **Phototherapy is stopped** when it is believed that the level is low enough to eliminate concern about the toxic effects of bilirubin, when the risk factors for toxic levels of bilirubin are gone, and when the baby is old enough to handle the bilirubin load. A bilirubin level is usually checked 12 to 24 hours after phototherapy is stopped. In a recent study of infants with nonhemolytic hyperbilirubinemia, phototherapy was discontinued at mean bilirubin levels of 13.0 ± 0.7 mg/dL in term and 10.7 ± 1.2 mg/dL in preterm infants. Rebound bilirubin levels 12 to 15 hours later averaged less than 1 mg/dL, and no infant required reinstitution of phototherapy.

11. **Home phototherapy** is effective and is cheaper than hospital phototherapy, and is easy to implement with the use of fiberoptic blankets. Most candidates for home phototherapy are breastfed infants whose bilirubin problems can be resolved with a brief interruption of breastfeeding and increased fluid intake. Constant supervision is required, and all the other details of phototherapy, such as temperature control and fluid intake, are also required. The American Academy of Pediatrics has issued guidelines for the use of home phototherapy.

12. It is contraindicated to put jaundiced infants under direct sunlight, as severe hyperthermia may result.

D. **Side effects of phototherapy**

1. **Insensible water loss** is increased in infants undergoing phototherapy, especially those under radiant warmers. The increase may be as much as 40% for term and 80 to 190% in premature infants. Incubators with servocontrolled warmers will decrease this water loss. Extra fluid must be given to make up for these losses (see Chap. 9, Fluid and Electrolyte Management of the Newborn).

2. **Redistribution of blood flow.** In **term** infants, left ventricular output and renal blood flow velocity decrease, while left pulmonary artery and cerebral blood flow velocity increase. All velocities return to baseline after discontinuation of phototherapy. In the **preterm** infant, cerebral blood flow velocity also increases and renal vascular resistance increases with a reduction of renal blood flow velocity. In ventilated preterm infants the changes in blood flow velocities do not return to baseline even after discontinuation of phototherapy. In addition, in preterm infants under conventional phototherapy, it has been shown that the usual postprandial

increase in superior mesenteric blood flow is blunted. Fiberoptic phototherapy did not seem to affect the postprandial response. Although, the changes in cerebral, renal, and superior mesenteric artery blood flow with phototherapy treatment in preterm infants is of potential concern, no detrimental clinical effects due to these changes have been determined.

3. **Watery diarrhea and increased fecal water loss** may occur. The diarrhea may be caused by increased bile salts and unconjugated bilirubin in the bowel.

4. **Low calcium** levels have been described in preterm infants under phototherapy.

5. **Retinal damage** has been described in animals whose eyes have been exposed to phototherapy lamps. The eyes should be shielded with eye patches. Follow-up studies of infants whose eyes have been adequately shielded show normal vision and electroretinography.

6. **Tanning** of the skin of black infants. Erythemia and increased skin blood flow may also be seen.

7. **"Bronze baby" syndrome** (see VII.B.3).

8. **Mutations, sister chromatid exchange, and DNA strand breaks** have been described in cell culture. It may be wise to shield the scrotum during phototherapy.

9. **Tryptophan is reduced in amino acid solutions** exposed to phototherapy. Methionine and histidine are also reduced in these solutions if multivitamins are added. These solutions should probably be shielded from phototherapy by using aluminum foil on the lines and bottles.

10. **No significant long-term developmental differences** have been found in infants treated with phototherapy compared with controls.

11. Phototherapy upsets **maternal–infant interactions** and therefore should be used only with adequate thought and explanation.

VIII. Exchange transfusion

A. **Mechanisms.** Exchange transfusion removes partially hemolyzed and antibody-coated RBCs as well as unattached antibodies and replaces them with donor RBCs lacking the sensitizing antigen. As bilirubin is removed from the plasma, extravascular bilirubin will rapidly equilibrate and bind to the albumin in the exchanged blood. Within half an hour after the exchange, bilirubin levels return to 60% of preexchange levels, representing the rapid influx of bilirubin into the vascular space. Further increases in postexchange bilirubin levels are due to hemolysis of antibody-coated RBCs sequestered in bone marrow or spleen, from senescent donor RBCs, and from early labeled bilirubin.

B. **Indications for exchange transfusion**

1. When phototherapy fails to prevent a rise in bilirubin to toxic levels (see VI and Figs. 18.2, 18.4, 18.5).

2. Correct anemia and improve heart failure in hydropic infants with hemolytic disease.

3. Stop hemolysis and bilirubin production by removing antibody and sensitized red blood cells (RBCs).

4. Figure 18.5 shows the natural history of bilirubin rise in infants with Rh sensitization without phototherapy. In hemolytic disease, immediate exchange transfusion is usually indicated if:

   a. The cord bilirubin level is over 4.5 mg/dL and the cord hemoglobin level is under 11 gm/dL.

   b. The bilirubin level is rising over 1 mg/dL per hour despite phototherapy.

   c. The hemoglobin level is between 11 and 13 g/dL and the bilirubin level is rising over 0.5 mg/dL per hour despite phototherapy.

   d. The bilirubin level is 20 mg/dL, or it appears that it will reach 20 mg/dL at the rate it is rising (see Fig. 18.5).

   e. There is progression of anemia in the face of adequate control of bilirubin by other methods (e.g., phototherapy).

5. Repeat exchanges are done for the same indications as the initial exchange. All infants should be under intense phototherapy while decisions regarding exchange transfusion are being made.

C. **Blood for exchange transfusion**

1. We use fresh (<7 days old) irradiated reconstituted whole blood (hematocrit 45 to 50) made from packed red blood cells (PRBCs) and fresh frozen plasma collected in citrate-phosphate-dextrose (CPD). Cooperation with the obstetrician and the blood bank is essential in preparing for the birth of an infant requiring exchange transfusion (see Chap. 26).

2. **In Rh hemolytic disease,** if blood is prepared before delivery, it should be type O Rh-negative cross-matched against the mother. If the blood is obtained after delivery, it also may be cross-matched against the infant.

3. **In ABO incompatibility,** the blood should be type O Rh-negative or Rh-compatible with the mother and infant, be cross-matched against the mother and infant, and have a low titer of naturally occurring anti-A or anti-B antibodies. Usually, type O cells are used with AB plasma to ensure that no anti-A or anti-B antibodies are present.

4. In other isoimmune hemolytic disease, the blood should not contain the sensitizing antigen and should be cross-matched against the mother.

5. In nonimmune hyperbilirubinemia, blood is typed and cross-matched against the plasma and red cells of the infant.

6. Exchange transfusion usually involves double the volume of the infant's blood and is known as a two-volume exchange. If the infant's blood volume is 80 mL/kg, then a two-volume exchange transfusion uses 160 mL/kg of blood. This replaces 87% of the infant's blood volume with new blood.

D. **Technique of exchange transfusion**

1. Exchange is done with the infant under a servocontrolled radiant warmer and cardiac and blood pressure monitoring in place. Equipment and personnel for resuscitation must be readily available, and an intravenous line should be in place for the administration of glucose and medication. The infant's arms and legs should be properly restrained.

2. An assistant should be assigned to the infant to record volumes of blood, observe the infant, and check vital signs.

3. The glucose concentration of CPD blood is about 300 mg/dL. After exchange, we measure the infant's glucose to detect rebound hypoglycemia.

4. Measurement of potassium and pH of the blood for exchange may be indicated if the blood is over 7 days old or if metabolic abnormalities are noted following exchange transfusion.

5. The blood should be warmed to 37°C.

6. Sterile techniques should be used. Old, dried umbilical cords can be softened with saline-soaked gauze to facilitate locating the vein and inserting the catheter. If a dirty cord was entered or there was a break in sterile technique, we treat with oxacillin and gentamicin for 2 to 3 days.

7. We do most exchanges by the **push-pull technique** through the umbilical vein inserted only as far as required to permit free blood exchange. A catheter in the heart may cause arrhythmias. (See Chap. 36 for insertion of an umbilical venous catheter.)

8. **Isovolumetric** exchange transfusion (simultaneously pulling blood out of the umbilical artery and pushing new blood in the umbilical vein) may be tolerated better in small, sick, or hydropic infants.

9. If it is not possible to insert the catheter in the umbilical vein, exchange transfusion can be accomplished through a central venous pressure line placed through the antecubital fossa or into the femoral vein via the saphenous vein.

10. In the push-pull method, blood is removed in aliquots that are tolerated by the infant. This usually is **5 mL** for infants under 1500 g, **10 mL** for infants 1500 to 2500 g, **15 mL** for infants 2500 to 3500 g, and **20 mL** for

infants over 3500 g. The rate of exchange and aliquot size have little effect on the efficiency of bilirubin removal, but smaller aliquots and a slower rate place less stress on the cardiovascular system. The recommended time for the exchange transfusion is 1 hour.

11. The blood should be gently mixed after every deciliter of exchange to prevent the settling of RBCs and the transfusion of anemic blood at the end of the exchange.

12. After exchange transfusion, phototherapy is continued and bilirubin levels are measured every 4 hours.

13. When the exchange transfusion is finished, a silk purse-string suture should be placed around the vein; the tails of the suture material should be left. This localization of the vein will facilitate the next exchange transfusion.

14. When the catheter is removed, the tie around the cord should be tightened snugly for about 1 hour. It is important to remember to loosen the tie after 1 hour to avoid necrosis of the skin.

E. Complications of exchange transfusions

1. **Hypocalcemia and hypomagnesemia.** The citrate in CPD blood binds ionic calcium and magnesium. Hypocalcemia associated with exchange transfusion may produce cardiac and other effects (see Chap. 29). We usually do not give extra calcium unless the electrocardiogram (ECG) and clinical assessment suggest hypocalcemia. The fall in magnesium associated with exchange transfusion has not been associated with clinical problems.

2. **Hypoglycemia.** The high glucose content of CPD blood may stimulate insulin secretion and cause hypoglycemia 1 to 2 hours after an exchange. Blood glucose is monitored for several hours after exchange and the infant should have an intravenous line containing glucose (see Chap. 29).

3. **Acid–base balance.** Citrate in CPD blood is metabolized to alkali by the healthy liver and may result in a late metabolic alkalosis. If the baby is very ill and unable to metabolize citrate, the citrate may produce significant acidosis.

4. **Hyperkalemia.** Potassium levels may be greatly elevated in stored PRBCs, but washing the cells before reconstitution with fresh frozen plasma removes this excess potassium. Washing by some methods (IBM cell washer) may cause hypokalemia. If blood is over 24 hours old, it is best to check the potassium level before using it (see Chap. 9).

5. **Cardiovascular.** Perforation of vessels, embolization (with air or clots), vasospasm, thrombosis, infarction, arrhythmias, volume overload, and arrest.

6. **Bleeding.** Thrombocytopenia, deficient clotting factors (see Chap. 26).

7. **Infections.** Bacteremia, hepatitis, CMV, HIV (AIDS), West Nile virus, and malaria (see Chap. 23).

8. **Hemolysis.** Hemoglobinemia, hemoglobinuria, and hyperkalemia caused by overheating of the blood have been reported. Massive hemolysis, intravascular sickling, and death have occurred from the use of hemoglobin SC (sickle cell) donor blood.

9. **Graft-versus-host disease.** This is prevented by using **irradiated blood.** Before blood was irradiated, a syndrome of transient maculopapular rash, eosinophilia, lymphopenia, and thrombocytopenia without other signs of immunodeficiency was described in infants receiving multiple exchange transfusions. This did not usually progress to graft-versus-host disease.

10. **Miscellaneous.** Hypothermia, hyperthermia, and possibly necrotizing enterocolitis.

IX. Other treatment modalities

A. **Increasing bilirubin conjugation. Phenobarbital,** in a dose of 5 to 8 mg/kg every 24 hours, induces microsomal enzymes, increases bilirubin conjugation and excretion, and increases bile flow. It is useful in treating the indirect hyperbilirubinemia of Crigler-Najjar syndrome type II (but not type I) and in the treatment of the direct hyperbilirubinemia associated with hyperalimentation. Phenobarbital given antenatally to the mother is effective in lowering bilirubin levels in erythroblastotic infants, but concerns about toxicity prevent its routine use in pregnant women in the United States. Phenobarbital does not augment the effects of phototherapy.

B. Decreasing enterohepatic circulation. In breastfed and formula-fed infants with bilirubins above 15 mg/dL, oral agar significantly increases the efficiency and shortens the duration of phototherapy. In fact, oral agar alone was as effective as phototherapy in lowering bilirubin levels. Although oral agar may prove to be an economical therapy for hyperbilirubinemia, we have limited experience with its use in our nurseries.

C. Inhibiting bilirubin production. Metalloprotoporphyrins (e.g., tin and zinc protoporphyrins) are competitive inhibitors of heme oxygenase, the first enzyme in converting heme to bilirubin. They have been used to treat hyperbilirubinemia in Coombs'-positive ABO incompatibility and in Crigler-Najjar type I patients. In addition, a single dose of tin mesoporphyrin given shortly after birth substantially reduced the development of hyperbilirubinemia and the duration of phototherapy in Greek preterm (30 to 36 weeks) infants. A follow-up study by the same research group demonstrated that a single dose of Sn-mesoporphyrin in G6PD-deficient newborns significantly reduced bilirubin levels and eliminated the need for phototherapy. However, these agents are still experimental and are not yet in routine use.

D. Inhibiting hemolysis. High-dose intravenous immune globulin (500–750 mg/kg IV over 2 to 4 hours) has been used to reduce bilirubin levels in infants with isoimmune hemolytic disease. The mechanism is unknown, but the immune globulin could act by occupying the Fc receptors of reticuloendothelial cells, thereby preventing them from taking up and lysing antibody-coated RBCs.

X. Direct or conjugated hyperbilirubinemia (CB) is due to failure to excrete CB from the hepatocyte into the duodenum. It is manifested by a CB level over 2.0 mL/dL or a CB level greater than 15% of the total bilirubin level. It may be associated with hepatomegaly, splenomegaly, pale stools, and dark urine. CB is found in the urine; unconjugated bilirubin (UCB) is not. The preferred term to describe it is cholestasis, which includes retention of conjugated bilirubin (CB), bile acids, and other components of bile.

A. Differential diagnosis

1. Liver cell injury (normal bile ducts)

   a. Toxic. Intravenous hyperalimentation in low-birth-weight infants is a major cause of elevated CB in the newborn intensive care unit. It appears to be unrelated to the parenteral use of lipid. Sepsis and ischemic necrosis may cause cholestasis.

   b. Infection. Viral: hepatitis (B, C), giant-cell neonatal hepatitis, rubella, cytomegalovirus, herpes, Epstein-Barr virus, coxsackievirus, adenovirus, echoviruses 14 and 19. Bacterial: syphilis, Escherichia coli, group B b-hemolytic streptococcus, listeria, tuberculosis, staphylococcus. Parasitic: Toxoplasma.

   c. Metabolic. Alpha-1-antitrypsin deficiency, cystic fibrosis, galactosemia, tyrosinemia, hypermethionemia, fructosemia, storage diseases (Gaucher's, Niemann-Pick, glycogenosis type IV, Wolman's), Rotor syndrome, Dubin-Johnson syndrome, Byler disease, Zellweger syndrome, idiopathic cirrhosis, porphyria, hemochromatosis, trisomy 18.

2. Excessive bilirubin load (inspissated bile syndrome). Seen in any severe hemolytic disease but especially in infants with erythroblastosis fetalis who have been treated with intrauterine transfusion. In addition, a self-limited cholestatic jaundice is frequently seen in infants supported on extracorporeal membrane oxygenation (ECMO) (see Chap. 24). The cholestasis may last as long as 9 weeks and is thought to be secondary to hemolysis during ECMO.

3. **Bile flow obstruction (biliary atresia, extrahepatic or intrahepatic).** The extrahepatic type may be isolated or associated with a choledochal cyst, trisomy 13 or 18, or polysplenia. The intrahepatic type may be associated with the Alagille syndrome, intrahepatic atresia with lymphedema (Aagenaes syndrome, nonsyndromic paucity of intrahepatic bile ducts, coprostanic acidemia, choledochal cyst, bile duct stenosis, rupture of bile duct, lymph node enlargement, hemangiomas, tumors, pancreatic cyst, inspissated bile syndrome, and cystic fibrosis).

4. In the newborn intensive care unit, the most common causes of elevated CB, in decreasing order of frequency, are parenteral nutrition, idiopathic hepatitis, biliary atresia, alpha-1-antitrypsin deficiency, intrauterine infection, choledochal cyst, galactosemia, and increased bilirubin load from hemolytic disease.

B. **Diagnostic tests and management**

1. Evaluate for hepatomegaly, splenomegaly, petechiae, chorioretinitis, and microcephaly.

2. Evaluate liver damage and function by measurement of serum glutamic oxaloacetic transaminase (SGOT) level, serum glutamic pyruvic transaminase (SGPT) level, alkaline phosphatase level, prothrombin time (PT), partial thromboplastin time (PTT), and serum albumin level.

3. Stop parenteral nutrition with amino acids. If this is the cause, the liver dysfunction will usually resolve.

4. Test for bacterial, viral, and intrauterine infections (see Chap. 23).

5. Serum analysis for alpha-1-antitrypsin deficiency.

6. Serum and urine amino acids determinations (see Chap. 29).

7. Urinalysis for glucose and reducing substances (see Chap. 29).

8. If known causes are ruled out, the problem is to differentiate idiopathic neonatal hepatitis from bile duct abnormalities such as intrahepatic biliary atresia or hypoplasia, choledochal cyst, bile plug syndrome, extrahepatic biliary atresia, hypoplasia, or total biliary atresia.

   a. Abdominal ultrasound should be done to rule out a choledochal cyst or mass.

   b. We use a hepatobiliary scan with technetium [99m Tc]diisopropyliminodiacetic (DISIDA) as the next step to visualize the biliary tree.

   c. Iodine-131–rose bengal fecal excretion test may be useful if the [99m Tc]DISIDA scan is not available.

   d. A nasoduodenal tube can be passed and fluid collected in 2-hour aliquots for 24 hours. If there is no bile, treat with phenobarbital, 5 mg/kg per day for 7 days, and repeat the duodenal fluid collection.

   e. If the duodenal fluid collections, scans, and ultrasound suggest no extrahepatic obstruction, the child may be observed with careful follow-up.

   f. If the ultrasound, scans, or fluid collections suggest extrahepatic obstruction disease, the baby will need an exploratory laparotomy, cholangiogram, and open liver biopsy to enable a definite diagnosis.

   g. If the diagnosis of extrahepatic obstruction disease cannot be ruled out, the baby must have the studies outlined, because surgical therapy for choledochal cyst is curative if done early and hepatoportoenterostomy has better results if done early.

XI. **Hydrops** is a term used to describe generalized subcutaneous edema in the fetus or neonate. It is usually accompanied by ascites and often by pleural and/or pericardial effusions. Hydrops fetalis is discussed here, because in the past, hemolytic disease of the newborn was the major cause of both fetal and neonatal hydrops. However, because of the decline in Rh sensitization, nonimmune conditions are now the major causes of hydrops in the United States.

A. **Etiology.** The pathogenesis of hydrops includes anemia, cardiac failure, decreased colloid oncotic pressure (hypoalbuminemia), increased capillary permeability, asphyxia, and placental perfusion abnormalities. There is a general, but not a constant, relationship between the degree of anemia, the serum albumin level, and the presence of hydrops. There is no correlation between the severity of hydrops and the blood volume of the infant. Most hydropic infants have normal blood volume (80 mg/kg).

1. **Hematologic** due to chronic *in utero* anemia (10% of cases). Isoimmune hemolytic disease (e.g., Rh incompatibility), homozygous alpha thalassemia, homozygous G6PD deficiency, chronic fetomaternal hemorrhage, twin-to-twin transfusion, hemorrhage, thrombosis, bone marrow failure (chloramphenicol, maternal parvovirus infection), bone marrow replacement (Gaucher's disease), leukemia.

2. **Cardiovascular** due to heart failure (20% of cases) (see Chap. 25).
   a. **Rhythm disturbances.** Heart block, supraventricular tachycardia, atrial flutter.
   b. **Major cardiac disease.** Hypoplastic left heart, Epstein's anomaly, truncus arteriosus, myocarditis (coxsackievirus), endocardial fibroelastosis, cardiac neoplasm (rhabdomyoma), cardiac thrombosis, arteriovenous malformations, premature closure of foramen ovale, generalized arterial calcification, premature restructure of the foramen ovale.

3. **Renal** (5% of cases). Nephrosis, renal vein thrombosis, renal hypoplasia, urinary obstruction.

4. **Infection** (8% of cases). Syphilis, rubella, cytomegalovirus, congenital hepatitis, herpes virus, adenovirus, toxoplasmosis, leptospirosis, Chagas' disease, parvovirus (see Chap. 23).

5. **Pulmonary** (5% of cases). Congenital chylothorax, diaphragmatic hernia, pulmonary lymphangiectasia, cystic adenomatoid malformations, intrathoracic mass.

6. **Placenta or cord** (rare cause). Chorangioma, umbilical vein thrombosis, arteriovenous malformation, chorionic vein thrombosis, true knot in umbilical cord, cord compression, choriocarcinoma.

7. **Maternal conditions** (5% of cases). Toxemia, diabetes, thyrotoxicosis.

8. **Gastrointestinal** (5% of cases). Meconium peritonitis, in utero volvulus, atresia.

9. **Chromosomal** (10% of cases). Turner syndrome; trisomy 13, 18, 21; triploidy; aneuploidy.

10. **Miscellaneous** (10% of cases). Cystic hygroma. Wilms' tumor, angioma, teratoma, neuroblastoma, central nervous system (CNS) malformations, amniotic band syndrome, lysosomal storage disorders, congenital myotonic dystrophy, skeletal abnormalities (osteogenesis imperfecta, achondrogenesis, hypophosphatasia, thanatophoric dwarf, arthrogryposis), Noonan syndrome, acardia, absent ductus venosus, renal venous thrombosis, cystic hygroma.

11. **Unknown** (20% of cases).

B. **Diagnosis.** A pregnant woman with polyhydramnios, severe anemia, toxemia, or isoimmune disease should undergo ultrasonic examination of the fetus. If the fetus is hydropic, a careful search by ultrasound and real-time fetal echocardiography may reveal the cause and may guide fetal treatment. The accumulation of pericardial or ascitic fluid may be the first sign of impending hydrops in a Rh-sensitized fetus. Investigations should be carried out for the causes of fetal hydrops mentioned in A. The usual investigation includes the following:

1. **Maternal** blood type and Coombs' test as well as red cell antibody titers, complete blood count and red blood cell indices, hemoglobin electrophoresis, Kleihauser-Betke stain of maternal blood for fetal red cells, tests for syphillis, studies for viral infection and toxoplasmosis (see Chap. 23), sedimentation rate, lupus tests.

2. **Fetal** echocardiography for cardiac abnormalities and ultrasound for other structural lesions.

3. **Amniocentesis** for karyotype, metabolic studies, fetoprotein, cultures and polymerase chain reaction (PCR) for viral infections and restriction endonucleases as indicated.

4. **Fetal blood sampling (PUBS)** (see Chap. 1). Karyotype, complete blood count (CBC), hemoglobin electrophoresis, cultures, and PCR, DNA studies, albumin.

5. **Neonatal.** Following delivery, many of the same studies may be carried out on the infant. A complete blood count, blood typing, and Coombs' test; ultrasound studies of the head, heart, and abdomen; and a search for the causes listed in XI.A should be done. Examination of pleural and/or ascitic fluid, liver function tests, urinalysis, viral titers, chromosomes, placental examination, and X rays may be indicated. If the infant is still-born or dies, a detailed autopsy should be done.

C. Management

1. A hydropic fetus is at great risk for intrauterine death. A decision must be made about intrauterine treatment if possible, for example, fetal transfusion in isoimmune hemolytic anemia (see Chap. 1) or maternal digitalis therapy for supraventricular tachycardia (see Chap. 25). If fetal treatment is not possible, the fetus must be evaluated for the relative possibility of intrauterine death versus the risks of premature delivery. If premature delivery is planned, pulmonary maturity should be induced with steroids if it is not present (see Chap. 24). Intrauterine paracentesis or thoracentesis just prior to delivery may facilitate subsequent newborn resuscitation.

2. Resuscitation of the hydropic infant is complex and requires advance preparation whenever feasible. Intubation can be extremely difficult with massive edema of the head, neck, and oropharynx and should be done by a skilled operator immediately after birth. (A fiberoptic scope may facilitate placement of the endotracheal tube.) A second individual should provide rapid relief of hydrostatic pressure on the diaphragm and lungs by paracentesis and/or thoracentesis with an 18- to 20-gauge angiocatheter attached to a three-way stopcock and syringe. After entry into the chest or abdominal cavity, the needle is withdrawn so that the plastic catheter can remain without fear of laceration. Cardiocentesis may also be required if there is electromechanical dissociation due to cardiac tamponade.

3. Ventilator management can be complicated by pulmonary hypoplasia, barotrauma, pulmonary edema, or reaccumulation of ascites and/or pleural fluid. If repeated thoracenteses cannot control hydrothorax, chest tube drainage may be indicated. Judicious use of diuretics (e.g., furosemide) is often helpful in reducing pulmonary edema. Arterial access is needed to monitor blood gases and acid-base balance.

4. Because hydropic infants have enormous quantities of extravascular salt and water, fluid intake is based on an estimate of the infant's "dry weight" (e.g., 50th percentile for gestational age). Free water and salt are kept at a minimum (e.g., 40 to 60 mL/kg per day as dextrose water) until edema is resolved. Monitoring the electrolyte composition of serum, urine, ascites fluid, and/or pleural fluid, and careful measurement of intake, output, and weight are essential for guiding therapy. Normoglycemia is achieved by providing glucose at a rate of 4 to 8 mg/kg per minute. Unless cardiovascular and/or renal function are compromised, edema will eventually resolve and salt and water intake can then be normalized.

5. If the hematocrit is under 30%, a partial exchange transfusion with 50 to 80 ml/kg packed red blood cells (hematocrit 70%) should be performed to raise the hematocrit and increase oxygen carrying capacity. If the problem is Rh isoimmunization, the blood should be type O Rh-negative. We often use O-negative cells and AB serum prepared before delivery and cross-matched against the mother. An isovolumetric exchange (simultaneous removal of blood from the umbilical artery while blood is transfused in the umbilical vein at 2 to 4 mL/kg per minute) may be better tolerated in infants with compromised cardiovascular systems.

6. Inotropic support (e.g., dopamine) may be required to improve cardiac output. Central venous and arterial lines are needed for monitoring pressures. Most hydropic infants are normovolemic, but manipulation of the

blood volume may be indicated after measurement of arterial and venous pressures and after correction of acidosis and asphyxia. If a low serum albumin level is contributing to hydrops, fresh-frozen plasma may help. Care must be taken not to volume-overload an already failing heart, and infusions of colloid may need to be followed by a diuretic.

7. Hyperbilirubinemia should be treated as in VI.
8. Many infants with hydrops will survive if aggressive neonatal care is provided.

XII. **Isoimmune hemolytic disease of the newborn**

A. **Etiology.** Maternal exposure (via blood transfusion, feto-maternal hemorrhage, amniocentesis, or abortion) to foreign antigens on fetal RBCs causes the production and transplacental passage of specific maternal IgG antibodies directed against the fetal antigens, resulting in the immune destruction of fetal RBCs. The usual antigen involved prenatally is the Rh(D) antigen, and postnatally, the A and B antigens. A positive Coombs' test result in an infant should prompt identification of the antibody. If the antibody is not anti-A or anti-B, then it should be identified by testing the mother's serum against a panel of red cell antigens or the father's red cells. This may have implications for subsequent pregnancies. Since the dramatic decline in Rh hemolytic disease with the use of Rhogam, maternal antibody against A or B antigens (ABO incompatibility) is now the most common cause of isoimmune hemolytic disease. In addition, other relatively uncommon antigens (Kell, Duffy, E, C, and c) now account for a greater proportion of cases of isoimmune hemolytic anemia (Tables 18.3, 18.4, 18.5). The **Lewis antigen** is a commonly found antigen, but this antigen does not cause hemolytic disease of the newborn. Most Lewis antibodies are of the IgM class (which do not cross the placenta) and the Lewis antigen is poorly developed and expressed on the fetal and/or neonatal erythrocytes.

B. **Fetal management.** All pregnant women should have blood typing, Rh determination, and an antibody screening performed on their first prenatal visit. This will identify the Rh-negative mothers and identify any antibody due to Rh or any rare antigen sensitization. In a Caucasian population in the United States, 15% of people lack the D antigen (dd). Of the remainder, 48% are heterozygous (dD) and 35% are homozygous (DD). Approximately 15% of matings in this population will result in a fetus with the D antigen and a mother without it.

1. If the mother is **Rh-positive** and her **antibody screening is negative,** it may be advisable to repeat the antibody screening later in pregnancy, but this will have a low yield.
2. If the mother is **Rh-negative/antibody screen negative** and the father of the fetus is Rh-negative, she should be retested at 28 and 35 weeks' gestation (see D for prenatal Rhogam). If the father is Rh-positive, she should be retested at 18 to 20 weeks and monthly thereafter. If the paternal phenotype is heterozygous for Rh(O) amniocentesis is used to determine the fetal blood type by polymerase chain reaction (PRC).
3. If the mother is **Rh-negative/antibody screen positive,** the antibody titer is repeated at 16 to 18 weeks, at 22 weeks, and every 2 weeks thereafter. Amniocentesis is usually done for antibody titers over 1:16 or at a level at which the local center has had a fetal demise (each center should have its own standards for action on various titers). Irrespective of antibody titers, if there is a prior history of a severely isoimmunized fetus, serial amniocentesis may be indicated beginning at 16 to 18 weeks to measure the optical density at a wavelength of 450 nm (bilirubin) to assess the risk for fetal death from hydrops. If the fetus is less than 24 weeks (optical density is less accurate) or if placental trauma is likely with amniocentesis, direct percutaneous fetal blood sampling for blood type, direct Coombs' test, hematocrit, CBC, and blood gases may be preferable. Doppler assessment of fetal middle cerebral artery peak blood flow velocity is emerging as an accurate tool to predict fetal anemia and may replace amniocentesis for evaluation of fetal anemia.

4. Fetuses at high risk for death may be treated by early delivery if the risk of fetal demise or intrauterine transfusion exceeds the risk of early delivery. In our institution, this is usually 30 weeks, but this requires careful fetal monitoring, induction of pulmonary maturity, and close cooperation between obstetrician and neonatologist. If the hydropic fetus is too immature for early delivery to be considered, **intrauterine transfusion is indicated.** Transfusion can be carried out by intraperitoneal or intravascular routes, although intravascular transfusion may be the only option in a moribund hydropic infant who has ascites, is not breathing, and is unable to absorb intraperitoneal blood. Intrauterine transfusions are repeated whenever fetal hemoglobin levels fall below about 10 g/dL. Following transfusion, serial ultrasound examinations are done to assess changes in the degree of hydrops and fetal well-being. Some infants who have undergone multiple intrauterine transfusions will be born with all adult O-negative RBCs because all the fetal cells are destroyed. Although one should be prepared, not all infants will need postnatal exchange transfusion. These infants are at risk to develop conjugated hyperbilirubinemia.

C. **Neonatal management.** About half the infants with a positive Coombs' test result from Rh hemolytic disease will have minimum hemolysis and hyperbilirubinemia (cord bilirubin level <4 mg/dL and hemoglobin level >14 g/dL). These infants may require no treatment or only phototherapy. One-fourth of infants with Rh hemolytic disease present with anemia, hemoglobin level less than 14 g/dL, and hyperbilirubinemia (cord bilirubin >4 mg/dL). They have increased nucleated red cells and reticulocytes on blood smear. These infants may have thrombocytopenia and a very elevated white blood cell count. They have an enlarged liver and spleen, and they require early exchange transfusion and phototherapy (see VI.B, VII, and VIII). Figure 18.5 and Table 18.3 can be used in deciding what treatment to use. Infants with isoimmune hemolytic anemia may develop an exaggerated physiologic anemia at 12 weeks of age, requiring blood transfusion. Erythropoietin is currently being evaluated for use in preventing this late anemia. High-dose intravenous immune gammaglobulin therapy 400–600 mg/kg IV is used for hemolytic disease. (See IX.D)

D. **Prevention.** Eliminating exposure of women to foreign red cell antigens will prevent immune hemolytic disease of the newborn. Avoiding unnecessary transfusions and medical procedures that carry the risk of transplacental passage of blood will help decrease sensitization. Rh hemolytic disease is now being prevented by the administration of **Rho(D) immune globulin (Rhogam)** to unsensitized Rh-negative mothers. This is usually done at 28 weeks' gestation and again within 72 hours after delivery. Other indications for Rho(D) immune globulin (or for using larger doses) are prophylaxis following abortion, amniocentesis, chorionic villus sampling, and transplacental hemorrhage. Interestingly, ABO incompatibility between mother and fetus protects against sensitization of an Rh-negative mother, probably because maternal antibodies eliminate fetal RBCs from the maternal circulation before they can encounter antibody-forming lymphocytes.

XIII. **ABO hemolytic disease of the newborn.** Since the introduction of Rh immune globulin, ABO incompatibility has been the most common cause of hemolytic disease of the newborn in the United States.

A. **Etiology.** The cause is the reaction of maternal anti-A or anti-B antibodies to the A or B antigen on the red blood cells of the fetus or newborn. It is usually seen only in type A or B infants born to type O mothers because these mothers make anti-A or anti-B antibodies of the immunoglobulin G (IgG) class, which cross the placenta, while mothers of type A or B usually make anti-A or anti-B antibodies of the immunoglobulin M (IgM) class, which do not cross the placenta. The combination of a type O mother and a type A or type B infant occurs in 15% of pregnancies in the United States. Only one-fifth of infants with this blood group setup (or 3% of all infants) will develop significant jaundice. Some bacterial vaccines, such as tetanus toxoid and pneumococcal vaccine, had A and B substance in the culture media and were associated with significant hemolysis in type A or type B neonates born to type O mothers who were given these vaccines. New preparations of the vaccine are said to be free of these A and B substances.

B. Clinical presentation. The situation is a type O mother with a type A or type B infant who becomes jaundiced in the first 24 hours of life. Approximately 50% of the cases occur in firstborn infants. There is no predictable pattern of recurrence in subsequent infants. **The majority of ABO-incompatible infants have anti-A or anti-B antibody on their red blood cells, yet only a small number have significant ABO hemolytic disease of the newborn.** Infants may have a low concentration of antibody on their red cells; consequently, their antibody will not be demonstrated by elution techniques or by a positive direct antiglobulin test (Coombs' test). As the antibody concentration increases, the antibody can be demonstrated first by elution techniques and then by the Coombs' test. Although all ABO-incompatible infants have some degree of hemolysis, significant hemolysis is usually associated only with a positive direct Coombs' test result on the infant's red cells. If there are other causes of neonatal jaundice, ABO incompatibility will add to the bilirubin production. In infants with significant ABO incompatibility, there will be many spherocytes on the blood smear and an elevated reticulocyte count. RBCs from infants with ABO incompatibility may have increased osmotic fragility and autohemolysis, as in hereditary spherocytosis (HS). The autohemolysis is not corrected by glucose, as in HS. The family history and long-term course will usually help with the diagnosis of HS.

C. Management. If blood typing and Coombs' test are done on the cord blood of infants born to type O mothers, these infants can have bilirubin levels monitored and therapy instituted early enough to prevent severe hyperbilirubinemia. However, this approach may not be cost-effective, because most infants do not develop significant jaundice and only 10% of infants with a positive direct Coombs' test result for ABO incompatibility will need phototherapy. In the absence of a routine test on all infants born to type O mothers, one must rely on clinical observation to notice the jaundiced infants. This will depend on the observation of the caregivers and may not be reliable in infants whose skin pigmentation makes the diagnosis of jaundice difficult. A bilirubin level at 12 hours of age, or cord blood typing and a Coombs' test on all black or Asian infants born to type O mothers, may be a reasonable compromise. Infants born to type O mothers who are to have an early discharge (within 24 hours) should be evaluated for ABO incompatibility, and the parents should be made aware of the possibility of jaundice. Many infants have an initial rise in bilirubin that quickly falls to normal levels. If the criteria for Rh disease are used, many will undergo unnecessary treatment. An approach to phototherapy and exchange transfusion management has been outlined in VI.B. IV gamma globulin to inhibit hemolysis can be considered (see IX.D). Kernicterus has been reported in ABO incompatibility. If exchange transfusion is necessary, it should be with type O blood that is of the same Rh type as the infant with a low titer of anti-A or anti-B antibody. We often use type O cells resuspended in type AB plasma. There is no need for prenatal diagnosis or treatment and no need for early delivery.

Suggested Readings

AAP. Practice parameter: Management of hyperbilirubinemia in the healthy term newborn. *Pediatrics* 1994;94:558.

Benders M.J., et al. The effect of phototherapy on cerebral blood flow velocity in preterm infants. *Acta Paediatr* 1998;87:786–791.

Benders M.J., et al. The effect of phototherapy on renal blood flow velocity in preterm infants. *Biol Neonate* 1998;73:228–234.

Bhutani V.K., et al. Jaundice technologies: Prediction of hyperbilirubinemia in term and near-term newborns. *J Perinatol* 2001;21 Suppl 1:S76–S82; discussion S83–S87.

Bhutani V.K., et al. Noninvasive measurement of total serum bilirubin in a multiracial predischarge newborn population to assess the risk of severe hyperbilirubinemia. *Pediatrics* 2000;106:E17.

Bhutani V.K., et al. Predictive ability of a predischarge hour-specific serum bilirubin for subsequent significant hyperbilirubinemia in healthy term and near-term newborns. *Pediatrics* 1999;103:6–14.

Caglayan S., et al. Superiority of oral agar and phototherapy combination in the treatment of neonatal hyperbilirubinemia. *Pediatrics* 1993;92:86–89.

Dennery P.A., et al. Neonatal hyperbilirubinemia. *N Engl J Med* 2001;344:581–590.

Gourley G.R. Breastfeeding, diet, and hyperbilirubinemia. *NeoReviews* 2000;1:e25–e30.

Hammerman C., et al. Recent developments in the management of neonatal hyperbilirubinemia. *NeoReviews* 2000;1:e19–e24.

Iolascon A., et al. UGT1 promoter polymorphism accounts for increased neonatal appearance of hereditary spherocytosis. *Blood* 1998;91:1093.

Kaplan M., et al. Gilbert's syndrome and hyperbilirubinaemia in ABO-incompatible neonates. *Lancet* 2000;356:652–653.

Kaplan M., et al. Glucose-6-phosphate dehydrogenase deficiency: A worldwide potential cause of severe neonatal hyperbilirubinemia. *NeoReviews* 2000;1:e32–e38.

Kaplan M. Genetic interactions in the pathogenesis of neonatal hyperbilirubinemia: Gilbert's Syndrome and glucose-6-phosphate dehydrogenase deficiency. *J Perinatol* 2001;21 Suppl 1:S30–S34; discussion S35–S39.

Kappas A., et al. A single dose of Sn-mesoporphyrin prevents development of severe hyperbilirubinemia in glucose-6-phosphate dehydrogenase-deficient newborns. *Pediatrics* 2001;108:25–30.

MacDonald M.G. Hidden risks: Early discharge and bilirubin toxicity due to glucose 6-phosphate dehydrogenase deficiency. *Pediatrics* 1995;96:734–738.

Maisels M.J., et al. Kernicterus in otherwise healthy, breastfed term newborns. *Pediatrics* 1995;96:730–733.

Maisels M.J., et al. Transcutaneous bilirubinometry decreases the need for serum bilirubin measurements and saves money. *Pediatrics* 1997;99:599–601.

Martinez J.C., et al. Hyperbilirubinemia in the breastfed newborn: a controlled trial of four interventions. *Pediatrics* 1993;91:470–473.

Maruo Y., et al. Association of neonatal hyperbilirubinemia with bilirubin UDP-glucuronosyltransferase polymorphism. *Pediatrics* 1999;103:1224–1227.

Maruo Y., et al. Prolonged unconjugated hyperbilirubinemia associated with breast milk and mutations of the bilirubin uridine diphosphate-glucuronosyltransferase gene. *Pediatrics* 2000;106:E59.

Monaghan G., et al. Gilbert's syndrome is a contributory factor in prolonged unconjugated hyperbilirubinemia of the newborn. *J Pediatr* 1999;134:441–446.

Moise K.J. Diagnosis and management of Rhesus (Rh) alloimmunization. December 2002. http://stone.utdol.com/APP/index.asp.

Newman T.B., et al. Neonatal hyperbilirubinemia and long-term outcome: another look at the Collaborative Perinatal Project. *Pediatrics* 1993;92:651–657.

Newman T.B., et al. Prediction and prevention of extreme neonatal hyperbilirubinemia in a mature health maintenance organization. *Arch Pediatr Adolesc Med* 2000; 154:1140–1147.

Peterec S.M. Management of neonatal Rh disease. *Clin Perinatol* 1995;22:561–592.

Pezzati M., et al. Changes in mesenteric blood flow response to feeding: conventional versus fiber-optic phototherapy. *Pediatrics* 2000;105:350–353.

Rubo J., et al. High-dose intravenous immune globulin therapy for hyperbilirubinemia caused by Rh hemolytic disease. *J Pediatr* 1992;121:93–97.

Stevenson D.K., et al. Prediction of hyperbilirubinemia in near-term and term infants. *Pediatrics* 2001;108:31–39.

Tan K.L. Decreased response to phototherapy for neonatal jaundice in breast-fed infants. *Arch Pediatr Adolesc Med* 1998;152:1187–1190.

Watchko J.F., et al. Kernicterus in preterm newborns: past, present, and future. *Pediatrics* 1992;90:707–715.

19. DRUG ABUSE AND WITHDRAWAL

Sylvia Schechner

I. **Maternal substance abuse.** In the epidemic of substance abuse in the United States, the drugs most often abused are cannabinoids, heroin, and cocaine, probably because of its inexpensive alkaloidal free-base form, "crack." There is a 15% overall prevalence of at least one of the above illicit substances in urine samples obtained during pregnancy. Intrauterine exposure to alcohol occurs more often than all the above listed illicit substances combined. Despite all the adverse publicity, tobacco use continues in approximately 25% of pregnancies. Iatrogenic neonatal abstinence syndrome may be seen in infants who required narcotics for sedation for surgery or other procedures.

A. **Take a comprehensive medical and psychosocial history** including a specific inquiry about maternal drug use as part of every prenatal and newborn evaluation, although accurate information regarding illicit drug use during pregnancy is often difficult to obtain.

  1. **Maternal associations with drug abuse**
     a. Poor or no prenatal care.
     b. Preterm labor.
     c. Placental rupture.
     d. Precipitous delivery.
     e. Frequent demands or requests for large doses of pain medication.
  2. **Signs of maternal drug abuse in the infant**
     a. Small for gestational age (SGA).
     b. Microcephaly.
     c. Neonatal stroke or any arterial infarction.
     d. Any of the symptoms in Table 19.1.

B. **Diagnostic tests.** Screen urine if drug withdrawal is a possibility. Meconium analysis by radioimmunoassay affords a longer view into the drug-use pattern, but is an expensive test. Hair analysis of the infant can reveal maternal drug use during the previous 3 months, but hair grows slowly and recent drug use may not be detected. Consider the implications of a positive test result. The following is our statement for testing:

Physician Guidelines for Testing, Reporting, and Care of Neonates Who May Have Been Exposed Prenatally to Controlled Substances
Brigham and Women's Hospital, Boston, MA
  1. **Testing**
     a. **Purpose.** A positive urine test for controlled substances can serve several purposes: (1) it may help to complete a diagnostic workup for an infant with symptoms of drug dependency or withdrawal (e.g., seizures or jitteriness); (2) it may serve as a marker for an infant at risk for developmental delay; and (3) it may indicate an at-risk family in need of social services. (A negative test result, however, cannot rule out any of these items.)
     b. **Symptomatic infants**
        (1) *Performance of a toxic screen is recommended for infants with any of the following symptoms: (a) severe intrauterine growth retardation (IUGR) which is defined as a birth weight below the third percentile; (b) symptoms consistent with neonatal drug dependency and withdrawal; (c) central nervous system (CNS) irritability; and (d) symptoms consistent with intracranial hemorrhage (ICH) such as focal seizures or paresis. These criteria are intended to serve as guidelines only. The attending physician must decide on a case-by-case basis whether a toxic screen is indicated.*

TABLE 19.1. REPORTED WITHDRAWAL SYNDROMES IN NEWBORNS AFTER MATERNAL DRUG INGESTION

	Lethargy	Poor state control	Fever	Diaphoresis	Tachycardia	Tachypnea	Cyanosis	High-pitched cry	Altered sleeping	Tremors	Hypotonicity	Hypertonicity	Hyperreflexia	Increased suck
Narcotics														
Heroin			X	X	X	X		X	X	X			X	X	X
Methadone			X	X	X	X		X	X	X			X	X	X
Propoxyphene				X	X	X		X			X		X	X	X
Pentazocine plus tripelennamine					X	X		X				X	X	X	X
("T's and Blues")						X		X						X	
Codeine	X									X		X	X	
Sedatives														
Barbiturates				X				±	X	X	X	X		
Butalbital (Fiorinal, Esgic)														
Chlordiazepoxide										X				
Diazepam					X	X				X			X	X
Diphenhydramine										X				
Ethanol				X						X	X			
Ethchlorvynol (Placidyl) (plus propoxyphene plus diazepam)				X							X			
Glutethimide (plus heroin)			X	X				X		X		X	X	
Hydroxyzine (Vistaril) (600 mg/day plus Pb)				X				X		X			X	
Stimulants														
Methamphetamine	X	X						X				X		
Phencyclidine											X	X	X	
Cocaine	X	X						X	X	X		X	X	X
Antidepressants														
Tricyclics				X	X	X	X			X	X	X	X	
Antipsychotics														
Phenothiazines								X		X		X	X	X

Key: X = symptom usually present; ± = symptom may be present, but not always;
Pb = phenobarbital.

(2) *It is hospital policy not to require a separate specific consent from the parents for a toxic screen on a symptomatic infant. As testing of symptomatic infants is done to assist in the medical diagnosis or treatment of the infant, the general parental consent obtained in the initial admission consent form is usually sufficient. Parents, however, should be informed by the responsible pediatrician (prior to the test if possible) of the purpose of the toxic screen, and that a pos-*

Ineffective suck	Irritability	Jitteriness	Seizures	Nasal congestion	Sneezing/yawning	Ravenous appetite	Vomiting	Excessive regurgitation	Diarrhea	Weight loss	Abdominal distention	Onset	Duration
	X	X	X	X	X	X	X	X	X	X		1–144 hours	7–20 days
	X	X	X	X	X	X	X	X	X	X		1–14 days	20–45 days
	X	X	X	X			X	X		X	±	3–20 hours	56 h–6 days
	X	X	X	X	X		X				X		
X	X	X											
X	X	X					X		X			0.5–30 hours	4–17 days
X	X	X	X		X	X	X	X	X	X		0.5 h–14 days	11 days–6 months
X	X	X	?	X								2 days	24 days
		X										21 days	37 days
X		X						X			X	2–6 hours	10 days–6 weeks
								X				5 days	10 days–5 weeks
	X	X	X		±					±	X	6–12 hours	
X	X	X					X	X				24 hours	9–10 days
	X								X			8 hours	45 days
X	X	X	X									15 minutes	156 hours
	X				X								5–24 hours
		X					X		X			18–20 hours	18 days–2 months
X			X	X	X							1–3 days	
X	X	X	X									5–12 hours	96 hours–30 days
X	X	X									X	21 days	>11 days–4 months

itive test will be included in any report to the State Department of Social Services. This discussion should be documented in the medical record. In the event that the parents, when informed, object to the performance of the toxic screen, the legal office should be contacted for consultation. The results of the test and any follow-up or treatment should also be discussed with the parents. The obstetrician should also be notified of all positive test results.

c. Asymptomatic infants

(1) *Specific parental consent must be obtained in order to perform a toxic screen on an asymptomatic infant. (The general admission consent form is not sufficient.) As part of the process of seeking consent, the parent or parents should be advised by the attending physician or the physician designee of the purpose of the test and that a positive test will likely result in a referral to the Department of Social Services. Documentation of this discussion and the oral parental response should be made in the infant's medical record. (A separate written consent form signed by the parent is not required.) The obstetrician should also be notified of all positive test results.*

(2) *Testing of an asymptomatic infant may be indicated by the following circumstances: (a) lack of adequate prenatal care; (b) past or present parental history or signs of substance abuse; or (c) abruptio placenta. These criteria are simply guidelines. It is the responsibility of the attending physician to determine on a case-by-case basis whether testing of an asymptomatic infant may be beneficial.*

2. Referral. *Physicians, nurses, social workers, and other patient-care employees are required by the State of Massachusetts' Protection and Care of Children Act (commonly known as 51A) to report to the Massachusetts Department of Social Services cases of suspected child abuse and neglect, including all infants "determined to be physically dependent upon an addictive drug at birth." Reports generated by this hospital are usually filed by the hospital Social Services Department. The hospital Social Services Department should therefore be notified of all infants with symptoms of physical dependency to an addictive drug so that a 51A report can be filed as legally required.*

The hospital Social Services Department should also be notified of all asymptomatic infants with a positive toxic screen and all infants believed to be at risk due to possible parental or family substance abuse. Such cases are not automatically required by law to be reported, and the hospital Social Services Department will conduct a further evaluation to determine whether a potential abuse or neglect situation exists. If such situation is believed to exist, a report will be made. Prior experience indicated that most situations involving an infant with a positive screen (regardless of whether the infant is asymptomatic) will warrant the filing of a report.

Drugs administered during labor may cause difficulty in interpreting urine results. The length of time during which results may be positive varies with the drug.

a. Cocaine: up to 4 days.

b. Heroin: 2 to 4 days.

c. PCP: 2 to 4 days.

d. Marijuana: 2 to 5 days.

If the drugs were taken before these times, negative results may be falsely reassuring.

C. A drug-addicted mother is at **increased risk for other diseases** such as sexually transmitted diseases, tuberculosis, hepatitis B and C, and acquired immondeficiency syndrome (AIDS), especially if she involves herself in intravenous drug use or prostitution. About 30% of pregnant intravenous drug users are seropositive for human immunodeficiency virus (HIV).

II. Withdrawal in the infant. The onset of symptoms for acute narcotic withdrawal varies from shortly after birth to 2 weeks of age, but symptoms usually begin in 24 to 48 hours, depending on the type of drug and when the mother took the last dose. Table 19.1 shows the withdrawal symptoms in newborns. Methadone, heroin, and cocaine are the most common reasons for withdrawal seen in our nurseries.

A. **The severity of withdrawal** depends on the drugs used. Withdrawal from polydrug use is more severe than from methadone, which is more severe than from opiates alone or cocaine alone.

B. **Methadone,** because of its ability to block the euphoric effects of heroin, is used in pregnancy to treat heroin addiction.

1. It can cause withdrawal in 75 to 90% of infants exposed in utero. Term infants have more severe abstinence symptoms than preterm infants.

2. The severity of the symptoms correlates with the maternal dose.

3. Maintaining a woman on less than 20 mg/day will minimize symptoms in the infant. Higher methadone doses may increase severity and prolong withdrawal.

4. Some infants have late withdrawal, which may be of two types:
   a. Symptoms appear shortly after birth, improve, and recur at 2 to 4 weeks.
   b. Symptoms are not seen at birth but develop 2 to 3 weeks later.

5. Effects in the infant exposed to methadone during pregnancy:
   a. Lower birth weight, length, and head circumference.
   b. Sleep disturbances.
   c. Depressed interactive behavior.
   d. Poor self-calming.
   e. Tremors.
   f. Increased tone.
   g. Abstinence-associated seizures.
   h. Abnormal pneumograms.
   i. Increased incidence of sudden infant death syndrome (SIDS).
   j. Follow-up studies reveal a higher incidence of hyperactivity, learning and behavior disorders, and poor social adjustment. This may be due more to environmental factors than as a consequence of in utero methadone exposure.

C. **Differential diagnosis.** Consider hypoglycemia, hypocalcemia, hypomagnesemia, sepsis, and meningitis even if the diagnosis of drug-addicted mother is certain.

III. **Treatment of infant narcotic withdrawal.** The goal is an infant who is not irritable, has no vomiting or diarrhea, can feed well and sleep between feedings, and yet is not heavy sedated (see Fig. 19.2).

Never give **Narcan** (naloxone) to these infants nor to one whose mother was on methadone; it may precipitate immediate withdrawal or seizures.

A. **Symptomatic treatment.** Forty percent need no medication. Symptomatic care includes tight swaddling, holding, rocking, placing in a slightly darkened quiet area, and hypercaloric formula (24 calories per 30 mL) as needed.

B. **Medication.** Infants who are unresponsive to symptomatic treatment will need medication. Base the decision to start medication on objective measurement of symptoms recorded on a withdrawal scoring sheet, such as the one shown in Fig. 19.1. A total abstinence score of 8 or higher for three consecutive scorings indicates a need for pharmacologic intervention. Once the infant scores 8 or higher, decrease the scoring interval from 4-hour to 2-hour intervals. Once the desired effect has been obtained for 72 hours, slowly taper the dose until it is discontinued. Observe the infant for 2 to 3 days prior to discharge.

Currently there is very little evidence regarding the efficacy of different pharmacologic therapeutic regimes for treating neonatal abstinence syndrome (NAS). More studies are required to produce the evidence to allow us a rational choice between treatment modalities. We use the following pharmacologic agents in our nurseries:

1. **Neonatal morphine solution (NMS).** This solution of morphine sulfate made up in a concentration of 0.4 mg/mL is our treatment of choice for narcotic withdrawal.
   a. It is a pharmacologic replacement.
   b. Controls all symptoms.
   c. Least impairs sucking.

DATE: _____

SYSTEM	SIGNS AND SYMPTOMS	SCORE	AM	PM	COMMENTS
CENTRAL NERVOUS SYSTEM DISTURBANCES	Excessive High-pitched (OR Other) Cry Continuous High-pitched (OR Other) Cry	2 3			Daily Weight:
	Sleeps < 1 Hour After Feeding Sleeps < 2 Hours After Feeding Sleeps < 3 Hours After Feeding	3 2 1			
	Hyperactive Moro Reflex Markedly Hyperactive Moro Reflex	2 3			
	Mild Tremors Disturbed Moderate-Severe Tremors Disturbed	1 2			
	Mild Tremors Undisturbed Moderate-Severe Tremors Undisturbed	3 4			
	Increased Muscle Tone	2			
	Excoriation (Specify Area): _____	1			
	Myoclonic Jerks	3			
	Generalized Convulsions	5			
METABOLIC/VASOMOTOR/RESPIRATORY DISTURBANCES	Sweating	1			
	Fever < 101 (99-100.8° F./37.2-38.2° C) Fever > 101 (38.4° C. and Higher)	1 2			
	Frequent Yawning (> 3-4 times/interval)	1			
	Mottling	1			
	Nasal Stuffiness	1			
	Sneezing (> 3-4 times/interval)	1			
	Nasal Flaring	2			
	Respiratory Rate > 60/Min. Respiratory Rate > 50/Min. with Retractions	1 2			

Guidelines for the use of neonatal abstinence scoring system

1. Record time of scoring (end of observation interval).
2. Give points for all behaviors or symptoms observed during the scoring interval, even though they may not be present at the time of recording. (For example, if the baby was diaphoretic at 11 A.M. and is "scored" at noon, when he or she is not, the baby still gets the "sweating" point.)
3. Awaken the baby to test reflexes. Calm before assessing muscle tone, respirations, or Moro reflex. Many of the signs of hunger can appear the same as withdrawal. Appearance after feeding gives a good idea of muscle activity.
4. Count respirations for a full minute. Always take temperature at the same site. The temperatures on the sheet are rectal levels; an axillary temperature that is 2 degrees cooler may also indicate withdrawal.
5. Do not give points for perspiration if it occurs due to swaddling.
6. A startle reflex should not be substituted for the Moro reflex.

GASTROINTESTINAL DISTURBANCES

Excessive Sucking	1
Poor Feeding	2
Regurgitation	2
Projectile Vomiting	3
Loose Stools	2
Watery Stools	3

TOTAL SCORE

INITIALS OF SCORER

7. Record doses administered (dose/time/initials) on sheet. One hour leeway is acceptable in dosing a fairly stable baby.
8. Record daily weight on graphic sheet.
9. Do not hesitate to get your experienced colleagues' opinions.

NO.	PHARMACOTHERAPY REGIMEN	STATUS OF PHARMACOTHERAPY	RX	STATUS	DOSE	TIME	STATUS	DOSE	TIME	STATUS	DOSE	TIME	STATUS	DOSE	TIME	STATUS
1	TITRATION REGIMENS	Indicate exact dose, time of administration & coded dosing status in the following blocks	#1													
		Dosing Code	#2													
2		Initiation (+) Maintenance (m)	#3													
		Increase (↑) Decrease (↓) Discontinuation (−)	#4													

(Time columns marked AM / PM)

Drug Administered:

SEROLOGIC QUANTITATION OF PHARMACOLOGIC AGENTS

* BEFORE BIRTH

− AFTER BIRTH

FIG. 19.1. Neonatal abstinence syndrome assessment and treatment. Guidelines for use of the neonatal abstinence scoring system are also included. (Adapted from Finnigan L.P., et al. A scoring system for evaluation and treatment of neonatal abstinence syndrome: A new clinical and research tool. In: Morselli P.L., Garattini S., Serini F. (Eds.) *Basic and Therapeutic Aspects of Perinatal Pharmacology.* New York: Raven Press, 1975.)

   d. Contains few additives.
   However, high doses are often necessary, and withdrawal is slow.
   This is the equivalent dose of morphine contained in neonatal opium solution (NOS) (see III.B.2). Since the only diluent is water, it avoids alcohol, preservatives, or camphor. Ours is made up in the hospital pharmacy. It has greater stability than deodorized tincture of opium (DTO), and if it is prepared properly there are no problems with overgrowth of mold or microorganisms. The dose is 0.05 mL/kg or 2 drops per kilogram every 4 to 6 hours, increased by 2 drops (or 0.05 mL/kg) at the end of each 4-hour period until the desired response is achieved.
   An alternative dosing scheme for NMS or NOS according to abstinence score is as follows:

Score	NMS or NOS
8–10	0.8 mL/kg/day divided q4h
11–13	1.2 mL/kg/day divided q4h
14–16	1.6 mL/kg per day divided q4h
17 or greater	2.0 mL/kg per day divided q4h; increase by 0.4-mL increments until controlled

   Add phenobarbital to control irritability when the NMS or NOS dose is greater than 2.0 mL/kg per day (see III.B.2). Some babies will need medication more often than every 4 hours.
   Once an adequate dose has been found, and infant scores have been less than 8 for 72 hours, wean by 10% (of total dose) daily. If weaning results in scores greater than 8, restart the last effective dose. Discontinue NMS or NOS when the daily dose is less than 0.3 mL/kg per day. The infant should be able to tolerate mild symptomatology during reduction.
   If the scores are low, make sure that the infant is not overdosed. Side effects include sleepiness, constipation, poor suck, and ultimately profound narcosis with obtundation, hypothermia, respiratory depression, apnea, and bradycardia. If these symptoms occur, stop the medication until the abstinence scores are over 8. Use Colace to treat constipation.
2. Neonatal opium solution (NOS) (DTO). If NMS is not available, use NOS for treatment of narcotic withdrawal. DTO is a hydroalcoholic solution containing 10% USP laudanum and is equal to morphine 1.0%. This is diluted 25-fold with sterile water to a concentration and potency equal to that of paregoric (0.4 mg/mL of morphine). The diluted mixture should be called NOS, as suggested in the Neonatal Drug Withdrawal Statement of the American Academy of Pediatrics' Committee on Drugs. The NOS dose is the same as that of NMS. This dilution is stable for 2 weeks. Keep the stock solution of tincture of opium in the pharmacy and dilute it there because of the possibility of giving the stronger mixture to the patient in error.
3. Paregoric contains opium 0.4%, equivalent to morphine 0.04% (0.4 mg/mL). It also contains anise oil, benzoic acid, camphor, and glycerin in an alcohol base. Dose as for NMS or NOS. Paregoric is readily available and has a long shelf life. Because of the unknown effects of many of the ingredients, we do not use it.
4. Phenobarbital, a loading dose of 10 mg/kg is given. A maintenance dose is given depending on the abstinence score.

Abstinence score	Maintenance Phenobarbital
8–10	6 mg/kg per day divided q8h
11–13	8 mg/kg per day divided q8h
14–16	10 mg /kg per day divided q8h
17 or greater	12 mg/kg per day divided q8h

The maintenance dose may be increased by 2 mg/kg per day until control is achieved. Phenobarbitol can be given PO or IM. Usually given PO. Taper by 10% each day after improvement of symptoms. Phenobarbital is the drug of choice if the infant is thought to be withdrawing from a nonnarcotic drug or from multiple drug use. In narcotic withdrawal, some prefer phenobarbital to NOS to discontinue exposing the developing neonatal brain to narcotics. The possible side effects of phenobarbital include sedation and poor sucking. It does not control the diarrhea that occurs with withdrawal. Using phenobarbital with NOS allows a lower dose of NOS and lessens the side effects. Phenobarbital elixir may contain 20% alcohol, and the parenteral form may contain propylene glycol, ethyl alcohol, and benzyl alcohol.

5. **Chlorpromazine** is no longer used by us because of its unacceptable side effects, including tardive dyskinesia. It is useful to control the vomiting and diarrhea that sometimes occur in withdrawal. The dosage is 1.5 to 3.0 mg/kg per day, administered in four divided doses, initially IM, then PO. Maintain this dose for 2 to 4 days and then taper as tolerated every 2 to 4 days.

6. **Methadone** is not routinely used by us for withdrawal from narcotics. Methadone is excreted in breast milk at a very low level. It is now considered safe for methadone-treated mothers to breast feed if there are no other contraindications. It has a prolonged plasma half-life (24 hours). Doses used are 0.5 to 1.0 mg/kg every 6 hours with increases of 0.05 mg/kg until symptoms are controlled. Weaning can then be attempted by giving methadone every 12 hours, then every 24 hours at the last dose used. Once the dose reached 0.05 mg/kg per day it could be discontinued. The oral formulation of methadone contains 8% ethanol.

7. **Morphine** in doses of 0.1 to 0.2 mg/kg can be effective in the emergency treatment of seizures or shock due to acute narcotic withdrawal.

8. We do not recommend **diazepam** (Valium), but it has been used for control of symptoms. Some hospitals use it in doses of 0.1 to 0.3 mg/kg IM until symptoms are controlled, halve the dose, then change to every 12 hours, and lower again. The major side effect is respiratory depression. Breakthrough symptoms, including seizures, respiratory depression, and bradycardia have been seen during diazepam use. Also, withdrawal has recurred after termination of therapy. The sodium benzoate included in parenteral diazepam may interfere with the binding of bilirubin to albumin. The manufacturer warns that the safety and efficacy of injectable diazepam have not been established in the newborn (see Appendix).

9. **Lorazepam** is often used for sedation by itself or with NMS or NOS. The parenteral preparation of lorazepam contains benzyl alcohol and polyethylene glycol. It is given as 0.05 to 0.1 mg/kg IV per dose. When used in conjunction with NOS, it may decrease the amount of NOS needed. Limited data are available about its use in newborns.

C. Closely monitor **fluid and electrolyte** intake and losses. Replace as needed.

D. The **narcotic abstinence scoring sheet** (see Fig. 19.1) will help establish objective criteria for weaning the infant from the medications. Irritability, tremors, and disturbance of sleeping patterns may last for up to 6 months and should not be a reason for continuing medication. For a general approach to management, see Fig. 19.2.

IV. **Maternal addiction to drugs other than narcotics.** Infants born to mothers using drugs other than narcotics may be symptomatic.

A. **Cocaine** has a potent anorexic effect and may cause prenatal malnutrition, an increased rate of premature labor, spontaneous abortion, placental abruption, fetal distress, meconium staining, and low Apgar scores. Cocaine increases catecholamines, which can increase uterine contractility and cause maternal hypertension and placental vasoconstriction with diminished uterine blood flow and fetal hypoxia.

1. The following are congenital anomalies associated with cocaine use during pregnancy: cardiac anomalies; genitourinary malformations; "prune

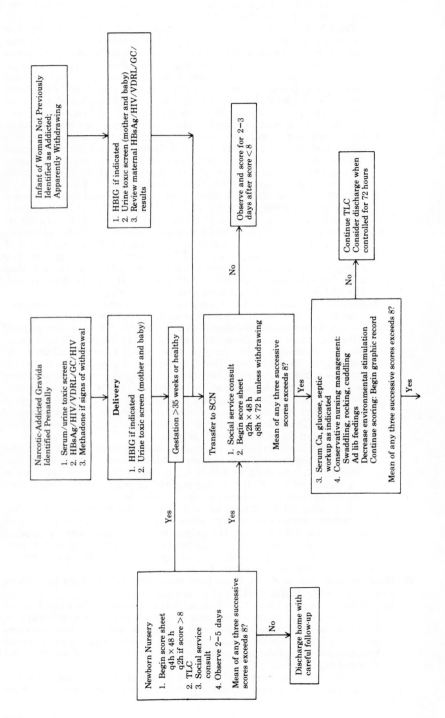

232

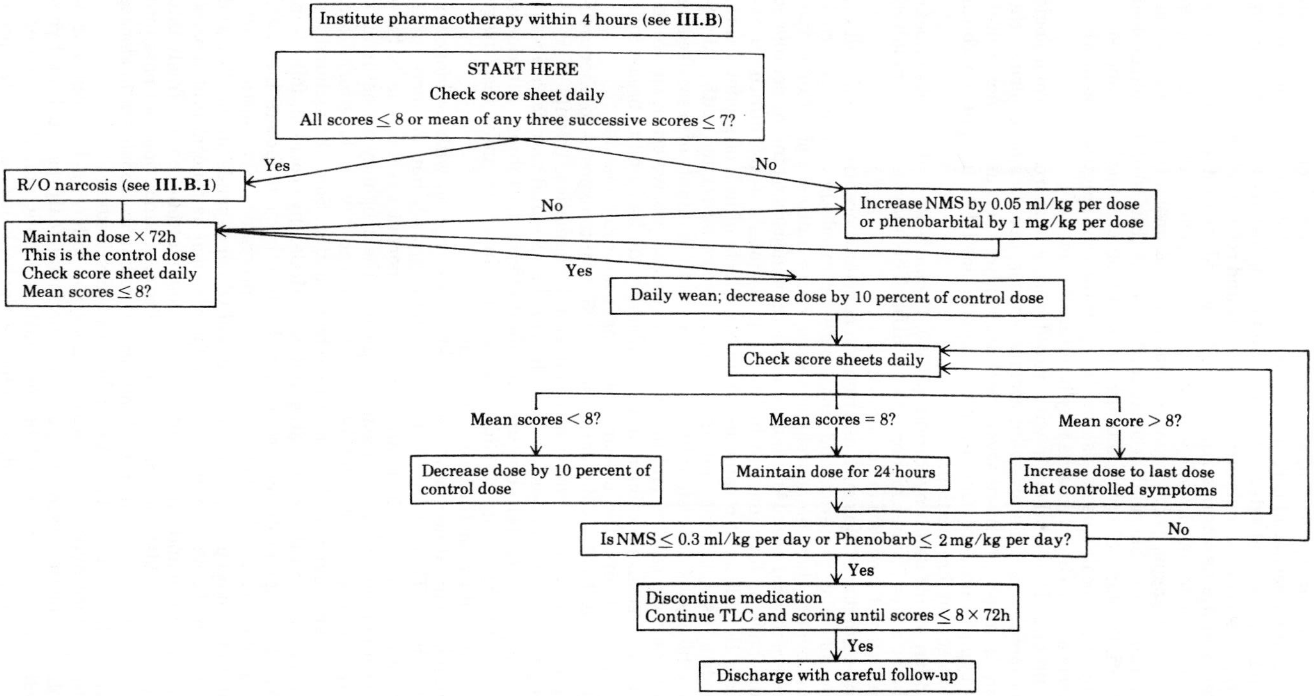

FIG. 19.2. General approach to management of a narcotic-addicted gravida identified antenatally and of a withdrawing infant of a woman not previously identified as addicted. HBsAG = hepatitis B surface antigen, VDRL = Venereal Disease Research Laboratory, TLC = tender loving care, NMS = neonatal morphine solution, RR = respiratory rate, HR = heart rate, GC = gonorrhea, HBIG = hepatitis B immune globulin, HIV = human immunodeficiency virus, SCN = special care nursery.

belly" syndrome; intestinal atresias; microcephaly with or without growth retardation, perinatal cerebral infarctions, usually in the distribution of the middle cerebral artery with resultant cystic lesions; early-onset necrotizing enterocolitis; and retinal dysgenesis and retinal coloboma.

2. **Effects in the newborns.** Although cocaine-addicted infants do not show the classic signs of narcotic withdrawal, they demonstrate abnormal sleep patterns, tremors, poor organizational response, inability to be consoled, and transiently abnormal electroencephalograms (EEGs) and visual evoked potentials. Many of these findings are also true of tobacco use and since many crack cocaine users also smoke cigarettes, the identification of which defects are specific to cocaine may be difficult to identify.

3. **Treatment.** The newborn's withdrawal rarely requires pharmacologic treatment. When the pregnant cocaine abuser also uses other drugs, the neonate may have more severe withdrawal; we then use phenobarbital.

   If symptomatic treatment is not adequate (see III.4), use phenobarbital or lorazepam for sedation.

4. **Sudden infant death syndrome (SIDS).** Cocaine-exposed infants appear to be at a 3 to 7 times higher risk for SIDS. This may be due to impaired regulation of respiration and arousal.

5. **Long-term disabilities** such as attention deficits, concentration difficulties, abnormal play patterns, and flat, apathetic moods have been reported. Some believe that the neurologic and cognitive outcomes of cocaine exposure are unclear because standard methods of measuring infant neurologic and behavioral functions are difficult to quantitate. It is also difficult to extricate the effects of cocaine use from the effects of lack of prenatal care, polydrug use, smoking, and the increased risks associated with a drug-using lifestyle. Convulsions have been seen both in infants of breastfeeding mothers using cocaine and in infants exposed to passive crack smoke inhalation. Because cocaine and its metabolites can be found in breast milk for up to 60 hours after use, breastfeeding is not recommended.

B. **Phencyclidine (PCP).** A metaanalysis of 206 infants exposed to phencyclidine prenatally did not show any congenital anomalies. Infants of PCP-abusing mothers are of normal size. Most of the neonatal manifestations of in utero exposure center on neurobehavioral effects (irritability, jitteriness, hypertonicity). Since phencyclidine is excreted in breast milk, discourage breastfeeding if the mother uses this drug.

C. **Marijuana.** Prenatal use may result in shorter gestation with prolonged or arrested labor. There may be decreased fetal growth but no increase in major or minor morphologic anomalies. No reported adverse effects have been documented with breastfeeding. However, the drug may persist in milk for days after exposure and become concentrated with long-term use. Encourage abstinence if the infant is to be breastfed. Some have found low Brazelton scores in these neonates and poor McCarthy scores on follow-up.

D. **Ethanol.** Teratogenic studies are confounded by other risk factors, but there is no established safe level of ethanol use in pregnancy. Symmetric growth retardation can occur in utero, the extent of which depends on the dose and duration of maternal use and on other factors such as concomitant tobacco or other drug use and overall nutrition. Although alcohol passes freely into breast milk, acetaldehyde, the toxic metabolite of ethanol, does not pass into milk. Therefore, the American Academy of Pediatrics considers moderate maternal ethanol use to be compatible with breastfeeding.

1. **Fetal alcohol syndrome (FAS)** includes the following features: microcephaly, growth retardation, dysmorphic facial features (such as hypoplastic midface, low nasal bridge, flattened philtrum, thinned upper vermilion, epicanthal fold, shortened palpebral fissure), cardiac problems, hydronephrosis, increased incidence of mental retardation, motor problems, and behavioral issues. Heavy prenatal alcohol exposure with or without physical features of FAS can lead to intelligence quotient (IQ) deficits. As is the case with other syndromes associated with craniofacial

anomalies and hearing impairments, speech and language pathologies may also occur in FAS babies.

E. Tobacco. Smoking by pregnant women is associated with a higher rate of spontaneous abortions. Placental vascular resistance is increased as a consequence of the effects of nicotine, with resultant chronic ischemia and hypoxia. Nicotine can enter breast milk in relatively low levels and is not well absorbed by the infant's intestinal tract. This does not negate the risks to the infant from passive exposure to smoke.

1. **Effects on newborn infants of regular smokers (1 pack per day)**
   a. Typically weigh 150 to 250 g less than the newborns of nonsmokers. The most pronounced effects of smoking on fetal growth occur after the second trimester. Fetuses may also be at risk by passive exposure.
   b. Increased tremors.
   c. Poor auditory responsiveness.
   d. Increased tone.
   e. No association has been found between maternal smoking during pregnancy and congenital anomalies.
   f. SIDS has been associated, in a dose-response manner, with maternal smoking, possibly secondary to passive exposure to smoke after birth.

V. Disposition. The major problems with infants of a drug-addicted mother are proper disposition and follow-up. Studies show a high incidence of abuse and violence in the childhood and lives of drug-abusing women. This, combined with their own drug use and chaotic lifestyles, places them at risk for inadequate parenting. These factors may be more important to the outcome of the child than the drug abuse. The health of the mother, especially if she has acquired immunodeficiency syndrome (AIDS), is significant for the ultimate well-being of the infant.

A. These infants are difficult to care for, as they are often irritable, have poor sleeping patterns, and will try the patience of any caregiver. They are at increased risk for child abuse. Infants of HIV-positive mothers should be followed up closely because of their increased risk of AIDS (see Chap. 23).

B. Coordination of plans with social service agencies, drug treatment centers, and the courts, when necessary, is essential for proper follow-up and disposition.

C. Many states require that infants who show signs of withdrawal be reported as battered children.

Suggested Readings

American Academy of Pediatrics. Neonatal Drug Withdrawal. *Pediatrics* 1998;101(6).

Frank D.A., et al. *Growth, Development and Behavior in Early Childhood Following Prenatal Cocaine Exposure: A Systematic Review. JAMA* 2001;285(12).

Kwang T.C., Shearer D. Substance abuse in pregnancy. *Clin Obstet Gynecol* 1998;25(1).

Philipp B.L., et al. Methadone and breast feeding: New horizons. *Pediatrics* 2003;111:1429–1430.

Rosen T.S., Bateman D.A. Infants of addicted mothers. In: Fanaroff A.A., Martin R.J. (Eds.). *Neonatal-Perinatal Medicine,* 7th ed. St. Louis: Saunders, 2002;56:661–673.

Smeriglio V.L., Wilson H.C. Prenatal Drug Exposure and Child Outcome. *Clin Perinatol* 1999;26(1).

Theis J.G. Current management of the neonatal abstinence syndrome: A critical analysis of the evidence. *Biol Neonate* 1997;71(6).

20. BIRTH TRAUMA

Elisa Abdulhayoglu

I. Background. Birth injury is defined by the National Vital Statistics Report as "an impairment of the infant's body or structure due to adverse influences, which occurred at birth." Injury may occur antenatally, intrapartum, or during resuscitation, and may be avoidable or unavoidable.

   A. Incidence. Mortality due to birth trauma is 3.7 deaths per 100,000 live births. The morbidity rate is higher, 2.9 per 1000 live births, and varies with the type of injury.

   B. Risk factors. When fetal size, immaturity, or malpresentation complicate delivery, the normal intrapartum compressions, contortions, and forces can lead to injury in the newborn, including hemorrhage and fracture. Obstetrical instrumentation may increase the mechanical forces, amplifying or inducing a birth injury. Breech presentation carries the greatest risk of injury. However, cesarean delivery without labor does not prevent all birth injuries. The following factors may contribute to an increased risk of birth injury:

   1. Primiparity.
   2. Small maternal stature.
   3. Maternal pelvic anomalies.
   4. Prolonged or unusually rapid labor.
   5. Oligohydramnios.
   6. Malpresentation of the fetus.
   7. Use of mid-forceps or vacuum extraction.
   8. Versions and extraction.
   9. Very low birth weight or extreme prematurity.
   10. Fetal macrosomia or large fetal head.
   11. Fetal anomalies.

   C. Evaluation. A newborn at risk for birth injury should have a thorough examination, including a detailed neurologic evaluation. Newborns who required resuscitation after birth should be evaluated, as occult injury may be present. Particular attention should be paid to symmetry of structure and function, cranial nerves, range of motion of individual joints, and integrity of the scalp and skin.

II. Types of birth trauma

   A. Head and neck injuries

   1. **Injuries associated with intrapartum fetal monitoring.** Placement of an electrode on the fetal scalp or presenting part for fetal heart monitoring occasionally causes superficial abrasions or lacerations. These injuries require minimal local treatment, if any. Facial or ocular trauma may result from a malpositioned electrode. Rarely, abscesses form at the electrode site. Hemorrhage is a rare complication of fetal blood sampling.

   2. **Extracranial hemorrhage**

   a. **Caput succedaneum**

   (1) Caput succedaneum is a commonly occurring subcutaneous, extraperiosteal fluid collection that is occasionally hemorrhagic. It has poorly defined margins and can extend over the midline and across suture lines. It typically extends over the presenting portion of the scalp, and is usually associated with molding.

   (2) The lesion usually resolves spontaneously without sequelae over the first several days after birth. It rarely causes significant blood loss or jaundice. There are rare reports of scalp necrosis with scarring.

   (3) **Vacuum caput** is a caput succedaneum with margins well demarcated by the vacuum cup.

   b. **Cephalohematoma**

(1) A **cephalohematoma** is a subperiosteal collection of blood resulting from rupture of the superficial veins between the skull and periosteum. The lesion is always confined by suture lines. It may occur in as many as 2.5% of live births.

(2) An extensive cephalohematoma can result in significant hyperbilirubinemia. Hemorrhage is rarely serious enough to necessitate blood transfusion. Infection is also a rare complication, and usually occurs in association with septicemia and meningitis. Skull fractures have been associated with 5 to 20% of cephalohematomas. A head computed tomography (CT) scan should be obtained if neurologic symptoms are present. Most cephalohematomas resolve within 8 weeks. Occasionally, calcification may persist for several months.

(3) Management is limited to observation in most cases. Incision and aspiration of a cephalohematoma may introduce infection and is contraindicated. Anemia or hyperbilirubinemia should be treated as needed.

c. **Subgaleal hematoma**

(1) Subgaleal hematoma is hemorrhage under the aponeurosis of the scalp. Because the subgaleal or subaponeurotic space extends from the orbital ridges to the nape of the neck and laterally to the ears, the hemorrhage can spread across the entire calvarium.

(2) The initial presentation typically includes pallor, poor tone, and a fluctuant swelling on the scalp. The hematoma may grow slowly or increase rapidly and result in shock. With progressive spread, the ears may be displaced anteriorly and periorbital swelling can occur. Ecchymosis of the scalp may develop. The blood is resorbed slowly and swelling gradually resolves. The mortality rate is 25% in newborns who require intensive care for this lesion.

(3) There is no specific therapy. The infant must be observed closely for signs of hypovolemia and blood volume should be maintained as needed with transfusions. Phototherapy should be provided for hyperbilirubinemia. An investigation for a bleeding disorder should be considered. Surgical drainage should be considered only for unremitting clinical deterioration. A subgaleal hematoma associated with skin abrasions may become infected; it should be treated with antibiotics and may need drainage.

3. Intracranial hemorrhage (see Chap. 27)

4. Skull fracture

a. Skull fractures may be either linear, usually involving the parietal bone, or depressed, involving the parietal or frontal bones. The latter are often associated with forceps use. Occipital bone fractures are most often associated with breech deliveries.

b. Most infants with linear or depressed skull fractures are asymptomatic unless there is an associated intracranial hemorrhage (e.g., subdural or subarachnoid hemorrhage). Occipital osteodiastasis is a separation of the basal and squamous portions of the occipital bone that often results in cerebellar contusion and significant hemorrhage. It may be a lethal complication in breech deliveries. A linear fracture that is associated with a dural tear may lead to herniation of the meninges and brain, with development of a leptomeningeal cyst.

c. Uncomplicated linear fractures usually require no therapy. The diagnosis is made by skull X ray. Head CT scan should be obtained if intracranial injury is suspected. Depressed skull fractures require neurosurgical evaluation. Some may be elevated using closed techniques. Comminuted or large skull fractures associated with neurologic findings need immediate neurosurgical evaluation. If leakage of cerebrospinal fluid from the nares or ears is noted, antibiotic therapy should be started and neurosurgical consultation obtained. Follow-up imaging should be performed at 8 to 12 weeks to evaluate possible leptomeningeal cyst formation.

5. **Facial or mandibular fractures**

   a. Facial fractures can be caused by numerous forces including natural passage through the birth canal, forceps use, or delivery of the head in breech presentation.

   b. Fractures of the mandible, maxilla, and lacrimal bones warrant immediate attention. They may present as facial asymmetry with ecchymoses, edema, and crepitance, or respiratory distress with poor feeding. Untreated fractures can lead to facial deformities with subsequent malocclusion and mastication difficulties. Treatment should begin promptly because maxillar and lacrimal fractures begin to heal within 7 to 10 days and mandibular fractures start to repair at 10 to 14 days. Treated fractures usually heal without complication.

   c. Airway patency should be closely monitored. A plastic surgeon or otorhinolaryngologist should be consulted immediately and appropriate radiographic studies obtained. Head CT or magnetic resonance imaging (MRI) may be necessary to evaluate for retro-orbital or cribriform plate disruption. Antibiotics should be administered for fractures involving the sinuses or middle ear.

6. **Nasal injuries**

   a. Nasal fracture and dislocation may occur during the birth process. The most frequent nasal injury is dislocation of the nasal cartilage, which may result from pressure applied by the maternal symphysis pubis or sacral promontory. The incidence of dislocation is 0.6 to 0.93%.

   b. Infants with significant nasal trauma develop respiratory distress. Similar to facial fractures, nasal fractures begin to heal in 7 to10 days and must be treated promptly. Rapid healing usually occurs once treatment is initiated. If treatment is delayed, deformities are common.

   c. A misshapen nose may appear dislocated. To differentiate dislocation from a temporary deformation, compress the tip of the nose. With septal dislocation, the nares collapse and the deviated septum is more apparent. With a misshapen nose, no nasal deviation occurs. Nasal edema from repeated suctioning may mimic partial obstruction. Patency can be assessed with a cotton wisp under the nares. Management involves protection of the airway and otorhinolaryngology consultation.

7. **Ocular injuries**

   a. Retinal and subconjunctival hemorrhages are commonly seen after vaginal delivery. They result from increased venous congestion and pressure during delivery. Malpositioned forceps can result in ocular and periorbital injury including hyphema, vitreous hemorrhage, lacerations, orbital fracture, lacrimal duct or gland injury and disruption of Descemet's membrane of the cornea (which can lead to astigmatism and amblyopia).

   b. Retinal hemorrhages usually resolve within 1 to 5 days. Subconjunctival hemorrhages resorb within 1 to 2 weeks. No long-term complications usually occur. For other ocular injuries, prompt diagnosis and treatment are necessary to ensure a good long-term outcome.

   c. Management. Prompt ophthalmologic consultation should be obtained.

8. **Ear injuries**

   a. Ears are susceptible to injury, particularly with forceps application. More significant injuries occur with fetal malposition. Abrasions, hematomas, and lacerations may develop.

   b. Abrasions generally heal well with local care. Hematomas of the pinna may lead to the development of a "cauliflower" ear; lacerations may result in perichondritis. Temporal bone injury can lead to middle and inner ear complications, such as hemotympanum and ossicular disarticulation.

   c. Hematomas of the pinna should be drained to prevent clot organization and development of cauliflower ear. If the cartilage and temporal bone are involved, an otolaryngologist should be consulted. Antibiotic therapy may be required.

9. Sternocleidomastoid (SCM) injury
   a. SCM injury is also referred to as congenital or muscular torticollis. The etiology is uncertain. The most likely cause is a muscle compartment syndrome resulting from intrauterine positioning. Torticollis can also arise during delivery as the muscle is hyperextended and ruptured, with development of a hematoma and subsequent fibrosis and shortening.
   b. Torticollis may present at birth with a palpable 1–2 cm mass in the SCM region and head tilt to the side of the lesion. More often it is noted at 2 to 3 weeks of age. Facial asymmetry may be present along with hemihypoplasia on the side of the lesion. Prompt treatment may lessen or correct the torticollis.
   c. Other conditions may mimic congenital torticollis and should be ruled out. These include cervical vertebral anomalies, hemangioma, lymphangioma, and teratoma.
   d. Treatment is initially conservative. Stretching of the involved muscle should begin promptly and be performed several times per day. Recovery typically occurs within 3 to 4 months in approximately 80% of cases. Surgery is needed if torticollis persists after 6 months of physical therapy.

10. Pharyngeal injury
   a. Minor submucosal pharyngeal injuries can occur with postpartum bulb suctioning. More serious injury, such as perforation into the mediastinal or pleural cavity, may result from nasogastric or endotracheal tube placement. Affected infants may have copious secretions and difficulty swallowing, and it may be difficult to advance a nasogastric tube.
   b. Mild submucosal injuries typically heal without complication. More extensive trauma requires prompt diagnosis and treatment for complete resolution.
   c. The diagnosis of a retropharyngeal tear is made radiographically using water-soluble contrast material. Infants are treated with antibiotics and feedings are withheld for 2 weeks. The contrast study is repeated to confirm healing before feedings are restarted. Infants with pleural effusions may require chest tube placement. Surgical consultation is obtained if the leak persists or the perforation is large.

B. Cranial nerve, spinal cord, and peripheral nerve injury
  1. Cranial nerve injuries
    a. Facial nerve injury (cranial nerve VII)
     (1) Injury to the facial nerve is the most common peripheral nerve injury in neonates. The exact incidence is unknown, as many cases are subtle and resolve readily. The incidence ranges from 1.8 to 7.5 per 1000 live births. The etiology includes compression of the facial nerve by forceps (particularly mid-forceps), pressure on the nerve secondary to the fetal face lying against the maternal sacral promontory, or, rarely, from pressure of a uterine mass (e.g., fibroid).
     (2) Facial nerve injury results in asymmetric crying facies.
      (a) Central facial nerve injury occurs less frequently than peripheral nerve injury. Paralysis is limited to the lower 1/2 to 2/3 of the contralateral side, which is smooth with no nasolabial fold present. The corner of the mouth droops. Movement of the forehead and eyelid is unaffected.
      (b) Peripheral injury involves the entire side of face and is consistent with a lower motor neuron injury. The nasolabial fold is flattened and the mouth droops on the affected side. The in-

fant is unable to wrinkle the forehead and close the eye completely. The tongue is not involved.

(c) Peripheral nerve branch injury results in paralysis that is limited to only one group of facial muscles: the forehead, eyelid, or mouth.

(3) Differential diagnosis includes Mobius syndrome (nuclear agenesis), intracranial hemorrhage, congenital hypoplasia of the depressor anguli oris muscle, congenital absence of facial muscles or nerve branches.

(4) The prognosis of acquired facial nerve injury is excellent with recovery usually complete by 3 weeks. Initial management is directed at prevention of corneal injuries by using artificial tears and protecting the open eye by patching. Electromyography may be helpful to predict recovery or potential residual effects. Because full recovery is likely, surgical intervention should not be considered within the first year.

b. Recurrent laryngeal nerve injury

(1) Unilateral abductor paralysis may be caused by recurrent laryngeal injury secondary to excessive traction on the fetal head during breech delivery or lateral traction on the head with forceps. The left recurrent laryngeal nerve is involved more often because of its longer course. Bilateral recurrent laryngeal nerve injury can be caused by trauma, but is usually due to hypoxia or brain-stem hemorrhage.

(2) A neonate with unilateral abductor paralysis is often asymptomatic at rest, but has hoarseness and inspiratory stridor with crying. Unilateral injury is occasionally associated with hypoglossal nerve injury, and presents with difficulty with feedings and secretions. Bilateral paralysis usually results in stridor, severe respiratory distress, and cyanosis.

(3) Differential diagnosis of symptoms similar to unilateral injury includes congenital laryngeal malformations. Particularly with bilateral paralysis, intrinsic central nervous system (CNS) malformations must be ruled out, including Chiari malformation and hydrocephalus. If there is no history of birth trauma, cardiovascular anomalies and mediastinal masses should be considered.

(4) The diagnosis can be made using direct or flexible fiberoptic laryngoscopy. A modified barium swallow and speech pathology consultation may be helpful to optimize feeding. Unilateral injury usually resolves by 6 weeks of age without intervention and treatment. Bilateral paralysis has a variable prognosis; tracheostomy may be required.

2. Spinal cord injuries

a. Vaginal delivery of an infant with a hyperextended head or neck, breech delivery, and severe shoulder dystocia are risk factors for spinal cord injury. However, significant spinal cord injuries are unusual. Injuries include spinal epidural hematomas, vertebral artery injuries, traumatic cervical hematomyelia, spinal artery occlusion, and transection of the cord.

b. Spinal cord injury presents in four ways;

(1) Some infants with severe high cervical or brain-stem injury present as stillborn or in poor condition at birth, with respiratory depression, shock, and hypothermia. Death generally occurs within hours of birth.

(2) Infants with an upper or midcervical injury present with central respiratory depression. They have lower extremity paralysis, absent deep tendon reflexes and absent sensation in the lower half of the body, urinary retention, and constipation. Brachial plexus injury may be present.

(3) Injury at the seventh cervical vertebra or lower may be reversible. However, permanent neurologic complications may result, including muscle atrophy, contractures, bony deformities, and constant micturition.

(4) Partial spinal injury or spinal artery occlusions may result in subtle neurologic signs and spasticity.

c. Differential diagnosis includes amyotonia congenita, myelodysplasia associated with spina bifida occulta, spinal cord tumors, and cerebral hypotonia.

d. The prognosis depends on the severity and location of the injury. If a spinal injury is suspected at birth, efforts should focus on resuscitation and prevention of further damage. The head and spine should be immobilized. Neurology and neurosurgical consultations should be obtained. Careful and repeated exams are necessary to help predict long-term outcome. Cervical spine radiographs, CT, and magnetic resonance imaging (MRI) may be helpful.

3. Cervical nerve root injuries

a. Phrenic nerve injury (C3, 4, or 5)

(1) Phrenic nerve damage leading to paralysis of the ipsilateral diaphragm may result from a stretch injury due to lateral hyperextension of the neck at birth. Risk factors include breech and difficult forceps deliveries. Injury to the nerve is thought to occur where it crosses the brachial plexus. Thus, at least 75% of patients also have brachial plexus injury. Occasionally, chest tube insertion or surgery injures this nerve.

(2) Respiratory distress and cyanosis are often seen. Some infants present with persistent tachypnea and decreased breath sounds at the lung base. There may be decreased movement of the affected hemithorax. Chest radiographs may show elevation of the affected diaphragm, although this may not be apparent if the infant is on continuous positive airway pressure (CPAP) or mechanical ventilation. If the infant is breathing spontaneously and not on CPAP, increasing atelectasis may develop. The diagnosis is confirmed by ultrasonography or fluoroscopy that shows paradoxical (upward) movement of the diaphragm with inspiration.

(3) Differential diagnosis includes cardiac, pulmonary, and other neurologic causes of respiratory distress. These can usually be evaluated by a careful exam and appropriate imaging. Congenital absence of the nerve is rare.

(4) The initial treatment is supportive. CPAP or mechanical ventilation may be needed, with careful airway care to avoid atelectasis and pneumonia. Most infants recover in 1 to 3 months without permanent sequelae. Diaphragmatic plication is considered in refractory cases. Phrenic nerve pacing is possible for bilateral paralysis.

b. Brachial plexus injury

(1) The incidence of brachial plexus injury is 0.6 to 2.5 per 1000 live births. The cause is excessive traction on the head, neck, and arm during birth. Risk factors include macrosomia, shoulder dystocia, and breech presentation. Injury usually involves the nerve root, especially where the roots come together to form the nerve trunks of the plexus.

(2) Duchenne-Erb's palsy involves the upper trunks (C5, C6, and occasionally C7) and is the most common type of brachial plexus injury. Total brachial plexus palsy occurs in some cases and involves all roots from C5 to T1. Klumpke's palsy involves C7/C8 to T1 and is the least common.

(a) Duchenne-Erb palsy. The arm is typically adducted and internally rotated at the shoulder. There is extension and pronation at the elbow and flexion of the wrist and fingers in the characteristic "waiter's tip" posture. The deltoid, infraspinatus, biceps, supinator and brachioradialis muscles, and the extensors of the wrist and fingers may be weak or paralyzed. The Moro, biceps, and radial reflexes are absent on the affected side. The grasp reflex is intact. Sensation is variably affected. Diaphragm paralysis occurs in 5% of cases.

    (b) **Total brachial plexus injury.** The entire arm is flaccid. All reflexes, including grasp, and sensation, are absent. If sympathetic fibers are injured at T1, Horner's syndrome may be seen.

    (c) **Klumpke's palsy.** The lower arm paralysis affects the intrinsic muscles of the hand and the long flexors of the wrist and fingers. The grasp reflex is absent. However, the biceps and radial reflexes are present. There is sensory impairment on the ulnar side of the forearm and hand. Because the first thoracic root is usually injured, its sympathetic fibers are damaged, leading to an ipsilateral Horner's syndrome.

  (3) Differential diagnosis includes a cerebral injury, which usually has other associated CNS symptoms. Injury of the clavicle, upper humerus, and lower cervical spine may mimic a brachial plexus injury.

  (4) Radiographs of the shoulder and upper arm should be performed to rule out bony injury. The chest should be carefully examined to detect diaphragm paralysis. Initial treatment is conservative. Physical therapy and passive range of motion exercises prevent contractures. These should be started at 7 to 10 days when the post-injury neuritis has resolved. "Statue of Liberty" splinting should be avoided as contractures in the shoulder girdle may develop. Wrist and digit splints may be useful.

  (5) The prognosis for full recovery varies with the extent of injury. If the nerve roots are intact and not avulsed, the prognosis for full recovery is excellent (>90%). Notable clinical improvement in the first 2 weeks after birth indicates that normal or near-normal function will return. Most infants recovery fully by 3 months of age. In those with slow recovery, electromyography and nerve-conduction studies may distinguish an avulsion from a stretch injury.

C. Bone injuries

  1. Clavicular fracture is the most commonly injured bone during delivery.

    a. These fractures are seen in vertex presentations with shoulder dystocia or in breech deliveries when the arms are extended. Macrosomia is a risk factor.

    b. A greenstick or incomplete fracture may be asymptomatic at birth. The first clinical sign may be a callus at 7 to 10 days of age. Signs of a complete fracture include crepitus, palpable bony irregularity, and spasm of the SCM. The affected arm may have a pseudoparalysis because motion causes pain.

    c. Differential diagnosis includes fracture of the humerus or a brachial plexus palsy.

    d. A **clavicular fracture** is confirmed by chest X ray. If arm movement is decreased, the cervical spine, brachial plexus, and humerus should be assessed. Therapy should be directed at decreasing pain with analgesics. The infant's sleeve should be pinned to the shirt to limit movement until the callus begins to form. Complete healing is expected.

  2. Long bone injuries

    a. Humeral fractures

      (1) Humeral fractures typically occur during a difficult delivery of the arms in the breech presentation and/or of the shoulders in vertex. Direct pressure on the humerus may also result in fracture.

      (2) A greenstick fracture may not be noted until the callus forms. The first sign is typically loss of spontaneous arm movement, followed by swelling and pain on passive motion. A complete fracture with displaced fragments presents as an obvious deformity. X ray confirms the diagnosis.

(3) Differential diagnosis includes clavicular fracture and brachial plexus injury.

(4) The prognosis is excellent with complete healing expected. Pain should be treated with analgesics.

   (a) A fractured humerus usually requires splinting for 2 weeks. Displaced fractures require closed reduction and casting. Radial nerve injury may be seen.

   (b) Epiphyseal displacement occurs when the humeral epiphysis separates at the hypertrophied cartilaginous layer of the growth plate. Severe displacement may result in significant compromise of growth. The diagnosis can be confirmed by ultrasonography because the epiphysis is not ossified at birth. Therapy includes immobilization of the limb for 10 to 14 days.

b. Femoral fractures

   (1) Femoral fractures usually follow a breech delivery. Infants with congenital hypotonia are at increased risk.

   (2) Physical exam usually reveals an obvious deformity of the thigh. In some cases, the injury may not be noted for a few days until swelling, decreased movement, or pain with palpation develop. The diagnosis is confirmed by X ray.

   (3) Complete healing without limb shortening is expected.

   (a) Fractures, even if unilateral, should be treated with traction and suspension of both legs with a spica cast. Casting is maintained for approximately 4 weeks.

   (b) Femoral epiphyseal separation may be misinterpreted as developmental dysplasia of the hip because the epiphysis is not ossified at birth. Pain and tenderness with palpation are more likely with epiphyseal separation than dislocation. The diagnosis is confirmed by ultrasonography. Therapy includes limb immobilization for 10 to 14 days and analgesics for pain.

D. Intra-abdominal Injuries. Intra-abdominal birth trauma is uncommon.

1. Hepatic injury

   a. The liver is the most commonly injured solid organ during birth. Macrosomia, hepatomegaly, and breech presentation are risk factors for hepatic hematoma and/or rupture. The etiology is thought to be direct pressure on the liver.

   b. Subcapsular hematomas are generally not symptomatic at birth. Nonspecific signs of blood loss such as poor feeding, pallor, tachypnea, tachycardia, and onset of jaundice develop during the first 1 to 3 days after birth. Serial hematocrits may suggest blood loss. Rupture of the hematoma through the capsule results in discoloration of the abdominal wall and circulatory collapse with shock.

   c. Differential diagnosis includes trauma to other intra-abdominal organs.

   d. Management includes restoration of blood volume, correction of coagulation disturbances, and surgical consultation for probable laparotomy. Early diagnosis and correction of volume loss increase survival.

2. Splenic injury

   a. Risk factors for splenic injury include macrosomia, breech delivery, and splenomegaly (e.g., congenital syphilis, erythroblastosis fetalis).

   b. Signs are similar to hepatic rupture. A mass is sometimes palpable in the left upper quadrant and the stomach bubble may be displaced medially on an abdominal radiograph.

   c. Differential diagnosis includes injury to other abdominal organs.

   d. Management includes volume replacement and correction of coagulation disorders. Surgical consultation should be obtained. Expectant management with close observation is appropriate if the bleeding has stopped and the patient has stabilized. If laparotomy is necessary, salvage of the spleen is attempted to minimize the risk of sepsis.

3. **Adrenal hemorrhage**

   a. The relatively large size of the adrenal gland at birth may contribute to injury. Risk factors are breech presentation and macrosomia. Ninety percent of adrenal hemorrhages are unilateral; 75% occur on the right.

   b. Findings on physical exam depend on the extent of hemorrhage. Classic signs include fever, flank mass, purpura, and pallor. Adrenal insufficiency may present with poor feeding, vomiting, irritability, listlessness, and shock. The diagnosis is made with abdominal ultrasound.

   c. Differential diagnosis includes other abdominal trauma. If a flank mass is palpable, neuroblastoma and Wilms' tumor should be considered.

   d. Treatment includes blood volume replacement. Adrenal insufficiency may require steroid therapy. Extensive bleeding that requires surgical intervention is rare.

E. Soft tissue injuries

1. **Petechiae and ecchymoses** are commonly seen in newborns. The birth history, location of lesions, their early appearance without development of new lesions, and the absence of bleeding from other sites help to differentiate petechiae and ecchymoses secondary to birth trauma from those caused by a vasculitis or coagulation disorder. If the etiology is uncertain, studies to rule out coagulopathies and infection should be performed. Most petechiae and ecchymoses resolve within 1 week. If bruising is excessive, jaundice and anemia may develop. Treatment is supportive.

2. **Lacerations and abrasions** may be secondary to scalp electrodes and fetal scalp blood sampling or injury during birth. Deep wounds (e.g., scalpel injuries during cesarean section) may require sutures. Infection is a risk, particularly with scalp lesions and an underlying caput succedaneum or hematoma. Treatment includes cleansing the wound and close observation.

3. **Subcutaneous fat necrosis** is not usually recognized at birth. It usually presents during the first 2 weeks after birth as sharply demarcated, irregularly shaped, firm, nonpitting subcutaneous plaques or nodules on the extremities, face, trunk, or buttocks. The injury may be colorless, or have a deep-red or purple discoloration. Calcification may occur. No treatment is necessary. Lesions typically resolve completely over several weeks to months.

Suggested Reading

Medlock M.D., Hanigan W.C. Neurologic birth trauma; intracranial, spinal cord, and brachial plexus injury. *Clin Perinatol* 1997;24:845.

21. DECISION-MAKING AND ETHICAL DILEMMAS

Tara K. Bastek

I. **Background.** Neonatal intensive care units (NICUs) necessitate decision-making. Routine decisions about fluids, nutrition, antibiotics, tests, and other specifics of patient care are made with relative ease. For these decisions, systems are in place; expectations are defined and shared by both professionals and families. However, this apparatus is stressed when decisions with ethical implications are required. These include decisions about instituting, withholding, or withdrawing life-supporting therapy, extreme prematurity, severe depression at birth, infants with multiple congenital anomalies, and infants with severe chronic conditions such as ventilator dependency.

   A. Competing **ethical principles** involved in NICU care decisions include beneficence and nonmaleficence, respect for autonomy, and justice. Caregivers and parents must balance choices that are in the infant's best interest (beneficence) against choices that minimize harm to the infant (nonmaleficence). Since they are incapable of making decisions for themselves, infants are owed special protections (respect for autonomy). Last, treatment decisions must be based on the infant's best interests, free from considerations of race, ethnicity, ability to pay, or other influences (justice).

   B. More and more frequently the debate between quality of life and sanctity of life enters into these difficult decisions as smaller or sicker infants are able to be sustained with improving medical technologies. Staff and parents often struggle with identifying the medical and moral choices and with making decisions based on those choices.

II. **Developing a process for ethical decision-making.** It is important for a NICU to define the decision-making process. Generating this process allows discussions among NICU personnel that incorporate ethical knowledge and values at a time and place distant from a specific patient. Ideally, this preparation will ease the stress when an actual decision needs to be made.

   A. **Develop a written set of guidelines** for addressing difficult decisions regarding patient care. Focus on process (who, when, where) as well as on substance (how). Identifying areas of frequent consensus and disagreement within a NICU and outlining a general approach to those situations can provide helpful guidance. The guidelines should be available in the NICU and discussed during the orientation of new personnel.

   B. **Identify common situations** (e.g., extreme prematurity, multiple congenital anomalies, severe asphyxia) and have a series of multidisciplinary discussions about these models. These conversations should include a review of the common underlying ethical principles likely to be in conflict and illuminate common areas of agreement or disagreement. These discussions help develop a consensus on group values, promote a tolerance for individual differences, and establish trust among professionals. The overall goal is to better prepare caregivers when actual situations arise.

   C. **Define and support the role of the parents,** who should be seen as the primary decision-makers unless they have indicated otherwise. The desired decision-making role of the parents should be explored with open and honest discussions with the parents on this matter. The ethical and legal presumption is that they will make decisions that are in the best interests of their child (best interests standard) and within the context of accepted legal and social boundaries. If the health-care providers believe that the parental choice is not in the child's best interest, then they have an obligation as an advocate for the infant to override the parental decision.

   D. **Develop consensus among the primary clinical team** prior to meeting with the parents. Team meetings prior to family meetings provide the opportunity for caregivers to clarify the dilemmas and options and, hopefully, to reach a consensus regarding recommendations. It also allows the team to establish who will communicate with the family to help maintain consistency during the discussion of complicated medical and ethical issues.

E. **Identify available resources.** Determine the roles of social service, chaplain, hospital attorney, and the hospital ethics committee. While a general knowledge of existing hospital policies on common situations such as "do not resuscitate" orders or withdrawal of life support should be included in the multidisciplinary discussions mentioned in the foregoing, the NICU should identify one or two key resource people who are easily accessible. These professionals should be familiar with hospital policies, the ethics codes of the hospital as well as those of national organizations such as the American Academy of Pediatrics or the American Medical Association, and applicable federal and state laws. In our institutions, this key resource person is a member of the hospital ethics committee who is available without pursuing a formal ethics consult.

F. **Base decisions on the most accurate, up-to-date medical information.** Good ethics starts with good facts. Take the time to accumulate the relevant data. Consultation services are likely to provide valuable input. Be wary of setting certainty as a goal, as it is almost never achievable in the NICU. Instead, a reasonable degree of medical certainty is often more achievable. As the weight of a decision's consequences increases, so does the rigor of the requirement for a reasonable degree of certainty and the importance of parental involvement in the decision-making process.

G. **People of good conscience can disagree.** Individual caregivers must feel free to remove themselves from patient care if their ethical sense conflicts with the decision of the primary team and parents. Parents and caregivers must be able to appeal decisions to an individual such as the NICU director or hospital attorney or to a group such as an ethics committee. No system will provide absolute certainty that the "right" decision will always be made. However, a system that is inclusive, systematic, and built on an approach that establishes a procedure for handling these difficult issues is most likely to produce acceptable decisions.

III. **Extremely premature infants.** Almost all NICUs have struggled with decisions about infants at the threshold of viability and the question of "how small is too small." The practice of some NICUs to resuscitate infants between 23 and 24 weeks' gestation presents difficult medical and ethical challenges. Current technology allows some of these extremely premature infants to survive, but with a great risk of substantial handicap. Parents increasingly ask neonatologists to pursue aggressive therapies despite poor prognoses. Neonatologists are concerned that instituting those therapies may not be the most appropriate course of action. The American Academy of Pediatrics statement on perinatal care at the threshold of viability stresses several key areas: (1) parents must receive adequate and current information about potential infant survival and short- and long-term outcomes; (2) physicians are obligated to be aware of the most current national and local survival data; and (3) parental choice should be respected as much as possible with joint decision-making by both the parents and the physicians as the standard. As more experience is gained with these very difficult situations, further debate and discussion are likely to lead to greater consensus in this area.

IV. **The decision to redirect life-sustaining care to comfort measures.** One of the most difficult issues is deciding when to withhold or withdraw life-sustaining therapies. Philosophies and approaches vary among caregivers and NICUs. The model we use emphasizes an objective interdisciplinary approach to determine the best course of action.

A. The goal of the process is to identify the action that is in the **baby's best interest.** The interests of others, including family and caregivers, are of less priority than are the baby's.

B. **Decision-making should be guided by data.** Caregivers should explore every reasonable avenue to maximize collection of data relevant to the ethical question at hand. Information about alternative therapies and prognosis should be sought. The objective data are evaluated in the context of the primary team's meetings. When relevant, subspecialty consultations should be obtained and included in the primary team's deliberations.

C. **Communication** among caregivers and parents is completely open. The primary care team should meet daily with the parents to discuss the baby's progress, current status, plan of care, and to summarize the team's medical and ethical discussions.

D. As the decision to withhold or withdraw life-sustaining medical treatment becomes the focus, the team discusses the data, their implications, and their degree of certainty. The goal should be to build a **consensus** regarding the best plan of care for the baby and/or recommendations for the parents. Sometimes there will be strong scientific support for a particular option. In other instances, the best course of action must be estimated. During this time, it is especially important to actively seek feedback from the parents regarding their thoughts, feelings, and understanding of the clinical situation.

E. **The parents' role as surrogate decision-makers is respected.** Parental views are always considered; they are most likely to influence decisions when it remains unclear which option (e.g., continuing versus discontinuing life-sustaining treatment) is in the child's best interest. Parents are not expected to evaluate clinical data in isolation. Even in instances of medical uncertainty, the primary team objectively assesses what is known as well as what remains uncertain about the baby's condition and/or prognosis. The team should provide the parents with this information as well as their best assessment and recommendation. In the face of substantial medical uncertainty, parental wishes should be supported in deference to those of the primary medical team.

F. There is agreement among ethical and legal scholars that there is no important distinction between **withholding or withdrawing life-sustaining treatments.** Amendments to the Child Abuse and Neglect Prevention and Treatment Act of 1984 established that medically indicated treatment can be withheld or withdrawn under the following conditions: (1) ongoing treatment is prolonging the baby's death, (2) the baby is in an irreversible coma, or (3) the underlying condition is so significant as to render ongoing treatment futile and inhumane. It has been argued that these conditions both protect the rights of children to treatment despite underlying conditions or potential handicaps and support the importance of quality of life determinations in the provision of care. Substantial conflict can arise if the caregivers and parents disagree about the goals of care. A NICU must be prepared for these circumstances.

G. The **hospital ethics committee** is helpful when the primary team is unable to reach consensus or disagrees with the parents' wishes. In our experience, consultation with the ethics committee helps encourage communication among all involved parties and improve collaborative decision-making. They can often ease tensions between parents and caregivers, allowing for a resolution to the dilemma.

Suggested Readings

Committee on the Fetus and Newborn. Perinatal care at the threshold of viability. *Pediatrics* 2002;110:5.

Campbell D.E., Fleischman A.R. Limits of viability: Dilemmas, decisions, and decision makers. *Am J Perinatol* 2001;18:3.

Committee on Bioethics. Ethics and the care of critically ill infants and children. *Pediatrics* 1996;98:1.

Committee on the Fetus and Newborn. The initiation or withdrawal of treatment for high-risk newborns. *Pediatrics* 1995;96:2.

Committee on Bioethics. Guidelines on foregong life-sustaining medical treatment. *Pediatrics* 1994;93:3.

Goldworth A., et al. (Eds.). *Ethics and Perinatology.* New York: Oxford University Press, 1995.

22. MANAGEMENT OF NEONATAL DEATH AND BEREAVEMENT FOLLOW-UP

Caryn Douma

I. **Introduction:** Neonatal death is traumatic for both families and caretakers. The goal of management is to establish and reinforce a memory of the infant to facilitate successful grieving. It is important for families to be cared for by a compassionate, knowledgeable staff that can provide a dignified, pain-free death for their child. Bereavement follow-up provides an important link that guides families toward recovery.

II. **Management of neonatal death**

  A. **Staff.** The primary team caring for an infant and the family usually consists of an attending physician, nurses, and a social worker. The team may also include a neonatology fellow, pediatric resident, respiratory therapist, and pediatric consultants. This multidisciplinary team supports the family and cares for the infant during the hospital course and bereavement period. End-of-life care is always challenging for caretakers. It is helpful to have guidelines that include a plan for discussing the withdrawal of life support, management of the dying infant, follow-up, and support for families and staff. Parents need consistent information presented in a concise, honest manner. It may be difficult for families to build close relationships with the entire team. Depending on individual circumstances, it may be more appropriate to choose one or two representatives to discuss the end-of-life decisions.

  B. **Relationship with the family.** Developing an honest, trusting relationship with families is crucial to the management of neonatal death and bereavement. Staff can facilitate this relationship in the following ways:

    1. Communicate with families through frequent meetings with the primary team.
    2. Encourage sibling visitation and extended family support.
    3. Encourage cultural and spiritual customs.
    4. Provide an environment that allows parents to develop a relationship with their infant, visiting and holding as often as medically indicated.

  C. **Decision-making.** End-of-life decisions are made collaboratively with parents through a series of meetings with the care team. Parents should not feel that they alone are responsible for any decisions made. When the primary team is in agreement that further intervention is not in the best interest of the infant, this information should be presented to the family. When meeting with the family it is important to:

    1. Meet in a quiet, private area and allow ample time for the family to understand the information presented and the recommendations of the team.
    2. Refer to the baby by name.
    3. Ask the parents how they feel and how they perceive the situation.
    4. The decision to redirect care away from supporting life to comfort measures must be accompanied by a discussion describing how intensive care support will be withdrawn. Be specific and involve parents in the plan.

  D. **Withdrawing life support.** Once a decision has been made to withdraw life support, the family should be provided an environment that is quiet, private, and will accommodate everyone the family wishes to include. Staffing should be arranged so that one nurse and one physician will be readily available to the family at all times. The following steps will help ensure that the family will feel supported during this difficult time:

    1. Allow parents ample time to create memories and become a family. Allow them to hold, take pictures, bathe, and dress their infant before, during, or after withdrawing mechanical ventilation or other life support.

2. Discuss the entire process with parents, including endotracheal tube removal and pain control. Gently describe how the infant will look and measures that the staff will take to provide the infant with a comfortable, pain-free death. Let them know that death will not always occur immediately.

3. Arrange for baptism and spiritual support if desired.

4. Anticipate medications that may be required, leaving IV access in place. Discontinue muscle relaxation before extubation. The goal of medication use should be to ensure that the infant is as comfortable as possible.

5. When the infant is extubated, discontinue all unnecessary intravenous catheters and equipment.

6. Allow parents to hold their infant for as long as they desire after withdrawing life support. The nurse and attending physician should be nearby to assist the family and assess heart rate and comfort of the infant.

7. Autopsy should be discussed before or after death at the discretion of the attending physician.

8. Create a memory box including crib cards, photographs, clothing, a lock of hair, footprints, handprints, and any other mementos accumulated during the infant's life. Keep them in a designated place if the family does not desire to see or keep them at the time of death. They often change their mind later.

9. Be sure photographs of the infant have been taken. It is helpful for the NICU to have a camera and the capability of making printed photographs.

III. **Bereavement follow-up.** Each NICU should have a bereavement follow-up program in place that provides continuing support to families as they begin the grieving process, assess their progress, and provide community referrals if necessary.

A. Before the family leaves the hospital they should understand that the staff will continue to support them through phone calls and follow-up meetings. They should understand the normal grieving process and what to expect in the following days and weeks.

B. Assistance in making burial or cremation arrangements should be offered.

C. The family's obstetrician, pediatrician, and other community supports should be notified of the infant's death.

D. A representative from the primary team should assume responsibility for coordinating bereavement follow-up. This person is responsible for arranging and documenting the following:

1. A phone call within the first few days after the infant's death.

2. A sympathy card, signed by members of the primary team sent to the family at home.

3. A follow-up meeting with the family approximately 4 to 6 weeks after the infant's death. Timing will depend on availability of autopsy results and the parents' preference.

4. Referrals to appropriate professionals or agencies including bereavement support groups.

5. Card and phone call at 1-year anniversary.

E. In some cases, the family will not want to return to the hospital or continue contact. The coordinator will be sure this is documented and arrange for the family to be followed through a primary-care provider or other community agency. Follow-up calls can still be made if the family consents.

Meetings with families can be in the hospital or another designated place that will be more comfortable. Meetings include the following:

1. Review of events that led to the infant's death.

2. Review of autopsy results or other studies, if available, including implications for future pregnancies.

3. Assessment of how well the family is coping and progressing through the grieving process.

4. Plan for future meetings if the family desires.

IV. Staff education and support. Caring for infants and families around the time of death is challenging and requires compassion and knowledge of the normal grieving process. Each NICU should create its own guidelines including orientation for all new staff, ongoing continuing education and conferences, designated staff members willing to mentor new staff, and a forum for discussing ethical issues.

Suggested Readings

Abe N., Catlin A., Mihara D. End of life in the NICU: A study of ventilator withdrawal. *MCN, Am J Matern Child Nurs* May/June 2001;26(3):141–146.

Chiswick M. Parents and end of life decisions in neonatal practice. *Arch Dis Child Fetal Neonatal Ed* July 1, 2001;85(1):F1–F3.

McHaffie H.E., Laing I.A., Lloyd D.J. Follow-up care of bereaved parents after treatment withdrawal from newborns. *Arch Dis Child Fetal Neonatal Ed* March 1, 2001;84(2):F125–128.

McHaffie H.E., Lyon A.J., Fowlie P.W. Lingering death after treatment withdrawal in the neonatal intensive care unit. *Arch Dis Child Fetal Neonatal Ed* July 1, 2001;85(1):F4–F7.

23. INFECTIONS

Viral Infections*

Sandra K. Burchett

I. **Introduction.** Vertically transmitted (mother-to-child) viral infections of the fetus and newborn can generally be divided into two major categories. The first is **congenital infections**, which are transmitted to the fetus in utero. The second is **perinatal infections**, which are acquired intrapartum or in the postpartum period. Infections acquired through breastfeeding are in the latter category. Classifying these infections into congenital and perinatal categories highlights aspects of their pathogenesis in the fetus and newborn infant. Generally, when these infections occur in children or adults, they are benign; however, if the host is immunocompromised or if the immune system is not yet developed, such as in the neonate, clinical symptoms may be quite severe or even fatal. Congenital infections can have clinical manifestations that are apparent antenatally by ultrasound or when the infant is born, whereas perinatal infections may not become clinically apparent until after the first few days or weeks of life. Although classically the congenital infections have gone by the acronym TORCH (T = toxoplasmosis, O = other, R = rubella, C = cytomegalovirus, H = herpes simplex virus), this term is now archaic and should be avoided. When congenital or perinatal infections are suspected, the diagnosis of each of the possible infectious agents should be considered separately and the most appropriate and rapid diagnostic test requested. Useless information is often obtained when the diagnosis is attempted by drawing a single serum sample to be sent for measurement of TORCH titers. These antibodies are acquired by passive transmission to the fetus and merely reflect the maternal serostatus. The following discussion is divided by pathogen as to the usual timing of acquisition of infection (congenital or perinatal) and in approximate order of prevalence.

II. **Cytomegalovirus (CMV: congenital and perinatal).** Disease manifestations are most commonly seen in neonates with congenital infection. CMV is a DNA virus; therefore infection is lifelong. It is a member of the herpesvirus family, is found only in humans, and derives its name from the histopathologic appearance of infected cells, which have abundant cytoplasm and both intranuclear and cytoplasmic inclusions. It is present in saliva, urine, genital secretions, breast milk, and blood/blood products of infected persons, and can be transmitted by exposure to any of these sources. Primary infection (when the host has just acquired infection) is usually asymptomatic in older infants, children, and adults, but may manifest with mononucleosislike symptoms, including a prolonged fever and a mild hepatitis. Latent infection is asymptomatic unless the host becomes immunocompromised. CMV infection is very common, with seroprevalence in the United States between 50 and 85% by age 40. Forty percent or more of pregnant women in the United States are infected, with the lowest infection prevalence in young primigravidas. Vertical transmission can occur at any time in gestation or in the perinatal period and is usually asymptomatic, especially if the mother was seropositive before pregnancy. However, there are reports that as many as 17% of all infants with symptomatic CMV are born to women with prior seropositivity.

    A. **Epidemiology.** Congenital CMV occurs in at least 1% of all live births in the United States each year and is the leading infectious cause of sensorineural hearing loss and developmental delay. Of these 40,000 CMV-infected infants, 10% will have symptomatic disease. Additionally, 10% of the asymptomatic infants will have significant sequelae. Therefore, at least 8000 infants are severely affected by or die from CMV infection in the United States each year. Primary (first episode) CMV infection occurs in 1 to 3% of pregnant

---

*This is a revision of Chapter 12 by Dr. Nicholas G. Guerina in the 3rd edition of the *Manual of Neonatal Care*.

women. It is estimated that 30 to 40% of fetuses of women with primary infection will become infected with CMV, and approximately 15% of these fetuses will develop significant disease. The risk of transmission to the fetus as a function of gestational age is uncertain, but infection during early gestation likely carries a higher risk of severe fetal disease.

B. Clinical manifestations. Symptomatic CMV infection of the fetus has two presentations.

1. **Early manifestations** can include a pattern consistent with an acute fulminant infection involving multiple organ systems and carries a high risk of mortality (as much as 30%). Findings with this presentation include petechiae or purpura (79%), hepatosplenomegaly (74%), jaundice (63%), and "blueberry muffin spots" consistent with extramedullary hematopoiesis. **Laboratory abnormalities** include elevated hepatic transaminase and bilirubin levels (as much as half is direct or conjugated), anemia, and thrombocytopenia. Hyperbilirubinemia may be present at birth or develop over time. It usually persists beyond the period of physiologic jaundice. About a third of these infants are preterm, and a third have intrauterine growth restriction (IUGR).

2. A second early presentation includes those infants who are symptomatic but without life-threatening complications. These babies may have intrauterine growth restriction or disproportionate microcephaly (48%) with or without intracranial calcifications. The calcifications may occur anywhere in the brain, but are classically found in the periventricular area. Other central nervous system (CNS) manifestations can include chorioretinitis in approximately 10 to 15% of infants. Babies with CNS abnormalities almost always have developmental abnormalities and neurologic dysfunction, ranging from IQ scores below 50, motor abnormalities, deafness, and visual problems to mild learning and language disability or mild hearing loss. Because sensorineural hearing loss is the most common sequela of CMV infection (60% in symptomatic and 5% in asymptomatic infants), any infant failing the newborn hearing screen should be quickly assessed for CMV infection. Infants with CMV infection should have hearing tested as neonates and young infants.

In contrast to symptomatic newborn infants, those with **asymptomatic infection** have no mortality, but 5 to 15% may have developmental abnormalities. These include hearing loss, mental retardation, motor spasticity, and microcephaly. Other problems that can be detected later in life include dental defects characterized by abnormal enamel production.

III. Perinatal infection. Perinatally acquired CMV infection may occur (1) from intrapartum exposure to the virus with in the maternal genital tract, (2) from postnatal exposure to infected breast milk, (3) from exposure to infected blood or blood products, or (4) nosocomially through urine or saliva. The incubation period varies from 4 to 12 weeks. Almost all term infants who acquire infection perinatally from infected mothers remain asymptomatic. Many of these infections arise from mothers with reactivated viral excretion. In these cases, long-term developmental and neurologic abnormalities are infrequently seen. However, symptomatic perinatally acquired infections may occur at a higher frequency in preterm infants. Hearing abnormalities may also be detected in infants with perinatal CMV infection; therefore, hearing should be assessed in infants documented to have acquired CMV.

IV. CMV pneumonitis. CMV has been associated with pneumonitis occurring in infants less than 4 months old. Symptoms and radiographic findings in CMV pneumonitis are similar to those seen in afebrile pneumonia of other causes in neonates and young infants, including *Chlamydia trachomatis, Ureaplasma urealyticum,* and respiratory syncytial virus. Symptoms include tachypnea, cough, coryza, and nasal congestion. Intercostal retractions and hypoxemia may be present, and apnea may occur. Radiographically, there is hyperinflation, diffuse increased pulmonary markings, thickened bronchial walls, and focal atelectasis. A small number of infants may have symptoms that are severe enough to require mechanical ventilation, and approximately 3% of infants die. Laboratory findings in CMV pneumonitis are nonspecific. Long-term sequelae include recurrent pulmonary problems, including wheezing, and, in some cases, repeated hospitalizations for respiratory distress. Whether this reflects congenital or perinatal CMV infection is unclear, but it does pose a risk, especially to the preterm infants. Conversely, merely finding CMV present in respiratory secretions of a preterm infant does not prove causality of symptomatology because CMV is present in saliva.

V. **Transfusion-acquired CMV infection.** In the past, significant morbidity and mortality could occur in newborn infants receiving CMV-infected blood or blood products. Those most severely affected were preterm, low-birth-weight infants born to CMV-seronegative women. Symptoms typically developed 4 to 12 weeks after transfusion, lasted for 2 to 3 weeks, and consisted of respiratory distress, pallor, and hepatosplenomegaly. Hematologic abnormalities were also seen, including hemolysis, thrombocytopenia, and atypical lymphocytosis. Mortality was estimated to be 20% in very-low-birth-weight infants. This is now rare, prevented by using blood/blood products from CMV seronegative donors or filtered, leuko-reduced products (see Chap. 26, Blood Products Used in the Newborn).

VI. **Diagnosis.** Congenital CMV infection should be suspected in any infant having typical symptoms of infection or if there is a maternal history of seroconversion or a mononucleosislike illness in pregnancy. The diagnosis is made if CMV is identified in urine, saliva, blood, or respiratory secretions and defines as *congenital* infection if found within the first 2 weeks of life and as *perinatal* infection if after 4 weeks of life. There are three rapid diagnostic techniques:

A. **Spin-enhanced culture or "shell vial."** Virus can be isolated from urine or saliva, but CMV is concentrated in high titers in urine. For this technique, urine (in which CMV is concentrated in high titer) should be maintained at 4°C (ice or refrigerator) for transport and storage. The urine is then placed in viral tissue culture medium containing a coverslip on which tissue culture cells have been grown. If CMV is present, it infects the cells, which 24 to 72 hours later are lysed and stained with antibody to CMV antigens. Virus can be detected with high sensitivity and specificity within 24 to 72 hours of inoculation. It is much more rapid than the standard tissue culture, which may take from 2 to 6 weeks for replication and identification.

B. **CMV antigen.** Peripheral blood can be centrifuged and the buffy coat spread on a slide. The neutrophils are then lysed and stained with an antibody to CMV pp65 antigen. Positive results confirm CMV infection and viremia; however, negative results do not rule out CMV infection. This test is usually used to follow efficacy of therapy.

C. **CMV PCR.** Commercial laboratories are beginning to offer polymerase chain reaction (PCR) to detect CMV in blood. The sensitivity of using this test as a diagnostic modality is unknown in neonatal CMV disease. The determination of serum antibody titers to CMV has limited usefulness for the neonate, although negative immunoglobulin G (IgG) titers in both maternal and infant sera are sufficient to exclude congenital CMV infection. The interpretation of a positive IgG titer in the newborn is complicated by the presence of transplacentally derived maternal IgG. Uninfected infants usually show a decline in IgG within 1 month and have no detectable titer by 4 to 9 months. Infected infants continue to produce IgG throughout the same time period. Tests for CMV-specific IgM have limitations but can help to elucidate infant infection.

If the diagnosis of congenital CMV infection is made, the infant should have a thorough physical and neurological exam, a computed tomography (CT) scan of the brain, an ophthalmologic exam, and a hearing test. Laboratory tests include a complete blood count, liver function tests, and cerebrospinal fluid (CSF) exam [if the CSF PCR is positive for CMV, the infant should be classified as having central nervous system (CNS) disease]. There are data from 56 CMV-infected infants with symptomatic disease that suggest that 90% of CMV-infected infants with an abnormal CT scan will have CNS sequelae; however, 29% of infants with a normal CT scan will also have sequelae.

VII. Treatment. Ganciclovir (9-[(13-dihydroxy-2-propoxy)methyl]guanine) and more recently valganciclovir have been effective in the treatment of and prophylaxis against dissemination of CMV in adult immunocompromised patients. In the earliest studies of ganciclovir treatment of infants with symptomatic CMV disease, the majority had thrombocytopenia and neutropenia during the course of therapy. Longer-term questions remain as to future reproductive system effects because ganciclovir has been found to cause testicular atrophy in animal studies. However, broader study of this agent is warranted for congenital CMV because in symptomatic disease, the majority of infants have poor neurodevelopmental outcome; early ganciclovir studies showed a trend toward efficacy as assessed by stabilization or improvement of sensorineural hearing loss. Additionally, although there have been no controlled trials, hyperimmune CMV immunoglobulin might conceivably benefit infants with congenital CMV, especially those with a fulminant presentation.

VIII. Prevention

  A. Screening. Because only 1 to 3% of women acquire acute primary CMV infection during pregnancy, with fetal infection in approximately 40% and with severe disease in 15% of the infected infants, the overall risk of symptomatic fetal infection is low (0.2%), and many do not recommend screening for women at risk of seroconversion. Isolation of virus from the cervix or urine of pregnant women cannot be used to predict fetal infection. In cases of documented primary maternal infection or seroconversion, some obstetric practices offer antenatal testing of amniotic fluid or fetal blood to determine whether the fetus acquired infection. However, counseling about a positive finding of fetal infection is difficult because 85% of infected fetuses will not have serious disease. Some investigators suggest that higher CMV viral loads from the amniotic fluid correlate with abnormal neurodevelopmental outcome, but this is not proven. Presently, there is not enough information about fetal transmission and outcome to provide guidelines for obstetric management. At this time, no recommendations for therapeutic abortion can be made, even if primary maternal CMV infection is documented. The Centers for Disease Control and Prevention recommends that (1) pregnant women practice hand-washing with soap and water after contact with diapers or oral secretions; (2) pregnant women who develop a mononucleosislike illness during pregnancy should be evaluated for CMV infection and counseled about risks to the unborn child; (3) antibody testing can confirm prior CMV infection; (4) recovery of CMV from the cervix or urine of women near delivery does not warrant a cesarean section; (5) the benefits of breastfeeding outweigh the minimal risk of acquiring CMV; (6) there is no need to screen for CMV or exclude CMV-excreting children from schools or institutions.

  B. Immunization. Passive immunization with hyperimmune anti-CMV immunoglobulin and active immunization with a live attenuated CMV vaccine represent attractive therapies for prophylaxis against congenital CMV infections. However, data from clinical trials are lacking. Immune globulin might be considered as prophylaxis of susceptible women against primary CMV infection in pregnancy. Two live attenuated CMV vaccines have been developed, but their efficacy has not been clearly established. The possibility of reactivation of vaccine-strain CMV in pregnancy with subsequent infection of the fetus must be considered carefully before adequate field trials can be completed in women of childbearing age.

  C. Breast milk restriction. Although breast milk is a common source for perinatal CMV infection in the newborn, symptomatic infection is rare, especially in term infants. In this setting, protection against disseminated disease may be provided by transplacentally derived maternal IgG or antibody in breast milk. However, there may be insufficient transplacental IgG to provide adequate protection in preterm infants. Although additional studies are needed, perhaps mothers of preterm infants should be screened for CMV seropositivity, and if positive, consideration should be given to alternatives or to pasteurizing or freezing breast milk at $-20°C$, which will reduce the titer of CMV although it will not eliminate active virus. At present there is no recommended method of minimizing the risk of exposure to CMV in infected breast milk.

D. Environmental restrictions. Day-care centers and hospitals are potential high-risk environments for acquiring CMV infection. Not surprisingly, a number of studies confirmed an increased risk for infection in day-care workers. However, there does not appear to be an increased risk for infection in hospital personnel. These studies demonstrated that good hand-washing and infection-control measures practiced in hospital settings may be sufficient to control the spread of CMV to workers. Unfortunately, such control may be difficult to achieve in day-care centers. Good hand-washing technique should be suggested to pregnant women with children in day care, especially if they are known to be seronegative. The determination of the CMV susceptibility of these women by serology may be useful for counseling.

E. Transfusion product restrictions. The risk of transfusion-acquired CMV infection in the neonate has been almost eliminated by the use of CMV antibody-negative donors, by freezing packed red blood cells (PRBCs) in glycerol, or by removing the white blood cells. It is particularly important to use blood from one of these sources in preterm, low-birth-weight infants (see Chap. 26, Blood Products Used in the Newborn).

IX. Herpes simplex virus (HSV: perinatal). HSV is a DNA virus with very common seroprevalence. There are two virologically distinct types of HSV: types 1 and 2. HSV-2 is the predominant cause of neonatal disease (75–80%), but both types produce clinically indistinguishable syndromes. At least 80% of the U.S. population is infected with HSV type 1, the cause of recurrent orolabial disease, and 40% are infected with HSV-2, the predominant cause of recurrent genital disease by older age. Infection in the newborn occurs as a result of direct exposure, most commonly in the perinatal period from maternal genital disease. The virus can cause localized disease of the skin, eye, or mouth, or may disseminate by cell-to-cell contiguous spread or viremia. After adsorption and penetration into host cells, viral replication proceeds, resulting in cellular swelling, hemorrhagic necrosis, formation of intranuclear inclusions, cytolysis, and cell death.

A. Epidemiology. Because HSV-2 is more likely to recur in the genital tract and therefore accounts for the majority of neonatal HSV infections, it is important to understand the potential for neonatal exposure to virus. The seroprevalence of HSV-2 varies according to locale in the United States, but is likely to be at least 30%. In a study of 779 women attending a sexually transmitted disease clinic, 47% had serologic evidence of HSV-2 infection, but only 22% had symptoms. The characteristic ulcerations of the genitalia were present only in two-thirds of the genital tracts from which HSV could be isolated, and the others had asymptomatic shedding or atypical lesions. It is estimated that 0.01 to 0.39% of all women shed virus at delivery, and approximately 1% of all women with a history of recurrent HSV infection asymptomatically shed HSV at delivery. However, when the birth canal is carefully visualized and those with asymptomatic lesions excluded, this rate of shedding may be nearer 0.5%. **It is critical to recognize that the majority of mothers of infants with neonatal HSV do not have a history of HSV.** Infants at greatest risk of acquisition of infection are those born to mothers with newly acquired HSV during pregnancy (primary infection), in whom the rate of transmission of HSV is estimated to be 50%. Additionally, one-third of infants born to mothers with newly acquired HSV-2, although already infected with HSV-1 (nonprimary, first episode), may acquire HSV infection. Infants born to HSV-2–seropositive mothers (recurrent) have an approximate 3% risk of acquiring infection. This may well be due to protective maternal type-specific antibodies in the infant's serum or the birth canal. The overall incidence of newborn infection with HSV is estimated to be 1:2000 to 1:20,000 per year, or 200 to 2000 infants.

B. Intrapartum transmission. This is the most common cause of neonatal HSV and is primarily associated with active shedding of virus from the cervix or vulva at the time of delivery. As many as 95% of newborn infections occur as a result of intrapartum transmission. Several factors have been identified that relate to intrapartum transmission. The amount and duration of maternal virus shedding is likely to be a major determinate of fetal transmission. These are greatest with primary maternal infections. Maternal antibody to HSV is also important and is associated with a decreased risk of fetal transmission. In fact, when maternal antibody is present, the risk of acquisition of HSV, even for the newborn exposed to HSV in the birth canal, is very low. The exact mechanism of action of maternal antibody in preventing perinatal infection is not known, but transplacentally acquired antibody has been shown to reduce the risk of severe newborn disease following postnatal HSV exposure. The risk of intrapartum infection increases with ruptured membranes, especially when ruptured longer than 4 hours. Finally, direct methods for fetal monitoring, such as with scalp electrodes, increase the risk of fetal transmission in the setting of active shedding. It is best to avoid these techniques in women with a history of recurrent infection or suspected primary HSV disease.

C. Antenatal transmission. In utero infection has been documented but is uncommon. Spontaneous abortion has occurred with primary maternal infection before 20 weeks' gestation, but the true risk to the fetus of early-trimester primary infection is not known. Fetal infections may occur by either transplacental or ascending routes and have been documented in the setting of both primary and recurrent maternal disease. There may be a wide range of clinical manifestations, from localized skin or eye involvement to multiorgan disease and congenital malformations. Chorioretinitis, microcephaly, and hydranencephaly may be found in a small number of patients.

D. Postnatal transmission. There is evidence that a percentage of neonatal HSV infections result from postnatal exposure. Potential sources include symptomatic and asymptomatic oropharyngeal shedding by either parent, hospital personnel, or other contacts; maternal breast lesions; and nosocomial spread. Measures to minimize exposure from these sources are discussed below.

E. Clinical manifestations. Data from the National Institute of Allergy and Infectious Diseases (NIAID) Collaborative Antiviral Study Group indicate that morbidity and mortality of neonatal HSV best correlates with three categories of disease. These are infection localized to the skin, eye, and/or mouth; encephalitis with or without localized mucocutaneous disease; and disseminated infection with multiple organ involvement. The NIAID Collaborative Antiviral Study Group reported on the outcome of 210 infants with HSV infection who were randomized to receive either acyclovir or vidarabine antiviral therapy. Eight babies had congenital infection with signs (chorioretinitis, skin lesions, hydrocephalus) at birth. The highest mortality (> 50%) was seen in infants having disseminated disease; hemorrhagic shock and pneumonitis were the principal causes of death. Of the survivors for whom follow-up was available, significant neurologic sequelae were seen in a high percentage of the infants with encephalitis and disseminated disease.

1. Skin, eye, and mouth infection. Approximately 50% of infants with HSV have disease localized to the skin, eye, or mucocutaneous membranes. Vesicles typically appear on the sixth to ninth day of neonatal life. A cluster of vesicles often develops on the presenting part of the body, where extended direct contact with virus may occur. Vesicles occur in 90% of infants with localized mucocutaneous infection, and recurrent disease is common. Furthermore, significant morbidity can occur in these infants despite the absence of signs of disseminated disease at the time of diagnosis; up to 10% of infants later show neurologic impairment, and infants with keratoconjunctivitis can develop chorioretinitis, cataracts, and retinopathy. Ophthalmologic and neurologic follow-up is important in all

infants with mucocutaneous HSV. Infants with three or more recurrences of vesicles have an increased risk of neurologic complications.
2. **CNS infection.** Approximately one-third of neonates with HSV present with encephalitis in the absence of disseminated disease, and from 40 to 60% of these infants do not have mucocutaneous vesicles. These infants usually become symptomatic at 10 to 14 days of life with lethargy, seizures, temperature instability, and hypotonia. In the setting of disseminated disease, HSV is thought to invade the CNS from hematogenous spread. However, CNS infection in the absence of disseminated disease probably results from retrograde axonal spread. The latter condition most often occurs in infants having transplacentally derived viral-neutralizing antibodies, which may protect against widespread dissemination but not influence intraneuronal viral replication. Mortality is high without treatment and is approximately 15% with treatment, and approximately two-thirds of surviving infants have impaired neurodevelopment. Long-term sequelae from acute HSV encephalitis include microcephaly, hydranencephaly, porencephalic cysts, spasticity, blindness, chorioretinitis, and learning disabilities.
3. **Disseminated infection.** This is the most severe form of neonatal HSV infection. It accounts for approximately 22% of all infants with neonatal HSV infection and ends in mortality for 57% of the infants with this presentation. Pneumonitis is associated with greatest mortality. Symptoms usually begin within the first week of neonatal life. The liver, adrenals, and multiple other visceral organs are usually involved. Approximately two-thirds of infants also have encephalitis. Clinical findings include seizures, shock, respiratory distress, disseminated intravascular coagulation (DIC), and pneumonitis. A typical vesicular rash may be absent in as many as 20% of infants. Forty percent of the infants who survive have morbidity.
F. **Diagnosis.** HSV infection should be considered in the differential diagnosis of ill neonates with a variety of clinical presentations. These include CNS abnormalities, fever, shock, DIC, and/or hepatitis. HSV also should be considered in infants with respiratory distress without an obvious bacterial cause or a clinical course and findings consistent with surfactant deficiency. The possibility of concomitant HSV infection with other commonly encountered problems of the preterm infant should be considered. Viral isolation or fluorescent antibody detection in the appropriate clinical setting remains critical to the diagnosis. Serology is of little value, because specific IgM may not be detected for up to 3 weeks. However, the number of different viral antigen-specific antibodies produced seems to correlate with the extent of disseminated disease, and the presence of certain antigen-specific antibodies may have long-term prognostic value. For the infant with mucocutaneous lesions, tissue should be scraped from vesicles, placed in the appropriate viral transport medium, and promptly processed for culture by a diagnostic virology laboratory. Alternatively, virus can be detected directly when tissue samples are swabbed onto a glass slide and evaluated by direct fluorescent antibody technique. Virus also can be isolated from the oropharynx and nasopharynx, conjunctivae, stool, and urine. In the absence of a vesicular rash, viral isolation from these sites may aid in the diagnosis of disseminated HSV or HSV encephalitis. With encephalitis, an elevated CSF protein level and pleocytosis are often seen, but initial values may be within normal limits. Thus serial CSF examinations may be very important. Electroencephalography and CT/magnetic resonance imaging are also useful in the diagnosis of HSV encephalitis. Viral isolation from CSF is reported to be successful in as many as 40% of cases, and rates of detection in CSF by PCR may reach close to 100%. Laboratory abnormalities seen with disseminated disease include elevated hepatic transaminase levels, direct hyperbilirubinemia, neutropenia, thrombocytopenia, and coagulopathy. A diffuse inter-

stitial pattern is usually observed on X ray films of infants with HSV pneumonitis.

G. **Treatment.** Effective antiviral therapy exists for HSV, but the timing of therapy is critical. Treatment is indicated for all forms of HSV disease. Previously, extensive studies were carried out with vidarabine, which reduced the morbidity and mortality for all forms of neonatal HSV. Unfortunately, with disseminated disease, very high mortality occurred despite therapy. In a collaborative study examining the efficacy of vidarabine in the treatment of neonatal HSV, therapy reduced the mortality from disseminated disease from 90 to 70%. The mortality with encephalitis was reduced from 50 to 15%. Recently the NIAID Collaborative Antiviral Study Group found that acyclovir may be as efficacious as vidarabine for the treatment of neonatal HSV. Furthermore, acyclovir is a selective inhibitor of viral replication with minimal side effects on the host. It can be administered in relatively small volumes over short infusion times. Thus acyclovir has become favored in the treatment of neonatal HSV. Doses of 45 or 60 mg/kg per day are being compared with the standard dose of 30 mg/kg per day. Early studies suggested tolerance and greater efficacy. At present, infants with skin, eye, and mouth disease should receive 10 to 15 mg acyclovir per kg every 8 hours for 10 to 14 days. Infants with CNS or disseminated disease should receive 10 to 15 mg acyclovir per kg every 8 hours for 21 days.

H. **Prevention.** Several trials have shown efficacy and safety of treating pregnant women with clinically symptomatic primary HSV infection with a 10-day course of acyclovir. Additionally, there is a suggestion that if a woman asymptomatically seroconverts during pregnancy that a course of acyclovir therapy beginning at 38 weeks' gestation might be helpful in prevention of active lesions at the time of delivery.

I. **Management of the newborn at risk for HSV** (Table 23.1). The principal problem in developing strategies for the prevention of HSV transmission is

TABLE 23.1. MANAGEMENT OF THE CHILD BORN TO A WOMAN WITH ACTIVE GENITAL HSV INFECTION

Maternal primary or first-episode infection:

- Consider offering an elective cesarean section, regardless of lesion status at delivery, or if membranes ruptured > 4 hours
- Swab infant's conjunctivae and nasopharynx, and possibly collect urine for direct fluorescent antibody (DFA) and culture to determine exposure to HSV
- Treat with acyclovir if DFA or culture positive or signs of neonatal HSV

If cesarean section performed after 24 hours of ruptured membranes or if vaginal delivery unavoidable:

- Swab infant's conjunctivae and nasopharynx, and collect urine for direct fluorescent antibody and culture to determine exposure to HSV
- Consider initiation of acyclovir while pending culture and DFA results or if signs of neonatal HSV

Recurrent infection, active at delivery:

- Cesarean section after 4 hours of ruptured membranes or unavoidable vaginal delivery
- Swab infant's conjunctivae and nasopharynx, and possibly collect urine for direct fluorescent antibody and culture to determine exposure to HSV
- Treat with acyclovir if culture positive or signs of HSV infection

DFA = direct fluorescent antibody; HSV = herpes simplex virus.

the inability to identify maternal shedding of virus at the time of delivery. Viral identification requires isolation in tissue culture, so any attempt to identify women who may be shedding HSV at delivery would require antenatal cervical cultures. Unfortunately, such screening cultures taken before labor fail to predict active excretion at delivery.

Until more rapid techniques are made available for the identification of HSV, the only clear recommendation that can be made is to deliver infants by cesarean section if genital lesions are present at the start of labor. The efficacy of this approach may diminish when membranes are ruptured beyond 4 hours. Nevertheless, it is generally recommended that cesarean section be considered even with membrane rupture of longer durations, although data showing efficacy beyond 4 hours are lacking. The upper time limit for membrane rupture has been suggested to be 12 hours to 24 hours. For women with a history of prior genital herpes, careful examination should be performed to determine whether lesions are present when labor commences. If lesions are observed, cesarean section should be carried out. If no lesions are identified, vaginal delivery is appropriate, but a cervical swab should be obtained for culture. At this time there are no data to support the prophylactic use of antiviral agents or immunoglobulin to prevent transmission to the newborn infant.

Infants inadvertently delivered vaginally in the setting of cervical lesions should be isolated from other infants in the nursery, and cultures should be obtained from the oropharynx/nasopharynx and conjunctivae. If the mother can be identified as having recurrent infection, the resultant neonatal infection rate is low, and parents should be instructed to consult their pediatrician when a rash or other clinical changes (lethargy, tachypnea, poor feeding) develop. Weekly pediatric follow-up during the first month is recommended. Infants with a positive culture from any site or the evolution of clinical symptomatology should immediately have cultures repeated and antiviral therapy started.

Before starting acyclovir therapy, the infant should have conjunctival, nasopharyngeal swabs for direct fluorescent antibody (DFA) and culture, urine for culture, and a CSF evaluation for pleocytosis and HSV DNA PCR. These infants should be evaluated for possible disseminated HSV, as well by liver function tests and possibly a chest radiograph.

J. Prevention. Infants and mothers with HSV lesions should be in contact isolation. Careful hand-washing and preventing the infant from having direct contact with lesions should be emphasized. Breastfeeding should be avoided if there are breast lesions, and women with oral HSV should wear a mask while breastfeeding. Hospital personnel with orolabial HSV infection represent a low risk to the newborn, although the use of face masks should be recommended if active lesions are present. Of course, hand-washing or use of gloves should again be emphasized. The exception to these guidelines is nursery personnel with herpetic whitlows. Because they have a high risk of viral shedding, and because transmission can occur despite the use of gloves, these individuals should not care for newborns.

X. Parvovirus (congenital). Parvoviruses are small, unenveloped single-stranded DNA viruses that range in size from 18 to 26 mm. Humans are the only known host.

A. Epidemiology. Parvovirus transmission results after contact with respiratory secretions, blood/blood products, or by vertical transmission. Cases can occur sporadically or in outbreak settings (especially in schools in late winter and early spring). Secondary spread occurs to at least half of susceptible household contacts. Infection is very common, such that 90% of elderly persons are seropositive. The prevalence of infection increases throughout childhood, such that about half of women of childbearing age are immune and half are susceptible to primary infection. The annual seroconversion rate in these women is 1.5%; however, because assessment of parvovirus infection status is not part of routine prenatal testing and because clinical infection is often asymptomatic, the rate of fetal infection in women who seroconvert during pregnancy is unknown. Women who are parents of young children, elementary school teachers, or childcare workers may be at greatest risk for exposure. Unfortunately, the time of greatest transmissibility is before the onset of symptoms or rash. Additionally, 50% of contagious contacts may not have a rash, and 20% may be asymptomatic. The incubation period is usually 4 to 14 days but can be as long as 21 days. Rash and joint symptoms occur 2 to 3 weeks after infection. The virus is probably spread by means of respiratory secretions, which clear in patients with typical erythema infectiosum at or shortly after the onset of rash. The overall rate of vertical transmission of parvovirus from the mother with primary infection to the fetus is approximately one-third. The overall risk of fetal loss is greatest when maternal infection occurs in the first half of pregnancy and is approximately 3 to 6%. Fetal death usually occurs within 6 weeks of maternal infection. The risk of fetal hydrops is approximately 1%. Therefore, parvovirus B19 could be causal of as many as 1400 cases of fetal death or hydrops fetalis each year in the United States.

B. Pathogenesis. The cellular receptor for parvovirus B19 is the P blood group antigen, which is found on erythrocytes, erythroblasts, megakaryocytes, endothelial cells, placenta, and fetal liver and heart cells. This tissue specificity correlates with sites of clinical abnormalities (which are usually anemia with or without thrombocytopenia and sometimes fetal myocarditis). Lack of the P antigen is extremely rare, but these persons are resistant to infection with parvovirus.

C. Clinical manifestations

1. **Disease in children.** Parvovirus B19 has been associated with a variety of rashes, including the typical "slapped cheek" rash of erythema infectiosum (fifth disease). In approximately 60% of school-age children with erythema infectiosum, fever occurs 1 to 4 days before the facial rash appears. Associated symptoms include myalgias, upper respiratory or gastrointestinal symptoms, and malaise, but these symptoms generally resolve with the appearance of the rash. The rash is usually macular, progresses to the extremities and trunk, and may involve the palms and soles. The rash may be pruritic and may recur. These children are likely most infectious before the onset of fever or rash. In group settings such as classrooms, the appearance of one clinically symptomatic child could reinforce the need for good hand-washing practices among potentially seronegative pregnant women.

2. **Disease in adults.** The typical school-age presentation of erythema infectiosum can occur in adults, but arthralgias and arthritis are more common. As many as 60% of adults with parvovirus B19 infection may have acute joint swelling, most commonly involving peripheral joints (symmetrically). Rash and joint symptoms occur 2 to 3 weeks after infection. Arthritis may persist for years and may be associated with the development of rheumatoid arthritis.

3. **Less common manifestations of parvovirus B19 infection**
   a. **Infection in patients with severe anemia or immunosuppression.** Parvovirus B19 has been clearly identified as a cause of persistent and profound anemia in patients with rapid red blood cell turnover such as in those with sickle-cell disease, hemoglobin SC disease, thalassemia, hereditary spherocytosis, and cellular enzyme deficits, such as pyruvate kinase deficiency. Parvovirus B19 also has been associated with acute and chronic red blood cell aplasia in immunosuppressed patients.
   b. **Fetal infection.** Although parvovirus B19 has genotypic variation, no antigenic variation between isolates has been demonstrated. Parvoviruses tend to infect rapidly dividing cells and can be transmitted across the placenta, posing a potential threat to the fetus. Based pri-

marily on the demonstration of viral DNA in fetal tissue samples, parvovirus B19 has been implicated in approximately 10% of cases of fetal nonimmune hydrops. The presumed pathogenic sequence is as follows:

Maternal primary infection → Transplacental transfer of B19 virus → Infection of red blood cell precursors → Arrested red blood cell production → Severe anemia (Hb < 8 g/dL) → Congestive heart failure → Edema

Furthermore, B19 DNA has been detected in cardiac tissues from aborted fetuses. It has been suggested that B19 may cause fetal myocarditis and that this may contribute to the development of hydrops. Finally, fetal hepatitis with severe liver disease has been documented. Although there have been rare case reports of infants with fetal anomalies and parvovirus infection, it is unlikely that parvovirus causes fetal anomalies; hence, therapeutic abortion should not be recommended, but rather the pregnancy should be followed carefully by frequent exam and ultrasound.

D. **Diagnosis.** Parvovirus B19 will not grow in standard tissue cultures because humans are the only host. Determination of serum IgG and IgM levels is the most practical test. Serum B19 IgG is absent in susceptible hosts, and IgM appears by day 3 of an acute infection. Serum IgM may be detected in as many as 90% of patients with acute B19 infection, and serum levels begin to fall by the second to third month after infection. Serum IgG appears a few days after IgM and may persist for years. Serum or plasma can also be assessed for viral DNA by PCR and defines recent infection. Viral antigens may be directly detected in tissues by radioimmunoassay, ELISA, immunofluorescence, *in situ* nucleic acid hybridization, or PCR. These techniques may be valuable for certain clinical settings, such as the examination of tissues from fetuses with nonimmune hydrops or determination of infection (PCR).

E. **Treatment.** Treatment is generally supportive. Intravenous immunoglobulin (IVIG) has been used with reported success in a limited number of patients with severe hematologic disorders related to persistent parvovirus infection. The rationale for this therapy stems from the observations that (1) the primary immune response to B19 infection is the production of specific IgM and IgG, (2) the appearance of systemic antibody coincides with the resolution of clinical symptoms, and (3) specific antibody prevents infection. However, no controlled studies have been undertaken to establish the efficacy of IVIG prophylaxis or therapy for B19 infections. There are no recommendations for use of IVIG in pregnancy.

In the carefully followed pregnancy in which hydrops fetalis is worsening, intrauterine blood transfusions may be considered, especially if the fetal hemoglobin is less than 8g/dL. The risk/benefit of this procedure to the mother and fetus will need to be assessed because some hydrops will improve without intervention, there is some tangible percentage of fetal demise associated with the procedure, and in some cases, if there is also fetal myocardopathy secondary to parvovirus infection, the cardiac function may be inadequate to handle transfusion. Attempts to identify other causes of fetal hydrops are obviously important. The possible contribution of cardiac dysfunction that may not respond to blood transfusions also should be considered.

F. **Prevention.** Three groups of pregnant women of interest when considering the potential risk of fetal parvovirus disease are those exposed to an infected household contact, schoolteachers, and health-care providers. In each, the measurement of serum IgG and IgM levels may be useful to determine who is at risk or acutely infected after B19 exposure. The risk of fetal B19 disease is apparently very small for asymptomatic pregnant women in communities where outbreaks of erythema infectiosum occur. In this setting, no special diagnostic tests or precautions may be indicated. However, household contacts with erythema infectiosum place pregnant women at increased risk for acute B19 infection. The estimated risk of B19 infection in a susceptible adult with a household contact is approximately 50%. Considering an estimated risk of 5% for severe fetal disease with acute maternal B19 infection, the risk of hydrops fetalis is approximately 2.5% for susceptible pregnant women exposed to an infected household contact during the first 18 weeks of gestation. Management of these women may include the following:

1. **Determination of susceptibility of acute infection** by serum IgG and IgM and PCR.
2. For susceptible or acutely infected women, **serial fetal ultrasound** to monitor fetal growth and the possible evolution of hydrops.
3. Serial determinations of **maternal serum alpha-fetoprotein (AFP)** (AFP may rise up to 4 weeks before ultrasound evidence of fetal hydrops), although this use is questioned.
4. Determination of **fetal IgM or DNA PCR** by percutaneous umbilical blood sampling (PUBS). The utility of this is questionable given the relatively high-risk–benefit ratio at present, especially because it is unclear that obstetric management will be altered by results. It may be useful to confirm B19 etiology when hydrops fetalis is present.

The epidemiology of community outbreaks of erythema infectiosum suggests that the risk of infection to susceptible schoolteachers is approximately 19% (compared with 50% for household contacts). This would lower the risk of B19 fetal disease in pregnant schoolteachers to less than 1%. It is not obvious that special precautions are necessary in this setting. In fact, there is likely to be widespread inapparent infection in both adults and children, providing a constant background exposure rate that cannot be altered. Considering the high prevalence of B19, the low risk of severe fetal disease, and the fact that attempts to avoid potential high-risk settings only reduce but do not eliminate exposure, exclusion of pregnant schoolteachers from the workplace is not recommended.

A similar approach may be taken for pregnant health-care providers where the principal exposure will be from infected children presenting to the emergency room or physician's office. However, in many cases, the typical rash of erythema infectiosum may already be present, at which time infectivity is low. Furthermore, precautions directed at minimizing exposure to respiratory secretions may be taken to decrease the risk of transmission. Particular care should be exercised on pediatric wards where there are immunocompromised patients or patients with hemolytic anemias in whom B19 disease is suspected. These patients may shed virus well beyond the period of initial clinical symptoms, particularly when presenting with aplastic crisis. In this setting, there may be a significant risk for the spread of B19 to susceptible health-care workers or other patients at risk for B19-induced aplastic crisis. To minimize this risk, patients with aplastic crises from B19 infections should be maintained on contact precautions, masks should be worn for close contact, and pregnant health-care providers should not care for these patients.

XI. **Human immunodeficiency virus (HIV: congenital and perinatal).** HIV is a cytopathic RNA retrovirus. HIV-1 is the principal cause of HIV infection in the United States and throughout the world. The virus binds to the host CD4+ cell. This virus/receptor complex then binds to a coreceptor, and the viral core enters the host cell cytoplasm. The virus uses reverse transcriptase to synthesize DNA from its viral RNA, and this viral DNA integrates into the host genome. Upon cell activation, the viral DNA is transcribed to RNA, and viral proteins are synthesized. The virion acquires its outer envelope coat upon budding from the host cell surface and is then infectious for other CD4+ cells. HIV contains genomic RNA within a core that is surrounded by an inner protein shell and an outer lipid envelope. The genome consists of the three genes found in all retroviruses (gag, pol, env), along with at least six additional genes, including gp120, which is necessary for the binding of virus to target cells, and p24, which is the major core protein.

A. **Epidemiology.** As of the end of 2001, 816,149 cases of the acquired immuno-deficiency syndrome (AIDS) in the United States, caused by HIV, have been reported to the Centers for Disease Control and Prevention. Approximately 58% of persons have died (467,910) since the beginning of the epidemic in the United States. Approximately 80,000 people died yearly from AIDS from 1993 to 1997, and about 15,000 to 20,000 died yearly since 1997. The decreased death rate is in large part attributed to access to more potent antiretroviral therapies since 1996. There are at least 360,000 persons living with AIDS in the United States, and some estimate as many as an additional 1 million persons who are HIV infected but without a diagnosis of AIDS. These estimates are difficult because only AIDS is mandatorily reported in all states. Additionally, many persons who are HIV infected will not have been tested and therefore do not know their infection status. Approximately 20% of persons living with AIDS are women, most of childbearing age. One percent of cases are in children younger than 13 years (n = 9074 as of the end of 2001), with at least 3923 more children reported as HIV infected. Approximately 175 to 200 infants and children are reported each year with AIDS. In women of childbearing age, the leading risk behavior is heterosexual contact with a known HIV-infected person or unknown risk behavior (presumably heterosexual contact with a person of unknown positive status). Previously, injection drug use accounted for the major risk behavior, but this is no longer the case.

The number of cases occurring in infants and children younger than 13 years rose rapidly until 1994. In that year, data from the Pediatric AIDS Clinical Trials Group Study 076 of the effectiveness of zidovudine (AZT) use antenatally, intrapartum, and for the neonate for the first 6 weeks of life became available. Currently, most states emphasize the importance of antenatal testing for HIV and offering zidovudine to reduce vertical transmission. At present, approximately 90% of HIV-infected pregnant women receive zidovudine at or before delivery. The epidemic in the United States has largely been curtailed in pediatrics; however, sub-Saharan Africa, India, Southeast Asia, Russia, and China continue to have uncontrolled epidemics. In some countries, 40% of women of childbearing age are seropositive for HIV. World Health Organization statistics estimate that by the end of 2002, there will be 42 million persons living with AIDS (19.2 million women, 3.2 million children younger 15 years). New HIV infections were estimated in 2002 to be 5 million (2 million in women, 800,000 in children). Deaths in 2002 were 3.1 million (1.2 million in women and 610,000 in children). Unquestionably, HIV poses one of the most serious and challenging health problems of the late twentieth and early twenty-first centuries.

B. **Pathogenesis.** When HIV-infected lymphocytes are activated, such as in intercurrent illnesses, many virions may be transcribed, and the cell can be lysed or apoptosis is enhanced, each resulting in host cell death. Because CD4+ lymphocytes are central to developing an appropriate immune response to almost all pathogens, the host with CD4+ counts below 200/mm^3 is susceptible to opportunistic infections and malignancies. In initial HIV infection, virus may first infect dendritic cells, viremia is present, and the lymphoid tissue is seeded. The host immune response is triggered, viremia is cleared, and 80% of patients become asymptomatic; for 20%, a rapidly progressive course ensues. In untreated asymptomatic patients, CD4+ cell loss progresses, with the median duration of the asymptomatic phase being approximately 10 years in adults. After this phase, the patient becomes symptomatic, generally with opportunistic infections, and death occurs within 5 years.

At present, prevention of horizontal transmission relies on barrier protection for known HIV-infected persons and on reduction of viral load in genital fluids with antiretroviral therapy. Many developing countries have not had access to any antiretroviral therapy; however, over the past few years, many governments and nongovernmental organizations are trying to offer HIV counseling and testing to pregnant women and offer intrapartum prophylactic therapy to positive women. Breastfeeding has been found to increase the rate of perinatal transmission by about 14%; however, infant mortality is approximately equal to that in nonbreastfed infants in developing countries. Trials of continued maternal and/or infant prophylaxis with antiretroviral therapy as well as with early weaning and alternatives to breastfeeding are continuing. Additionally, some countries are able to offer antiretroviral therapy to HIV-infected women postpartum and the fathers of these babies, recognizing that even if the infant escapes HIV infection, he or she may become orphaned and thus have a lower life expectancy unless the parents are treated. Contributions from wealthy foundations and governments in developed countries such as the United States are helping to put these treatment programs in place. Expansion of the monies needed for antiretroviral therapy has been seen by using generically manufactured drugs.

Infants with HIV infection have an initially high viral load, which declines over the first 5 years of life as the immune system develops. Current U.S. guidelines suggest treating all infants diagnosed with HIV infection in the first year of life so that the immune system can develop normally. After 1 year of age, suggestions for initiation of therapy based on CD4+ cell count and HIV viral load are less specific. Therapy should be implemented for children with symptomatic infection and for those with the lowest CD4+ cell percentages, regardless of age. Issues of when to initiate antiretroviral therapy must be individualized, and willingness of the care provider to assure the infant or child receives every dose every day is a critical component of success.

C. **Transmission.** There are three principal routes for HIV transmission: sexual contact, parenteral inoculation, and maternal-fetal or maternal-newborn transfer.

1. **Sexual contact.** This remains the principal mode of transmission of HIV worldwide. In the United States, sexual contact is the major risk behavior for men who have sex with men, but the rate of heterosexual transmission has increased considerably. Both semen and vaginal secretions have been found to contain HIV. The principal risk behavior for mothers of children reported with AIDS is heterosexual contact.

2. **Parenteral transmission.** Parenteral transmission of HIV results from the direct inoculation of infected blood or blood products. The groups affected have been intravenous drug users and patients receiving transfusions or factor concentrates. Careful screening of blood donors for risk factors for infection, universal HIV antibody and p24 antigen testing of donated blood, and the special preparation of clotting factor to eliminate the risk of viral contamination have greatly reduced the incidence of transfusion-acquired HIV. The most likely reason for false-negative HIV serology is the seronegative window that occurs between the time of initial infection and the production of antiviral antibody. The odds of transfusion-acquired HIV infection from the transfusion of a single unit of tested blood have been estimated to be from 1:250,000 to 1:150,000 (see Chap. 26, Blood Products Used in the Newborn).

3. **Congenital and perinatal transmission.** In utero and intrapartum transmissions from infected mothers constitute the principal modes of HIV infection in the pediatric population. Breast milk can contribute an additional 14%. Approximately 90% of pediatric AIDS cases have resulted from maternal transmission. The rate of transmission of HIV from infected mothers to their fetuses and newborn infants has been estimated to be between 15 and 40%. Prospective studies before February 1994 suggested that the overall risk for transmission in untreated persons may be closer to 25%. Transmission can occur throughout gestation, at birth, or postnatally through breast milk. HIV has been isolated from cord blood speci-

mens, and products of conception have demonstrated HIV infection as early as 14 to 20 weeks' gestation; however, it is now believed that the majority of infection is transmitted in late third trimester or at delivery. The mechanism of transplacental transfer of HIV is not known, but HIV can infect trophoblast and placental macrophage (Hofbauer) cell lines. Neither infection of nor quantity of virus present in the placenta correlate with congenital infection. This may suggest that the placenta in general acts as a protective barrier to transmission or conversely as a focus of potential transmission.

In a study of 100 sets of twins delivered to HIV-infected mothers, twin A was infected in 50% delivered vaginally and 38% delivered by cesarean. Twin B was infected in 19% of both vaginal and cesarean deliveries. This study—as well as the Women and Infants Transmission study and a meta-analysis of transmission studies—suggest that intrapartum infection occurs as a correlate of duration of ruptured membranes and that elective (without onset of labor) cesarean section deliveries may be preventive, especially if the HIV viral load is not controlled by antiretrovirals at delivery. Infants who are culture or DNA PCR or high-level RNA PCR positive in the first 3 days of life are considered to have been infected in utero; infants who test negative in the first 3 days and positive for HIV thereafter are considered to have peripartum-acquired HIV. This differentiation is relevant because offering potent antiretroviral therapy at the time of delivery, even in undiagnosed and/or untreated mothers, may be highly effective in reducing vertical transmission. Studies of rapid diagnostic testing for HIV in previously untested women at presentation for delivery with institution of prophylactic therapy are under way. Based on this kind of information, investigators are targeting the intrapartum interval to offer preventive treatments such as antiretroviral therapy (especially using nevirapine) or birth canal washes. Intrapartum transmission is likely to account for at least 50% of HIV infections in infants.

Any instrumentation, including fetal scalp electrodes and pH sampling, during the intrapartum period that would expose the fetus to maternal blood and secretions should be avoided in HIV-positive women. Postpartum, the mother should be advised to avoid allowing her infant to contact her blood or secretions.

Studies have also suggested that in countries where breastfeeding is almost exclusively practiced, the transmission rate may be as much as 14% over the presumed rate seen that is due to in utero or intrapartum transmission. In studies of women in endemic areas who were not HIV infected at the time of delivery but who seroconverted postpartum, some infants seroconverted almost simultaneously with their mothers. Several investigators reported on infants born to women who were not HIV infected, but who were breastfed by an HIV-infected wet nurse and subsequently acquired HIV infection. It may be that infants who do not have maternally derived, passively transferred antibody to HIV or those infants whose mothers acquire primary HIV infection during lactation are at a higher risk of acquisition of HIV exposure through breast milk than are those who are probably exposed to virions and antibody together. Therefore breastfeeding is contraindicated in countries in which formula preparations are safe and nutritionally replete.

D. **HIV in pregnancy.** The HIV-infected pregnant woman should be counseled that completion of pregnancy probably does not worsen her prognosis. HIV-infected women should be carefully screened for other sexually transmitted diseases (gonorrhea, herpes, chlamydia, hepatitis B and C, and syphilis), as well as being tested for antibody to CMV and toxoplasmosis. The mother should also have a tuberculin skin test and, when appropriate, be offered hepatitis B, pneumococcal, and influenza vaccines. If the CD4+ count is below 350 per µL, she should be offered antiretroviral therapy, including zidovudine, for her own health care. Additionally, guidelines suggest that pregnant women should be treated with the same antiretroviral combinations and with the same goal of suppression of HIV viral load and maintenance or increase of CD4+ lymphocytes as nonpregnant women. Exceptions to these recommendations are twofold. First, efavirenz has shown teratogenic effects in animal studies, and the combination of didanosine and stavudine has been associated with rare cases of maternal hepatic steatosis and death, precluding use of efavirenz or the combination of didanosine/stavudine in pregnancy. Second, all HIV-infected pregnant women should be offered at least zidovudine throughout pregnancy, even if the HIV viral load and CD4+ cell count would not warrant initiation of therapy for their own health care. Currently in the United States, the rate of vertical transmission is less than 2% in women who are diagnosed and take antiretroviral therapy before delivery. This rate is less than 1% when the HIV viral load is suppressed at delivery. This essentially makes perinatal transmission of HIV a preventable disease when women have antenatal counseling and testing and receive zidovudine for themselves and their infants. HIV testing is not mandatory component of antenatal care; hence every obstetric provider and pediatrician should offer testing and counseling to all pregnant women so they may consider therapeutic options for themselves and prophylactic options for their fetuses. New York and Connecticut are the only two states in which infants born to untested women are assessed for HIV exposure immediately after birth. Since this policy has been instituted, New York has seen an increase in antenatal testing and a decrease in vertical transmission. Data have shown that instituting the zidovudine regimen antenatally, intrapartum, or even neonatally reduces transmission compared with that seen (approximately 25%) when no antiretroviral therapy is received by the mother or the infant.

Pneumocystis carinii and possibly *Mycobacterium avium* intracellulare prophylaxis should be considered. Currently, prospective studies on HIV in pregnancy, such as through the Pediatric AIDS Clincal Trials Group or the Women and Infants Transmission Study, which are multicenter National Institutes of Health–sponsored investigations, are under way.

E. HIV infection in children. The majority of pediatric AIDS cases occurs in infants and young children, reflecting the preponderance of congenital and perinatally acquired infections. Fifty percent of pediatric AIDS cases are reported in the first year of life, and approximately 80% are reported by the age of 3 years. Of these patients, HIV-related symptoms occur in more than 80% in the first year of life (median age at onset of symptoms is 9 months). It is estimated that 20% of infants with congenital/perinatal HIV infection will die within the first year of life, and 60% will have severe symptomatic disease by the age of 18 months. These patients are defined as "rapid progressors." These statistics reflect only pediatric AIDS cases reported to the Centers for Disease Control and Prevention and may reflect only the part of the spectrum of disease that is identified. Statistics are also heavily influenced by the natural disease progression in untreated children or those treated with one or two drug therapies with the nucleoside analogue reverse transcriptase inhibitors only. It is possible that many infected children are undiagnosed and remain asymptomatic for years (7 to 15 years). There is no data for long-term outcome recently because more potent therapies have been available since 1996, both for mothers and infants.

F. Clinical manifestations. The clinical presentation differs in children compared with adults. The HIV-infected newborn is usually asymptomatic, but may present with lymphadenopathy and/or hepatosplenomegaly. Generally the infant infected peripartum does not develop signs or symptoms until after the first 2 weeks of life. These include lymphadenopathy and hepatosplenomegaly (as in adults), poor weight gain as might be found in chronic viral infection, and occasionally neuromotor abnormalities or encephalopathy. Before antiretroviral therapy was available to children, 50 to 90% of HIV-infected children had CNS involvement characterized by an encephalopathy that was often clinically devastating. Although the clinical presentation may vary, developmental delay or loss of developmental milestones and diminished cognitive function are common features. All too often an infant is diagnosed with AIDS between the ages of 2 to 6 months when he or she presents with *Pneumocystis carinii* pneumonia (PCP). This is an interstitial pneumonia often without ascultatory findings. Patients present with low-grade fever, tachypnea, and often, tachycardia. Progressive hypoxia ensues and may result in mortality as high as 90%. PCP is the AIDS-defining illness at presentation in 37% of pediatric patients, with a peak incidence at the age of 4 months. Treatment is intravenous trimethoprim-sulfamethoxazole and steroids. Prophylaxis to prevent such life-threatening possibilities is of course preferable to acquisition of disease. Based on adult studies, early on the Centers for Disease Control and Prevention recommended offering PCP prophylaxis to HIV-infected infants based on CD4+ lymphocyte number and percent by age. The majority of infants with PCP in the first year of life had CD4+ cell counts lower than 1500 per μL. It was recognized that fully 50% of infants presenting with PCP had either no CD4+ cell assessment available or the count was above the 1500/μL guideline. It is now recommended by the Public Health Service that all infants born to HIV-infected mothers be started on PCP prophylaxis at the age of 1 month until the infection and immune status of that infant is known.

A second condition possibly unique to pediatric AIDS is the development of chronic interstitial lung disease, referred to as lymphoid interstitial pneumonitis (LIP). LIP is characterized by a diffuse lymphocytic and plasma cell infiltrate. The clinical course of LIP is quite variable but may be progressive, resulting in marked respiratory distress (tachypnea, retractions, wheezing, hypoxemia). There is an association with Epstein-Barr virus infection, but the significance of this is uncertain. After the initial presentation, the prognosis appears to be more favorable for children with symptomatic HIV infection when the AIDS-defining illness is LIP. In addition to LIP, recurrent bacterial infections are a frequent feature of pediatric AIDS, owing in part to the early occurrence of B-cell dysfunction with dysfunctional hypergammaglobulinemia. Both focal and disseminated infections are encountered, with sepsis being most common. The organism usually isolated from the bloodstream is *Streptococcus pneumoniae*, but a variety of other bacteria have been recovered, especially from hospitalized patients. It will be interesting to see if this epidemiology holds true now that conjugated pneumococcal vaccines are standard of care for infants in the first 6 months of life. Other manifestations of HIV infection that may be more common in children are parotitis and cardiac dysfunction. Older children present with the more typical AIDS-defining opportunistic infections, as do adults when the CD4+ count wanes.

G. Diagnosis. The diagnosis of HIV infection in adults is made by the detection of specific antibody by an enzyme-linked immunosorbent assay (ELISA) with confirmation by Western blot analysis. Testing should be offered to anyone engaging in risk behaviors for HIV transmission. Testing requires counseling and informed consent. Serology is of limited value in diagnosing vertically transmitted HIV infection in infants less than 15 months old, because maternal IgG crosses the placenta and can persist in infants throughout the first year or more of life. In the presence of an AIDS-defining illness and a positive antibody test, the diagnosis is made even if the infant is less than 15 months of age. However, the picture is less clear in infants with minimal or no symptomatology. Thus viral detection tests must be used to identify infected infants born to HIV-seropositive mothers. These include the following:

1. PCR to detect viral DNA in peripheral blood cells.

2. PCR for viral RNA in plasma (must be > 10,000 copies/mL to be diagnostic.

3. *In vitro* cell culture of mononuclear cells.

The blood samples for these tests should be collected in anticoagulant, but not heparin. Sometimes the diagnosis is made with a positive p24 antigen detection in peripheral blood or *in situ* hybridization to detect HIV-specific DNA in infected cells.

Culture is sensitive and specific but is expensive, is technically difficult, and may require weeks before results are obtained. PCR generally correlates with cell culture and may be more quickly obtained. The mainstays of early viral diagnostic testing of the infant born to an HIV-infected mother remain HIV culture and PCR to detect both viral RNA and DNA. The p24 antigen assay suffers from a lack of sensitivity, particularly in infants, and can be replaced by acid-dissociated p24 antigen detection, which has a much greater sensitivity. The importance of obtaining an early diagnosis is clear: to provide even very young infants the benefit of antiretroviral therapy, which is hoped to reduce viral load and possibly prevent or reduce the viral burden at sites such as the CNS, as well as to maintain normal numbers of CD4+ cells.

H. Treatment. The major part of the management of HIV infection is antiretroviral therapy. This should be offered to all symptomatic patients regardless of CD4+ cell count. At present, there is no cure for HIV infection, but the goal of antiretroviral therapy is to suppress the HIV viral load to nondetectable and to maintain or reconstitute CD4+ cell numbers to greater than 25%. Generally, these agents are of three classes:

1. Nucleoside or nucleotide analogue reverse transcriptase inhibitors (NRTIs: e.g., zidovudine/AZT). These agents prevent viral RNA from being reverse-transcribed to DNA; therefore, infection of cells can be aborted.

2. Non-nucleoside analogue reverse transcriptase inhibitors (NNRTIs: e.g., nevirapine). These agents also act to prevent reverse transcription, but at a slightly different site on the enzyme. They are generally more potent than the NRTIs, but resistance can develop rapidly if the viral load is not controlled.

3. Protease inhibitors (PIs) act to prevent processing of viral proteins. These agents are quite potent.

Generally, initial therapy is with two NRTIs and a PI or an NNRTI. Other possible therapies being investigated include other sites of action in the retroviral life cycle as well as immune-based therapies.

Optimization of nutrition, immunizations, prophylaxis against opportunistic infections (most notably PCP), and the prompt recognition and treatment of HIV-related complications (e.g., opportunistic infections, cardiac dysfunction) are paramount to the improvement in the longevity and the quality of life for HIV-infected patients. In the newborn, special attention should be given to the possibility of congenitally and perinatally transmitted pathogens, such as tuberculosis, toxoplasmosis, and sexually transmitted diseases, which may have a relatively high prevalence in HIV-infected adults.

I. Prevention. In February 1994, a large clinical trial conducted by the AIDS Clinical Trials Group was closed early owing to astonishing results. HIV-infected pregnant women with more than 200 CD4+ T cells were randomized to receive zidovudine (at 100 mg five times/day) or placebo, beginning at 14 weeks' gestation. The mothers randomized to receive zidovudine also received intrapartum zidovudine intravenously at 2 mg/kg for the first hour of labor followed by 1 mg/kg/h until delivery, and their infants orally received zidovudine syrup at 2 mg/kg every 6 hours for the first 6 weeks of life. This trial (PACTG 076) closed when approximately 183 babies had been born to each cohort and had been assessed for HIV infection. Only 13 babies (8.3%) in the ziduovudine-receiving group were infected, whereas 40 babies (25.5%) in the placebo group were infected. As of February 1994, it has been the standard of care to offer zidovudine to pregnant HIV-infected women with more than 200 CD4+ T cells following the 076 algorithm. The infection rate of babies born to mothers with fewer than 200 CD4+ T cells is also decreased with zidovudine use, as shown in PACTG 185. Current standard of care in the United States is to reduce maternal viral load to nondetectable during pregnancy (and after pregnancy to optimize the maternal health care) using combination of the approved agents to treat HIV infection, except efavirenz, which showed teratogenicity in preclinical trials. An equally exciting trial in Uganda (HIVNET 012) offered a single dose of nevirapine to HIV-infected women in labor and followed this with a single dose of nevirapine at 3 days of life to the infants. Approximately 10% of these infants were already HIV infected in utero; however, the rate of perinatal transmission was markedly reduced. Nevirapine was found to readily cross the placenta, and with the two-dose regimen for the mother-infant pair, the nevirapine level in the infant's blood is above the level needed to reduce HIV viral load for at least a week. Unfortunately, by 18 months of age, the infant mortality in the nevirapine-treated group equaled that in the other group, most likely because of HIV transmission from breast-milk feeding, which was essentially universal. Implementation of the two-dose nevirapine regimen is ongoing in developing countries, as are studies designed to prevent breastmilk transmission of HIV.

When these treatments are instituted, the rate of transmission is less than 1% for women with a nondetectable viral load. Clearly these data challenge all health-care providers to participate in offering testing and counseling to all pregnant women, especially those who have engaged in high-risk behaviors. Frequently mothers may learn for the first time that they are HIV infected during their pregnancy. The appropriate social, nonjudgmental support network must be effectively in place to achieve the best pregnancy outcome possible. The mother's health, both medical and emotional, should not be subjugated to that of the fetus; rather, optimization of the mother-baby pair is key in effecting the best possible outcome.

Several studies suggested that maternal viral load, along with lower CD4+ T cell counts, is a strong correlate of vertical transmission. Assessment of viral load might also allow for targeting the pregnancies at highest risk of transmission to selected therapeutic strategies. Because HIV may be transmitted at the time of delivery, there has been speculation as to whether the risk of fetal infection may be reduced by cesarean section. Trials have been initiated to test this notion. No recommendations concerning mode of delivery can be made at this time.

Further strategies targeted to reduce the rate of vertical transmission even in the setting of zidovudine use are being planned. It is estimated that persons newly infected with HIV will acquire a zidovudine-resistant strain approximately 15% of the time; therefore, studies of other antiretroviral agents such as didanosine are being conducted in pregnancy. Resistance develops quickly to other agents such as NNRTIs (e.g., nevirapine), but these agents may be quite efficacious in decreasing the viral load at critical time periods, such as the intrapartum interval. Hyperimmune gamma globulin, prepared from healthy HIV-infected volunteers, is also under study to reduce the rate of transmission. Active immunity has also been an avenue of pursuit with vaccines to the surface glycoprotein of HIV (gp120). Infants will also be offered both active and passive immunity with vaccine and gamma globulin, much along the hepatitis B model. Birth canal washes with a virostatic agent have also been proposed, as HIV administered by gavage has been found to infect infant monkeys. It is hoped that combinations of these approaches or newer ones will be able to reduce the anticipated 15% rate of transmission of HIV to infants of infected mothers of any CD4+ count, even if receiving zidovudine.

Education plays an important role in the prevention of the spread of HIV infection. Informing the public about high-risk behaviors, such as intravenous drug use and unprotected sexual contact, is critical in curtailing this epidemic. The health-care provider should take advantage of every patient contact to provide preventive education. Eliminating unwarranted fears about casual contact with HIV-infected individuals is also within the purview of the provider.

J. HIV and the health-care worker. The transmission of HIV from patients to health-care providers is very uncommon, as is transmission from care providers to patients. The greatest risk for transmission is from parenteral inoculation of infected blood by inadvertent needle sticks or cuts with contaminated sharp instruments. To minimize the risk of transmission of HIV, universal precautions have been recommended for all hospital environments. Particular emphasis in perinatal/neonatal medicine should be placed on the avoidance of blood and bloody secretions in the delivery room by the wearing of gowns, gloves, and eye protection (preferably goggles with side shields). Meconium and gastric aspirates should never be suctioned by mouth; special meconium suction adapters and catheters that can be attached to wall suction are generally available. Of special concern in the nursery is the recapping of needles after drawing blood from umbilical lines. If recapping is required, it is best to use cap-holding devices to avoid needle sticks. Also, syringes should not be tapped or "flicked" to remove air when obtaining arterial blood gas samples. Specific guidelines have been suggested for the recognition and management of occupational exposures to HIV. Types of exposures include percutaneous injury (needle sticks, cuts with sharp instruments), mucous membrane contact, and skin contact (particularly from skin with cuts, abrasions, or dermatitis, or for prolonged exposure or over a large area) with potentially infectious tissues or body fluids. The guidelines recommend procedures for serologic testing in the worker and the patient contact. The use of zidovudine for postexposure prophylaxis is also discussed. Review of these guidelines is recommended for all individuals at risk for occupational exposure to HIV. The average risk of contracting HIV per episode of percutaneous exposure to HIV-infected blood is estimated to be approximately 0.3%. It is unknown if postexposure zidovudine will further reduce this risk.

XII. Hepatitis. Acute viral hepatitis is defined by the following clinical criteria: (1) symptoms consistent with viral hepatitis, (2) elevation of serum aminotransaminase levels to more than 2.5 times the upper limit of normal, and (3) the absence of other causes of liver disease. At least five agents have been identified as causes of viral hepatitis: hepatitis A virus (HAV); hepatitis B virus (HBV); hepatitis D virus (HDV); hepatitis C virus (HCV) (posttransfusion non-A, non-B hepatitis virus [NANB]); and hepatitis E virus (HEV) (enteric, epidemic NANB hepatitis virus). HDV, also referred to as the delta agent, is a defective virus that requires coinfection or superinfection with HBV. HDV is coated with hepatitis B surface antigen (HBsAg). Specific antibodies to HDV can be detected in infected individuals, but there is no known therapy to prevent infection in exposed HBsAg-positive patients. For the newborn, therapy directed at the prevention of HBV infection also should prevent HDV infection, because coinfection is required.

A. Hepatitis A virus (HAV: no vertical transmission). This RNA virus is spread by the fecal-oral route and can be detected by the presence of hepatitis A antigen in stool or by the presence of anti-HAV antibody. Anti-HAV IgG is present very early in infection, and levels may already be significantly elevated at the time of clinical diagnosis. Thus a fourfold rise in IgG, ordinarily diagnostic of acute infection, may be difficult to demonstrate. However, specific IgM can be determined. The usual incubation period for HAV is approximately 4 weeks (range 15–50 days). Symptoms include fever, malaise, anorexia, nausea, abdominal discomfort, dark urine, and jaundice. Infectivity typically diminishes rapidly. Immunization or prophylaxis against HAV is recommended primarily for travelers to developing countries or individuals at risk from personal contact with infected patients.

Studies of acute hepatitis during pregnancy failed to demonstrate fetal transmission of HAV, although an increase in preterm deliveries may occur. Nevertheless, acute maternal HAV infection near the peripartum period poses a threat to the neonate. It is recommended that infants born to a mother who developed acute HAV infection within 2 weeks of delivery receive an intramuscular injection of 0.5 mL of immune serum globulin. Measures also should be taken to minimize fecal-oral spread of virus from the infected mother to her newborn and within the nursery. Of particular importance here are the appropriate disposal of contaminated materials and good hand-washing practices. Blood transfusion is a rare cause of HAV infection.

B. Hepatitis B virus (HBV: perinatal and congenital). This DNA virus is one of the most common causes of acute and chronic hepatitis worldwide. In endemic populations, the carrier state is high, and perinatal transmission is a common event. The risk of chronic infection is inversely proportional to age, with a 90% carriage rate following infection in neonates. The overall incidence of HBV infections in the United States is relatively low but still substantial. There are estimates of approximately 300,000 infections yearly, with 250 deaths from fulminate disease. As many as 1 million individuals are chronic carriers, approximately 25% of whom develop chronic active hepatitis. Patients with chronic active hepatitis are at increased risk for developing cirrhosis and hepatocellular carcinoma, and approximately 5000 of these patients die each year from HBV-related hepatic complications (primarily cirrhosis). The incubation period for HBV infection is approximately 120 days (range 45–160 days). Transmission occurs by percutaneous or permucosal routes from infected blood or body fluids. Symptoms include anorexia, malaise, nausea, vomiting, abdominal pain, and jaundice.

1. **High-risk groups for HBV infection** in the United States include the following:
    a. **Persons born in endemic areas.** Alaskan natives and Pacific Islanders and natives of China, Southeast Asia, most of Africa, parts of the Middle East, and the Amazon basin; descendants of individuals from endemic areas.
    b. **Persons with high-risk behavior.** Men who have sex with men, intravenous drug use, and multiple sex partners.
    c. **Close contacts with HBV-infected persons** (sex partners, family members).
    d. **Selected patient populations,** particularly those receiving multiple blood or blood product transfusions.
    e. **Selected occupational groups,** including health-care providers.
2. **Diagnosis.** The diagnosis is made by specific serology and by the detection of viral antigens. The specific tests are as follows:
    a. **HBsAg determination.** Usually found 1 to 2 months after exposure and lasts a variable period of time.
    b. **Anti-HB surface antigen (anti-HBs).** Appears after resolution of infection or immunization and provides long-term immunity.
    c. **Anti-HB core antigen (anti-HBc).** Present with all HBV infections and lasts for an indefinite period of time.
    d. **Anti-HBc IgM.** Appears early in infection, is detectable for 4 to 6 months after infection, and is a good marker for acute or recent infection.
    e. **HB e antigen (HbeAg).** Present in both acute and chronic infections and correlates with viral replication and high infectivity.
    f. **Anti-HB e antigen (anti-HBe).** Develops with resolution of viral replication and correlates with reduction in infectivity.

   Infectivity correlates best with HBeAg positivity, but any patient positive for HBsAg is potentially infectious. Acute infection can be diagnosed by the presence of clinical symptoms and a positive HBsAg or anti-HBc IgM. The chronic carrier state is defined as the presence of HBsAg on two occasions, 6 months apart, or the presence of HBsAg without anti-HBc IgM.
3. **Prevention.** The transmission of HBV from infected mothers to their newborns is thought to result primarily from exposure to maternal blood at the time of delivery. Transplacental transfer appears to occur in Taiwan,

but this has not been found in other parts of the world, including the United States. In Taiwan there is a high chronic carrier rate that may be related to the transplacental transfer observed in that country. When acute maternal HBV infection occurs during the first and second trimesters of pregnancy, there generally is little risk to the newborns, because antigenemia is usually cleared by term and anti-HBs is present. Acute maternal HBV infection during late pregnancy or near the time of delivery, however, may result in a 50 to 75% transmission rate.

The principal strategy for the prevention of neonatal HBV disease has been to use immunoprophylaxis for newborns at high risk for infection. Vaccination of these infants is also an important part of perinatal prevention and safeguards against postnatal exposure as well. Immunization of infants effectively reduced the risk of chronic HBV infection in Taiwan. Universal immunization of infants promises to be one of the best options for disease control in the United States and is now recommended for all infants born to HBsAg-negative mothers. Three doses before the age of 18 months should be given. High-risk populations, such as Alaskan natives, Pacific Islanders, and infants of immigrant mothers from areas where HBV is endemic, should receive the three-dose series by the age of 6 to 9 months. The recommended schedule is begun during the newborn period or by the age of 2 months; the second dose is given 1 to 2 months later; and the third dose is given at the age of 6 to 18 months. The preterm infant should be started on the immunization series at discharge or at approximately 2 months of age, unless born to an HBsAg-positive mother, in which case immunization and treatment with hepatitis B immune globulin (HBIG) should begin immediately (see Table 23.2). Other methods of disease control have been considered and include delivery by cesarean section. In one study in Taiwan, cesarean delivery in conjunction with maternal immunization dramatically reduced the incidence of perinatally acquired HBV from highly infective mothers. These results are promising and may offer a potential adjunctive therapy for very high-risk situations (e.g., HBsAg/HBe-positive women). Currently, no specific recommendations can be made regarding mode of delivery.

It is recommended that all pregnant women be screened for HBsAg. Screening should be done early in gestation. If the test result is negative, no further evaluation is recommended unless there is a potential exposure history. When there is any concern about a possible infectious contact, development of acute hepatitis, or high-risk behavior in a nonimmunized woman, testing should be repeated. All infants born to mothers confirmed to be positive for HBsAg should receive HBIG in addition to recombinant

TABLE 23.2. DOSES OF HEPATITIS B VACCINES IN NEONATES*

	Active immunization: Either		Passive immunization HBIG
	Recombivax HB Merck	Engerix-B SmithKline Beecham	
Infants of HBsAg-negative mothers	5 μg (0.5 mL)	10 μg (0.5 mL)	
Infants of HBsAg-positive mothers	5 μg (0.5 mL)	10 μg (0.5 mL)	0.5 mL

HBIg = hepatitis B immunoglobulin; HBsAg = hepatitis B surface antigen.
*Both vaccine regimens use a three-dose schedule.

hepatitis B vaccine. The first immunization and HBIG are given within the first 12 hours of life, and the vaccine is repeated at the ages of 1 and 6 months. If the mother has immigrated from an endemic area, HBIG also should be given unless the mother is found to be HBsAg-negative.

Postnatal transmission of HBV by the fecal-oral route probably occurs, but the risk appears to be small. Nevertheless, this possibility adds further support to the need for the immunization of infants born to HBsAg-positive women. Another potential route of infection is by means of breast milk. This mode of transmission appears to be very uncommon in developed countries; there has been no documented increase in the risk of HBV transmission by breastfeeding mothers who are HBsAg-positive. This is true even though HBsAg can be detected in breast milk. Recommendations regarding breast-feeding in developed countries should be individualized, depending on how strongly breastfeeding is desired by the mother. The risk is certain to be negligible in infants who have received HBIG and hepatitis vaccine.

4. **Prevention of nosocomial spread.** HBsAg-positive infants pose a definite risk for nosocomial spread in the nursery. To minimize this risk, nursery personnel are advised to wear gloves and gowns when caring for infected infants. Of course, current universal precautions should be in effect in all nurseries, so the risk of exposure to blood and body secretions already should be minimized. Immunization of health-care workers is also strongly recommended, but if exposure should occur in a nonimmunized person, blood samples should be sent for hepatitis serology and HBIG administered as soon as possible unless the individual is known to be anti-HBs–positive. This should apply to personnel having close contact without appropriate precautions, as well as those exposed parenterally (e.g., from a contaminated needle).

C. **Hepatitis C virus (HCV: perinatal and congenital).** Hepatitis C is the agent responsible for the majority of NANB hepatitis in transfusion or organ transplant recipients and is a single-strand RNA virus related to the Flavivirus family.

1. **Epidemiology.** At least five HCV subtypes have been characterized based on sequence heterogeneity of the viral genome. HCV is found worldwide, and different subtypes have been identified from the same area. Subtype 1 is the most common in the United States and has a poorer prognosis than other subtypes.

   a. **Horizontal transmission.** Injection drug use is now the most common risk behavior for infection. In addition to injection drug users and transfusion recipients, dialysis patients and sexual partners of HCV-infected persons may also be infected, but 50% of identified persons are unable to define a risk factor.

   b. **Vertical transmission.** Overall rate of transmission is approximately 5% from known hepatitis C–infected women to their infants. The transmission rate may well be much higher and may approach 70% when the pregnant mother has a high viral load as assessed by semiquantitative PCR. HCV is transmitted at a higher frequency if the mother is also HIV infected, but this has not been assessed in women with a controlled HIV viral load and lower semiquantitative HCV viral load. The mode of transmission is also unknown. Detection of HCV by RNA PCR in cord blood would suggest that at least in some cases, in utero transmission occurs. There is also a case report of one infant having been infected with an HCV strain different from all maternal strains at the time of delivery, suggesting in utero transmission. Conversely, PCR-negative infants at birth may develop PCR positivity later in infancy, suggesting perinatal infection. One study found 50% of vaginal samples collected at 30 weeks' gestation from HCV-positive mothers to contain HCV, suggesting the possibility of infection by passage through the birth canal. The potential risk of breastfeeding is not well defined. HCV has been detected in breast milk by PCR, but vertical transmission rates in breast-fed and bottlefed infants are similar. The Centers for Disease Control and Prevention currently states that maternal HCV infection is not a contraindication to breastfeeding. The decision to breastfeed should be discussed with the mother on an individual basis.

2. **Clinical manifestations.** HCV accounts for 20 to 40% of viral hepatitis in the United States. The incubation period is 40 to 90 days after exposure, and manifestations often present insidiously. Serum transaminase levels may fluctuate or remain chronically elevated for as long as 1 year. Chronic disease may result in as many as 60% of community-acquired HCV infections. Cirrhosis may result in as many as 20% of chronic disease cases, but may be less likely in pediatric patients.

3. **Diagnosis.** The ELISA detects antibodies to three proteins (c100–3, c22–3, and c33c) that are components of HCV. This test may be able to detect infection as early as 2 weeks after exposure. Another serologic assay with even greater sensitivity is the radioimmunoblot assay, which detects antibodies to the three antigens detected by the ELISA and a fourth antigen, 5–5–1. Infants born to HCV-infected mothers will show evidence of passively acquired maternal antibody; therefore, to determine infection in the infant, RNA PCR, which detects the viral genome itself, must be performed. This assay can detect viremia within 1 week of infection in adults. In adults, approximately 70% of samples with detectable antibody will also be positive by PCR. This is a curious finding in that a serologic response does not provide adequate protection. Persons who have had an acute infection that resolves will become antibody negative. Infants born to known seropositive women should be tested for HCV antibody and HCV RNA by PCR at 1 year of age, and possibly by RNA PCR earlier to determine which infants to follow more closely.

4. **Treatment.** Clinical trials suggest that symptomatic persons with chronic HCV infection may benefit from treatment with alpha interferon and ribavirin, given for as long as a year. Side effects of this therapy include fever and myalgias, and the risk-benefit ratio must be carefully weighed.

5. **Prevention.** Blood products are screened for antibody to HCV. Presence of the antibody likely also indicates presence of virus, and the unit is discarded if antibody positive. Before blood products were screened and before the recognition that viremia often accompanied antibody positivity, some had recommended the use of immune globulin for prophylaxis for individuals exposed to HCV. This concept had transcended to the infant of the HCV-infected mother. There is *no* benefit to immune globulin given to the exposed infant or to the needle-stick recipient, as products containing antibody are excluded from the lot.

D. **Hepatitis E virus (HEV).** Enterically transmitted NANB viral hepatitis (HEV) is a single-stranded RNA virus that is similar to a calcivirus. It is primarily spread by fecal-contaminated water supplies. Epidemics have been documented in parts of Asia, Africa, and Mexico, and shellfish have been implicated as sources of infection. Incubation is 15 to 60 days. The clinical picture in infected individuals is similar to that of HAV infection, with fever, malaise, jaundice, abdominal pain, and arthralgia. HEV infection has an unusually high incidence of mortality in pregnant women. Treatment is supportive. The efficacy of immunoglobulin prophylaxis against this form of hepatitis is unknown, but because the infection is not endemic in the United States, commercial preparations in the United States would not be expected to be helpful.

E. **Hepatitis G virus (HGV).** Hepatitis G virus is a single-stranded RNA virus in the Flaviviridae family that shares 27% homology with HCV. HGV can be found worldwide and is found in about 1.5% of blood donors in the United States. Coinfection with HBV or HCV may be as much as 20%, suggesting common routes of transmission, such as transfusion or organ transplantation. Transplacental transmission is probably rare and may be associated with higher maternal viral loads. HGV is diagnosed by RNA PCR in research settings, and there is no current treatment or prophylactic therapy.

XIII. Varicella-zoster virus (V-Z virus: congenital or perinatal). The causative agent of varicella (chickenpox) is a DNA virus member of the herpesvirus family. The same agent is responsible for herpes zoster (shingles); hence, this virus is referred to as varicella-zoster virus (V-Z virus). Chickenpox results from primary V-Z virus infection, following which the virus may remain latent in sensory nerve ganglia. Zoster results from reactivation of latent virus later in life or if the host becomes immunosuppressed.

A. Epidemiology. Before the use of varicella vaccine, there were approximately 3 million cases of varicella yearly in the United States, primarily occurring in school-age children. The majority of adults have antibodies to V-Z virus, indicating prior infection, even when there is thought to be no history of chickenpox. It follows that varicella is an uncommon occurrence in pregnancy. The precise incidence of gestational varicella is uncertain, but is certainly less than it was before widespread use of varicella vaccine. There are recommendations to immunize nonimmune adults who are at high risk of infection unless they are pregnant. Alternatively, zoster is primarily a disease of adults. The incidence of zoster in pregnancy is also unknown, but the disease is likely to be uncommon as well. The overall risk of the congenital varicella syndrome following maternal infection in the first trimester is 2%, 0.4% in the first 12 weeks of pregnancy, and 2% from 13 to 20 weeks' gestation. It is primarily seen with gestational varicella but may occur with maternal zoster. It appears that the primary mode of transmission of V-Z virus is through respiratory droplets from patients with chickenpox. Spread through contact with vesicular lesions also can occur. Typically, individuals with chickenpox are contagious from 1 to 2 days before and 5 days after the onset of rash. Conventionally, a patient is no longer considered contagious when all vesicular lesions have dried and crusted over. The incubation period for primary disease extends from 10 to 21 days, with most infections occurring between 13 and 17 days. Transplacental transfer of V-Z virus may take place, presumably secondary to maternal viremia, but the frequency of this event is unknown.

Varicella occurs in approximately 25% of newborns whose mothers developed varicella within the peripartum period. The onset of disease usually occurs 13 to 15 days after the onset of maternal rash. When the rash develops in the newborn within 10 days, it is presumed to result from in utero transmission. The greatest risk for severe disease is seen when maternal varicella occurs within 5 days before or 2 days after delivery. In these cases there is insufficient time for the fetus to acquire transplacentally derived V-Z virus–specific antibodies. Symptoms generally begin 5 to 10 days after delivery, and the expected mortality is approximately 30%.

When in utero transmission of V-Z virus occurs before the peripartum period, there is no obvious clinical impact in the majority of fetuses; however, congenital varicella syndrome can occur.

B. Clinical manifestations

   1. Congenital varicella syndrome. There is a strong association between gestational varicella and a spectrum of congenital defects comprising a unique syndrome. Characteristic findings include cicatricial skin lesions, ocular defects, CNS abnormalities, intrauterine growth restriction, and early death. The syndrome most commonly occurs with maternal V-Z virus infection in weeks 7 to 20 of gestation.

   2. Zoster. Zoster is uncommon in young infants but may occur as a consequence of in utero fetal infection with V-Z virus. Similarly, children who develop zoster but have no history of varicella most likely acquired V-Z virus in utero. Zoster in childhood is usually self-limiting, with only symptomatic therapy indicated in otherwise healthy children.

3. **Postnatal varicella.** Varicella acquired in the newborn period as a result of postnatal exposure is generally a mild disease. Rarely, severe disseminated disease occurs in newborns exposed shortly after birth. In these instances, treatment with acyclovir may be beneficial. Varicella has been detected in breast milk by PCR; therefore, it may be prudent to defer breastfeeding at least during the period of time in which the mother is likely to be viremic and/or infectious.

C. **Diagnosis.** Infants with congenital varicella resulting from in utero infection occurring before the peripartum period do not shed virus, and the determination of V-Z virus–specific antibodies is often confusing. Thus the diagnosis is made on the basis of clinical findings and maternal history. With neonatal disease, the presence of a typical vesicular rash and a maternal history of peripartum varicella or postpartum exposure are all that is required to make the diagnosis. Laboratory confirmation can be made by (1) culture of vesicular fluid, although the sensitivity of this method is not optimal because the virus is quite labile; (2) demonstration of a fourfold rise in V-Z virus antibody titer by the fluorescent antibody to membrane antigen (FAMA) assay or by ELISA. Antigen also can be detected from cells at the base of a vesicle by immunofluorescent antibody detection. The latter is sensitive, specific, and rapid and should be the preferred method of diagnosis when vesicles are present.

D. **Treatment.** Infants with congenital infection, resulting from in utero transmission before the peripartum period, are unlikely to have active viral disease, so antiviral therapy is not indicated. However, infants with perinatal varicella acquired from maternal infection near the time of delivery are at risk for severe disease. In this setting, therapy with acyclovir is generally recommended. Data are not available on the most efficacious and safe dose of acyclovir for the treatment of neonatal varicella, but minimal toxicity has been shown with the administration of 60 mg/kg divided every 8 hours for the treatment of neonatal HSV infection.

At the present time, there is no established immunotherapy for the treatment of V-Z virus infections, but varicella-zoster immune globulin (VZIG) may be of prophylactic value. When administered within 72 hours of exposure, VZIG is effective in preventing or attenuating V-Z virus infection. The dose for newborns is 125 units intramuscularly.

E. **Prevention**

1. **Vaccination** of women who are not immune to varicella should decrease the incidence of congenital and perinatal varicella. Women should not receive the vaccine if they are pregnant or within 3 months before pregnancy. If this inadvertently occurs, the women should be enrolled in the National Registry. Additionally, acyclovir should also be considered for seronegative women exposed to varicella during pregnancy beginning 7 to 9 days postexposure and continuing 7 days. Women who acquire primary varicella during pregnancy should be treated with acyclovir for their own health as well as to prevent fetal infection.

2. **Management of varicella in the nursery.** The risk of horizontal spread of varicella following exposure in the nursery appears to be low, possibly because of a combination of factors, including (1) passive protection resulting from transplacentally derived antibody in infants born to varicella-immune mothers; (2) brief exposure with a lack of intimate contact. Nevertheless, nursery outbreaks do occur, so steps should be taken to minimize the risk of nosocomial spread. The infected infant should be isolated in a separate room, and visitors and caregivers should be limited to individuals with a history of varicella. A new gown should be worn upon entering the room, and good hand-washing technique should be used. Bedding and other materials should be bagged and sterilized. VZIG can be given to all other exposed neonates, but this can be withheld from full-term infants whose mothers have a history of varicella. Neonates at less than 28 weeks' gestation should be given VZIG postexposure regardless

of maternal status. Exposed personnel without a history of varicella should be tested for V-Z virus antibodies, and patient care by these individuals should be restricted as outlined below.

In the regular nursery, all exposed infants will ordinarily be discharged home before they could become infectious. Occasionally, an exposed infant needs to remain in the nursery for more than 8 days, and in this circumstance, isolation may be required. In the neonatal intensive care unit, exposed neonates are generally cohorted and isolated from new admissions within 8 days after exposure. If there is antepartum exposure within 21 days before hospital admission for a mother without a history of varicella, the mother and infant should be discharged as soon as possible from the hospital. If the exposure was from a household contact with current disease, VZIG should be administered to both mother and infant before discharge. Alternatively, arrangements to isolate the infectious household contact from the mother and infant may be done before discharge. If the exposure occurred 6 days or less before admission and the mother is discharged within 48 hours, no further action is required. Otherwise, mothers hospitalized between 8 to 21 days after exposure should be kept isolated from the nursery and other patients.

Personnel without a history of varicella should be kept from contact with a potentially infectious mother. If such an individual is inadvertently exposed, serologic testing (FAMA or ELISA) should be performed to determine susceptibility, and further contact should be avoided until immunity is proved. If the mother at risk for infection has not developed varicella 48 hours after the staff member was exposed, no further action is required. Alternatively, if a susceptible staff member is exposed to any individual with active varicella lesions or in whom a varicella rash erupts within 48 hours of the exposure, contact with any patients should be restricted for that staff member from day 8 through day 21 after exposure. Personnel without a history of varicella should have serologic testing, and if not immune, they should be vaccinated.

For mothers in whom varicella has occurred within 21 days before delivery, if there were resolution of the infectious stage before hospitalization, maternal isolation is not required. The newborn should be isolated from other infants (room in with mother). If the mother has active varicella lesions on admission to the hospital, isolate the mother and administer VZIG (125 units intramuscularly) to the newborn if maternal disease began less than 5 days before delivery or within 2 days postpartum (not 100% effective, and may consider acyclovir in addition). The infant should be isolated from the mother until she is no longer infectious. If other neonates were exposed, VZIG may be administered; these infants may require isolation if they are still hospitalized by day 8 after exposure.

XIV. Enteroviruses (congenital). The enteroviruses are RNA viruses belonging to the Picornaviridae family. They are classified into four major groups: coxsackieviruses group A, coxsackieviruses group B, echoviruses, and polioviruses. All four groups cause disease in the neonate. Infections occur throughout the year, with a peak incidence between July and November. The viruses are shed from the upper respiratory and gastrointestinal tracts. In most children and adults, infections are asymptomatic or produce a nonspecific febrile illness.

   A. Epidemiology. Most infections in newborns are caused by coxsackieviruses B and echoviruses. The mode of transmission appears to be primarily transplacental, although this is less well understood for echoviruses. Clinical manifestations are most commonly seen with transmission in the perinatal period.

   B. Clinical manifestations. Symptoms in the newborn often appear within the first week postpartum. Clinical presentations vary from a mild nonspecific febrile illness to severe life-threatening disease. There are three major clinical presentations in neonates with enterovirus infections. Approximately 50% have meningoencephalitis, 25% have myocarditis, and 25% have a sepsislike illness. The mortality (approximately 10%) is lowest for the group with meningoencephalitis. With myocarditis, there is a mortality of approximately 50%. The mortality from the sepsislike illness is essentially 100%. The majority (70%) of severe enteroviral infections in neonates are caused by echovirus 11.

C. **Diagnosis.** The primary task in symptomatic enterovirus infections is differentiating between viral and bacterial sepsis and meningitis. In almost all cases, presumptive therapy for possible bacterial disease must be initiated. Obtaining a careful history of a recent maternal viral illness, as well as that of other family members, particularly young siblings, and especially during the summer and fall months, may be helpful. The principal diagnostic laboratory aid generally available at this time is viral culture. Material for cultures should be obtained from the nose, throat, stool, blood, urine, and CSF. Usually, evidence of viral growth can be detected within 1 week, although a longer time is required in some cases. PCR is also available.

D. **Treatment.** In general, treatment of symptomatic enteroviral disease in the newborn is supportive only. There are no approved specific antiviral agents known to be effective against enteroviruses. However, protection against severe neonatal disease appears to correlate with the presence of specific transplacentally derived antibody. Furthermore, the administration of immune serum globulin appears to be beneficial in patients with agammaglobulinemia who have chronic enteroviral infection. Given these observations, it has been recommended that high-dose immune serum globulin be given to infants with severe, life-threatening enterovirus infections. It may also be beneficial to delay the time of delivery if acute maternal enteroviral infection is suspected, provided there are no maternal or fetal contraindications. The clinical presentation in infants with a sepsislike syndrome frequently evolves into shock, fulminant hepatitis with hepatocellular necrosis, and DIC. This expectation dictates close monitoring with early interventions for any signs of cardiovascular instability and coagulopathy. In the initial stages of treatment, broad-spectrum antibiotic therapy is indicated for possible bacterial sepsis. Later, with the recognition of progressive viral disease, some form of antibiotic prophylaxis to suppress intestinal flora may be helpful. Neomycin (25 mg/kg every 6 hours) has been recommended. A drug designed to prevent attachment of enterovirus to the host cell called pleconaril may be available in the future for severe neonatal disease.

XV. **Rubella (congenital).** This human-specific RNA virus is a member of the Togavirus family. It causes a mild self-limiting infection in susceptible children and adults, but its effects on the fetus can be devastating.

A. **Epidemiology.** Before widespread immunization beginning in 1969, rubella was a common childhood illness: 85% of the population was immune by late adolescence and nearly 100% by ages 35 to 40 years. Epidemics occurred every 6 to 9 years, with pandemics arising with a greater and more variable cycle. During pandemics, susceptible women were at significant risk of exposure to rubella, resulting in a high number of fetal infections. A worldwide epidemic from 1963 to 1965 accounted for an estimated 11,000 fetal deaths and 20,000 cases of congenital rubella syndrome (CRS). Childhood immunization has dramatically reduced the number of cases of rubella in the United States. In fact, some states have omitted rubella serologic screening from standard antenatal diagnostic recommendations because the very few cases of congenital rubella syndrome in recent years have been reported from unimmunized immigrants. The relative risk of fetal transmission and the development of CRS as a function of gestational age have been studied. With maternal infection in the first 12 weeks of gestation, the rate of fetal infection was 81%. The rate dropped to 54% for weeks 13 to 16, 36% for weeks 17 to 22, and 30% for weeks 23 to 30. During the last 10 weeks of gestation, the rate of fetal infection again rose: 60% for weeks 31 to 36 and 100% for weeks 36 and beyond. Fetal infection can occur at any time during pregnancy, but early-gestation infection may result in multiple organ anomalies. When maternofetal transmission occurred during the first 10 weeks of gestation, 100% of the infected fetuses had cardiac defects and deafness. Deafness was found in one-third of fetuses infected at 13 to 16 weeks, but no abnormalities were found when fetal infection occurred beyond the twentieth week of gestation. There are also case reports of vertical transmission with maternal reinfection.

B. Clinical manifestations. Classically, CRS is characterized by the constellation of cataracts, sensorineural hearing loss, and congenital heart disease. The most common cardiac defects are patent ductus arteriosus and pulmonary artery stenosis. Common early features of CRS are intrauterine growth restriction, retinopathy, microphthalmia, meningoencephalitis, electroencephalographic abnormalities, hypotonia, dermatoglyphic abnormalities, hepatosplenomegaly, thrombocytopenic purpura, radiographic bone lucencies, and diabetes mellitus. The onset of some of the abnormalities of CRS may be delayed months to years. Many additional rare complications have been described, including myocarditis, glaucoma, microcephaly, chronic progressive panencephalitis, hepatitis, anemia, hypogammaglobulinemia, thymic hypoplasia, thyroid abnormalities, cryptorchidism, and polycystic kidney disease. A 20-year follow-up study of 125 patients with congenital rubella from the 1960s epidemic found ocular disease to be the most common disorder (78%), followed by sensorineural hearing deficits (66%), psychomotor retardation (62%), cardiac abnormalities (58%), and mental retardation (42%).

C. Diagnosis

   1. Maternal infection. The diagnosis of acute rubella in pregnancy requires serologic testing. This is necessary because the clinical symptoms of rubella are nonspecific and can be seen with infection by other viral agents (e.g., enteroviruses, measles, human parvovirus). Furthermore, a large number of individuals may have subclinical infection. Several sensitive and specific assays exist for the detection of rubella-specific antibody. Viral isolation from the nose, throat, and/or urine is possible, but this is costly and not practical in most instances. **Symptoms** typically begin 2 to 3 weeks after exposure and include malaise, low-grade fever, headache, mild coryza, and conjunctivitis occurring 1 to 5 days before the onset of rash. The rash is a salmon-pink macular or maculopapular exanthem that begins on the face and behind the ears and spreads downward over 1 to 2 days. The rash disappears within 5 to 7 days from onset, and posterior cervical lymphadenopathy is common. Approximately one-third of women may have arthralgias without arthritis. In women suspected of having acute rubella infection, confirmation can be made by demonstrating a fourfold or higher rise in serum IgG titers when measured at the time of symptoms and approximately 2 weeks later. The results of some assays may not directly correlate with a fourfold rise in titer, so other criteria for a significant increase in antibody may be required. When there is uncertainty about the interpretation of assay results, advice should be obtained from the laboratory running the test and an infectious diseases consultation.

   2. Recognized or suspected maternal exposure. Any individual known to have been immunized with rubella vaccine after his or her first birthday is generally considered immune. However, it is best to determine immunity by measuring rubella-specific IgG, which has become a standard of practice in obstetric care. If a woman exposed to rubella is known to be seropositive, she is immune, and the fetus is considered not to be at risk for infection. Reinfections in previously immune women have been rarely documented, but the risk of fetal damage appears to be very small. If the exposed woman is known to be seronegative, a serum sample should be obtained 3 to 4 weeks after exposure for determination of titer. A negative titer indicates that no infection has occurred, whereas a positive titer indicates infection. Women with an uncertain immune status and a known exposure to rubella should have serum samples obtained as soon as possible after exposure. If this is done within 7 to 10 days of exposure, and the titer is positive, the patient is rubella immune and no further testing is required. If the first titer is negative or was determined on serum taken more than 7 to 10 days after exposure, repeat testing (approximately 3 weeks later) and careful clinical follow-up are necessary. When both the immune status and the time of exposure are uncertain, serum samples for titer determination should be obtained 3 weeks apart. If both titers are negative, no infection has occurred. Alternatively, infection is confirmed if seroconversion or a fourfold increase in titer is observed. Further testing and close clinical follow-up are required if titer results are inconclusive. In this situation, specific IgM determination may be helpful. It should be emphasized that all serum samples should be tested simultaneously by the same laboratory when one is determining changes in titers with time. This can be accomplished by saving a portion of each serum sample before sending it for titer determination. The saved portion can be frozen until convalescent serum samples have been obtained.

   3. **Congenital rubella infection**
      a. **Antenatal diagnosis.** The risk of severe fetal anomalies is highest with acute maternal rubella infection during the first 16 weeks of gestation. However, not all early-gestation infections result in adverse pregnancy outcomes. Approximately 20% of fetuses may not be infected when maternal rubella occurs in the first 12 weeks of gestation, and as many as 45% of fetuses may not be infected when maternal rubella occurs closer to 16 weeks of gestation. Unfortunately, there is no foolproof method of determining infected from uninfected fetuses early in pregnancy, but in utero diagnosis is being investigated. One method that has been used with some success is the determination of specific IgM in fetal blood obtained by PUBS. Direct detection of rubella antigen and RNA in a chorionic villous biopsy specimen also has been used successfully. Although these techniques offer promise, their use may be limited by sensitivity and specificity or the lack of widespread availability.
      b. **Postnatal diagnosis.** Guidelines for the establishment of congenital rubella infection or CRS in neonates have been summarized by the Centers for Disease Control and Prevention. The diagnosis of congenital infection is made by one of the following:
         (1) **Isolation of rubella virus** (oropharynx, urine). Notify the laboratory in advance as special culture medium needs to be prepared.
         (2) **Detection of rubella-specific IgM** in cord or neonatal blood.
         (3) **Persistent rubella-specific titers over time** (i.e., no decline in titer as expected for transplacentally derived maternal IgG). If, in addition, there are congenital defects, the diagnosis of CRS is made.

   D. **Treatment.** There is no specific therapy for either maternal or congenital rubella infection. Maternal disease is almost always mild and self-limiting. If primary maternal infection occurs during the first 5 months of pregnancy, termination options should be discussed with the mother. More than one-half of newborns with congenital rubella may be asymptomatic at birth. If infection is known to have occurred beyond the twentieth week of gestation, it is unlikely that any abnormalities will develop, and parents should be reassured. Nevertheless, hearing evaluations should be repeated during childhood. Closer follow-up is required if early-gestation infection is suspected or the timing of infection is unknown. This is true for asymptomatic infants as well as those with obvious CRS. The principal reason for close follow-up is to identify delayed-onset abnormalities or progressive disorders. In some cases, early interventions, such as therapy for glaucoma, may be critical. Unfortunately, there is no specific therapy to halt the progression of most of the complications of CRS.

   E. **Prevention.** The primary means of prevention of CRS is by immunization of all susceptible persons. Immunization is recommended for all nonimmune individuals 12 months or older. Documentation of maternal immunity is an important aspect of good obstetric management. When a susceptible woman is identified, she should be reassured of the low risk of contracting rubella, but she should also be counseled to avoid contact with anyone known to have acute or recent rubella infection. Individuals with postnatal infection typically shed virus for 1 week before and 1 week after the onset of rash. On the other hand, infants with congenital infection may shed virus for many months, and contact should be avoided during the first year. Unfortunately, once exposure has occurred, little can be done to alter the chances of maternal and subsequently fetal disease. Although hyperimmune globulin has not been shown to diminish the risk of maternal rubella following exposure or the rate of fetal transmission, it should be given in large doses to any woman who is exposed to rubella and who does not wish to interrupt her pregnancy. The lack of proven efficacy must be emphasized in these cases.

Susceptible women who do not become infected should be immunized soon after pregnancy. There have been reports of acute arthritis occurring in women immunized in the immediate postpartum period, and a small percentage of these women developed chronic joint or neurologic abnormalities or viremia. Vaccine-strain virus also may be shed in breast milk and transmitted to breastfed infants, some of whom may develop chronic viremia. Thus it may be best to avoid breastfeeding in women receiving rubella vaccine. Conception also should be avoided for 3 months following immunization. Immunization during pregnancy is not recommended because of the theoretical risk to the fetus. Inadvertent immunizations during pregnancy have occurred, and fetal infection has been documented in a small percentage of these pregnancies. However, no cases of CRS have been identified. In fact, the rubella registry at the Centers for Disease Control and Prevention has been closed, with the following conclusions: The number of inadvertent immunizations during pregnancy is too small to be able to state with certainty that no adverse pregnancy outcomes will occur, but these would appear to be very uncommon. Thus it is still recommended that immunization not be carried out during pregnancy, but when this has occurred, reassurance of little risk to the fetus can be given.

XVI. Respiratory syncytial virus (RSV: neonatal). Respiratory syncytial virus (RSV) is an enveloped RNA paramyxovirus that is the leading cause of bronchiolitis and can cause severe or even fatal lower respiratory tract disease, especially in preterm infants. Conditions that increase the risk of severe disease include cyanotic or complicated congenital heart disease, pulmonary hypertension, bronchopulmonary dysplasia, and immune-compromised states.

A. Epidemiology. Humans are the only source of infection, spread by respiratory secretions as droplets or fomites, which can survive on environmental surfaces for hours. Spread by hospital workers to infants occurs, especially in the winter and early spring months in temperate climates. Viral shedding is 3 to 8 days, but in very young infants may take weeks. The incubation period is 2 to 8 days.

B. Diagnosis. Rapid diagnosis is made by immunofluorescent antigen testing of respiratory secretions. This test can have up to 95% sensitivity and is quite specific. Viral culture usually requires 3 to 5 days.

C. Treatment. Treatment is largely supportive, with hydration, supplemental oxygen, and mechanical ventilation as needed. Controversy exists as to whether albuterol nebulized therapy is beneficial. Ribavirin has been marketed for treatment of infants with RSV infection because it does have *in vitro* activity; however, efficacy has never been repeatedly proven in randomized trials. This makes the risk of ribavirin (aerosol route, potentially toxic side effects to health-care personnel, and high cost) important to consider on a case-by-case basis.

D. Prevention. Respiratory syncytial virus immune globulin (RSV-IG, Respigam[R]) prepared from donors with high titers, to RSV and palivizumab (Synagis[R]), a humanized mouse monoclonal antibody given intramuscularly, have been approved by the Food and Drug Administration for prevention of RSV disease in children younger than 2 years of age with bronchopulmonary dysplasia (BPD) or who were less than 35 weeks' gestation. Neither has been approved for treatment. Generally palivizumab is preferred because of the ease of administration and low volume of product required. RSV-IG and palivizumab are given just before and monthly throughout the RSV season (typically mid-November to March/April). RSV-IG is given as 750 mg/kg intravenously over 4 hours. RSV-IG is supplied intravenously in 2.5 g/50 mL vials and 1 g/20 cc vials. Palivizumab is given as 15 mg/kg intramuscularly monthly. Because the drug supply is limited, its protection incomplete, the administration of RSV-IG difficult, and each is costly, the American Academy of Pediatrics has made recommendations regarding which high-risk infants should receive RSV-IG intravenously.:

1. **Infants who have required therapy for chronic lung disease** within 6 months of the RSV season.
2. **Infants who are born at less than 32 weeks' gestation** without chronic lung disease: up to 12 months of age if born at 28 weeks' gestation or less; up to 6 months of age if born at 29 to 32 weeks' gestation.
3. **Preterm infants 32 to 35 weeks** < 6 months of age who have two or more of the following risk factors: attending day care, with school-aged siblings in household, exposure to environmental pollutants, congenital abnormalities of the airways, or severe neuromuscular disease.

   If an RSV outbreak is documented in a high-risk unit (e.g., pediatric intensive-care unit), primary emphasis should be placed on proper infection-control practices. The need for and efficacy of antibody prophylaxis in these situations has not been documented. Each unit should evaluate the risk to its exposed infants and decide on the need for treatment. If the patient stays hospitalized, this may only require one dose.
4. Children who are 24 months of age or younger with hemodynamically significant cyanotic or acyanotic congenital heart disease.

E. **Antibody preparations are not recommended for:**
   1. Healthy preterm babies greater than 32 weeks' gestation without other risk factors.
   2. Patients with hemodynamically significant heart disease.

   Palivizumab does not interfere with the routine immunization schedule; however, if RSV-IG is given, measles-mumps-rubella vaccine should be deferred for 9 months.

Suggested Readings

American Academy of Pediatrics, Committee on Infectious Diseases, *2003 Red Book: Report of the Committee on Infectious Diseases,* 25th Ed. 2003; Elk Grove Village, Ill: American Academy of Pediatrics.

Bopanna S.B., et al. Intrauterine transmission of cytomegalovirus to infants of women with preconceptual immunity. *N Engl J Med* 2001;1366–1371.

Fowler K.B., et al. The outcome of congenital CMV infection in relation to maternal antibody status. *N Engl J Med* 1992;326:663–667.

Guidelines for Perinatal HIV and for Antiretroviral Therapy for Children. http://www.aidsinfo.nih.gov/.

Kimberlin D.W., et al. Natural history of neonatal herpes simplex virus infections in the acyclovir era. *Pediatrics* 2001;108:223–229.

Mofenson L.M., et al. Risk factors for perinatal transmission of human immunodeficiency virus type 1 in women treated with zidovudine. *N Engl J Med* 1999;341: 385–393.

Palumbo P., Burchett S.K. Diagnosis of HIV infection and markers of disease progression in infants and children. In: Pizzo, PA and Wilfert, CM (Eds.) *Pediatric AIDS: The Challenge of HIV Infection in Infants, Children, and Adolescents,* 3rd Ed. 1998; Philadelphia: Lippincott Williams & Wilkins, 67–88.

Sperling R.S., et al. Reduction of maternal-infant transmission of HIV type 1 with zidovudine treatment. *N Engl J Med* 1994;331:1173–1180.

Whitley R.J., et al. Predictors of morbidity and mortality in neonates with herpes simplex virus infections. The National Institute of Allergy and Infectious Diseases Collaborative Antiviral Study Group. *N Engl J Med* 1991;324:450–454.

Bacterial and Fungal Infections

Karen M. Puopolo

I. Bacterial sepsis and meningitis

A. Introduction. Bacterial sepsis and meningitis continue to be major causes of morbidity and mortality in newborns, particularly in low-birth-weight infants. In the 1990s, improvements in neonatal intensive care have decreased the morbidity and mortality from early-onset sepsis (EOS) in term infants. Preterm infants, however, remain at high risk for both EOS and its sequelae. They are also at risk for nosocomially acquired sepsis. Neonatal survivors of sepsis can have severe neurologic sequelae due to central nervous system (CNS) infection, as well as from secondary hypoxemia resulting from septic shock, persistent pulmonary hypertension, and severe parenchymal lung disease.

B. Epidemiology of early-onset sepsis. Several studies report the rate of early-onset sepsis to vary from 1 to 4 cases per 1000 live births. Recent data from the Centers for Disease Control shows that the incidence of Group B Streptococcus (GBS) EOS has decreased with the implementation of recommendations for intrapartum antibiotic prophylaxis (IAP) against GBS. However, the incidence of non-GBS EOS is unchanged among overall births; the incidence of non-GBS EOS is increasing among very-low-birth weight (<1500 g) infants.

C. Risk factors for EOS. Maternal and infant characteristics associated with the development of EOS have been most rigorously studied with respect to GBS EOS. Maternal factors predictive of GBS disease include intrapartum fever (>37.5°C), chorioamnionitis, and prolonged rupture of membranes (ROM) (>18 hours). Neonatal risk factors include prematurity (<37 weeks' gestation) and low birth weight (<2500 g). The incidence of EOS is nearly 10 times higher in infants with a birth weight less than 1000 g than that for infants with normal birth weight.

D. Clinical presentation of EOS. Early-onset disease can manifest as asymptomatic bacteremia, generalized sepsis, pneumonia, and/or meningitis. The clinical signs of EOS are usually apparent in the first hours of life; 90% of infants are symptomatic by 24 hours of age. Respiratory distress is the most common presenting symptom. Respiratory symptoms can range in severity from mild tachypnea and grunting, with or without a supplemental oxygen requirement, to respiratory failure. Persistent pulmonary hypertension of the newborn (PPHN) can also accompany sepsis. Other less specific signs of sepsis include irritability, lethargy, temperature instability, poor perfusion, and hypotension. Disseminated intravascular coagulation (DIC) with purpura and petechiae can occur in more severe septic shock. Gastrointestinal symptoms can include poor feeding, vomiting, and ileus. Meningitis may present with seizure activity, apnea, and depressed sensorium, but may complicate sepsis without specific neurologic symptoms, underscoring the importance of the lumbar puncture in the evaluation of sepsis.

Other diagnoses to be considered in the immediate newborn period in the infant with signs of sepsis include transient tachypnea of the newborn, meconium aspiration syndrome, intracranial hemorrhage, congenital viral disease, and congenital cyanotic heart disease. In infants presenting at more than 24 hours of age, closure of the ductus arteriosus in the setting of a ductal-dependent cardiac anomaly (such as critical coarctation of the aorta or hypoplastic left heart syndrome) can mimic sepsis. Other diagnoses that should be considered in the infant presenting beyond the first few hours of life with a sepsislike picture include bowel obstruction, necrotizing enterocolitis (NEC), and inborn errors of metabolism.

E. **Evaluation of the symptomatic infant for EOS.** Laboratory evaluation of the symptomatic infant suspected of EOS includes at minimum a complete blood count (CBC) with differential and blood culture. An elevated white blood cell count (WBC) with a predominance of immature granulocytes (PMN), a depressed total WBC (<5000) and absolute neutropenia (PMN < 1500) are commonly found. However, a normal WBC and differential can be initially seen; a second WBC performed at 12 to 24 hours of age can be helpful in making a clinical diagnosis of infection. Other laboratory abnormalities can include hyperglycemia and metabolic acidosis. Thrombocytopenia as well as evidence of DIC [elevated prothrombin time (PT), partial thromboplastin time (PTT), and international normalized ratio (INR); decreased fibrinogen] can be found in more severely ill infants. For infants with a strong clinical suspicion of sepsis, a lumbar puncture for cerebrospinal fluid (CSF) cell count, protein and glucose concentration, gram stain, and culture should be performed prior to the administration of antibiotics if the infant is clinically stable. The lumbar puncture may be deferred until after the institution of antibiotic therapy if the infant is clinically unstable, or if later culture results or clinical course demonstrate that sepsis was present.

Infants with respiratory symptoms should have a **chest radiograph** as well as other indicated evaluation such as arterial blood gas measurement. Radiographic abnormalities caused by retained fetal lung fluid or atelectasis, usually resolve within 48 hours. **Neonatal pneumonia** will present with persistent focal or diffuse radiographic abnormalities and variable degrees of respiratory distress. Neonatal pneumonia (particularly that caused by GBS) can be accompanied by primary or secondary surfactant deficiency.

F. **Treatment of EOS.** Empiric **antibiotic therapy** includes broad coverage for organisms known to cause EOS, usually a beta-lactam antibiotic and an aminoglycoside. In our institutions, we use ampicillin (150 mg/kg per dose q12h) and gentamicin (3 to 4 mg/kg per dose q24h). We add a third-generation cephalosporin (cefotaxime or ceftazidime) to the empiric treatment of critically ill infants for whom there is a strong clinical suspicion for sepsis because of a recent increased incidence of ampicillin-resistant *Escherichia coli* EOS infections. See Tables 23.3 and 23.4 for treatment recommendations. **Supportive treatments for sepsis** include the use of mechanical ventilation; exogenous surfactant therapy for pneumonia and respiratory distress syndrome (RDS); volume and pressor support for hypotension and poor perfusion; sodium bicarbonate for metabolic acidosis; and anticonvulsants for seizures. **Echocardiography** may be of benefit in the severely ill, cyanotic infant to determine if significant pulmonary hypertension or cardiac failure is present. Infants born at ≥34 weeks with symptomatic pulmonary hypertension may benefit from treatment with inhaled nitric oxide (**iNO**). Extra-

TABLE 23.3. SUGGESTED ANTIBIOTIC REGIMENS FOR SEPSIS AND MENINGITIS*

Organism	Antibiotic	Bacteremia	Meningitis
GBS	Ampicillin or penicillin G	10–14 days	21 days
E. coli,	Cefotaxime or ampicillin and gentamicin	14 days 14 days	21 days 21 days
CONS	Vancomycin	7 days	—
Enterobacter, Klebsiella†	Cefotaxime or cefipime or meropenem and gentamicin	14 days	21 days
Enterococcus‡	Ampicillin or vancomycin and gentamicin	10 days	21 days
Listeria	Ampicillin and gentamicin	10–14 days	21 days
Pseudomonas	Ceftazidime or piperacillin/ tazobactam and gentamicin or tobramycin	14 days	21 days
S. aureus§	Nafcillin	10–14 days	21 days

*All treatment courses are counted from the first documented negative blood culture and assume that antibiotic sensitivity data are available for the organisms. In late-onset infections, all treatment courses assume central catheters have been removed. With CONS and enterococcal infections, the clinician may choose to retain the catheter during antibiotic treatment, but if two to three cultures remain positive, the catheters must be removed.
†Cefipime (a fourth-generation cephalosporin) is reported to induce cephalosporinases in *Enterobacter* species with lesser frequency than third-generation cephalosporins. However, there are now reports of cefipime resistance in the literature. Meropenem therapy is reserved for cephalosporin-resistant strains of *Enterobacter*.
‡Enterococci are resistant to all cephalosporins. Ampicillin-resistant strains of enterococci are common, and require treatment with vancomycin. Treatment of vancomycin resistant strains (VRE) require consultation with an infectious disease specialist.
§*S. aureus* bacteremia may be treated for only 10 days if central catheters have been removed. Deep infections such as osteomyelitis or infectious arthritis often require surgical drainage and treatment for 3 to 4 weeks.

corporeal membrane oxygenation (**ECMO**) can be offered to these infants if respiratory and/or circulatory failure occurs despite all conventional measures of intensive care.

A variety of **adjunctive immunotherapies** for sepsis have been trialed since the 1980s to address deficits in immunoglobulin and neutrophil number and function. Double-volume exchange transfusions, granulocyte infusions, the administration of intravenous immunoglobulin (IVIG), and treatment with granulocyte-colony stimulating factor and granulocyte-macrophage stimulating factor (G-CSF and GM-CSF) have all been investigated with variable results.

TABLE 23.4. NEONATAL DOSING OF COMMON INTRAVENOUS ANTIBIOTICS

Antibiotic	Dosing Regimen	
Ampicillin*	≤7 days	150 mg/kg per dose q12h
	>7 days and <1200 g	50–150 mg/kg per dose q12h
	>7 days and 1200 g–2000 g	25–50 mg/kg per dose q8h
	>7 days and >2000 g	25–50 mg/kg per dose q8h
In each case, lower dosing for sepsis alone and higher dosing for meningitis		
Cefotaxime	≤7 days: 50 mg/kg per dose q12h	
	>7 days: 50 mg/kg per dose q8h	
Cefipime	50 mg/kg per dose q8h	
Ceftazidime†	≤7 days: 50 mg/kg per dose q12h	
	> 7 days: 50 mg/kg per dose q8h	
Clindamycin	≤29 weeks: 7.5 mg/kg per dose q12h	
	>29 weeks: 7.5 mg/kg per dose q8h	
Gentamicin‡	<35 weeks: 3 mg/kg per dose q24h	
	≥35 weeks: 4 mg/kg per dose q24h	
Meropenem	Sepsis: 20 mg/kg per dose q12h	
	Meningitis: 40 mg/kg per dose q8h	
Nafcillin	≤7 days and < 2 kg	25 mg/kg per dose q12h
	≤7 days and ≥ 2 kg	25 mg/kg per dose q8h
	>7 days and <1200 g	25 mg/kg per dose q12h
	>7 days and 1200–2000 g	25 mg/kg per dose q8h
	>7 days and >2000 g	25 mg/kg per dose q6h
Penicillin G	GBs sepsis: 200,000 U/kg/day ÷ q8h	
	GBs meningitis: 400,000 U/kg/day ÷ q8h	
Vancomycin§	≤7 days and <1.2 kg	15 mg/kg per dose q24h
	≤7 days and 1.2 – 2.0 kg	10 mg/kg per dose q12h
	≤7 days and > 2.0 kg	15 mg/kg per dose q12h
	>7 days and <1.2 kg	15 mg/kg per dose q24
	>7 days and 1.2 –2.0 kg	15 mg/kg per dose q12h
	>7 days and > 2 kg	10 mg/kg per dose q8h

GA, gestational age; PNA, postnatal age.
*At our institution, we use ampicillin 150 mg/kg/dose q12h and gentamicin as empiric therapy for EOS.
†For meningitis, ceftazidime should be given at 50 mg/kg per dose q8h regardless of age.
‡Gentamicin levels: Trough < 1.5 µg/ml Peak 6–15 µg/ml.
§Vancomycin levels: Trough 5–15 µg/ml We no longer monitor vancomycin peak levels at our institution.
See Appendix A for administrative guidelines.

1. **Double-volume exchange transfusion and granulocyte infusion:** Several small trials have been conducted to assess the efficacy of repleting neutrophils in neutropenic septic infants. This can be achieved by: (1) double-volume exchange transfusion with fresh whole blood, (2) infusion of fresh buffy-coat preparations, or (3) infusion of granulocytes collected by leukopheresis. Double-volume exchange with whole blood also provides platelets and removes bacteria, bacterial toxins, and circulating inflammatory molecules. Case reports from the early 1980s suggested a

benefit from this procedure in profoundly ill neonates. A 1993 report of exchange transfusion with whole blood in 30 neutropenic infants with (largely gram-negative) sepsis reported a 50% reduction in mortality in the infants undergoing exchange, and demonstrated increases in neutrophil number and improvement in neutrophil function in the exchanged infants. A recent meta-analysis of granulocyte transfusion studies concluded that when given in adequate dose (>1 x 10^9 neutrophils/kg) these infusions were of significant survival benefit to neonates. Both whole blood exchange transfusion and granulocyte infusion do present significant risks, including graft-versus-host disease; blood-group sensitization; and transmission of infections such as CMV, HIV, and viral hepatitis. In addition, the availability of these blood products (especially leukopheresed granulocytes) in an emergent fashion is limited in most centers. We do not currently use either of these treatments in the treatment of early- or late-onset sepsis.

2. **Intravenous immune globulin (IVIG).** The use of IVIG in the acute treatment of neonatal sepsis is controversial. It is likely that any efficacy of IVIG would be highest in early-onset sepsis, which in the United States is largely due to the encapsulated organisms GBS and *E. coli* K1, and in premature infants, who are most likely to have inadequate immunoglobulin reserves. A 1997 meta-analysis of three studies of the use of IVIG in the acute treatment of neonatal sepsis showed a sixfold decrease in mortality. Each of the included studies were prospective and randomized, and included mostly preterm infants. Interestingly, none of the studies individually demonstrated a statistically significant survival benefit. Each used a different dosing regimen and/or immunoglobulin preparation. IVIG is expensive and has potential infectious risks, and most authorities have not endorsed the routine use of IVIG in the treatment of neonatal sepsis. However, in light of this meta-analysis, a single dose of IVIG at 750 mg/kg per dose for preterm infants (1 g/kg for term infants) with overwhelming sepsis is a reasonable adjunctive therapy in the seriously ill infant.

3. **Cytokines.** Recombinant G-CSF and GM-CSF have been shown to restore neutrophil levels in small studies of neutropenic growth-restricted infants, ventilator-dependent neutropenic infants born to mothers with preeclampsia, and in neutropenic infants with sepsis. A rise in the absolute neutrophil count above 1500/mm^3 occurred in 24 to 48 hours. However, two randomized trials of these cytokines in the treatment of EOS did not show significant effect on morbidity or mortality.

G. **Evaluation of the asymptomatic infant at risk for EOS.** There are a number of clinical factors that place infants at risk for EOS. These factors also identify a group of asymptomatic infants who may have colonization or bacteremia that places them at risk for the development of symptomatic EOS. These infants include those born to mothers who have received inadequate IAP for GBS (see below) and those born to mothers with suspected chorioamnionitis. Blood cultures are the definitive determination of bacteremia. A number of laboratory tests have been evaluated for their ability to predict which of the at-risk infants will go on to develop symptomatic or culture-proven sepsis, but no single test has adequate sensitivity and specificity.

1. **Blood culture.** With advances in the development of computer-assisted, continuous-read culture systems, most blood cultures will be positive within 24 to 36 hours of incubation if organisms are present. Most institutions, including ours, empirically treat infants for sepsis for a minimum of 48 hours with the assumption that true positive cultures will turn positive within that period. At least 0.5 mL (and preferably 1 mL) of blood should be placed in most pediatric blood culture bottles. We use two culture bottles, one aerobic and one anaerobic. Certain organisms causing EOS [such as *Bacteroides fragilis* (*B. fragilis*)] will only grow under anaer-

obic conditions. GBS, Staphylococcus species, and many gram-negative organisms grow in a facultative fashion, and the use of two culture bottles increases the likelihood of detecting low-level bacteremia with these organisms.

2. **White blood count (WBC).** A total WBC < 5000; an absolute neutrophil count (ANC) <1000; and an immature to total neutrophil count (I:T ratio) > 0.2 have all been correlated with the presence of bacterial infection. An elevated WBC (>20,000) is not predictive in newborn infants. The overall positive predictive value of WBC values is poor, as there are a number of neonatal conditions that result in neutrophilia and an elevated I:T ratio including maternal fever, neonatal asphyxia, meconium aspiration syndrome, pneumothorax, and hemolytic disease. Maternal pregnancy-induced hypertension and preeclampsia are associated with neonatal neutropenia as well as thrombocytopenia. WBC values can be useful, however, when placed in the clinical context and used as part of an algorithm to evaluate infants for sepsis risk. In addition, a repeat WBC obtained at 12 to 24 hours of age is more predictive of infection than a single determination at birth. Some centers use a "sepsis screen" (for example, the use of an algorithm incorporating total WBC, I/T ratio, total band count, with or without C-reactive protein values) to guide treatment decisions.

3. **C-reactive protein.** CRP is a nonspecific marker of inflammation or tissue necrosis. Elevations in CRP are found in bacterial sepsis and meningitis. A single determination of CRP at birth lacks both sensitivity and specificity for infection, but serial CRP determinations at birth, and at 12 hours and beyond have been used to manage infants at risk for sepsis. We do not use CRP measurements in the evaluation of infants at risk for sepsis.

4. **Cytokine measurements.** Advances in the understanding of the immune responses to infection and in the measurement of small peptide molecules have allowed investigation into the utility of these inflammatory molecules in predicting infection in neonates at risk. Serum levels of interleukin-6, interleukin-8, granulocyte-colony stimulating factor (G-CSF), TNF-alpha and interleukin-1 beta have each been correlated with both culture-proven and clinical sepsis. Noninfection-related illness severity, however, has been shown to influence IL-6 levels. Studies of cord blood interleukin-6 and interleukin-8, do show some promise in predicting early-onset infection. One recent study of the use of cord blood IL-6 and IL-8 levels in premature infants reported 96% sensitivity and 95% specificity for IL-6 and 87% sensitivity, 94% specificity for IL-8 in predicting culture-proven sepsis.

The need for serial measurements and the availability of the specific assays so far limit the use of cytokine markers in diagnosing neonatal infection. In addition, most studies have been performed on infants who are symptomatic and being evaluated for sepsis. These measurements may be most useful in making judgments about empiric treatment of sepsis in the absence of a positive blood culture. It remains to be seen what value cytokine determinations alone will be in the evaluation of the asymptomatic infant at risk for sepsis.

5. **Other strategies. Gram stain of gastric aspirate contents** for bacteria and PMNs was once used to predict the presence of early onset infection but has fallen out of use due to poor specificity and sampling error. **Urine latex particle agglutination testing for GBS** remains available at some institutions; we have given up use of this test due to very poor predictive value. Latex particle testing of CSF for both GBS and *E. coli* K1 can be of use in evaluating CSF after the institution of antibiotic treatment.

6. **Lumbar puncture.** The use of routine lumbar puncture (LP) in the evaluation of **asymptomatic neonates** at risk for EOS remains controversial. A retrospective review of infants with culture-positive CSF taken from a population of 169,849 infants identified 8 infants with culture-positive CSF, but with negative blood cultures and no CNS symptoms. They con-

cluded that the selective use of LP in the evaluation of EOS may lead to missed diagnoses of meningitis. However, these infants were not all evaluated for sepsis in the absence of symptoms, and this study was complicated by a large number of hospitals and likely disparate culture systems. Another study reviewed the results of sepsis evaluations in a population of 24,452 infants from a single institution. This study found 11 cases of meningitis, all in symptomatic infants; 10 of 11 corresponding blood cultures were positive for the same organism. No cases of meningitis were found in 3423 asymptomatic infants evaluated with lumbar puncture.

Beginning in 1994, we stopped the routine use of lumbar puncture for the evaluation of **asymptomatic term infants** at risk for EOS. A review of our own data from 1996–2001, a period during which IAP for GBS was implemented using a screening-based approach, revealed 12 cases of culture-positive meningitis from a population of over 40,000 deliveries. Only two cases occurred in term infants; both infants grew GBS from both blood and CSF cultures and both infants were symptomatic.

It is our current policy to perform lumbar punctures only on (1) infants with positive blood cultures and (2) symptomatic infants with negative blood cultures who are treated empirically for the clinical diagnosis of sepsis. Whenever clinically feasible, lumbar punctures are performed on symptomatic infants with a high suspicion for sepsis before administering antibiotics. When lumbar punctures are performed after the administration of antibiotics, a clinical evaluation of the presence of meningitis is made, taking into account the blood culture results, the CSF cell count, protein, and glucose levels as well as the clinical scenario. Whenever the CSF is being examined after the administration of antibiotics, we recommend sending two separate CSF samples for cell count from the same lumbar puncture, to account for the role of possible fluctuation in CSF cell count measurements.

Normal CSF WBC counts in term, noninfected infants are variable, with most studies reporting a mean of less than 20 cells/mm^3, with ranges of up to 90 cells, and widely varying levels of polymorphonuclear cells on the differential. One recent study defined "noninfected" infants by negative bacterial blood, CSF and urine cultures, and negative viral CSF culture as well as negative enteroviral CSF PCR. This study reported a mean CSF WBC 7.3 (+/-14)/mm^3 with a range of 0 to 130 cells. The presence of blood in the CSF, due to subarachnoid or intraventricular hemorrhage, or to blood contamination of CSF samples by "traumatic" lumbar punctures, can yield abnormal cell counts that may be due to the presence of blood in the CSF rather than true infection. All these considerations emphasize the need for clinical judgment in the diagnosis of blood and CSF culture-negative meningitis.

H. Algorithm for the evaluation of the infant born at $\geq$ 35 weeks' gestation at risk for EOS. At the Brigham and Women's Hospital, we have recently revised our guidelines for the evaluation of asymptomatic, $\geq$35-week-gestation infants who are at risk for developing EOS. Our guidelines incorporate both the evaluation of infants based on maternal GBS colonization, and an evaluation of infants at risk of EOS due to maternal intrapartum risk factors (Figure 23.1). We use a total WBC < 5000 or an immature to total neutrophil ratio (I/T ratio) > 0.2 to guide treatment decisions in the evaluation of the well-appearing infant at risk for sepsis. A single WBC determination is used in most cases to avoid multiple blood draws from otherwise asymptomatic infants (although significantly abnormal values are usually confirmed within 12 to 24 hours). We also take into account the impact of a clustering of risk factors for sepsis to guide treatment decisions. These guidelines are based on a delivery service for which a screening-based approach to GBS prophylaxis has been in place since 1996, and for which approximately 90% of vaginal deliveries involve epidural placement (which alone can cause low-grade intrapartum fever). We use a

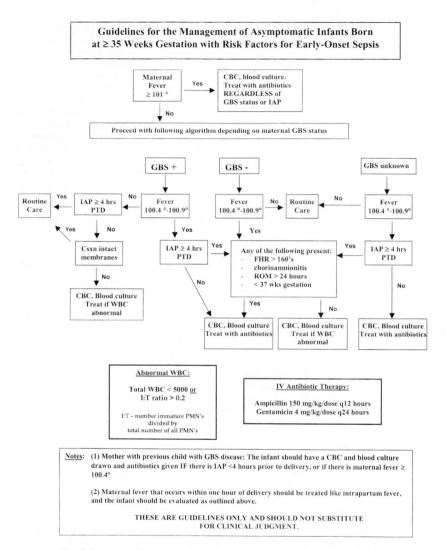

FIG. 23.1. Guidelines for the evaluation of asymptomatic infants at risk for EOS.

fever threshold of 100.4°F (38°C) for evaluation in accordance with CDC and other published recommendations.

I. Specific organisms causing EOS. The bacterial species responsible for EOS vary by locality and time period. In the United States since the 1980s, GBS has been the leading cause of neonatal EOS. Despite the implementation of IAP against GBS, it remains the leading cause of EOS in term infants. However, coincident with the increased use of intrapartum IAP for GBS, gram-negative enteric bacteria have become the leading cause of EOS in preterm infants. Enteric bacilli causing EOS include *E. coli, Bacteroides fragilis,* and *Enterobacter* species. Less common organisms that can cause serious early-onset disease include *Listeria monocytogenes* and *Citrobacter diversus*. Staphylococci and enterococci can be found in EOS but are more commonly causes of nosocomial sepsis and are discussed under that heading below. Fungal species can cause EOS primarily in preterm infants; this is also discussed separately below.

1. Group B streptococcus. GBS (*Streptococcus agalactiae*) frequently colonizes the human genital and gastrointestinal tracts, and the upper respiratory tract in young infants. In addition to causing neonatal disease, GBS is a frequent cause of urinary-tract infection, chorioamnionitis, postpartum endometritis, and bacteremia in pregnant woman. There is some evidence suggesting that vaginal colonization with a high inoculum of GBS during pregnancy contributes to premature birth.

   a. Microbiology. GBS are facultative diplococci that are easily cultivated in selective laboratory media. GBS are primarily identified by the Lancefield group B carbohydrate antigen, and are further subtyped into nine distinct serotypes (types Ia, Ib, II–VIII) by analysis of capsular polysaccharide composition. Most neonatal disease in the United States was originally caused by types Ia, Ib, II, and III; type V GBS have caused an increasing proportion of neonatal disease in the 1990s and are of importance since this type is frequently resistant to penicillin-alternate medications such as clindamycin, erythromycin, and tetracycline. Type III GBS are associated with the development of meningitis and are commonly a cause of late-onset GBS disease.

   b. Pathogenesis. Neonatal GBS infection is acquired in utero or during passage through the birth canal. Because not all women are colonized with GBS, documented colonization with GBS is the strongest predictor of GBS EOS. Approximately 20 to 30% of American women are colonized with GBS. A recent longitudinal study of GBS colonization in a cohort of primarily young, sexually active women demonstrated that 45% of initially GBS-negative women acquired colonization at some time over a 12-month period. In the absence of IAP, approximately 50% of infants born to mothers colonized with GBS are found to be colonized with this organism at birth, and 1 to 2% of colonized infants develop invasive GBS disease. Lack of maternally derived, protective capsular polysaccharide-specific antibody is associated with the development of invasive GBS disease. Other factors predisposing the newborn to GBS disease are less well understood, but relative deficiencies in complement, neutrophil function and innate immunity may be important.

   c. Clinical risk factors for GBS EOS. Heavy maternal colonization [vaginal inoculum >10^5 colony forming units (cfu)/mL] with GBS is associated with a higher risk of invasive disease. GBS bacteriuria during pregnancy is associated with heavy colonization of the rectovaginal tract, and is considered a significant risk factor for EOS. Black race and maternal age <20 years are associated with higher rates of GBS EOS, although it is not entirely clear whether this reflects only higher rates of GBS colonization in these populations. The odds ratios for the development of GBS EOS by specific risk factor are shown in Table 23.5. Although multiple gestation has been reported as a risk factor GBS EOS, when controlled for disease concordance between twins and the effect of low birth weight, it is **not** an independent risk factor for the development of GBS disease.

   d. Prevention of GBS infection. Since the 1980s, a number of antibiotic-based strategies have been proposed to prevent neonatal GBS disease. These include (1) antenatal treatment of pregnant women to eliminate colonization; (2) treatment of all women during labor who have specific risk factors for early-onset GBS infection (the "risk factor–based approach"); (3) screening pregnant women for GBS colonization and antibiotic treatment during labor for those colonized (the "screening-based approach."). Antepartum treatment of colonized women was shown

TABLE 23.5. RISK FACTORS FOR EARLY-ONSET GBS SEPSIS IN THE ABSENCE OF IAP

Risk Factor	Odds Ratio (95% CI)
Maternal GBS colonization	204 (100–419)
BW < 1000 g	24.8 (12.2–50.2)
BW < 2500 g	7.37 (4.48–12.1)
Prolonged ROM > 18 h	7.28 (4.42–12.0)
Chorioamnionitis	6.42 (2.32–17.8)
Intrapartum fever >37.5°C	4.05 (2.17–7.56)

CI, confidence interval; ROM, rupture of membranes.
Adapted from Benitz W.E., Gould J.B., Druzin M.M.L. Risk factors for early-onset group B streptococcal sepsis: Estimation of odds ratios by critical literature review. *Pediatrics* 1999;103(6):e77.

to be ineffective in preventing GBS EOS, but multiple trials demonstrated that the use of intrapartum penicillin or ampicillin significantly reduced the rate of neonatal colonization with GBS and the incidence of early-onset GBS disease. In 1996, the Centers for Disease Control (CDC) published consensus guidelines for the prevention of neonatal GBS disease that endorsed the use of **either** a risk factor-based or screening based approach. These guidelines were endorsed by the American Academy of Pediatric (AAP) and American Academy of Obstetricians and Gynecologists (ACOG) and led to the widespread implementation of IAP.

Active surveillance by the CDC revealed that with the use of IAP, the incidence of GBS EOS fell from 1.7 cases per 1000 births in 1993 to 0.6 cases per 1000 births in 1998. In July 2002, the CDC published the results of a retrospective cohort study of 629,912 births comparing the use of the risk factor-based approach to the screening approach in preventing GBS EOS. This study demonstrated that the screening-based approach prevented more cases of GBS disease than did the risk factor–based approach. With this information, as well as with the knowledge gained from multiple epidemiologic studies of IAP implementation and its clinical and microbiological consequences, the CDC issued revised guidelines for the prevention of early onset GBS disease in August 2002. These guidelines, "Preventon of Perinatal Group B Streptococcal Disease," (*MMWR* 1 Vol. 51, No. RR11:1–22, 08/16/2002) can be accessed on the Internet at http://www.cdc.gov/mmwr/preview/mmwrhtml/rr5111a1.htm or in PDF form at http://www.cdc.gov/mmwr/PDF/RR/RR5111.pdf. The highlight of the revised guidelines is the recommendation of **universal screening of pregnant women for GBS by rectovaginal culture are 35 to 37 weeks' gestation and management of IAP based on screening results** (Figure 23.2). There are two exceptions to the recommendation for universal screening. Pregnant women with documented GBS bacteriuria during pregnancy or who previously delivered an infant who developed invasive GBS disease need not be screened as these women should be given IAP **regardless of current GBS colonization status.** Recommendations were also made for the use of GBS prophylaxis in women experiencing threatened preterm labor (Figure 23.3).

The revised guidelines addressed concerns over the documented emergence of GBS resistance to erythromycin and clindamycin, antibiotics frequently used for IAP in the penicillin-allergic woman. The

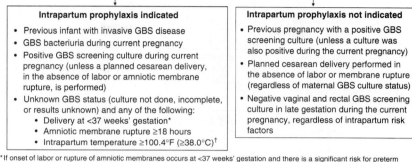

Intrapartum prophylaxis indicated	Intrapartum prophylaxis not indicated

• Previous infant with invasive GBS disease
• GBS bacteriuria during current pregnancy
• Positive GBS screening culture during current pregnancy (unless a planned cesarean delivery, in the absence of labor or amniotic membrane rupture, is performed)
• Unknown GBS status (culture not done, incomplete, or results unknown) and any of the following:
  • Delivery at <37 weeks' gestation*
  • Amniotic membrane rupture ≥18 hours
  • Intrapartum temperature ≥100.4°F (≥38.0°C)†
	• Previous pregnancy with a positive GBS screening culture (unless a culture was also positive during the current pregnancy)
	• Planned cesarean delivery performed in the absence of labor or membrane rupture (regardless of maternal GBS culture status)
	• Negative vaginal and rectal GBS screening culture in late gestation during the current pregnancy, regardless of intrapartum risk factors

*If onset of labor or rupture of amniotic membranes occurs at <37 weeks' gestation and there is a significant risk for preterm delivery (as assessed by the clinician), a suggested algorithm for GBS prophylaxis management is provided (Figure 3).

†If amnionitis is suspected, broad-spectrum antibiotic therapy that includes an agent known to be active against GBS should replace GBS prophylaxis.

FIG. 23.2. *2002 CDC Revised Guidelines for the Prevention of Early Onset GBS Disease.* Indications for intrapartum antibiotic prophylaxis to prevent perinatal GBS disease under a universal prenatal screening strategy based on combined vaginal and rectal cultures collected at 35 to 37 weeks' gestation from all pregnant women.

CDC continues to recommend penicillin or ampicillin for IAP. In the penicillin-allergic woman, it is now recommended that any GBS isolates identified on screening be tested for antibiotic susceptibility. For the woman deemed to be **not at high risk** for penicillin anaphylaxis, cefazolin is recommended for IAP; for the woman deemed to be at high risk for anaphylaxis, clindamycin or erythromycin are recommended for sensitive strains; vancomycin is recommended if resistance is documented or susceptibility data is unavailable. No data on the efficacy of any antibiotic other than ampicillin or penicillin in preventing neonatal GBS colonization or disease are available.

The development of a **vaccine for GBS** could eliminate the need for most IAP. Capsular polysaccharide-based vaccines alone and polysaccharide-tetanus toxoid vaccines have been developed and tested in phase I and II trials. For greatest efficacy, the development of a multivalent vaccine (serotypes Ia, Ib, II, III, and V) or the inclusion of a GBS protein common to most serotypes will be needed.

e. **Evaluation of infants after maternal GBS IAP.** The revised guidelines include a recommended algorithm for the evaluation of infants born to mothers exposed to IAP. **We have incorporated these guidelines into our policy for the evaluation of the asymptomatic (≥ 35-week) infant at risk for early-onset sepsis** (Figure 23.1).

f. **Treatment of infants with invasive GBS disease.** When GBS is identified as the sole causative organism in EOS, empiric antibiotic treatment should be narrowed to ampicillin (200 to 300 mg/kg per day) penicillin G (200,000 to 400,000 U/kg per day) alone, with the higher dosing reserved for cases complicated by meningitis. The total duration of therapy should be at least 10 days for sepsis without a focus, 21 days for meningitis, and 28 days for osteomyelitis. Bone and joint

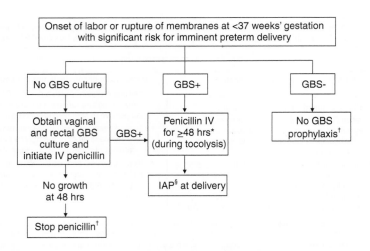

* Penicillin should be continued for a total of at least 48 hours, unless delivery occurs sooner. At the physician's discretion, antibiotic prophylaxis may be continued beyond 48 hours in a GBS culture-positive woman if delivery has not yet occurred. For women who are GBS culture positive, antibiotic prophylaxis should be reinitiated when labor likely to proceed to delivery occurs or recurs.
† If delivery has not occurred within 4 weeks, a vaginal and rectal GBS screening culture should be repeated and the patient should be managed as described, based on the result of the repeat culture.
§ Intrapartum antibiotic prophylaxis.

FIG. 23.3. *2002 CDC Revised Guidelines for the Prevention of Early Onset GBS Disease.* Sample algorithm for GBS prophylaxis for women with threatened preterm delivery. This algorithm is not an exclusive course of management. Variations that incorporate individual circumstances or institutional preferences may be appropriate.

infections that involve the hip or shoulder require surgical drainage in addition to antibiotic therapy.

    g. Recurrent GBS infection. Recurrent GBS infections are infrequent, with reported incidences ranging from 1 to 6%. Infants usually fail to have a specific antibody response after infection with GBS, and GBS can be isolated from mucosal surfaces of infants even after appropriate antibiotic treatment for invasive disease. Occasionally reinfection with a new strain of GBS occurs. Treatment of recurrent GBS infections is the same as for primary infection except that susceptibility testing of the GBS strain to penicillin is recommended if not routinely performed. Rifampin, which eliminates colonization in other infections such as meningococcal disease, does not reliably eradicate mucous membrane colonization with GBS.

  2. *Escherichia coli* and other enteric gram-negative bacilli. Before the widespread implementation of IAP against GBS, *E. coli* was the second leading cause of EOS bacteremia and sepsis among both term and preterm infants. With the implementation of IAP against GBS, the incidence of EOS with gram-negative enteric bacilli may be increasing, particularly among very-low-birth-weight (VLBW) infants.

    Ampicillin-resistant *E. coli* infections are increasing among preterm infants. In a recent study of EOS in VLBW infants, the reduction in the incidence of EOS caused by GBS (from 5.9 to 1.7/1000 live births) was accompanied by an absolute increase in the incidence of *E. coli* EOS (3.2 to 6.8/1000 live births). Eighty-five percent of the cases of *E. coli* EOS were caused by organisms that were ampicillin-resistant. More exposure to maternal antibiotics before delivery was observed in the infants with ampicillin-resistant infections. Large-scale multicenter studies confirm smaller reports of an increase in ampicillin-resistant *E. coli* isolates accompanying the implementation of IAP against GBS. An analysis of our own data from 1996–2001 also reveals an increase in EOS caused by ampicillin-resistant gram-negative organisms among preterm infants.

a. **Microbiology and pathogenesis.** *E. coli* are aerobic gram-negative rods found universally in the human intestinal tract and commonly in the human vagina and urinary tract. There are hundreds of different LPS, flagellar, and capsular antigenic types of *E. coli*, but EOS *E. coli* infections, particularly those complicated by meningitis, are primarily due to strains with the K1-type polysaccharide capsule. *E. coli* with the K1 antigen are resistant to the bacteriocidal effect of normal human serum; strains that possess both a complete LPS and K1 capsule have been shown to specifically evade both complement-mediated bacteriolysis and neutrophil-mediated killing. The K1 antigen has been shown to be a primary factor in the development of meningitis in a rat model of *E. coli* infection. The K1 capsule is a poor immunogen, however, and despite widespread carriage of this strain in the population, there is usually little protective maternal antibody available to the infant. In addition to the K1 antigen, surface fimbriae or pili are have been associated with adherence to vaginal and uroepithelial surfaces and may also function as a virulence mechanism in EOS.

b. **Treatment.** As noted above, when there is a strong clinical suspicion for sepsis in a critically ill infant, the possibility of ampicillin-resistant *E. coli* must be considered. The addition of a third-generation cephalosporin such as cefotaxime or ceftazidime is recommended in this setting. *E. coli* bacteremia should be treated with a total of 14 days of antibiotic according to the identified sensitivities. *E. coli* meningitis is treated with a 21-day course of cefotaxime (see Tables 23.3 and 23.4).

3. **Listeria monocytogenes.** Although uncommon, *Listeria monocytogenes* deserves special note due to its unique role in pregnancy. *Listeria monocytogenes* are gram-positive, beta-hemolytic, motile bacteria that frequently cause disease in animals, and most commonly infect humans via the ingestion of contaminated food. These bacteria do not cause significant disease in immunocompetent adults, but can cause severe illness in the immunocompromised (i.e., renal transplant patients), in pregnant women and their fetuses, and in newborns. There is human epidemiologic evidence and evidence in animal models of listeriosis that indicate that *L. monocytogenes* is particularly virulent in pregnancy. The bacteria readily invades the placenta and can infect the developing fetus either by ascending infection, direct tissue invasion or hematogenous spread, causing spontaneous abortion or preterm labor and delivery, and often fulminant early-onset disease. Like GBS, *L. monocytogenes* can also cause late-onset neonatal infection, the pathogenesis of which is not fully understood. Over 90% of late-onset infections are complicated by meningitis.

The true incidence of listeriosis in pregnancy is difficult to determine because many cases are undiagnosed when they result in spontaneous abortion of the previable fetus. The incidence of EOS due to *L. monocytogenes* is often quoted as 13 cases per 100,000 live births; the incidence in the recent CDC active surveillance effort in Atlanta and San Francisco was 2.4 cases per 100,000 live births. Listeriosis can result from ingestion of contaminated food such as soft cheeses, deli meat, and hot dogs. Infection in pregnant woman may not be recognized, or may cause a mild febrile illness with or without gastrointestinal symptoms before resulting in pregnancy loss or preterm labor. Epidemic outbreaks of listerosis affecting both pregnant and nonpregnant adults are reported. Epidemic outbreaks in the United States in 2000 and 2002 were linked to turkey deli meat; an outbreak in 2001 linked to homemade, unpasteurized Mexican-style cheese

that resulted in five stillbirths, three premature deliveries, and two infected newborns among ten infected pregnant women.
  a. **Microbiology and pathogenesis.** L. *monocytogenes* are distinguished
     from other gram-positive rods by tumbling motility that is most promi-
     nent at room temperature. The organisms can be gram-variable and
     depending on growth stage, can also appear coccilike, and can thus be ini-
     tially misdiagnosed on gram stain. L. *monocytogenes* is an intracellular
     pathogen that can invade cells as well as persist in phagocytic cells
     (monocytes, macrophages.) *Listeria* possess a variety of virulence fac-
     tors, including surface proteins that promote cellular invasion, and en-
     zymes (listeriolysin O, phospholipase) that enhance the ability of the
     organism to persist intracellularly. On pathologic examination of tis-
     sues infected with *Listeria*, miliary granulomas and areas of necrosis
     and suppuration are seen. The liver is prominently involved. Both T-cell-
     mediated killing as well as immunoglobulin M (IgM)-complement-medi-
     ated killing are involved in host response to listeriosis. Deficiencies in
     both of these arms of the newborn immune system may contribute to the
     virulence of L. *monocytogenes* in the neonate; similarly, it is hypothesized
     that local downregulation of the immune response in the pregnant
     uterus may account for proliferation of the bacteria in the placenta.
  b. **Treatment.** EOS due to L. *monocytogenes* is treated with ampicillin and
     gentamicin for 14 days; meningitis is treated for 21 days. L. *monocyto-
     genes* is resistant to cephalosporins. In the case of meningitis, it is recom-
     mended that lumbar punctures be repeated daily until sterilization of
     the CSF is achieved. Additional therapy with rifampin or trimethoprim-
     sulfamethoxazole, as well as cerebral imaging is recommended if the or-
     ganism persists in the CSF for longer than 2 days. We have noted that
     L. *monocytogenes* can persist in the stool of preterm infants even after ad-
     equate systemic treatment of the infection. Proper infection control mea-
     sures must be observed to prevent nosocomial spread of the organism.
4. **Other organisms responsible for EOS.** Bacteria causing EOS vary with
   time and locality. Beyond GBS and *E. coli*, there are a number of pathogens that cause EOS in the United States in the era of IAP for GBS.
   Viridans streptococci (species such as *Streptococcus mitis, Streptococcus
   oralis, and Streptococcus sanguis*, which are part of the oral flora), Enterococci and *Staphylococcus aureus* are next in frequency. *Listeria*, a variety of gram-negative organisms (*Klebsiella, Hemophilus, Enterobacter,
   Pseudomonas* species) and the anaerobe *Bacteroides fragilis* cause most
   of the remaining infections. Gram-negative organisms, especially *H. influenzae* and *Klebsiella*, predominate in some Asian and South American
   countries.
J. **Late-onset sepsis.** Late-onset neonatal sepsis (LOS) is defined as occurring
   from 8 to 90 days of life. LOS can be divided into two distinct entities: disease occurring in otherwise healthy term infants in the community, and disease affecting premature infants in the neonatal intensive care unit (NICU).
   The latter is often referred to as nosocomial sepsis, as the risk factors for
   LOS in premature infants are related to the necessities of their care (i.e., the
   presence of central lines) and the bacteria that cause LOS are often acquired
   in the NICU.
     This section is largely devoted to LOS in the NICU population, but disease
   in **healthy term infants** deserves mention. In these infants, LOS is largely
   caused by GBS and gram-negative species such as *E. coli* and *Klebsiella*
   species. Causes of bacteremia in older infants (such as *Streptococcus pneumoniae, and Neisseria meningitidis*) occur less frequently.
     The **risk factors for late-onset GBS disease** are not as well defined as for
   early-onset disease, but like early-onset disease are related to colonization
   of the infant from maternal (or less commonly, hospital) sources and lack of
   maternally derived protective antibody. The use of IAP for GBS has had
   no significant impact on late-onset disease; the rate of LOS due to GBS has

remained constant at from 1990–1998 at approximately 0.3–0.5 cases per 1000 live births. Late-onset GBS disease is more often complicated by meningitis that early-onset disease, and is predominantly caused by polysaccharide serotype III strains. Research suggests that both inherent characteristics of the type III polysaccharide capsule as well as other virulence factors specific to type III strains account for the predominance of these strains in late-onset disease. Mortality from GBS meningitis is reported in older case series as 20 to 25%, and sequelae in survivors can be severe, ranging from hearing loss to severe global brain damage. **Gram-negative bacteremia** is often associated with urinary-tract infection (UTI). Different series report 20 to 30% of UTIs in infants under a month old are complicated by bacteremia. Mortality is low if promptly treated, and sequelae are few unless meningitis occurs. *Listeria monocytogenes* can also cause late-onset disease, with onset commonly by 30 days of life, and can account for up to 20% of LOS in some centers. Late-onset listeriosis is frequently complicated by meningitis, but unlike late-onset GBS meningitis, the morbidity and long-term sequelae are infrequent if the disease is diagnosed and treated in timely fashion.

Term infants with LOS generally present with fever and/or poor feeding and lethargy to the private pediatrician or emergency department. Evaluation in the infant less than 3 months old in most centers includes at minimium a CBC, urinalysis, CSF cell count, glucose and protein and cultures of blood, urine, and CSF. Infants under a month old are generally hospitalized for empiric IV therapy that includes coverage for GBS, *Listeria*, and gram-negative organisms (commonly ampicillin and cefotaxime); over a month of age, management varies in different centers.

K. Epidemiology of LOS in premature infants. The majority of late-onset sepsis occurs in the NICU among low-birth-weight infants. The National Institute of Child Health and Human Development (NICHD) Neonatal Research Network data from 1998–2000 revealed that 21% of their VLBW cohort had at least one episode of blood-culture-proven sepsis beyond 3 days of life. The Network data demonstrate no significant change in mortality statistics over these periods. Overall mortality was 17 to 18% of infected infants versus 7% of uninfected infants in both cohorts. The mortality among infants with gram-negative infections was about 40%, and 30% with fungal infections.

L. Risk factors for LOS. A number of clinical factors are associated with an increased risk of late-onset sepsis (Table 23.6). The incidence of LOS is inversely related to birth weight. The risk of developing LOS associated with central catheters, hyperalimentation, and mechanical ventilation are all increased with longer duration of these therapies.

M. Microbiology of late-onset sepsis. Nearly half of the cases of LOS are caused by coagulase-negative staphylococci (CONS). In the NICHD study, 22% of cases of LOS were caused by other gram-positive organisms (GBS, *S. aureus*, Enterococcus); 18% by gram-negative organisms (*E. coli, Klebsiella, Pseudomonas, Enterobacter, Serratia*), and 12 % by fungal species (*Candida albicans* and *Candida parapsilosis*).

  1. Coagulase-negative staphylococcus (CONS). CONS are a heterogeneous group of gram-positive organisms with a structure similar to *S. aureus*, but these organisms lack protein A and have different cell wall components. *Staphylococcus epidermidis* is the primary cause of NICU disease. CONS universally colonize the skin of NICU patients. They are believed to cause bacteremia by first colonizing the surfaces of central catheters. A polysaccharide surface adhesin (PSA), as well as several other surface components have been implicated in adherence to and colonization of the catheter surface; subsequent biofilm and slime production inhibit the ability of the host to eliminate the organism. Most CONS are resistant to penicillin, semisynthetic penicillins, and gentamicin, and empiric treatment for LOS in the NICU usually includes vancomycin. CONS disease is rarely fatal even to the VLBW infant, and rarely if ever causes

TABLE 23.6. RISK FACTORS FOR LATE-ONSET SEPSIS IN INFANTS WITH BIRTH WEIGHT <1500 G

Birth weight < 750 g

Presence of central venous catheters (umbilical, percutaneous, and tunneled)

Delayed enteral feeding

Prolonged hyperalimentation

Mechanical ventilation

Complications of prematurity
  Patent ductus arteriosus
  Bronchopulmonary dysplasia
  Necrotizing enterocolitis (NEC)

Adapted from Stoll B.J., et al. Late onset sepsis in very low birth weight neonates: The experience of the NICHD Neonatal Research Network. *Pediatrics* 2002;110(2): 285–291 and Makhoul I.R., et al. Epidemiological, clinical and microbiological characteristics of late-onset sepsis among very low birth weight infants in Israel: A national survey. *Pediatrics* 2002;109(1): 34–39.

meningitis or site-specific disease. However, CONS disease can cause systemic instability resulting in temporary cessation of enteral feeding and/or escalation of ventilatory support, and is associated with prolonged hospitalization and poorer overall outcome.

2. **Staphylococcus aureus.** *S. aureus* is an encapsulated gram-positive organism that elaborates multiple adhesins, virulence-associated enzymes, and toxins to cause a wide range of serious disease, including bacteremia, meningitis, cellulitis, omphalitis, osteomyelitis, and arthritis. *S. aureus* is distinguished from CONS by the production of coagulase, and by the presence of protein A, a component of the cell wall that contributes to virulence by binding to the Fc portion of immunoglobulin G (IgG) antibody and blocking opsonization. LOS caused by *S. aureus* can be result in significant morbidity. Disease complicated by deep tissue infection is often marked by persistent bacteremia despite antibiotic administration. Joint infections often require open surgical drainage and can lead to joint destruction and permanent disability. The treatment of *S. aureus* requires the use of semisynthetic penicillins such as nafcillin or oxacillin. Methicillin-resistant organisms (MRSA) are an increasing problem in both neonatal and adult intensive-care units and require treatment with vancomycin. MRSA can be spread within the NICU in epidemic and endemic fashion. Infection control measures including identification of colonized infants by routine surveillance and cohorting and isolation of colonized infants may be required to prevent spread and persistence of the organism.

3. **Enterococci.** Formerly categorized as members of Group D Streptococci, both *Enterococcus faecalis* and *Enterococcus faecium* cause LOS in premature infants. These organisms are associated with indwelling catheters; they are encapsulated organisms that produce both biofilm and slime and can adhere to and persist on catheter surfaces as described above for CONS. Although disease can be complicated by meningitis and is sometimes associated with necrotizing enterocolitis (NEC), enterococcal LOS is associated with low overall mortality. Enterococci are resistant to cephalosporins and often resistant to penicillin G and ampicillin; treatment requires the synergistic effect of an aminoglycoside with ampicillin or vancomycin. Vancomycin-resistant enterococci (VRE) present a significant problem in adult intensive-care settings, and outbreaks have occurred in NICUs as well. VRE

of *faecium* origin can be treated with Synercid (quinupristin/dalfopristin) but this combination is not effective against *Enterococcus faecalis*. VRE outbreaks may also require the institution of infection control measures (surveillance to identify colonized infants, isolation and cohorting of those colonized) to control spread and persistence of the organism.

4. **Gram negative organisms:** LOS caused by gram-negative organisms is complicated by a 40% mortality rate in the NICHD cohort. *E. coli* were discussed under EOS (see I.1.2).

   a. ***Pseuodomonas aeruginosa.*** Mortality associated with *P. aeruginosa* sepsis in low-birth-weight infants is high–(76% in the NICHD cohort). A number of bacterial factors, including lipopolysaccharide (LPS), mucoid capsule, adhesins, invasins, and toxins (notably exotoxin A) contribute to its extreme virulence in premature infants as well as in debilitated adults and burn victims. Both LPS and the mucoid capsule help the organism avoid opsonization and secreted proteases inactivate complement, cytokines, and immunoglobulin. The lipid A moiety of LPS (endotoxin) causes the typical aspects of gram-negative septicemia (i.e., hypotension, DIC). Exotoxin A is antigenically distinct from diptheria toxin, but acts by the same mechanism: adenovirus death protein (ADP)-ribosylation of eukaryotic elongation factor 2 results in inhibition of protein synthesis and cell death. *P. aeruginosa* is present in the intestinal tract of approximately 5% of healthy adults, but colonizes premature infants at much higher rates due to nosocomial acquisition of the bacteria. Selection of the bacteria, likely due to the resistance of *Pseudomonas* to most common antibiotics, also plays a role in colonization; prolonged exposure to intravenous antibiotics is an identified risk factor for LOS with *Pseudomonas. Pseudomonas* can be found in environmental reservoirs in ICUs (i.e., sinks, respiratory equipment), and outbreaks of nosocomial disease have been linked to both environmental sources and spread by the hands of healthcare workers.

   Treatment requires a combination of two agents active against *Pseudomonas*, such as ceftazidime, piperacillin/tazobactam, gentamicin, or tobramycin. Generally a beta-lactam–based antibiotic combined with an aminoglycoside is preferred. A survey of neonatologists' practices in the treatment of LOS reveals that the most common antibiotics empirically used are vancomycin and gentamicin. When an infant presents as severely ill, or when the infant becomes acutely sicker during or after standard antibiotic treatment, consideration should be given to empiric coverage for *Pseudomonas* until blood culture results are available.

   b. ***Enterobacter species:*** Like *E. coli, Enterobacter* species are LPS-containing, gram-negative rods that are normal constituents of colonic flora that can cause overwhelming sepsis in low-birth-weight infants. The most common isolates are *Enterobacter cloacae* and *Enterobacter aerogenes. Enterobacter sakazakii* has received recent publicity due to outbreaks of disease caused by contamination of powdered infant formulas with this organism. *Enterobacter* species contain chromosomally encoded, inducible beta-lactamases and treatment with cephalosporins, even if the initial isolate appears to be sensitive to cephalosporins, can result in the emergence of cephalosporin-resistant organisms. Expression of a multidrug efflux pump in *Enterobacter* has also been reported. Since 1990, there are multiple reports of increases in the proportion of LOS attributable to *Enterobacter*, and as well as epidemic outbreaks of resistant *Enterobacter* in NICUs. Infection control measures and restriction of cephalosporin use, are effective in controlling outbreaks of resistant organisms. The fourth-generation cephalosporin cefipime was initially thought to be less likely to induce cephalosporin resistance, but cefipime resistance has now been reported. Despite these known characteristics of *Enterobacter*, most authorities endorse the treatment of infants with beta-lactam antibiotics (including cephalosporins), guided by the resistance profile of the isolate. Meropenem and an aminoglycoside are often effective in treatment of cephalosporin-resistant isolates.

N. **Symptoms and evaluation of LOS.** The spectrum of symptoms in LOS ranges from a mild increase in apnea to fulminant sepsis. Lethargy, an increase in the number or severity of apneic spells, feeding intolerance, temperature instability, and/or an increase in ventilatory support all may be early signs of LOS—or may be part of the variability in the course of the VLBW infant. The difficulty in distinguishing between these two in part explains the frequency of evaluation for LOS; in the NICHD study, 62% of VLBW infants had at least one blood culture drawn after day of life 3. With mild symptoms and a low suspicion for the presence of sepsis, it is reasonable to draw a CBC with differential and a blood culture and wait for the results of the CBC (while monitoring the infant's symptoms closely) before beginning empiric antibiotic therapy. If the CBC is abnormal or the infant's status worsens, empiric antibiotic therapy should be started. If the suspicion for sepsis is still low, and/or the clinical impression is that a CONS infection is likely, it is not unreasonable to obtain a blood culture only. Ideally cultures of urine and CSF should also be obtained prior to antibiotic therapy, both to guide empiric therapy and to ensure proper follow-up (such as renal imaging if a UTI is present.) If a previously well, convalescing premature infant presents primarily with increased apnea with or without UTI symptoms, consideration should be given to a viral source of infection as well. Tracheal or nasal aspirate should be sent for rapid analysis and culture to rule out respiratory syncytial virus (RSV), parainfluenze, and influenzae A and B if seasonally appropriate.

O. **Treatment of LOS.** Tables 23.3 and 23.4 list suggested antibiotic regimens for selected organisms. Note that for many antibiotics dosing is dependent on gestational and postnatal age (see also Appendix A). A recent study addressed the issue of **central line removal** in culture-proven LOS. This study demonstrated that bacteremic infants experience fewer complications of infection if central lines are removed promptly upon identification of a positive culture. This was particularly true for infections caused by *S. aureus* and gram-negative organisms.

P. **Prevention of LOS.** In addition to significant mortality, LOS is associated with prolonged hospitalization and overall poorer outcome in VLBW infants compared to those that remain uninfected. A number of strategies to lower rates of LOS have been studied.

1. **Intravenous immunoglobulin.** Multiple studies have been conducted using prophylactic administration of IVIG to address the relative deficiency of immunoglobulin in low-birth-weight infants and prevent LOS. A meta-analysis of these 19 trials revealed that although the use of IVIG to prevent LOS resulted in a 3 to 4% decrease in LOS, IVIG was not associated with a decrease in mortality or other serious outcomes and is generally not recommended.

2. **Granulocyte-stimulation colony factor.** GCSF has been shown to resolve preeclampsia–associated neutropenia, and may thus decrease the rate of LOS in this population of infants. One trial of GM-CSF in premature neonates with the clinical diagnosis of early-onset disease did not improve mortality but was associated with acquiring fewer nosocomial infections over the subsequent 2 weeks.

3. **Antibiotic restriction.** Limitation of the use of broad-spectrum antibiotics in neonatal, pediatric and adult ICUs has been inconsistently associated with decreases rates of patient colonization with antibiotic-resistant organisms. This practice is reported to be successful in case reports of outbreaks of specific antibiotic-resistant organisms, but has failed in other reports to reduce overall acquisition of antibiotic-resistant organisms. Cy-

cling of antibiotics used for empiric treatment has not been successful in preventing LOS. However, other studies suggest that substitution of oxacillin for vancomycin in the empiric treatment of LOS is not likely to cause significant morbidity in VLBW infants because of the low virulence of the organism, and may decrease the acquisition and spread of VRE and other antibiotic-resistant organisms.

4. **Hygiene practices.** Reinforcement of hand-washing policies, use of waterless hand disinfectants, restriction of artificial fingernails and nail polish, and cohorting and isolation of patients colonized with resistant organisms, have all been reported to decrease the risk of LOS.

5. **Prophylactic vancomycin.** A meta-analysis of several trials of low-dose vancomycin administration to VLBW infants demonstrated that the administration of prophylactic vancomycin reduced the incidence of both total LOS and CONS-associated infections, but did not improve mortality or length of hospitalization. Prophylactic vancomycin IV lock solution has been studied with some success in decreasing CONS infection. Antibiotic-impregnated catheters are not currently available for VLBW infants. There is concern that widespread use of vancomycin in these ways will lead to the increased emergence of vancomycin-resistant organisms.

6. **Establishment of early enteral feedings** in VLBW infants may have the greatest effect on reducing LOS by reducing exposure to hyperalimentation and allowing for decreased use of central catheters. **Breast-milk** feeding may also help decrease nosocomial infection rates among VLBW infants, both by its numerous infection-protective properties [i.e., secretory immunoglobulin A (IgA), lactoferrin, lysozyme] and by aiding in the establishment of enteral feeds. A retrospective cohort study of 212 VLBW infants from a single center revealed lower rates of LOS in infants receiving breast milk (29%) versus infants receiving formula (47%).

II. **Anaerobic Bacterial Infections.** Anaerobic bacteria comprise a significant portion of the oral, vaginal, and gastrointestinal flora. Although many anaerobes are of low virulence, a few anaerobic organisms can cause both EOS and LOS. These organisms include *Bacteroides fragilis, Peptostreptococcus,* and *Clostridia perfringens.* Necrotizing entercolitis and/or bowel perforation can be complicated by anaerobic sepsis alone or in a polymicrobial infection. In addition to bacteremia, *B. fragilis* can cause abdominal abscesses, meningitis, omphalitis, cellulitis at the site of fetal scalp monitors, endocarditis, osteomyelitis and arthritis in the neonate.

A. **Treatment of anaerobic infections.** Bacteremia and/or meningitis are treated with intravenous antibiotics; abscesses and other focal infections often require surgical drainage. *B. fragilis* is a gram-negative rod, and although oral *Bacteroides* species are sensitive to penicillin, *B. fragilis* usually requires treatment with drugs such as metronidazole, chloramphenicol, clindamycin, cefoxitin, or imipenem. Occasional strains of *B. fragilis* are also resistant to clindamycin, cefoxitin and/or imipenem. Most other cephalosporins and vancomycin are ineffective against *B. fragilis. Peptostreptococcus* and *Clostridia* are gram-positive organisms that are sensitive to penicillin G. NEC and intestinal perforations are treated with ampicillin, gentamicin, and clindamycin to provide coverage for the spectrum of organisms that can complicate these illnesses.

B. **Neonatal tetanus.** This syndrome is caused by the effect of a neurotoxin produced by the anaerobic bacterium *Clostridium tetani.* It is a significant cause of neonatal mortality in developing countries. In 1993, the World Health Organization (WHO) estimated that 515,000 neonatal deaths were caused by neonatal tetanus for a global mortality rate of 4.1 deaths per 1000 live births. Infection can occur by invasion of the umbilical cord due to unsanitary childbirth or cord care practices. Due to maternal immunization and sanitary health practices, this disease is virtually nonexistent in the United States. The last reported case of neonatal tetanus in the United States is from 1998, and was caused by the application of cosmetic clay to the umbilical stump of an infant born to an unvaccinated mother. Infected infants develop hypertonia and muscle spasms including trismus and consequent inability to feed. Treatment consists of the administration of tetanus toxoid (500 U IM) and penicillin G (100 to 300,000 U/kg per day for 10 to 14 days) as well as supportive care with mechanical ventilation, sedatives, and muscle relaxants. Neonatal tetanus does not result in immunity to tetanus and infants require standard tetanus immunizations after recovery.

III. **Fungal Infections**
  A. **Mucocutaneous candidiasis.** Fungal infections in the well term infant are generally limited to mucocutaneous disease involving *Candida albicans*. *Candida* species are normal commensal flora beyond the neonatal period and rarely cause serious disease in the immunocompetent host. Immaturity of host defenses and colonization with *Candida* prior to complete establishment of normal intestinal flora probably contribute to the pathogenicity of *Candida* in the neonate. Oral and gastrointestinal colonization with *Candida* occurs prior to the development of oral candidiasis (thrush) or diaper dermatitis. *Candida* can be acquired via the birth canal, or via the hands or breast of caretakers. Nosocomial transmission in the nursery setting has been documented, as has transmission from feeding bottles and pacifiers.

  Oral candidiasis in the young infant is treated with a nonabsorbable oral antifungal medication, which has the advantages of little systemic toxicity and concomitant treatment of the intestinal tract. **Nystatin** oral suspension (100,000 U/mL) is standard treatment (1 mL is applied to each side of the mouth every 6 hours, for a minimum of 10 to 14 days). Ideally treatment is continued for several days after lesions resolve. **Gentian violet** (1%, applied once or twice) remains an approved and effective treatment for thrush, but it does not eliminate intestinal fungal colonization. This topical dye has fallen out of favor in the United States; it stains skin and clothing, can irritate the mucosa with prolonged use, and has been shown to be mutagenic *in vitro*. **Miconazole** oral gel (20 mg/g) is more effective than nystatin, but is not available in the United States. Systemic **fluconazole** is highly effective in treating chronic mucocutaneous candidiasis in the immunocompromised host. A recent small pilot study demonstrated the superiority of oral fluconazole over nystatin suspension in curing thrush in otherwise healthy infants, but fluconazole is not currently approved for this use. Infants with chronic, severe thrush refractory to treatment should be evaluated for an underlying congenital or acquired immunodeficiency.

  Oral candidiasis in the **breastfed infant** is often associated with superficial or ductal candidiasis in the mother's breast. Concurrent treatment of both the mother and infant is necessary to eliminate continual cross-infection. Breastfeeding of term infants can continue during treatment. Mothers with breast ductal candidiasis who are providing expressed breast milk for VLBW infants should be advised to withhold expressed milk until treatment has been instituted. Freezing does not eliminate *Candida* from expressed breast milk.

  Candidal diaper dermatitis is effectively treated with topical agents such as 2% nystatin ointment, 2% miconazole ointment, or 1% clotrimazole cream. Concomitant treatment with oral nystatin to eliminated intestinal colonization is often recommended, but not well studied. It is reasonable to use simultaneous oral and topical therapy for refractory candidal diaper dermatitis.

  B. **Systemic candidiasis.** Systemic candidiasis is a serious form of nosocomial infection in VLBW infants. Recent data on late-onset sepsis from the NICHD Neonatal Research Network showed that 12% of cases of late-onset sepsis were caused by fungal species, primarily *Candida albicans* and *Candida parapsilosis*, and one-third of those infants died. Invasive candidiasis is associated with overall poorer neurodevelopmental outcomes and higher rates of threshold retinopathy of prematurity, compared to matched VLBW control infants. Gastrointestinal tract colonization of the low-birth-weight infants often precedes invasive infection, and **risk factors for colonization and invasive disease** are similar. Epidemiologic factors include birth weight <1000 g and gestational age <32 weeks; clinical factors include markers of illness severity such as 5-minute Apgar <5, shock, disseminated intravascular coagulation (DIC), prolonged intubation, delayed introduction of enteral feeding, and the presence of central venous catheters. The administration of parenteral nutrition and intralipid infusions and the use of H2-blockers, systemic steroids, and third-generation cephalosporins have also been identified as independent risk factors for the development of invasive fungal infection.

1. **Microbiology.** Disseminated candidiasis is primarily caused by *Candida albicans* in preterm infants, but infection with *Candida parapsilosis, Candida tropicalis, Candida pseudotropicalis, Candida lusitaniae,* and *Candida glabrata* has been described. The pathogenicity of *C. albicans* is associated with the variable production of a number of toxins, including an endotoxin. *C. parapsilosis* has emerged as the second most common cause of disseminated neonatal candidiasis in recent years. *C. albicans* can be acquired perinatally as well as postnatally. Studies suggest that *C. parapsilosis* is primarily a nosocomial pathogen, in that it is acquired at a later age than *C. albicans*, and is associated with colonization of healthcare workers' hands. Overall, *C. parapsilosis* causes less severe disease than *C. albicans* and is associated in most studies with lower mortality rates. One recent study attributed a mortality rate from *C. parapsilosis* equal to that of *C. albicans* to a delay in central venous catheter removal when the organism was first identified.

2. **Clinical manifestations.** Candidiasis due to in utero infection can occur. Congenital cutaneous candidiasis can present with severe, widespread, and desquamating skin involvement. Pulmonary candidiasis can occur in isolation or with disseminated infection and presents as a severe pneumonia. Most cases of systemic candidiasis, however, present as late-onset sepsis in VLBW infants, most often after the third week of life. The initial clinical features of **late-onset invasive candidiasis** are often nonspecific, and can include lethargy, increased apnea or need for increased ventilatory support, poor perfusion, feeding intolerance, and hyperglycemia. Hyperthermia can be present, an otherwise unusual sign of sepsis in the low-birth-weight infant. Both the total WBC and the differential can be normal early in the course of infection, and although thrombocytopenia is a consistent feature, it is not universally found at presentation. The clinical picture is initially difficult to distinguish from sepsis caused by CONS infection, and contrasts with the abrupt onset of septic shock that often accompanies late-onset sepsis caused by gram-negative organisms. Candidemia can be complicated by meningitis and brain abscess, as well as end-organ involvement of the kidneys, heart, joints, and eyes (endophthalmitis). The fatality rate of disseminated candidiasis is high relative to that found in CONS infections, and increases in the presence of CNS involvement.

3. **Diagnosis.** *Candida* can be cultured from standard pediatric blood culture systems; the time to identification of a positive culture is usually by 48 hours, although late identification (beyond 72 hours) does occur more frequently than with bacterial species. Specialized fungal isolator tubes can aid in the identification of fungal infection if it is suspected by allowing for direct culture on selective media. Both fungal culture and fungal staining (KOH preparation) of urine obtained by suprapubic aspiration (SPA) can be helpful in making the diagnosis of systemic candidiasis. Specimens obtained by bag urine collection or bladder catheterization are difficult to interpret as they can be readily contaminated with colonizing species. We have obtained urine by SPA from VLBW infants under bedside ultrasound guidance for maximal safety. Before the initiation of antifungal therapy, CSF should be obtained for cell count and fungal culture.

4. **Treatment.** Systemic candidiasis is treated with **amphotericin B**, 0.5 to 1 mg/kg per day for durations of 7 to 14 days after a documented negative blood culture and for longer periods if specific end organ infection is present. This medication is associated with a variety of dose-dependent immediate and delayed toxicities in older children and adults and can cause phlebitis at the site of infusion. Febrile reactions to the infusion do not usually occur in the low-birth-weight infant (although renal and electrolyte disturbances can occur) and we start infants at the higher 1 mg/kg dose from the beginning of treatment. The medication is given slowly (over 4 to 6 hours) to minimize the risk of seizures and arrhythmias during the infusion. There is increased experience in VLBW babies with **liposomal preparations of amphotericin B.** Doses up to 5 mg/kg per day have been used without toxicity, and the medication can be given over 1 to 2 hours with less irritation at the site of infusion. Treatment of CNS disease requires the use of an additional second agent, commonly **5'-fluorocytosine (flucytosine 5:FC) (100 to 150 mg/kg per day) or fluconazole (6 mg/kg per day).** Flucytosine achieves good CNS penetration, and appears to be safe in infants. Bone marrow and liver toxicity has occurred in adults, however, and correlates with elevated serum levels of the medication. Serum levels can be monitored (< 100 µg/mL is desirable.) Fluconazole is safe for use in infants, and has occasionally been used when amphotericin B has failed to eradicate candidemia.

   Removal of central catheters in place when candidemia is identified is essential to the eradication of the infection. Delayed catheter removal is associated with persistent candidemia and increased mortality.

   Further evaluation of the infant with invasive candidiasis should include renal and brain ultrasonography to rule out fungal abscess formation and opthalmologic examination to rule out enopthalmitis. In infants who are persistently fungemic despite catheter removal and appropriate therapy, an echocardiogram to rule out endocarditis or vegetation formation is warranted.

5. **Prevention.** Minimizing use of broad-spectrum antibiotics (particularly cephalosporins) and H2-blockers may be helpful in preventing disseminated candidiasis. The CDC recommends changing infusions of lipid suspensions every 12 hours to minimize microbial contamination; solutions of parenteral nutrition and lipid mixtures should be changed every 24 hours. Two randomized trials of prophylactic fluconazole administration have been recently published. One trial used prophylactic fluconazole in 100 infants with BW < 1500 g [median gestational age (GA) 28 weeks, median birth weight (BW) 919–992 g] and demonstrated a 67% decrease in rectal colonization with fungal species, with no statistically significant effect on invasive disease. Another trial enrolled infants with BW <1000 g (median GA 25.5 weeks, median BW 700 to 740 g). This trial demonstrated a 63% decrease in colonization and statistically significant decrease in invasive fungal disease (from 20% in placebo group to 0% in treatment group), with no adverse effects. Although neither trial demonstrated an overall effect on mortality, a meta-analysis of the two trials suggests that the relative risk of death in the fluconazole-treated group was 0.44 (95% confidence interval 0.21, 0.91). These results will need to be confirmed with larger trials targeting infants with BW <1000 g. The widespread implementation of this strategy, however, may be limited by the emergence of azole-resistant fungal species.

C. **Malassezia furfur.** This organism is a lipophilic dermatophyte that readily colonizes infants in neonatal units, and is found in 30 to 60% of neonates over time. *M. furfur* requires exogenous long-chain fatty acids for growth and readily contaminates and proliferates in intravenous lipid preparations as well as on the catheters used for administration of lipids. It causes a nonspecific sepsis syndrome. *M. furfur* grows poorly in standard pediatric blood culture bottles, but isolation is optimized by the addition of a lipid source to the bottles, or by the use of fungal isolator systems and the addition of sterile olive oil to the selective media. In most reported cases, removal of the contaminated central catheter results in cure; amphotericin B is effective when catheter removal alone does not resolve the fungemia.

IV. Focal Bacterial Infections

A. Skin Infections. The newborn may develop a variety of rashes associated with both systemic and focal bacterial disease. Responsible organisms include all of the usual causes of EOS (GBS, enteric gram-negative rods, and anaerobes) as well as gram-positive organisms that specifically colonize the skin—staphylococci and other streptococci. Colonization of the newborn skin occurs with organisms acquired from vaginal flora as well as from the environment. **Sepsis** can be accompanied by skin manifestations such as maculopapular rashes, erythema multiforme, and petechiae or purpura. **Localized infections** can arise in any site of traumatized skin: in the scalp at lesions caused by intrapartum fetal monitors or blood gas samples; in the penis and surrounding tissues due to circumcision; in the extremities at sites of venipuncture or IV placement; in the umbilical stump (omphalitis.) Generalized pustular skin infections can occur due to S. aureus, occasionally in epidemic fashion.

1. Cellulitis usually occurs at traumatized skin sites as noted above. Localized erythema and/or drainage in a term infant (e.g., at a scalp electrode site) can be treated with careful washing and local antisepsis with antibiotic ointment (bacitracin or mupirocin ointment) and close monitoring. Cellulitis at sites of intravenous access or venipuncture in premature infants must be addressed in a more aggressive fashion due to the risk of local and systemic spread, particularly in the VLBW infant. If the premature infant with a localized cellulitis is well appearing, a CBC and blood culture should be obtained and intravenous antibiotics administered to provide coverage primarily for skin flora (i.e., oxacillin or nafcillin and gentamicin). If MRSA is a concern in a particular setting, vancomycin should be substituted for nafcillin. If blood cultures are negative, the infant can be treated for a total of 5 to 7 days with resolution of the cellulitis. If an organism grows from the blood culture, a lumbar puncture should be performed to rule out meningitis and careful physical examination should be performed to rule out accompanying osteomyelitis or septic arthritis. Therapy is guided by the organism identified (see Tables 23.3 and 23.4).

2. Pustulosis. Infectious pustulosis is usually caused by S. aureus and must be distinguished from the benign neonatal rash erythema toxicum and transient pustular melanosis (see Chap. 34, Skin Care). The pustules are most commonly found in the axillae, groin, and periumbilical area; both erythema toxicum and transient pustular melanosis have a more generalized distribution. Lesions can be unroofed after cleansing in sterile fashion with betadine or 4% chlorhexidene, and contents aspirated and analyzed by gram stain and culture. Gram stain of infectious pustules will reveal neutrophils and gram-positive cocci, whereas Wright stain of erythema toxicum lesions will reveal predominantly eosinophils and no (or a few contaminating) organisms. Gram stain of transient pustular melanosis lesions will reveal neutrophils but no organisms. Cultures of the benign rashes will be sterile or grow contaminating organisms such as S. epidermidis. Treatment of pustulosis caused by S. aureus is tailored to the degree of involvement and condition of the infant. A few lesions in a healthy term infant may be treated with topical mupirocin and oral therapy with medications such as amoxicillin/clavulonate, dicloxacillin, or cephalexin. More extensive lesions, systemic illness, or pustulosis occurring in the premature infant requires intravenous therapy with nafcillin or oxacillin.

Some strains of S. aureus produce toxins that can cause **bullous lesions or scalded skin syndrome.** The cutaneous changes are due to local and systemic spread of toxin. Although blood cultures may be negative, intravenous antibiotics should be given (nafcillin or oxacillin) until the progression of disease stops and skin lesions are healing.

Pediatricians who diagnose infectious pustulosis in an infant under 2 weeks of age should report the case to the birth hospital; **epidemic outbreaks due to nosocomial acquistion in newborn nurseries** are often recognized in this way since the rash may not occur until after hospital discharge. When such outbreaks are recognized in the nursery or NICU, hospital infection control experts should be consulted. Appropriate steps may include surveillance cultures of staff members and newborns and cohorting of colonized infants.

3. **Omphalitis.** Omphalitis is characterized by erythema and/or induration of the periumbilical area with purulent discharge from the umbilical stump. The infection can progress to widespread abdominal wall cellulitis or necrotizing fasciitis; complications such as peritonitis, umbilical arteritis or phlebitis, hepatic vein thrombosis, and hepatic abscess have all been described. Responsible organisms include both gram-positive and gram-negative species. Treatment consists of a full sepsis evaluation (CBC, blood culture, lumbar puncture) and empiric intravenous therapy with oxacillin or nafcillin and gentamicin. With serious disease progression, broader-spectrum gram-negative coverage with a cephalosporin or piperacillin/tazobactam should be considered. As noted in II.A, Treatment of Anaerobic Infections, invasion of the umbilical stump by *Clostridia tetani* under conditions of poor sanitation can result in neonatal tetanus in the infant of an unimmunized mother.

B. **Conjunctivitis (ophthalmia neonatorum).** This condition refers to inflammation of the conjunctiva within the first month of life. Causative agents include topical medications (chemical conjunctivitis), bacteria, and herpes simplex viruses. Chemical conjunctivitis is most commonly seen with silver nitrate prophylaxis, requires no specific treatment, and usually resolves within 48 hours. Bacterial causes include *Neisseria gonorrhoeae,* and *Chlamydia trachomatis,* as well as staphylococci, streptococci, and gram-negative organisms. In the United States where routine birth prophylaxis against opthalmia neonatorum is practiced, the incidence of this disease is reported to be approximately 1.6%. In developing countries in the absence of prophylaxis, the incidence is 20 to 25% and remains a major cause of blindness.

1. **Prophylaxis against infectious conjunctivitis.** One percent silver nitrate solution (1 to 2 drops to each eye), 0.5% erythromycin opthlamic ointment (1-cm strip to each eye), and 2.5% povidone-iodine solution (1 drop to each eye) administered within 1 hour of birth are all effective in the prevention of opthalmia neonatorum. In a trial comparing the use of these three agents conducted in Kenya, povidone-iodine was shown to be slightly more effective against both *C. trachomatis* and other causes of infectious conjunctivitis, and equally effective against *N. gonorrhoeae* and *Staphylococcus aureus.* Povidone-iodine was associated with less noninfectious conjunctivitis and is less costly than the other two agents; in addition, this agent is not associated with the development of bacterial resistance. In our institution, where most mothers receive prenatal care and the incidences of chlamydia and gonorrhea are low, we use erythromycin ointment, primarily because the medication does not stain. Silver nitrate or povidone-iodine are the preferred agents in areas where the incidence of penicillinase-producing *N. gonorrhoeae* is high.

2. ***N. gonorrhoeae.*** Pregnant women should be screened for *N. gonorrhoeae* as part of routine prenatal care. High-risk women or women without prenatal care should be screened at delivery. If a mother is known to have untreated *N. gonorrhoeae* infection, the infant should receive **ceftriaxone 25 to 50 mg/kg IV or IM (not to exceed 125 mg) at birth.**

Gonococcal conjunctivitis presents with chemosis, lid edema, and purulent exudate beginning 1 to 4 days after birth. Clouding of the cornea or pan-ophthalmitis can occur. Gram stain and culture of conjunctival scrapings will confirm the diagnosis. The treatment of infants with uncomplicated gonococcal conjunctivitis requires only a single dose of ceftriaxone (25 to 50 mg/kg IV or IM, not to exceed 125 mg). Additional topical treatment is unnecessary. However, infants with gonococcal conjunctivitis should be hospitalized and screened for invasive disease (i.e., sepsis, meningitis, arthritis). Scalp abscesses can result from internal fetal monitoring. Treatment of these complications is ceftriaxone (25 to 50 mg/kg per day IV or IM q24h) or cefotaxime (25 mg/kg IV or IM q12h) for 7 to 14 days (10 to 14 days for meningitis). The infant and mother should be screened for coincident chlamydial infection.

3. *C. trachomatis.* Pregnant women should be screened for *C. trachomatis* as part of routine prenatal care. Prophylaxis for infants born to mothers with untreated chlamydial infection is not indicated. Chlamydial conjunctivitis is the most common identified cause of infectious conjunctivitis in the United States. It presents with variable degrees of inflammation, yellow discharge, and eyelid swelling 5 to 14 days after birth. Conjunctival scarring can occur, although the cornea is usually not involved. Examination of conjunctival scrapings for chlamydia by DNA probe testing is currently used for diagnosis of chlamydia at our institution. Direct fluorescent-antibody and enzyme-linked immunoassay (ELISA)-based detection methods are also available, but culture-based detection is technically involved and takes several days to complete. Chlamydial conjunctivitis is treated with **erythromycin base or ethylsuccinate 50 mg/kg per day divided into 4 doses for 14 days.** Topical treatment alone is not adequate, and is unnecessary when systemic therapy is given. An association of oral erythromycin therapy and infantile hypertrophic pyloric stenosis has been reported in infants less than 6 weeks of age. Infants should be monitored for this condition. The efficacy of treatment is approximately 80%, and infants must be evaluated for treatment failure and the need for a second course of treatment. Infants should also be evaluated for the concomitant presence of chlamydial pneumonia. The treatment for pneumonia is the same as for conjunctivitis, in addition to necessary supportive respiratory care.

4. **Other bacterial conjunctivitis.** Other causes are generally diagnosed by culture of eye exudate. *S. aureus, E. coli,* and *Hemophilus influenzae* can cause conjunctivitis that is usually easily treated with local ophthalmic ointments (erythromycin or gentamicin) without complication. Very severe cases caused by *H. influenzae* may require parenteral treatment and evaluation for sepsis and meningitis. *Pseudomonas aeruginosa* can cause a rare and devastating form of conjunctivitis that requires parenteral treatment.

C. **Pneumonia.** The diagnosis of **neonatal pneumonia** is challenging. It is difficult to distinguish primary (occurring from birth) neonatal bacterial pneumonia clinically from sepsis with respiratory compromise, or radiographically from other causes of respiratory distress (hyaline membrane disease, retained fetal lung fluid, meconium aspiration, amniotic fluid aspiration). Persistent focal opacifications on chest radiograph due to neonatal pneumonia are uncommon and their presence should prompt some consideration of noninfectious causes of focal lung opacification (such as congenital cystic lesions or pulmonary sequestration). The causes of neonatal bacterial pneumonia are the same as for early-onset sepsis, and antibiotic treatment is generally the same as for sepsis. The infant's baseline risk for infection, radiographic and laboratory studies, and most important, the clinical progression must all be taken into account when making the diagnosis of neonatal pneumonia.

The diagnosis of **nosocomial, or ventilator-associated pneumonia** in neonates who are ventilator-dependent due to chronic lung disease or other illness, is equally challenging. Culture of tracheal secretions in infants who are chronically ventilated can yield a variety of organisms, including all the causes of EOS and LOS as well as (often antibiotic-resistant) gram-negative organisms that are endemic within a particular NICU. A distinction must be made between colonization of the airway and true tracheitis or pneumonia. Culture results must be taken together with the infant's respiratory and systemic condition, as well as radiographic and laboratory studies when making the diagnosis of nosocomial pneumonia.

Ureaplasma urealyticum deserves mention with respect to chronically ventilated infants. This mycoplasmal organism frequently colonizes the vagina of pregnant women, and has been associated with chorioamnionitis, spontaneous abortion and premature delivery, and infection of the premature infant. Infection with *Ureaplasma* has been studied as a contributing factor to the development of chronic lung disease, but the role of the organism and the value of diagnosis and treatment is unclear. *Ureaplasma* requires special culture conditions and will grow within 2 to 5 days. It will not be identified on routine bacterial culture. It is sensitive to erythromycin, but can be difficult to eradicate, and few data are available on the dosing, treatment duration, and efficacy of treatment when this organism is found in tracheal secretions.

D. Urinary tract infection. The incidence of urinary-tract infections (UTI) in the first month of life is reported to range from 0.1 to 1%, but is perhaps higher in preterm infants. UTIs may occur secondary to bacteremia, or bacteremia may occur secondary to primary UTI. The incidence is higher in male infants than female infants. The most common causative organisms are gram-negative, such as *E. coli*, but enterococci can also cause UTI. Culture of urine is not routinely recommended as part of the evaluation for EOS, but is an essential part of the evaluation for LOS (see earlier section on Late Onset Sepsis). The most common presenting symptoms in term and older preterm infants are fever, lethargy, and poor feeding; younger preterm infants will present as for LOS. Diagnosis is made by urinalysis and urine culture. Culture of urine obtained from a bag collection or diaper is of little value as it will commonly be contaminated with skin and fecal flora. Specimens should be obtained by bladder catheterization or suprapubic aspiration with sterile technique. Ultrasound guidance can be useful in performing suprapubic aspiration in the VLBW infant. Empiric treatment in term and preterm infants is as for LOS (see I.J); antibiotic choice and treatment duration is guided by blood, urine, and CSF culture results. If the urine culture **alone** is positive in a term infant, treatment is completed with oral therapy once the infant is afebrile. Treatment duration in the absence of a positive blood or CSF culture is 10 to 14 days. It is recommended that infants with UTI undergo renal ultrasound and vesicourethrocytogram (VCUG) imaging to identify any underlying anatomic or functional abnormalities (i.e. reflux) that may have contributed to the development of the UTI. Infants should receive UTI prophylaxis with amoxicillin (10 to 20 mg/kg once per day) after completing UTI treatment until imaging studies are performed.

E. Osteomyelitis and septic arthritis. These focal infections are rare in newborns, and may result from hematogenous seeding in the setting of bacteremia, or direct extension from a skin source of infection. The most common organisms are *S. aureus,* GBS, and gram-negative organisms including *Neisseria gonorrhoeae*. Symptoms include localized erythema, swelling, and apparent pain or lack of spontaneous movement of the involved extremity. The hip, knee, and wrist are commonly involved in septic arthritis, and the femur, humerus, tibia, radius, and maxilla are the most common bone sites of infection. The evaluation should be as for sepsis, including blood, urine, and CSF culture, and culture of any purulent skin lesions. Needle aspiration of an infected joint is sometimes possible, and plain film and ultrasound can aid in diagnosis. Empiric treatment is with nafcillin or oxacillin and gentamicin, and is later tailored to any identified organisms. Joint infections commonly require surgical drainage; material can be sent for gram stain and culture at surgery. Duration of therapy is 3 to 4 weeks. Significant disability can result from joint or growth plate damage.

Suggested Readings

Hyde T.B., et al. Trends in incidence and antimicrobial resistance of early-onset sepsis: Population-based surveillance in San Francisco and Atlanta. *Pediatrics* 2002 Oct;110(4):690–695.

Isenberg S.J., Apt L., Wood M. A controlled trial of povidone-iodine as prophylaxis against ophthalmia neonatorum. *N Engl J Med* 1995 Mar 2;332(9):562–566.

Kaufman D., et al. Fluconazole prophylaxis against fungal colonization and infection in preterm infants. *N Engl J Med* 2001 Dec 6;345(23):1660–1666.

Schrag S.J., et al. Group B streptococcal disease in the era of intrapartum antibiotic prophylaxis. *N Engl J Med* 2000 Jan 6;342(1):15–20.

Stoll B.J., et al. Late-onset sepsis in very low birth weight neonates: The experience of the NICHD Neonatal Research Network. *Pediatrics* 2002 Aug;110(2 Pt 1): 285–291.

Stoll B.J., et al. Changes in pathogens causing early-onset sepsis in very-low-birth-weight infants. *N Engl J Med* 2002 Jul 25;347 (4):240–247.

Tuberculosis

Dara D. Brodsky and John P. Cloherty

I. **Incidence** The World Health Organization (WHO) estimates that one-third of the world's population is infected by the acid-fast bacillus *Mycobacterium tuberculosis* with 8 million new cases each year and 2 million deaths per year (1,2). Between 1985 and 1992, there was a 20% increase in reported cases of **tuberculosis (TB)** in the United States (1). This increase was greatest in young adults and children and has been attributed to five factors: the human immunodeficiency virus (HIV) epidemic; recent immigration to the United States from areas with a high prevalence of TB; increased transmission in high-risk facilities (prisons, hospitals, nursing homes, and homeless shelters); development of multidrug-resistant TB; and the decrease in public health TB services (3).

Intensified strategic measures initiated in 1989 have reduced the incidence of TB in the United States by 45% since the epidemic peak in 1992 (1). Indeed, there were only 16,377 cases reported in the United States in 2000 (1). However, the Centers for Disease Control's (CDC) goal of eliminating TB from the United States by 2010 remains a challenge because of reports of TB still occurring in every state and the continued increase among foreign-born persons (4,5). The increase in TB among foreign-born persons is due to increased immigration to the United States and emigration from countries with higher rates of TB (6).

The rate of decline of TB in the pediatric population has not been as significant as in adults (4). Indeed, foreign-born children younger than 5 years of age had the highest rate of TB between 1993 and 1998 among different age groups (4). Since the highest risk group for mortality from TB is in patients under 5 years of age, and untreated TB in the newborn is fatal in ~40 to 50% of cases, pediatricians and neonatologists should maintain a high index of suspicion for this disease.

II. **Transmission and Pathogenesis.** Tuberculosis is transmitted by respiratory droplets, which can remain viable in the air for several hours. The risk of infectivity increases if: a cough is present, the sputum has low-viscosity, the sputum smear is positive for acid-fast bacillus (AFB) in addition to a positive culture, or there is a prolonged period of symptoms without treatment (7). The **preinfectious stage** occurs after a person has had close contact with someone suspected or confirmed to have had contagious pulmonary TB (3). During this stage, the tuberculin skin test or purified protein derivative (PPD) and the chest X ray (CXR) are negative. The groups that have a greater risk for exposure to TB include: substance abusers; foreign-born persons from areas with a high incidence of TB (Asia, Africa, Latin America, Eastern Europe, Russia); homeless persons; shelter dwellers; migrant workers; residents of institutions or prisons; and health-care workers in high-risk areas (5).

Following exposure, the smaller respiratory droplets may travel to the alveoli where they are ingested by alveolar macrophages; the majority of the bacilli are destroyed while the remaining bacilli multiply. Following cellular death, the organisms are released and can spread to the regional lymph nodes and the bloodstream. During this **infection stage**, adults may have a positive PPD, while neonates and children may take up to 3 months to test positive (3). In all age groups, the CXR may be normal or demonstrate enlarged lymph nodes or focal infiltrates (3). It is critical to initiate treatment at this stage to prevent future disease with the treatment protocol depending on the presence or absence of radiographic findings.

Two to 10 weeks after infection, the immune response destroys most of the bacilli, preventing further hematogenous spread. If this defense system is unsuccessful, TB infection progresses to the **disease stage**. There is greater likelihood of progression to disease if a person is immunosuppressed (HIV seropositive, neonate, chronic steroid therapy); is infected with TB within the past 2 years (particularly neonates and young children); has a history of inadequately treated TB; or has an underlying illness (5). Although TB disease primarily involves the lungs, TB may also affect the brain, kidneys, bones and joints, or lymphatic system. Extrapulmonary manifestations of TB are more common in immunosuppressed patients and occur in 25 to 35% of infants and young children with disease (6). Patients who are immunosuppressed, including neonates, may have a negative PPD despite disease.

III. **Diagnosis**

A. **Maternal tuberculosis**

1. **PPD.** Early diagnosis and treatment of TB in pregnant women is the most efficient method of preventing TB in the newborn. Since the majority of pregnant women infected with TB are asymptomatic or have minimal disease, there should be a low threshold for obtaining a PPD in pregnant women. Skin testing should be done on all pregnant women who: are exposed to a person with TB; are immigrants from areas with a high incidence of TB; have increased susceptibility to TB because of HIV infection, diabetes, gastrectomy; live in a high prevalence area; or work in a profession with a high probability of exposure (8). Pregnancy does not alter the response to a tuberculin skin test, and there have been no adverse effects on women or their infants from tuberculin testing (3).

A positive PPD reaction in an asymptomatic woman is the most common method of diagnosing TB infection during pregnancy in the United

States. Forty-eight to 72 hours after placement of a PPD (5 units), a positive result is defined as induration:

   a. ≥5mm if person is immunosuppressed (e.g., HIV seropositive), has close contact with person(s) who have infectious TB disease, or has radiographic fibrotic pulmonary lesions.

   b. ≥10 mm if person is an intravenous drug user, has an underlying medical disorder (including chronic renal failure, diabetes mellitus, malnutrition, leukemia, gastrectomy), is foreign-born from high TB prevalence area, resident of long-term facility or shelter, lives in a medically underserved region, or is a health-care worker in high-risk areas.

   c. ≥15 mm without risk factors (3,8).

2. Chest radiography. If the tuberculin skin test is positive or there is clinical evidence of TB, a CXR should be obtained to determine if there is active disease. An abdominal shield is required to protect the fetus from the X ray. Radiographic findings consistent with active disease include adenopathy, focal or multinodular infiltrates, cavitation, and decreased expansion of the upper lobes of the lung (8). Since radiographic findings may be normal despite TB disease, further evaluation (e.g., sputum cultures) is necessary if symptoms are present.

3. Maternal signs and symptoms. The clinical manifestations of TB during pregnancy are identical to those in nonpregnant women. Although many women may be asymptomatic, possible symptoms include cough (74%), weight loss (41%), fever (30%), malaise and fatigue (30%), or hemoptysis (20%) (9). Malaise, fatigue, and vomiting can often be mistaken for other pregnancy-associated conditions. Extrapulmonary involvement can lead to mastitis, miliary tuberculosis, tuberculosis meningitis, and more commonly, involvement of the lymph nodes, bones, or kidneys.

   Any pregnant woman suspected of having TB (positive PPD reaction, suspicious or positive CXR and/or clinical manifestations), should have three early-morning sputum samples obtained for acid-fast staining, culture (isolation can take up to 6 weeks), and susceptibility testing (6,9). Since 5 to 10% of pregnant women with TB exhibit extrapulmonary disease, a complete evaluation is essential, and if indicated, lymph node or liver biopsies should be obtained for staining and culture. A peritoneal fibrinous exudate at cesarean section or an infected placenta may assist in the diagnosis of TB in the mother and/or neonate. If there is evidence of active TB, close contacts should be tested for the disease. Active TB during pregnancy is not an indication for a therapeutic abortion, however, since therapies for the disease are available.

B. Tuberculosis of the fetus or newborn

1. Pathogenesis (6,8,10). Although **congenital TB** is rare (~300 reported cases), it can be acquired by:

   a. Hematogenous spread through the umbilical vein from an infected placenta to the fetal liver, and lungs (can also involve the gastrointestinal tract, bone marrow, skin, or mesenteric nodes).

   b. Aspiration or ingestion of infected amniotic fluid, in utero or at the time of birth, leading to primary infection in the lungs or gastrointestinal tract. The diagnosis of congenital TB requires the presence of TB lesions in the first week of life, primary hepatic lesions, maternal placental or genital TB, or exclusion of postnatal transmission after an extensive investigation. If none of these findings are present, the infection was probably acquired **postnatally** by:

      (1) Inhalation (most common) or ingestion of infected respiratory droplets.

      (2) Contamination of traumatized skin or mucous membranes.

2. Neonatal signs and symptoms (3). The clinical manifestations of TB in the neonate vary in relation to the duration, mechanism, and location of the infection in the infant. Although symptoms may be present at birth, they are more commonly observed in the second or third week of life. Clinical manifestations are often nonspecific and include hepatic and splenic enlargement (76%); respiratory distress (72%); fever (48%); lymphadenopathy (38%); abdominal distension (24%); lethargy and irritability (21%); ear discharge (17%); and skin papules (14%). In addition, apnea, failure to thrive, jaundice, and central nervous system signs can occur. Infection is more likely to disseminate in neonates compared with older children and adults.

The majority of infected infants will have an abnormal CXR (infiltrates or miliary pattern in 50%), and almost all infected infants will have an initial negative PPD. The PPD (5 units, 0.1 cc) is more likely to be positive (defined in children < 4 years of age as ≥10 mm) if infection has been present for 4 to 6 months. Stains for acid-fast bacilli (AFB) and cultures should be performed on blood, urine, three early morning gastric aspirates, tracheal aspirates, and CSF. Abnormal liver function tests suggest disseminated disease. Tissue from lymph nodes, liver, lung, bone marrow, skin lesions, and the placenta may reveal organisms on pathologic examination and culture. Drug sensitivities should be performed on any organism grown from these cultures as well as organisms grown from maternal isolates. If all direct smears are negative and the infant is ill, antituberculosis therapy should be started until the diagnosis of TB is excluded. HIV testing should be done on all neonates with TB since the treatment regimen is longer for coinfection.

IV. **Management** (5,6,11) (refer to Fig. 23.4)
   A. **Pregnant women with active TB.** If active TB is diagnosed during pregnancy (positive culture, clinical or radiographic evidence), prompt initial therapy with isoniazid (INH), rifampin (RIF), and ethambutol (EMB) is recommended. Pyridoxine (50 mg daily) is added to this regimen because of the increased requirement of this vitamin (B_6) during pregnancy and because it might help prevent INH-related neuropathy. The length of therapy of each drug is dependent upon the sensitivity results of the organism. If the bacilli are sensitive to INH and RIF, EMB should be discontinued and INH and RIF continued for 9 months. If the bacilli are sensitive to only one medication (INH or RIF), that drug and EMB are required for 12 to 18 months. If extrapulmonary manifestations are present, prolonged therapy may be warranted. All patients with active TB should be isolated in a room with an independent air-handling system and negative air pressure. Notify the local health department so that a contact investigation can be done.

   INH, RIF, and EMB appear to be relatively safe for the fetus, and the benefit of treatment outweighs the potential risk to the fetus. While streptomycin (STREP) is often used to treat TB, it is contraindicated in pregnant women since it can cause ototoxicity in the fetus. There are no data on the effects of pyrazinamide (PZA) in pregnancy, so it should be avoided if possible. Consult an expert if a pregnant woman has multidrug-resistant TB and thus requires treatment with medications that are usually contraindicated in pregnancy or have unknown fetal effects. Although anti-TB medications pass through breast milk, the amount transmitted is low and there is little effect on the neonate.
   B. There is some debate about whether to treat **asymptomatic pregnant women who have a positive PPD, negative sputum, and normal CXR** (11). Since treatment with INH is associated with hepatitis during pregnancy, therapy should be delayed until after delivery if the woman is immunocompetent, does not have a known TB exposure, and is otherwise healthy. On the other hand, a pregnant woman who is a recent converter (within the past 2 years), has had recent contact with an infectious person, or is immunosuppressed (e.g., HIV seropositive), should receive INH and pyridoxine for 9 months beginning in the second trimester.
   C. **Management of congenital TB** (6,11) (refer to Fig. 23.4 and Table 23.7). Initiate treatment of the neonate with INH, RIF, PZA, and either STREP, or

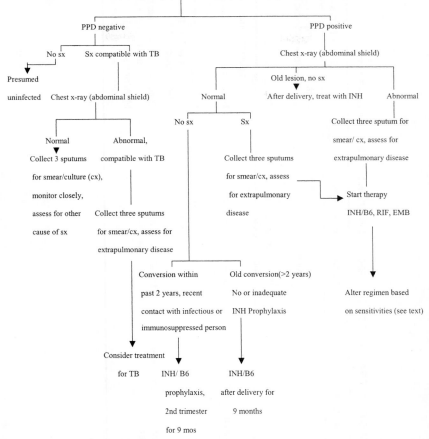

FIG. 23.4. Diagnosis and treatment of tuberculosis in the pregnant woman. (Modified from refs. 3,8,9.)

EMB. This initial regimen provides broad coverage, since neonates are at greater risk of developing extrapulmonary TB (e.g., meningitis, miliary TB, bone and joint disease). If extrapulmonary TB is diagnosed, the infant should receive 2 months of this broad therapy followed by 7 to 10 months of INH and RIF. Corticosteroids should be added if TB meningitis is confirmed. If the infant has multidrug-resistant TB, a prolonged (12 to 18 months) four-drug regimen is often recommended in consultation with a TB specialist. Since the yield of culturing bacilli in the neonate is low, the clinician may need to rely on the mother's susceptibilities to determine treatment. In contrast to older children who have adequate pyridoxine levels, infants who are breastfeeding and receiving INH should be supplemented with pyridoxine due to relatively low levels of this vitamin in breast milk. Consider isolating

TABLE 23.7. COMMONLY USED MEDICATIONS FOR TREATMENT OF TB INFECTION IN NEONATES AND CHILDREN [11]

Drug	Activity	Dosage (mg/kg/day)	Side Effects
Isoniazid (INH) Tablets (100 or 300 mg) (syrup unstable), also IM	Bactericidal	10–15 (or 20–30 mg/kg twice weekly)	Peripheral neuropathy, hepatotoxic, allergic reactivity
Rifampin (RIF) Capsules (150 or 300 mg) (syrup unstable), also IV	Bactericidal	10–20 (or 10–20 mg/kg twice weekly)	Orange discoloration of body fluids, hepatotoxic, vomiting, thrombocytopenia
Pyrazinamide (PZA) Tablets (500 mg)	Bactericidal	20–40 (or 50 mg/kg twice weekly)	Hepatotoxic, hyperuricemia
Streptomycin (STREP) 400 mg/ml in 2.5 ml vials	Bactericidal	20–40 IM (12 weeks maximal use)	Ototoxic, nephrotoxic, rash Monitor renal function and hearing screens
Ethambutol (EMB) Tablets (100 or 400 mg)	Bacteriostatic, bactericidal (higher doses)	15–25 (or 50 mg/kg twice weekly)	Optic neuritis, allergic reactivity, gastrointestinal symptoms Monitor visual fields, acuity, and color discrimination.

infants with congenital TB since they typically have a high inoculum of organisms in their tracheal aspirates. Consult a TB specialist during neonatal therapy.

D. **Asymptomatic neonate, active infection in the mother** (6,12). Assess the infant for clinical evidence of TB, place a PPD, obtain a CXR, send three gastric aspirates for smear and culture, perform a lumbar puncture, and examine the placenta for organisms. If there is evidence of neonatal disease, treat as in congenital TB (see IV.C); if there is no evidence of neonatal disease, the infant is at high risk and should receive daily INH. If the bacillus is INH-resistant, give RIF for 6 months. If the bacilli is INH and RIF-resistant, consult a specialist.

Continue INH therapy in the infant until the mother is culture negative for 2 to 3 months. At that time, if the neonate has a positive PPD without evidence of clinical or radiographic TB, continue INH for a total of 9 months (12 months if infant is HIV seropositive). In contrast, if the neonate has a negative PPD, INH can be discontinued if the mother is adherent and there is adequate clinical response to therapy. Repeat skin testing at 3 months and if positive, reevaluate the infant for disease. In all scenarios, close clinical monitoring of the neonate is necessary.

As soon as a mother is diagnosed with active TB, notify the local health department, so that a contact investigation can be performed and separate the infant from the mother. Once the infant is receiving chemotherapy, further isolation is not required unless the mother is severely ill, noncompliant, or has multidrug-resistant TB. When the infant and mother are reunited, breastfed infants should receive pyridoxine.

E. **Asymptomatic neonate, mother with positive PPD and abnormal CXR** (11,12). Separate the infant and mother until the mother has been evaluated. If the mother has active TB, follow protocol as in D (see above). If the mother has inactive pulmonary disease, the infant is at low risk of infection and does not require therapy. If the mother has not been treated in the past, however, she requires therapy to prevent reactivation. Evaluate household members for TB. Closely monitor neonate with PPD (testing every 3 months for 1 year, yearly thereafter) and frequent clinical evaluations.

F. **Asymptomatic neonate, mother with positive PPD, negative sputum and normal CXR** (6,12). In this situation, the infant is not separated from the mother. While the mother requires INH postpartum, the infant does not need therapy. Evaluate household members for TB. If disease cannot be excluded in household members, or if disease is found in the family, further skin testing in the neonate is required.

G. **Neonate with TB exposure in the nursery** (6). Although neonates exposed to TB in the nursery have a low risk for acquiring disease, infection can occur. If the exposure is considered to be significant, the infant should be skin tested and, even if negative, treated with INH for 3 months. The skin test should then be repeated; if it is still negative, therapy can be stopped. If the skin test is positive, the infant should be treated with INH for 9 months with close clinical monitoring. To prevent transmission of TB in the nursery, personnel should be skin tested yearly.

V. **Bacillus Calmette-Guerin (BCG)** (11,13). BCG is a live, attenuated vaccine prepared from *Mycobacterium bovis*. While BCG vaccination has recently been shown to prevent serious forms of TB in children, its efficacy in the prevention of pulmonary disease in adolescents and adults remains uncertain. Although vaccination is required in more than 60 countries, the indications in the United States are limited to select groups that meet defined criteria: (1) infants and children (PPD-negative and HIV seronegative) with prolonged exposure to untreated, ineffectively treated contagious persons, or multidrug-resistant contagious persons if removal from the source is not possible; or (2) nontuberculin reactors working in homeless shelters or health-care facilities in high-risk multidrug-resistant TB areas (provided infection-control precautions have not been successful).

Before administering the BCG vaccine, consult a local TB specialist. When BCG is given, closely follow the instructions on the insert. Infants less than 2 months old do not need tuberculin testing, while older children typically require a negative PPD before receiving BCG. Infants less than 30 days of age should receive one-half the recommended dose. If the indications for vaccination persist after 1 year of age, they should receive a full vaccine dose if their PPD is < 5 mm. Preliminary data suggest that BCG may have minimal effectiveness in premature infants. Patients with burns or generalized skin infection should not receive BCG. In the United States, BCG is also contraindicated in HIV-infected persons, infants of HIV-infected mothers and persons receiving high-dose corticosteroids. Outside the United States, the WHO recommends that asymptomatic HIV-infected children living in areas with a high incidence of TB should receive BCG. Due to the unknown effects of BCG on the fetus, the vaccine is not recommended during pregnancy.

Following BCG vaccination, pustular formation often occurs at the injection site within 3 weeks and often leads to a permanent scar. Other complications are infrequent but may include ulceration at the injection site, lymphadenitis, and possible osteomyelitis; disseminated BCG may occur in severely immunodeficient patients. Adverse reactions can be treated with anti-TB medications in consultation with a TB expert. Report all adverse reactions to the manufacturer.

It is recommended that tuberculin reactivity following BCG vaccination should be documented. Initial testing should be performed 3 months after injection and induration size should be documented. In the future, if the PPD induration increases ($\geq$10 mm if <35 years of age; $\geq$15 mm if $\geq$35 years of age), newly acquired TB infection should be suspected. Although BCG administration may limit the future diagnostic utility of the PPD, studies have shown that most children who receive BCG in infancy have a negative PPD at 5 years of age.

Acknowledgments

The authors would like to thank Robert N. Husson, MD (Assistant Professor of Pediatrics, Boston Children's Hospital) and Elsa Villarino, MD (Department of Health and Human Services, Centers for Disease Control and Prevention) for their critical review of this manuscript.

References

1. Small P.M., Fujwara P.I. Management of TB in the US. *N Engl J Med* 2001; 345(3):189.
2. Dye C., et al. Global burden of tuberculosis. *JAMA* 1999; 282:677.
3. Starke J.R. Tuberculosis. *Clin Perinatol* 1997; 24(1):107.
4. Talbot E.T., et al. Tuberculosis among foreign-born persons in the US, 1993–1998. *JAMA* 2000; 284(22):2894.
5. Centers for Disease Control and Prevention. Core curriculum on TB. Available at: http://www.cdc.gov/nchstp/tb/pubs/corecurr/.
6. Starke J.R., Smith, M.D. Tuberculosis. In: Remington J.S., Klein J.O. (Eds.). *Infectious Diseases of the Fetus and Newborn Infant*, 5th ed. Philadelphia: Saunders, 2001.
7. Abernathy R.S. Tuberculosis: An update. *Pediatr Rev* 1997; 18(2):50.
8. Riley L. Pneumonia and TB in pregnancy. *Infect Dis Clin North Am* 1997;11 (1):119.
9. Jacobs R.F., Abernathy, R.S. Management of TB in pregnancy and the newborn. *Clin Perinatol* 1988; 15(2):305.
10. Cantwell M.F., et al. Congenital tuberculosis. *N Engl J Med* 1994;330(15):1051.
11. American Academy of Pediatrics. Tuberculosis. In: Pickering L.K. (Ed.). *2000 Red Book: Report of the Committee on Infectious Diseases,* 25th ed. Elk Grove Village, Ill.: American Academy of Pediatrics; 2000:593.
12. Mallory M.D., Jacobs R.F. Congenital T.B. *Semin Pediatr Infect Dis* 1999; 10(3):177.

13. Centers for Disease Control and Prevention. The role of BCG vaccine in the prevention and control of TB in the US. *MMWR* 1996; 45 (No. RR-4).

Syphilis*

Louis Vernacchio

I. Pathophysiology (3)

A. Acquired syphilis is a sexually transmitted infection caused by the spirochete *Treponema pallidum*. The incubation period is typically about 3 weeks but ranges from 9 to 90 days. The disease has three clinically recognizable stages.

    1. Primary syphilis is manifest by one or more chancres (painless indurated ulcers) at the site of inoculation, typically the genitalia, anus, or mouth. It is often accompanied by regional lymphadenopathy.

    2. Secondary syphilis occurs 3 to 6 weeks after the appearance of the chancre, often after the chancre has resolved. The secondary stage is characterized by a polymorphic rash, most commonly maculopapular, generalized, and involving the palms and soles. Sore throat, fever, headache, diffuse lymphadenopathy, myalgias, arthralgias, alopecia, condylomata lata, and mucous membrane plaques may also be present. The symptoms resolve without treatment. Some patients develop recurrences of the manifestations of secondary syphilis.

    3. Latent syphilis is defined as those periods of time with no clinical symptoms but positive serologic evidence of infection. A variable latent period usually follows the manifestations of secondary syphilis, sometimes interrupted by recurrences of the secondary symptoms.

    4. Tertiary syphilis usually occurs 4 to 12 years after the secondary stage and is characterized by gummata—nonprogressive, localized lesions that may occur in the skin, bones, or viscera. These lesions are thought to be due to pronounced immunologic reaction. The tertiary stage can also be marked by cardiovascular syphilis, especially inflammation of the great vessels.

    5. Neurosyphilis may occur at any stage of the disease. Early manifestations include meningitis, and neurovascular disease. Late manifestations include dementia, posterior column disease (tabes dorsalis), and seizures, among others.

B. Congenital syphilis results from transplacental passage of *Treponema pallidum*. The risk of transmission to the fetus correlates largely with the duration of maternal infection—the more recent the maternal infection, the more likely transmission to the fetus will occur. During the primary and secondary stages of syphilis, the likelihood of transmission from an untreated women to her fetus is extremely high, approaching 100%. After the secondary stage, the likelihood of transmission to the fetus declines steadily until it reaches approximately 10 to 30% in late latency. Although transplacental transmission has generally been thought to occur during the second and third trimesters of pregnancy, more recent data suggest that transmission may occur in the first trimester as well.

    Congenital infection may result in stillbirth, hydrops fetalis, or premature delivery. Most affected infants will be asymptomatic at birth, but clinical signs usually develop within the first 3 months of life. The most common signs of early congenital syphilis include hepatomegaly, skeletal abnormalities (osteochondritis, periostitis, pseudoparalysis), skin and mucocutaneous lesions, jaundice, pneumonia, splenomegaly, anemia, and snuffles. If un-

---

*See (ref. 1,2).

treated, late manifestations appear after 2 years of age and may include neurosyphilis, bony changes (frontal bossing, short maxilla, high palatal arch, Hutchinson teeth, saddle nose), interstitial keratitis, and eighth nerve deafness, among others (4).

II. Epidemiology

The incidence of primary and secondary syphilis in the United States, which had increased significantly throughout the 1980s and early 1990s, underwent a dramatic decline in the late 1990s. The overall U.S. incidence of primary and secondary syphilis cases as reported by the Centers for Disease Control and Prevention (CDC) was 20.3/100,000 in 1990, but only 2.5/100,000 in 1999 (5). Rates are significantly higher among African-Americans (15.2/100,000 in 1999), in urban areas, and in the Southeastern United States.

Along with the decreasing incidence of primary and secondary syphilis, the number of cases of congenital syphilis reported by the CDC likewise declined throughout the 1990s from a high of 4408 cases in 1992 to 529 cases in 2000 (13.4/100,000 live births) (6).

The most important risk factors for congenital syphilis are lack of prenatal health care and maternal illicit drug use, particularly cocaine use (7,8). Clinical scenarios that contribute to the occurrence of congenital syphilis include: lack of prenatal care; no serologic test for syphilis (STS) performed during pregnancy; a negative STS in the first trimester, without repeat test later in pregnancy; a negative maternal STS around the time of delivery in a woman who was recently infected with syphilis but had not converted her STS yet; laboratory error in reporting STS results; delay in treatment of a pregnant woman identified as having syphilis; and failure of treatment in an infected pregnant woman.

III. Diagnosis of syphilis (1,9)

A. Serologic tests for syphilis

1. **Nontreponemal tests** include the rapid plasma reagin test (RPR), the venereal disease research laboratory test (VDRL), and the automated reagin test (ART). These tests measure antibodies directed against a cardiolipin-lecithin-cholesterol antigen from *T. pallidum* and/or its interaction with host tissues. These antibodies give quantitative results, are helpful indicators of disease activity, and are useful for follow-up after treatment. Titers usually rise with each new infection and fall after effective treatment. A sustained fourfold decrease in titer of the nontreponemal test with treatment demonstrates adequate therapy; a similar increase after treatment suggests reinfection.

    Nontreponemal tests will be positive in approximately 75% of cases of primary syphilis, nearly 100% of cases of secondary syphilis, and 75% of cases of latent and tertiary syphilis. In secondary syphilis, the RPR or VDRL is usually positive in a titer greater than 1:16. In the first attack of primary syphilis, the RPR or VDRL will usually become nonreactive 1 year after treatment while in secondary syphilis, the test will usually become nonreactive about 2 years after treatment. In latent or tertiary syphilis, the RPR or VDRL may become nonreactive 4 or 5 years after treatment, or and may never turn completely nonreactive. A notable cause of false-negative nontreponemal tests is the prozone phenomenon, a negative or weakly positive reaction that occurs with very high antibody concentrations. In this case, dilution of the serum will result in a positive test.

    One percent of the time, the positive RPR or VDRL is not caused by syphilis. This has been called a biologic false positive (BFP) reaction and is probably related to tissue damage from various causes. Acute BFPs, which usually resolve in about 6 months, may be caused by certain viral infections (particularly infectious mononucleosis, hepatitis, measles, and varicella), endocarditis, intravenous drug abuse, and mycoplasma or protozoa infections. Rarely, BFPs are seen as a result of pregnancy alone. Patients with BFPs usually have low titers (1:8 or less) and nonreactive treponemal tests. Chronic BFPs may be seen in chronic hepatitis, cirrhosis, tuberculosis, extreme old age, malignancy (if associated with excess gamma globulin), connective tissue disease, or autoimmune disease. Patients with systemic lupus erythematosus may have a positive RPR or VDRL. The titer is usually 1:8 or less.

2. **Treponemal tests** include the fluorescent treponemal antibody absorption test [fluorescent treponemal antibody absorption test (FTA-ABS)] and the *T. pallidum* particle agglutination test (TP-PA). Although these tests are more specific than nontreponemal tests, they are also more expensive and labor-intensive and thus are not used for screening. Rather, they are used to confirm positive nontreponemal tests. The treponemal tests correlate poorly with disease activity and usually remain positive for life, even after successful therapy, and therefore should not be used to assess treatment response.

False-positive treponemal tests occur occasionally, particularly in other spirochetal diseases such as Lyme disease, yaws, pinta, leptospirosis, and rat-bite fever; nontreponemal tests should be negative in these situations. Also, in some cases where antibodies to DNA are present, such as in systemic lupus erythematosus, rheumatoid arthritis, polyarteritis, and other autoimmune diseases, a false-positive FTA-ABS may occur. Rarely, pregnancy itself will cause a false-positive treponemal test.

B. **Cerebrospinal fluid** (CSF) testing for neurosyphilis should be done by VDRL. A cell count and protein concentration should also be performed. A positive CSF VDRL is diagnostic of neurosyphilis, but a negative CSF VDRL does not exclude neurosyphilis. The FTA-ABS is recommended by some experts for CSF testing because it is more sensitive than the VDRL; however, contamination with blood during the lumbar puncture may result in a false-positive CSF FTA-ABS (9). A negative CSF FTA-ABS test is good evidence against neurosyphilis. The RPR should not be used for CSF testing.

C. **New tests** under investigation for the diagnosis of syphilis include:

1. **FTA-ABS 19S Immunoglobulin M (IgM) test.** This test detects antitreponemal IgM antibodies. Since IgM does not cross the placenta, a positive test in newborn serum should indicate congenital syphilis. This test represents an advance over previous antitreponemal IgM tests that were very nonspecific; however, due to continued problems with diagnostic accuracy, it is not currently recommended for clinical use (9).

2. **IgM imunnoblotting of serum** identified all infants who had *T. pallidum* infection of the central nervous system (CNS) in a recent study (10).

3. **Polymerase chain reaction (PCR).** PCR can detect the presence of the *T. pallidum* genome in a clinical specimen and thus should be helpful in diagnosing congenital syphilis and neurosyphilis. PCR is not yet widely available for clinical use but may become more so in the near future (9–11).

IV. **Screening and treatment of pregnant women for syphilis** (1,2)

A. **All pregnant women should be screened for syphilis with a nontreponemal STS.** Testing should be performed at the first prenatal visit and, in high-risk populations, should also be repeated at 28 weeks and at delivery. When a woman presents in labor with no history of prenatal care or if results of previous testing are unkown, a STS should be performed at delivery and the infant should not be discharged from the hospital until the test results are known. In women at very high risk, consideration should be given to a repeat STS 1 month postpartum to capture the rare patient who was infected just prior to delivery but had not yet seroconverted. All positive nontreponemal STS in pregnant women should be confirmed with a treponemal test.

B. **Pregnant women with a reactive nontreponemal STS confirmed by a reactive treponemal STS should be treated unless previous adequate treatment**

is clearly documented and follow-up nontreponemal titers have declined at least fourfold. Treatment depends on the stage of infection:

1. **Primary and secondary syphilis.** Benzathine penicillin G 2.4 million units IM. Some experts recommend a second dose 1 week later.
2. **Early latent syphilis (without neurosyphilis).** Treatment is the same as in primary and secondary syphilis.
3. **Late latent syphilis over 1 year duration or syphilis of unknown duration (without neurosyphilis).** Benzathine penicillin G in a total dose of 7.2 million units given as 2.4 million units IM weekly for 3 weeks.
4. **Tertiary syphilis (without neurosyphilis).** Benzathine penicillin G in a total dose of 7.2 million units given as 2.4 million units IM weekly for 3 weeks.
5. **Neurosyphilis.** Aqueous crystalline penicillin G 18 to 24 million units daily administered as 3 to 4 million units IV every 4 hours for 10 to 14 days. If compliance can be assured, an alternative regimen of procaine penicillin 2.4 million units IM daily plus probenecid 500 mg orally 4 times a day for 10 to 14 days may be used. At the end of these therapies, some experts recommend benzathine penicillin G 2.4 million units IM weekly for up to 3 weeks.
6. **Penicillin-allergic patients.** There are no proven alternatives to penicillin for the prevention of congenital syphilis. If an infected pregnant woman has a history of penicillin allergy, she should be skin-tested against the major and minor penicillin determinants. If these tests are negative, penicillin may be given under medical supervision. If the tests are positive, the patient should be desensitized and then given penicillin. Desensitization should be done in consultation with an expert and in a facility where emergency treatment is available (1).
7. **Human immunodeficiency virus (HIV)-infected pregnant women** receive the same treatment as HIV-negative pregnant women, except that treatment for primary and secondary syphilis and early latent syphilis may be extended to three weekly doses of benzathine penicillin G 2.4 million units IM per week.
8. **The Jarisch-Herxheimer reaction**—the occurrence of fever, chills, headache, myalgias, and exacerbation of cutaneous lesions—may occur after treatment of pregnant women for syphilis. Fetal distress, premature labor, and stillbirth are rare but possible.
9. If a mother is treated for syphilis in pregnancy, **monthly follow-up should be provided.** A sustained fourfold decrease in nontreponemal titer should be seen with successful treatment. All patients with syphilis should be evaluated for other sexually transmitted diseases, such as chlamydia, gonorrhea, herpes, and HIV.

V. **Evaluation and treatment of infants for congenital syphilis** (2): No newborn should be discharged from the hospital until the mother's serologic syphilis status is known. Screening of newborn serum or cord blood in place of screening maternal blood is not recommended because of potential false-negative results.

A. Any infant born to a mother with a reactive nontreponemal test confirmed by a treponemal test should be evaluated with the following:
1. **Complete physical examination** looking for evidence of congenital syphilis (see I.B).
2. **Quantitative nontreponemal test (RPR or VDRL).** This test should be performed on infant serum, not on cord blood because of potential false-negatives and false-positives (12). Since IgG is readily transported across the placenta, the infant's serum RPR or VDRL will be positive even if the infection was not transmitted. The infant's titer should begin to fall by 3 months and become nonreactive by 6 months if the antibody is passively acquired. If the baby was infected, the titer will not fall and may rise. The tests may be negative at birth if the infection was acquired late in pregnancy. In this case, repeating the test later will confirm the diagnosis.

3. **Pathological examination** of the placenta or umbilical cord using specific fluorescent antitreponemal antibody staining, if available.
4. **Darkfield microscopic examination** of direct fluorescent antibody staining of any suspicious lesions or body fluids (e.g., nasal discharge).
5. New tests such as **PCR and immunoglobulin M (IgM)** immunoblotting may identify infants with CNS infections (10).

B. The CDC recommends classifying infants evaluated for congenital syphilis into one of the following four scenarios:

1. **Scenario One**
   a. **Any** of the following are evidence of **proven or highly probable disease:**
      (1) **Abnormal physical examination** consistent with congenital syphilis.
      (2) **Nontreponemal titer** that is **fourfold higher** than the mother's titer (*Note:* the absence of a fourfold or greater titer does not exclude congenital syphilis).
      (3) **Positive darkfield** or **fluorescent antibody test** of body fluid(s).
   b. Further evaluation of infants with proven or highly probable disease should include:
      (1) **CSF analysis for VDRL, cell count, and protein concentration.** Note that in the neonatal period, interpretation of CSF values may be difficult. Normal values of protein and white blood cells (WBC) are higher in preterm infants. Values up to 25 WBC/mm^3 and 150 mg protein/dL may be normal (see Table 36.1).
      (2) **Complete blood count** with differential and platelet count.
      (3) **Other tests** as clinically indicated, including long-bone radiographs, chest radiograph, liver function tests, cranial ultrasound, ophthalmologic exam, and auditory brainstem responses.
   c. Treatment for infants with proven or highly probable disease should consist of either:
      (1) **Aqueous crystalline penicillin G** 100,000 to 150,000 units/kg/day IV, divided every 12 hours during the first 7 days and every 8 hours thereafter for a total of 10 to 14 days or;
      (2) **Procaine penicillin G** 50,000 units/kg per dose IM daily in a single dose for 10 days.

2. **Scenario Two**
   a. Infants who have a normal physical exam and a serum quantitative nontreponemal titer the same or less than fourfold the maternal titer and **any of** the following:
      (1) **Maternal treatment not given,** inadequate, or not documented.
      (2) **Maternal treatment with erythromycin** or any other **nonpenicillin** regimen.
      (3) **Maternal treatment** administered less than **4 weeks before delivery.**
      (4) **Mother** with early syphilis **whose nontreponemal titer has not decreased fourfold,** or **has increased fourfold.**
   b. Such infants should be evaluated with:
      (1) **Complete blood count** with differential and platelet count.
      (2) **CSF analysis for VDRL, cell count, and protein concentration.**
      (3) **Long-bone radiographs.**
   c. Treatment of such infants should consist of either:
      (1) **Aqueous crystalline penicillin G** 100,000 to 150,000 units/kg per day IV, divided every 12 hours during the first 7 days and every 8 hours thereafter for a total of 10 to 14 days or;
      (2) **Procaine penicillin G** 50,000 units/kg per dose IM daily in a single dose for 10 to 14 days or;
      (3) If the complete evaluation is normal (CBC with differential and platelets, CSF analysis with VDRL, cell count, and protein concentration, and long-bone radiographs) and follow-up is certain, **a single dose of benzathine penicillin G** 50,000 units/kg IM **may be substituted for the full 10-day course.** If any part of the evaluation is abnormal or uninterpretable (e.g., CSF sample contaminated with

blood), or if follow-up is not certain, then the full 10 day course of parenteral therapy should be given.

3. Scenario Three

    a. Infants who have a normal physical exam and a serum quantitative nontreponemal titer the same or less than fourfold the maternal titer and **all of** the following:

        (1) Maternal treatment during pregnancy with a penicillin regimen appropriate for the stage of infection, and more than 4 weeks prior to delivery.

        (2) Maternal nontreponemal titer decreased fourfold after therapy if early syphilis, or remained stable and low for late syphilis.

        (3) no evidence of maternal reinfection or relapse.

    b. Such infants require no evaluation.

    c. Such infants should be treated with a **single dose of benzathine penicillin G** 50,000 units/kg IM.

4. Scenario Four

    a. Infants who have a normal physical exam and a serum quantitative nontreponemal titer the same or less than fourfold the maternal titer and **both of** the following:

        (1) Adequate maternal treatment before pregnancy.

        (2) Maternal nontreponemal titer remained low and stable before and during pregnancy and at delivery (VDRL $\leq$ 1:2 or RPR $\leq$ 1:4).

    b. Such infants require no evaluation.

    c. No treatment is recommended; however some experts administer a single dose of benzathine penicillin G 50,000 units/kg IM, particularly if follow-up is uncertain.

C. Evaluation and treatment of infants and children **over 1 month of age**.

Children identified as having a reactive STS after the neonatal period should have maternal serology and treatment records reviewed to determine if the child has congenital or acquired syphilis.

  1. If the child is at risk for congenital syphilis, **evaluation should include:**

    a. Complete blood count with differential and platelet count.

    b. CSF analysis for VDRL, cell count, and protein concentration.

    c. Other tests as clinically indicated, including long-bone radiographs, chest radiograph, liver function tests, cranial ultrasound, ophthalmologic exam, and auditory brainstem responses.

  2. Treatment should consist of aqueous crystalline penicillin G 200,000 to 300,000 units/kg per day IV divided every 4 to 6 hours for 10 days. Some experts also suggest administering a single dose of benzathine penicillin G 50,000 units/kg IM following the 10-day course of IV therapy.

D. Some would treat all newborns with a positive serolgic test for syphilis because it may be difficult to document that the mother has had adequate treatment and falling serologic titers, a low titer may be present in latent maternal syphilis, infected newborns may have no clinical signs at birth, and follow-up/compliance may be difficult in the population at risk for congenital syphilis. If the mother has received an appropriate regimen of penicillin therapy more than 1 month before delivery, the infant's clinical and laboratory examination are normal, and follow-up is assured, some would follow the infant without treatment (1).

VI. Follow-up of infants treated for congenital syphilis. All seroreactive infants should have a physical examination and nontreponemal titer every 2 to 3 months until the test becomes nonreactive or the titer decreases fourfold. If the titer is found to increase or remain reactive at 6 to 12 months, the infant should undergo reevaluation for signs of active syphilis and retreatment should be seriously considered. Infants with possible neurosyphilis (abnormal or uninterpretable CSF results at the time of initial diagnosis) should undergo repeat CSF examination at 6-month intervals until the CSF is normal. If the CSF VDRL remains positive at any 6-month interval, retreatment is recommended. If the CSF VDRL is negative, but the CSF cell count and/or protein concentration are not declining or remain abnormal at 2 years, retreatment is recommended.

VII. Infection control. Nasal secretions and open syphilitic lesions are highly infectious. Strict bodily fluid precautions should be taken. Health-care personnel as well as family members and other visitors should wear gloves when handling infants with congenital syphilis until therapy has been administered for at least 24 hours. Those who have close contact with an infected infant or mother before precautions were taken should be examined and tested for infection and treatment should be considered.

A. Infants and their mothers at risk for or infected with syphilis should be evaluated for other sexually transmitted diseases such as herpes, gonorrhea, chlamydia, and HIV.

B. Assistance and guidance in syphilis testing and treatment are available from the Centers for Disease Control and Prevention, Atlanta, Georgia, and state health departments.

References

1. Syphilis. In: Pickering L.K., ed. *2000 Red Book: Report of the Committee on Infectious Diseases.* 25th ed. Elk Grove Village, Ill.: American Academy of Pediatrics; 2000:547–559.
2. Centers for Disease Control and Prevention. Sexually Transmitted Diseases Treatment Guidelines 2002. *MMWR* 2002;51:18–30.
3. Wicher V., Wicher K. Pathogenesis of maternal-fetal syphilis revisited. *Clin Infect Dis* 2001;33:354–363.
4. Gutman L.T. Syphilis. In: Feigin R.D., Cherry J.D., (Ed.). *Textbook of Pediatric Infectious Diseases.* 4th ed. Philadelphia: W.B. Saunders:1998:1543–1556.
5. Centers for Disease Control and Prevention. Primary and secondary syphilis—United States 1999. *MMWR* 2001;50:113–117.
6. Centers for Disease Control and Prevention. Congenital syphilis—United States, 2000. *MMWR* 2001;50:573–557.
7. Webber M.P., et al. Maternal risk factors for congenital syphilis: A case-control study. *Am J Epidemiol* 1993;137:415–422.
8. Ricci J.M., et al. Congenital syphilis: the University of Miami/Jackson memorial Medical Center experience 1986–88. *Obstet Gynecol* 1989;74:687–693.
9. Wicher K., et al. Laboratory methods of diagnosis of syphilis for the beginning of the third millennium. *Microbes Infect* 1999;1:1035–1049.
10. Michelow I.C., et al. Central nervous system infection in congenital syphilis. *N Engl J Med* 2002; 346:1792–1798.
11. Sanchez P.J. Laboratory tests for congenital syphilis. *Pediatr Infect Dis J* 1998; 17:70–71.
12. Chhabra R.S., et al. Comparison of maternal sera, cord blood, and neonatal sera for detecting congenital syphilis: relationship with maternal treatment. *Pediatrics* 1993;91:88–91.

Lyme Disease

John A.F. Zupancic and John P. Cloherty

I. Lyme disease (Lyme borreliosis) (1,3) is the most common vector-borne disease in the United States. The causative organism is the spirochete *Borrelia burgdorferi,* which is transmitted to humans through the bite of a tick of the Ixodid species. White-footed mice and deer are important in the life cycle of the tick. Distribution of Lyme disease correlates with the distribution of these hosts. Most cases in the United States are clustered in the Northeast from Massachusetts to Maryland, in the Midwest in Wisconsin and Minnesota, or in California.

There have been cases reported from all states, Canada, Europe, China, Japan, and Russia. Humans are the most likely to be infected in June, July, and August. Clinical manifestations of Lyme disease are noted in Table 23.8.

Early case reports (5,8,12) and case series (3,7) confirmed that transplacental transmission of *B. burgdorferi* was possible and raised concerns about a congenital Lyme disease syndrome analagous to that seen with other spirochetal infections such as syphilis. A wide variety of clinical manifestations were noted, but initial concerns were focused on congenital cardiac malformations and fetal death. However, epidemiologic studies have not supported an association between congenital infection and adverse fetal or neonatal outcomes. A prospective study of 2014 pregnant women showed no association between seropositivity or history of tick bite and congenital malformations, low birth weight, or fetal death (11). A report by the same authors compared 2504 infants born in an endemic region to 2507 delivered in a nonendemic region (13). This study showed a significant increase in the rate of congenital cardiac malformations in the endemic compared to the nonendemic region, but notably no association within the endemic region between seropositivity and cardiac malformation. Similarly, in a retrospective case-control study of 796 patients with congenital heart disease and 704 control infants, there was no association between cardiac anomalies and clinical evidence of Lyme disease during pregnancy (10). Although these studies were limited by the low prevalence of Lyme disease, it appears from available evidence that any increased risk for adverse neonatal effects of prenatal Lyme borreliosis are likely to be small (4,9).

There is no evidence that *B. burgdorferi* is transmitted in human milk (1).

II. **Diagnosis** (1). Lyme disease may be diagnosed by the appearance of a typical rash (erythema migrans) in women living in or visiting an area where cases of Lyme disease have been previously reported. However, the spectrum of clinical symptoms may be quite variable (see Table 23.8). As discussed, there is no accepted syndrome of congenital Lyme borreliosis. Serologic testing begins with acute and convalescent enzyme immunoassay (EIA) or immunofluoresence assay (IFA) to detect IgM antibodies against *B. burgdorferi*. The immunoglobulin M (IgM) titer peaks at 3 to 6 weeks after infection, and may be negative for patients with isolated erythema migrans, those who are pregnant (6) or those who have been treated early. In addition, false-positive EIA and IFA results occur secondary to cross-reaction with other spirochetal and viral infections and autoimmune disease. Therefore, positive or equivocal EIA or IFA test results should be confirmed with Western immunoblot. If central nervous system involvement is suspected, spinal fluid serology should also be obtained. Polymerase chain reaction for detection of *B. burgdorferi* is currently investigational.

III. **Treatment of mothers and the newborn** (1,12,14). Patients known to have Lyme disease or who are suspected of having Lyme disease during pregnancy should be treated. The treatment is the same as for nonpregnant persons except that doxycycline is contraindicated (14).

A. **Tick bite.** Prophylactic treatment of tick bites in endemic areas is not recommended.

B. **Localized early Lyme disease** (see stage 1, Table 23.8). Amoxicillin 500 mg po TID for 14 to 21 days or cefuroxime axetil 500 mg po BID for 14 to 21 days. For penicillin-allergic patients, erythromycin 500 mg po QID for 14 to 21 days is an alternative; however, macrolides appear to be less effective, and these patients should therefore be closley followed (14).

C. **Disseminated early Lyme disease or any manifestations of late disease.** Ceftriaxone 2 g IV once daily for 14 to 28 days or penicillin G 18 to 24 million units IV q day divided q4h. Patients with isolated cranial nerve palsy, first- or second-degree heart block, or arthritis without neurological manifestations may be treated with oral therapy as for localized early Lyme disease.

D. **Newborn of mother with confirmed Lyme disease in pregnancy.** The relative risk of fetal transmission as a function of severity of maternal disease, chronicity of maternal disease, or choice of antibiotic and route of adminis-

TABLE 23.8. MANIFESTATIONS OF LYME DISEASE BY STAGE*

| System[†] | Early Infection | | Late Infection (Persistent [Stage 3]) |
	Localized (Stage 1)	Disseminated (Stage 2)	
Skin	Erythema migrans	Secondary annular lesions, malar rash, diffuse erythema or urticaria, evanescent lesions, lymphocytoma	Acrodermatitis chronica atrophicans, localized sclerodermalike lesions
Musculoskeletal system		Migratory pain in joints, tendons, bursae, muscle, bone; brief arthritis attacks; myositis;[†] osteomyelitis;[‡] panniculitis[‡]	Prolonged arthritis attacks, chronic arthritis, peripheral enthesopathy, periostitis or joint subluxations below lesions of acrodermatitis
Neurologic system		Meningitis, cranial neuritis, Bell's palsy, motor or sensory radiculoneuritis, subtle encephalitis, mononeuritis multiplex, myelitis,[‡] chorea,[‡] cerebellar ataxia[‡]	Chronic encephalomyelitis, spastic paraparesis, ataxic gait, subtle mental disorders, chronic axonal polyradiculopathy, dementia[‡]
Lymphatic system	Regional lymphadenopathy	Regional or generalized lymphadenopathy, splenomegaly	
Heart		Atrioventricular nodal block, myopericarditis, pancarditis	
Eyes		Conjunctivitis, iritis,[‡] choroiditis,[‡] retinal hemorrhage or detachment,[‡] panophthalmitis[‡]	Keratitis
Liver		Mild or recurrent hepatitis	
Respiratory system		Nonexudative sore throat, nonproductive cough, adult respiratory distress syndrome[‡]	
Kidney		Microscopic hematuria or proteinuria	
Genitourinary system		Orchitis[‡]	
Constitutional symptoms	Minor	Severe malaise and fatigue	Fatigue

*The classification by stages provides a guideline for the expected timing of the illness's manifestations, but this may vary from case to case.
[†]Systems are listed from the most to the least commonly affected.
[‡]The inclusion of this manifestation is based on one or a few cases.

329

tration is not known. Similarly, data are lacking on the optimal therapy for the newborn infant with symptoms of acute Lyme disease. In the study by Markowitz et al. (7), a 38-week fetus born to a mother who developed acute Lyme disease 1 week prior to delivery developed petechiae and a vesicular rash that resolved with the intravenous administration of penicillin G for 10 days. If an infant is thought to have Lyme disease, treatment with penicillin or ceftriaxone intravenously should be given for 14 to 21 days after studies are taken from blood and spinal fluid. If a mother was treated for Lyme disease with erythromycin during pregnancy, consideration should be given to treatment of the infant with penicillin or ceftriaxone.

   E. Prevention of Lyme disease. A recombinant vaccine against the outer surface protein of *B. burgdorferi* was licensed by the Food and Drug Administration (FDA) in 1998 for individuals between 15 and 70 years of age (2). It was not recommended for use in pregnant women (1). The vaccine was withdrawn from the market in 2002 by the manufacturer due to lack of demand.

References

1. American Academy of Pediatrics. Lyme disease. In: Pickering L.K., ed. *2000 Red Book: Report of the Committee of Infectious Disease.* 25th ed. 2000; Elk Grove Village, Ill.: American Academy of Pediatrics, p. 374.
2. American Academy of Pediatrics. Committee on Infectious Diseases. Prevention of Lyme disease. *Pediatrics* 2000;105;142.
3. Ciesielski C.A., et al. Prospective study of pregnancy outcome in women with Lyme disease. Interscience Conference on Antimicrobial Agents and Chemotherapy, New York, 1987 (Abstract No. 39).
4. Elliott D.J., et al. Teratogen update: Lyme disease. *Teratology* 2001;64:276–281.
5. MacDonald A.B., et al. Stillbirth following maternal Lyme disease. *N Y J Med* 1987;87:615.
6. MacDonald A.B. Gestational Lyme borreliosis: Implications for the fetus. *Rheum Dis Clin North Am* 1989;15:657.
7. Markowitz L.E., et al. Lyme disease during pregnancy. *JAMA* 1986;255:3394.
8. Schlesinger P.A., et al. Maternal-fetal transmission of the Lyme disease spirochete. *Ann Intern Med* 1985;103:67.
9. Silver H.M. Lyme disease during pregnancy. *Infect Dis Clin North Am* 1997;11:93.
10. Strobino B., et al. Maternal Lyme disease and congenital heart disease: A case-control study in an endemic area. *Am J Obstet Gynecol* 1999;180:711.
11. Strobino B.A., et al. Lyme disease and pregnancy outcome: a prospective study of two thousand prenatal patients. *Am J Obstet Gynecol* 1993:169:367.
12. Weber K., et al. B. burgdorferi in a newborn despite oral penicillin for Lyme disease during pregnancy. *Pediatr Infect Dis J* 1988;7:286.
13. Williams C.L., et al. Maternal Lyme disease and congenital malformations: A cord blood serosurvey in endemic and control areas. *Paediatr Perinat Epidemiol* 1995;9:320.
14. Wormser G.P., et al. Practice guidelines for the treatment of Lyme disease. *Clin Infect Dis* 2000;31(suppl 1):1.

Toxoplasmosis

Nicholas G. Guerina

   I. *Toxoplasma gondii* is an obligate, intracellular protozoan parasite that is well recognized as an important human pathogen. This is particularly true for the fetus, newborn infant, and immunocompromised adults. Many animals may become infected, but the cat is the only definitive host. During an acute infection the cat may shed up to 1 million oocysts in the stool per day for up to 2 weeks or longer (19,20,26). These oocysts may remain viable in soil for many months depending upon climactic conditions. Susceptible farm animals become infected by ingesting the oocysts resulting in localization of viable organisms in muscle cysts. Principal modes of transmission to humans beyond the newborn period is by the ingestion of the cysts in undercooked meat, or by the direct ingestion of oocysts. Transmission following the transfusion of whole blood or leukocytes may occur, but the risk is unknown. Normal children and adults are susceptible to acute infection if they lack specific antibody to the organism. Both humoral and cell-mediated immunity are important in the control of infection. Following an acute parasitemia, the organism invades tissues where cysts are formed. The cysts persist in multiple organs, probably for life. Most often these are of little consequence to the normal host, but progressive localized, or reactivated disease may occur in a subset of patients.

II. **Diagnosis.** A number of methods may be employed in the diagnosis of congenital toxoplasma infection (31). These include isolation or histologic demonstration of the organism; detection of toxoplasma antigens in tissues and body fluids; detection of toxoplasma nucleic acid by polymerase chain reaction (PCR); and serological tests. Of these, serological tests are most frequently used and are often critical in diagnosing acute maternal and congenital infections. In addition, the PCR appears to be very sensitive and specific in determining fetal infection.

Toxoplasma-specific immunoglobulin G (IgG) appears within 1 to 2 weeks following acute infection, peaks at 1 to 2 months, and persists throughout life. Many commercial laboratories now offer a toxoplasma-specific IgG and immunoglobulin M (IgM) testing, as well as PCR on amniotic and spinal fluid. **It is strongly recommended that all positive IgM test results be confirmed by a toxoplasma reference laboratory, and PCR testing should only be performed in a reference laboratory.** All of the serologic tests discussed in this section are performed by the Toxoplasma Serology Laboratory at the Palo Alto Medical Foundation, Ames Bldg, 795 El Camino Real, Palo Alto, CA 94301 (*Tel: (650) 853–4828 Fax: (650) 614–3292 Email:* toxolab@pamf.org). Test descriptions, specimen collection and handling instructions, and specimen requisition forms are available at http://www.pamf.org/serology.

A. **Sabin-Feldman dye test.** This test makes use of the uptake by toxoplasma tachyzoites of the dye methylene blue (organisms appear swollen and blue). The tachyzoite membranes lyse in the presence of complement and specific antibody (primarily IgG) resulting in a thin, unstained appearance to the organisms. There is extensive experience with the use of this test, and it is particularly useful as an antenatal screening test for maternal seroconversion in pregnancy (31).

B. **Enzyme-linked immunosorbent assay (ELISA).** This test has been adapted for the detection of toxoplasma-specific IgG, IgM, immunoglobulin A (IgA), and immunoglobulin E (IgE). The IgG test is readily available in most commercial laboratories but has limited utility in the determination of acute infection in both pregnant women and newborn infants. A double-sandwich toxoplasma-specific IgM-ELISA (DS-IgM-ELISA) has been developed, which greatly aids in the diagnosis of congenital toxoplasma infection (31). Maternal IgM may remain elevated from months to many years so the test may not help in determining recent maternal infection. Since IgM does not cross the placenta, however, the test may be very useful in determining congenital infection.

Enzyme-linked immunosorbent assays have also been developed for measuring toxoplasma-specific IgA and IgE (31). Like IgM antibody, IgA antibody rises rapidly following an acute infection, and it may persist for more than 1 year. The test may have greater sensitivity for newborn infants compared to IgM assays, so it may aid in the early postnatal diagnosis of congenital infection. Toxoplasma-specific IgE levels usually do not persist as long as IgM and IgA, so this assay may be useful in the diagnosis of recently acquired infection.

C. **Immunosorbent agglutination assay (ISAGA).** This test measures toxoplasma-specific antibody captured from sera by the agglutination of a particulate antigen preparation (31). Assays for detecting IgM and IgA have been developed and both tests may be complementary to ELISA procedures in determining congenital infection.

D. **Differential agglutination test.** This test compares agglutination titers for sera against formalin-fixed tachyzoites (HS antigen) with those against acetone- or methanol-fixed tachyzoites (AC antigen) (31). The different test preparations display antigens present at different times in infection so the relative titers with each preparation may be indicative of acute versus remote infection.

E. **IgG avidity.** Toxoplasma-specific IgG antibodies produced early in infection have low avidity, but the avidity increases over time. High-avidity IgG antibodies against toxoplasma have been shown to exclude infection occuring within the preceding 3 months (18,27). When used in conjunction with other toxoplasma serologies, IgG avidity may help deliniate recently acquired from remote infection in pregnant women.

F. **Polymerase chain reaction (PCR).** This test has been adapted for the identification of *T. gondii* in amniotic fluid specimens obtained on women with acquired toxoplasma in pregnancy. The potential sensitivity and specificity of this procedure was determined in a comparison study (16) using amniotic fluid PCR compared to ultrasonographic screening with studies on fetal blood obtained by percutaneous umbilical blood sampling (6). Congenital infection was identified in 34 of 339 fetuses by ultrasound/fetal blood testing, but all of these cases were also identified by amniotic fluid PCR. In addition, three infants who were missed by ultrasound or fetal blood testing were identified by PCR. There was only one false-negative and no false-positive PCR result. A lower sensitivity for the amniotic fluid PCR assay has also been reported (28), emphasizing the need to extend until delivery antenatal maternal therapy directed at the prevention or treatment of fetal infection. It is highly recommended that this test be performed by a toxoplasma reference laboratory.

III. **Epidemiology and clinical manifestations**

A. **Maternal infection.** The prevalence of toxoplasma antibody varies with age and geographic location. In the United States, 50 to 85% of women of childbearing age are at risk for acute toxoplasmosis in pregnancy. Seroprevalence data from New York City has shown that approximately16% of childbearing women ages 15 years to 19 years are seropositive (7), but the seroprevalence increases to approximately 50% for >35 years old. Universal screening of newborn infants for toxoplasma-specific IgM has been conducted for the past 8 years in Massachusetts (13). The screening is carried out on filter paper-dried–blood-spot specimens, which are routinely sent to Public Health State Laboratories for screening for metabolic and endocrine abnormalities in all newborn infants. Over a 1-year period, screening for toxoplasma-specific IgG was also conducted. Since maternal IgG readily crosses the placenta, the prevalence of specific IgG in the newborn reflects the overall seroprevalence in childbearing women. It was found that 17% of 90,000 newborn specimens tested had IgG to *T. gondii* indicating that 83% of mothers were at risk for acute infection. Data from the National Collaborative Perinatal Project (National Institutes of Health) showed a toxoplasma seroprevalence rate of 38.7% for 22,000 women in the United States, and the estimated incidence of acute maternal infection in pregnancy was 1.1 per 1000 (29).

Symptoms of acute toxoplasma infection in pregnant women may be transient and nonspecific, and most cases go undiagnosed in the absence of universal antibody screening. When symptoms are present they usually are limited to lymphadenopathy and fatigue; adenopathy may persist for months and a single lymph node may be involved. Less commonly, a mononucleosis-like syndrome characterized by fever, malaise, sore throat, headache, myalgia, and an atypical lymphocytosis has been described.

B. Congenital infection. Previous estimates of the incidence of congenital toxoplasma infection in certain areas of the United States have been as high as 1/1000 to 2/1000 births, but more recent studies suggest a lower incidence (1,6,8,9). For example, cord blood screening for toxoplasma-specific IgM showed a decreasing incidence from 2/1000 to 0.1/1000 births (17,26). An incidence of approximately 0.1/1000 births was also found for infected newborn identified through a newborn screening program in Massachusetts over a 6.5-year period beginning in January 1986 (13).

Vertical transmission of *T. gondii* from mother to fetus occurs at an average rate of 30 to 40%, but the rate varies with the gestational age at which acute maternal infection occurs (8). The average transmission rate is 15 percent for the first trimester but increases to 60% for the third trimester; transmission appears to correlate well with placental blood flow and may approach 90% at term. The severity of fetal disease is inversely proportional to gestational age. In the absence of toxoplasma-specific chemotherapy, most fetuses infected in the first trimester die in utero or in the neonatal period, or have severe central nervous system and ophthalmologic disease. Conversely, most fetuses infected in the second trimester, and all infants infected in the third trimester, have mild or subclinical disease in the newborn period.

Infants with congenital toxoplasma infection may present with one of four recognized patterns (Table 23.9): (1) symptomatic neonatal disease; (2) symptomatic disease occurring in the first months of life; (3) sequelae or relapse in infancy, or later childhood, of previously undiagnosed infection; and (4) subclinical infection (1). The principal clinical findings for infants presenting with severe disease were described in the classic report of Eichenwald (10). These infants invariably had some degree of central nervous system (CNS) involvement and often had significant retinal disease. The infants appeared to fall into one group who primarily had marked CNS and retinal disease or one group with generalized clinical and laboratory abnormalities in addition to retinal disease and somewhat less prominent CNS findings. Infants with primary neurologic disease typically had intracranial calcifications, abnormal cerebrospinal fluid (CSF) profiles, chorioretinitis, and convulsions. Infants with signs and symptoms of generalized disease had hepatosplenomegaly, lymphadenopathy, jaundice and anemia, in addition to CSF abnormalities and chorioretinitis. More recently, McAuley et al. (24) reported the clinical presentations and treatment outcomes for infants with congenital toxoplasma infection followed in the Chicago collaborative treatment trial. Thirty-five of the infants were diagnosed at 2 months of age, and nearly all of them were diagnosed because of clinical findings indicating they had symptomatic congenital infection. These infants had clinical findings comparable to those described by Eichenwald (10) except that there was considerable overlap in the clinical presentations of generalized and neurologic disease.

It is important to note that 80 to 90% of infants with congenital toxoplasma do not have overt signs of infection at birth (1,2,13,26). Nevertheless, these infants may have retinal and CNS abnormalities when further testing is performed. In addition, these infants remain at risk for severe long-term ophthalmologic and neurologic sequelae. In the New England Regional Newborn Screening program, filter paper–dried–blood-spot specimens are screened for toxoplasma-specific IgM (13). Confirmation IgM and IgG tests are performed on a repeat blood sample from each infant with a positive screening test, and on a serum sample from each infant's mother. Infants with confirmed infection have an ophthalmologic examination, intracranial imaging [head computed tomography (CT scan)], and cerebrospinal fluid (CSF) examination performed. Over a 6.5-year period starting January

TABLE 23.9. FREQUENCIES FOR INITIAL CLINICAL AND LABORATORY ABNORMALITIES IN INFANTS WITH CONGENITAL TOXOPLASMA INFECTION FROM THE CHICAGO COLLABORATIVE TREATMENT TRIAL* AND THE NEW ENGLAND REGIONAL NEWBORN SCREENING PROGRAM†

Clinical/Laboratory Finding	No. Infants with Specific Finding (%)	
	Chicago Study	New England Study
Generalized abnormalities		
Fever	4/35 (11)	0/54 (0)
Respiratory illness	8/35 (23)	0/54 (0)
Splenomegaly	20/35 (57)	0/54 (0)
Hepatomegaly	18/35 (51)	1/54 (2)
Jaundice	23/35 (66)	1/54 (2)
Thrombocytopenia	14/35 (40)	0/54 (0)
Neurologic abnormalities		
Intracranial calcifications	25/35 (71)	13/50 (26)
Elevated CSF protein	19/33 (56)	11/35 (31)
Hydrocephalus	15/35 (43)	4/50 (8)
Seizures‡	6/35 (17)	1/54 (2)
Microcephaly	5/35 (14)	1/54 (2)
Motor deficit	21/35 (60)	7/54 (13)
Ophthalmologic abnormalities		
Peripheral retinal scars only	3/35 (9)	2/54 (4)
Macular lesions	21/35 (60)	11/54 (20)
Visual impairment‡	15/35 (43)	11/54 (20)

*From McAuley J., et al. *Clin Infect Dis* 1994;18(1):38; includes only infants 2 months of age at initial presentation.
†From Guerina N. G., et al. *N Engl J Med* 1994;330:1858.
‡Abnormality at or shortly after initial presentation.
Source: Guerina N. G. Management strategies for infectious diseases in pregnancy. *Semin Perinatol* 1994;18:305.

1986, 52 of 635,000 infants screened were identified with congenital toxoplasma, and 50 of these infants were identified solely through newborn screening; all 50 were term, had normal routine physical examinations, and were discharged home for routine newborn follow-up. After congenital infection was confirmed by follow-up serologic testing, additional studies revealed abnormalities of either the CNS or retina in 19 of 48 (40%) infants examined. Table 23.9 summarizes the clinical and laboratory findings for infants with congenital toxoplasma infection identified through the New England Newborn Screening Program compared with those from the Chicago collaborative treatment trial. Since infants from the New England Newborn Screening Program were identified by statewide universal serologic screening, the clinical presentations of this group more accurately reflect the expected incidence of abnormalities.

1. **Sequelae of congenital toxoplasma infection in the absence of extended chemotherapy.** Several prospective studies have been conducted to determine the frequency of adverse outcomes in infants with subclinical congenital toxoplasma infection. Koppe et al. (21,22) prospectively followed 11 infants with congenital toxoplasma infection and found that 9 (82%) developed chorioretinitis over a 20-year follow-up period. Four of these infants developed severe visual impairment and 3 had unilateral blindness. These infants either received no treatment (7 infants) or treat-

ment was limited to a 3-week course of pyrimethamine and sulfadiazine (4 infants). Wilson et al. (30) reported similar results for 23 infants with congenital toxoplasma infection. Thirteen of these infants had no clinical evidence of disease at birth and were diagnosed solely by the presence of toxoplasma-specific IgM in cord blood specimens. As in the Koppe et al. study, infants received either no treatment or a brief course (1 month) of pyrimethamine and sulfadiazine. On follow-up over several years, 11 (85%) children developed chorioretinitis, including 3 with unilateral blindness.

Although the patients followed by Koppe et al. (21,22) were reported to have had normal school performance (based on parental reporting), the children described by Wilson et al. (30) were found to develop significant neurologic complications; of the 13 infants with subclinical infection identified through cord blood serologic screening, one child developed psychomotor retardation, microcephaly, and seizures; two children had delayed psychomotor development (reported to eventually become normal); and 2 children had persistent cerebellar dysfunction. Three children developed sensorineural hearing loss. The mean IQ for all 13 children was 88 with 2 children reported to be severely affected with IQ values of 36 and 62. Furthermore, six children who had a mean IQ score of 97 on initial testing had a significant drop in their mean score to 74 when retested 5.5 years later. Neurologic complications were also reported in the study by Sever et al. (29). In their follow-up over a 7-year period of mother–infant pairs in the Collaborative Perinatal Project, deafness occurred in infants born to mothers with toxoplasma-specific IgG. In addition, infants born to mothers with toxoplasma-specific titers suggestive of acute infection in pregnancy had a 60% increase in the incidence of microcephaly, and a 30% increase in the occurrence of low IQ scores (<70). These studies demonstrate the risk for long-term ophthalmologic and neurologic abnormalities in infants with congenital toxoplasma infection despite their initial clinical presentation.

IV. Treatment

A. Management of the at-risk and infected fetus.

The risk of vertical transmission of *T. gondii* from an acutely infected mother to her fetus may be significantly diminished by maternal treatment with spiramycin (9). The drug is currently available in the United States through an investigational new drug (IND) number issued by the Food and Drug Administration (FDA). The results of toxoplasma serology must be reviewed with the Toxoplasma Serology Laboratory, Palo Alto Medical Foundation (650-853-4828). Confirmatory testing may be required. The dose is 1 g every 8 hours. Although this drug reduces the incidence of vertical transmission, the severity of disease when fetal infection occurs may not be altered (9). Thus, when acute maternal infection is determined, it is important to evaluate the fetus for possible infection, in addition to initiating maternal spiramycin therapy. In early studies, Daffos et al. (6) evaluated an antenatal screening and treatment program in which women were screened for acute infection by serial antibody assays. When a woman seroconverted, indicating acute infection, she was started on spiramycin, and fetal infection was assessed by amniotic fluid culture, fetal blood studies (percutaneous umbilical blood sampling for culture, specific IgM, total IgM, and blood chemistries), and fetal ultrasound surveys. When fetal infection was confirmed either elective pregnancy termination was carried out, or maternal treatment was changed to combination anti-toxoplasma chemotherapy; the therapeutic regimen was pyrimethamine plus sulfonamide alternating every 3 weeks with spiramycin beginning at the 24th week of gestation. Folinic acid was also added to help prevent the potentially toxic side effects of pyrimethamine. Of 746 documented maternal infections, 42 cases of congenital infections were observed, 39 of which were identified by the antenatal screening tests. Twenty-four pregnancies were terminated. The remaining 15 pregnancies were carried to term and at 3 months follow-up, 13 of 15 remain asymptomatic. The other two infants were diagnosed with chorioretinitis. A more recent study reported the outcome of infants with congenital toxoplasma born to mothers diagnosed with acute infection by seroconversion between 8 and 26 weeks' gestation (3). One hundred and sixty-three women were diagnosed and treated with spiramycin. The fetuses of these women were evaluated for evidence of infection by cordocentesis and serial ultrasounds, and 23 of the women were treated with pyrimethamine and sulfadiazine. Three fetuses died and 27 of 162 liveborn infants had confirmed congenital infection. Ten of the infected infants had clinical signs of infection with intracranial calcifications (5 infants), moderate ventricular dilation (2 infants), and peripheral chorioretinitis (7 infants). All 27 infants are reported to be free from symptoms at 15 to 71 months of age. The investigators conclude that pregnancy termination may not be necessary for acquired toxoplasma in the first and second trimester, provided anti-toxoplasma chemotherapy is given and repeated fetal ultrasounds remain normal.

The benefits of antenatal screening for acute maternal toxoplasma infection seem apparent, but universal testing has been controversial in the United States. The major concerns have included the cost of serial tests in a relatively low incidence population, and the reliability of commercially available screening assays. These are not insurmountable obstacles and universal maternal screening should probably be performed. Wong and Remington (31) have recommended antenatal maternal screening for pregnant women in the United States using the Sabin-Feldman dye test (or equivalent assay) at 12 weeks with retesting at 20 to 22 weeks and again near term. The dye test is available through the Toxoplasma Serology Laboratory, Palo Alto Medical Foundation (650-853-4828; http://www.pamf.org/serology). Commercial laboratories offer other serologic tests but sensitivity and specificity vary and inconsistent results are sometimes obtained. If the dye test is not readily available, maternal toxoplasma-specific IgG ELISA and double-sandwich IgM ELISA may be requested. A positive IgG and negative IgM indicates remote infection (no risk to fetus if mother does not have immunodeficiency). If the IgM test is positive on the initial screen, additional testing may be required to help determine the likelihood of a recent infection.

If seroconversion is documented during pregnancy, acute maternal infection should be assumed and infectious disease consultation obtained. The timing of antenatal treatment with respect to acute maternal infection may be important to fetal infection (11). Some question has also been raised as to the intensity of antenatal treatment required to impact on fetal transmission and the severity of fetal disease (12). It is well recognized, however, that the timing from maternal infection to fetal transmission may be delayed for many weeks (26), and it is recommended that antenatal treatment be initiated promptly upon the identification of acute maternal infection irrespective of any delay that may have occurred in the diagnosis. Testing for fetal infection (amniotic fluid PCR) should be attempted in all women with confirmed acute toxoplasma in pregnancy, provided testing can be done with minimal risks. In confirmed cases of fetal infection, or in cases where amniotic fluid testing cannot be performed, pyrimethamine (50 mg twice each day for 2 days, then once each day), folinic acid (10 to 20 mg each day), and sulfadiazine (2 g twice each day) should be given beginning near the end of the second trimester (20,26). This regimen may be altered with spiramycin every 3 weeks.

B. Treatment and follow-up of the infected newborn infant (Table 23.10). Since many infants who develop long-term complications have no overt disease at birth, postnatal sequelae appear to result, at least in part, from ongoing insult or reactivated disease after delivery. Current treatment options do not eradicate T. gondii from infected hosts so investigators have attempted to control the infection in young infants by extended anti-toxoplasma drug regimens. The benefits of extended therapy was first suggested by the studies by

TABLE 23.10. SUGGESTED EVALUATION AND TREATMENT PROGRAM FOR INFANTS WITH CONGENITAL TOXOPLASMA INFECTION*

Initial evaluation:

Complete physical examination
Cranial CT scan
CSF protein, glucose, cell count
Complete eye examination by a pediatric ophthalmologist
Complete blood count, liver function tests (especially ALT, bilirubin)
Serum glucose-6-phosphate dehydrogenase screen (prior to initiating sulfadiazine)

Pediatric neurology assessment if apparent symptomatic CNS disease

Follow-up evaluation:

Complete blood counts to monitor for drug toxicity:*
    1–2 times/week while on daily pyrimethamine
    1–2 times/month while on every other day pyrimethamine

Complete pediatric examination, including neurodevelopmental assessment every month

Pediatric ophthalmology examination every 3 months until 18 months of life, then yearly thereafter[†]

Pediatric neurology examination every 3–6 months until 1 year of age[‡]

Treatment regimen:

Pyrimethamine 1 mg/kg daily for 2–6 months, then 1 mg/kg every other day to complete 1 year of therapy
Sulfadiazine 100 mg/kg in 2 divided doses each day for 1 year
Folinic acid (leukovorin) 10 mg 3 times/week with dose increased as needed for pyrimethamine toxicity

ALT, alinine aminotransferase test.
*Counts should be done at the more frequent interval if there is an intercurrent illness or any occurrence of neutropenia. Folinic acid (leucovorin) dose should be increased 10 mg each day if the absolute neutrophil count (ANC) falls below 1000, and pyrimethamine may need to be briefly withheld if the ANC falls below 500. Persistent neutropenia despite withholding of pyrimethamine may be caused by sulfadiazine. Measurement of serum ALT and creatinine, and obtaining a urinalysis every 3 months may be useful in monitoring for side effects of sulfadiazine.
[†]Frequency of examinations adjusted as needed if retinal disease present.
[‡]Frequency and duration of pediatric neurology follow-up determined by the presence of neurologic abnormalities.
Source: From Guerina N.G. Congenital infection with Toxoplasma gondii. *Pediatr Ann* 1994;23:138.

Couvreur and colleagues (4,5) who prospectively followed infants diagnosed with congenital toxoplasma infection by postnatal serology. Follow-up on a portion of these infants over several years showed an 8% incidence of new-onset retinal disease in untreated infants compared with no new retinal lesions in treated infants. There also appeared to be an inverse relationship between the duration of therapy and the incidence of disease.

More recent studies have further demonstrated the benefit of extended therapy for both symptomatic and subclinical congenital infection. In the Chicago collaborative treatment trial (24) a total of 44 infected infants were followed during a 10-year period from 1981 to 1991. As noted previously, the majority of infants in this study were identified because they had clinical symptoms suspicious for congenital infection. Many of these infants had significant clinical and laboratory abnormalities on initial presentation (see Table 23.9). A total of 37 infants were entered into a 1-year treatment program, 35 of whom were 2 months of age when therapy was initiated. Most of the infants received sulfadiazine 50 mg/kg twice a day and pyrimethamine 1 mg/kg each day for 2 months followed by 1 mg/kg every other day for the remaining 10 months. Folinic acid (leucovorin) 5 to 10 mg 3 times each week was given to help prevent side effects of pyrimethamine. Ophthalmologic follow-up revealed new retinal lesions in 8% of treated infants (mean age 3.4 years) compared with 29% of untreated controls (mean age 5.6 years). Twenty-one (57%) of the 37 treated infants had motor abnormalities or seizures on initial evaluation, but on follow-up only 8 (24%) of 34 infants tested had significant neurologic complications. In contrast, there was no improvement in the neurologic status of untreated infants. In this study the untreated "controls" were a small number of infants who were referred beyond the treatment enrollment period, and thus they do not represent a randomized control population. They also were older with a longer period of follow-up. Nevertheless, these results were encouraging and demonstrate that even infants with significant disease from in utero infection may benefit from treatment. The most pronounced risk factors associated with poor outcomes were a delay in initiation of treatment (delay in diagnosis), prolonged concomitant neonatal hypoxemia and hypoglycemia, prolonged uncorrected hydrocephalus, and severe visual impairment. Of 19 infants without hydrocephalus nearly all were developmentally normal (IQ scores 85 to 140) whereas severe disabilities occurred in 8 of 10 infants who had hydrocephalus at birth, and 2 of 8 infants who were diagnosed with hydrocephalus in the first months of life.

Infants followed in the New England Newborn Screening Program (13) were also treated with a 1-year course of combination anti-toxoplasma chemotherapy. Most infants were treated with sulfadiazine/ pyrimethamine/ folinic acid as in the Chicago study except the pyrimethamine dose was 1 mg/kg every other day, and during the final 6 months, pyrimethamine administration was given every other month. Thirty-nine infants had ophthalmologic follow-up from 1 to 6 years (number of person-years of follow-up: 115 years total and 3 years median). In 9 infants who had retinal disease at birth, only one had new retinal lesions noted on follow-up (small peripheral scars first noted at 6 years of age). New retinal lesions were found in 3 other infants who initially had no evidence of disease at birth, but only one of these infants had a clinically significant lesion; a macular scar with unilateral visual impairment. Thus, a total of 4 of 39 (10%) of infants had new retinal disease. Only one of 46 infants had a persistent neurologic deficit (hemiplegia attributable to a cerebral lesion present at birth). Because of the expected high incidence of long-term sequelae in untreated infants, no controls were used in this study. Nevertheless, the excellent clinical outcomes for these children indicate a likely benefit for extended therapy.

Table 23.10 outlines treatment guidelines for infants diagnosed with congenital toxoplasma infection. The principal side effect of therapy is neutropenia, which primarily results from pyrimethamine treatment. For this reason close monitoring of blood counts is required. In the Chicago collaborative treatment trial, 21 (58%) of 36 infants developed neutropenia, usually in conjunction with a viral illness (24). The incidence in the New England study (13) was lower, possibly due to the greater interval used for pyrimethamine dosing. Neutropenia less commonly can result from sulfadiazine. In general, increasing the dose of folinic acid (leucovorin) can reverse the neutropenia associated with pyrimethamine, but temporary cessation of therapy or dose modification may be required. Published information on pyrimethamine levels in infants indicate that the serum half-life is approximately 33 hours with steady-state levels being nearly twice as high with daily dosing compared to every other day dosing (25). Both dosing regimens produced serum and CSF levels in the concentration range that is active against T. gondii in vitro, but CSF levels were only 10 to 25% of serum levels.

Based upon this information, as well as the minimal and reversible side effects that have been reported thus far, it is reasonable to maximize levels with daily pyrimethamine dosing for some initial period of treatment.

V. Prevention. The best way to prevent congenital toxoplasma is by preventing acute maternal infection in pregnancy. At present, this requires the appropriate education of pregnant women about simple procedures that may minimize exposure (19,20,26). These include the following:

A. Cats
1. Keep indoors.
2. Empty litter every day (avoid if pregnant or wear gloves).
3. Feed cats only dry, canned, or cooked food.

B. Meat
1. Avoid eating undercooked meat in pregnancy.
2. Wear gloves when handling, or wash hands thoroughly after handling.
3. Keep cutting boards, utensils thoroughly cleaned.

C. Vegetables
1. Wear gloves when gardening.
2. Wash vegetables thoroughly before eating.
3. Wear gloves when handling, or wash hands thoroughly after handling.

D. Other, potentially more preventive measures are being investigated, including vaccine development for immunization of cats and possibly intermediate hosts.

References

1. Alford C. A., Jr., et al. Subclinical central nervous system disease of neonates: A prospective study of infants born with increased levels of IgM. *J Pediatr* 1969;75: 1167.
2. Alford C. A., Jr., et al. Congenital toxoplasmosis: Clinical, laboratory and therapeutic considerations, with special reference to subclinical disease. *Bull NY Acad Med* 1974;50:160.
3. Berrebi A., et al. Termination of pregnancy for maternal toxoplasmosis. *Lancet* 1994;344:36.
4. Couvreur J., et al. Etude d'une serie homogene de 210 cases de toxoplasmose congenitale chez des nourrissons ages de 0 a 11 mois et depistes de facon prospective. *Ann Pediatr (Paris)* 1984;31:815.
5. Couvreur J., et al. Le prognostic oculaire de la toxoplasmose congenitale: Role du traitement. *Ann Pediatr (Paris)* 1984;31(10):855.
6. Daffos F., et al. Prenatal management of 746 pregnancies at risk for congenital toxoplasmosis. *N Engl J Med* 1988;318:271.
7. Desmonts G., et al. Toxoplasmosis in pregnancy and its transmission to the fetus. *Bull NY Acad Med* 1974;50:146.
8. Desmonts G., et al. Congenital toxoplasmosis: A prospective study of the offspring of 542 women who acquired toxoplasmosis during pregnancy. Pathophysiology of congenital disease. In: Thalhammer O., Baumgarten K., Pollak A. (Eds.). *Perinatal Medicine,* 6th European Congress. 1979; Stuttgart: Georg Thieme Publishers, p. 51.
9. Desmonts G., et al. Immunoglobulin M-immunosorbent agglutination assay for diagnosis of infectious diseases: Diagnosis of acute congenital and acquired toxoplasma infections. *J Clin Microbiol* 1981;14(5):486.
10. Eichenwald H. A. study in congenital toxoplasmosis. In Siim J. C. (Ed.). *Human Toxoplasmosis.* 1959; Copenhagen: Williams & Wilkins, p. 41.
11. Gilbert R. E., et al. Effect of prenatal treatment on mother to child transmission of Toxoplasma gondii: retrospective cohort study of 554 mother-child pairs in Lyon, France. *Int J Epidemiol* 2001;30(6):1303.
12. Gilbert R., et al. Ecological comparison of the risks of mother-to-child transmission and clinical manifestations of congenital toxoplasmosis according to prenatal treatment protocol. *Epidemiol Infect* 2001;127(1):113.

13. Guerina N. G., et al. Neonatal serologic screening and early treatment of congenital Toxoplasma gondii infection. *N Engl J Med* 1994;330:1858.
14. Guerina N. G. Congenital infection with Toxoplasma gondii. *Pediatr Ann* 1994;23: 138.
15. Guerina N. G. Management strategies for infectious diseases in pregnancy. *Semin Perinatol* 1994;18:305.
16. Hohlfeld P., et al. Prenatal diagnosis of congenital toxoplasmosis with a polymerase-chain-reaction test on amniotic fluid. *N Engl J Med* 1994;331:695.
17. Hunter K., et al. Prenatal screening of pregnant women for infections caused by cytomegalovirus, Epstein-Barr virus, herpesvirus, rubella, and Toxoplasma gondii. *Am J Obstet Gynecol* 1983;145:269.
18. Liesenfeld O., et al. Effect of testing for IgG avidity in the diagnosis of Toxoplasma gondii infection in pregnant women: Experience in a US reference laboratory. *J Infect Dis* 2001;183(8):1248.
19. Lynfield R., Guerina, N. G. Toxoplasmosis. *Pediatr Rev* 1997;18(3):75.
20. Lynfield R., Guerina N. G. Toxoplasmosis. In: DeAngelis C. D., Feigin R. D., McMillan J. A., Warshaw J. B. (Eds.). *Oski's Pediatrics: Principles and Practice* (3rd Ed.). 1999; Philadelphia: Lippincott-Raven, p. 1184.
21. Koppe J. G., et al. Toxoplasmosis and pregnancy, with a long-term follow up of the children. *Eur J Obstet Gynecol Reprod Biol* 1974;4:101.
22. Koppe J. G., et al. Results of 20 year follow-up of congenital toxoplasmosis. *Lancet* 1986;1:254.
23. Matsui D. Prevention, diagnosis and treatment of fetal toxoplasmosis. *Clin Perinatol* 1994;21:675.
24. McAuley J., et al. Early and longitudinal evaluations of treated infants and children and untreated historical patients with congenital toxoplasmosis: The Chicago collaborative treatment trial. *Clin Infect Dis* 1994;18(1):38.
25. McLeod R., et al. Levels of pyrimethamine in sera and cerebrospinal and ventricular fluids from infants treated for congenital toxoplasmosis. *Antimicrob Agents Chemother* 1992;36(5):1040.
26. Remington J. S., et al. Toxoplasmosis. In: Remington J. S., Klein J. O. (Eds.). *Infectious Diseases of the Fetus and Newborn Infant* (4th Ed.). Philadelphia: Saunders, 1994, p. 140.
27. Roberts A., et al. Multicenter evaluation of strategies for serodiagnosis of primary infection with Toxoplasma gondii. *Eur J Clin Microbiol Infect Dis* 2001;20(7): 467.
28. Romand S., et al. Prenatal diagnosis using polymerase chain reaction on amniotic fluid for congenital toxoplasmosis. *Obstet Gynecol* 2001;97(2):296.
29. Sever J. L., et al. Toxoplasmosis: Maternal and pediatric findings in 23,000 pregnancies. *Pediatrics* 1988;82(2):181.
30. Wilson C. B., et al. Development of adverse sequelae in children born with subclinical congenital toxoplasma infection. *Pediatrics* 1980;66:767.
31. Wong S. Y., et al. Toxoplasmosis in pregnancy. *Clin Infect Dis* 1994;18:853.

24. RESPIRATORY DISORDERS

Respiratory Distress Syndrome

Dynio Honrubia and Ann R. Stark

The primary cause of respiratory distress syndrome (RDS), also known as hyaline membrane disease, is inadequate pulmonary surfactant due to preterm birth. The manifestations of the disease are caused by the resultant diffuse alveolar atelectasis, edema, and cell injury. Subsequently, serum proteins that inhibit surfactant function leak into the alveoli. The increased water content, immature mechanisms for clearance of lung liquid, lack of alveolar-capillary apposition, and low surface area for gas exchange typical of the immature lung also contribute to the disease. Significant advances made in the management of RDS include the development of prenatal diagnosis to identify infants at risk, prevention of the disease by antenatal administration of glucocorticoids, improvements in perinatal care, advances in respiratory support, and surfactant replacement therapy. As a result, the mortality from RDS has decreased. However, the survival of increasing numbers of extremely immature infants has provided new challenges, and RDS remains an important contributing cause of neonatal mortality and morbidity.

I. **Identification**

    A. **Perinatal risk factors**

        1. Factors that affect the state of lung development at birth include prematurity, maternal diabetes, and genetic factors (white race, history of RDS in siblings, male sex). Thoracic malformations that cause lung hypoplasia, such as diaphragmatic hernia, may also increase the risk for surfactant deficiency. Surfactant protein B deficiency, a genetic disorder of surfactant production, causes congenital alveolar proteinosis that in its early stages can resemble RDS and is usually lethal.

        2. Factors that may acutely impair surfactant production, release, or function include perinatal asphyxia in premature infants and cesarean section without labor. Infants delivered before labor starts do not benefit from the adrenergic and steroid hormones released during labor, which increase surfactant production and release.

    B. **Prenatal prediction**

        1. **Assesment of fetal lung maturity.** Prenatal prediction of lung maturity can be made by testing amniotic fluid obtained by amniocentesis.

            a. The **lecithin-sphingomyelin (L/S) ratio** is performed by thin-layer chromatography. Specific techniques vary among laboratories and may affect the results. In general, the risk of RDS is very low if the L/S ratio is greater than 2.0. Exceptions to the prediction of pulmonary maturity with an L/S ratio greater than 2.0 are infants of diabetic mothers (IDMs), intrapartum asphyxia, and erythroblastosis fetalis. Possible exceptions are intrauterine growth restriction (IUGR), abruptio placentae, preeclampsia, and hydrops fetalis. Contaminants, such as blood and meconium, affect the interpretation of results. Blood and meconium tend to elevate an immature L/S ratio and depress a mature L/S ratio. As a result, an L/S ratio over 2.0 in a contaminated specimen is probably mature, and a ratio under 2.0 is probably immature.

            b. The **TDx-Fetal Lung Maturity (FLM II)** measures the surfactant-albumin ratio using fluorescent polarization technology. Reference values used at Brigham and Women's Hospital are immature, less than 40 mg/g; indeterminate, 40 to 59 mg/g; and mature, greater or equal to 60 mg/g. These are more conservative than published values. Contamination with blood or meconium may interfere with interpretation of this test, although the extent and direction are uncertain.

2. Antenatal corticosteroid therapy should be given to pregnant women 24 to 34 weeks' gestation with intact membranes or with preterm rupture of the membranes (ROM) without chorioamnionitis, who are at high risk for preterm delivery within the next 7 days. Treatment should occur regardless of gender or race. This strategy induces sufactant production and accelerates maturation of the lungs and other fetal tissues, resulting in a substantial reduction of RDS, intraventricular hemorrhage, and perinatal mortality. A full course consists of two doses of betamethasone (12 mg IM) separated by a 24-hour interval, or four doses of dexamethasone (6 mg IM) at 12-hour intervals, although incomplete courses may improve outcome. Contraindications to treatment include chorioamnionitis or other indications for immediate delivery.

C. Postnatal diagnosis. A premature infant with RDS has clinical signs shortly after birth. These include tachypnea, retractions, flaring of the nasal alae, grunting, and cyanosis. The classic radiographic appearance is of low-volume lungs with a diffuse reticulogranular pattern and air bronchograms.

II. Management. The keys to the management of infants with RDS are (1) to prevent hypoxemia and acidosis (this allows normal tissue metabolism, optimizes surfactant production, and prevents right-to-left shunting); (2) to optimize fluid management (avoiding hypovolemia and shock, on the one hand, and edema, particularly pulmonary edema, on the other); (3) to reduce metabolic demands; (4) to prevent worsening atelectasis and pulmonary edema; (5) to minimize oxidant lung injury; and (6) to minimize lung injury caused by mechanical ventilation.

A. Surfactant replacement therapy has been shown in numerous clinical trials to be successful in ameliorating RDS. These trials have examined the effects of surfactant preparations delivered through the endotracheal tube either within minutes of birth (prophylactic treatment) or after the symptoms and signs of RDS are present (selective or "rescue" treatment). Surfactant of human, bovine, or porcine origin or synthetic preparations have been studied. In general, these studies have shown improvement in oxygenation and decreased need for ventilator support lasting hours to days after treatment and, in many of the larger studies, decreased incidence of air leaks and death. Survanta (a bovine lung extract), Infasurf (a calf lung extract), and Curosurf (a porcine lung extract) are currently available in the United States.

1. Timing. Prophylactic treatment of surfactant deficiency, before lung injury occurs, results in better distribution and less lung injury than supplementation once respiratory failure is severe. "Early rescue" (prior to 2 hours of age) is preferable to delayed treatment, although whether prophylactic treatment is better than early treatment is uncertain. In general, we administer early rescue surfactant as soon as the diagnosis of RDS is made and after adequate oxygenation, ventilation, perfusion, and monitoring have been established, usually within 1 to 2 hours of age. Prophylactic therapy is justifiable in very premature infants who have a high incidence of RDS, in centers that have several skilled staff available to attend each delivery, so that resuscitation is not delayed by surfactant administration. Local conditions such as equipment to provide warmed, humidified, blended air/oxygen, and full monitoring facilities in the delivery room will also influence the decision.

2. The **response** to surfactant therapy varies from baby to baby. The causes of this variability include timing of treatment and patient factors such as other concurrent illnesses and degree of lung immaturity. Delayed resuscitation, insufficient lung inflation, improper ventilator strategies, and excessive fluid administration may negate the benefits of surfactant therapy. The combined use of antenatal corticosteroids and postnatal surfactant when indicated improves neonatal outcome more than postnatal surfactant therapy alone.

In infants with established RDS, repeated surfactant treatment results in greater improvement in oxygenation and ventilation, a decreased risk of pneumothorax, and a trend toward improved survival when compared to single-dose therapy. However, there is no clear benefit to more than 4 doses of Survanta or Infasurf or 3 doses of Curosurf. Whether all infants should be retreated, or only those who meet certain criteria for severity of illness at the recommended intervals for retreatment is unresolved. We generally retreat infants who still require mechanical ventilation with mean airway pressures above 7 cm H_2O and fractional concentration of inspired oxygen (FiO_2) over 0.30 up to the maximum number of doses, although the majority of infants require only one or two doses.

3. **Administration.** The Survanta dose is 4 mL (100 mg phospholipid) per kg of body weight. It is administered during brief disconnection from the ventilator, in quarter doses via a feeding tube that is cut to a length just slightly longer than that of the endotracheal tube. The baby is ventilated for at least 30 seconds, or until stable between quarter doses. Changes in positioning of the infant during administration are routine and intended to facilitate distribution. However, studies suggest that other strategies of administration, such as omitting the position changes, do not result in loss of efficacy, although delivery that is too slow does. Careful observation is necessary during treatment. Desaturation, bradycardia, and apnea are frequent adverse effects. Administration should be adjusted according to the infant's tolerance. Apnea commonly occurs at slow ventilation rates, so the rate should be at least 30 breaths per minute during administration. In addition, some infants respond rapidly and need careful adjustment of ventilator settings to prevent hypotension or pneumothorax secondary to sudden improvement in compliance. Others become transiently hypoxic during treatment and require additional oxygen. Subsequent doses of Survanta, if needed, are given at 6-hour intervals.

The initial dose of Infasurf is 3 mL/kg (105 mg/kg phospholipid), divided into two aliquots; subsequent doses are given at 12-hour intervals, if needed. The initial dose of Curosurf is 2.5 mL/kg (200 mg/kg phospholipid); subsequent doses of 1.25 mL/kg are given at 12-hour intervals, if needed. Specific instructions about administration of these preparations are available on the package insert.

4. **Complications.** Pulmonary hemorrhage is an infrequent adverse event after surfactant therapy. It most commonly occurs in extremely low-birth-weight (ELBW) infants, in males, and in infants who have clinical evidence of patent ductus arteriosus (PDA). The risk is decreased by antenatal glucocorticoid therapy and by early postnatal treatment of PDA with indomethacin.

Surfactant treatment has not consistently reduced the incidence of intraventricular hemorrhage, necrotizing enterocolitis (NEC), and retinopathy of prematurity. Although these disorders tend to be associated with severe RDS, they are primarily caused by immaturity of other organs. Likewise, most studies have not demonstrated a reduced incidence of bronchopulmonary dysplasia (BPD) particularly in the smallest infants, who are at the highest risk. However, the reduction in mortality attributable to surfactant therapy has not typically been associated with a large increase in rates of BPD, suggesting that surfactant therapy prevents BPD in some infants. No significant difference has been shown in infants treated with surfactant versus placebo with regards to both neurodevelopmental outcomes and physical growth.

B. **Oxygen**
1. **Delivery of oxygen** should be sufficient to maintain arterial tensions at 50 to 80 mm Hg, a range generally sufficient to meet metabolic demands. Higher than necessary FiO_2 levels should be avoided because of the danger of potentiating the development of lung injury and retinopathy of prematurity. The oxygen is warmed, humidified, and delivered through an air-oxygen blender that allows precise control over the oxygen concentration. For infants with acute RDS, oxygen is ordered by concentration to be delivered to the infant's airway, not by flow, and oxygen concentration is checked at least hourly. When ventilation with an anesthesia bag is re-

quired during suctioning of the airway, during insertion of an endotracheal tube, or for an apneic spell, the oxygen concentration should be similar to that before bagging to avoid hyperoxia and should be adjusted in response to continuous monitoring.

2. **Blood gas monitoring** (see Blood Gas and Pulmonary Graphic Monitoring). During the acute stages of illness, frequent sampling may be required to maintain arterial blood gases within appropriate ranges. Arterial blood gases [arterial oxygen tension (PaO_2), arterial carbon dioxide tension ($PaCO_2$), and pH] should be measured 30 minutes after changes in respiratory therapy, such as alteration in the FiO_2, ventilator pressures, or rate. We use indwelling arterial catheters for this purpose. To monitor trends in oxygenation continuously, we use pulse oximeters. In more stable infants, capillary blood from warmed heels may be adequate for monitoring $PaCO_2$ and pH.

C. **Continuous positive airway pressure (CPAP)**

1. **Indications.** We begin CPAP therapy as soon as possible after birth in infants (see Mechanical Ventilation) with RDS who have mild respiratory distress, require an FiO_2 below 0.4 to maintain a PaO_2 of 50 to 80 mm Hg, and have $PaCO_2$ less than 55 mm Hg. Early CPAP therapy may reduce the need for mechanical ventilation and the incidence of long-term pulmonary morbidity. In infants with RDS, CPAP appears to help prevent atelectasis, thus minimizing lung injury and preserving the functional properties of surfactant, and allowing reduction of oxygen concentration as the PaO_2 rises. In each infant, however, the relative benefits of endotracheal intubation and mechanical ventilation in order to administer artificial surfactant should be weighed. It is uncertain whether brief intubation and administration of surfactant followed by extubation to CPAP is comparable to surfactant treatment with continued mechanical ventilation and extubation from low levels of support. We use the latter strategy for surfactant administration.

   If CPAP enables the infant to inspire on a more compliant portion of the pressure–volume curve, $PaCO_2$ may fall. However, minute ventilation may decrease on CPAP, particularly if the distending pressure is too great. We obtain a chest radiograph before or soon after starting CPAP to confirm the diagnosis of RDS and to exclude disorders in which this type of therapy should be approached with caution, such as air leak.

2. **Methods of administering CPAP.** We usually begin CPAP via nasal prongs or nasopharyngeal tubes using a continuous flow ventilator. We generally start at 5 to 7 cm H_2O pressure, using a flow high enough to avoid rebreathing (5 to 10 L/min), then adjust the pressure in increments of 1 to 2 cm H_2O to a maximum of 8 cm H_2O, observing the baby's respiratory rate and effort and monitoring oxygen saturation. A nasogastric tube is always placed to decompress swallowed air.

3. **Problems encountered with CPAP**

   a. CPAP may interfere with venous return to the heart and thus decrease cardiac output. Positive pressure may be transmitted to the pulmonary vascular bed, raising pulmonary vascular resistance and thereby promoting right-to-left shunting. The risk of these phenomena increases as lung compliance increases, as RDS resolves. In this circumstance, reduction of the CPAP may improve oxygenation.

   b. Hypercarbia may indicate that CPAP is too high and tidal volume is thereby reduced.

   c. The use of nasal prongs or nasopharyngeal tubes may be unsuccessful if crying or mouth opening prevents adequate transmission of pressure or if the infant's abdomen becomes distended despite insertion of a nasogastric tube. In these situations, endotracheal intubation is often necessary.

4. **Weaning.** As the infant improves, we begin by reducing the FiO_2 in decrements of 0.05. Generally, when FiO_2 is less than 0.30, CPAP can be reduced to 5 cm H_2O, following oxygen saturation. Physical examination will provide ev-

idence of respiratory effort during weaning, and chest radiographs may help estimate lung volume. Lowering of the distending pressure should be attempted with caution if the lung volumes appear low and alveolar atelectasis persists. We generally discontinue CPAP if there is no distress and the FiO_2 remains less than 0.3.

D. Mechanical ventilation (see Mechanical Ventilation)

1. The initiation of ventilator therapy is influenced by the decision to administer surfactant (see II.A). The goals, once mechanical ventilation is initiated, are to limit tidal volume without losing lung volume or promoting atelectasis and to wean to extubation as soon as possible. Indications to start ventilation are a respiratory acidosis with a $PaCO_2$ greater than 55 mm Hg or rapidly rising, a PaO_2 less than 50 mm Hg or oxygen saturation less than 90% with an FiO_2 above 0.50, or severe apnea. The actual levels of PaO_2 and $PaCO_2$ necessitating intervention depend on the course of the disease and the size of the infant. For example, a high $PaCO_2$ early in the course of RDS will generally indicate the need for ventilator support, while the same $PaCO_2$ when the infant is recovering might be managed, after careful evaluation, by observation and repeated sampling before any intervention is made.

2. **Ventilators.** A continuous-flow, pressure-limited, time-cycled ventilator is useful for ventilating newborns because pressure waveforms, inspiratory and expiratory duration, and pressure can be varied independently and because the flow of gas permits unobstructed spontaneous breathing.

   High-frequency oscillatory ventilation (HFOV) may be useful to minimize lung injury in very small and/or sick infants who require very high peak inspiratory pressures and oxygen concentration to maintain adequate gas exchange and to manage infants in whom air leak syndromes complicate RDS.

   a. **Initial settings.** We generally start mechanical ventilation with a peak inspiratory pressure of 20 to 25 cm H_2O, positive end-expiratory pressure (PEEP) of 4 to 6 cm H_2O, frequency of 25 to 30 breaths per minute, inspiratory duration of 0.3 to 0.4 seconds, and the previously required FiO_2 (usually 0.50 to 1.00). It is useful to ventilate the infant first by hand, using an anesthesia bag and manometer to determine the actual pressures required. The infant should be observed for color, chest motion, and respiratory effort, and the examiner should listen for breath sounds and observe changes in oxygen saturation. Adjustments in ventilator settings may be required on the basis of these observations or arterial blood gas results.

   b. **Adjustments** (see Mechanical Ventilation). $PaCO_2$ should be maintained in the range of 45 to 55 mm Hg. Acidosis may exacerbate RDS. Thus, if relative hypercapnia is accepted to minimize lung injury, meticulous control of any metabolic acidosis is necessary. Rising $PaCO_2$ levels may indicate the onset of complications, including atelectasis, air leak, or symptomatic PDA. PaO_2 usually rises in response to increases in FiO_2 or mean airway pressure. Infants who remain hypoxemic despite these measures sometimes improve with sedation or muscle relaxants. Some infants have pulmonary hypertension resulting in right-to-left shunting through fetal pathways; in these infants, interventions to reduce pulmonary vascular resistance may improve oxygenation (see Persistent Pulmonary Hypertension of the Newborn). More commonly, premature infants remain hypoxemic because of shunting through atelectic lung and respond to measures that improve lung recruitment.

3. **Care of the infant** receiving ventilator therapy includes scrupulous attention to vital signs and clinical condition. FiO_2 and ventilator settings must be checked frequently. Oxygen saturation should be monitored continuously. Blood gas levels should be checked at least every 4 to 6 hours during the acute illness, or more frequently if the infant's condition is

changing rapidly, and 30 minutes following changes in ventilator settings. Airway secretions may require periodic suctioning.

4. Danger signs

a. If an infant receiving CPAP or mechanical ventilation deteriorates, the following should be suspected:

(1) Blocked or dislodged endotracheal tube.

(2) Malfunctioning ventilator.

(3) Air leak.

b. Remedial action. The infant should be removed from the ventilator and ventilated with an anesthesia bag, which should be immediately available at the bedside. An appropriate suction catheter is passed to determine patency of the tube, and the tube position is checked by auscultation of breath sounds or by laryngoscopy. If there is any doubt, the tube should be removed and the infant should be ventilated by bag and mask pending replacement of the tube. The ventilator should be checked to ensure that FiO_2 settings are appropriate. The baby's chest is auscultated and transilluminated to check for pneumothorax (see Air Leak). If pneumothorax is suspected, chest radiographs should be obtained, but if the infant's condition is critical, immediate aspiration by needle is both diagnostic and therapeutic. Hypotension secondary to hemorrhage, capillary leak, or myocardial dysfunction also can complicate RDS and should be treated by blood volume expansion or pressors or both. Pneumopericardium and pulmonary or intraventricular hemorrhage also can cause a sudden deterioration. Immediate attention to treatable conditions is appropriate.

5. Weaning. As the infant shows signs of improvement, weaning from the ventilator should be attempted. Specific steps to reduce inspiratory pressure, PEEP, rate, and FiO_2 depend on the infant's blood gases, physical examination, and responses.

a. The settings at which mechanical ventilation can be successfully discontinued will vary with the size, condition, respiratory drive, and individual pulmonary mechanics of the infant. Infants weighing less than 2 kg are usually best weaned to ventilator rates of about 10 to 15 breaths per minute and then extubated if they are stable on FiO_2 less than 0.30 and peak inspiratory pressure less than 18 cm H_2O. Larger infants may tolerate extubation from higher settings. We frequently use CPAP via nasal prongs or nasopharyngeal tubes to stabilize lung volumes after extubation.

b. Failure to wean may result from a number of causes, of which the following is a partial list.

(1) Pulmonary edema may be present owing to capillary leak during acute stages of the illness or may develop secondary to patency of the ductus arteriosus.

(2) Recovery of the lung from RDS is not uniform, and segmental or lobar atelectasis, edema, or interstitial emphysema may delay weaning.

(3) As the infant's lungs become more compliant, the inspiratory and expiratory times may have to be increased to allow optimal inflation and deflation of the lungs.

(4) Other reasons include onset of BPD or of apnea of prematurity. We frequently begin caffeine therapy before extubation in infants less than 30 weeks' gestation to improve respiratory drive and prevent apnea (see Apnea). Glottic or subglottic edema resulting in obstruction may respond to inhaled racemic epinephrine; a brief course of systemic glucocorticoids may rarely be needed.

E. Supportive therapy

1. Temperature (see Chap. 12, Temperature Control). Temperature control is crucial in all low-birth-weight infants, especially in those with respiratory disease. If the infant's temperature is too high or low, metabolic demands increase considerably. If oxygen uptake is limited by RDS, the increased demand cannot be met. An incubator or a radiant warmer must be used to maintain a neutral thermal environment for the infant.

2. **Fluids and nutrition** (see Chaps. 9 and 10).

   a. Infants with RDS initially require intravascular administration of fluids. We generally start fluid therapy at 60 to 80 mL/kg per day, using dextrose 10% in water. Very-low-birth-weight (VLBW) infants in whom poor glucose tolerance and large transcutaneous losses are expected are usually started at 100 to 120 mL/kg per day. Extremely low-birth-weight (ELBW) infants may be started as high as 120 to 140 mL/kg/day. Phototherapy, skin trauma, and radiant warmers increase insensible losses. Excessive fluid administration may cause pulmonary edema and increases the risk for a symptomatic PDA. The key to fluid management is careful monitoring of serum electrolytes and body weight, and frequent adjustments in fluids as indicated. Fluid retention is common in infants with RDS. However, extremely immature infants often lack renal concentration efficiency and have enormous evaporative losses.

   b. By the second day, we usually add sodium (2 mEq/kg per day), potassium (1 mEq/kg per day), and calcium (100 to 200 mg/kg per day) to the fluids. If it seems unlikely that adequate enteral nutrition will be achieved within several days, we add an amino acid solution and intravenous fat solution by the first or second day.

   c. In most infants with RDS, spontaneous diuresis occurs on the second to fourth day, preceding improvement in pulmonary function. If diuresis and improvement in lung disease do not occur by 1 to 2 weeks of age, this may indicate the onset of BPD (see Bronchopulmonary Dysplasia, chronic lung disease).

3. **Circulation** is assessed by monitoring the heart rate, blood pressure, and peripheral perfusion. Judicious use of blood or a volume expander (normal saline) may be necessary, and pressors may be used to support the circulation. In general, we attempt to limit crystalloid administration (attempting to avoid both capillary leak of fluid into inflamed lung parenchyma and the excessive administration of sodium from repeated boluses of saline). We often use dopamine (starting at 5 µg/kg per minute) to maintain adequate blood pressure and cardiac output and ensure improved tissue perfusion and urine output, and avoid metabolic acidosis. After the first 12 to 24 hours, hypotension and poor perfusion can also result from a large left-to-right shunt through a PDA, so careful assessment is warranted. The volume of blood drawn should be monitored and, in very-low-birth-weight infants who are sick with RDS, generally should be replaced by packed red blood cell (PRBCs) transfusion when the hematocrit falls below 35 to 40%.

4. **Possible infection.** Since pneumonia can duplicate the clinical signs and radiographic appearance of RDS, we obtain blood cultures and complete blood counts with differential from all infants with RDS and treat with broad-spectrum antibiotics (ampicillin and gentamicin) for at least 48 hours.

F. **Acute complications**

1. **Air leak** (see Air Leak). Pneumothorax, pneumomediastinum, pneumopericardium, or interstitial emphysema should be suspected when an infant with RDS deteriorates, typically with hypotension, apnea, bradycardia, or persistent acidosis.

2. **Infection** (see Chap. 23) may accompany RDS and may present in a variety of ways. Also, instrumentation, such as catheters or respiratory equipment, provides access for organisms to invade the immunologically immature preterm infant. Whenever there is suspicion of infection, appropriate cultures should be obtained and antibiotics administered promptly.

3. **Intracranial hemorrhage** (see Chap. 27). Infants with severe RDS are at increased risk for intracranial hemorrhage and should be monitored with cranial ultrasound examinations.
4. **Patent ductus arteriosus (PDA)** (see Chap. 25, Cardiac Disorders) frequently complicates RDS. PDA typically presents as pulmonary vascular pressures begin to fall. If untreated, it may result in increasing left-to-right shunt and ultimately cause heart failure, manifested by respiratory decompensation and cardiomegaly. The systemic consequences of the shunt may include low mean blood pressure, metabolic acidosis, decreased urine output, and worsening jaundice due to impaired organ perfusion. We generally treat infants, especially those weighing less than 1500 g, with intravenous indomethacin if they develop any signs of a symptomatic PDA, such as a systolic or continuous murmur, hyperdynamic precordium, bounding pulses, or widened pulse pressure. In infants who weigh less than 1000 g, we treat with indomethacin when a PDA first becomes clinically apparent (i.e., presence of ductal murmur without the signs or symptoms of a large left-to-right shunt). We reserve surgical ligation for infants in whom indomethacin is contraindicated (e.g., those with renal failure or necrotizing enterocolitis) or those in whom two courses of indomethacin have failed. In larger infants who are improving steadily despite PDA and who have no evidence of heart failure, mild fluid restriction and time may result in closure.

G. **Long-term complications** include BPD (see Bronchopulmonary Dysplasia), and other complications of prematurity, including neurodevelopmental impairment and retinopathy of prematurity. The risk of these complications increases with decreasing birth weight and gestational age.

Suggested Readings

Crowley P. Prophylactic corticosteroids for preterm birth *Cochrane Database Syst Rev* 2000;(2)CD000065.

Jobe A.H., Ikegami M. Biology of surfactant. *Clin Perinatol* Sept. 2001;28: 655–667.

Richardson D.K., Heffner L.J. Fetal-lung maturity: Tests mature, interpretations not. *Lancet* 2001;358: 684–686.

Suresh G.K., Soll R.F. Current surfactant use in premature infants. *Clin Perinatol* 2001; 28: 671–694.

Mechanical Ventilation

Eric C. Eichenwald

I. **General principles.** Mechanical ventilation is an invasive life support procedure with many effects on the cardiopulmonary system. The goal is to optimize both gas exchange and clinical status at minimum FiO_2 and ventilator pressures/tidal volume. The ventilator strategy employed to accomplish this goal depends, in part, on the infant's disease process. In addition, recent advances in technology have brought more options for ventilatory therapy of newborns.
II. **Types of ventilatory support**
   A. **Continuous positive airway pressure (CPAP)**
      1. CPAP is usually administered by means of a ventilator. Any system used to deliver CPAP should allow continuous monitoring of the delivered pres-

sure, and be equipped with safety alarms to indicate when the pressure is above or below the desired level. Alternatively, CPAP may be delivered by a simplified system providing blended oxygen flowing past the infant's airway with the end of the tubing submerged in 0.25% acetic acid in sterile water solution to the desired depth to generate pressure ("bubble CPAP").

2. General characteristics. A continuous flow of heated, humidified gas is circulated past the infant's airway at a set pressure of 3 to 8 cm H_2O, maintaining an elevated end-expiratory lung volume while the infant breathes spontaneously. The air–oxygen mixture and airway pressure can be adjusted. CPAP is usually delivered by means of nasal prongs or a nasopharyngeal tube. Prolonged endotracheal CPAP is not used because the high resistance of the endotracheal tube increases the work of breathing, especially in small infants. Positive-pressure hoods and continuous-mask CPAP are not recommended.

3. Advantages
  a. CPAP is less invasive than mechanical ventilation and causes less barotrauma.
  b. When used early in infants with RDS, it can help prevent alveolar and airway collapse, which might result in deterioration of PaO_2, and thus reduce the need for mechanical ventilation.
  c. CPAP decreases the frequency of obstructive and mixed apneic spells in some infants.

4. Disadvantages
  a. CPAP does not improve ventilation and may worsen it.
  b. CPAP provides inadequate respiratory support in the face of severe changes in pulmonary compliance and resistance.
  c. Maintaining nasal or nasopharyngeal CPAP in large, active infants may be technically difficult.
  d. Swallowed air can elevate the diaphragm and must be removed by a gastric tube.

5. Indications
  a. Early treatment of mild RDS.
  b. Moderately frequent apneic spells.
  c. After recent extubation.
  d. Weaning chronically ventilator-dependent infants.
  e. Early treatment to prevent atelectasis in premature infants with minimal respiratory distress and minimal need for supplemental oxygen.

B. Pressure-limited, time-cycled, continuous-flow ventilators are used most frequently in newborns with respiratory failure.

1. General characteristics. A continuous flow of heated and humidified gas is circulated past the infant's airway; the gas is a selected mixture of air with oxygen. Maximum inspiratory pressure (Pi), positive end-expiratory pressure (PEEP), and respiratory timing (rate and duration of inspiration and expiration) are selected.

2. Advantages
  a. The continuous flow of fresh gas allows the infant to make spontaneous respiratory efforts between ventilator breaths (intermittent mandatory ventilation, IMV).
  b. Good control is maintained over respiratory pressures.
  c. Inspiratory and expiratory time can be independently controlled.
  d. The system is relatively simple and inexpensive.

3. Disadvantages
  a. Tidal volume is poorly controlled.
  b. The system does not respond to changes in respiratory system compliance.
  c. Spontaneously breathing infants who breathe out of phase with too many IMV breaths ("bucking" or "fighting" the ventilator) may receive inadequate ventilation and are at increased risk for air leak.

    4. Indications. Useful in any form of lung disease in infants.

C. Synchronized and patient-triggered (assist/control, or pressure support) ventilators are adaptations of conventional pressure-limited ventilators used for newborns.

    1. General characteristics. These ventilators combine the features of pressure-limited, time-cycled, continuous-flow ventilators with an airway pressure, air flow, or respiratory movement sensor. By measuring inspiratory flow or movement, these ventilators deliver intermittent positive-pressure breaths at a fixed rate in synchrony with the baby's inspiratory efforts ("synchronized IMV," or SIMV). During apnea, SIMV ventilators continue to deliver the set IMV rate. In patient-triggered ventilation, a positive pressure breath is delivered with every inspiratory effort. As a result, the ventilator delivers more frequent positive pressure breaths, usually allowing a decrease in the peak inspiratory pressure needed for adequate gas exchange. During apnea, the ventilator in patient-triggered mode delivers an operator-selected IMV ("control") rate. Ventilators equipped with a flow sensor can also be used to monitor delivered tidal volume continuously by integration of the flow signal.

    2. Advantages

      a. Synchronizing the delivery of positive-pressure breaths with the infant's inspiratory effort reduces the phenomenon of breathing out of phase with IMV breaths ("fighting" the ventilator). This may decrease the need for sedative medications and aid in weaning mechanically ventilated infants.

      b. Pronounced asynchrony with ventilator breaths during conventional IMV has been associated with the development of air leak and intraventricular hemorrhage. Whether the use of SIMV or assist/control ventilation reduces these complications is not known.

    3. Disadvantages

      a. Under certain conditions, the ventilators may inappropriately trigger a breath because of artifactual signals, or fail to trigger because of problems with the sensor.

      b. Few data are available on the effects of patient-triggered ventilation in newborns. Pressure support ventilation may not be appropriate for small premature infants with irregular respiratory patterns and frequent apnea because of the potential for significant variability in ventilation.

      c. It is more expensive and complicated to use than a conventional pressure-limited device.

    4. Indications. SIMV can be used when a conventional pressure-limited ventilator is indicated. If available, it may be the preferable mode of ventilator therapy in infants who are breathing spontaneously while on IMV. The indications for assist/control ventilation have not been established.

D. Volume-cycled ventilators are rarely used in newborn infants, although recent advances in technology have renewed interest in this mode of ventilation in selected situations. Only volume-cycled ventilators specifically designed for newborns should be used.

    1. General characteristics. Volume-cycled ventilators are similar to pressure-limited ventilators except that the operator selects the volume delivered, rather than the peak inspiratory pressure.

    2. Advantages. The pressure automatically varies with respiratory system compliance to deliver the selected tidal volume, theoretically minimizing variability in minute ventilation.

    3. Disadvantages

      a. The system is complicated and requires more skill to operate.

      b. Because tidal volumes in infants are small, most of the tidal volume selected is lost in the ventilator circuit or from air leaks around uncuffed endotracheal tubes. A separate in-line tidal volume monitor may be helpful.

      c. It is more expensive than a pressure-limited device.

    4. Indications. May be useful if lung compliance is rapidly changing.

E. The **high-frequency ventilator (HFV)** is an important adjunct to conventional mechanical ventilation in newborns. The recommended uses and the ventilatory strategies employed with high frequency ventilators continue to evolve with clinical experience. Three types of high-frequency ventilators are approved for use in newborns: a **high-frequency oscillator (HFO), a high-frequency flow interrupter (HFFI), and a high-frequency jet ventilator (HFJ)**.

1. **General characteristics.** Available HFVs are similar despite considerable differences in design. All HFVs are capable of delivering extremely rapid rates (300 to 1500 breaths per minute, 5 to 25 Hz; 1 Hz = 60 breaths per minute) with tidal volumes equal to or smaller than anatomical dead space. These ventilators apply continuous distending pressure to maintain an elevated lung volume; small tidal volumes are superimposed at a rapid rate. HFJ ventilators are paired with a conventional pressure-limited device, which is used to deliver intermittent "sigh" breaths to help prevent atelectasis. "Sigh" breaths are not used with HFO ventilation. Expiration is passive (i.e., dependent on chest wall and lung recoil) with HFFI and HFJ machines, while it is active with HFO. The mechanisms of gas exchange with HFV are incompletely understood.

2. **Advantages**
   a. HFVs can achieve adequate ventilation while avoiding the large swings in lung volume required by conventional ventilators and associated with lung injury. Because of this, they may be useful in pulmonary air leak syndromes (pulmonary interstitial emphysema, pneumothorax).
   b. HFV allows the use of a high mean airway pressure (MAP) for alveolar recruitment and resultant improvement in ventilation-perfusion matching. This may be advantageous in infants with severe respiratory failure requiring high MAP to maintain adequate oxygenation on a conventional mechanical ventilator.

3. **Disadvantages.** Despite theoretical advantages of HFV, no significant benefit of this method has been demonstrated in routine clinical use over more conventional ventilators. Only one rigorously controlled study found a small reduction in BPD in infants at high risk treated with HFOV as the primary mode of ventilation. This experience is likely not generalizable, however, as other studies have shown no difference. These ventilators are more complex and expensive, and there is less long-term clinical experience. The initial studies with HFO suggested an increased risk of significant intraventricular hemorrhage, although this complication has not been observed in recent clinical trials. Studies comparing the different types of HFVs are unavailable; thus, the relative advantages or disadvantages of HFO, HFFI, and HFJ, if any, are not characterized.

4. **Indications.** HFVs are primarily used as a rescue therapy for infants failing conventional ventilation. Both HFJ and HFO ventilators have been shown to be superior to conventional ventilation in infants with air leak syndromes, especially pulmonary interstitial emphysema. Because of the potential for complications, we do not use high-frequency ventilation as the primary mode of ventilatory support in infants.

F. **Negative pressure.** These infant versions of the adult "iron lung" are rarely used because nursing access is limited by the negative-pressure cylinder and because the neck seal makes them feasible only for large babies. Their use is restricted to older infants with neuromuscular problems who can thus be ventilated without an endotracheal tube.

III. **Indications for respiratory support.** See Chapter 36 for intubation procedures and proper selection of endotracheal tube sizes.

A. **Indications for continuous positive airway pressure (CPAP)** in the preterm infant with RDS include:
   1. Recently delivered premature infant with minimal respiratory distress and low supplemental oxygen requirement (to prevent atelectasis).
   2. Respiratory distress and requirement of FiO_2 above 0.30 by hood.

   3. FiO_2 above 0.40 by hood.
   4. Clinically significant retractions and/or distress after recent extubation.
   5. In general, infants with RDS who require FiO_2 above 0.35 to 0.40 on
      CPAP should be intubated, ventilated, and given surfactant replacement
      therapy. In some neonatal intensive care units (NICUs), CPAP is used in
      infants with RDS after intubation for surfactant therapy followed by im-
      mediate extubation to CPAP. This method of surfactant delivery requires
      more investigation before it is routinely recommended. We use mechani-
      cal ventilation for all infants who are given surfactant.
   B. Relative indications for mechanical ventilation in any infant include
      1. Frequent intermittent apnea unresponsive to drug therapy.
      2. Early treatment when use of mechanical ventilation is anticipated be-
         cause of deteriorating gas exchange.
      3. Relieving "work of breathing" in an infant with signs of respiratory diffi-
         culty.
      4. Administration of surfactant therapy in infants with RDS.
   C. Absolute indications for mechanical ventilation
      1. Prolonged apnea.
      2. PaO_2 below 50 mm Hg or FiO_2 above 0.80. This indication may not apply
         to the infant with cyanotic congenital heart disease.
      3. $PaCO_2$ above 60 mm Hg with persistent acidemia.
      4. General anesthesia.
IV. How ventilator changes affect blood gases
   A. Oxygenation (Table 24.1)
      1. FiO_2. The goal is to maintain adequate tissue oxygen delivery. Generally,
         this can be accomplished by achieving a PaO_2 of 50 to 70 mm Hg. This re-

TABLE 24.1. VENTILATOR MANIPULATIONS TO INCREASE OXYGENATION

Parameter	Advantage	Disadvantage
↑ FiO_2	Minimizes barotrauma Easily administered	Fails to affect V̇/Q̇ matching Direct toxicity, especially >0.60
↑ Pi	Critical opening pressure Improves V̇/Q̇	Barotrauma: air leak, BPD

↑ PEEP	Maintains FRC/prevents collapse
	
	Splints obstructed airways
	Regularizes respiration
		Shifts to stiffer compliance
		  curve
		Obstructs venous return
		Increases expiratory work and
		  CO_2
		Increases dead space

↑ Ti	Increases MAP without
	  increase Pi
	"Critical opening time"
		Necessitates slower rates,
		  higher Pi
		Lower minute ventilation for
		  given Pi-PEEP combination

↑ Flow	Square wave—maximizes MAP	Greater shear force, more
		  barotrauma
		Greater resistance at greater
		  flows

↑ Rate	Increases MAP while using
	  lower Pi
		Inadvertent PEEP with high
		  rates or long-term constants

Note: All manipulations (except FiO_2) result in higher mean airway pressure (MAP).

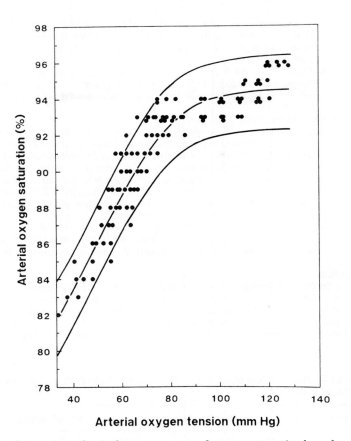

FIG. 24.1. Comparison of paired measurements of oxygen saturation by pulse oximetry and of oxygen tension by indwelling umbilical artery oxygen electrode. The lines represent ± 2 standard deviations. (Modified from Wasunna A., Whitelaw A. G., Pulse oximetry in preterm infants. *Arch Dis Child* 1987;62:957.)

sults in a hemoglobin saturation of 89 to 95% (see Fig. 24.1). Increasing inspired oxygen is the simplest and most direct means of improving oxygenation. In premature infants, the risk of retinopathy and pulmonary oxygen toxicity argue for minimizing PaO_2. For infants with other conditions, the optimum PaO_2 may be higher. Direct pulmonary oxygen toxicity begins to occur at FiO_2 values greater than 0.60 to 0.70.

2. **Mean airway pressure (MAP)**
   a. MAP is the average area under the curve of the pressure waveform. Many ventilators now display MAP or can be equipped with a device to do so. MAP is increased by increases in PEEP, inspiratory pressure (Pi), inspiratory time (Ti), rate, and flow rate. All these changes lead to higher PaO_2, but each has different effects on $PaCO_2$. For a given rise in MAP, increasing PEEP gives the greatest improvement in PaO_2. Other ways to raise MAP are to increase Pi and prolong Ti.
   b. Optimum MAP results from a balance between optimizing PaO_2, minimizing direct oxygen toxicity, minimizing barotrauma, achieving ade-

quate ventilation, and minimizing adverse cardiovascular effects. Ventilator-induced lung injury is probably most closely related to peak-to-peak swings in lung volume, although changes in airway pressure are also implicated.

   c. MAP as low as 5 cm H_2O may be sufficient in infants with normal lungs, whereas 20 cm H_2O or more may be necessary in severe RDS. Excessive MAP may impede venous return and adversely affect cardiac output.

3. **Ventilation** (Table 24.2)

   a. **CO_2** elimination depends on minute ventilation. Since minute ventilation is the product of respiratory rate and tidal volume, increases in ventilator rate will lower $PaCO_2$. Increases in tidal volume can be achieved by increasing the Pi on pressure-cycled ventilators or by increasing volume on volume-limited machines. Because tidal volume is a function of the difference between Pi and PEEP, a reduction in PEEP also improves ventilation. At very low tidal volumes, the volume of dead space becomes important and may lead to CO_2 retention.

   b. **Optimal $PaCO_2$** varies according to disease state. For very immature infants or infants with air leak, a $PaCO_2$ of 50 to 60 mm Hg may be tolerated to minimize ventilator-induced lung injury, provided pH is greater than 7.25.

V. **Disease States**

   A. **Effects of diseases.** Respiratory failure can result from numerous illnesses through a variety of pathophysiologic mechanisms. Optimal ventilatory strategy must take into account the pathophysiology, expected time course, and particular vulnerabilities of the patient.

   B. **Pulmonary mechanics** influence the ventilator strategy selected.

TABLE 24.2. VENTILATOR MANIPULATIONS TO INCREASE VENTILATION AND DECREASE $PaCO_2$

Parameter	Advantage	Disadvantage
↑ Rate	Easy to titrate Minimizes barotrauma	Maintains same dead space/tidal volume May lead to inadvertent PEEP
↑ Pi	Better bulk flow (improved dead space/tidal volume)	More barotrauma Shifts to stiffer compliance curve
↓ PEEP	Widens compression pressure Decreases dead space Decreases expiratory load Shifts to steeper compliance curve	Decreases MAP Decreases oxygenation/alveolar collapse Stops splinting obstructed/closed airways
↑ Flow	Permits shorter Ti, longer Te	More barotrauma
↑ Te	Allows longer time for passive expiration in face of prolonged time constant	Shortens Ti Decreases MAP Decreases oxygenation

MAP = mean airway pressure; ↑ = increase; ↓ = decrease; Ti = inspiratory time; Te = expiratory time; Pi = peak inspiratory pressure; PEEP = positive end-expiratory pressure; FiO_2 = fractional concentration of inspired oxygen.

1. **Compliance** is the stiffness or distensibility of the lung and chest wall, that is, the change in volume (ΔV) produced by a change in pressure (ΔP), or $\Delta V/\Delta P$. It is decreased with surfactant deficiency, excess lung water, and lung fibrosis. It is also decreased when the lungs are hyperexpanded.

2. **Resistance** is the impediment to airflow due to friction between gas and airways (airway resistance) and between tissues of the lungs and chest wall (viscous tissue resistance). Almost half of airway resistance is in the upper airways, including the endotracheal tube when in use. Resistance is high in diseases characterized by airway obstruction, such as meconium aspiration and bronchopulmonary dysplasia (BPD). Resistance can change rapidly if, for example, secretions partially occlude the endotracheal tube.

3. **Time constant** is the product of compliance and resistance. This is a measure of the time it takes to equilibrate pressure between the proximal airway and the alveoli. Expiratory time constants are somewhat longer than inspiratory ones. When time constants are long, as in meconium aspiration, care must be taken to set ventilator inspiratory times and rates that permit adequate inspiration to deliver the required tidal volume and adequate expiration to avoid inadvertent PEEP.

4. **Functional residual capacity (FRC)** is a measure of the volume of the lungs at end-expiration. FRC is decreased in diseases that permit alveolar collapse, particularly surfactant deficiency.

5. **Ventilation-perfusion matching ($\dot{V}/\dot{Q}$).** Diseases that reduce alveolar surface area (through atelectasis, inflammatory exudates, or obstruction) permit intrapulmonary shunting of desaturated blood. The opposite occurs in persistent pulmonary hypertension, when extrapulmonary shunting diverts blood flow away from the ventilated lung. Both mechanisms result in systemic recirculation of desaturated blood.

6. **Work of breathing** is especially important in the smallest infants and those with chronic lung disease, whose high airway resistance, decreased lung compliance, compliant chest wall, and weak musculature may overwhelm their metabolic energy requirements and impede growth.

C. **Specific disease states.** Several of the more common neonatal disease processes are described below and are presented in Table 24.3 along with the optimal ventilatory strategies. Before initiating ventilatory support, however, clinicians must evaluate for mechanical causes of distress, including pneumothorax or airway obstruction.

1. **Respiratory distress syndrome** (RDS) (see Respiratory Distress Syndrome)

   a. **Pathophysiology.** RDS is caused by surfactant deficiency, which results in a severe decrease in compliance (stiff lung). This causes diffuse alveolar collapse with $\dot{V}/\dot{Q}$ mismatching and increased work of breathing.

   b. **Surfactant replacement.** The availability of exogenous surfactant therapy for the treatment of RDS has changed ventilatory management of the disease. We recommend intubation and initiation of mechanical ventilation early in the course of the disease in order to provide surfactant therapy promptly. The distinctive time course of escalation, plateau, and weaning in classic RDS has changed with the use of surfactant therapy. Ventilatory strategy should anticipate the increased risk of pneumothorax as compliance increases and time constants lengthen, especially with the rapid improvements that can be seen after surfactant administration. In all approaches, a $PaCO_2$ value higher than the physiologic value is acceptable to minimize ventilator-induced lung injury.

   c. **Ventilator strategy**

      (1) **CPAP.** In mildly affected infants who may not require intubation and surfactant administration, CPAP is used early in the disease course to prevent further atelectasis. CPAP is initiated at 5 to 6 cm H_2O, and increased to a maximum of 7 to 8 cm H_2O. CPAP is

TABLE 24.3. NEONATAL PULMONARY PHYSIOLOGY BY DISEASE STATE

Disease	Compliance ml/cm H_2O	Resistance cm H_2O/ml/s	Time Constant (s)	FRC (ml/kg)	$\dot{V}/\dot{Q}$ Matching	Work
Normal term	4–6	20–40	0.25	30 ml/kg	—	—
RDS	↓↓	—	↓↓	↓	↓↓↓	↑
Meconium aspiration	—/↓	↑/↑↑	↑	↑/↑↑	↓↓	↑
BPD	↑/↓	↑↑	↑	↑↑	↓↓/↓	↑↑
Air leak	↓↓	—/↑	—/↑	↑↑	↓↓↓	↑↑
VLBW apnea	↓	—	↓↓	—/↓	↓/—	—/↑

↑ = increase; ↓ = decrease; — = little or no change; / = either/or.

titrated by clinical assessment of retractions and respiratory rate and by observation of O_2 saturation. Alternatively, in infants with slightly more severe RDS, consideration may be given to intubation for surfactant administration, a short period of mechanical ventilation, followed by CPAP.

(2) **Mechanical ventilation** is used when ventilation perfusion scan ($\dot{V}/\dot{Q}$) mismatching is so severe that increased FiO_2 and CPAP are inadequate, or in infants who tire from the increased work of breathing. Recent data suggest that a ventilator strategy that avoids large changes in tidal volume (V_T) may reduce ventilator-induced lung injury. The objective of all strategies of assisted ventilation in the infant with RDS should be to provide the lowest level of ventilatory support possible to support adequate oxygenation and ventilation while attempting to reduce acute and chronic lung injury secondary to barotrauma/volutrauma and oxygen toxicity. Our preferred approach is to maintain the appropriate MAP with a Ti initially set at 0.3 second and rate of approximately 20 to 40 breaths/min. Rarely, a longer Ti is required to provide adequate oxygenation. This ventilatory approach requires a moderate Pi to provide adequate minute ventilation and to maintain alveolar recruitment.

(3) **Pi and PEEP.** Pi, applied to recruit alveoli, is initially estimated by good chest excursion and is usually 20 to 25 cm H_2O. PEEP is set at 4 to 5 cm H_2O and may go up to 6 cm H_2O. Higher PEEP may interfere with cardiac output and should be avoided in acute RDS.

(4) **Flow.** Flow rates of 7 to 12 L/min are needed to provide a relatively square pressure waveform. Higher flows may be required at very high Pi (>35 cm H_2O).

(5) **Rates** are generally set initially at 20 to 40 breaths per minute, and adjusted by blood gas results.

(6) **Weaning.** When the patient becomes stable, FiO_2 and Pi are weaned first, alternating with rate, in response to assessment of chest excursion, oxygen saturation, and blood gas results. Extubation is usually successful when ventilator rates are about 15 breaths per minute. Caffeine citrate may be used to facilitate spontaneous breathing prior to extubation and may increase the success rate of extubation in very-low-birth-weight infants.

(7) **Advantages and disadvantages.** This ventilatory strategy maximizes alveolar recruitment, but with a potential for greater barotrauma secondary to the higher Pi and volutrauma secondary to higher V_T.

(8) **Alternative ventilator strategies.** An alternative approach to mechanical ventilation in RDS relies on high rates to maintain MAP while reducing Pi and V_T to minimize barotrauma/volutrauma. Rates of 60 to 80 breaths per minute are used, with Ti as low as 0.2 second. Inadvertent PEEP is not encountered because the time constant in RDS may be as short as 0.05 second. Pi is set as low as 12 to 18 cm H_2O, with PEEP of 4 to 5 cm H_2O. Initial settings are based on auscultation of good breath sounds and are increased as needed to maintain adequate minute ventilation and oxygenation. In general, pressure is weaned first, while the rate remains high, or by 10% drops in rate alternating with pressure, as tolerated. This ventilator strategy may minimize barotrauma due to Pi and utilizes lower V_T, with the disadvantage of less alveolar recruitment and consequent need for higher FiO_2 to maintain adequate oxygen saturation.

High-frequency ventilation may be initiated if conventional ventilation fails to maintain adequate gas exchange. High-frequency ventilation should be used only by clinicians familiar with its use. We consider the use of HFV when the MAP required for adequate gas exchange exceeds 10 to 11 cm H_2O in small infants and 12 cm

H_2O in larger infants, or if air leak occurs. Strategies differ depending on whether HFJ, HFO, or HFFI is used. We prefer HFOV over other available HFV because of its ease of use and applicability in a wide range of pulmonary diseases and infant weights.

(a) **High-frequency jet ventilation.** HFJ requires a special adapter for a standard endotracheal tube to allow connection to the jet port of the ventilator.

   (i) **Pi and PEEP.** Peak pressures on the jet ventilator are initially set approximately 20% lower than on those being used with conventional ventilation, and adjusted to provide adequate chest vibration assessed clinically and by blood gas determinations. Pi, PEEP, and FiO_2 are adjusted as needed to maintain oxygenation. CO_2 elimination is dependent on the pressure difference (Pi − PEEP). Because of the lower peak pressures required to ventilate, PEEP may be increased to 8 to 10 cm H_2O if needed to improve oxygenation.

   (ii) **Rate.** The frequency is usually set at 420 breaths per minute, with an inspiratory jet valve on-time of 0.02 second.

   (iii) **Conventional ventilator settings.** Once the HFJ is properly adjusted, the conventional ventilator rate is decreased to 2 to 10 breaths per minute to help maintain alveolar recruitment, with Pi set at 2 to 3 cm H_2O lower than the jet Pi. In air leak syndromes, it may be advantageous to provide no sigh breaths from the conventional ventilator as long as the PEEP is set high enough to maintain lung volume.

   (iv) **Weaning** from HFJ ventilation is accomplished by decreasing the jet Pi in response to blood gas determinations and the FiO_2. PEEP is weaned as tolerated if pressures higher than 4 to 5 cm H_2O are used. Frequency and jet valve on-time are generally not adjusted.

   (v) Similar strategies outlined for the HFJ apply in use of the HFFI.

(b) **High-frequency oscillatory ventilation.** With HFO, operator-selected parameters include MAP, frequency, and piston amplitude.

   (i) **Mean airway pressure.** In RDS, the initial MAP selected is usually 2 to 5 cm H_2O higher than that being used on the conventional ventilator to enhance alveolar recruitment. MAP used with HFO is titrated to O_2 requirement and to provide adequate lung expansion on chest X ray. Care must be exercised to avoid lung hyperinflation, which might adversely affect oxygen delivery by reducing cardiac output.

   (ii) **Frequency** is usually set at 10 to 15 Hz. Inspiratory time is set at 33%.

   (iii) **Amplitude.** Changes in piston amplitude primarily affect ventilation. It is set to provide adequate chest vibration, assessed clinically and by blood gas determinations.

   (iv) **Flow** rates of 8 to 15 L/min are usually adequate.

   (v) **Weaning.** In general, FiO_2 is weaned first, followed by MAP in decrements of 1 to 2 cm H_2O once the FiO_2 falls below 0.6. Piston amplitude is adjusted by frequent assessment of chest vibration and blood gas determinations. Frequency is usually not adjusted. In both HFJ and HFO, we usually wean to extubation after transfer back to conventional ventilation, although infants can be extubated directly from HFV.

2. **Meconium aspiration syndrome** (MAS) (see Meconium Aspiration)

   a. **Pathophysiology.** MAS results from aspiration of meconium-stained amniotic fluid. The severity of the syndrome is related to the associated asphyxial insult and the amount aspirated. The aspirated meconium causes acute airway obstruction, marked airway resistance, scattered atelectasis with V̇/Q̇ mismatching, and hyperexpansion due to obstructive ball-valve effects. The obstructive phase is followed by an inflammatory phase 12 to 24 hours later that results in further alveolar involvement. Aspiration of other fluids (such as blood or amniotic fluid) has similar but milder effects.

   b. **Ventilator strategy.** Because of the ball-valve effects, the application of positive pressure may result in pneumothorax or another air leak, so initiating mechanical ventilation requires careful consideration of the risks and benefits. Low levels of PEEP (4 to 5 cm H_2O) are helpful in splinting open partially obstructed airways and equalizing V̇/Q̇ matching. Higher levels may lead to hyperinflation. If airway resistance is high and compliance is normal, a slow-rate, moderate-pressure strategy is needed. If pneumonitis is more prominent, more rapid rates can be used. Sedation or muscle relaxation may be used to minimize the risks of air leak in severe MAS because of the high transpulmonary pressures these large infants can generate when "fighting" the ventilator and the ball-valve hyperexpansion caused by their disease. Use of synchronized IMV may be helpful. Weaning may be rapid if the illness is primarily related to airway obstruction or prolonged if complicated by barotrauma and severe inflammation. The use of surfactant therapy in more severe cases of MAS may improve lung compliance and oxygenation, and should be considered.

   High-frequency ventilation has also been successfully used in infants with MAS who are failing conventional ventilation or who have suffered air leak. The strategies are similar to those described above. During HFO, slower frequencies (8 to 10 Hz) may be useful to improve oxygenation in severe cases.

3. **Bronchopulmonary dysplasia (BPD)** (see Bronchopulmonary Dysplasia)

   a. **Pathophysiology.** BPD results from injury to the alveoli and airways. Bleb formation may lead to poor recoil. Fibrosis and excess lung water may cause stiffer compliance. Airways may be narrowed and fibrotic or hyperreactive. The upper airways may be overdistended and conduct airflow poorly. BPD is marked by shifting focal atelectasis, hyperinflation with V̇/Q̇ mismatching, chronic and acute increases in airway resistance, and a significant increase in the work of breathing.

   b. **Ventilator strategy.** The optimal strategy is to wean infants off the ventilator as soon as possible to prevent further barotrauma and oxygen toxicity. If this is not feasible, ventilator settings should be minimized to permit tissue repair and long-term growth. Rates as low as 10 to 15 breaths per minute should generally be avoided to prevent increased work of breathing, but longer Ti (0.4 to 0.6 second) may be used to maintain FRC. Higher pressures are sometimes required (20 to 30 cm H_2O) because of the stiff lungs, although the high resistance prevents transfer of most of this to the alveoli. Oxygenation should be maintained (saturations of 90 to 92%), but higher $PaCO_2$ values can be permitted (55 to 65 mm Hg), provided the pH is normal. Acute decompensations can result from bronchospasm and interstitial fluid accumulation. These must be treated with adjustment of Pi, bronchodilators, and diuretics. Acute BPD "spells" in which oxygenation and airway resistance worsen rapidly are due to larger airway collapse, and may be treated succesfully with higher PEEP (7 to 8 cm H_2O). Frequent rapid desaturations secondary to acute decreases in FRC with crying or infant movement respond to changes in FiO_2, but may also be partially ameliorated by using higher PEEP. Weaning is a slow and difficult process, decreasing rate by 1 to 2 breaths per minute or 1-cm H_2O decrements in Pi every day when tolerated. Fortunately, with improved medical and ventilatory care of these infants, it is rare for infants with BPD to require tracheostomy for chronic ventilation.

4. **Air leak** (see Pulmonary Air Leak)
   a. **Pathophysiology.** Pneumothorax and pulmonary interstitial emphysema (PIE) are the two most common air leak syndromes. **Pneumothorax** results when air ruptures into the pleural space. In **PIE**, the interstitial air substantiallly reduces tissue compliance as well as recoil. In addition, peribronchial and perivascular air may compress the airways and vascular supply, causing "air block."
   b. **Ventilator strategy.** Since air is driven into the interstitium throughout the ventilatory cycle, the primary goal is to reduce MAP through any of its components (Pi, Ti, PEEP) and to rely on increased FiO_2 to provide oxygenation. This strategy holds for all air leak syndromes. If dropping the MAP is not tolerated, other techniques may be tried. Because the time constants for interstitial air are much longer than those for the alveoli, we sometimes use very rapid conventional rates (up to 60 breaths per minute), which may preferentially ventilate the alveoli.

   High-frequency ventilation is an important alternative therapy for severe air leak and, if available, may be the ventilatory treatment of choice. HFV strategies for air leak differ from those used in diffuse alveolar disease. As described for conventional ventilation, the ventilatory goal in air leak syndromes is to decrease MAP, relying on FiO_2 to provide oxygenation. With HFJ and HFFI, PEEP is maintained at lower levels (4 to 6 cm H_2O), and few to no sigh breaths provided. With HFO, the MAP initially used is the same as that being used on the conventional ventilator, and the frequency set at 15 Hz. While weaning, MAP is decreased progressively, tolerating higher FiO_2 in the attempt to limit the MAP exposure.

5. **Apnea** (see Apnea)
   a. **Pathophysiology.** Occasionally, apnea is severe enough to warrant ventilator support, even in the absence of pulmonary disease. This may result from apnea of prematurity, during or following general anesthesia, or from neuromuscular paralysis.
   b. **Ventilator strategy.** For infants completely dependent on the ventilator, the goal should be to provide "physiologic" ventilation using moderate PEEP (3 to 4 cm H_2O), low gas flow, and normal rates (30 to 40 breaths per minute), with Pi adjusted to prevent hyperventilation (10 to 18 cm H_2O). Prolonged Ti is unnecessary. For infants requiring a ventilator because of intermittent but prolonged apnea, low rates (12 to 15 breaths per minute) may be sufficient.

VI. Adjuncts to mechanical ventilation

A. **Sedation** can be used when agitation or distress is associated with excessive lability of oxygenation and hypoxemia. Although this problem is more common in the neonate receiving long-term ventilation, acutely ill newborns may occasionally benefit from sedation. Morphine (0.05 to 0.1 mg/kg) or fentanyl (1 to 3 μg/kg) can be used but may cause neurologic depression. Prolonged use may lead to dependence. Lorazepam (0.05 to 0.1 mg/kg per dose given every 4 to 6 hours) has been used in more mature infants and in more chronic situations because of its long duration of action. In preterm infants, nonpharmacologic methods, such as limiting environmental light and noise and providing behavioral supports, may help decrease agitation and limit the need for sedative medications. As discussed, synchronized IMV or ventilation may also help diminish agitation and ventilatory lability.

B. Muscle relaxation with pancuronium bromide (0.1 mg/kg per dose, repeated as needed) is rarely used, but may be indicated in some infants who continue to breathe out of phase with the ventilator after attempts at finding appropriate settings and sedation have failed. High FiO_2 requirement (over 0.75) or peak inspiratory pressure (over 30 cm H_2O) are also relative indications for muscle relaxation. Although unequivocal data are not available, gas exchange may be improved in some infants following muscle relaxation, and the occurrence of chronic lung disease may be reduced. Prolonged muscle relaxation leads to fluid retention and may result in deterioration in compliance. Sedation is routinely administered to infants receiving muscle relaxants.

C. Blood gas monitoring (see Blood Gas and Pulmonary Graphic Monitoring). All infants receiving mechanical ventilation require continuous monitoring of oxygen saturation and intermittent blood gas measurements.

VII. Complications and sequelae. As a complex and invasive technology, mechanical ventilation can result in numerous adverse outcomes, both iatrogenic and unavoidable.

A. Barotrauma/volutrauma and oxygen toxicity

    1. Bronchopulmonary dysplasia (BPD) is related to increased airway pressure and changes in lung volume, although oxygen toxicity, anatomic and physiologic immaturity, and individual susceptibility also contribute.

    2. Air leak is directly related to increased airway pressure. Risk is increased at MAPs in excess of 14 cm H_2O.

B. Mechanical

    1. Obstruction of endotracheal tubes may result in hypoxemia and respiratory acidosis.

    2. Equipment malfunction, particularly disconnection, is not uncommon and requires functioning alarm systems and vigilance.

C. Complications of invasive monitoring

    1. Peripheral arterial occlusion with infarction (see Chap. 26)

    2. Aortic thrombosis from umbilical arterial catheters, occasionally leading to renal impairment and hypertension.

    3. Emboli from flushed catheters, particularly to the lower extremities, the splanchnic bed, or even the brain.

D. Anatomic

    1. Subglottic stenosis.

    2. Palatal grooves from prolonged orotracheal intubation.

    3. Vocal cord damage.

Suggested Reading

Carlo W. Assisted ventilation. In: Klaus M.H., Fanaroff A.A. (Eds.). *Care of the High Risk Neonate,* 5th ed. 2001; Philadelphia: Saunders.

Blood Gas and Pulmonary Graphic Monitoring

Michael R. Jackson and John Chuo

I. General principles. The purpose of blood gas monitoring is to ensure adequate gas exchange while avoiding the risks of excessive or inadequate oxygenation and ventilation. Oxygenation and ventilation should be monitored in all infants with cardiopulmonary disorders. Monitoring can be invasive or noninvasive, depending on factors such as the severity and anticipated duration of lung disease, the patient's clinical stability, and availability of arterial access. Monitoring should be intensified during transitions in care, such as initiation of mechanical ventilation, changes in ventilator settings, during transport, during weaning from the ventilator, and after extubation.

II. **Blood gas analysis.** Intermittent measurement of arterial blood gases (ABGs) is the gold standard for assessing the adequacy of oxygen delivery, ventilation, and pH. All noninvasive methods should be correlated with ABGs.

  A. **ABGs** are usually measured every q1–6h when acute respiratory support is needed and less frequently with stable respiratory illness. Percutaneous arterial puncture is preferred when sampling is infrequent or the course is expected to be short. Indwelling arterial catheters are used when multiple samples are needed and the course is expected to be at least several days.

   1. Measurements will be affected by noxious stimuli including recent airway care and arterial puncture, which can cause drops in oxygenation, especially in chronically ill infants with little pulmonary reserve.

   2. Heparin in the sample may also affect measurements. Since heparin solutions equilibrate with room air, excessive liquid heparin in the syringe used for blood sampling may raise PO_2 and lower PCO_2, similar to the effect of air bubbles. Samples diluted with infused solutions will also cause erroneous measurements. Extreme hypothermia or hyperthermia may lead to overestimates or underestimates, respectively, of arterial oxygention.

  B. **Capillary or venous blood gas measurements** can be used if arterial samples cannot be readily obtained or if measurements of PCO_2 and pH are needed to supplement noninvasive oxygen monitoring.

   1. A **capillary blood gas** is relatively easy to obtain. When obtained with free flow of blood from a warm and well-perfused extremity (usually the heel), it provides a good estimate of arterial PCO_2. However, it is traumatic to the heel, and may be inaccurate if obtained under conditions where perfusion is poor, such as hypotension or hypothermia.

   2. **Venous blood** can also be used to monitor PCO_2. Venous PCO_2 is usually 6 to 10 mm Hg higher and pH values are 0.02 to 0.04 lower than arterial samples, although this relationship varies depending on cardiac output and metabolic demands.

  C. **Continuous blood gas analysis.** Continuous in-line monitoring of blood PO_2, PCO_2, and pH is useful for the rapid evaluation of changes in clinical status. This technique also reduces the volume of blood withdrawn for sampling. Use is limited by reliability and cost.

III. **Noninvasive continuous monitoring.** Noninvasive continuous monitoring is useful for the rapid evaluation of changes in clinical status, such as apnea or pneumothorax. It provides immediate feedback after changes in ventilator settings. Noninvasive monitoring has little risk to the patient.

  A. **Pulse oximetry**

   1. **General characteristics.** Oximeters depend on the fact that reduced hemoglobin absorbs more red than infrared light, and oxygenated hemoglobin absorbs more infrared than red. The oximeter detects the difference in transmission of red and infrared light through tissue. The proportion of oxygenated to reduced hemoglobin is calculated and displayed as the percent oxygen saturation.

   2. **Measurements.** The PaO_2 at any given arterial oxygen saturation (SaO_2) is a function of the oxyhemoglobin dissociation curve (see Fig. 24.1). Because SaO_2 increases little as the PaO_2 increases at the flat upper end of the curve, oximetry poorly distinguishes high normal oxygen tensions (80 to 100 mm Hg) from dangerously hyperoxic ones (200 to 400 mm Hg). This poor discrimination at the upper end of the curve is accentuated by any shifts in the curve itself. A shift to the right means less saturation at a given PaO_2. Higher concentrations of adult hemoglobin, increases in $PaCO_2$ or temperature, and acidosis shift the dissociation curve to the right.

   3. **Calibration and maintenance.** The photosensors do not need calibration. However, it is useful to compare PaO_2 obtained by ABG with saturation measurement ($StcO_2$, transcutaneous oxygen saturation) so that the O_2 dissociation curve can be estimated for an individual infant.

4. **Interpretation.** Different models of oximeters use different sensors and computation programs. These may result in different baseline saturation readings. Bright ambient light may interfere with the measurement but shielding the sensor may minimize this. Motion artifacts can be a problem in active infants.

    a. **High and low values.** Because of the unpredictable location of the upper end of the O_2 dissociation curve, a measured $StcO_2$ of 97% might correspond to a PaO_2 ranging from 90 to 135 mm Hg. In preterm infants with predominantly fetal hemoglobin, saturations of 86 to 92% correspond to PaO_2 values of 37 to 97 mm Hg, respectively. Thus, for a premature baby receiving oxygen or ventilator support, PaO_2 should also be monitored when the $StcO_2$ is greater than 90%. At the lower end of the curve, the effects of shifts in the curve are more evident in saturation than in PaO_2. For example, at a PaO_2 of 45 mm Hg, saturation may decrease from about 88% at pH 7.4 (which is satisfactory) to about 80% at pH 7.25 (which may be inadequate for tissue oxygenation). In general, saturation above 88% is adequate, and below 80% is inadequate. $StcO_2$ between 80 and 88% may be adequate if the PaO_2 is greater than 45 mm Hg. These values assume normal cardiac output and hemoglobin concentration.

5. **Alarm settings.** Monitor alarm settings should allow for the expected variation in O_2 saturation while protecting babies from extreme values. Narrow setting ranges lead to nuisance alarms and detract from caregiver responses. The optimal settings are controversial. For infants with birthweight < 1250g or gestational age < 28 weeks, the target range is SaO_2 of 90–92%. The alarm limits are set to 85 and 95%. At a postmenstrual age of 32 weeks, we set the alarm limits at 87 to 97%. The range is adjusted for the particular clinical situation. Although monitoring saturation is useful at lower levels, it must be remembered that partial pressure determines the rate of oxygen transferred to the tissues and also muscle tone in the wall of the ductus arteriosus and pulmonary arterioles.

6. **Advantages of oximetry**
    a. Saturation is the basic physiologic determinant of tissue oxygen delivery.
    b. No warm-up or equilibration time.
    c. Immediate readouts permit spot monitoring and shared equipment.
    d. Pulse-by-pulse detection of rapid or transient changes in saturation (e.g., apneic spells).
    e. Relatively low maintenance and technician costs.

7. **Disadvantages of oximetry**
    a. Risk of hyperoxia at saturations between 94 and 100%.
    b. Variability in hemoglobin saturation curve during the first weeks makes estimates of PaO_2 unpredictable. This variability is affected by pH and the relative amounts of adult and fetal hemoglobin.
    c. Motion and light artifacts may disrupt monitoring.
    d. Function is reduced with poor perfusion or marked edema and may be unreliable immediately after birth.
    e. Does not account for reduced oxygen-carrying capacity with anemia.
    f. May provoke evaluation and treatment of transient, clinically insignificant, or falsely detected desaturations.
    g. Supplemental O_2 may be weaned too slowly because high PaO_2 is not recognized.

B. **Transcutaneous oxygenation ($PtcO_2$)** measures oxygen tension based on local tissue perfusion. Values are similar to arterial samples.
1. **General characteristics.** $PtcO_2$ monitoring uses a sensor that is applied to the skin on an occlusive contact medium. The heated sensor causes localized hyperemia, which maximizes capillary blood flow under the sensor. Tissue oxygen diffuses across the skin to the sensor membrane. A 10- to 15-minute equilibration time after sensor application is needed before the readings become reliable. Transcutaneous oxygen sensors have been supplanted by pulse oximetry for continuous monitoring, although they can

be used to perform noninvasive hyperoxia tests to evaluate infants suspected to have cyanotic congenital heart disease (see Chap. 25).

C. **Noninvasive PCO$_2$ monitoring** is available although rarely used. Although this method allows continuous monitoring of PCO$_2$, many limitations exist. The slow response time makes it less useful for detecting acute rises in PaCO$_2$. Decreased perfusion increases the gradient between arterial and transcutaneous values. Prolonged placement of the electrode may irritate skin. The electrodes are costly and fragile, and membranes need periodic replacement. Thus, we prefer intermittent blood gas sampling to monitor PCO$_2$.

D. **Capnography** (end-tidal CO$_2$) uses infrared spectroscopy or mass spectrometry readings of expired gas to analyze CO$_2$ content. An end-tidal CO$_2$ plateau is needed in order to estimate alveolar CO$_2$; the typical respiratory rate and expiratory flow make this difficult to achieve in newborns. The usefulness of this technique is therefore limited by the poor correlation with PaCO$_2$, as well as the additional dead space introduced by the airway adapter.

IV. **Pulmonary graphic monitoring** is available with some infant ventilators. Measurements of air flow (measured with a pneumotachometer or a hot wire anemometer), tidal volume (integrated from the air flow measurement), and driving pressure are displayed over time. Alternatively, two values can be displayed (e.g., pressure-volume loop). Although some measurements may be helpful in the management of mechanically ventilated infants, routine use of graphic monitoring has not been shown to affect outcome.

A. **Tidal volume.** We use tidal volume measurements to supplement clinical assessment and blood gas determinations. This is often helpful to adjust mechanical ventilator settings, especially during weaning. Although the appropriate tidal volume is controversial and depends on an individual infant's clinical condition, we often aim for a measurement of 4 to 6 mL/kg in preterm infants with RDS.

B. **Synchronous breathing.** A graphical display of volume changes can show whether an infant's intermittent efforts are asynchronous with the ventilator breaths. This approach may be useful to assess the effect of interventions to improve synchronous breathing, such as swaddling or sedation.

C. **Pressure-volume curves** can be used to help select an appropriate level of positive end-expiratory pressure. However, this process is complex and should only be used by clinicians experienced with the procedure.

Suggested Readings

American Association for Respiratory Care (AARC) Clinical Practice Guideline (http://www.aarc.org).

Bhutani V.K., Sivieri E.M. Clinical use of pulmonary mechanics and waveform graphics. *Clin Perinatol* 2001;28:487.

Namasivayam A., Carlo W.A. Hypocapnia and hypercapnia in respiratory management of newborn infants. *Clin Perinatol* 2001;28:487.

Poets C.F., Southall D.P. Noninvasive monitoring of oxygenation in infants and children: Practical considerations and areas of concern. *Pediatrics* 1994;93:737.

ECMO

Mehrengise Cooper and John Arnold

I. **Background.** Extracorporeal membrane oxygenation (ECMO) is a life support technique used for profound cardiorespiratory failure in neonates who fail to

TABLE 24.4. ECLS, JULY 2001, PUBLISHED BY EXTRACORPOREAL LIFE SUPPORT ORGANIZATION, ANN ARBOR, MICHIGAN

Neonatal	Total Patients	Survived ECLS	Survival to Discharge
Respiratory	16,488	14,125 (86%)	12,876 (78%)
Cardiac	1505	836 (56%)	582 (39%)
ECPR	62	36 (58%)	25 (40%)

Neonatal categories	Total runs	% survival
CDH	3699	54
MAS	5831	94
PPHN/PFC	2382	79
RDS	1318	84
Sepsis	2223	75
Pneumonia	215	59
Air leak syndrome	83	70
Other	930	66

CDH, Congenital diaphragmatic hernia; MAS, meconium aspiration syndrome; PFC, persistent fetal circulation; PPHN, persistent pulmonary hypertension of the newborn.

respond to conventional therapy (Table 24.4). The use of ECMO has been extended from neonates to adults with the best survival in the neonatal population.the efficacy of extracorporeal life support (ECLS) is supported by two prospective randomized trials of newborns with respiratory failure associated with persistent pulmonary hypertension. Continued excellent results with ECMO have solidified its role in the treatment of respiratory failure in newborns. Technologies such as high-frequency oscillatory ventilation and inhaled nitric oxide have appropriately reduced the need for ECMO.

II. Physiology

A. Theory. While pulmonary function is inadequate, ECMO provides effective gas exchange, including oxygenation and removal of carbon dioxide. ECMO allows "lung rest"; the lungs are protected from further injury due to barotrauma or oxygen, since lower ventilator settings can be used.

B. Method. Extracorporeal life support (ECLS) is provided by draining blood from the venous circulation, adding oxygen, and removing carbon dioxide via an artificial lung (membrane oxygenator). Blood is returned to either the venous or the arterial circulation.

C. Veno-arterial (V-A) ECMO. In veno-arterial ECMO, the oxygenated blood is returned to the systemic circulation. Partial cardiac bypass is created in that the circuit blood returned to the patient is mixed with blood from the patient's own cardiac output. The total cardiac output (CO) is thus the sum of the native cardiac output and the output (pump flow) generated by the circuit:

$$CO_{total} = CO_{native} + CO_{circuit}$$

Increasing the bypass flow decreases the cardiac preload and results in a decrease in the ventricular stroke volume and ventricular output. The total cardiac output, however, remains unchanged. Assuming there is no myocardial damage, these changes in native contractility and cardiac output resolve after cessation of ECMO. Monitoring pH and PO_2 of a mixed venous sample (preoxygenator blood sample) can assess adequate perfusion and oxygen delivery.

D. Veno-venous (V-V) ECMO. Oxygenated blood from the circuit in veno-venous bypass is returned to the right atrium, where it mixes with blood returning from the systemic circulation. Thus, the oxygen content of mixed venous blood increases while the carbon dioxide content is reduced. Some of this blood is recirculated in the ECMO circuit, and the rest goes to the right ventricle, through the pulmonary vascular bed, to the left side of the heart, and into the systemic circulation. Since the volume of blood removed from the venous circulation for ECLS is equal to the volume returned, the preload and thus the native cardiac output remain unchanged during veno-venous ECMO. ECMO flow rate, therefore, has no effect on cardiac output during veno-venous ECMO. Measuring the mixed venous sample is not very reliable in V-V ECMO as recirculation may lead to falsely elevated PO_2; it is more useful to follow other markers such as those indicating persistent metabolic acidosis, seizures, elevated liver function tests, oliguria and hypotension. Converting to veno-arterial (V-A) ECMO is considered if there is hypoxemia, hypotension, metabolic acidosis, or inability to generate adequate circuit flow.

E. Oxygen delivery. Oxygen delivery is the product of cardiac output and arterial oxygen content. During extracorporeal life support, many factors contribute to the delivery of oxygen. They include gas exchange in the membrane oxygenator, rate of flow through the ECMO circuit, gas exchange from the infant's lung, and cardiac output from the infant's heart. The $PaCO_2$ and $SaCO_2$ in the systemic circulation measured by arterial blood gas are a function of total gas exchange. Membrane and pulmonary gas exchange, as well as ECMO flow rate and native cardiac output, contribute to arterial oxygen saturation. At a constant ECLS flow rate and sweep gas, an improvement in the $PaCO_2$ signifies an improvement in pulmonary gas exchange. Alternatively, a deterioration in $PaCO_2$ may signify increase pulmonary blood flow without improvement in oxygen diffusion.

F. CO_2 removal. Carbon dioxide removal is extremely efficient in the membrane lung. The amount of CO_2 removed is dependent on the PCO_2 of blood circulating in the membrane, the surface area of the membrane, and the gas flow through the membrane lung (sweep gas flow). In ECLS, blood and sweep gas flow in opposite directions, setting up a countercurrent exchange of CO_2 in the membrane. The PCO_2 of the blood decreases as it travels through the membrane. The exchange of CO_2 occurs maximally in the blood inlet region and decreases as it reaches the outlet. As physiologic pulmonary function and tidal volume improve, the $PaCO_2$ decreases. The sweep gas can be adjusted by adding CO_2 to the sweep or decreasing sweep flow rate in order to prevent respiratory alkalosis.

G. Renal perfusion. Blood flow through an ECMO circuit is maintained by a nonpulsatile pump. In veno-arterial ECMO, as flow through the ECMO circuit increases, more and more blood is directed to the circuit. With increasing flows, the patient's heart contributes less to the total cardiac output. The pulse pressure eventually becomes dampened with increased flows and can flatten when maximal bypass is reached. At least one side effect of this nonpulsatile flow is an increase in renin production by the kidney. Although the mean arterial pressure may be normal, the kidneys produce renin in response. This can result in renal insufficiency. Hemodynamics during venovenous ECMO are unchanged and therefore have no effect on the systemic pulsatile flow.

H. Blood-prosthetic interaction. During ECLS, blood is in continuous contact with the prosthetic surface of the ECMO circuit. This blood-prosthetic surface interaction results in activation of both the complement and clotting cascades and the production of fibrin, lymphokines, and cytokines. Blood flowing through the extracorporeal circuit has a tendency toward clot formation. This is a result of fibrinogen binding to the circuit surface and activation of the clotting cascade. Once activated, fibrin formation results in the accumulation of platelets and the formation of a clot, which can trap red blood cells.

I. Heparin/ACT. Heparin is used to inhibit the intrinsic clotting cascade and to prevent fibrin formation. Heparin infusion is adjusted according to blood activated clotting time (ACT). The ACT is maintained in the range of 180 to 200 seconds. Unfortunately, in an effort to prevent clot formation, heparin infusion may result in bleeding. Bleeding is the most significant complication of ECMO. Heparin-induced thrombocytopenia (HIT) can also occur, leading to multiple platelet transfusions. It can be diagnosed by measuring levels of HIT antibodies. However, experience with non-heparin anticoagulation is limited.

J. Free radicals and cytokines. Before beginning ECLS, patients are generally hypoxemic. The characteristic changes that occur after initiation of ECLS are consistent with hypoxemia and shock followed by reperfusion. These changes include the production of oxygen-free radicals and other cytokines. The effect of these substances on the outcome of ECMO patients is poorly understood and difficult to separate from existing pathophysiological disturbances.

K. Edema. Total body water and extracellular fluid increase during ECMO and resolve with its discontinuation. The resolution of lung "whiteout" that occurs during ECMO correlates with improvement in pulmonary gas exchange and discontinuation of ECLS. These findings result from the reperfusion injury that occurs when ECLS support is begun for an infant in shock. This reperfusion injury results in pulmonary edema and diffuse capillary leak syndromes.

III. Indications

A. Indications. The indications for neonatal ECLS are (1) reversible respiratory failure and (2) a predicted mortality rate with conventional therapy great enough to warrant the risks of ECMO. ECMO is also considered in patients with life-threatening air leak and acute clinical deterioration in spite of optimal ventilatory and cardiovascular management. A relative criterion to initiate ECMO is failure to respond to treatment, including the inability to wean from high MAP over a prolonged period, failure to wean inspired oxygen concentration to 0.60 or less, or profound hypotension.

Defining the appropriate mortality rate is difficult, however, and varies with the primary disease. In two studies, an alveolar–arterial oxygen gradient (A–a)DO$_2$ greater than 600 torr for 12 hours was associated with 94% mortality and an (A–a)DO$_2$ greater than 610 torr for 8 hours was associated with 79% mortality.

B. Oxygenation index (OI) is calculated as:

$$OI = \frac{MAP \times FiO_2}{PaO_2} \times 100$$

where MAP equals mean airway pressure, the FiO$_2$ equals inspired oxygen concentration, and PaO$_2$ equals partial pressure of arterial oxygen. We generally consider ECMO in newborns with an OI greater than 0.6 on high-frequency oscillatory ventilation (HFOV) for 1 hour, or an OI greater than 0.4 on conventional ventilation from two consecutive arterial blood gases within 1 hour, or an OI greater than 0.4 from one arterial blood gas in a patient with cardiovascular instability. In addition, an OI >25 at 72 hours following initiation of HFOV +/– inhaled nitric oxide therapy has been shown to predict later deterioration leading to a need for ECMO. Thus, ECMO may be considered earlier in infants receiving these treatments without improvement.

C. Contraindications. The relative contraindications for ECMO in newborns include 10 or more days of mechanical ventilation, grade II or larger intraventricular hemorrhage, body weight less than 1.5 kg, or gestational age less than

34 weeks. The absolute contraindications for ECLS in our institution include significant intraventricular or parenchymal hemorrhage, weight < 1.5 kg, lethal congenital abnormality, and continuous cardiopulmonary resuscitation (CPR) for 1 hour prior to the initiation of ECMO.

IV. **Management strategies**

A. **Basic.** When a patient has met a center's criteria for ECMO, consent is obtained and cannulation of the blood vessels is performed. If the infant's condition allows, we perform head ultrasound examination and echocardiogram to exclude large intracranial hemorrhages and congenital heart defects that require surgical intervention.

B. **Circuit priming.** The appropriate circuit for a neonate is assembled using a 0.8 m^2 or 1.5 m^2 membrane oxygenator. The circuit is first primed with carbon dioxide, evacuated, and then primed with saline. After debubbling the circuit prior to use, albumin is added. The saline/albumin prime is then displaced with 500 mL of CMV-negative packed red blood cells, 200 mL of fresh frozen plasma, tromethamine (THAM), heparin, calcium gluconate, and sodium bicarbonate. Circuit pH, ionized calcium, and electrolytes are checked before ECMO is started. Once ECMO flow commences following cannulation, 2 units of concentrated platelets and 2 units of cryoprecipitate are given.

C. **Cannulation.** Anesthesia is administered using narcotics, benzodiazepines, and paralytic agents. We try to use veno-venous (V-V) ECMO whenever possible. A 12-French double-lumen cannula (DLC) is used for V-V ECMO. Patients who require multiple inotropic infusions for blood pressure support, or CPR, require V-A ECMO. A jugular vein not large enough to accommodate a 12F cannula may also preclude the use of V-V ECMO. In order to maximize venous drainage in V-A ECMO, the largest venous cannula that the jugular vein can accommodate is used. Similarly, the largest arterial cannula is used for the carotid artery to maximize flow capability and to prevent high postmembrane pressures.

D. **Circuit upkeep.** Circuits are examined every 4 hours for clots. The circuit tubing is shifted in the roller pump at 120 hours of ECLS. Elective circuit changes are made only if one of the following indications is met: (1) excessive clotting in the circuit; (2) elevation of the premembrane pressure (>350 mmHg), indicating membrane clotting and failure; (3) membrane failure proved by inadequate change from pre- to postmembrane PaO_2 and $PaCO_2$; (4) excessive platelet consumption not attributable to the patient; and (5) an uncorrectable coagulopathy that is thought to be caused by the circuit/membrane. If a circuit needs to be changed, a new circuit is primed, the patient is cycled off of ECLS, the old circuit is cut away, and the new circuit is connected, with care being taken to keep air out of the system. A new circuit may help correct a persistent coagulopathy and/or platelet consumption.

E. **Blood product evaluation.** Heparin is used in all patients to prevent clot formation. The whole blood-activated clotting time (ACT) is used to monitor heparin infusion and avoid hemorrhagic complications. We optimize other factors and keep ACT at 180 to 200 seconds. Prothrombin time is maintained at less than 17 seconds using fresh frozen plasma, fibrinogen is kept above 150 mg/dL using cryoprecipitate, and the platelet count is maintained above 150,000 using concentrated platelets. The hematocrit is kept above 35% to facilitate oxygen delivery. A whole blood exchange may be considered in conditions of sepsis with coagulopathy pre-ECMO, suspected sepsis (where a reduction in heparin requirement has been noted), and vasomotor instability.

F. **ε-Aminocaproic acid (Amicar)** lowers the incidence of hemorrhagic complications associated with ECMO, including intracranial and postoperative hemorrhage. Patients who are considered to be at high risk for bleeding complications are given Amicar. They include infants who (1) are in the perioperative period; (2) are less than 37 weeks' gestational age; (3) have sepsis; (4) have prolonged hypoxia or acidosis (pH 7.1) before ECMO; or (5) have grade I or II intraventricular hemorrhage. A loading dose of Amicar (100 mg/kg) is given, followed by a 30 mg/kg/hour infusion. After 72 hours of Amicar, the patient is assessed for further risks of bleeding complications. If these risks still exist, Amicar is continued and the circuit is changed at 120 hours. Otherwise, the Amicar infusion is discontinued.

G. Medications. Standard medications for ECMO patients in addition to heparin include broad-spectrum antibiotics (ampicillin, oxacillin, cefotaxmine), inotropes for blood pressure support (primarily V-V ECMO), narcotic analgesics, and sedatives. In order to maximize mobilization of extracellular fluid, we try to avoid muscle relaxation, but it may be necessary in acute situations where patient movement intereferes with venous return.

H. Nutrition. Nutrition is provided with parenteral alimentation. A total of 80 to 100 mL/kg/day of fluid is generally given, excluding blood products. Lipid is administered up to 2 mg/kg per day and the circuit is closely observed for evidence of lipid accumulation.

I. Fluid management. In order to maximize diuresis during ECLS, patients are given loop diuretics (as bolus doses or in an infusion) and low-dose dopamine. Hemofiltration is used in parallel with the circuit when excessive extracellular fluid is present (>500 mL positive fluid balance in preceding 24 hours), while maintaining a urine output of at least 1 mL/kg per hour.

J. Neurologic evaluation. Head ultrasound examinations are performed within 24 hours following cannulation, and every other day while the patient is receiving ECMO. Electroencephalograms (EEGs) are perfomed when seizure activity is suspected. Small intracranial hemorrhages are managed by optimizing clotting factors and using Amicar. Larger intracranial hemorrhages may force premature discontinuation of ECMO.

K. Ventilator management. While receiving ECMO, patients are maintained on "resting" ventilator settings with peak inspiratory pressure (PIP) = 25 cm H_2O, positive end-expiratory pressure (PEEP) = 5 cm H_2O, rate = 10, inspiratory time 1.0 seconds, and FiO_2 = 0.4. With a patient on V-A ECMO for active airleaks, apneic oxygenation should be considered starting at CPAP settings of 12 cm H_2O and decreasing until no further air leaks are present. Use of higher PEEP (12 to 14 cm H_2O) during ECMO, as advocated by others, may help prevent deterioration of pulmonary function and result in more rapid lung recovery. During ECMO, lung function is assessed as follows: (1) As lungs improve, CO_2 removal and oxygen content of the native cardiac output improve, resulting in improved PaO_2 and $PaCO_2$. Sweep gases can be adjusted accordingly. (2) Chest radiographs show gradual resolution of pulmonary edema. (3) As pulmonary edema resolves, lung mechanics improve and expired tidal volumes increase.

L. Cycling and decannulation. When expired tidal volumes reach approximately 5 to 7 cc/kg (in the nonparalyzed patient), attempts are made at cycling by temporarily clamping the ECMO circuit and obtaining blood gas determinations. Comparisons to previous cycling attempts are used to assess a patient's progress. Our criteria for decannulation are as follows: PIP = 30 cm H_2O; PEEP = 5 cm H_2O; rate = 25 breaths/minute; and FiO_2 = 0.35: PaO_2 over 60 mm Hg; $PaCO_2$ = 40 to 50 mm Hg; pH < 7.50.

When these criteria are used, patients rarely require recannulation. At the time of decannulation from V-A ECMO, we attempt to reconstruct the common carotid artery. The jugular vein is routinely ligated. Two units of concentrated platelets are given following decannulation.

Discontinuation of ECMO support is also considered in the following situations: when the disease process becomes irreversible, failure to wean successfully, neurological events (devestating neurological examination, significant intracranial hemorrhage), or multiorgan failure.

V. Complications

A. Mechanical. Hypovolemia can lead to poor venous return to the circuit and therefore poor pump flow. Other causes must be sought before administering fluids. This includes small venous catheter diameter, excessive catheter length, kinked tubing, poor catheter positioning, insufficient hydrostatic column length (height of patient above pump head) and improper setup of the venous control module system. Following this assessment, fluids may then be administered; however, fluid overload may result secondary to the combination of capillary leak and muscle relaxation, leading to poor chest wall compliance and compromised gas exchange.

B. Neurological. Sequelae resulting in neurological damage often originate from acidosis and hypoxia prior to commencement of ECMO.

VI. Follow-up

A. Pulmonary. One study found that 25% of former ECMO patients required hospitalization within the first year because of pulmonary complications. This compares to a hospitalization rate of 10 to 36% in newborns with similar lung disease treated conventionally. Other studies have shown less-chronic lung disease in patients who received ECMO compared to conventional treatment (12% versus 25%). In contrast, healthy infants with no previous history of respiratory disease have a 20 to 25% incidence of lower respiratory tract infections during the first 2 years of life with less than 1% requiring hospitalization. The UK collaborative randomized trial of neonatal ECMO followed children to 4 years of age, and found intermittent attacks of wheezing in more children with conventional treatment than ECMO (77% versus 42%); more conventionally treated children received regular bronchodilator treatment.

B. Neurodevelopment. Developmental outcome following ECMO appears to improve with age and is similar to newborns with similar lung disease treated conventionally. The initial diagnosis does not relate to neurodevelopment at 3.5 years. Studies of ECMO graduates have shown a 79 to 90% incidence of normal cognitive development. In comparison, adverse neurologic outcomes occurred in 25 to 60% of neonates with similar lung disease treated conventionally. In one follow-up study of ECMO survivors, cognitive development was normal in 90% of school-age children, 70% of preschoolers, and 57% of infants. Neurodevelopmental morbidity included seizures, cerebral palsy, and mild developmental delay. EEG abnormalities are commonly seen in ECMO survivors and do not appear to correlate with neurodevelopmental outcome. The abnormalities are bilateral and not predominantly in the right hemisphere, suggesting that ligation of the right common carotid artery does not produce a lateralized brain injury.

C. Hearing. Sensorineuronal hearing loss occurs in 4 to 21% of infants treated with ECMO, with a tendency for thresholds to be worse toward the higher

TABLE 24.5. OVERALL STATUS BY 4 YEARS

	ECMO (n = 93)		Conventional (n = 92)	
Deaths	31	33%	45	59%
Unable to allocate overall outcome	2	2%	3	3%
Severe disability	3	3%	0	
Moderate disability	9	10%	10	11%
Mild disability	18	19%	12	13%
Impairment only	18	19%	9	10%
No abnormal signs / disability	12	13%	4	4%
No disability	30/60	50%	13/35	37%

From UK collaborative randomized trial of neonatal ECMO—follow-up to age 4 years. *Lancet* 2001;357:1094–1096.

sound frequencies. Hearing loss occurred in 20 to 52% of infants with persistent pulmonary hypertension of the newborn (PPHN) who received conventional therapy. Hearing loss in PPHN has been attributed to hyperventilation with resultant cerebral vasoconstriction and decreased cerebral perfusion. The use of furosemide and gentamicin may also contribute.

D. **Intracranial hemorrhage.** Intracranial hemorrhage is a major factor in the morbidity and mortality following ECLS. In one study of 42 infants requiring ECLS, 12% had major hemorrhage and 17% had minor hemorrhage. The ELSO registry reports a 12% incidence of infarction. One study reports a higher incidence of right-sided brain lesions followed veno-arterial ECMO as a result of right common carotid artery ligation, although this has not been seen by others.

E. **Behavioral difficulties.** Children treated with conventional therapies appear to have an excess of problems reported using standardised questionnaires. Hyperactivity and conduct difficulties have been reported in up to one-third of ECMO survivors.

F. **Nutrition and growth.** Feeding problems have been reported in up to one-third of ECMO-treated infants. Possible causes include CNS dysfunction, tachypnea, reduced hunger drive, poor oral-motor coordination; it may also be in part related to the initial diagnosis. Somatic growth is normal. However, children treated with ECMO have an increased incidence of head circumference less than fifth percentile.

Suggested Reading
Bennett C. C., et al. for the UK Collaborative ECMO Trial Group. UK collaborative randomised trial of neonatal extracorporeal membrane oxygenation: follow-up to age 4 years. *Lancet* 2001;357:1094.

Pulmonary Air Leak

Mark T. Ogino

I. **Background**
A. **Incidence and risk factors.** Risk factors for air leak in premature infants include respiratory distress syndrome (RDS), mechanical ventilation, sepsis, and pneumonia. Surfactant therapy has markedly decreased the incidence of pneumothorax. Risk factors in term infants are aspiration of meconium, blood, or amniotic fluid; pneumonia; congenital malformations; and mechanical ventilation.

B. **Pathogenesis.** Air leak syndromes arise via a common mechanism. Transpulmonary pressures that exceed the tensile strength of the noncartilagenous terminal airways and alveolar saccules can damage the respiratory epithelium. Loss of epithelial integrity permits air to enter the interstitium, causing pulmonary interstitial emphysema. Persistent elevation in transpulmonary pressure facilitates the dissection of air toward the visceral pleura and/or the hilum via the peribronchial and perivascular spaces. In rare circumstances, air can enter the pulmonary veins and result in an air embolus. Rupture of the pleural surface allows the adventitial air to decompress into the pleural space, causing pneumothorax. Following a path of least resistance, air can dissect from the hilum and into the mediastinum, resulting in pneumomediastinum, or into the pericardium, resulting in pneumopericardium. Air in the mediastinum can decompress into the pleural space, the fascial planes of the neck and skin (subcutaneous emphysema), or the retroperitoneum. In turn, retroperitoneal air can rupture into the peritoneum (pneumoperitoneum) or dissect into the scrotum or labial folds.

1. Elevations in transpulmonary pressure can occur during the infant's first breaths when negative inspiratory pressure can approach 100 cm H_2O. Uneven ventilation due to atelectasis, surfactant deficiency, pulmonary hemorrhage, or retained fetal lung fluid can increase transpulmonary pressure. In turn, this leads to alveolar overdistention and rupture. Similarly, aspiration of blood, amniotic fluid, or meconium can facilitate alveolar overdistention by a ball-valve mechanism.

2. In the presence of underlying pulmonary conditions, positive pressure ventilation increases the risk of air leak. The high airway pressure required to achieve adequate oxygenation and ventilation in infants with poor pulmonary compliance (e.g., pulmonary hypoplasia, RDS, inflammation, pulmonary edema) further increases this risk. Excessive transpulmonary pressures can occur when ventilator pressures are not decreased as pulmonary compliance improves. This situation sometimes occurs in infants with RDS who improve rapidly after surfactant treatment. Mechanically ventilated preterm infants who make expiratory efforts against ventilator breaths are also at increased risk for pneumothorax.

3. Direct trauma to the airways can also cause air leak. Laryngoscopes, endotracheal tubes, suction catheters, and malpositioned feeding tubes can damage the lining of the airways and provide a portal for air entry.

II. Types of air leaks

A. Pneumothorax. Spontaneous pneumothoraces have been observed in 0.07% of otherwise healthy appearing neonates. One in 10 of these infants is symptomatic. The high inspiratory pressures and uneven ventilation that occur in the initial stages of lung inflation may contribute to this phenomenon. Pneumothorax is more common in newborns treated with mechanical ventilation for underlying pulmonary disease. Clinical signs of pneumothorax range from insidious changes in vital signs to the complete cardiovascular collapse that frequently accompanies a tension pneumothorax. As intrathoracic pressure rises, there is decreased lung volume, mediastinal shift, compression of the large intrathoracic veins, and increased pulmonary vascular resistance. The net effect is an increase in central venous pressure, a decrease in preload, and, ultimately, diminished cardiac output. A pneumothorax must be considered in mechanically ventilated infants who develop unexplained alterations in hemodynamics, pulmonary compliance, or oxygenation and ventilation.

1. Diagnosis

a. Physical examination

(1) Signs of respiratory distress include tachypnea, grunting, flaring, and retractions.

(2) Cyanosis.

(3) Chest asymmetry with expansion of the affected side.

(4) Episodes of apnea and bradycardia.

(5) Shift in the point of maximum cardiac impulse.

(6) Diminished or distant breath sounds on the affected side.

(7) Abdominal distension from displacement of the diaphragm.

(8) Alterations in vital signs. With smaller collections of extrapulmonary air, compensatory increases may occur in heart rate and blood pressure. As the amount of air in the pleural space increases, however, central venous pressure rises and severe hypotension, bradycardia, apnea, hypoxia, and hypercapnia may occur.

b. Arterial blood gases. Changes in arterial blood gas measurements are nonspecific and demonstrate a decreased PO_2 and increased PCO_2 (and decreased pH).

c. Chest radiographs. Anteroposterior (AP) views can show a hyperlucent hemithorax, a separation of the visceral from the parietal pleura, flattening of the diaphragm, and mediastinal shift. Smaller collections of intrapleural air can be detected beneath the anterior chest wall by obtaining a cross-table lateral view; however, an AP view is needed to identify the affected side. The lateral decubitus view, with the side of suspected pneumothorax up, may be helpful in detecting a small pneumothorax and may help differentiate skin folds, congenital lobar emphysema, cystic adenomatoid malformations, and surface blebs that occasionally give the appearance of intrapleural air.

   d. Transillumination with a high-intensity fiberoptic light source may demonstrate a pneumothorax. This technique is less sensitive in infants with chest-wall edema or severe pulmonary interstitial edema (PIE), in extremely small infants with thin chest walls, or in full-term infants with thick chest walls or dark skin. We often obtain a baseline transillumination in infants at high risk for air leak.

   e. Needle aspiration. In a rapidly deteriorating clinical situation, thoracentesis may confirm the diagnosis and be therapeutic (see II.2.b).

2. Treatment

   a. Conservative therapy. Close observation may be adequate for infants who have no underlying lung disease or complicating therapy (such as mechanical ventilation), are in no significant respiratory distress, and have no continuous air leak. The extrapulmonary air will usually resolve in 24 to 48 hours. Although some of these infants may require an increase in their ambient O_2 concentration, we do not routinely administer 100% oxygen.

   b. Needle aspiration. Thoracentesis with a "butterfly" needle or intravenous catheter with an inner needle can be used to treat a symptomatic pneumothorax. Needle aspiration may be curative in infants not receiving mechanical ventilation and is frequently a temporizing measure in mechanically ventilated infants. In infants with severe hemodynamic compromise, thoracentesis may be a life-saving procedure.

   (1) Attach a 23- or 25-gauge butterfly needle or 22- or 24-guage intravenous catheter to a 10- to 20-cc syringe previously fitted with a three-way stopcock.

   (2) Identify the second or third intercostal space in the midclavicular line, and prepare the overlying skin with an antibacterial solution.

   (3) Insert the needle firmly into the intercostal space and pass it just above the top of the third rib. This will minimize the chance of lacerating an intercostal artery, as these vessels are located on the inferior surface of the ribs. As the needle is inserted, have an assistant apply continuous suction with the syringe. A rapid flow of air into the syringe occurs when the needle enters the pleural space. Once the pleural space has been entered, stop advancing the needle. This will reduce the risk of puncturing the lung while the remaining air is evacuated.

   (4) A continuous air leak can be aspirated while a chest tube is being inserted (see II.2.c). The "butterfly" needle can be left in place and if an intravenous catheter is used, the needle can be removed and the plastic catheter left in place for further aspiration. A short piece of IV extension tubing, for example, a "T" connector, attached to the intravenous catheter hub will allow flexibility during repeated aspirations. Otherwise, withdraw the needle after the air flow has ceased.

   c. Chest tube drainage. Chest tube drainage is generally needed to evacuate pneumothoraces that develop in infants receiving positive pressure ventilation. Frequently, these air leaks are continuous and will result in severe hemodynamic compromise if left untreated.

   (1) Insertion of a chest tube

      (a) Select a chest tube of the appropriate size—no. 10 (smaller) and no. 12 (larger) French catheters are adequate for most infants.

(b) Prepare the chest area with an antibacterial solution. Infiltrate the subcutaneous tissues overlying the fourth to sixth rib at the midaxillary line with a 1% lidocaine solution. We administer an appropriate dose of narcotic for pain management.

(c) In the midaxillary line in the sixth intercostal space (ICS), parallel to the rib, make a small incision (1.0 to 1.5 cm) through the skin. Incisions of breast tissue should be avoided by locating the position of the nipple and surrounding tissue.

An alternative site is in the anterior-superior portion of the chest wall; however, due to the possible complications of injury to the internal mammary artery and other regional vessels, we do not routinuely use this approach.

(d) With a small curved hemostat, dissect the subcutaneous tissue overlying the rib. Make a subcutaneous track to the fourth ICS. Care should be taken to avoid the nipple area, the pectoralis muscle, and the axillary artery.

(e) Enter the pleural space in the fourth ICS at the intersection of the nipple line just anterior to the midclavicular line with the closed hemostat. Guide the tip over the top of the rib to avoid trauma to the intercostal artery. Push the hemostat through the intercostal muscles and parietal pleura. Listen for a rush of air to indicate pleural penetration. Spread the tips to widen the opening and leave the hemostat in place. We rarely use trochars since the use of these instruments may increase the risk of lung perforation.

(f) Grasp the end of the chest tube with the tips of the mosquito hemostat. The chest tube and the hemostat should be in a parallel orientation. Direct the chest tube through the skin incision, into the pleural opening, and between the opened tips. After the pleural space has been entered, direct the chest tube anteriorly and cephalad by rotating the curved points of the hemostat. Release the hemostat and advance the chest tube a few centimeters. Be certain that the side ports of the chest tube are in the pleural space.

(g) The chest tube will "steam up" once it has been placed into the pleural space.

(h) Direct the chest tube to the location of the pleural air. The anterior pleural space is generally most effective for infants in the supine position.

(i) Palpate the chest wall around the entry site to confirm that the chest tube is not in the subcutaneous tissues.

(j) Attach the chest tube to a Heimlich valve (for transport) or an underwater drainage system such as a Pleur-evac. Apply negative pressure (10 to 20 cm H_2O) to the underwater drainage system.

(k) Using 3-0 or 4-0 silk, close the skin incision. We place a purse-string suture around the tube or a single interrupted suture on either side of the tube. Secure the chest tube by wrapping and then tying the skin suture tails around the tube. A second loop may be placed around the chest tube at a position 2 to 4 cm from the skin surface.

(l) Cover the insertion site with petrolatum gauze and a small, clear, plastic, adhesive surgical dressing. We avoid extensive taping or large dressings, as they interfere with chest examination and may delay the discovery of a displaced chest tube.

(m) AP and lateral chest radiographs are obtained to confirm tube position and ascertain drainage of the pleural air.

(n) Radiographs may reveal chest tubes that are ineffective in evacuating extrapulmonary air. The most common cause of failure is tube placement in the posterior pleural space or the subcutaneous tissue. Other causes for ineffective drainage are tubes that perforate the lung, diaphragm, or mediastinum. Extrapulmonary air not in the pleural space, such as a pneumomediastinum or a subpleural pulmonary pseudocyst, will not be drained by a chest tube. Complications of chest tube insertion include hemorrhage, lung perforation, cardiac tamponade, and phrenic nerve injury.

    (2) Removal of a chest tube. When the infant's lung disease has improved and the chest tube has not drained air for 24 to 48 hours, we discontinue suction and leave the tube under water seal. If radiographic examination shows no reaccumulation of extrapulmonary air in the next 12 to 24 hours, the chest tube is removed. A narcotic is given for pain control prior to the chest tube removal. To reduce the chance of introducing air into the pleural space, cover the chest wound with a small occlusive dressing while removing the tube. Remove the chest tube during expiration in spontaneously breathing infants and during inspiration in mechanically ventilated infants. A manual mechanical or bagged breath can insure removing the chest tube during the inspiratory phase.

  d. Persistent pneumothorax refractory to routine measures may improve with high-frequency oscillation ventilation (HFOV); some infants require ECMO (see I).

    We sometimes place catheters under ultrasound or fluoroscopic guidance to drain air collections that are inaccessible by standard techniques.

    We often initiate HFOV to minimize mean airway pressure and resolve airleaks in mechanically ventilated infants. In patients with severe air leaks, oxygen supplementation is often increased so that mean airway pressure can be minimized.

3. Complications
  a. Profound ventilatory and circulatory compromise can occur and, if untreated, result in death.
  b. Intraventricular hemorrhage may result, possibly secondary to a combination of fluctuating cerebrovascular pressures, impaired venous return, hypercapnia, hypoxia, and acidosis.
  c. Inappropriate antidiuretic hormone secretion may occur.

B. Pulmonary interstitial emphysema (PIE). PIE occurs most often in mechanically ventilated, extremely preterm infants with RDS or sepsis. Interstitial air can be localized or can spread to involve significant portions of one or both lungs. Interstitial air can dissect toward the hilum and the pleural surface via the adventitial connective tissue surrounding the lymphatics and pulmonary vessels. This can compromise lymphatic drainage and pulmonary blood flow. Furthermore, PIE alters pulmonary mechanics by decreasing compliance, increasing residual volume and dead space, and enhancing ventilation/perfusion mismatch. Rupture of interstitial air into the pleural space and mediastinum can result in pneumothorax and pneumomediastinum, respectively.

1. Diagnosis
  a. PIE frequently develops in the first 48 hours of life.
  b. PIE may be accompanied by hypotension, bradycardia, hypercarbia, hypoxia, and acidosis.
  c. PIE has two radiographic patterns: cystlike and linear. Linear lucencies radiate from the lung hilum. Occasionally, large cystlike blebs give the appearance of a pneumothorax.

2. Treatment
  a. If possible, attempt to decrease mean airway pressure by lowering peak inspiratory pressure, PEEP, and inspiratory time. We generally use high-frequency oscillatory ventilation in infants with PIE to avoid large swings in lung volume.

    b. Unilateral PIE may improve if the infant is positioned with the affected lung dependent. Endotracheal suctioning and manual positive pressure ventilation should be minimized. Severe localized PIE that has failed to improve with conservative management may require collapse of the affected lung by selective bronchial intubation or occlusion or, rarely, surgical resection.

  3. Complications

    a. PIE may precede more severe complications such as pneumothorax, pneumopericardium, or an air embolus.

C. Pneumomediastinum. Mediastinal air can develop when pulmonary interstitial air dissects into the mediastinum or when direct trauma occurs to the airways or the posterior pharynx.

  1. Diagnosis

    a. Physical examination. Heart sounds may appear distant.

    b. Chest radiograph. Air collections are central and usually elevate or surround the thymus. This results in the characteristic "spinnaker sail" sign. A pneumomediastinum is best seen on a lateral view.

  2. Treatment

    a. Pneumomediastinum is of little clinical importance, and specific drainage procedures are usually unnecessary. Rarely, cardiorespiratory compromise may develop if the air is under tension and does not decompress into the pleural space, the retroperitoneum, or the soft tissues of the neck. This situation may require mediastinostomy drainage.

    b. If the infant is mechanically ventilated, reduce mean airway pressure if possible.

  3. Complications

    a. Observe for other air leaks.

D. Pneumopericardium. Pneumopericardium is the least common form of air leak in newborns but the most common cause of cardiac tamponade. Asymptomatic pneumopericardium is occasionally detected as an incidental finding on a chest radiograph. Most cases occur in preterm infants with RDS treated with mechanical ventilation, preceded by PIE and pneumomediastinum. The mortality rate for critically ill infants who develop pneumopericardium is 70 to 80%.

  1. Diagnosis. Pneumopericardium should be considered in mechanically ventilated newborn infants who develop acute or subacute hemodynamic compromise.

    a. Physical examination. Although infants may initially have tachycardia and decreased pulse pressure, hypotension, bradycardia, and cyanosis may ensue rapidly. Auscultation reveals muffled or distant heart sounds. A pericardial knock (Hamman sign) or a characteristic millwheel-like murmur (bruit de moulin) may be present.

    b. Chest radiograph. Anteroposterior views show air surrounding the heart. Air under the inferior surface of the heart is diagnostic.

    c. Transillumination. A high-intensity fiberoptic light source may illuminate the substernal region. Flickering of the light with the heart rate may help differentiate pneumopericardium from pneumomediastinum or a medial pneumothorax.

    d. Electrocardiogram (ECG). Decreased voltages, manifest by a shrinking QRS complex, are consistent with pneumopericardium.

  2. Treatment

    a. Conservative management. Asymptomatic infants not receiving positive pressure ventilation can be managed expectantly. Vital signs are closely monitored (especially changes in pulse pressure), and frequent chest radiographs are obtained until the pneumopericardium resolves.

    b. Needle aspiration. Cardiac tamponade is a life-threatening event that requires immediate pericardiocentesis.

      (1) Prepare the subxiphoid area with antibacterial solution.

(2) Attach a 20- to 22-gauge intravenous catheter with an inner needle to a short piece of IV extension tubing that, in turn, is connected to a three-way stopcock and a 20-cc syringe. In the subxiphoid space, insert the catheter at a 30 to 45 degree angle and toward the infant's left shoulder. Have an assistant aspirate with the syringe as the catheter is advanced. Once air is aspirated, stop advancing the catheter. Slide the plastic catheter over the needle and into the pericardial space. Remove the needle, reattach the IV tubing to the hub of the plastic catheter, evacuate the remaining air, and withdraw the catheter. If air leak persists, prepare for pericardial tube placement. If blood is aspirated, immediately withdraw the catheter to avoid lacerating the ventricular wall. The complications of pericardiocentesis include hemopericardium and laceration of the right ventricle or left anterior descending coronary artery.

    c. Continuous pericardial drainage. Because pneumopericardium often progresses to cardiac tamponade and may recur following aspiration, a pericardial tube may be needed for continuous drainage. We manage the pericardial tube like a chest tube, although less negative pressure (5 to 10 cm H_2O) is used for suction.

  3. Complications. Ventilated infants who have a pneumopericardium drained by needle aspiration frequently (80%) have a recurrence. Recurrent pneumopericardium can occur days after apparent resolution of the initial event.

E. Other types of air leaks

  1. Pneumoperitoneum. Intraperitoneal air may result from extrapulmonary air that decompresses into the abdominal cavity. Usually the pneumoperitoneum is of little clinical importance, but it must be differentiated from intraperitoneal air resulting from a perforated viscus. Rarely, pneumoperitoneum can impair diaphragmatic excursion and compromise ventilation. In these cases, continuous drainage may be necessary.

  2. Subcutaneous emphysema. Subcutaneous air can be detected by palpation of crepitus in the face, neck, or supraclavicular region. Large collections of air in the neck, although usually of no clinical significance, can partially occlude or obstruct the compressible, cartilaginous trachea of the premature infant.

  3. Systemic air embolism. An air embolism is a rare but usually fatal complication of pulmonary air leak. Air may enter the vasculature either by disruption of the pulmonary venous system or by inadvertent injection through an intravascular catheter. The presence of air bubbles in blood withdrawn from an umbilical artery catheter can be diagnostic.

Persistent Pulmonary Hypertension of the Newborn

Linda J. Van Marter

I. Definition. Persistent pulmonary hypertension of the newborn (PPHN) is the result of disruption in the normal perinatal fetal-neonatal circulatory transition. The disorder is characterized by sustained elevation in pulmonary vascular resistance (PVR) at birth. Improved ventilator management, treatment with inhaled nitric oxide (iNO), and extracorporeal membrane oxygenation (ECMO) have led to improved survival among infants with PPHN. Survivors of PPHN are at risk of adverse sequelae include chronic pulmonary disease, neurodevelopmental disabilities, hearing impairment, and intracranial hemorrhage or infarction.

A. **Perinatal circulatory transition.** The normal perinatal circulatory transition is characterized by a rapid fall in PVR accompanying the first breath and a marked rise in systemic vascular resistance (SVR) with the clamping of the umbilical cord. These events raise SVR relative to PVR and result in the functional closure of the foramen ovale. Humoral mediators released in response to the rise in arterial oxygen content and change in pH cause constriction of the ductus arteriosus. These events signal the change in the pulmonary and systemic circulations from functionally parallel to series circuits. PPHN physiology mimics the fetal circulation in which PVR exceeds SVR and right-to-left hemodynamic shunting occurs through the foramen ovale or ductus arteriosus. Before birth, this circulatory configuration results in systemic delivery of oxygenated blood from the placental circulation; in postnatal life it causes diminished pulmonary perfusion and hypoxemia.

II. **Epidemiologic associations.** PPHN occurs at a rate of 1 to 2 per 1000 live births and is most common among full-term and post-term infants. Perinatal risk factors reported in association with PPHN include meconium-stained amniotic fluid and neonatal conditions such as fever, anemia, and pulmonary disease. A case-control study evaluating antenatal risk factors for PPHN among infants hospitalized at several thousand hospitals revealed associations between PPHN and fewer years of maternal education, maternal diabetes mellitus, urinary tract infection during pregnancy, and aspirin and nonsteroidal anti-inflammatory drug consumption during pregnancy. Although mechanisms of antenatal pathogenesis remain under investigation, there are a number of perinatal and neonatal conditions with well-established links with PPHN.

A. **Intrauterine or perinatal asphyxia** is the most common associated diagnosis. Prolonged fetal stress and hypoxemia might result in remodeling and abnormal muscularization of the smallest pulmonary arteries. Acute birth asphyxia also causes release of vasoconstricting humoral factors and suppression of pulmonary vasodilators, possibly inducing pulmonary vasospasm.

B. **Pulmonary parenchymal disease,** including respiratory distress syndrome (RDS), pneumonia, and aspiration syndromes, especially meconium aspiration, can cause hypoxia-induced pulmonary vasospasm or may be associated with the characteristic pulmonary vascular remodeling. Mechanisms leading to associated pulmonary hypertension appear to be more prominent when the fetus is of more advanced gestational age.

C. **Abnormalities of pulmonary development,** including alveolar capillary dysplasia, congenital diaphragmatic hernia, and parenchymal hypoplasia, are often associated with PPHN.

D. **Myocardial dysfunction,** myocarditis, intrauterine constriction of the ductus arteriosus, and a number of forms of congenital heart disease, including left- and right-sided obstructive lesions, lead to pulmonary hypertension.

E. **Pneumonia and/or sepsis** of bacterial or viral origin can initiate PPHN. Underlying pathophysiologic mechanisms that contribute to pulmonary hypertension in this clinical setting include suppression of nitric oxide production, endotoxin-mediated myocardial depression, and pulmonary vasoreactivity associated with release of thromboxanes and leukotrienes.

F. **Genetic predisposition** might influence PPHN risk. Infants with PPHN have low plasma levels of arginine and nitric oxide metabolites and have a greater likelihood of specific polymorphisms at position 1405 of the carbamoyl-phosphate synthetase gene.

III. **Pathology and pathophysiology**

A. **Pulmonary vascular remodeling** is pathognomonic of idiopathic PPHN and has been reported among infants dying of PPHN following meconium aspiration. Abnormal muscularization of the normally nonmuscular intraacinar arteries, with increased medial thickness of the larger muscular arteries, results in a decreased cross-sectional area of the pulmonary vascular bed and elevated PVR. Mechanisms leading to vascular remodeling are under investigation. One possibility is that pulmonary vascular remodeling is the result of intrauterine hypoxemia. This mechanism is biologically plausible since humoral growth factors released by hypoxia-damaged endothelial cells promote vasoconstriction and muscular overgrowth. Laboratory and limited clinical data suggest that vascular changes also may occur following fetal exposure to nonsteroidal anti-inflammatory agents (i.e., prostaglandin synthetase inhibitors), which cause constriction of the fetal ductus arteriosus and secondary pulmonary hypertension.

B. **Pulmonary hypoplasia** affects both alveolar and pulmonary arterial development. It may be seen as an isolated anomaly or with congenital diaphragmatic hernia (see Chap. 33), oligohydramnios syndrome, renal agenesis (i.e., Potter syndrome), or abnormalities associated with decreased fetal breathing.

C. **Pulmonary vasospasm** is suspected in infants with reversible PPHN. The underlying disease process, the associated conditions, and the maturity of the host each appear to modulate the pathophysiologic response. Hypoxia induces profound pulmonary vasoconstriction and this response is exaggerated by acidemia. Neural and humoral vasoactive substances each might contribute to the pathogenesis of PPHN, the response to hypoxemia, or both. These include factors associated with platelet activation and production of arachidonic acid metabolites. Suppression of endogenous nitric oxide, prostacyclin, or bradykinin production and release of thromboxanes (A_2 and its metabolite, B_2), leukotrienes (C_4 and D_4), endothelin and platelet-derived growth factor likely mediate the increased PVR seen with sepsis and/or hypoxemia.

D. **Myocardial dysfunction with elevated PVR**

1. **Right ventricular (RV) dysfunction** can be caused by intrauterine closure of the ductus arteriosus, which results in altered fetal hemodynamics, postnatal pulmonary hypertension, RV failure, and a right-to-left shunt at the atrial level. RV failure resulting in altered diastolic compliance can cause right-to-left atrial shunting even in the absence of elevated PVR.

2. **Left ventricular (LV) dysfunction** causes pulmonary venous hypertension and reflex pulmonary arterial hypertension, often to suprasystemic levels. Right-to-left hemodynamic shunting through the ductus arteriosus subsequently occurs. Treating this form of pulmonary hypertension requires approaches aimed at improving LV function, rather than simply lowering PVR.

E. **Mechanical factors** that influence PVR include cardiac output and blood viscosity. Low cardiac output recruits fewer arteriolar channels and may raise PVR by this mechanism as well as by its primary effect of lowering mixed venous oxygen content. Hyperviscosity, associated with polycythemia, reduces pulmonary microvasculature perfusion. Pulmonary microthrombi have been observed in autopsies of some infants with intractable PPHN.

IV. **Diagnosis.** PPHN should be considered routinely in evaluating the cyanotic newborn.

A. Among cases of suspected PPHN, the most common **alternative diagnoses** are uncomplicated severe pulmonary parenchymal disease, sepsis, and congenital heart disease.

B. The **physical examination** is generally less remarkable for PPHN than for signs of associated diagnoses. Among infants with PPHN, the cardiac examination is notable for a prominent precordial impulse, a single or narrowly split and accentuated second heart sound, and/or a systolic murmur consistent with tricuspid regurgitation, especially when a hypoxic-ischemic perinatal insult precedes PPHN.

C. **A gradient in oxygenation between simultaneous preductal (right upper extremity or head) and postductal (lower extremity or abdomen) arterial blood gas (ABG) values** or transcutaneous oxygen saturation measurements documents the presence of a ductus arteriosus right-to-left hemodynamic shunt. A 10% or greater pre/post ductal difference in oxygen saturation in the absence of structural heart disease suggests PPHN. A subset of infants with PPHN have hemodynamic shunting only at the level of the foramen ovale. Therefore, the absence of a significant ductal shunt does not exclude pulmonary hypertension associated with an isolated atrial right-to-left hemodynamic shunt.

D. The **chest radiograph** usually appears normal or shows associated pulmonary parenchymal disease or air leak. The cardiothymic silhouette is normal or borderline enlarged; pulmonary blood flow is normal or diminished.

E. The **ECG** most commonly shows RV predominance that is within the range considered normal for age. Less commonly, the ECG might reveal signs of myocardial ischemia or infarction or findings consistent with structural heart disease.

F. An **echocardiographic study** should be performed in all infants with suspected PPHN to evaluate hemodynamic shunting, ventricular function, and to exclude cyanotic congenital heart disease. Color Doppler examination is useful to assess the presence of intracardiac or ductal shunting. Additional echocardiographic markers, such as flattened or left-bowed septum, suggest pulmonary hypertension. Pulmonary artery pressure can be estimated using continuous-wave Doppler sampling of the velocity of the tricuspid regurgitation jet, if present.

G. Other diagnostic considerations. A number of disorders, some of which are associated with secondary pulmonary hypertension, are misdiagnosed as PPHN. Therefore, an important aspect of the evaluation of the infant with presumed PPHN is the effort to rule out competing conditions, including:

1. Structural cardiovascular abnormalities associated with right-to-left ductal or atrial shunting include the following:

a. Obstruction to pulmonary venous return. Infradiaphragmatic total anomalous pulmonary venous return, hypoplastic left heart, cor triatriatum, congenital mitral stenosis.

b. Myopathic LV disease. Endocardial fibroelastosis, Pompe's disease.

c. Obstruction to LV outflow. Critical aortic stenosis, supravalvar aortic stenosis, interrupted aortic arch, coarctation of the aorta.

d. Obligatory left-to-right shunt. Endocardial cushion defect, arteriovenous malformation, hemitruncus, coronary arteriovenous fistula.

e. Miscellaneous disorders. Ebstein anomaly, transposition of the great arteries.

2. Left or right ventricular dysfunction associated with right-to-left shunting. LV dysfunction, due to ischemia or obstruction caused by myopathic LV disease or obstruction to LV outflow, sometimes presents with a right-to-left ductal shunt. RV dysfunction may be associated with right-to-left atrial shunting as a result of decreased diastolic compliance and elevated end-diastolic pressure. These diagnoses must be differentiated from PPHN caused by pulmonary vascular abnormalities.

H. Signs favoring cyanotic congenital cardiac disease over PPHN include cardiomegaly, weak pulses, active precordium, pulse differential between upper and lower extremities, pulmonary edema, grade 3+ murmur, and persistent arterial oxygen tension (PaO_2) at or below 40 mm Hg (see Chap. 25).

V. Management. The cyanotic newborn is a medical emergency. Immediate, appropriate intervention aims to prevent or ameliorate PPHN and is critical in the effort to avoid or minimize hypoxic-ischemic end-organ injury. Initial goals of therapy are to reverse hypoxemia and restore normal oxygenation. Normal oxygenation and acid-base balance facilitate the normal perinatal circulatory transition. Therefore, the goals of treatment are to optimize cardiorespiratory function; specifically, to reduce elevated PVR, improve oxygenation and optimize systemic blood pressure. Once stability is achieved, weaning should be accomplished conservatively with careful attention to the infant's tolerance of each step that tapers cardiorespiratory support.

A. Supplemental oxygen. Hypoxemia is one of the most powerful pulmonary vasoconstrictors. Therefore, the use of supplemental oxygen to achieve normal or elevated arterial oxygen tension is the most important therapy used to reduce abnormally elevated PVR. In the presence of hypoxemia, 100% oxygen should be administered to any near-term or full-term cyanotic newborn. After 10 minutes, the effects of oxygen therapy should be evaluated with a postductal ABG analysis. If the postductal PaO_2 is less than 100 mm Hg in 100% oxygen, or oxygen saturation is less than 90%, simultaneous preductal and postductal ABG analyses or oxygen saturation levels are performed to assess transductal shunting. Continuous noninvasive monitoring allows detection of rapid changes in oxygenation.

B. Intubation and mechanical ventilation. Respiratory support is instituted when hypoxemia persists despite maximal administration of oxygen by hood or PaO_2 is borderline despite supplementation with 100% oxygen. Specific approaches to respiratory support and mechanical ventilation vary across medical centers (see Mechanical Ventilation). We recommend an approach that maintains adequate oxygenation and mild hyperventilation, initially attempting to keep the PaO_2 greater than 80 mm Hg, arterial carbon dioxide tension ($PaCO_2$) at 35 to 45 mm Hg, and pH at 7.35 to 7.45. After 12 to 24 hours of stability, these parameters can be gradually modified to accept oxygen saturation values greater than 90 to 92%, $PaCO_2$ values of 45 to 55 mm Hg, and a less alkalotic pH, with careful attention to the infant's physiologic responses.

1. The nature of the underlying pulmonary parenchymal abnormality, if any, and the infant's clinical lability or stability are important factors to consider when choosing the specific respiratory management strategy.

2. In the absence of alveolar disease, high mean airway pressure may impede cardiac output and elevate PVR. We use a strategy of rapid, low-pressure, short-inspiratory-time mechanical ventilation designed to minimize mean airway pressure. Typical ventilator settings are rate, 30 to 60 breaths per minute; peak inspiratory pressure (PIP), 20 to 25 cm H_2O; positive end-expiratory pressure (PEEP), 3 to 4 cm H_2O; and inspiratory duration, 0.3 to 0.4 seconds. High gas flow (20 to 30 L/min) might be required, and large-diameter ventilator tubing is used to maintain PEEP at low levels in the presence of high flow rates.

3. When PPHN complicates parenchymal pulmonary disease, appropriate ventilator strategies address the primary pulmonary disease. High-frequency oscillatory ventilation (HFOV) is often useful in treating infants whose PPHN is associated with severe pulmonary parenchymal disease.

C. Inhaled nitric oxide (iNO). iNO administered by conventional or high-frequency ventilation in doses of 5 to 40 parts per million selectively decreases PVR. Nitric oxide (NO) is a naturally occurring substance produced by endothelial cells. Whether produced by pulmonary endothelium or delivered via the ventilator circuit, NO diffuses into smooth muscle cells, increases intracellular cyclic guanosine monophosphate (cGMP), relaxes the actin-myosin complex, and causes pulmonary vasodilation. In the circulation, NO is bound by hemoglobin and, thus, causes little or no systemic vasodilation or hypotension. Meta-analysis by the Cochrane Collaborative deemed iNO useful in reducing the need for ECMO among term infants with severe respiratory failure.

1. We consider iNO in infants ≥ 34 weeks' gestation with PPHN confirmed by echocardiogram who have a persistent oxygenation index ≥ 25 after lung recruitment and other therapies have been optimized. Inhaled NO is most effective when administered after adequate alveolar recruitment. This can be accomplished among infants with diffuse pulmonary disease by the concomitant use of HFOV and/or surfactant treatment.

2. We start iNO at a dose of 20 ppm and anticipate an improvement in oxygenation or a decrease in lability within 15 to 20 minutes.

3. As oxygenation improves, we gradually decrease the inspired oxygen concentration. If the FiO2 is <0.6 and PaO_2 is ≥ 60 and $SaCO_2$ is > 90%, we

decrease iNO to 10 ppm. If the increased oxygenation is sustained, we gradually decrease iNO from 10 to 5 to 1 ppm. This usually occurs over 3 to 4 days, but may take longer in severe cases.

4. Caution must be taken in weaning iNO to avoid potential rebound hypoxemia. When FiO_2 is ≤ 0.4 and oxygenation is maintained with iNO 1 ppm, we transiently increase the FiO_2 to 0.6 and discontinue iNO. If oxygenation decreases and FiO_2 is > 0.6, iNO is restarted at 1 ppm, and discontinuation is attempted again in 4 to 8 hours.

5. A potential toxicity of iNO is methemoglobinemia. Therefore, methemoglobin levels must be monitored daily in infants receiving iNO.

6. Because not all infants with PPHN respond to iNO (approximately 40% in two large trials) and some may deteriorate rapidly, we recommend treatment of critically ill infants at a center where ECMO is readily accessible.

D. Extracorporeal membrane oxygenation (ECMO). ECMO is a lifesaving therapy for infants with PPHN who fail conventional management and/or iNO treatment (see ECMO).

E. Sedation and analgesia. Because catecholamine release activates pulmonary alpha-adrenergic receptors, thereby potentially raising PVR, a narcotic analgesic, such as morphine sulfate (0.1 mg/kg every 2 to 4 hours PRN) or fentanyl (3 to 8 µg/kg per hour) is a useful adjunct therapy. Fentanyl is a potent, short-acting narcotic that reduces pain and discomfort and minimizes sympathetic nervous system activity. In rare instances, we use neuromuscular blockade with pancuronium (0.1 mg/kg per dose; every 1 to 3 hours PRN) to accomplish muscle relaxation to completely synchronize the infant's breathing with mechanical ventilation.

F. Metabolic alkalosis. Correction of acidosis is second in importance only to oxygenation in the treatment of PPHN. Alkalosis, rather than hypocarbia is the physiologic stimulus that reduces PVR. Alkalosis can be achieved by gentle hyperventilation, optimizing blood pressure and perfusion, and/or metabolic therapy with sodium bicarbonate. In infants with PPHN, we recommend maintaining the pH at 7.35 to 7.45.

G. Hemodynamic support. Adequate cardiac output is necessary to maximize tissue oxygenation and mixed venous oxygen content. Optimizing systemic blood pressure to override the elevated PVR, effectively reducing or eliminating the right-to-left hemodynamic shunt, is a short-term treatment goal. Because many infants with PPHN have PVR that is at or near normal systemic blood pressures, it is reasonable to set initial treatment goals of raising systemic blood pressure to levels of 60 to 80 mm Hg (systolic) and 50 to 60 mm Hg (mean).

1. In the clinical setting of PPHN, volume resuscitation and pressors, such as dopamine, dobutamine, and/or epinephrine, often are necessary to achieve adequate cardiac output (see Chap. 17). When cardiac function is very poor, cardiotonic medications such as milrinone are sometimes useful.

2. Intravascular volume support with normal saline (0.9% NS) or packed red blood cells may be important adjunct therapies for infants with pathophysiologic conditions associated with intravascular volume depletion (e.g., hemorrhage, hydrops, capillary leak) or decreased SVR (e.g., septic shock) or systemic hypotension.

H. Correction of metabolic abnormalities. Biochemical abnormalities might contribute to right-to-left shunting through impaired cardiac output. Correction of hypoglycemia and hypocalcemia is especially important in treating infants with PPHN in order to provide adequate substrates for myocardial function and response to pharmacologic agents (e.g., pressors).

I. Correction of polycythemia. Hyperviscosity, associated with polycythemia, increases PVR and is associated with release of vasoactive substances through platelet activation. Partial exchange transfusion to reduce the hematocrit to 50 to 55% should be considered in the infant with PPHN whose central hematocrit exceeds 65% (see Chap. 26).

J. Additional pharmacologic agents. Complementary pharmacologic therapy is directed at the simultaneous goals of optimizing cardiac output, enhancing systemic blood pressure, and reducing PVR. Consideration of associated and differential diagnoses and the known or hypothetical pathogenesis of the right-to-left shunt may prove helpful in selecting the best agent or combination of agents for a particular infant.

1. At the present time, data are insufficient to support the use of other proposed medical therapies for PPHN, including magnesium sulfate infusion, inhaled prostacyclin, or inhaled ethyl nitrite.
2. Phosphodiasterase inhibitors, such as sildenafil, that increase the concentration of cyclic GMP by reducing its degradation, are under investigation.

K. Treatment controversies. There is substantial interinstitutional variation in approaches to diagnosis and management of PPHN. Some centers report successful treatment of PPHN without the use of mechanial ventilation, iNO, or ECMO.

L. Outcome. The availability of iNO and ECMO has been associated with reductions in PPHN-associated mortality from 25 to 50% to 10 to 15%. Survivors of PPHN remain at substantial risk of medical and neurodevelopmental sequelae. Controlled clinical trials suggest that the risk of morbid sequelae is not affected by specific PPHN treatment(s). Survivors of PPHN have a risk of rehospitalization within one year of discharge of approximately 20%, and have a 20 to 46% risk of audiologic, neurodevelopmental, or cognitive impairments.

Suggested Readings

Finer N.N., Barrington K.J. Nitric oxide for respiratory failure in infants born at or near term. *Cochrane Library* 2002; 4: CD000509.

Kinsella J.P., Abman S.H. Inhaled nitric oxide: Current and future uses in neonates. *Semin Perinatol* 2000; 24: 387–395.

Lipkin P.H., et al. I-NO/PPHN Study Group. Neurodevelopmental and medical outcomes of persistent pulmonary hypertension in term newborns treated with nitric oxide. *J Pediatr* 2002; 140: 306–310.

Walsh M.C., Stork E.K. Persistent pulmonary hypertension of the newborn: Rational therapy based on pathophysiology. *Clin Perinatol* 2001; 28: 609–627.

Transient Tachypnea of the Newborn

Nancy A. Louis*

I. **Definition.** Transient tachypnea of the newborn (TTN), also known as "wet lung," is a relatively mild, self-limited disorder, usually affecting infants who are born at or near term gestation. TTN is characterized by tachypnea with signs of mild respiratory distress including retractions, and mild cyanosis, usually alleviated with a supplemental oxygen requirement of FiO_2 less than 0.40.

II. **Pathophysiology.** TTN is characterized by a transient pulmonary edema resulting from delayed clearance of fetal lung liquid. Potential causes include conditions that elevate central venous pressure, leading to delayed clearance of fluid by the thoracic duct or the pulmonary lymphatic system. Retained fluid accumulates in the peribronchiolar lymphatics and bronchovascular spaces, causing compression and bronchiolar collapse with areas of air trapping and

---

*This is a revision of a chapter in the 4th edition originally written by Mark E. Lawson.

hyperinflation. These changes decrease lung compliance, leading to tachypnea to counter the resultant increased respiratory work.

III. Risk factors. Premature birth, precipitous birth, and operative birth without labor have all been associated with an increased risk of TTN. This has been attributed to impaired fluid clearance possibly due to the absence of "thoracic squeeze" normally contributed by passage through the birth canal. Delayed cord clamping or cord milking, promoting placental–fetal transfusion, leads to an elevation in the infant's central venous pressure and is also associated with an increase in TTN. Additional risk factors include male gender and birth to an asthmatic mother. The mechanism for the latter associations is uncertain, although it may be related to an altered sensitivity to catecholamines, which may delay clearance of lung fluid. Additional risk factors include macrosomia and multiple gestations. The associations between TTN and other obstetric factors such as excessive maternal sedation, prolonged labor, and complications resulting in administration of large amounts of intravenous fluids to the mother have been less consistent.

IV. Clinical presentation. Affected term or near-term infants typically present within the first 6 hours after birth with tachypnea (respiratory rate > 80 breaths per minute). In preterm infants, retained lung fluid may complicate surfactant deficiency and contribute to greater requirements of respiratory support.

The infant with TTN usually has mild to moderate respiratory distress with tachypnea, cyanosis, subcostal retractions, nasal flaring, and increased anteroposterior diameter of the chest secondary to air trapping. Expiratory grunting is common. Auscultation usually reveals good air entry, and crackles may be audible. TTN usually occurs in the absence of cardiac, central nervous system (CNS), hematologic, infectious, or metabolic disorders. However, it is important to exclude these potential sources of respiratory distress, which require more targeted and aggressive intervention. Signs of TTN usually persist for 12 to 24 hours in cases of mild disease, but can last up to 48 to 72 hours in more severe cases.

V. Differential diagnosis. TTN is a diagnosis of exclusion and other potential etiologies of respiratory distress must be ruled out.

A. Pneumonia/sepsis. The infant should be evaluated for sepsis risk factors and signs of infection. If risk factors or laboratory signs suggest sepsis, or if the infant's respiratory distress does not improve within 4 to 6 hours, we treat with broad-spectrum antibiotics.

B. Cyanotic congenital heart disease. If suspected, evaluation should include a hyperoxia test.

C. RDS. Infants with RDS are preterm or have risk factors for pulmonary immaturity, and usually have a characteristic chest X ray. Infants with RDS usually have more severe respiratory distress and a greater need for supplemental oxygen than those with TTN.

D. Central hyperventilation. This disorder may be seen in term infants with birth asphyxia, who typically have tachypnea without respiratory distress. Chest x-ray findings are usually minimal, and blood gas analysis usually shows respiratory alkalosis.

E. Other conditions that may cause tachypnea and should be excluded are pulmonary hypertension, meconium aspiration, and polycythemia.

VI. Diagnosis

A. Laboratory studies. CBC and differential can provide information concerning possible infection and also exclude polycythemia. **Arterial blood gas analysis** may show a mild respiratory acidosis and mild hypoxemia. These usually resolve within 24 hours. Infants with profound hypoxemia should be evaluated for congenital heart disease, myocardial failure, and/or pulmonary hypertension. A **blood culture** should be obtained if sepsis is suspected.

B. Chest radiograph. Radiographic findings include:

1. Prominent perihilar streaking due to engorgement of periarterial lymphatics with accumulation of interstitial fluid along the bronchovascular spaces.

2. Mild to moderate cardiomegaly.
3. Coarse, fluffy densities due to liquid-filled alveoli.
4. Fluid in the minor fissure, pleural effusions, and widening of the interlobar fissures.
5. Hyperinflation with flattening of the diaphragm due to air trapping secondary to bronchiolar collapse.

These radiographic abnormalities usually show evidence of clearing by 12 to 18 hours, with complete resolution by 48 to 72 hours. Rapid clearance of these findings help distinguish TTN from bacterial pneumonia and meconium aspiration. Increased pulmonary vascularity in the absence of cardiomegaly may be seen in a preterm infant with patent ductus arteriosus or a term infant with total anomalous pulmonary venous return.

VII. **Management.** Management is mainly supportive. Supplemental oxygen is provided to keep arterial oxygen saturation >90%. In some infants, continuous positive airway pressure (CPAP) may support lung expansion. Despite the role of fluid retention in the pathogenesis of TTN, diuretic therapy does not affect the clinical course. Infants with sustained respiratory rates greater than 60 breaths/minute should not be fed orally and are given intravenous fluids. Some infants with mild tachypnea (60 to 80 breaths/minute) may be fed with an orogastric feeding tube.

VIII. **Complications.** Complications are uncommon. The risk of air leak may be increased. Delayed initiation of oral feedings may interfere with parental bonding and establishment of breastfeeding, and prolong hospital stay.

IX. **Prognosis.** TTN is a self-limited process and the prognosis is excellent, with no residual pulmonary effects.

Pulmonary Hemorrhage

Nancy A. Louis*

I. **Definition.** Pulmonary hemorrhage is defined on pathologic examination as the presence of erythrocytes in the alveoli, interstitial spaces, or both. Infants who survive longer than 24 hours have predominantly interstitial hemorrhage. Confluent hemorrhages involving at least two lobes of the lungs are termed massive pulmonary hemorrhage. There is no uniformly accepted clinical definition of pulmonary hemorrhage. We generally define pulmonary hemorrhage as the presence of hemorrhagic fluid in the trachea that is accompanied by a respiratory decompensation requiring increased respiratory support or intubation within 60 minutes of the appearance of the fluid.

II. **Epidemiology.** Accurate incidence rates are difficult to ascertain as the clinical definition is unclear and definitive diagnosis requires pathological examination. The latter is often unavailable either because the event is not fatal or because permission for autopsy is not obtained. The rate of clinically apparent pulmonary hemorrhage has been estimated at 1 to 12 per 1000 live births. In high-risk groups such as premature and growth-restricted infants, the incidence increases to as many as 50 per 1000 live births. In autopsy studies, pulmonary hemorrhage of any degree is much more prevalent. Some studies demonstrated hemorrhage in up to 68% of autopsied neonates, with severe pulmonary hemorrhage occurring in 19% of infants dying in the first week after birth. In the majority of cases, death occurred 2 to 4 days after birth. Massive pulmonary hemorrhage was observed in between 1.7 and 28% of infants in large autopsy studies. It was only infrequently suspected prior to death.

III. **Pathogenesis.** The underlying mechanism of pulmonary hemorrhage is uncertain. The hematocrit in lung effluents obtained from infants with pulmonary

*Revised from chapter by Thomas M. Berger and Shoo Lee in the Fourth Edition.

hemorrhage was relatively low compared to whole blood, suggesting that the disorder is due to hemorrhagic pulmonary edema rather than direct hemorrhage into the lung. Acute left ventricular failure, often caused by hypoxia and acidosis, may lead to increased pulmonary capillary pressure with rupture of some blood vessels and transudation from others. This may be the final common pathway of many of the conditions associated with pulmonary hemorrhage. Factors that alter the integrity of the epithelial-endothelial barrier in the alveolus or that change the filtration pressure across these membranes could predispose infants to pulmonary hemorrhage (Fig. 24.2).

IV. **Risk factors** include conditions predisposing the infant to increased left ventricular filling pressure, increased pulmonary blood volume, compromised pulmonary venous drainage, or poor cardiac contractility. In retrospective autopsy surveys, pulmonary hemorrhage has been associated with conditions including respiratory distress syndrome, intrauterine growth restriction, intrauterine and intrapartum asphyxia, infection, congenital heart disease, oxygen toxicity, maternal blood aspiration, diffuse pulmonary emboli, and urea cycle defects accompanied by hyperammonemia. Increased pulmonary blood flow and compromised ventricular function accompanying a symptomatic patent ductus arteriosus in a preterm infant is a significant risk factor. Thrombocytopenia and vascular leak accompanying conditions such as sepsis appears to increase the risk. Coagulopathy is also associated with the occurrence of pulmonary hemorrhage, although it is unclear whether it is an inciting factor or a result of the hemorrhage.

V. **Surfactant replacement as a potential risk factor.** It is controversial whether surfactant replacement therapy increases the risk of pulmonary hemorrhage. In *in vitro* studies, erythrocyte lysis is increased with exposure to artificial surfactant. In addition, a meta-analysis of 11 surfactant trials, which prospectively reported the clinical occurrence of pulmonary hemorrhage, showed that exogenous surfactant increased the risk of pulmonary hemorrhage by approximately 50%. This resulted mainly from a significant increase in pulmonary hemorrhage in infants treated with synthetic surfactants using a prevention strategy. The risk of pulmonary hemorrhage was not increased in infants treated with either synthetic surfactant using a rescue strategy or natural surfactant with either strategy. In pooled data from five synthetic surfactant trials, the incidence of pulmonary hemorrhage at autopsy was not different for infants treated with synthetic surfactant or air placebo. The previously reported increase in pulmonary hemorrhage may result from surfactant-associated changes in hemodynamics and lung compliance resulting in increased pulmonary perfusion in the setting of compromised left ventricular function, rather than an effect of surfactant on the integrity of the pulmonary endothelial barrier. It has been suggested that the risk of pulmonary hemorrhage following surfactant therapy can be reduced by judicious use of fluids and by closure of the ductus arteriosus.

VI. **Diagnosis.** The clinical diagnosis of pulmonary hemorrhage is made when sudden cardiorespiratory decompensation occurs in association with hemorrhagic fluid in the upper respiratory tract. Only a small proportion of pulmonary hemorrhages observed at autopsy are evident clinically. This is most likely due to the difficulty in diagnosing hemorrhage confined to the interstitial space without spread to the airways. In the absence of hemorrhagic secretions, respiratory deterioration is usually attributed to other causes.

Radiographic changes may support the diagnosis. These changes are acute, though nonspecific, and consist of diffuse opacification of one or both lungs accompanied by air bronchograms.

Laboratory studies may reflect the accompanying cardiorespiratory decompensation with a metabolic or mixed acidosis. There may be a drop in hematocrit or evidence of coagulopathy. In most cases, the coagulopathy is probably a result of the hemorrhage rather than a precipitating factor.

VII. **Treatment.** Because the underlying pathogenesis is unclear, treatment is supportive. The general approach involves clearing the airway of hemorrhagic fluid and restoring adequate ventilation. Use of elevated positive end-expiratory pressure (PEEP) of 6 to 8 cm H_2O helps to decrease the efflux of

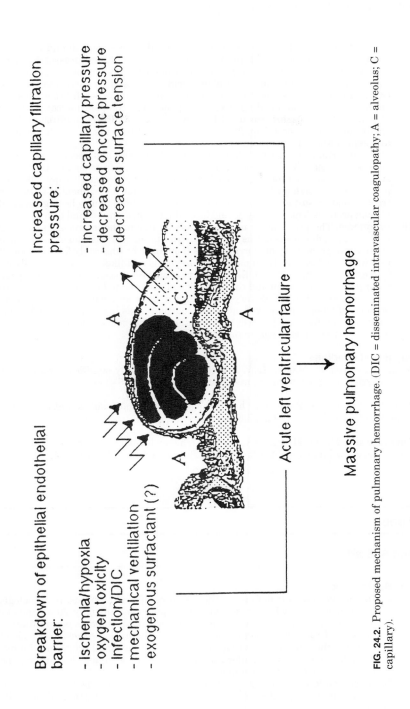

Breakdown of epithelial endothelial barrier:

- Ischemia/hypoxia
- oxygen toxicity
- Infection/DIC
- mechanical ventilation
- exogenous surfactant (?)

Increased capillary filtration pressure:

- increased capillary pressure
- decreased oncotic pressure
- decreased surface tension

Acute left ventricular failure

Massive pulmonary hemorrhage

FIG. 24.2. Proposed mechanism of pulmonary hemorrhage. (DIC = disseminated intravascular coagulopathy; A = alveolus; C = capillary).

interstitial fluid into the alveolar space. Circulatory status should be stabilized with infusions of fluid, red blood cell replacement, and pressor support, as needed. Acidosis should be corrected through restoration of adequate ventilation and blood pressure. Metabolic acidosis should be corrected with bicarbonate therapy, as needed. Echocardiography may be helpful to assess left ventricular function, need for pressor support, and the possible contribution of a patent ductus arteriosus (PDA). A hemodynamically significant PDA should be closed (see Chap. 25). Other abnormalities, such as coagulopathy and sepsis, should be treated.

It is uncertain whether high-frequency ventilation with high mean airway pressure is more effective than conventional ventilation in minimizing further interstitial and alveolar fluid accumulation. A role for surfactant therapy following pulmonary hemorrhage has been suggested for continued treatment of RDS or to treat secondary surfactant deficiency resulting from inhibition by hemoglobin and plasma proteins. This therapy should be evaluated on an individual basis.

VIII. **Prognosis.** The prognosis is uncertain, in part due to the imprecision involved in the clinical diagnosis of this condition. Prior to the introduction of mechanical ventilation, pulmonary hemorrhage was thought to be uniformly fatal, although this was based primarily on pathologic diagnosis and likely excluded mildly affected infants who survived. Early reports of survivors stressed the role of positive pressure ventilation and the correction of acidosis and clotting disorders. In a retrospective study of 58 very-low-birth-weight infants with pulmonary hemorrhage, of whom 29 survived, although mortality was high, pulmonary hemorrhage did not increase the risk of pulmonary or neurodevelomental disabilities at 20 months corrected age among survivors.

Suggested Readings

Berger T., Allred E., Marter, L. V. Antecedents of clinically significant pulmonary hemorrhage among newborn infants. *J Perinatol* 2000;5:295–300.

Raju T, Langenberg P. Pulmonary hemorrhage and exogenous surfactant therapy: A meta-analysis. *J Pediatr* 1993;123:603.

Tomaszewska M., et al. Pulmonary hemorrhage: Clinical course and outcomes among very-low-birth-weight infants. *Arch Pediatr Adolesc Med* 1999;153:715–721.

Apnea

Ann R. Stark

I. **Background**
   A. **Definition.** Apnea is defined as the cessation of airflow. Apnea is pathologic (an apneic spell) when absent airflow is prolonged (usually 20 seconds or more) or accompanied by bradycardia (heart rate <100 beats per minute) or cyanosis. Bradycardia and cyanosis are usually present after 20 seconds of apnea, although they can occur more rapidly in the small premature infant. After 30 to 45 seconds, pallor and hypotonia are seen, and infants may be unresponsive to tactile stimulation.
   B. **Classification** of apnea is based on whether absent air flow is accompanied by continued inspiratory efforts and upper airway obstruction. Most spells are central or mixed apnea.
      1. **Central apnea** occurs when inspiratory efforts are absent.
      2. **Obstructive apnea** occurs when inspiratory efforts persist. Airway obstruction is present.

3. **Mixed apnea** occurs when airway obstruction with inspiratory efforts precedes or follows central apnea.
C. **Incidence.** Apneic spells occur frequently in premature infants. The incidence of apnea increases with decreasing gestational age. As many as 25% of all premature infants who weigh less than 1800 g (about 34 weeks' gestational age) have at least one apneic episode. Essentially all infants less than 28 weeks' gestational age have apnea.
   1. **Onset.** Apneic spells generally begin at 1 or 2 days after birth; if they do not occur during the first 7 days, they are unlikely to occur later.
   2. **Duration.** Apneic spells persist for variable periods postnatally and usually cease by 37 weeks' gestational age. In infants born before 28 weeks' gestation, however, spells often persist beyond term gestational age. In a study in which infants were monitored at home, significant apnea and/or bradycardia were recorded up to 43 weeks' gestational age in 20% of preterm infants who were free of spells for at least 5 days before discharge and in 33% of those who had spells observed during that period. The clinical significance of these events is uncertain.
   3. **Term infants.** Apneic spells occurring in infants at or near term are always abnormal and are nearly always associated with serious, identifiable causes, such as birth asphyxia, intracranial hemorrhage, seizures, or depression from medication. Failure to breathe at birth in the absence of drug depression or asphyxia is generally caused by irreversible structural abnormalities of the central nervous system.
II. **Pathogenesis.** Several mechanisms have been proposed to explain apnea in premature infants. Many clinical conditions also have been associated with apneic spells, and some may be causative.
   A. **Developmental immaturity** of central respiratory drive is a likely contributing factor, since apneic spells occur more frequently in immature infants.
      1. The occurrence of apnea may correlate with brainstem neural function. The frequency of apnea decreases over a period in which brainstem conduction time of the auditory evoked response shortens as gestational age increases.
      2. Breathing in infants is strongly influenced by sleep state. Active or rapid-eye-movement (REM) sleep is marked by irregularity of tidal volume and respiratory frequency. REM sleep predominates in preterm infants, and apneic spells occur more frequently in this state than in quiet sleep.
   B. **Chemoreceptor response**
      1. In preterm infants, hypoxia results in transient hyperventilation, followed by hypoventilation and sometimes apnea, in contrast to the response in adults. In addition, hypoxia makes the premature infant less responsive to increased levels of carbon dioxide. Thus, hypoxemia may be involved in the pathogenesis of some apneic spells.
      2. The ventilatory response to increased carbon dioxide is decreased in preterm infants with apnea compared with a matched group without apnea, which suggests that abnormal respiratory control may contribute to the pathogenesis of apnea.
   C. **Reflexes.** Active reflexes invoked by stimulation of the posterior pharynx, lung inflation, fluid in the larynx, or chest wall distortion can precipitate apnea in infants. These reflexes may be involved in the apnea that is sometimes associated, for example, with vigorous use of suction catheters in the pharynx or with fluid in the upper airway during feeding.
   D. **Respiratory muscles.** Ineffective ventilation may result from impaired coordination of the inspiratory muscles (diaphragm and intercostal muscles) and the muscles of the upper airway (larynx and pharynx).
      1. **Airway obstruction** contributes to mixed and obstructive apneic spells. The site of this obstruction is usually the upper pharynx, which is vulnerable because of poor muscle tone, especially in REM sleep. Passive neck flexion, pressure on the lower rim of a face mask, and submental pressure (all encountered during nursery procedures) can obstruct the airway in

infants and lead to apnea, especially in a small premature infant. Spontaneously occurring airway obstruction is seen more frequently when preterm infants assume a position of neck flexion.

2. **Nasal obstruction** can lead to apnea, especially in preterm infants, who usually do not switch to oral breathing after nasal occlusion.

E. **Gastroesophageal reflux** is common in preterm infants. However, no association has been demonstrated between apnea of prematurity and gastroesophageal reflux.

III. **Monitoring and Evaluation.** All infants less than 35 weeks' gestational age should be monitored for apneic spells for at least the first week after birth because of the risk of apneic spells in this group. Monitoring should continue until no significant apneic episode has been detected for at least 5 days. Since impedance apnea monitors may not distinguish respiratory efforts during airway obstruction from normal breaths, heart rate should be monitored in addition to, or instead of, respiration. Even with careful monitoring, some prolonged spells of apnea and bradycardia may not be recognized.

A. **When a monitor alarm sounds,** one should remember to **respond to the infant,** not the monitor, checking for bradycardia, cyanosis, and airway obstruction.

B. **Most apneic spells** in premature infants **respond to tactile stimulation.** Infants who fail to respond to stimulation should be ventilated during the spell with bag and mask, generally with a fractional concentration of inspired oxygen (FiO_2) of under 0.40 or equal to the FiO_2 prior to the spell to avoid marked elevations in arterial oxygen tension (PO_2).

C. After the first apneic spell, **the infant should be evaluated for a possible underlying cause** (Table 24.5); if a cause is identified, specific treatment can then be initiated. One should be particularly alert to the possibility of a precipitating cause in infants who are more than 34 weeks' gestational age. Evaluation should include a history and physical examination, arterial blood gas measurement with continuous oxygen saturation monitoring, complete blood count, and measurement of blood glucose, calcium, and electrolyte levels.

TABLE 24.6. EVALUATION OF AN INFANT WITH APNEA

Potential Cause	Associated History or Signs	Evaluation
Infection	Feeding intolerance, lethargy, temperature instability	Complete blood count, cultures, if appropriate
Impaired oxygenation	Cyanosis, tachypnea, respiratory distress	Continuous oxygen monitoring, arterial blood gas measurement, chest x-ray examination
Metabolic disorders	Jitteriness, poor feeding, lethargy, CNS depression, irritability	Glucose, calcium, eletrolytes
Drugs	CNS depression, hypotonia, maternal history	Magnesium, screen for toxic substances in urine
Temperature instability	Lethargy	Monitor temperature of patient and environment
Intracranial pathology	Abnormal neurologic examination, seizures	Cranial ultrasound examination

IV. Treatment. When apneic spells are repeated and prolonged (i.e., more than two to three times per hour) or when they require frequent bag and mask ventilation, treatment should be initiated in order of increasing invasiveness and risk.

A. General measures

1. Specific therapy should be directed at an underlying cause, if one is identified.

2. In general, oxygen saturation should be maintained between 88 and 92%, with supplemental oxygen provided if needed.

3. Care should be taken to avoid reflexes that may trigger apnea. Suctioning of the pharynx should be done carefully, and oral feedings should be avoided.

4. Positions of extreme flexion or extension of the neck should be avoided, to reduce the likelihood of airway obstruction.

5. Decreasing the environmental temperature to the low end of the neutral thermal environment range may lessen the number of spells. Avoiding swings in environmental temperature may prevent apnea.

6. Whether blood transfusion reduces the frequency of apneic spells in some infants is controversial. We consider a transfusion of packed red blood cells (PRBCs) if the hematocrit is less than 25% and the infant has episodes of apnea and bradycardia that are frequent or severe while methylxanthine levels are therapeutic (see Chap. 26).

B. Nasal continuous positive airway pressure (CPAP) at low levels (4 to 6 cm H_2O) can reduce the number of mixed and obstructive apneic spells. It is especially useful in infants less than 32 to 34 weeks' gestational age and those with residual lung disease.

C. Methylxanthine therapy markedly reduces the number of apneic spells and the need for mechanical ventilation. Mechanisms by which methylxanthines may decrease apnea include (1) respiratory center stimulation; (2) antagonism of adenosine, a neurotransmitter that can cause respiratory depression; and (3) improvement of diaphragmatic contractility

1. We treat frequent and/or severe apnea with **caffeine citrate**. We use a loading dose of 20 mg/kg of caffeine citrate (10 mg/kg caffeine base) orally or intravenously over 30 minutes, followed by maintenance doses of 5 to 8 mg/kg (2.5 to 5.0 mg/kg caffeine base) in one daily dose beginning 24 hours after the loading dose.

   a. If apnea continues, we give an additional dose of 10 mg/kg caffeine citrate, and increase the maintenance dose by 20%.

   b. Caffeine serum levels of 5 to 20 μg/mL are considered therapeutic. We do not routinely measure serum drug concentration because of the wide therapeutic index and the lack of an established dose-response relationship. However, we measure drug concentration in infants with signs of toxicity or liver dysfunction, and sometimes in those with persistent apnea.

   c. Caffeine is generally discontinued at 34 to 36 weeks' gestational age if no apneic spells have occurred for 5 to 7 days. The effect of caffeine likely remains for approximately 1 week after it has been discontinued. We continue monitoring until no apnea has been detected for at least 5 days after that period.

2. **Theophylline** is sometimes used to treat apnea, if a short-term effect is desired. A loading dose of 5 to 7 mg/kg aminophylline given intravenously over 30 minutes will rapidly achieve a steady-state concentration. This is followed by a maintenance dose of intravenous aminophylline or oral theophylline in a dose of 1.5 to 2.0 mg/kg every 6 to 8 hours. The steady-state level is measured 0.5 to 1 hour after any succeeding IV dose or 1 to 2 hours after any oral dose. We generally maintain levels at 7 to 12μg/mL.

3. **Side effects** of methylxanthines include tachycardia and signs of gastrointestinal dysfunction, including abdominal distention, feeding intolerance, or vomiting. Jitteriness and irritability may be seen. Seizures may occur at extremely high levels of theophylline. Caffeine appears to be

less toxic than theophylline. There may be no change in heart rate in infants treated with caffeine, in contrast to the tachycardia often associated with theophylline therapy. Diuresis and urinary calcium excretion occur with both drugs. Metabolic changes, including increased glucose and insulin levels, occur following a theophylline loading dose in some infants. Despite the theoretical risks related to decreased cerebral blood flow, retarded neuronal growth, and inhibition of constriction of the ductus arteriosus, no long-term sequelae have been demonstrated following methylxanthine treatment in infants.

4. **We do not use doxapram,** a respiratory stimulant that may reduce apnea if methylxanthine therapy has failed. Side effects of doxapram include hyperactivity, jitteriness, seizures, hyperglycemia, mild liver dysfunction, and hypertension. In addition, benzyl alcohol is used as a preservative.

D. **Mechanical ventilation** may be required if the other interventions are unsuccessful.

V. **Persistent apnea.** In some infants, especially those born at less than 28 weeks' gestation, apneic spells may persist at 37 to 40 weeks' gestational age, when the infant may be otherwise ready for discharge home from the nursery. There is no consensus yet on the appropriate management of these infants, but efforts are directed at reducing the risk of apneic spells so that the child can be cared for at home.

A. Recordings of **impedance pneumography** and **ECGs for 12 to 24 hours** ("pneumograms") **can be used** to document the occurrence of apnea and bradycardia during that time period, but they do not predict the risk of sudden infant death syndrome (SIDS).

B. **Continued use of caffeine may be helpful** in infants whose spells recur when the drug is discontinued. Attempts to withdraw the drug can be made at intervals of approximately 2 months while the child is closely monitored.

C. Some infants are cared for with **cardiorespiratory monitoring at home,** although few data are available on its effectiveness. Extensive psychosocial support must be provided for the parents, who should be skilled in cardiopulmonary resuscitation (CPR) and in the use of the monitor. Routine home monitoring of asymptomatic preterm infants is not indicated.

VI. **Strategies to prevent SIDS.** Although the peak incidence of SIDS occurs after the newborn period, parents frequently express concern about their child's risk. Although SIDS occurs more frequently in premature or low-birth-weight infants, a history of apnea of prematurity does not increase this risk. We encourage strategies that may reduce the risk of SIDS.

A. **Sleeping position.** Prone sleeping position increases the risk of SIDS, and sleeping on the back or side reduces the risk. In general, babies should be placed on their back or side to sleep. The exceptions include preterm infants with respiratory disease, infants with symptomatic gastroesophageal reflux, and infants with craniofacial abnormalities or evidence of upper airway obstruction. For these infants, soft bedding should be avoided.

B. **Smoking.** Infants exposed to maternal smoking during pregnancy and postnatally have a higher risk of SIDS. Smoking should be avoided by parents, and infants should not be exposed to smoke.

C. **Overheating.** Infants exposed to excessively high room temperatures or overheating from excess wrapping have an increased risk of SIDS. Caregivers should avoid practices that result in overheating.

D. **Breastfeeding.** Infants who were never breastfed have a higher risk of SIDS than do breastfed infants. We encourage breastfeeding for many reasons (see Chap. 11).

Suggested Readings

Eichenwald E.C., et al. Apnea frequently persists beyond term gestation in infants delivered at 24 to 28 weeks. *Pediatrics* 1997; 100:354.

Ramanathan R, et al. Cardiorespiratory events recorded on home monitors. *JAMA* 2001; 285:2199.

Bronchopulmonary Dysplasia/Chronic Lung Disease

Richard B. Parad

I. **Definition.** Infants born at <32 weeks' gestation who need supplemental oxygen at 36 weeks' gestational age and those born at ≥32 weeks' gestation who need additional oxygen after 28 postnatal days are defined as having bronchopulmonary dysplasia (BPD) or chronic lung disease (CLD, a more general term). The latter group can include term babies with meconium aspiration syndrome, pneumonia, and certain cardiac and GI anomalies that require chronic ventilatory support. This definition is associated with the development of long-term pulmonary problems. Lung parenchyma usually appears abnormal on chest radiographs.

II. **Epidemiology.** Approximately 3000 to 7000 cases of CLD are estimated to occur in the United States each year. Infants < 1250 g birth weight are most susceptible to developing CLD. Differences in populations (race/ethnicity/socioeconomic status), clinical practices, and definitions account for a wide variation in the incidence reported among centers. The risk is decreased in African-Americans and girls.

III. **Pathogenesis**

A. **Acute lung injury** is caused by the combination of oxygen toxicity, barotrauma, and volutrauma from mechanical ventilation. Cellular and interstitial injury results in the release of proinflammatory cytokines [interleukin-1β (IL-1β), IL-6, IL-8, tumor necrosis α (TNFα)] that cause secondary changes in alveolar permeability and recruit inflammatory cells into interstitial and alveolar spaces; further injury from proteases, oxidants, and additional chemokines and chemoattractants cause ongoing inflammatory cell recruitment and leakage of water and protein. Airway and vascular tone may be altered. Alveolar development is interrupted and parenchma is destroyed leading to emphysematous changes. Sloughed cells and accumulated secretions not cleared adequately by the damaged mucociliary transport system cause inhomogeneous peripheral airway obstruction that leads to alternating areas of collapse and hyperinflation and proximal airway dilation. Bombesin-like protein, a proinflammatory peptide produced by neuroendocrine cells, has been shown to be elevated in the urine of infants who subsequently develop CLD.

B. In the **chronic phase** of lung injury, the interstitium may be altered by fibrosis and cellular hyperplasia that results from excessive release of growth factors and cytokines, leading to insufficient repair. Interstitial fluid clearance is disrupted, resulting in pulmonary fluid retention. Airways develop increased muscularization and hyperreactivity. The physiologic effects are decreased lung compliance, increased airway resistance, and impaired gas exchange with resulting ventilation-perfusion mismatching and air trapping.

C. **Factors that may contribute to the development of CLD** include the following:
1. **Immature lung substrate.** The lung is most susceptible before alveolar formation begins. Injury at this stage may cause an arrest of alveolarization.
2. **Inadequate activity of the antioxidant enzymes** superoxide dismutase, catalase, glutathione peroxidase, and/or **deficiency of free-radical sinks** such as vitamin E, glutathione, and ceruloplasmin may predispose the lung to oxygen toxicity. Similarly, **inadequate antiprotease protection** may predispose the lung to injury from the unchecked proteases released by recruited inflammatory cells.

3. **Excessive early intravenous fluid administration** and persistent left-to-right shunt through the **patent ductus arteriosus (PDA).** Although prophylactic PDA ligation does not prevent CLD, persistent left-to-right shunt may still be a contributing factor.

4. **Intrauterine or perinatal infection** may contribute to the etiology of CLD or modify its course. Ureaplasma urealyticum has been associated with CLD in premature infants, although it remains unclear whether this relationship is causal. Chlamydia trachomatis and cytomegalovirus can cause gradually developing pneumonitis.

5. **Familial airway hyperreactivity.**

6. **Increased inositol clearance,** leading to diminished plasma inositol levels and decreased surfactant synthesis or impaired surfactant metabolism.

7. **An increase in vasopressin** and a **decrease in atrial natriuretic peptide release** may alter pulmonary and systemic fluid balance in the setting of obstructive lung disease.

IV. **Clinical presentation**

A. **Physical examination typically** reveals tachypnea, retractions, and rales on auscultation.

B. **Arterial blood gas (ABG)** analysis shows hypoxemia and hypercarbia with eventual metabolic compensation for the respiratory acidosis.

C. **The chest radiograph appearance changes** as the disease progresses. In early descriptions of BPD, stage I had the same appearance as RDS, stage II showed diffuse haziness with increased density and normal to low lung volumes, stage III demonstrated streaky densities with bubbly lucencies and early hyperinflation, and stage IV showed hyperinflation with larger hyperlucent areas interspersed with thicker, streaky densities. Not all infants progressed to stage IV, and some transitioned directly from stage I to stage III. Radiographic abnormalities often persisted into childhood. "New BPD," a term coined to distinguish the different histology and radiographic findings of the most immature VLBW infants, is often associated with stage II changes.

D. **Cardiac evaluation.** Nonpulmonary causes of respiratory failure should be excluded. ECG can show persistent or progressive right ventricular hypertrophy if cor pulmonale develops. Left ventricular hypertrophy may develop with systemic hypertension. Two-dimensional echocardiography may be useful in excluding left-to-right shunts (see Chap. 25). Biventricular failure is unusual when good oxygenation is maintained and the development of pulmonary hypertension is avoided.

E. **Pulmonary function testing,** if done, will show increased respiratory system resistance (Rrs) and decreased dynamic compliance (Crs).

F. **Pathologic changes** are detectable in severe cases by the first few days after birth. By the end of the first week, necrotizing bronchiolitis, obstruction of small airway lumens by debris and edema, and areas of peribronchial and interstitial fibrosis are present. Emphysematous changes and significant impairment in alveolar development result in diminished surface area for gas exchange. Changes in both large airways (glandular hyperplasia) and small airways (smooth muscle hyperplasia) likely form the histologic basis for reactive airway disease. Pulmonary vascular changes associated with pulmonary hypertension may be seen. Arrest of alveolariztion is more significant at lower gestational ages.

V. **Inpatient treatment.** The goals of treatment during the neonatal intensive care unit (NICU) course are to minimize further lung injury (baro- and volutrauma, oxygen toxicity, inflammation), maximize nutrition, and diminish oxygen consumption.

A. **Mechanical ventilation**

1. **Acute phase.** Ventilator adjustments are made to minimize airway pressures while providing adequate gas exchange (see Mechanical Ventilation).

In most circumstances, we avoid hyperventilation [keeping arterial carbon dioxide tension ($PaCO_2$) at >55 mm Hg, with pH >7.25] and maintain oxygen saturation (SaO_2) at 90 to 95% [arterial oxygen tension (PaO_2) 60 to 80 mm Hg. We do not routinely use high-frequency oscillatory ventilation because most available evidence suggests that this technique does not prevent CLD in high-risk infants.

2. **Chronic phase.** Once baseline ventilator settings are established with an arterial carbon dioxide tension ($PaCO_2$) not higher than 65 mm Hg, we maintain the ventilator rate without weaning until a pattern of steady weight gain is established.

B. **Supplemental oxygen** is supplied to maintain the PaO_2 >55 mm Hg at all times. The SaO_2 should be correlated with PaO_2 in each infant. In general, SaO_2 should be maintained between 90 and 95% to reach this goal. When <30% oxygen concentration is required by hood, we supply oxygen by nasal cannula. If adequate SaO_2 cannot be maintained on <1 L/min of flow, hood oxygen should be restored. We use a flowmeter that is accurate at low rates, and gradually decrease the flow of 100% oxygen while maintaining the appropriate SaO_2. Alternatively, flow can be decreased to the lowest marking on the flowmeter, as tolerated, and then oxygen concentration can be decreased. Hypopharyngeal FiO_2 can be estimated from that delivered by nasal cannula (Fig. 24.3). SaO_2 should remain >90% during sleep, feedings, and active periods before supplemental oxygen is discontinued.

C. **Surfactant replacement therapy** decreases the combined outcome of CLD or death at 28 days of age, although it has made little or no impact on the overall incidence of CLD. Meta-analyses suggest the incidence is decreased in larger premature infants, but is higher in smaller premature infants who would have died without surfactant therapy.

D. **Aggressive early management of a hemodynamically significant PDA** is recommended (see Chap. 25).

E. **Monitoring** (see Blood Gas and Pulmonary Graphic Monitoring)
   1. **ABG analysis** is used to monitor gas exchange and confirm noninvasive monitoring values.
   2. We use **continuous pulse oximetry** for long-term monitoring of infants with CLD, maintaining SaO_2 between 90 and 95% with the goal of keeping the corresponding PaO_2 > 55 mm Hg.
   3. **Capillary blood gas (CBG)** values are useful to monitor pH and PCO_2. Since pH and PCO_2 sometimes vary from central values, we compare them with ABG values. If CBG and ABG values are similar, we monitor stable ventilator-dependent infants with pulse oximetry and one or two CBG analyses per day; less frequent CBG tests are obtained for patients receiving oxygen by nasal cannula.
   4. **Pulmonary function testing** is used in some centers to document functional responses to trials of bronchodilators, and diuretics. (see V.G.1–4).

F. **Fluid management.** Fluid intake is limited to the minimum required. Initially, we provide intake adequate to maintain urine output at least 1 mL/kg per hour and serum sodium concentration of 140 to 145 mEq/L. Subsequently, we provide 130 to 150 mL/kg per day to supply sufficient calories for growth. We regularly recalculate fluid intake for weight gain, once it is above birth weight. Later, when respiratory status is stable, fluid restriction is gradually released.

G. **Drugs.** When the infant remains ventilator-dependent on restricted fluid intake in the absence of PDA or intercurrent infection, additional pharmacotherapeutic trials (usually >24 hours) should be considered.
   1. **Prevention.** In multicenter randomized clinical trials:
      a. **Vitamin A** (5000 U IM, 3 times weekly for the first 28 days of age) reduced the incidence of CLD in ELBW infants by 10%. We routinely treat ELBW infants with vitamin A.
      b. In <27-week infants, intratracheal **recombinant human Cu/Zn superoxide dismutase** administered intratracheally every 48 hours while

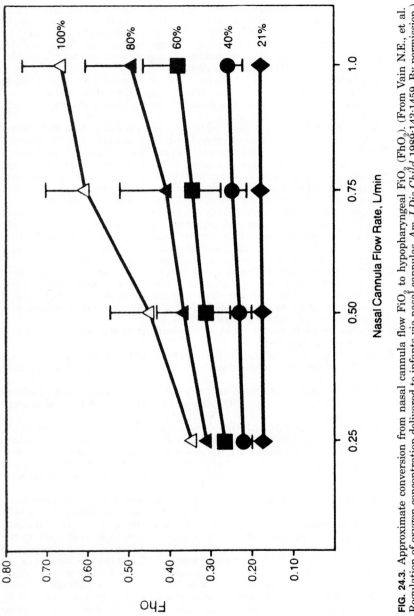

FIG. 24.3. Approximate conversion from nasal cannula flow FiO$_2$ to hypopharyngeal FiO$_2$ (FhO$_2$). (From Vain N.E., et al. Regulation of oxygen concentration delivered to infants via nasal cannulas. *Am J Dis Child* 1989;143:1459. By permission.)

intubated resulted in an approximately 50% reduction in use of asthma medictions, emergency room visits, and hospitalizations in the first year of life. This treatment remains investigational.

2. **Pulmonary fluid retention** is treated with **diuretics.** Diuretics indirectly attenuate symptoms of respiratory distress and result in decreased Rrs and increased Crs; gas exchange is variably affected. An acute clinical response may be seen within 1 hour, although maximal effect may not be achieved until 1 week of therapy. The clinical improvement is likely due to decreased lung water content, with decreased interstitial and peribronchial fluid resulting in less resistance and better compliance. The mechanisms of action may be due to either diuresis or nondiuretic effects.

   a. **Furosemide** is used initially at a dose of 0.5 to 1.0 mg/kg intravenously one to two times daily. The dose may be given at the time of blood transfusions if these have been associated with increased pulmonary fluid and respiratory distress. Immature infants are at increased risk of toxicity from larger or more frequent doses because of the prolonged drug half-life. Side effects include hypercalciuria, nephrocalcinosis, ototoxicity, electrolyte imbalance, and nephrolithiasis. We use lower doses or combine furosemide with other diuretics to avoid the need for compensation with electrolyte supplementation (see G.8). Alternate-day furosemide therapy may be effective in the chronic stage of the disease with fewer side effects.

   b. **Chlorothiazide.** An alternative to furosemide is treatment with chlorothiazide (20 to 40 mg/kg per day orally, divided BID). Chlorothiazide decreases calcium excretion and, if used in combination with furosemide, may minimize calcium loss and reverse nephrocalcinosis due to furosemide. The combination also allows the use of a lower furosemide dose.

3. **Bronchodilators.** Acute obstructive episodes or chronically increased resistance may be related to increased airway tone or bronchospasm and may respond to bronchodilator therapy. Infants with developing CLD may benefit as early as the second week of age.

   a. **Administration of nebulized beta-adrenergic agonists (BAAs)** results in decreased Rrs and increased Crs. Tachycardia is the major limiting side effect. Newer agents have increased beta-2 specificity with less beta-1 toxicity. We use an albuterol **metered-dose inhaler (MDI)** with a spacer device (1 puff) or nebulized 0.5% solution (5 mg/mL) 0.02 to 0.04 mL/kg (up to 0.1 mL total in 2 mL of normal saline solution) every 6 to 8 hours. In ventilated infants, for efficiency, our preference is an MDI with a spacer device placed in line with the ventilator near the endotracheal tube.

   b. **Muscarinic agents.** MDI (1 puff) or nebulized (25 mg/kg per dose) ipratropium bromide increases Crs and decreases Rrs. Combination MDI containing both BAAs and muscarinic agents may provide a synergistic effect, but this has not been studied in preterm infants.

   c. Theophylline is infrequently used as a bronchodilator because most infants with BPD are treated with **caffeine citrate** for apnea. Although not well studied, infants treated with caffeine for apnea may have improved Crs.

4. **Postnatal corticosteroids.** In early trials, treatment with glucocorticoids (usually dexamethasone) in infants who remained ventilator-dependent for 2 to 3 weeks resulted in increased Crs, decreased Rrs, diminished oxygen requirement, and earlier extubation. However, treatment with glucocorticoids does not appear to have a substantial impact on long-term pulmonary outcomes, such as duration of supplemental oxygen requirement, length of hospital stay, or mortality. Subsequent trials of earlier treatment, recurrent pulses, and lower doses have yielded inconsistent results as either a prophylactic or attenuating agent. Randomized trials

of inhaled glucocorticoids also did not demonstrate improved pulmonary outcome. In addition to short-term side effects, including hypertension, hyperglycemia, and spontaneous gastrointestinal performation, long-term follow-up of infants treated with postnatal corticosteroids has raised concerns about delays in neurodevelopment and growth. Because of this potential harm and lack of well-established long-term benefit, routine use of corticosteroids is discouraged, and reserved only for infants with progressive respiratory failure that is refractory to all other therapies. If treatment with glucocorticoids is undertaken, we discuss the potential neurodevelopmental harm with parents prior to use. Although this regimen has not been tested in clinical trials, we use a short course and relatively low dose of dexamethasone to reduce ventilator settings and facilitate extubation (see Table 24.6).

   a. Common acute complications of dexamethasone include glucose intolerance, systemic hypertension, and transient catabolic state. Total neutrophil counts, band counts, and platelet counts increase during steroid treatment. Hypertrophic cardiomyopathy sometimes occurs, but is transient and does not appear to affect cardiac function. Gastrointestinal perforation and gastric ulcerations can occur. Adrenal suppression is transient.

   b. Postextubation airway edema, with stridorous obstruction (see VI.A) leading to respiratory failure, may be attenuated with dexamethasone, 0.25 mg/kg per dose every 12 hours starting 8 to 12 hours before the next extubation. Edema also may be acutely diminished with nebulized racemic epinephrine.

5. **Cromolyn** acts on both airway and pulmonary vascular tone. Prophylactic treatment of reactive airways attenuates symptoms in infants with CLD who develop asthma during the first year of life. Use in the NICU setting has not been well evaluated. Dosing can be either with MDI and spacer, or nebulized (10 to 20 mg q6–8h).

6. **Inhaled nitric oxide (iNO).** In animal models of CLD, iNO may act to relax airway and pumonary vascular tone, and dimish lung inflammation. A multicenter clinical trial is underway to assess the potential efficacy of iNO in attenuating or preventing CLD.

7. **Pain management.** Pain managment and sedation are used for physical or autonomic signs of pain or discomfort. These responses may interfere

TABLE 24.7. SUGGESTED COURSE OF DEXAMETHASONE TREATMENT FOR SEVERE BPD

Length of Course	Day	Dose
Short	1	0.1 mg/kg q12h
	2	0.075 mg/kg q12h
	3	0.05 mg/kg q12h
	May repeat weekly, if necessary	
Long	1 and 2	0.1 mg/kg q12h
If no response after 48–72 h of this dosing, stop.		
If response:		
	3 and 4	0.075 mg/kg q12h
	5, 6, and 7	0.05 mg/kg q12h
	8	OFF
	9	0.05 mg/kg q12h
	10	END

with the ability to ventilate and oxygenate. Oral sucrose, morphine sulfate or fentanyl, phenobarbital, short-acting benzodiazepines, or chloral hydrate are used (see Chapter 37).

8. **Electrolyte supplements.** Hyponatremia, hypokalemia, and hypochloremia with secondary hypercarbia are common side effects of chronic diuretic therapy that are corrected by lowering the diuretic dose or adding NaCl and KCl supplements. Adequate sodium intake should be provided. Serum sodium level can fall below 130 mEq/L before intervention is required. Although hypochloremia may occur with compensated respiratory acidosis, low serum chloride concentration from diuretic-induced loss and inadequate intake can cause metabolic alkalosis and $PaCO_2$ elevation. Hypochloremia may also contribute to poor growth. Chloride deficit can be corrected with potassium chloride. Monitoring should be carried out at regular intervals until equilibrium is reached.

H. **Nutrition** (see Chap. 10)

1. Metabolic rate and energy expenditure are elevated in CLD while caloric intake is poor. **Providing more calories by** the administration of lipids instead of carbohydrates lowers the respiratory quotient, thus diminishing CO_2 production. **To optimize growth,** wasteful energy expenditure should be minimized and **caloric intake maximized.** Prolonged parenteral nutrition is often required. As enteral feeding is started, we feed by orogastric or nasogastric tube and limit oral feeding to avoid tiring the infant. We generally advance to 30 cal/oz formula, supplemented with additional protein.

2. **Vitamin, trace element, and other dietary supplementation.** Vitamin E and antioxidant enzymes diminish oxidant toxicity, although vitamin E supplementation does not prevent CLD. Vitamin A may promote epithelial repair and minimize fibrosis. Selenium, zinc, and copper are trace elements vital to antioxidant enzyme function, and inadequate intake may interfere with protection.

I. **Blood transfusions.** We generally maintain hematocrit approximately 30 to 35% (hemoglobin 8–10 g/dL) as long as supplemental oxygen is needed. Fluid-sensitive patients may benefit from furosemide given immediately following the transfusion. Improved oxygen delivery may allow better reserves for growth in the infant with increased metabolic demands.

J. **Behavioral factors.** As with all sick infants, care is best provided with individualized attention to behavioral and environmental factors (see Chap. 14).

VI. **Associated complications**

A. **Upper airway obstruction.** Trauma to the nasal septum, larynx, trachea, or bronchi is common after prolonged or repeated intubation and suctioning. Abnormalities include: laryngotracheobronchomalacia; granulomas; vocal cord paresis; edema; ulceration with pseudomembranes; subglottic stenosis; and congenital structural anomalies. Stridor may develop when postextubation edema is superimposed on underlying stenosis. Abnormalities are not excluded by the absence of stridor and may be asymptomatic, becoming symptomatic at the time of a viral upper respiratory tract infection. Flexible fiberoptic bronchoscopy should be used to evaluate stridor, hoarseness, persistent wheezing, recurrent obstruction, or repeated extubation failure.

B. **Cor pulmonale.** Pulmonary hypertension may have reversible and fixed components. Chronic hypoxemia leads to hypoxic vasoconstriction, pulmonary hypertension, and eventual right ventricular hypertrophy and failure. Decrease in cross-sectional perfusion area and abnormal muscularization of more peripheral vessels have been documented. Left ventricular function also can be affected. The ECG should be followed. Supplemental oxygen is used to maintain the $PaO_2 > 55$ mm Hg. Further studies may be required to define the dysfunction and evaluate therapy. Pulmonary vasodilators including hydralazine and nifedipine have variable efficacy and should only be tried during pulmonary artery pressure and PaO_2 monitoring. Echocardiographic studies can exclude structural heart disease, assess left ventricular function, and estimate pulmonary vascular resistance and right ventricular function.

C. Systemic hypertension, sometimes with left ventricular hypertrophy, may develop in CLD infants receiving prolonged O_2 therapy.

D. Systemic-to-pulmonary shunting. Left-to-right shunt through collateral vessels (e.g., bronchial arteries) can occur in CLD. The risk factors include chest tube placement, thoracic surgery, and pleural inflammation. When left-to-right shunt is suspected and echocardiography fails to show intracardiac or PDA shunting, collaterals may be demonstrated by angiography. Occlusion of large vessels has been associated with clinical improvement.

E. Metabolic imbalance secondary to diuretics (see V.G.2 and 8)

F. Infection. Because these chronically ill and malnourished infants are at increased risk, episodes of pulmonary and systemic decompensation should be evaluated for infection. Monitoring by gram stain of tracheal aspirates may help distinguish endotracheal tube colonization from tracheobronchitis or pneumonia (presence of organisms and neutrophils). Viral and fungal infections should be considered when fevers or pneumonia develop. In infants with more severe clinical courses, we frequently culture tracheal aspirates for possible infection with Ureaplasma sp. and Mycoplasma hominis and may treat with erythromycin if these organisms are identified.

G. CNS dysfunction. A neurologic syndrome presenting with extrapyramidal signs has been described in infants with CLD.

H. Hearing loss. Ototoxic drugs (furosemide, gentamicin) and ischemic or hypoxemic CNS injury increase the risk for sensorineural hearing loss. Screening with auditory brainstem responses should be performed at discharge (see Chap. 35).

I. Retinopathy of prematurity (ROP) (see Chap. 35). ELBW infants with CLD are at highest risk for developing ROP. The use of phenylephrine-containing eyedrops prior to eye examinations can cause an increase in airway resistance in some infants with CLD.

J. Nephrocalcinosis is frequently documented on ultrasound examination and has been linked to the use of furosemide and possibly steroids. Hematuria and passage of stones may occur. Most infants are asymptomatic, with eventual spontaneous resolution, but **renal function should be followed** (see Chap. 31).

K. Prematurity, inadequate calcium and phosphorus retention, and prolonged immobilization can lead to osteoporosis. Calcium loss due to furosemide and corticosteroids also may contribute. Supplementation with vitamin D, calcium, and phosphorus should be optimized (see Chap. 29).

L. Gastroesophageal reflux. We try to document and treat GER when reflux or aspiration may contribute to pulmonary decompensation, apnea, or feeding intolerance with poor growth.

M. The incidence of **inguinal hernia** is increased by the presence of the patent processus vaginalis in VLBW infants, particularly boys, with CLD. If the hernia is reducible, surgical correction should be delayed until respiratory status is improved. Spinal rather than general anesthesia avoids reintubation and postoperative apnea.

N. Early growth failure may result from inadequate intake and excessive energy expenditure and may persist after clinical resolution of pulmonary disease. Premature withdrawal of supplemental oxygen should be avoided because it may contribute to slowing of growth.

VII. Discharge planning. The timing of discharge depends on the availability of home-care support systems and parental readiness (see Chap. 16).

A. Weight gain and oxygen therapy. Supplemental oxygen should be weaned when the SaO_2 is maintained >94%, no significant periods of desaturations occur during feedings and/or sleep, good weight gain has been established, and respiratory status is stable (see V.B and VI.N). We prefer to delay discharge until oxygen has been discontinued. However, if long-term oxygen

supplementation seems likely in an infant who is stable, growing, and has capable caretakers, we offer the option of home oxygen therapy.
B. **Teaching.** The involvement of parents in caregiving is vital to the smooth transition from hospital to home care. Parents should be taught CPR and early signs of decompensation. Teaching about equipment use, medication administration, and nutritional guidelines should begin when discharge planning is initiated.
C. **Baseline values.** Baseline values of vital signs, daily weight gain, discharge weight and head circumference, blood gases, SaO_2, hematocrit, electrolytes, and the baseline appearance of the chest radiograph and ECG must be documented at discharge. This information is useful to evaluate subsequent changes in clinical status. An eye examination and hearing screening should be performed prior to discharge.

VIII. **Outpatient therapy**
A. **Oxygen.** Supplemental oxygen can be delivered by tanks or oxygen concentrator. Portable tanks allow mobility. Weaning is based on periodic assessment of SaO_2.
B. **Medications.** Infants receiving diuretics require monitoring of electrolytes. When the infant is stable, we allow him or her to outgrow the diuretic dose by 50% before discontinuing the drug. Bronchodilators are tapered when respiratory status is stable in room air. Nebulized medications are tapered last. Discontinued medications should remain available for early use when symptoms recur.
C. **Immunizations.** In addition to standard immunizations, infants with CLD should receive pneumococcal and influenza vaccines and Synagis (see Chap. 23).
D. **Nutrition.** Weight gain is a sensitive indicator of well-being and should be closely monitored. Caloric supplementation is often required to maintain good growth after discharge. At discharge, we supplement calories in a premature-to-term transitional formula.
E. **Passive smoke exposure.** Because smoking in the home increases respiratory tract illness in children, parents of CLD infants should be discouraged from smoking and should minimize the child's exposure to smoke-containing environments.

IX. **Outcome**
A. **Mortality.** Mortality is estimated at 10 to 20% during the first year of life. The risk increases with duration of oxygen exposure and level of ventilatory support. Death is frequently caused by infection. The risk of sudden unexpected death may be increased, but the cause is unclear.
B. **Long-term morbidity**
   1. **Pulmonary.** Tachypnea, retractions, dyspnea, cough, and wheezing can be seen for months to years in seriously affected children. Although complete clinical recovery can occur, underlying pulmonary function, gas exchange, and radiographic abnormalities may persist beyond adolescence. The impact of persistent minor abnormalities of function and growth on long-term morbidity and mortality is not known. Reactive airway disease occurs more frequently, and infants with CLD are at increased risk for bronchiolitis and pneumonia. The rehospitalization rate for respiratory illness during the first 2 years of life is approximately twice that of matched control infants.
   2. **Neurodevelopmental delay/neurologic deficits.** CLD is not clearly an independent predictor of adverse neurologic outcome. Early behavioral differences do exist, however, between VLBW infants with CLD and RDS controls. Later outcome varies widely; one-third to two-thirds of infants with CLD are normal by 2 years, and subsequent improvement may occur in some of the remaining infants. Our experience suggests specific motor coordination delays and visual-perceptual impairment may occur, rather than overall lower IQ, with resulting mean Bayley scores 1 standard deviation below the normal mean by ages 4 to 6 years.

3. **Growth failure.** The degree of long-term growth delay is inversely proportional to birth weight and probably is influenced by the severity and duration of CLD. Weight is most affected, and head circumference is least affected. Delayed growth occurs in one-third to two-thirds of these infants at 2 years. One-third of our school-age population is 3 standard deviations below the mean for height and weight.

Suggested Readings

AAP Policy Statement Postnatal Corticosteroids to Treat or Prevent Chronic Lung Disease in Preterm Infants. *Pediatrics* 2002;109:330–338.

Clark R.H., et al. Lung injury in neonates: Causes, strategies for prevention, and long-term consequences. *J Pediatr* 2001;239:478–486.

Davis J.M., et al. Pulmonary outcome at 1 year corrected age in premature infants treated at birth with recombinant human CuZn SOD. *Pediatrics* 2003;111:469–476.

Davis J.M., et al. Drug therapy for bronchopulmonary dysplasia. *Pediatr Pulmonol* 1990;8:117.

Ehrenkrantz R.A., Mercurio M.R. Bronchopulmonary dysplasia. In: Sinclair, JC and Bracken, MB (Eds.), *Effective Care of the Newborn Infant.* 1992. New York: Oxford University Press, 399–424.

Holtzman R.B., Frank L. (Guest Eds.). *Clin Perinatol* 19, 1992 (entire issue).

Northway W.H., Rosan R.C., Porter D.Y. Pulmonary disease following respirator therapy of hyaline-membrane disease. *N Engl J Med* 1967;276:357.

Jobe A.H., Bancalari E. Bronchopulmonary dysplasia. *Am J Respir Crit Care Med* 2001;163:1723–1729.

Meconium Aspiration

Jane S. Lee and Ann R. Stark

I. Background

A. **Cause.** Acute or chronic hypoxia can result in the passage of meconium in utero. In this setting, gasping by the fetus or newly born infant can cause aspiration of amniotic fluid contaminated by meconium. Meconium aspiration before or during birth can obstruct airways, interfere with gas exchange, and cause severe respiratory distress (Fig. 24.4).

B. **Incidence.** Meconium-stained amniotic fluid complicates delivery in approximately 9 to 15% of live births. Meconium-stained fluid is rarely seen prior to 37 weeks' gestation but may occur in more than 30% of pregnancies that continue past 42 weeks' gestation. Infants born through meconium-stained amniotic fluid frequently have had antepartum or intrapartum asphyxia. The timing of the insult may be suggested by the color of the fluid; yellow meconium is usually old, whereas green meconium suggests a more recent insult.

Suctioning of the mouth and oropharynx before delivery of the shoulders and direct suctioning of meconium from the trachea in depressed infants favorably affect the clinical course. Adequate airway management, however,

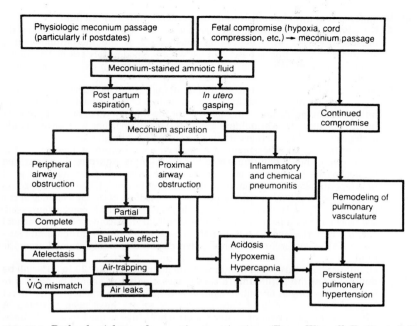

FIG. 24.4. Pathophysiology of meconium aspiration. (From Wiswell T., Bent R.C. Meconium staining and the meconium aspiration syndrome: Unresolved issues. *Pediatr Clin North Am* 1993;40:955. By permission.)

cannot prevent meconium aspiration altogether, since meconium may be aspirated by the fetus prior to delivery (see Chap. 4).

Of infants delivered through meconium-stained amniotic fluid, 5 to 33% develop respiratory symptoms and radiographic changes of meconium aspiration syndrome (MAS). Up to 50% of these infants require mechanical ventilation. Approximately one-third develop persistent pulmonary hypertension (PPHN), which contributes to the mortality associated with this syndrome (see Persistent Pulmonary Hypertension of the Newborn). Approximately 5% of survivors require supplemental oxygen at 1 month of age, and a substantial proportion may have abnormal pulmonary function, including increased functional residual capacity, airway reactivity, and higher incidence of pneumonia.

II. **Prevention of passage of meconium in utero.** Mothers at risk for uteroplacental insufficiency include those with preeclampsia or increased blood pressure, chronic respiratory or cardiovascular disease, poor uterine growth, post-term pregnancy, or heavy smokers. These women should be carefully monitored during pregnancy, and the fetal heart rate should be monitored during labor, with fetal scalp blood samples obtained for pH determination when indicated.

A. **Amnioinfusion.** The use of transcervical amnioinfusion with normal saline solution in women whose labor is complicated by meconium-stained amniotic fluid and repetitive fetal heart rate decelerations may reduce the incidence of meconium aspiration.

B. **Timing and mode of delivery.** In pregnancies that continue past the due date, induction as early as 41 weeks may help prevent MAS by avoiding passage of meconium. Delivery mode does not appear to significantly impact the risk of aspiration.

III. **Management of infants delivered through meconium-stained fluid**
   A. **Consistency of meconium.** Occurrence of MAS and other respiratory ill-
      nesses increases with increasing consistency of the meconium. Thinly
      stained amniotic fluid is described as "watery," moderately stained amniotic
      fluid as opaque without particles, and thick meconium as "pea soup" with
      particles.
   B. American Academy of Pediatrics/American College of Obstetrics and Gynecol-
      ogy guidelines recommend that when meconium of any consistency is present
      intrapartum, the obstetrician should **clear the infant's nose and oropharynx
      before delivery of the shoulders or chest.** This can be done with either a bulb
      syringe or a De Lee suction catheter, which are equally effective.
   C. During the initial assessment at a delivery complicated by meconium, the
      pediatrician should **determine whether the infant is vigorous,** demonstrated
      by heart rate >100 beats per minute, spontaneous respirations, and good
      tone (spontaneous movement or some degree of flexion). If the infant appears
      vigorous, routine care should be provided, regardless of the consistency of the
      meconium. If respiratory distress develops or the infant becomes depressed,
      the trachea should be intubated under direct laryngoscopy and intratracheal
      suctioning performed. In questionable cases, it is safer to intubate and suc-
      tion, as MAS can occur in infants delivered through thinly stained amniotic
      fluid.
   D. Of infants born through meconium-stained amniotic fluid, **20 to 30% will be
      depressed at the perineum.** In these cases, the infant should be handed to
      the anesthesiologist or pediatrician who intubates the trachea under direct
      laryngoscopy, preferably before inspiratory efforts have been initiated. A
      3.0- or 3.5-mm internal-diameter endotracheal tube is used in term infants.
      After intubation, the tube is attached to wall suction at a pressure of 80 to
      100 mm Hg by means of a plastic adapter (Neotech. Meconium Aspirator,
      Neotech Products, Chatsworth, CA). Continuous suction is applied as the
      tube is being withdrawn; the procedure is repeated until the trachea is
      cleared or resuscitation needs to be initiated. Visualization of the cords with-
      out suctioning is not adequate because significant meconium may be present
      below the cords. Positive pressure ventilation should be avoided, if possible,
      until tracheal suctioning is accomplished. Emptying of any gastric contents
      should also be postponed until the infant has stabilized.
   E. Although complication rates are low, **the infant's general condition must not
      be ignored in persistent attempts to clear the trachea.** This procedure
      should be accomplished rapidly, and ventilation with oxygen should be initi-
      ated before significant bradycardia occurs. Because a few inspiratory efforts
      by the infant will move the meconium from the trachea to the smaller air-
      ways, exhaustive attempts to remove it are unwise. Other reported compli-
      cations include bleeding, laryngospasm, stridor, apnea, and cyanosis.
IV. **Management of MAS.** Infants who are depressed at birth and have had meconium suctioned from the trachea are at risk for meconium aspiration pneumonia
   and should be observed closely for respiratory distress. A chest radiograph may
   help determine which infants are most likely to develop respiratory distress, although a significant number of asymptomatic infants will have an abnormal-
   appearing chest film. Monitoring of oxygen saturation during this period aids
   assessment of the severity of the infant's condition and avoids hypoxemia.
   A. **Routine care.** The thermal environment of all infants at risk for MAS
      should be watched closely. Tactile stimulation should be minimized. The use
      of sedation and muscle relaxation may be warranted in those who require
      mechanical ventilation. Blood glucose and calcium levels should be assessed
      and corrected if necessary. In addition, severely depressed infants may have
      significant metabolic acidosis that should be corrected. These infants may
      also require specific therapy for hypotension and poor cardiac output, in-
      cluding cardiotonic medications such as dopamine. Fluids should be re-
      stricted as much as possible to prevent cerebral and pulmonary edema.

Renal function should be continuously monitored (see Chap. 27, Perinatal Asphyxia).

B. Obstruction. In infants with significant meconium aspiration, mechanical obstruction of both large and small airways can occur, as well as chemical pneumonitis (see Fig. 24.4). Atelectasis and ongoing inflammation with the development of extrapulmonary shunting worsen the ventilation-perfusion mismatch, leading to severe arterial hypoxemia.

C. Hypoxemia. Management of hypoxemia should be accomplished by increasing the inspired oxygen concentration and by monitoring blood gases and pH. An indwelling arterial catheter is usually required for blood sampling and infusion. It is crucial to provide sufficient oxygen, because repeated hypoxic insults may result in ongoing pulmonary vasoconstriction and contribute to the development of PPHN.

If FiO_2 requirements exceed 0.40, a trial of continuous positive airway pressure (CPAP) may be considered. CPAP is often helpful, and the appropriate pressures must be individualized for each infant. In some instances, CPAP may aggravate air trapping and should be instituted with caution if hyperinflation is apparent clinically or radiographically.

D. Mechanical ventilation. Hypercapnia may become a problem in infants with very severe disease. For severe carbon dioxide retention ($PaCO_2 > 60$ mm Hg) or for persistent hypoxemia ($PaO_2 < 50$ mm Hg), mechanical ventilation is indicated. In these infants, higher inspiratory pressures (about 30 to 35 cm H_2O) are more often required than in infants with respiratory distress syndrome; the positive end-expiratory pressure (PEEP) selected (usually 3 to 6 cm H_2O) should depend on the individual's response. Adequate expiratory time should be permitted to prevent air trapping behind partly obstructed airways. Useful starting points are an inspiratory time of 0.4 to 0.5 seconds at a rate of 20 to 25 breaths per minute. Some infants may respond better to conventional ventilation at more rapid rates with inspiratory times as short as 0.2 seconds. High-frequency ventilation with jet or oscillatory ventilators may be successful in infants with severe MAS who fail to improve with conventional ventilation, and in those who develop air leak syndromes. There are no prospective, randomized controlled trials comparing the efficacy of the various ventilator modes in MAS.

E. Drug therapy

1. **Antibiotics.** Differentiating between bacterial pneumonia and meconium aspiration by clinical course and chest x-ray findings may be difficult. Although few infants with MAS have documented infections, the use of broad-spectrum antibiotics (e.g., ampicillin and gentamicin) is usually indicated in infants when an infiltrate is seen on chest radiograph. Blood cultures should be obtained to identify bacterial disease, if present, and to determine length of antibiotic course.

2. **Surfactant.** Endogenous surfactant activity may be inhibited by meconium. Surfactant treatment of MAS may improve oxygenation and reduce pulmonary complications and the need for ECMO. We do not routinely use surfactant to treat infants with MAS. However, in those infants whose clinical status continues to deteriorate and who require escalating support, surfactant may be helpful.

3. **Corticosteroids.** We do not recommend the use of corticosteroids in MAS, although this approach has been proposed to reduce inflammation induced by meconium and minimize prostaglandin-mediated pulmonary vasoconstriction.

V. Acute complications

A. Air leak. Pneumothorax or pneumomediastium occurs in approximately 10 to 20% of patients with MAS. Air leaks occur more frequently with mechanical ventilation, especially in the setting of air trapping. A high index of suspicion for air leak is necessary. Equipment should be available to evacuate a pneumothorax promptly (see Air Leak).

B. **Pulmonary hypertension.** PPHN occurs in 1:600 to 1:1500 live births, and is associated with MAS in approximately 35% of cases. Depending on the extent of hypoxemia, echocardiography should be performed to ascertain the degree to which the right-to-left shunting is contributing to the infant's overall hypoxemia and to exclude congenital heart disease as the etiology (see Persistent Pulmonary Hypertension of the Newborn). In severely ill infants with MAS and PPHN, inhaled nitric oxide reduces the need for ECMO.

Suggested Readings

Fuloria M., Wiswell T.E. Managing meconium aspiration. *Contemp Pediatr* 2000; 17:125–139.

Wiswell T.E. Advances in the treatment of the meconium aspiration syndrome. *Acta Pediatr Suppl* 2001; 90:28–30.

Wiswell T.E., et al. Delivery room management of the apparently vigorous meconium-stained neonate: Results of the multicenter, international collaborative trial. *Pediatrics* 2000; 105:1–7.

25. CARDIAC DISORDERS

Stephanie Burns Wechsler and Gil Wernovsky

I. **Introduction.** At the turn of the century, Dr. William Osler wrote in his textbook of medicine that congenital heart disease was of "limited clinical interest as in a large proportion of cases the anomaly is not compatible with life, and in others, nothing can be done to remedy the defect or even relieve the symptoms." In the years since 1938, when Dr. Robert Gross first successfully ligated a patent ductus arteriosus in a 7-year-old girl at Children's Hospital, Boston (with a 17-day postoperative stay, 12 of which were for "general interest in the case") the outlook for children with congenital heart disease has improved dramatically. This remarkable progress has been due to synergistic advances in pediatric and fetal cardiology, cardiac surgery, neonatology, cardiac anesthesia, intensive care, and nursing.

In critical lesions, the ultimate prognosis for the patient depends in part on (1) a timely and accurate assessment of the structural anomaly and (2) the evaluation and resuscitation of secondary organ damage. It is thus crucial that pediatricians and neonatologists be able to rapidly evaluate and participate in the initial medical management of neonates with congenital heart disease. A multidisciplinary approach involving several subspecialty services is frequently required, especially since one-fifth of patients with severe congenital heart disease may be premature and/or weigh less than 2500 g at birth (13). Although neonates (as a group) may have a slightly higher surgical mortality than term infants (13), the secondary effects of the unoperated lesion on the heart, lung, and brain may be quite severe. These secondary changes may include chronic congestive heart failure, failure to thrive, frequent infections, irreversible pulmonary vascular changes, delayed cognitive development or focal neurologic deficits. For these reasons, at Children's Hospital in Boston primary surgical correction in carried out early in life, often in the neonatal period (7). This chapter is intended as a practical guide for the initial evaluation and management, by pediatricians and neonatologists, of neonates and infants suspected of having congenital heart disease. For detailed discussion of the individual lesions, the clinician should consult current textbooks of pediatric cardiology and cardiac surgery (4,7,14, 15,19).

II. **Incidence and survival.** The incidence of moderate to severe structural congenital heart disease in live born infants is 6 to 8 per 1000 live births (18). This incidence has been relatively constant over the years and in different areas around the world. More recent higher incidence figures appear to be due to the inclusion of more trivial forms of congenital heart disease, such as tiny ventricular septal defects that are detected more frequently by highly sensitive echocardiography. Data from the New England Regional Infant Cardiac Program suggest that approximately 3 per 1000 live births have heart disease that results in death or requires cardiac catheterization or surgery during the first year of life (13). The majority of these infants with congenital heart disease are identified by the end of the neonatal period (13). The most common congenital heart lesions presenting in the first weeks of life are summarized in Table 25.1. Recent advances in diagnostic imaging, cardiac surgery, and intensive care have reduced the operative risks for many complex lesions; the hospital mortality following all forms of neonatal cardiac surgery has significantly decreased in the past decade.

III. **Clinical presentations of congenital heart disease in the neonate.** The timing of presentation and accompanying symptomatology depends on (1) the nature and severity of the anatomic defect, (2) the in utero effects (if any) of the structural lesion, and (3) the alterations in cardiovascular physiology secondary to the effects of the transitional circulation: **closure of the ductus arteriosus** and

TABLE 25.1. TOP FIVE DIAGNOSES PRESENTING AT DIFFERENT AGES*

Diagnosis	Percentage of Patients
Age on admission: 0–6 days (n = 537)	
D-Transposition of great arteries	19
Hypoplastic left ventricle	14
Tetralogy of Fallot	8
Coarctation of aorta	7
Ventricular-septal defect	3
Others	49
Age on admission: 7–13 days (n = 195)	
Coarctation of aorta	16
Ventricular septal defect	14
Hypoplastic left ventricle	8
D-Transposition of great arteries	7
Tetralogy of Fallot	7
Others	48
Age on admission: 14–28 days (n = 177)	
Ventricular septal defect	16
Coarctation of aorta	12
Tetralogy of Fallot	7
D-Transposition of great arteries	7
Patent ductus arteriosus	5
Others	53

*Reprinted with permission from Flanagan M.F., Yeager S.B., Weindling S.N. Cardiac disease. In: Avery M.A., Fletcher M.G., MacDonald M.G. (Eds.), *Neonatology: Pathophysiology and Management of the Newborn,* 5th ed. 1999. Philadelphia: Lippincott Williams & Wilkins.

the **fall in pulmonary vascular resistance.** This chapter focuses primarily on cardiovascular abnormalities with critical effects in the neonatal period.

In the first few weeks of life, the many heterogeneous forms of heart disease present in a surprisingly limited number of ways (in no particular order nor mutually exclusive): (1) cyanosis; (2) congestive heart failure (with the most extreme presentation being cardiovascular collapse or shock); (3) an asymptomatic heart murmur; and (4) arrhythmia. With increasing frequency, neonates with congenital heart disease have been diagnosed prior to delivery by fetal echocardiography (2) and thus are born with a presumptive diagnosis into an expectant team of physicians and nurses. In many neonates, however, congenital heart disease is not suspected until after birth. The clinician may be diverted away from a diagnosis of heart disease because of the report of a "normal" prenatal ultrasound performed for screening purposes. Finally, the diagnosis of "heart disease" should never divert the clinician from a complete noncardiac evaluation with a thorough search for additional or secondary medical problems—occasionally the neonate with complex congenital heart disease and hypoxemia has inadequate attention paid to an initial and continued assessment of an adequate airway and ventilation.

A. Cyanosis

   1. **Clinical findings.** Cyanosis (bluish tinge of the skin and mucus membranes) is one of the most common presenting signs of congenital heart disease in the neonate. Although cyanosis usually indicates underlying hypoxemia

(diminished level of arterial oxygen saturation), there are a few instances when cyanosis is associated with a normal arterial oxygen saturation. Depending on the underlying skin complexion, clinically apparent cyanosis is usually not visible until there is more than 3 gm/dL of **desaturated** hemoglobin in the arterial system. Thus, the degree of visible cyanosis depends on both the severity of hypoxemia (which determines the percent of oxygen saturation) as well as the hemoglobin concentration. For example, consider two infants with similar degrees of hypoxemia—each having an arterial oxygen saturation of 85%. The polycythemic newborn (hemoglobin of 22 gm/dL) will have 3.3 gm/dL (15% of 22) desaturated hemoglobin and be more easily appreciated to be cyanotic than the anemic infant (hemoglobin of 10 gm/dL) who will only have 1.5 gm/dL (15% of 10) desaturated hemoglobin. An additional note, true central cyanosis should be a generalized finding (i.e., not acrocyanosis, blueness of the hands and feet only, which is a normal finding in a neonate).

2. **Differential diagnosis.** Differentiation of cardiac from respiratory causes of cyanosis in the NICU is a common problem. Pulmonary disorders frequently are the cause of cyanosis in the newborn due to intrapulmonary right-to-left shunting. Primary lung disease (pneumonia, hyaline membrane disease, pulmonary arteriovenous malformations, etc.); pneumothorax; airway obstruction; extrinsic compression of the lungs (congenital diaphragmatic hernia, pleural effusions, etc.); and central nervous system abnormalities may produce varying degrees of hypoxemia manifesting as cyanosis in the neonate. For a more complete differential diagnosis of pulmonary causes of cyanosis in the neonate see Chapter 24. Finally, clinical cyanosis may occur in an infant without hypoxemia in the setting of methemoglobinemia or pronounced polycythemia. Table 25.2 summarizes the differential diagnosis of cyanosis in the neonate.

Cyanosis due to congenital heart disease can be broadly grouped into those lesions with (1) decreased pulmonary blood flow and intracardiac right-to-left shunting and (2) normal to increased pulmonary blood flow with intracardiac mixing (complete or incomplete) of the systemic and pulmonary venous return. Specific lesions and lesion specific management are covered in more detail in section V.

B. **Congestive heart failure**

1. **Clinical findings.** Congestive heart failure in the neonate (or in a patient of any age) is a **clinical** diagnosis made on the basis of the existence of certain signs and symptoms rather than on radiographic or laboratory findings (though these may be supportive evidence for the diagnosis). Signs and symptoms of congestive heart failure occur when the heart is unable to meet the metabolic demands of the tissues. Clinical findings are frequently due to homeostatic mechanisms attempting to compensate for this imbalance. In early stages, the neonate may be tachypneic and tachycardiac with an increased respiratory effort, rales, hepatomegaly, and delayed capillary refill. In contrast to adults, edema is rarely seen. Diaphoresis, feeding difficulties, and growth failure may be present. Finally, congestive heart failure may present acutely with cardiorespiratory collapse, particularly in "left-sided" lesions (see V.A). Hydrops fetalis is an extreme form of intrauterine congestive heart failure.

2. **Differential diagnosis.** The age when congestive heart failure develops depends on the hemodynamics of the responsible lesion. When heart failure develops in the first weeks of life, the differential diagnosis includes (1) a structural lesion causing severe pressure and/or volume overload; (2) a primary myocardial lesion causing myocardial dysfunction; or (3) arrhythmia. Table 25.3 summarizes the differential diagnoses of congestive heart failure in the neonate.

C. **Heart murmur.** Heart murmurs are not uncommonly heard when examining a newborn. The estimates of the prevalence of heart murmurs in neonates range from 1% to 70% depending on the study (1,5).

TABLE 25.2. DIFFERENTIAL DIAGNOSIS OF CYANOSIS IN THE NEONATE

Primary cardiac lesions
  Decreased pulmonary blood flow, intracardiac right-to-left shunt
    Critical pulmonary stenosis
    Tricuspid atresia
    Pulmonary atresia/intact ventricular septum
    Tetralogy of Fallot
    Ebstein anomaly
    Total anomalous pulmonary venous connection with obstruction
  Normal or increased pulmonary blood flow, intracardiac mixing
    Hypoplastic left heart syndrome
    Transposition of the great arteries
    Truncus arteriosus
    Tetralogy of Fallot/pulmonary atresia
    Complete common atrioventricular canal
    Total anomalous pulmonary venous connection without obstruction
    Other single-ventricle complexes

Pulmonary lesions (intrapulmonary right-to-left shunt) (see Chap. 24)
  Primary parenchymal lung disease
    Aspiration syndromes (e.g., meconium and blood)
    Respiratory distress syndrome
    Pneumonia
  Airway obstruction
    Choanal stenosis or atresia
    Pierre Robin syndrome
    Tracheal stenosis
    Pulmonary sling
    Absent pulmonary valve syndrome[a]
  Extrinsic compression of the lungs
    Pneumothorax
    Pulmonary interstitial or lobar emphysema
    Chylothorax or other pleural effusions
    Congenital diaphragmatic hernia
    Thoracic dystrophies or dysplasia
  Hypoventilation
    Central nervous system lesions
    Neuromuscular diseases
    Sedation
    Sepsis
  Pulmonary arteriovenous malformations

Persistent pulmonary hypertension (see Chap. 24)

Cyanosis with normal PO_2
  Methemoglobinemia
  Polycythemia[b]

[a]Typically associated with tetralogy of Fallot with intracardiac shunt as well.
[b]In the case of polycythemia, these infants have plethora and venous congestion in the distal extremities, which gives the appearance of distal cyanosis; these infants actually are not hypoxemic (see text).

Pathologic murmurs tend to appear at characteristic ages. Stenotic (systolic ejection murmurs) and atrioventricular valvar insufficiency (systolic regurgitant murmurs) tend to be noted very shortly after birth, on the first day of life. In contrast, murmurs due to left-to-right shunt lesions (systolic regurgitant ventricular septal defect murmur or continuous patent ductus arteriosus murmur) may not be heard until the second to fourth week of life, when the pulmo-

TABLE 25.3. DIFFERENTIAL DIAGNOSIS OF CONGESTIVE HEART FAILURE IN THE NEONATE

Pressure overload
  Aortic stenosis
  Coarctation of the aorta

Volume overload
  Left-to-right shunt at level of great vessels
    Patent ductus arteriosus
    Aorticopulmonary window
    Truncus arteriosus
    Tetralogy of Fallot, pulmonary atresia with multiple aorticopulmonary
      collaterals
  Left-to-right shunt at level of ventricles
    Ventricular septal defect
    Common atrioventricular canal
    Single ventricle without pulmonary stenosis (includes hypoplastic left heart
      syndrome)
  Arteriovenous malformations

Combined pressure and volume overload
  Interrupted aortic arch
  Coarctation of the aorta with ventricular septal defect
  Aortic stenosis with ventricular septal defect

Myocardial dysfunction
  Primary
    Cardiomyopathies
      Inborn errors of metabolism
      Idiopathic
    Myocarditis
  Secondary
    Sustained tachyarrhythmias
    Perinatal asphyxia
    Sepsis
    Severe intrauterine valvar obstruction (e.g., aortic stenosis)
    Premature closure of the ductus arteriosus

nary vascular resistance has decreased and the left-to-right shunt increases. Thus the **age of the patient** when the murmur is first noted and the **character of the murmur** provide important clues to the nature of the malformation.

  D. **Arrhythmias.** See VIII, Arrhythmias of this chapter for a detailed description of identification and management of the neonate with an arrhythmia.

  E. **Fetal echocardiography.** It is increasingly common for infants to be born with a diagnosis of probable congenital heart disease due to the widespread use of obstetrical ultrasound and fetal echocardiography. This may be quite valuable to the team of physicians caring for mother and baby, guiding plans for prenatal care, site and timing of delivery, as well as immediate perinatal care of the infant. The recommended timing for fetal echocardiography is 18 to 20 weeks' gestation although reasonable images can be obtained as early as 16 weeks, and transvaginal ultrasound may be used for diagnostic purposes in fetuses in the first trimester. Indications for fetal echocardiography are summarized in Table 25.4. Most severe forms of congenital heart disease can be accurately diagnosed by fetal echocardiography (3). Coarctation of the aorta, small ventricular and atrial septal defects, total anomalous pulmonary

TABLE 25.4. INDICATIONS FOR FETAL ECHOCARDIOGRAPHY

Fetus-related indications
  Suspected congenital heart disease on screening ultrasound
  Fetal chromosomal anomaly
  Fetal extracardiac anatomic anomaly
  Fetal cardiac arrhythmia
    Persistent bradycardia
    Persistent tachycardia
    Irregular rhythm
  Nonimmune hydrops fetalis

Mother-related indications
  Congenital heart disease
  Maternal metabolic disease
    Diabetes mellitus
    Phenylketonuria
  Maternal rheumatic disease (such as systemic lupus erythematosus)
  Maternal environmental exposures
    Alcohol
    Cardiac teratogenic medications
      Amphetamines
      Anticonvulsants
        Phenytoin
        Trimethadione
        Carbamazepine
        Valproate
      Isotretinoin
      Lithium carbonate
    Maternal viral infection
      Rubella

Family-related Indications
  Previous child or parent with congenital heart disease
  Previous child or parent with genetic disease associated with congenital heart
    disease

---

venous return, and mild aortic or pulmonary stenosis are abnormalities that may be missed by fetal echocardiography. In general, in complex congenital heart disease, the main abnormality is noted; however, the full extent of cardiac malformation may be better determined on postnatal examinations.

Finally, fetal tachy- or bradyarrhythmias (intermittent or persistent) may be detected on routine obstetrical screening ultrasound examinations; this should prompt more complete fetal echocardiography to rule out associated structural heart disease and further define the arrhythmia.

IV. Evaluation of the neonate with suspected congenital heart disease. As noted, the suspicion of congenital heart disease in the neonate typically follows one of a few clinical scenarios. Circulatory collapse is, unfortunately, not an uncommon means of presentation for the neonate with congenital heart disease. It must be emphasized that **emergency treatment of shock precedes definitive anatomic diagnosis.** Although sepsis may be suspected and treated, the signs of low cardiac output should always alert the examining physician to the likely possibility of congenital heart disease.

  A. Initial evaluation
    1. Physical exam. A complete physical exam provides important clues to the anatomic diagnosis. Inexperienced examiners frequently focus solely on the presence or absence of cardiac murmurs, but much more additional

information should be obtained during a complete examination. A great deal may be learned from simple visual inspection of the infant. Cyanosis may first be apparent on inspection of the mucous membranes and/or nailbeds (see III. A.1). Mottling of the skin and/or an ashen, gray color are important clues to severe cardiovascular compromise and incipient shock. While observing the infant, particular attention should be paid to the pattern of respiration including the work of breathing and use of accessory muscles.

Prior to auscultation, palpation of the distal extremities with attention to temperature and capillary refill is imperative. The cool neonate with delayed capillary refill should always be evaluated for the possibility of severe congenital heart disease. While palpating the distal extremities, note the presence and character of the distal pulses. Diminished or absent distal pulses are highly suggestive of obstruction of the aortic arch. Palpation of the precordium may provide an important clue to the presence of congenital heart disease. The presence of a precordial thrill usually indicates at least moderate pulmonary or aortic outflow obstruction, though a restrictive ventricular septal defect with low right ventricular pressure may present with a similar finding. A hyperdynamic precordium suggests a sizeable left-to-right shunt.

During auscultation, the examiner should first pay particular attention to the heart rate, noting its regularity and/or variability. The heart sounds, particularly the second heart sound, can be helpful clues to the ultimate diagnosis as well. A split second heart sound is a particularly important marker of the existence of two semilunar valves. Differentiating an S3 from an S4 heart sound is challenging in a tachycardic newborn; however, a gallop rhythm of either type is unusual and suggests the possibility of a significant left-to-right shunt or myocardial dysfunction. Ejection clicks suggest pulmonary or aortic valvar stenosis.

The presence and intensity of systolic murmurs can be very helpful in suggesting the type and severity of the underlying anatomic diagnosis; systolic murmurs are usually due to (1) semilunar valve or outflow tract stenosis, (2) atrioventricular valve regurgitation, or (3) shunting through a septal defect. Diastolic murmurs are **always** indicative of cardiovascular pathology. For a more complete description of auscultation of the heart, refer to one of the cardiology texts mentioned in section I.

A careful search for other anomalies is essential, since congenital heart disease is accompanied by at least one extracardiac malformation 25% of the time (14). Table 25.5 summarizes common malformation and chromosomal syndromes associated with congenital heart disease.

2. **Four-extremity blood pressure.** Measurement of blood pressure should be taken in both arms and both legs. Usually an automated Dynamapp is used, but in a small neonate with pulses that are difficult to palpate, manual blood pressure measurement with Doppler amplification may be necessary for an accurate measurement. A systolic pressure that is more than 10 mm Hg higher in the upper body compared to the lower body is abnormal and suggests coarctation of the aorta, aortic arch hypoplasia, or interrupted aortic arch. It should be noted that a systolic blood pressure gradient is quite specific for an arch abnormality but not sensitive; a systolic blood pressure gradient will not be present in the neonate with an arch abnormality in whom the ductus arteriosus is patent and nonrestrictive. Thus, the lack of a systolic blood pressure gradient in newborn does **not** conclusively rule out coarctation or other arch abnormalities, but the presence of a systolic pressure gradient is diagnostic of an aortic arch abnormality.

3. **Chest X ray.** A frontal and lateral view (if possible) of the chest should be obtained. In infants, particularly newborns, the size of the heart may be difficult to determine due to overlying thymus. Nevertheless, useful infor-

TABLE 25.5. COMMON CHROMOSOMAL ANOMALIES, SYNDROMES, AND ASSOCIATIONS ASSOCIATED WITH CONGENITAL HEART DISEASE

	Approximate Incidence or Mode of Inheritance	Extracardiac Features	Cardiac Features
CHROMOSOMAL ANOMALIES			
Trisomy 13 (Patau syndrome)	1/22,500	SGA, facies (midfacial hypoplasia, cleft lip and palate, microphthalmia coloboma, low-set ears); brain anomalies (microcephaly holoprosencephaly); aplasia cutis congenita of scalp; polydactyly	≥80% have cardiac defects, VSD most common
Trisomy 18 (Edward syndrome)	1/7500 (female-male = 3 : 1)	SGA; facies (dolicocephaly, prominent occiput, short palpebral fissures, low-set posteriorly rotated ears, small mandible); short sternum; rocker-bottom feet; overlapping fingers with "clenched fists"	≥95% have cardiac defects, VSD most common (sometimes multiple); redundant valvar tissue with regurgitation often affecting more than one valve (polyvalvar disease)
Trisomy 21 (Down syndrome)	1/850	Facies (brachycephaly, flattened occiput, midfacial hypoplasia, mandibular prognathism, upslanting palpebral fissures, epicanthal folds, Brushfield spots, large tongue); simian creases, clinodactyly with short fifth finger; pronounced hypotonia	40–50% have cardiac defects, CAVC, VSD most common, also TOF, ASD, PDA; complex congenital heart disease is very rare

Monosomy X (Turner's syndrome)	1/4000	Lymphedema of hands, feet; short stature; short webbed neck; facies (triangular with downslanting palpebral fissures, low-set ears); shield chest	25–45% have cardiac defects, coarctation, bicuspid aortic valve most common
SINGLE-GENE DEFECTS			
Noonan syndrome	AD	Facies (hypertelorism, epicanthal folds, downslanting palpebral fissures, ptosis); low-set ears; short webbed neck with low hairline; shield chest, cryptorchidism in males	≥50% have cardiac defect, usually valvar pulmonary stenosis, also ASD, hypertrophic CM
Holt-Oram syndrome	AD	Spectrum of upper limb and shoulder girdle anomalies	≥50% have cardiac defect, usually ASD or VSD
Ellis-van Creveld syndrome	AR	Short distal extremities, polydactyly; hypoplastic nails; dental anomalies	Approximately 50% have cardiac defect, usually ASD or common atrium
Alagille syndrome	AD	Cholestasis; facies (micrognathism, broad forehead, deep-set eyes); vertebral anomalies, ophthalmologic abnormalities	Cardiac findings in 90%. Peripheral pulmonic stenosis most common
GENE DELETION SYNDROMES			
Williams syndrome	Deletion 7q11	SGA, FTT; facies ("elfin" with short palpebral fissures, periorbital fullness or puffiness, flat nasal bridge, stellate iris, long philtrum, prominent lips); fussy infants with poor feeding, friendly personality later in childhood; characteristic mental deficiency (motor more reduced than verbal performance)	50–70% have cardiac defect, most commonly supravalvar aortic stenosis; other arterial stenoses also occur, including PPS, CoA, renal artery and coronary artery stenoses

(continues)

TABLE 25.5. *(continued)*

	Approximate Incidence or Mode of Inheritance	Extracardiac Features	Cardiac Features
DiGeorge syndrome	Deletion 22q11	Thymic hypoplasia/aplasia; parathyroid hypoplasia/aplasia; cleft palate or velopharyngeal incompetence	IAA and conotruncal malformations including truncus, TOF
ASSOCIATIONS VACTERL		Vertebral defects; anal atresia; TE fistula; radial and renal anomalies; limb defects	Approximately 50% have cardiac defect, most commonly VSD
CHARGE		Coloboma; choanal atresia; growth and mental deficiency; genital hypoplasia (in males); ear anomalies and/or deafness	50–70% have cardiac defect, most commonly conotruncal anomalies (TOF, DORV, truncus arteriosus)

VSD = ventricular septal defect; SGA = small for gestational age; CAVC = complete atrioventricular canal; TOF = tetralogy of Fallot; ASD = atrial septal defect; PDA = patent ductus arteriosus; AD = autosomal dominant; AR = autosomal recessive; CM = cardiomyopathy; FTT = failure to thrive; PPS = peripheral pulmonary stenosis; CoA = coarctation of the aorta; TEF = tracheoesophageal fistula; DORV = double outlet right ventricle; IAA = interrupted aortic arch.

mation can be gained from the chest X ray. In addition to heart size, notation should be made of visceral and cardiac situs (dextrocardia and situs inversus are frequently accompanied by congenital heart disease.) The aortic arch side (right or left) can frequently be determined; a right-sided aortic arch is associated with congenital heart disease in over 90% of patients (4). Dark or poorly perfused lung fields suggests decreased pulmonary blood flow while diffusely opaque lung fields may represent increased pulmonary blood flow or significant left atrial hypertension.

4. **Electrocardiogram (ECG).** The neonatal ECG reflects the hemodynamic relationships that existed in utero, thus the normal ECG is notable for right ventricular predominance. As many forms of congenital heart disease have minimal prenatal hemodynamic effects, the ECG is frequently "normal for age" despite significant structural pathology (e.g., transposition of the great arteries, tetralogy of Fallot, etc.). Throughout the neonatal period, infancy, and childhood, the ECG will evolve due to the expected changes in physiology and the resulting changes in chamber size and thickness that occur. Since the majority of findings on a neonate's ECG would be abnormal in an older child or adult, it is essential to refer to age-specific charts of normal values for most ECG parameters. Refer to Tables 25.6 and 25.7 for normal ECG values in term and premature neonates.

When interpreting an ECG, the following determinations should be made: (1) rate and rhythm; (2) P, QRS, and T axes; (3) intracardiac conduction intervals; (4) evidence for chamber enlargement or hypertrophy; (5) evidence for pericardial disease, ischemia, infarction, or electrolyte abnormalities; and (6) if the ECG pattern fits with the clinical picture. When the ECG is abnormal, one should also consider incorrect lead placement; a simple confirmation of lead placement may be done by comparing QRS complexes in limb lead I and precordial lead V_6—each should have a similar morphology if the limb leads have been properly placed. The ECG of the premature infant is somewhat different from that of the term infant (see Table 25.7).

5. **Hyperoxia test.** In **all** neonates with suspected critical congenital heart disease (not just those who are cyanotic), a hyperoxia test should be performed. **This single test is perhaps the most sensitive and specific tool in the initial evaluation of the neonate with suspected recent disease.**

To investigate the possibility of a fixed, intracardiac right-to-left shunt, the arterial oxygen tension should be measured in room air (if tolerated) followed by repeat measurements with the patient receiving 100% inspired oxygen (the "hyperoxia test"). If possible, the arterial partial pressure of oxygen (PO_2) should be measured directly via arterial puncture, though properly applied transcutaneous oxygen monitor (TCOM) values for PO_2 are also acceptable. **Pulse oximetry cannot be used** for documentation; in a neonate given 100% inspired oxygen, a value of 100% oxygen saturation may be obtained with an arterial PO_2 ranging from 80 torr (abnormal) to 680 torr (normal, see III.A.1).

Measurements should be made (by arterial blood gas or TCOM) at both "preductal" and "postductal" sites and the exact site of PO_2 measurement must be recorded, since some congenital malformations with desaturated blood flow entering the descending aorta through the ductus arteriosus may result in "differential cyanosis" (as seen in persistent pulmonary hypertension of the newborn). A markedly higher oxygen content in the upper versus the lower part of the body can be an important diagnostic clue to such lesions, including all forms of critical aortic arch obstruction or left ventricular outflow obstruction. There are also the rare cases of "reverse differential cyanosis" with elevated lower-body saturation and lower upper-body saturation. This occurs only in children with transposition of the great arteries with an abnormal pulmonary artery to aortic shunt due to coarctation, interruption of the aortic arch, or suprasystemic pulmonary vascular resistance ("persistent fetal circulation").

TABLE 25.6. ECG STANDARDS IN NEWBORNS

Measure	Age (Days)			
	0–1	1–3	3–7	7–30
Term infants				
Heart rate (beats/min)	122 (99–147)	123 (97–148)	128 (100–160)	148 (114–177)
QRS axis (degrees)	135 (91–185)	134 (93–188)	133 (92–185)	108 (78–152)
PR interval, II (sec)	0.11 (0.08–0.14)	0.11 (0.09–0.13)	0.10 (0.08–0.13)	0.10 (0.08–0.13)
QRS duration (sec)	0.05 (0.03–0.07)	0.05 (0.03–0.06)	0.05 (0.03–0.06)	0.05 (0.03–0.08)
V_1, R amplitude (mm)	13.5 (6.5–23.7)	14.8 (7.0–24.2)	12.8 (5.5–21.5)	10.5 (4.5–18.1)
V_1, S amplitude (mm)	8.5 (1.0–18.5)	9.5 (1.5–19.0)	6.8 (1.0–15.0)	4.0 (0.5–9.7)
V_6, R amplitude (mm)	4.5 (0.5–9.5)	4.8 (0.5–9.5)	5.1 (1.0–10.5)	7.6 (2.6–13.5)
V_6, S amplitude (mm)	3.5 (0.2–7.9)	3.2 (0.2–7.6)	3.7 (0.2–8.0)	3.2 (0.2–3.2)
Preterm infants				
Heart rate (beats/min)	141 (109–173)	150 (127–182)	164 (134–200)	170 (133–200)
QRS axis (degrees)	127 (75–194)	121 (75–195)	117 (75–165)	80 (17–171)
PR interval (sec)	0.10 (0.09–0.10)	0.10 (0.09–1.10)	0.10 (0.09–0.10)	0.10 (0.09–0.10)
QRS duration (sec)	0.04	0.04	0.04	0.04
V_1, R amplitude (mm)	6.5 (2.0–12.6)	7.4 (2.6–14.9)	8.7 (3.8–16.9)	13.0 (6.2–21.6)
V_1, S amplitude (mm)	6.8 (0.6–17.6)	6.5 (1.0–16.0)	6.8 (0.0–15.0)	6.2 (1.2–14.0)
V_6, R amplitude (mm)	11.4 (3.5–21.3)	11.9 (5.0–20.8)	12.3 (4.0–20.5)	15.0 (8.3–21.0)
V_6, S amplitude (mm)	15.0 (2.5–26.5)	13.5 (2.6–26.0)	14.0 (3.0–25.0)	14.0 (3.1–26.3)

Sources: Term infant values from Davignon A. et al., *Pediatr Cardiol* 1979–1980;1:123. Preterm infant values from Streenivasan V. V. et al., *Am J Cardiol* 1973;31: 57.

TABLE 25.7. ECG FINDINGS IN PREMATURE INFANTS (COMPARED TO TERM INFANTS)

Rate
    Slightly higher resting rate with greater activity-related and circadian variation (sinus bradycardia to 70, with sleep not uncommon)
Intracardiac conduction
    PR and QRS duration slightly shorter
    Maximum QT_c <0.44 second (longer than for term infants, QT_c <0.40 second)
QRS complex
    QRS axis in frontal plane more leftward with decreasing gestational age
    QRS amplitude lower (possibly due to less ventricular mass)
    Less right ventricular predominance in precordial chest leads

Source: Reproduced with permission from Thomaidie C., Varlamis G., Karemperis S. *Acta Paediatr Scand* 1988;77:653.

When a patient breathes 100% oxygen, an arterial PO_2 of greater than 250 torr in both upper and lower extremities virtually eliminates critical structural cyanotic heart disease (a "passed" hyperoxia test.) An arterial PO_2 of less than 100 in the absence of clear-cut lung disease (a "failed" hyperoxia test) is most likely due to intracardiac right-to-left shunting and is virtually diagnostic of cyanotic congenital heart disease. Patients who have an arterial PO_2 between 100 and 250 **may** have structural heart disease with complete intracardiac mixing and greatly increased pulmonary blood flow, as is occasionally seen with single-ventricle complexes such as hypoplastic left heart syndrome. **The neonate who "fails" a hyperoxia test is very likely to have congenital heart disease involving ductal-dependent systemic or pulmonary blood flow, and should receive prostaglandin E1 until anatomic definition can be accomplished** (see IV.b.2).

B. **Stabilization and transport.** On the basis of the initial evaluation, if an infant has been identified as likely to have congenital heart disease, further medical management must be planned as well as arrangements made for a definitive anatomic diagnosis. This may involve transport of the neonate to another medical center where a pediatric cardiologist is available.

1. **Initial resuscitation.** For the neonate who presents with evidence of decreased cardiac output or shock, initial attention is devoted to the basics of advanced life support. A stable airway must be established and maintained as well as adequate ventilation. Reliable vascular access is essential, usually including an arterial line. In the neonate, this can most reliably be accomplished via the umbilical vessels. Volume resuscitation, inotropic support, and correction of metabolic acidosis are required with the goal of improving cardiac output and tissue perfusion (see Chap. 17, Shock).

2. **Prostaglandin E$_1$ (PGE$_1$).** The neonate who "fails" a hyperoxia test (or has an equivocal result in addition to other signs or symptoms of congenital heart disease) as well as the neonate who presents in shock within the first 3 weeks of life is highly likely to have congenital heart disease. These neonates are very likely to have congenital lesions that include anatomic features with ductal-dependent systemic or pulmonary blood flow, or in whom a patent ductus arteriosus will aid in intercirculatory mixing.

PGE$_1$, administered as a continuous intravenous infusion, has important side effects that must be anticipated. PGE$_1$ causes apnea in 10 to 12% of neonates, usually within the first 6 hours of administration. Thus, the infant who will be transferred to another institution while receiving PGE_1 should be intubated for maintenance of a stable airway prior to leaving the referring hospital. In infants who will not require transport, intubation may not be required but continuous cardiorespiratory monitoring is essential. In addition, PGE_1 typically causes peripheral vasodilation and subsequent hypotension in many infants. A separate intravenous line should be secured for volume administration in any infant receiving PGE_1, especially those who require transport.

Other adverse reactions to PGE_1 include: fever (14%); cutaneous flushing (10%); bradycardia (7%); seizures (4%); tachycardia (3%); cardiac arrest (1%); and edema (1%). Specific information regarding dose and administration of PGE1 is in section VII.A.

The authors cannot overemphasize the need to begin PGE_1 in **any** neonate in whom congenital heart disease is strongly suspected [i.e., a failed hyperoxia test and/or severe, acute congestive heart failure (CHF)]. In the neonate with ductal-dependant pulmonary blood flow, oxygen saturation will typically improve and the pulmonary blood flow remain secure until an anatomic diagnosis and plans for surgery are made. In neonates with transposition of the great arteries, maintenance of a patent ductus improves intercirculatory mixing. Most important, **neonates who present in shock in the first few weeks of life have duct-dependent systemic blood flow until proven otherwise;** resuscitation will not be successful unless the ductus in opened. In these cases, it is appropriate to begin an infusion of PGE1 even **before** a precise anatomic diagnosis can be made by echocardiography.

It is prudent to remeasure arterial blood gases and reassess perfusion, vital signs and acid-base status within 15 to 30 minutes of starting a PGE_1 infusion. Rarely, patients may become more unstable after beginning PGE_1. This is usually due to lesions with obstruction to left atrial return (hypoplastic left heart syndrome with restrictive patent foramen ovale, subdiaphragmatic total anomalous pulmonary venous return, mitral atresia with restrictive patent foramen ovale, transposition of the great arteries with intact ventricular septum, and restrictive patent foramen ovale). In these lesions, deterioration on PGE_1 is often a helpful diagnostic finding, and **urgent** plans for echocardiography and possible interventional catheterization or surgery should be made.

3. **Inotropic agents.** Continuous infusions of inotropic agents, usually the sympathomimetic amines, can improve myocardial performance as well as perfusion of vital organs and the periphery. Care should be taken to replete intravascular volume before institution of vasoactive agents. **Dopamine** is a precursor of norepinephrine and stimulates beta-1, dopaminergic, and alpha-adrenergic receptors in a dose-dependent manner. Dopamine can be expected to increase mean arterial pressure, improve ventricular function, and improve urine output with a low incidence of side effects at doses less than 10 μg/kg per minute. **Dobutamine** is an analogue of dopamine, with predominantly beta-1 effects and relatively weak beta-2 and alpha-receptor stimulating activity. In comparison with dopamine, dobutamine lacks renal vasodilating properties, has less chronotropic effect (in adult patients), and does not depend on norepinephrine release from peripheral nerves for its effect. There are few published data available concerning the use of dobutamine in neonates, although clinical experience has been favorable. A combination of low-dose dopamine (up to 5 μg/kg per minute) and dobutamine may be used to minimize the potential peripheral vasoconstriction induced by high doses of dopamine while maximizing the dopaminergic effects on the renal circulation. See VII.B for details of administration of inotropic agents, and additional pharmacologic agents (see Chap. 17).

4. **Transport.** After initial stabilization, the neonate with suspected congenital heart disease often needs to be transferred to an institution that

provides subspecialty care in pediatric cardiology and cardiac surgery. A successful transport actually involves two transitions of care for the neonate: (1) from the referring hospital staff to the transport team; (2) from the transport team staff to the accepting hospital staff. The need for accurate, detailed, and complete communication of information between all these teams cannot be overemphasized. If possible, the pediatric cardiologist who will be caring for the patient should be included in the discussions of care while the neonate is still at the referring hospital.

Reliable **vascular access** should be secured for the neonate receiving continuous infusions of PGE_1 or inotropic agents. Umbilical lines placed for resuscitation and stabilization should be left in place for transport; the neonate with congenital heart disease may potentially require cardiac catheterization via this route.

Particular attention should be paid to the patient's airway and respiratory effort before transport. In general, all neonates receiving a PGE_1 infusion should be **intubated for transport** (see IV.B.2). Neonates with probable or definite congenital heart disease will most likely require surgical or interventional catheterization management during the hospitalization; thus, it is likely that they will be intubated at some point. Since there is real risk in not intubating these infants, as a general rule, all should be intubated for transport unless there is a compelling reason not to do so. All intubated patients should have gastric decompression by nasogastric or orogastric tube.

Acid-base status and oxygen delivery should be checked with an arterial blood gas prior to transport. Although most noncardiac patients are transported receiving supplemental oxygen at or near 100%, this is often **not** the inspired oxygen concentration of choice for the neonate with congenital heart disease (see V for details of lesion-specific care). This management decision for transport is particularly important for those infants with duct-dependent systemic blood flow and complete intracardiac mixing with single ventricle physiology, and emphasizes the need to consult with a pediatric cardiologist **prior** to transport to achieve optimal intratransport patient care.

Finally, it is important to remember in neonates that **hypotension** is a late finding in shock. Thus other signs of incipient decompensation, such as persistent tachycardia and poor tissue perfusion, are important to note and treat before transport. Before leaving the referring hospital, the patient's current hemodynamic status (distal perfusion, heart rate, systemic blood pressure, acid-base status, etc.) should be reassessed and relayed to the receiving hospital team.

C. Confirmation of the diagnosis

1. **Echocardiography.** Two-dimensional echocardiography, supplemented with Doppler and color Doppler has become the primary diagnostic tool for anatomic definition in pediatric cardiology. Echocardiography provides information about the structure and function of the heart and great vessels in a timely fashion. Though not an invasive test per se, a complete echocardiogram on a newborn suspected of having congenital heart disease may take an hour or more to perform, and thus may not be well tolerated by a sick and/or premature newborn. Temperature instability due to exposure during this extended time of examination may be a problem in the neonate. Extension of the neck for suprasternal notch views of the aortic arch may be problematic, particularly in the neonate with respiratory distress or with a tenuous airway. Thus, in sick neonates, **close monitoring by a medical staff person other** than the one performing the echocardiogram is recommended, with attention to vital signs, respiratory status, temperature, etc.

2. **Cardiac catheterization**

   a. **Indications** (See Table 25.8). Over the past 10 years, neonatal cardiac catheterization has changed a great deal in its focus. In the current

TABLE 25.8. INDICATIONS FOR NEONATAL CATHETERIZATION

Interventions
  Therapeutic*
    Balloon atrial septostomy
    Balloon pulmonary valvuloplasty
    Balloon aortic valvuloplasty
    Balloon angioplasty of native coarctation of the aorta
    Coil embolization of abnormal vascular communications
  Diagnostic
    Endomyocardial biopsy

Anatomic definition (not visualized by echocardiography)
  Coronary arteries
    Pulmonary atresia/intact ventricular septum
    Transposition of the great arteries
    Tetralogy of Fallot
  Aortic to pulmonary artery collateral vessels
    Tetralogy of Fallot
  Distal pulmonary artery anatomy

Hemodynamic measurements

*All of these interventions have alternative surgical options and are controversial based on institutional experience (see text).

era, it is rarely necessary to perform a cardiac catheterization for anatomic definition of intracardiac structures (though catheterization is still necessary for definition of the distal pulmonary arteries, aortic-pulmonary collaterals, and certain types of coronary artery anomalies) or for physiologic assessment as Doppler technology has assumed an increasingly important role in this regard. Increasingly, catheterization is performed for catheter-directed therapy of congenital lesions (4). See Figure 25.1 for normal newborn oxygen saturation and pressure measurements obtained during cardiac catheterization.

  b. Interventional catheterization. Since the first balloon dilation of the pulmonary artery reported by Kan in 1982, balloon valvuloplasty has become the procedure of choice in many types of valvar lesions, even extending to critical lesions in the neonate (21). At Children's Hospital, balloon valvuloplasty is considered the initial treatment of choice for both pulmonary and aortic stenosis, with a greater than 90% immediate success rate in the neonate (10,11). The application of balloon dilation of native coarctation of the aorta is controversial (see below).

  c. Preparation for catheterization. Since catheterization in the neonate is not without its attendant risks, careful preparation may minimize the complication rate. In one survey, the risk of a complication in children undergoing catheterization, including neonates and infants, was 9% (22). With appropriate anticipatory care, complications can be minimized. In addition to basic medical stabilization (see IV.B), specific attention to airway management is crucial. Sedation and analgesia are necessary, but will depress the respiratory drive in the neonate. When catheterizing a neonate, intubation and mechanical ventilation should be strongly considered, especially if an intervention is contemplated. In our institution, a **separate staff person not performing the catheterization** is present during the study, dedicated to the supervision of the infant's overall hemodynamic and respiratory status.

Normal Newborn

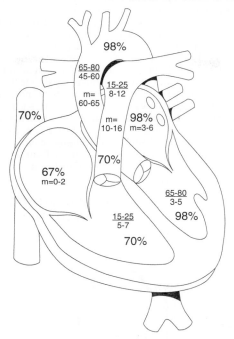

FIG. 25.1. Typical hemodynamic measurements obtained at cardiac catheterization in a newborn, term infant without congenital or acquired heart disease. In this (and subsequent diagrams), oxygen saturations are shown as percentages, and typical hemodynamic pressure measurements in mm Hg are shown. In this example, the transition from fetal to infant physiology is complete; the pulmonary vascular resistance has fallen, the ductus arteriosus has closed, and there is no significant shunt at the foramen ovale. M = mean value.

Supervision of the neonate undergoing catheterization should also include periodic evaluation of the patient's body temperature, acid-base status, serum glucose and monitoring of blood loss. All infants undergoing interventional catheterization should have 10 to 25 mL/kg packed red blood cells (PRBCs) typed and crossmatched *in the cath lab* during the procedure. Intravenous lines are recommended in the upper extremities or head (since the lower body will be draped and inaccessible during the case) in order to provide unobstructed access for medications, volume infusions, etc. Finally, the neonate may have the catheterization performed via umbilical vessels that were previously utilized for the administration of fluid, glucose, PGE_1, inotropic agents, or blood administration. Thus, a peripheral line should be started and medications changed to that site prior to transfer of the neonate to the cardiac catheterization laboratory.

Consultation with the pediatric cardiologist who will be performing the case beforehand will help clarify these issues and allow the infant to be well prepared and monitored during the case.

V. "Lesion-specific" care following anatomic diagnosis

A. Duct-dependent systemic blood flow.
Commonly referred to as **left-sided obstructive lesions,** this group of lesions includes a spectrum of hypoplasia of left-sided structures of the heart ranging from isolated coarctation of the aorta to hypoplastic left heart syndrome. These infants typically present in cardiovascular collapse as the ductus arteriosus closes, with resultant systemic hypoperfusion; they may also present more insidiously with symptoms of congestive heart failure (see III.B). Although all infants with significant left-sided lesions and duct-dependent systemic blood flow require prostaglandin-induced patency of the ductus arteriosus as part of the initial management, additional care varies somewhat with each lesion.

1. **Aortic stenosis** (see Fig. 25.2). Morphologic abnormalities of the aortic valve may range from a bicuspid, nonobstructive, functionally normal valve to a unicuspid, markedly deformed and severely obstructive valve, which greatly limits systemic cardiac output from the left ventricle. By convention, "severe" aortic stenosis is defined as a peak systolic gradient

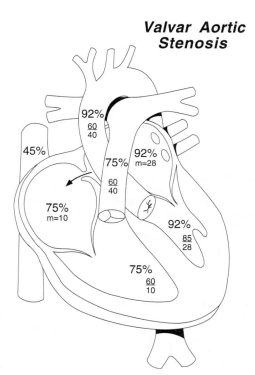

Valvar Aortic Stenosis

FIG. 25.2. Critical valvar aortic stenosis with a closed ductus arteriosus. Typical anatomic and hemodynamic findings include: (1) a morphologically abnormal, stenotic valve; (2) poststenotic dilatation of the ascending aorta; (3) elevated left ventricular end diastolic pressure and left atrial pressures contributing to pulmonary edema (mild pulmonary venous and arterial desaturation); (4) a left-to-right shunt at the atrial level (note increase in oxygen saturation from superior vena cava to right atrium); (5) pulmonary artery hypertension (also secondary to the elevated left atrial pressure); (6) only a modest (25 mm Hg) gradient across valve. The low measured gradient (despite severe anatomic obstruction) across the aortic valve is due to a severely limited cardiac output, as evidenced by the low mixed venous oxygen saturation (45%) in the superior vena cava.

from left ventricle to ascending aorta of at least 60 mm Hg. "Critical" aortic stenosis results from severe anatomic obstruction with accompanying left ventricular failure and/or shock. Patients with critical aortic stenosis have severe obstruction present *in utero* (usually due to a unicuspid, "plate-like" valve), with resultant left ventricular hypertrophy and, frequently, endocardial fibroelastosis. Associated left-sided abnormalities such as mitral valve disease and coarctation are not uncommon. Following closure of the ductus, the left ventricle must supply all of the systemic cardiac output. In cases of severe myocardial dysfunction, clinical congestive heart failure or shock will become apparent.

Initial management of the severely affected infant includes treatment of shock, stable vascular access, airway management and mechanical ventilation, sedation and muscle paralysis, inotropic support and institution of PGE_1. Positive end-expiratory pressure (PEEP) is helpful to overcome pulmonary venous desaturation from pulmonary edema secondary to left atrial hypertension. For a patient with critical aortic stenosis to benefit from a PGE_1 infusion, there must be a small patent foramen ovale to allow effective systemic blood flow (pulmonary venous return) to cross the atrial septum and ultimately enter the systemic vascular bed through the ductus. Inspired oxygen should be limited to a fractional concentration of inspired oxygen (FiO_2) of 0.5 to 0.6 unless severe hypoxemia is present.

Following anatomic definition of left ventricular size, mitral valve and aortic arch anatomy by echocardiography, cardiac catheterization or surgery should be performed as soon as possible to perform aortic valvotomy. With either type of therapy, patient outcome will depend largely on (1) the degree of relief of the obstruction; (2) the degree of aortic regurgitation; (3) associated cardiac lesions (especially left ventricular size); and (4) the severity of end-organ dysfunction secondary to the initial presentation (e.g., necrotizing enterocolitis or renal failure). All patients with critical aortic stenosis will require life-long follow-up, as stenosis frequently recurs. Multiple procedures in childhood are common.

2. **Coarctation of the aorta** (see Fig. 25.3) is an anatomic narrowing of the descending aorta, most commonly at the site of insertion of the ductus arteriosus (i.e.,"juxtaductal"). Additional cardiac abnormalities are common, including bicuspid aortic valve (which occurs in 80% of patients) and ventricular septal defect (which occurs in 40% of patients). In addition, hypoplasia or obstruction of other left-sided structures including the mitral valve, the left ventricle, and the aortic valve are not uncommon and must be evaluated during the initial echocardiographic evaluation.

In utero, systemic blood flow to the lower body is via the patent ductus arteriosus. Following ductal closure in the newborn with a critical coarctation, the left ventricle must suddenly generate adequate pressure and volume to pump the entire cardiac output past a significant point of obstruction. This sudden pressure load may be poorly tolerated by the neonatal myocardium and the neonate may become rapidly and critically ill because of lower body hypoperfusion.

As in critical aortic stenosis, initial management of the severely affected infant includes treatment of shock, stable vascular access, airway management and mechanical ventilation, moderate supplemental oxygen, sedation and muscle paralysis, inotropic support and institution of PGE_1. PEEP is helpful to overcome pulmonary venous desaturation from pulmonary edema secondary to left atrial hypertension. In some infants, PGE_1 is unsuccessful in opening the ductus.

In infants with symptomatic coarctation, surgical repair is performed as soon as the infant has been resuscitated and medically stabilized. Usually the procedure is performed through a left lateral thoracotomy incision. In infants with symptomatic coarctation and a large, coexisting ventricular septal defect, consideration should be given to repair both defects in the initial procedure via a median sternotomy. Balloon dilation of

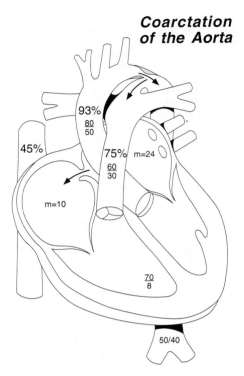

Coarctation of the Aorta

FIG. 25.3. Coarctation of the aorta in a critically ill neonate with a nearly closed ductus arteriosus. Typical anatomic and hemodynamic findings include: (1) "juxtaductal" site of the coarctation; (2) a bicommissural aortic valve (seen in 80% of patients with coarctation); (3) narrow pulse pressure in the descending aorta and lower body; (4) a bidirectional shunt at the ductus arteriosus. As in critical aortic stenosis (see Fig. 25.2) there is an elevated left atrial pressure, pulmonary edema, a left-to-right shunt at the atrial level, pulmonary artery hypertension, and only a moderate (30 mm Hg) gradient across the arch obstruction. The low measured gradient (despite severe anatomic obstruction) across the aortic arch is due to low cardiac output.

native coarctation is not routinely done at our institution because of the high incidence of restenosis and aneurysm formation, especially given the safe and effective surgical alternative.

3. **Interrupted aortic arch** (see Fig. 25.4) consists of complete atresia of a segment of the aortic arch. There are three anatomic subtypes of interrupted aortic arch based on the location of the interruption: distal to the left subclavian artery (type A); between the left subclavian artery and the left carotid artery (type B); and between the innominate artery and the left carotid artery (type C). Type B is the most common variety. Over 99% of these patients have a ventricular septal defect; abnormalities of the aortic valve and narrowed subaortic regions are associated anomalies.

Infants with interrupted aortic arch are completely dependent on a patent ductus arteriosus for lower body blood flow thus become critically ill when the ductus closes. Immediate management is similar to that described for coarctation (see V.A.2); PGE_1 infusion is essential. All other resuscitative measures will be ineffective if blood flow to the lower body is not restored. Oxygen saturations should be measured in the upper body;

Interrupted
Aortic Arch

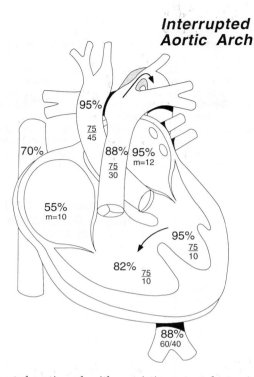

FIG. 25.4. Interrupted aortic arch with restrictive patent ductus arteriosus. Typical anatomic and hemodynamic findings include: (1) atresia of a segment of the aortic arch between the left subclavian artery and the left common carotid (the most common type of interrupted aortic arch—"type B"); (2) a posterior malalignment of the conal septum resulting in a large ventricular septal defect and a narrow subaortic area; (3) a bicuspid aortic valve occurs in 60% of patients; (4) systemic pressure in the right ventricle and pulmonary artery (due to the large, nonrestrictive ventricular septal defect); (5) increased oxygen saturation in the pulmonary artery due to left-to-right shunting at the ventricular level; (6) "differential cyanosis" with a lower oxygen saturation in the descending aorta due to a right-to-left shunt at the patent ductus. Note the lower blood pressure in the descending aorta due to constriction of the ductus; opening the ductus with PGE1 results in equal upper and lower extremity blood pressures, but continued "differential cyanosis."

pulse oximetry readings in the lower body are reflective of the pulmonary artery oxygen saturation, and are typically lower than that distributed to the central nervous system and coronary arteries. High concentrations of inspired oxygen may result in low pulmonary vascular resistance, a large left-to-right shunt, and a "run-off" during diastole from the lower body into the pulmonary circulation. Inspired oxygen levels should therefore be minimized, aiming for normal (95%) oxygen saturations in the **upper** body.

Surgical reconstruction should be performed as soon as metabolic acidosis (if present) has resolved, end-organ dysfunction is improving, and the patient is hemodynamically stable. The repair typically entails a corrective approach via a median sternotomy, with arch reconstruction (usually an end-to-end anastomosis) and closure of the ventricular septal defect. Arch reconstruction and a pulmonary artery band (via a lateral thoracotomy) are generally not recommended, typically reserved for patients with multiple ventricular septal defects.

4. **Hypoplastic left heart syndrome** (see Figs. 25.5A and 25.5B) represents a heterogeneous group of anatomic abnormalities in which there is a small or absent left ventricle with hypoplastic or atretic mitral and aortic valves. Prior to surgery, the right ventricle supplies both the pulmonary and systemic blood flows (via the patent ductus arteriosus), the proportion of cardiac output going to either circuit is dependent on the relative resistances of these vascular beds.

As the pulmonary vascular resistance begins to fall (Fig. 25.5A), blood flow is preferentially directed to the pulmonary circulation at the expense of the systemic circulation. As systemic blood flow decreases, stroke volume and heart rate increase as a mechanism to preserve systemic cardiac

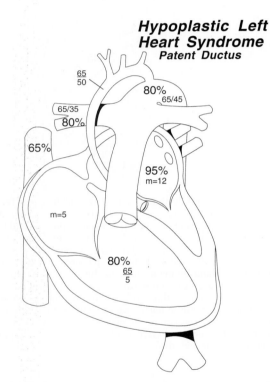

Hypoplastic Left Heart Syndrome
Patent Ductus

FIG. 25.5. **A**. Hypoplastic left heart syndrome in a 24-hour-old patient with falling pulmonary vascular resistance and a nonrestrictive ductus arteriosus. Typical anatomic and hemodynamic findings include: (1) atresia or hypoplasia of the left ventricle, mitral, and aortic valves; (2) a diminutive ascending aorta and transverse aortic arch, usually with an associated coarctation; (3) coronary blood flow is usually *retrograde* from the ductus arteriosus through the tiny ascending aorta; (4) systemic arterial oxygen saturation (in FiO_2 of 0.21) of 80%, reflecting relatively balanced systemic and pulmonary blood flows—the pulmonary artery and aortic saturations are equal (see text); (5) pulmonary hypertension secondary to the nonrestrictive ductus arteriosus; (6) minimal left atrial hypertension; (7) normal systemic cardiac output (note superior vena cava oxygen saturation of 65%) and blood pressure (65/45).

(continues)

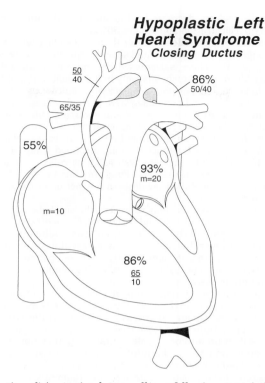

Hypoplastic Left Heart Syndrome
Closing Ductus

FIG. 25.5 B. *(continued)* Acute circulatory collapse following constriction of the ductus arteriosus in hypoplastic left heart syndrome. These neonates are typically in shock with poor perfusion, tachycardia, acidosis, and in respiratory distress. The anatomic features are similar to those in Fig. 25.5A, with the exception of the narrowed ductus arteriosus. Note (1) the low cardiac output (as evidenced by the low mixed venous oxygen saturation in the superior vena cava of 55%); (2) narrow pulse pressure; (3) elevated atrial and ventricular end-diastolic pressure—elevated left atrial pressure may cause pulmonary edema (note left atrial saturation of 93%); (4) significantly increased pulmonary blood flow, as reflected in an arterial oxygen saturation (in FiO_2 of 0.21) of 86%.

output. The right ventricle becomes progressively volume overloaded with mildly elevated end-diastolic and left atrial pressures. The infant may be tachypneic or in respiratory distress, hepatomegaly may be present. The greater proportion of pulmonary venous return in the mixed ventricular blood results in a mildly decreased systemic arterial oxygen saturation (80%), and visible cyanosis may be mild or absent. Not infrequently, these infants are discharged from the nursery as normal newborns.

At this point the continued fall in pulmonary vascular resistance results in a progressive increase in pulmonary blood flow and relative decrease in systemic cardiac output. As the total right ventricular output is limited by heart rate and stroke volume, there is the onset of clinically apparent congestive heart failure, right ventricular dilation and dysfunction, progressive tricuspid regurgitation, poor peripheral perfusion with metabolic acidosis, decreased urine output, and pulmonary edema. Arterial oxygen saturation approaches 90%.

Alternatively, a sudden deterioration takes place with rapidly progressive congestive heart failure and shock as the ductus arteriosus constricts (see Fig. 25.5B). There is decreased systemic perfusion and increased pulmonary blood flow, which is largely independent of the pulmonary vascular resistance. The peripheral pulses are weak to absent. Renal, hepatic, coronary, and central nervous system perfusion is compromised, possibly resulting in acute tubular necrosis, necrotizing enterocolitis, or cerebral infarction or hemorrhage. A vicious cycle may also result from inadequate retrograde perfusion of the ascending aorta (coronary blood supply), with further myocardial dysfunction and continued compromise of coronary blood flow. The pulmonary to systemic flow ratio approaches infinity as systemic blood flow nears zero. Thus, one has the paradoxical presentation of profound metabolic acidosis in the face of a relatively high PO_2 (70 to 100 mm Hg).

The arterial blood gas may represent the single best indicator of hemodynamic stability. Low arterial saturation (75 to 80%) with normal pH indicates an acceptable balance of systemic and pulmonary blood flow with adequate peripheral perfusion, while elevated oxygen saturation (>90%) with acidosis represents significantly increased pulmonary and decreased systemic flow with probable myocardial dysfunction and secondary effects on other organ systems.

Resuscitation of these neonates involves pharmacologic maintenance of ductal patency with PGE_1 and ventilatory maneuvers to **increase** pulmonary resistance. In our experience, a mild respiratory alkalosis (e.g., pH 7.35) is appropriate for most of these infants. It is important to note that **hyperventilation and/or supplemental oxygen is usually of no significant benefit and may be harmful** by causing excessive pulmonary vasodilation and pulmonary blood flow at the expense of the systemic blood flow.

Hypotension in these infants is more frequently caused by increased pulmonary blood flow (at the expense of systemic flow) rather that due to intrinsic myocardial dysfunction. Although small to moderate doses of inotropic agents are frequently beneficial, **large doses of inotropic agents may have a deleterious effect,** depending on the relative effects on the systemic and pulmonary vascular beds. Preferential selective elevations of systemic vascular tone will secondarily increase pulmonary blood flow, and careful monitoring of mean arterial blood pressure and arterial oxygen saturation is warranted.

Similar to the patient with critical aortic stenosis, in order for the neonate with hypoplastic left heart syndrome to benefit from a PGE_1 infusion, there must be at least a small patent foramen ovale to allow effective systemic blood flow (pulmonary venous return) to cross the atrial septum and ultimately enter the systemic vascular bed through the ductus. An infant with hypoplastic left heart syndrome and a severely restrictive or absent patent foramen ovale will be critically ill with profound cyanosis (oxygen saturation <60 to 65%), and will not improve after the institution of PGE_1. **In these neonates, emergent balloon dilation of the atrial septum may be necessary.**

Medical therapy may be briefly palliative; however, surgical therapy is necessary for survival of infants with hypoplastic left heart syndrome. After a period of medical stabilization and support to allow recovery of ischemic organ system injury (particularly of the kidneys, liver, central nervous system, and the heart itself), surgical relief of left-sided obstruction is required. Surgical intervention involves either staged reconstruction (with a neonatal Norwood procedure followed by a Fontan operation later in childhood) or neonatal cardiac transplantation. Recent results from both reconstructive surgery and transplantation have vastly improved the outlook for infants born with this previously 100% fatal condition.

B. Duct-dependent pulmonary blood flow. This underlying physiology is shared by a diverse group of lesions with the common finding of restricted pulmonary blood flow due to severe pulmonary stenosis or complete pulmonary atresia. Closure of the ductus arteriosus results in marked cyanosis.

   1. **Pulmonary stenosis** (see Fig. 25.6) with obstruction to pulmonary blood flow may occur at several levels: (1) within the body of the right ventricle; (2) at the pulmonary valve (see Fig. 25.7); (3) in the peripheral pulmonary arteries. Valvar pulmonary stenosis with an intact ventricular septum is the second most common form of congenital heart disease; "critical" obstruction occurs more rarely. Grading of the degree of pulmonary stenosis is similar to that of aortic stenosis (see V.A.1) with severe pulmonary stenosis defined as a peak systolic gradient from right ventricle to pulmonary artery of 60 mm Hg or more. By convention, "critical" pulmonary stenosis is defined as severe valvar obstruction with associated hypoxemia due to a right-to-left shunt at the foramen ovale. Critical pulmonary stenosis may be associated with hypoplasia of the right ventricle and/or

Valvar Pulmonary Stenosis

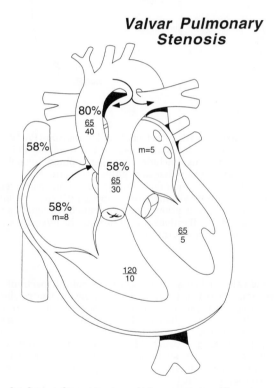

FIG. 25.6. Critical valvar pulmonary stenosis in a neonate with a nonrestrictive patent ductus arteriosus while receiving PGE_1. Typical anatomic and hemodynamic findings include: (1) thickened, stenotic pulmonary valve; (2) poststenotic dilatation of the main pulmonary artery with normal-sized branch pulmonary arteries; (3) right ventricular hypertrophy with suprasystemic pressure; (4) a right-to-left shunt at the atrial level via the patent foramen ovale with systemic desaturation (80%); (5) suprasystemic right ventricular (RV) pressure with a 55 mm Hg peak systolic ejection gradient; (6) systemic pulmonary artery pressure (due to the nonrestrictive patent ductus).

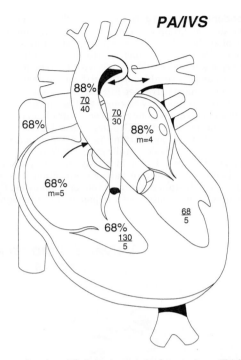

FIG. 25.7. Pulmonary atresia with intact ventricular septum (PA/IVS) in a neonate with a nonrestrictive patent ductus arteriosus while receiving PGE_1. Typical anatomic and hemodynamic findings include: (1) hypertrophied, hypoplastic right ventricle; (2) hypoplastic tricuspid valve and pulmonary annulus; (3) atresia of the pulmonary valve with no antegrade flow; (4) suprasystemic right ventricular pressure; (5) pulmonary blood flow via the patent ductus; (6) right-to-left shunt at the atrial level with systemic desaturation. Many patients have significant coronary abnormalities with sinusoidal or fistulous connections to the hypertensive right ventricle or significant coronary stenoses (not shown).

tricuspid valve and significant right ventricular hypertrophy. The pressure in the right ventricle is often higher than the left ventricular pressure (i.e., suprasystemic) in order to eject blood past the severe narrowing. Due to the longstanding (in utero) increased right ventricular pressure, there is typically a hypertrophied, noncompliant right ventricle with a resultant increase in right atrial filling pressure. When right atrial pressure exceeds left atrial pressure, a right-to-left shunt at the foramen ovale results in cyanosis and hypoxemia. There may be associated right ventricular dysfunction and/or tricuspid regurgitation.

After initial stabilization of the patient and definitive diagnosis by echocardiography, transcatheter balloon valvotomy has become the treatment of choice for this lesion, though surgical valvotomy may be utilized in specific cases. Despite successful relief of the obstruction during catheterization, cyanosis is usually not completely relieved, but rather resolves gradually over the first weeks of life as the right ventricle becomes more compliant and tricuspid regurgitation lessens. Successful balloon valvuloplasty is associated with excellent clinical results among patients; the need for repeat procedures is quite low.

2. **Pulmonary atresia with intact ventricular septum ("hypoplastic right heart syndrome", see Fig. 25.7)** is comparable to hypoplastic left heart syndrome in that there is atresia of the pulmonary valve with varying degrees of right ventricular and tricuspid valve hypoplasia. Perhaps the most important associated anomaly is the presence of coronary artery–myocardial–right ventricular sinusoidal connections. The coronary arteries may be quite abnormal, including areas of stenoses or complete atresia. Myocardial perfusion may therefore be dependent on a hypertensive right ventricle to supply the distal coronary arteries; surgical relief of the pulmonary atresia (with a right ventricular-to-pulmonary artery connection) may lead to myocardial infarction and death. The presence of sinusoidal connections between the right ventricle and the coronary arteries is associated with poorer long-term survival in all studies (14). Because there is no outlet of the right ventricle, there is typically suprasystemic pressure in the right ventricle and some tricuspid regurgitation. There is an obligatory right-to-left shunt at the atrial level and pulmonary blood flow is entirely dependent on a patent ductus arteriosus.

   Although the cornerstone of initial management is PGE_1 infusion to maintain ductal patency, a more permanent and reliable form of pulmonary blood flow must be surgically created for the infant to survive. Surgical management is often preceded by catheterization to define the coronary artery anatomy. In patients without significant coronary abnormalities, pulmonary blood flow is established by creating an outflow for the right ventricle by pulmonary valvotomy and/or right ventricular outflow tract augmentation. Usually at the time of this procedure, a systemic-to-pulmonary artery shunt (most often a Blalock-Taussig shunt) is constructed to also augment pulmonary blood flow. In patients with "right ventricular dependent" coronary arteries, a systemic-to-pulmonary artery shunt is the typical procedure performed in the neonate.

3. **Tricuspid atresia** (see Fig. 25.8) involves complete absence of the tricuspid valve and thus no direct communication from right atrium to right ventricle. The right ventricle may be severely hypoplastic or completely absent. More than 90% of patients have an associated ventricular septal defect, allowing blood to pass from the left ventricle to the right ventricular outflow and pulmonary arteries. The majority of patients have some form of additional pulmonary stenosis. In 70% of cases the great arteries are normally aligned with the ventricle; however, in the remaining 30% the great arteries are transposed. An atrial level communication is necessary for blood to exit the right atrium; there is an obligatory right-to-left shunt at this level. In patients with normally related great arteries, pulmonary blood flow is derived from the right ventricle; if the right ventricle (or its connection with the left ventricle via a ventricular septal defect) is severely diminutive, the pulmonary blood flow may be duct-dependent; closure of the ductus leads to profound hypoxemia and acidosis.

   Immediate medical management is primarily aimed at maintenance of adequate pulmonary blood flow. In the usual case of severe pulmonary stenosis and limited pulmonary blood flow, PGE_1 infusion maintains pulmonary blood flow via the ductus arteriosus. Surgical creation of a more permanent source of pulmonary blood flow (usually a Blalock-Taussig shunt) is undertaken as soon as possible. More complex cases (e.g. with transposition) may require more extensive palliative procedures (7).

4. **Tetralogy of Fallot** (see Fig. 25.9) consists of right ventricular outflow obstruction, a ventricular septal defect (of the anterior malalignment variety), "overriding" of the aorta over the ventricular septum, and hypertrophy of the right ventricle. There is a wide spectrum of anatomic variation encompassing these findings, depending particularly on the site and severity of the right ventricular outflow obstruction. The severely cyanotic neonate with tetralogy most likely has severe right ventricular outflow tract obstruction and a large right-to-left shunt at the ventricular level via the

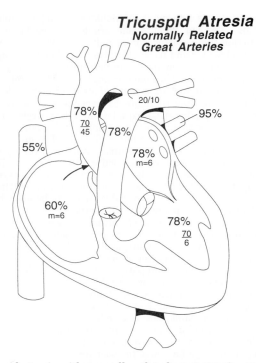

Tricuspid Atresia
Normally Related
Great Arteries

FIG. 25.8. Tricuspid atresia with normally related great arteries and a small patent ductus arteriosus. Typical anatomic and hemodynamic findings include: (1) atresia of the tricuspid valve; (2) hypoplasia of the right ventricle; (3) restriction to pulmonary blood flow at two levels: a (usually) small ventricular septal defect and a stenotic pulmonary valve; (4) all systemic venous return must pass through the patent foramen ovale to reach the left ventricle; (5) complete mixing at the left atrial level, with systemic oxygen saturation of 78% (in FiO_2 of 0.21), suggesting balanced systemic and pulmonary blood flow ("single ventricle physiology"—see text).

large ventricular septal defect. Pulmonary blood flow may be duct-dependent.

Immediate medical management involves establishing adequate pulmonary blood flow usually with PGE_1 infusion, though some have attempted balloon dilation of the right ventricular outflow tract. Detailed anatomic definition particularly regarding coronary artery anatomy, the presence of additional ventricular septal defects, and the sources of pulmonary blood flow (systemic to pulmonary collateral vessels) is necessary prior to surgical intervention. If echocardiography is not able to fully show these details, then diagnostic catheterization is performed. Surgical repair of the **asymptomatic** child with tetralogy of Fallot is usually recommended within the first 6 months of life. The **symptomatic** (i.e., severely cyanotic) neonate should have operative intervention. Complete repair is generally performed at our institution, though a systemic-to-pulmonary artery shunt is sometimes employed in cases of multiple ventricular septal defects or in patients with origin of the left anterior descending coronary artery from the right coronary artery (in whom the left anterior descending crosses the right ventricular outflow tract).

Tetralogy of Fallot

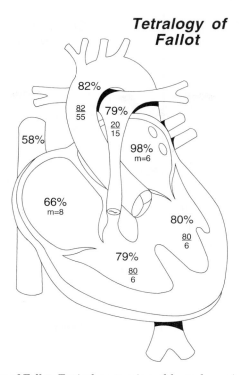

FIG. 25.9. Tetralogy of Fallot. Typical anatomic and hemodynamic findings include: (1) an anteriorly displaced infundibular septum, resulting in subpulmonary stenosis, a large ventricular septal defect, and overriding of the aorta over the muscular septum; (2) hypoplasia of the pulmonary valve, main, and branch pulmonary arteries; (3) equal right and left ventricular pressures; (4) a right-to-left shunt at ventricular level, with a systemic oxygen saturation of 82%.

5. **Ebstein anomaly** (see Figs. 25.10A and 25.10B) is an uncommon but grave anatomic lesion when presenting in the neonatal period. Anatomically there is "downward displacement" of the tricuspid valve into the body of the right ventricle. The tricuspid valve is frequently regurgitant resulting in marked right atrial enlargement and a large right-to-left shunt at the atrial level; there is little forward flow out the right ventricular outflow tract into the pulmonary circulation. The prognosis for neonates presenting with profound cyanosis due to Ebstein anomaly is quite grave. Surgical options are controversial and generally reserved for the severely symptomatic child. Further complicating the medical condition, Ebstein anomaly is often associated with Wolff-Parkinson-White syndrome and supraventricular tachycardia.

Medical management is aimed at supporting the neonate through the initial period of transitional circulation. Because of elevated pulmonary vascular resistance, pulmonary blood flow may be quite severely limited with profound hypoxemia and acidosis as a result. PGE_1 is used to maintain a patent ductus arteriosus; other measures to decrease pulmonary vascular resistance and promote antegrade pulmonary blood flow (such as a high level of supplemental oxygen and maintaining a mild respiratory alkalosis) are helpful. Recently, nitric oxide has been utilized with

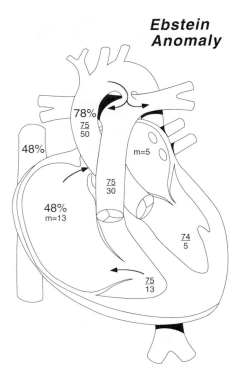

FIG. 25.10. A. Ebstein anomaly (with large nonrestrictive ductus arteriosus). Typical anatomic and hemodynamic findings include: (1) inferior displacement of the tricuspid valve into the right ventricle, which may also cause subpulmonary obstruction; (2) diminutive muscular right ventricle; (3) marked enlargement of the right atrium due to "atrialized" portion of right ventricle as well as tricuspid regurgitation; (4) right-to-left shunting at the atrial level (note arterial oxygen saturation of 78%); (5) a left-to-right shunt and pulmonary hypertension secondary to a large patent ductus arteriosus supplying the pulmonary blood flow; (6) low cardiac output (note low mixed venous oxygen saturation in the superior vena cava).

(continues)

limited success. An important contributor to the high mortality rate in the neonate with severe Ebstein anomaly is the associated pulmonary hypoplasia that is present (due to the massively enlarged right heart in utero, see Fig. 25.11).

C. Parallel circulation/transposition of the great arteries (see Fig. 25.11). Transposition of the great arteries is defined as an aorta arising from the morphologically right ventricle and the pulmonary artery from the morphologically left ventricle. Approximately one-half of all patients with transposition have an associated ventricular septal defect.

In the usual arrangement this creates a situation of "parallel circulations" with systemic venous return being pumped via the aorta back to the systemic circulation, and pulmonary venous return being pumped via the pulmonary artery to the pulmonary circulation. Following separation from the placenta, neonates with transposition are dependent on mixing between the parallel systemic and pulmonary circulations in order for them to survive. In patients with an intact ventricular septum, this communication exists through the patent ductus arteriosus and the patent foramen ovale. These

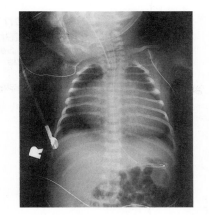

FIG. 25.10 B *(continued)*. Chest radiograph in a neonate with severe Ebstein anomaly and no significant pulmonary blood flow from the ductus arteriosus. The cardiomegaly is due to marked dilation of the right atrium. The pulmonary vascular markings are diminished due to the decreased pulmonary blood flow. Hypoplasia of the lungs is common due to the large heart causing a "space-occupying lesion".

patients are usually clinically cyanotic within the first hours of life leading to their early diagnosis. Those infants with an associated ventricular septal defect typically have somewhat improved mixing between the systemic and pulmonary circulations and may not be as severely cyanotic.

In neonates with transposition of the great arteries and an intact ventricular septum, a very low arterial PaO_2 (15 to 20 torr) with high $PaCO_2$ (despite adequate chest motion and ventilation) and metabolic acidosis are markers for severely decreased effective pulmonary blood flow and need urgent attention. The initial management of the severely hypoxemic patient with transposition includes (1) **ensure adequate mixing** between the two parallel circuits and (2) **maximize mixed venous oxygen saturation.**

In patients who do not respond with an increased arterial oxygen saturation to the opening of the ductus arteriosus with prostaglandin (usually these neonates have very restrictive atrial defects and/or pulmonary hypertension), **the foramen ovale should be emergently enlarged by balloon atrial septostomy.** Hyperventilation and treatment with sodium bicarbonate are important maneuvers to promote alkalosis, lower pulmonary vascular resistance, and increase pulmonary blood flow (which increases atrial mixing following septostomy).

In transposition of the great arteries, the majority of systemic blood flow is recirculated systemic venous return. In the presence of poor mixing, much can be gained by increasing the mixed venous oxygen saturation, which is the **major determinant of systemic arterial oxygen saturation.** These maneuvers include (1) decreasing the whole body oxygen consumption (muscle relaxants, sedation, mechanical ventilation) and (2) improving oxygen delivery (increase cardiac output with inotropic agents, increase oxygen-carrying capacity by treating anemia). Coexisting causes of pulmonary venous desaturation (e.g., pneumothorax) should also be sought and treated. Increasing the FiO_2 to 100% will have little effect on the arterial PO_2, unless it serves to lower pulmonary vascular resistance and increase pulmonary blood flow.

In the current era, definitive management is surgical correction with an arterial switch operation in the early neonatal period (7). If severe hypox-

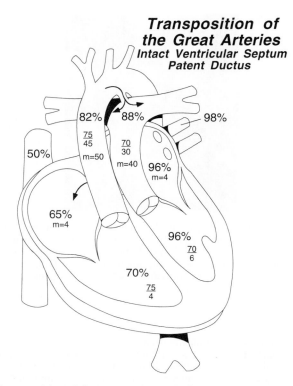

FIG. 25.11. Transposition of the great arteries with an intact ventricular septum, a large patent ductus arteriosus (on PGE_1) and atrial septal defect (status post balloon atrial septostomy). Note the following: (1) The aorta arises from the anatomic right ventricle, and the pulmonary artery from the anatomic left ventricle; (2) "transposition physiology," with a higher oxygen saturation in the pulmonary artery than in the aorta; (3) "mixing" between the parallel circulations (see text) at the atrial (after balloon atrial septostomy) and ductal levels; (4) shunting from the left atrium to the right atrium via the atrial septal defect (not shown) with equalization of atrial pressures; (5) shunting from the aorta to the pulmonary artery via the ductus arteriosus; (6) pulmonary hypertension due to a large ductus arteriosus.

emia persists despite medical management, mechanical support with extracorporeal membrane oxygenation (ECMO) or an urgent arterial switch operation may be indicated [9].
D. Lesions with complete intracardiac mixing
    1. Truncus arteriosus (see Fig. 25.12) consists of a single great artery arising from the heart, which gives rise to (in order) the coronary arteries, the pulmonary arteries, and the brachiocephalic arteries. The truncal valve is often anatomically abnormal (only 50% are tricuspid), and is frequently thickened, stenotic, and/or regurgitant. A coexisting ventricular septal defect is present in >98% of cases. The aortic arch is right-sided in approximately one-third of cases; other arch anomalies such as hypoplasia, coarctation and interruption are seen in 10% of cases. Extracardiac anomalies are present in 20 to 40% of cases. In a recent study, 34.5% of patients with truncus arteriosus had a small deletion of chromosome 22 at 22q11 (17).

Truncus Arteriosus
with Right Aortic Arch

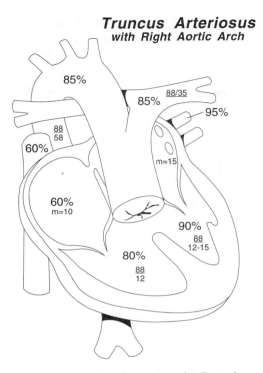

FIG. 25.12. Truncus arteriosus (with right aortic arch). Typical anatomic and hemodynamic findings include: (1) a single artery arises from the conotruncus giving rise to coronary arteries (not shown), pulmonary arteries, and brachiocephalic vessels; (2) abnormal truncal valve (quadricuspid shown) with stenosis and/or regurgitation common; (3) right-sided aortic arch (occurs in ≈30% of cases); (4) large conoventricular ventricular septal defect; (5) pulmonary artery hypertension with a large left-to-right shunt (note superior vena cava oxygen saturation of 60% and pulmonary artery oxygen saturation of 85%); (6) complete mixing (of the systemic and pulmonary venous return) occurs at the great vessel level.

The overwhelming majority of infants with truncus arteriosus present with symptoms of congestive heart failure in the first weeks of life. The infants may be somewhat cyanotic, but congestive heart failure symptoms and signs are usually dominant. The pulmonary blood flow is increased, with significant pulmonary hypertension common. The natural history of truncus arteriosus is quite bleak. Left unrepaired, only 15 to 30% survive the first year of life. Furthermore, in survivors of the immediate neonatal period, the occurrence of accelerated irreversible pulmonary vascular disease is common, making surgical repair in the neonatal period (or as soon as the diagnosis is made) the treatment of choice. "Medical management" of heart failure would be considered only a temporizing measure until surgical correction can be accomplished.

2. **Total anomalous pulmonary venous connection** (see Figs. 25.13A and 25.13B) occurs when all pulmonary veins drain into the systemic venous system with complete mixing of pulmonary and systemic venous return usually in the right atrium. The systemic blood flow is thus dependent on

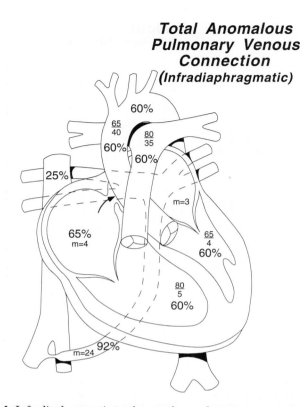

Total Anomalous Pulmonary Venous Connection
(Infradiaphragmatic)

FIG. 25.13. A. Infradiaphragmatic total anomalous pulmonary venous connection. Note the following: (1) pulmonary venous confluence does not connect with the left atrium, but descends to connect with the portal circulation below the diaphragm. This connection is frequently severely obstructed; (2) obstruction to pulmonary venous return results in significantly elevated pulmonary venous pressures, decreased pulmonary blood flow, pulmonary edema, and pulmonary venous desaturation (92%); (3) systemic to suprasystemic pressure in the pulmonary artery (in the absence of a patent ductus arteriosus, pulmonary artery pressures may exceed systemic pressures when severe pulmonary venous obstruction is present); (4) all systemic blood flow must be derived via a right-to-left shunt at the foramen ovale; (5) nearly equal oxygen saturations in all chambers of the heart (i.e., complete mixing at right atrial level), with severe hypoxemia (systemic oxygen saturation 60%) and low cardiac output (mixed venous oxygen saturation 25%).

(continues)

an obligate shunt through the patent foramen ovale into the left heart. The anomalous connections of the pulmonary veins may be (1) supracardiac (usually into the right superior vena cava or to the innominate vein via a persistent vertical vein); (2) cardiac (usually to the right atrium or coronary sinus); (3) subdiaphragmatic (usually into the portal system); or (4) mixed drainage.

In patients with total connection below the diaphragm, the pathway is frequently obstructed with severely limited pulmonary blood flow, pulmonary hypertension, and profound cyanosis. This form of total anomalous pulmonary venous connection is a surgical emergency, with minimal beneficial effects from medical management. Although PGE$_1$ will maintain ductal

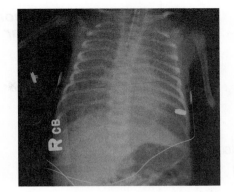

FIG. 25.13 B. *(continued)* Chest radiograph in a 16-hour-old neonate with severe infra-diaphragmatic obstruction to pulmonary venous return. Note the pulmonary edema, small heart, and hyperinflated lungs (on mechanical ventilation). Despite high inflating and positive end-expiratory pressures and an FiO_2 of 1.0, the arterial blood gas revealed a pH of 7.02, arterial carbon dioxide tension ($PaCO_2$) of 84, and an arterial oxygen tension (PaO_2) of 23 torr. Emergent surgical management is indicated.

patency, the limitation of pulmonary blood flow in these patients is **not** due to limited antegrade flow into the pulmonary circuit, but rather due to outflow obstruction at the pulmonary veins. In the current era of prostaglandin, ventilatory support, and advanced medical intensive care, obstructed total anomalous pulmonary venous connection represents one of the few remaining lesions that requires emergent, "middle of the night" surgical intervention. Early recognition of the problem (see Fig. 25.13B) and prompt surgical intervention (surgical anastomosis of the pulmonary venous confluence to the left atrium) are necessary in order for the infant to survive. Patients with a mild degree of obstruction typically have minimal symptoms, with many neonates escaping recognition until later in infancy.

3. **Complex single ventricles.** There are multiple complex anomalies that share the common physiology of complete mixing of the systemic and pulmonary venous return, frequently with anomalous connections of the systemic and/or pulmonary veins, and with obstruction to one of the great vessels (usually the pulmonary artery). In cases with associated polysplenia or asplenia and abnormalities of visceral situs, the term "heterotaxy syndrome" is frequently applied. It is beyond the scope of this chapter to define this heterogeneous group of patients, though all will fail a hyperoxia test, most have significantly abnormal ECGs, and the diagnosis of complex congenital heart disease is rarely in doubt (even before anatomic confirmation with echocardiography). As there is complete mixing of venous return and essentially a single pumping chamber, initial management is similar to that described for hypoplastic left heart syndrome (see V.A.4).

E. **Left-to right-shunt lesions.** For the most part, infants with pure left-to-right shunt lesions are not diagnosed because of severe systemic illness, but rather due to the finding of a murmur or symptoms of congestive heart failure usually occurring in the late neonatal period or beyond. The lesion of this group most likely to require attention in the neonatal nursery is that of a patent ductus arteriosus.

1. **Patent ductus arteriosus** is not particularly common in term newborns and rarely causes congestive heart failure. However, the frequency that a premature neonate will develop a hemodynamically significant left-to-

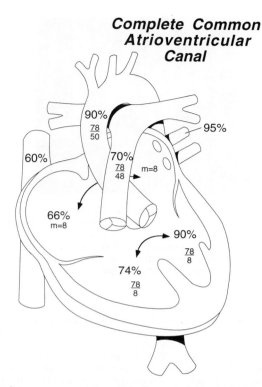

Complete Common Atrioventricular Canal

FIG. 25.14. Complete common atrioventricular canal. Typical anatomic and hemodynamic findings include: (1) large atrial and ventricular septal defects of the endocardial cushion type; (2) single, atrioventricular valve; (3) pulmonary artery hypertension (due to large ventricular septal defect); (4) bidirectional shunting (with mild hypoxemia) at atrial and ventricular level when pulmonary vascular resistance is elevated in the initial neonatal period. With subsequent fall in pulmonary vascular resistance, the shunt becomes predominantly left-to-right with symptoms of congestive heart failure.

right shunt through a patent ductus arteriosus is inversely proportional to advancing gestational age and weight (12).

The typical presentation of a patent ductus arteriosus begins with a harsh systolic ejection murmur heard over the entire precordium, but loudest at the left upper sternal border and left infraclavicular areas. As the pulmonary vascular resistance decreases, the intensity of the murmur increases and later becomes continuous (i.e., extends through the second heart sound). The peripheral pulses increase in amplitude ("bounding pulses"), the pulse pressure widens to greater than 25 mm Hg, the precordial impulse becomes hyperdynamic, and the patient's respiratory status deteriorates (manifesting as tachypnea or apnea, carbon dioxide retention, and an increasing mechanical ventilation requirement). Serial chest X rays show an increase in heart size and the lungs may appear more radiopaque.

It is important to remember that this typical progression of clinical signs is **not specific** only for a hemodynamically significant patent ductus arteriosus. Other lesions may produce bounding pulses, a hyperdynamic precordium, and cardiac enlargement (e.g., an arteriovenous fistula or an aorticopulmonary window). Generally, however, the clinical assessment of a premature infant with the typical findings of a hemodynamically significant ductus is adequate to guide therapeutic decisions. If the diagnosis is in doubt, an echocardiogram will clarify the anatomic diagnosis.

Initial medical management includes increased ventilatory support, fluid restriction, and diuretic therapy. In symptomatic patients, indomethacin is initially used for nonsurgical closure of patent ductus arteriosus in the premature neonate, and is effective in approximately 80% of case (16). Birth weight does not affect the efficacy of indomethacin, and there is no increase in complications associated with surgery after unsuccessful indomethacin therapy (16). In asymptomatic patients, the efficacy of prophylactic administration of indomethacin is controversial. Adverse reactions to indomethacin include transient oliguria, electrolyte abnormalities, decreased platelet function, and hypoglycemia. Contraindications to use of indomethacin and dosing information is noted in the Appendix.

Indications for closure of a patent ductus arteriosus vary from institution to institution. In general, we recommend treatment for mechanically ventilated premature infants weighing less than 1000 g when a patent ductus first becomes apparent, regardless of the presence of signs or symptoms of a significant left-to-right shunt. For infants larger than 1000 g, we recommend treatment with indomethacin only after cardiovascular or respiratory signs of a hemodynamically significant ductus develop. Some infants who fail to respond to the first course of treatment with indomethacin may respond to a second course.

Symptomatic patients who do not respond to a second treatment with indomethacin should undergo surgical ligation following echocardiographic documentation of the patent ductus. Although ligation through a left lateral thoracotomy remains the standard surgical approach, recent reports of minimally invasive, video-assisted thoracoscopic techniques show promise in selected newborns (6).

2. **Complete atrioventricular canal** (see Fig. 25.14) consists of a combination of defects in the (1) endocardial portion of the atrial septum, (2) the inlet portion of the ventricular septum, and (3) a common, single atrioventricular valve. Because of the large net left-to-right shunt, which increases as the pulmonary vascular resistance falls, these infants typically present early in life with congestive heart failure. There may be some degree of cyanosis as well, particularly in the immediate neonatal period before the pulmonary vascular resistance has fallen. In the absence of associated right ventricular outflow tract obstruction, pulmonary artery pressures are at systemic levels; pulmonary vascular resistance is frequently elevated, particularly in patients with Trisomy 21.

Nearly 70% of infants with complete atrioventricular canal have Trisomy 21; notation of the phenotypic findings of Down syndrome often lead to evaluation of the patient for possible congenital heart disease (see Table 25.5). In the immediate neonatal period, these infants may have an equivocal hyperoxia test since there may be some right to left shunting through the large intracardiac connections. Symptoms of congestive failure ensue during the first weeks of life as the pulmonary vascular resistance falls and the patient develops a marked left-to-right shunt. These patients have a characteristic ECG finding of a "superior axis" (QRS axis from 0 to −180 degrees; see Fig. 25.15) which can be a useful clue for the presence of congenital heart disease in an infant with Trisomy 21.

Most patients with complete atrioventricular canal will require medical treatment for symptomatic congestive heart failure with Digoxin and diuretics, though prolonged medical therapy in patients with failure to thrive and symptomatic heart failure is not warranted. Complete surgical

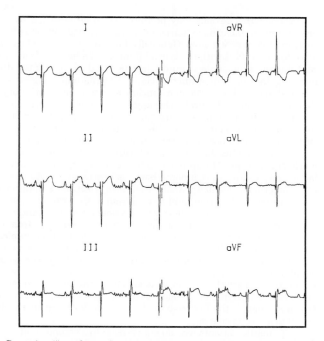

FIG. 25.15. Superior ("northwest") axis as seen on the electrocardiogram (only frontal plane leads shown) in a newborn with complete atrioventricular canal. Note the initial upward deflection of the QRS complex (and subsequent predominantly negative deflection) in leads I and aVF. A superior axis (0 to 180 degrees) is present in 95% of patients with endocardial cushion defects.

repair is undertaken electively in the first year of life, with earlier repair in symptomatic patients. In our experience, corrective surgery for complete atrioventricular canal can be performed successfully in early infancy with good results (7).

3. **Ventricular septal defect** is the most common cause of congestive heart failure after the initial neonatal period. Moderate to large ventricular septal defects become hemodynamically significant as the pulmonary vascular resistance decreases and pulmonary blood flow increases due to a left-to-right shunt across the defect. As this usually takes 2 to 4 weeks to develop, term neonates with ventricular septal defect and symptoms of congestive heart failure should be investigated for coexisting anatomic abnormalities, such as left ventricular outflow tract obstruction, coarctation of the aorta, or patent ductus arteriosus. Premature infants, who have a lower initial pulmonary vascular resistance, may develop clinical symptoms of heart failure earlier or require longer mechanical ventilation compared with term infants.

Ventricular septal defects may occur anywhere in the ventricular septum and are usually classified by their location (see Fig. 25.16). Defects in the membranous septum are the most common type. The diagnosis of ventricular septal defect is usually initially suspected on physical exam of the infant; echocardiography confirms the diagnosis and localizes the defect in the ventricular septum. Since a large number (as many as 50% depending on the anatomic type) of ventricular septal defects may close spontaneously in the first months of life, surgery is usually deferred be-

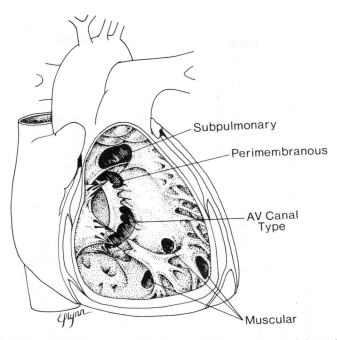

Subpulmonary

Perimembranous

AV Canal
Type

Muscular

FIG. 25.16. Diagram of types of ventricular septal defects as viewed from the right ventricle. (From Fyler D.C. *Nadas' Pediatric Cardiology,* with permission).

yond the neonatal period. In large series, only 15% of all patients with ventricular septal defects ever become clinically symptomatic. Medical management of congestive heart failure includes digoxin, diuretics, and caloric supplementation. Growth failure is the most common symptom of congestive heart failure not fully compensated by medical management. When it occurs, failure to thrive is an indication for surgical repair of the defect.

F. **Cardiac surgery in the neonate.** In the past, because of the perceived high risk of open heart surgery early in life, critically ill neonates were mostly subjected to palliative procedures or prolonged medical management. The unrepaired circulation and residual hemodynamic abnormalities frequently resulted in secondary problems to the heart, lungs, brain, as well as more nonspecific problems of failure to thrive, frequent hospitalizations, and infections. In addition, there are difficult to quantitate psychological burdens to the family of a chronically ill infant.

Low birth weight should not be considered an absolute contraindication for surgical repair. In a recent series, prolonged medical therapy in low-birth-weight infants to achieve further weight gain in the presence of a significant hemodynamic burden did not appear to improve the survival rate, and prolonged intensive-care management was associated with nosocomial complication (8). We feel that the symptomatic neonate with congenital heart disease should be repaired as early as possible, to prevent the secondary sequelae of the congenital lesion on the heart, lungs, and brain (7).

Recently, improvements in surgical techniques, cardiopulmonary bypass, and intensive care of the neonate and infant have resulted in significant improvements in surgical mortality and quality of life in the survivors. It is beyond the scope of this chapter to describe the multiple surgical procedures

TABLE 25.9. COMMON NEONATAL OPERATIONS AND THEIR EARLY SEQUELAE

Lesion	Surgical Repair (Eponym)	Early Postoperative Sequelae	
		Common	Rare
Corrective procedures			
TGA	Arterial switch procedure (Jatene) 1. Division and reanastomosis of PA and aorta to anatomically-correct ventricle 2. Translocation of coronary arteries 3. Closure of septal defects if present	Transient decrease in cardiac output 6–12 hours after surgery	Coronary ostial stenosis or occlusion/sudden death Hemidiaphragm paresis Chylothorax
	Atrial switch procedure (Senning or Mustard) 1. Intraatrial baffling of systemic venous return to LV (to PA) and pulmonary venous return to RV (to AO) 2. Closure of septal defects if present	Supraventricular tachycardia Sick sinus syndrome Tricuspid regurgitation	Pulmonary or systemic venous obstruction
TOF	1. Patch closure of VSD via ventriculotomy or right atrium 2. Enlargement of RVOT with infundibular patch or muscle bundle resection 3. ±Pulmonary valvotomy 4. ±Transannular RV to PA patch 5. ±RV to PA conduit	Pulmonary regurgitation (if transannular patch, valvotomy, or nonvalved conduit) Transient RV dysfunction Right-to-left shunt via PFO, usually resolves postoperatively as RV function improves	Residual left-to-right shunt at VSD patch Residual RVOT obstruction Junctional ectopic tachycardia Complete heart block

446

Lesion	Procedure	Physiologic consequences	Complications
COA	Resection with end-to-end anastomosis, or Subclavian flap (Waldhaussen), or Patch augmentation	Systemic hypertension Absent left-arm pulse (if Waldhaussen)	Ileus Hemidiaphragm paresis Vocal cord paresis Chylothorax
PDA	Ligation (±division) of PDA using open thoracotomy and direct visualization or video-assisted thoracoscopic visualization	—	Hemidiaphragm paresis Vocal cord paresis Chylothorax Interruption of left PA or descending aorta
TAPVC	1. Reanastomosis of pulmonary venous confluence to posterior aspect of left atrium 2. Division of connecting vein	Pulmonary hypertension Transient low cardiac output	Residual pulmonary venous obstruction
Truncus arteriosus	1. Closure of VSD; baffling LV to truncus (neoaorta) 2. Removal of PAs from truncus 3. Conduit placement from RV to PAs	Reactive pulmonary hypertension Transient RV dysfunction with right-to-left shunt via PFO Hypocalcemia (DiGeorge syndrome)	Truncal valve stenosis or regurgitation Residual VSD Complete heart block
Palliative procedures HLHS*	Stage I (Norwood) 1. Connection of main PA to aorta with reconstruction of aortic arch 2. Systemic-to-pulmonary shunt 3. Atrial septectomy	Low systemic cardiac output due to excessive pulmonary blood flow	Aortic arch obstruction Restrictive atrial septal defect
Complex lesions with decreased pulmonary blood flow*	Systemic-to-pulmonary shunt (using prosthetic tube = modified Blalock-Taussig shunt; using subclavian artery = classic Blalock-Taussig shunt)	Excessive pulmonary blood flow and mild congestive heart failure	Hemidiaphragm paresis Vocal cord paralysis Chylothorax Seroma

(continues)

TABLE 25.9. *(Continued)*

Lesion	Surgical Repair (Eponym)	Early Postoperative Sequelae	
		Common	Rare
Complex lesions with excessive pulmonary blood flow*	Ligation of main PA, creation of systemic-to-pulmonary shunt PA band (prosthetic or Silastic constriction of main PA)	—	PA distortion Aneurysm of main PA

TGA = transposition of the great arteries; LV = left ventricle; PA = pulmonary artery; RV = right ventricle; AO = aorta; TOF = tetralogy of Fallot; VSD = ventricular septal defect; RVOT = right ventricular outflow tract; PFO = patent foramen ovale; COA = coarctation of the aorta; PDA = patient ductus arteriosus; TAPVC = total anomalous pulmonary venous connection; HLHS = hypoplastic left heart syndrome.

*In patients with a single ventricle, the goal is to separate pulmonary and systemic venous return, rerouting systemic venous blood directly to pulmonary arteries (Fontan operation) though this is done in late infancy or early childhood.

Source: Adapted from Wernovsky G., Erickson L. C., Wessel D. L., Cardiac Emergencies. In: May H. L. (Ed.), *Emergency Medicine.* 1992; Boston: Little, Brown.

currently employed in the management of congenital heart disease; the reader is referred to Table 25.11 and general texts of cardiac surgery (7,19).

VI. **Acquired heart disease**

   A. **Myocarditis** may occur in the neonate as an isolated illness or as a component of a generalized illness with associated hepatitis and/or encephalitis. Myocarditis is usually the result of a viral infection (coxsackie, rubella, and varicella are most common), though other infectious agents such as bacteria and fungi as well as noninfectious conditions such as autoimmune diseases also may cause myocarditis. Although the clinical presentation (and in some cases endomyocardial biopsy) makes the diagnosis, specific identification of the etiologic agent is currently not made in most cases. However, recent improvements in molecular biology techniques (polymerase chain reactions for viral-specific RNA) may improve the frequency of accurate identification of viral pathogens in the future.

   The infant with acute myocarditis presents with signs and symptoms of congestive heart failure (see III.B.1) or arrhythmia (see VIII). The course of the illness is frequently fulminant and fatal; however, full recovery of ventricular function may occur if the infant can be supported and survive the acute illness. Supportive care including supplemental oxygen, diuretics, inotropic agents, afterload reduction, and mechanical ventilation is frequently used. In severe cases, mechanical support of the myocardium with extracorporeal membrane oxygenation or ventricular assist devices can be considered. Care should be used when administering digoxin, due to the potential for the potentiation of arrhythmias or complete heart block.

   B. **Transient myocardial ischemia** with myocardial dysfunction may occur in any neonate with a history of perinatal asphyxia. Myocardial dysfunction may be associated with maternal autoimmune disease such as systemic lupus erythematosus. A tricuspid or mitral regurgitant murmur is often heard. An elevated serum creatine kinase MB fraction or cardiac troponin level may be helpful in determining the presence of myocardial damage. Supportive treatment is dictated by the severity of myocardial dysfunction.

   C. **Hypertrophic and dilated cardiomyopathies** represent a rare and multifactorial complex of diseases, complete discussion of which is beyond the scope of this chapter. The differential diagnoses includes primary diseases (e.g., metabolic and storage disorders, "idiopathic") or secondary diseases (e.g., end-stage infection, ischemic, endocrine, neuromuscular, nutritional, drugs, etc.) The reader is referred to texts of pediatric cardiology (4,15).

   The most common hypertrophic cardiomyopathy presenting in neonates is that type seen in **infants born to diabetic mothers.** Echocardiographically and hemodynamically, these infants are indistinguishable from patients with the familial form of hypertrophic cardiomyopathy. They are different in one important respect: their cardiomyopathy will completely resolve in 6 to 12 months. Noting a systolic ejection murmur, with or without congestive heart failure, in the infant of a diabetic mother should raise the question of congenital heart disease including hypertrophic cardiomyopathy. Treatment is supportive addressing the infant's particular symptoms of congestive heart failure. Propranolol has been used successfully in some patients with severe obstruction. Most patients require no specific care and no long-term cardiac follow-up.

VII. **Pharmacology**

   A. **Prostaglandin E$_1$.** PGE$_1$ has been used since the late 1970s to pharmacologically maintain patency of the ductus arteriosus in patients with duct-dependent systemic or pulmonary blood flow. PGE$_1$ must be administered as a continuous parenteral infusion. The usual starting dose is 0.05 to 0.1 µg/kg per minute. Once a therapeutic effect has been achieved, the dose may often be decreased to as low as 0.025 µg/kg per minute without loss of therapeutic effect. The response to PGE$_1$ is often immediate if patency of the ductus is important for the hemodynamic state of the infant. Failure to respond to PGE$_1$ may mean that the initial diagnosis was incorrect, the ductus is unresponsive to PGE_1 (usually only in an older infant), or the ductus is absent. The infusion site has no significant effect on the ductal response to PGE_1. Adverse reactions to PGE_1 include apnea (10 to 12%), fever (14%), seizures (4%), cutaneous flushing (10%), bradycardia (7%), tachycardia (3%), cardiac arrest (1%), and edema (1%). See Table 25.10 for recommended mixing and dosing protocol for PGE_1.

B. **Sympathomimetic amine infusions** are the mainstay of pharmacologic therapies aimed at improving cardiac output and are discussed in detail elsewhere. Catecholamines, endogenous (dopamine, epinephrine), or synthetic (dobutamine, isoproterenol), achieve an effect by stimulating myocardial and vascular adrenergic receptors. These agents must be given as a continuous parenteral infusion. They may be given in combination to the critically ill neonate in an effort to maximize the positive effects of each agent while minimizing the negative effects. While receiving catecholamine infusions, patients should be closely monitored, usually with an electrocardiographic monitor and an arterial catheter. Prior to beginning sympathomimetic amine infusions, intravascular volume should be repleted if necessary, though this may further compromise a congenital lesion with coexisting volume overload. Adverse reactions to catecholamine infusions include tachycardia (which increases myocardial oxygen consumption), atrial and ventricular arrhythmias, and increased afterload due to peripheral vasoconstriction (which may decrease cardiac output). See Table 25.11 for recommended mixing and dosing of the sympathomimetic amines.

C. **Afterload reducing agents**

1. **Phosphodiesterase inhibitors** such as **amrinone** and **milrinone** are **bipyridine** compounds that selectively inhibit cyclic nucleotide phosphodiesterase. These nonglycosidic and nonsympathomimetic agents exert their effect on cardiac performance by increasing cyclic adenosine monophosphate (cAMP) in the myocardial and vascular muscle, but do so independently of β-receptors. Cyclic AMP promotes improved contraction via calcium regulation through two mechanisms: (1) activation of protein kinase [which catalyzes the transfer of phosphate groups from adenosine triphosphate (ATP)] leading to faster calcium entry through the calcium channels, and (2) activation of calcium pumps in the sarcoplasmic reticulum resulting in release of calcium.

There are three major effects of phosphodiesterase inhibitors: (1) increased inotropy, with increased contractility and cardiac output as a result of cAMP-mediated increase in trans-sarcolemmal calcium flux; (2) vasodilatation, with increase in arteriolar and venous capacitance as a result of cAMP-mediated increase in uptake of calcium and decrease in calcium available for contraction; and (3) increased lusitropy, or improved

TABLE 25.10. SUGGESTED PREPARATION OF PROSTAGLANDIN E$_1$

Add 1 Ampule (500 μg) to:	Concentration (μg/ml)	ml/hr × Weight (kg), Needed to infuse 0.1 μg/kg/min
200 ml	2.5	2.4
100 ml*	5	1.2
50 ml	10	0.6

*Usually the most convenient dilution, provides one-fourth of maintenance fluid requirement. Usually mix in dextrose-containing solution for newborns.
Source: Adapted from Warnovsky G., Erickson L. C., Wessel D. L. Cardiac Emergencies. In: May H. L. (Ed.), *Emergency Medicine.* 1992; Boston: Little, Brown.

TABLE 25.11. SYMPATHOMIMETIC AMINES

Drug	Usual Dose (μg/kg/min)	Effect
Dopamine	1–5	↑ urine output,↑ HR (slightly), ↑ contractility
	6–10	↑ HR, ↑ contractility,↑ BP
	11–20	↑ HR, ↑ contractility, ↑ SVR, ↑ BP
Dobutamine	1–20	↑ HR (slightly), ↑ contractility, ↓ SVR
Epinephrine	0.05–0.50	↑ HR, ↑ contractility, ↑ SVR, ↑ BP
Isoproterenol	0.05–1.00	↑ HR,↑ contractility, ↓ SVR, ↓ PVR

These infusions may be mixed in intravenous solutions containing dextrose and/or saline. For neonates, dextrose-containing solutions with or without salt should usually be chosen. Calculation for convenient preparation of IV infusions:

$$6 \times \frac{\text{desired dose } (\mu g/kg/min)}{\text{desired rate (ml/hr)}} \times \text{weight (kg)} = \frac{\text{mg drug}}{100 \text{ ml fluid}}$$

HR = heart rate; BP = blood pressure; SVR = systemic vascular resistance; PVR = pulmonary vascular resistance.

relaxation properties during diastole. There appear to be differences between the immature and adult myocardium in the handling of amrinone. One study suggested that neonates and infants require a higher loading dose (3 to 4.5 mg/kg) than adults to achieve adequate serum levels (20). Clinical experience with amrinone suggests that a continuous infusion of 5 to 15 ug/kg per minute is effective.

Indications include low cardiac output with myocardial dysfunction and elevated systemic vascular resistance not accompanied by severe hypotension. Side effects have been minimal and are typically (1) the need for volume infusions (5 to 10 cc/kg) following bolus (>2 mg/kg) administration and (2) occasional thrombocytopenia following prolonged amrinone (>7 to 10 days) use.

The use of phosphodiesterase inhibitors after cardiac surgery in the pediatric patient population has been shown to increase cardiac index and decrease systemic vascular resistance without a significant increase in heart rate. Despite successful application of amrinone treatment in adults and children with myocardial failure, some have avoided its use due to concerns of potential side effects and its relatively long biologic half-life. However, following successful clinical trials, phosphodiesterase inhibitors have now become the second line drug (after dopamine) in the treatment of low cardiac output in neonates, infants, and children following cardiopulmonary bypass in our institution.

2. **Other vasodilators** improve low cardiac output principally by decreasing impedance to ventricular ejection; these effects are especially helpful after cardiac surgery in children and in adults when systemic vascular resistance is particularly elevated.

Sodium nitroprusside is the most widely used afterload reducing agent. It acts as a nitric oxide donor, increasing intracellular cyclic guanosine monophosphate (cGMP), which effects relaxation of vascular smooth muscle in both arterioles and veins. The overall effect is a decrease in atrial filling pressure and systemic vascular resistance with a concomitant increase in cardiac output. The vasodilatory effects of nitroprusside occur within minutes with intravenous administration. The principal metabolites of sodium nitroprusside are thiocyanate and cyanide; thiocyanate toxicity is unusual in children with normal hepatic and renal function, and monitoring of cyanide and thiocyanate concentrations in children may not be correlated with clinical signs of toxicity.

In neonates with low cardiac output, there may be an increase in urine output and improvement in perfusion with institution of nitroprusside, but there can also be a significant drop in blood pressure necessitating care in its use.

Many other agents have been used as arterial and venous vasodilators to treat hypertension, reduce ventricular afterload and systemic vascular resistance (SVR), and improve cardiac output. A second nitrovasodilator, **nitroglycerine**, principally **a venous dilator**, also has rapid onset of action and a short half-life (about 2 minutes). Tolerance may develop after several days of continuous infusion. Nitroglycerine is used extensively in adult cardiac units for patients with ischemic heart disease; experience in pediatric patients is more limited. **Hydralazine** is more typically used for acute hypertension; its relatively long half-life limits its use in postoperative patients with labile hemodynamics. The angiotensin converting enzyme inhibitor **enalaprilat** similarly has a relatively long half-life (2 to 4 hours) which limits its use in the acute setting. **Beta-blockers** (e.g., propranolol, esmolol, labetolol), although excellent in reducing blood pressure, may have deleterious effects on ventricular function. **Calcium channel blockers** (e.g., verapamil) may cause acute and severe hypotension and bradycardia in the neonate and should **rarely be used.** All intravenous vasodilators must be used cautiously in patients with moderate to severe lung disease; their use has been associated with increased intrapulmonary shunting and acute reductions of PaO_2.

D. **Digoxin** (See Appendix A) remains important for the treatment of congestive heart failure. Term infants can begin initial treatment (a "digitalizing dose") with a total dose of 30 μg/kg in 24 hours; premature infants can usually be effectively digitalized with a total dose of 20 μg/kg in 24 hours. One-half of this **total digitalizing dose (TDD)** may be given IV, IM, or PO, followed by one-fourth of the TDD every 8 to 12 hours for the remaining two doses. An initial maintenance dose of one-fourth to one-third of the TDD (range 5 to 10 μg/kg per day) may then be adjusted according to the patient's clinical response, renal function, and tolerance for the drug (see Table 25.12). Alternatively, infants with mild symptoms, primary myocardial disease, renal dysfunction, or the potential for atrioventricular block may be digitalized using only the maintenance dose (omitting the loading dose).

Digoxin toxicity most commonly manifests with gastrointestinal upset, somnolence, and sinus bradycardia. More severe digoxin toxicity may cause high-grade atrioventricular block and ventricular ectopy. Infants suspected of having digoxin toxicity should have a digoxin level drawn and further doses withheld. The therapeutic level is <1.5 ng/mL with probable toxicity occurring at levels >4.0 ng/mL. In infants particularly, however, digoxin levels do not always correlate well with therapeutic efficacy nor with toxicity.

Digoxin toxicity in neonates is usually manageable by withholding further doses until the signs of toxicity resolve and by correcting electrolyte abnormalities (such as hypokalemia), which can potentiate toxic effects. Severe ventricular arrhythmias associated with digoxin toxicity may be managed

TABLE 25.12. DIGOXIN DOSAGE

	Total Digitalizing Dose	Maintenance[a]
Premature infants	20 μg/kg	5 μg/kg/day
Term infants	30 μg/kg	3–10 μg/kg/day

[a]Usually the maintenance dose is divided into equal twice-daily doses 12 hours apart.

with phenytoin, 2 to 4 mg/kg over 5 minutes, or lidocaine, 1 mg/kg loading dose, followed by an infusion at 1 to 2 mg/kg per hour. Atrioventricular block is usually unresponsive to atropine. Severe bradycardia may be refractory to these therapies and require temporary cardiac pacing.

The use of digoxin-specific antibody Fab (antigen-binding fragments) preparation (Digibind; Burroughs Wellcome) is reserved for those patient with evidence of severe digoxin intoxication and clinical symptoms of refractory arrhythmia and/or atrioventricular block; in these patients it is quite effective (23). Calculation of the Digibind dose in milligrams is as follows: (serum digoxin concentration in nanograms per milliliter × 5.6 × the body weight in kilograms/1000) × 64. The dose is given as a one-time intravenous infusion. A second dose of Digibind may be given in those patients who continue to have clinical evidence of residual Digoxin toxicity. Skin testing for hypersensitivity is recommended prior to the first dose.

E. **Diuretics** (see Appendix A) are frequently used in patients with congestive heart failure usually in combination with Digoxin. **Furosemide,** 1 to 2 mg/kg per dose, usually results in a brisk diuresis within an hour of administration. If no response is noted in an hour, a second dose (double the first dose) may be given. Chronic use of furosemide may produce urinary-tract stones as a result of its calciuric effects. A more potent diuretic effect may be achieved using a combination of a thiazide and a "loop" diuretic such as furosemide. Combination diuretic therapy may be complicated by hyponatremia and hypokalemia. Oral or intravenous potassium supplementation (3 to 4 mEq/kg per day) or an aldosterone antagonist usually should accompany the use of thiazide or "loop" diuretics to avoid excessive potassium wasting. It is important to carefully monitor serum potassium and sodium levels when beginning or changing the dose of diuretic medications. When changing from an effective parenteral to oral dose of furosemide, the dose should be increased by 50 to 80%. Furosemide may increase the nephro- and ototoxicity of concurrently used aminoglycoside antibiotics. Detailed discussion of alternative diuretics (e.g., chlorothiazide, spironolactone, etc.) is found elsewhere in the text (see Appendix A).

VIII. **Arrhythmias**
A. **Initial evaluation.** When evaluating any infant with an arrhythmia it is essential to simultaneously assess the electrophysiology and hemodynamic status. If the baby is poorly perfused and/ or hypotensive, reliable intravenous access should be secured and a level of resuscitation employed appropriate for the degree of illness. As always, **emergency treatment of shock should precede definitive diagnosis.** It should be emphasized, however, there is **rarely** a situation in which it is justified to omit a 12-lead ECG from the evaluation of an infant with an arrhythmia, the exceptions being ventricular fibrillation or torsade de pointes with accompanying hemodynamic instability. These arrhythmias frequently require immediate defibrillation but are extremely rare arrhythmias in neonates and young infants.

In nearly all circumstances, appropriate therapy (short- and long-term) depends on an accurate electrophysiologic diagnosis. Determination of the mechanism of a rhythm disturbance is most often made from a 12-lead ECG in the abnormal rhythm compared to the patient's baseline 12-lead ECG in sinus rhythm. Although rhythm strips generated from a cardiac monitor can be helpful supportive evidence of the final diagnosis, they are typically **not** diagnostic and should **not** be the only documentation of arrhythmia if at all possible.

The three broad categories for arrhythmias in neonates are (1) tachyarrhythmias, (2) bradyarrhythmias, and (3) irregular rhythms. An algorithm for approaching the differential diagnosis can be consulted (see Fig. 25.17) in most cases. When analyzing the ECG for the mechanism of arrhythmia, a stepwise approach should be taken in three main areas: (1) **rate** (variability, too fast, or too slow); (2) **rhythm** (regular or irregular, paroxysmal or gradual); and (3) *QRS morphology.*

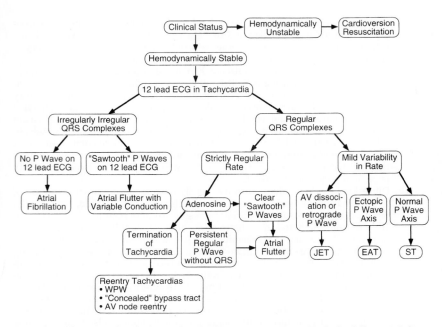

FIG. 25.17. Algorithm for analysis of arrhythmias in neonates. Bedside differential diagnosis of narrow complex tachycardias in neonates, the most common type of arrhythmia in this age group. Note that, regardless of the mechanism of tachycardia, if the patient is hemodynamically unstable, immediate measures to resuscitate the infant including cardioversion are required. Also, treatment with adenosine is helpful therapeutically as well as diagnostically. In general, tachycardias that terminate (even briefly) after adenosine are of the reentry type. JET = junctional ectopic tachycardia; EAT = ectopic atrial tachycardia; ST = sinus tachycardia; WPW = Wolff-Parkinson-White syndrome.

B. Differential diagnosis and initial management
1. Narrow QRS complex tachycardias
a. Supraventricular tachycardias (SVT) are the most common symptomatic arrhythmias in all children including neonates. SVTs usually have (1) a rate greater than 200 beats per minute, frequently "fixed" with no beat-to-beat variation in rate; (2) rapid onset and termination (in reentrant rhythms); and (3) normal ventricular complexes on the surface ECG. The infant may initially be asymptomatic, but later may become irritable, fussy, and refuse feedings. Congestive heart failure usually does not develop prior to 24 hours of continuous SVT; however, heart failure is seen in 20% of patients after 36 hours and in 50% after 48 hours.

SVT in the neonate is almost always "reentrant," involving either an accessory atrioventricular pathway and the atrioventricular node, or due to atrial flutter. About half of these patients will manifest preexcitation (delta wave) on the ECG when not in tachycardia [Wolff-Parkinson-White (WPW) syndrome, Fig. 25.18]. In rarer cases, the reentrant circuit may be within the atrium itself (atrial flutter) or within the atrial ventricular (A-V) node (A-V node reentrant tachycardia). Patients with SVT may have associated structural heart disease; evaluation for structural heart disease should be considered in all neonates with SVT. Another rare cause of supraventricular tachycardias in a neonate is ectopic atrial

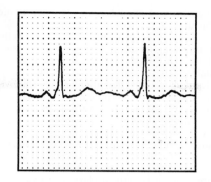

FIG. 25.18. Wolff-Parkinson-White syndrome. Note the characteristic "slurred" initial QRS deflection and short PR interval in leads I, Avr, and aVL in this electrocardiogram (frontal leads only pictured).

tachycardia, in which the distinguishing features are an abnormal P wave axis, normal QRS axis, and significant variability in the overall rate.

Long-term medical therapy for SVT in the neonate is based on the underlying electrophysiologic diagnosis. For patients without demonstrable WPW syndrome, **digoxin** is the initial therapy in patients without congestive heart failure. Parenteral digitalization is described in section VII.D. During digitalization, vagal maneuvers (facial/malar ice wrapped in a towel to elicit the "diving reflex") may be tried in stable neonates. Direct pressure over the eyes should be avoided. Parenteral digitalization usually abolishes the arrhythmia within 10 hours. If digoxin successfully maintains the patient in sinus rhythm, it typically is continued for 6 to 12 months. Although digoxin has long been the mainstay of treatment for SVT, reliance on this drug acutely has decreased, as more efficacious and faster-acting agents have become available.

Digoxin is avoided in chronic management of WPW syndrome because of its potential for enhancing antegrade conduction across the accessory pathway. **Propranolol** is used as the initial and chronic drug therapy for patients with SVT due to the WPW syndrome, to avoid the potential facilitation of antegrade (atrioventricular) conduction through the accessory pathway. Treatment with propranolol may be associated with apnea and hypoglycemia; thus neonates started on propranolol, especially premature infants, should be observed on a continuous cardiac monitor and have serial serum glucose checks for several days.

The addition or substitution of other antiarrhythmic drugs such as sotalol, flecainide, quinidine, or amiodarone alone or in combination may be necessary and should be done only in consultation with a pediatric cardiologist. In neonates, **verapamil should only rarely be used** because it has been associated with sudden death in babies.

In utero SVT may be suspected when a very rapid fetal heart rate is noted by the obstetrician during prenatal care. The diagnosis is confirmed by fetal echocardiography. At that time, an initial search for congenital heart disease and fetal hydrops may be made. In utero treatment of the immature fetus with SVT may be accomplished by treatment of the mother with antiarrhythmic drugs that cross the placenta. Digoxin, propranolol, procainamide, quinidine, and verapamil have been successful therapies. Failure to control the fetal SVT in the presence of fetal hydrops is an indication for delivery. Cesarean delivery of an infant in persistent SVT may be necessary, as the fetal heart rate will not be a reliable indicator of fetal distress.

b. Sinus tachycardia in the neonate is defined as persistent heart rate greater than 2 standard deviations above the mean for age with normal ECG complexes including a normal P wave morphology and axis. Sinus tachycardia is common and occurs particularly in response to systemic events such as anemia, stress, fever, high levels of circulating catecholamines, hypovolemia, and xanthine (e.g., aminophylline) toxicity. An important clue to the existence of sinus tachycardia, in addition to its normal ECG morphology, is that the rate is not fixed but rather will vary by 10 to 20% over time. Medical management consists of identifying and treating the underlying cause.

2. Wide-complex tachycardias

a. Ventricular tachycardia in the neonate is relatively rare and is usually associated with severe medical illnesses including hypoxemia, shock, electrolyte disturbances, digoxin toxicity, and catecholamine toxicity. It may rarely be due to an abnormality of the electrical conducting system of the heart such as prolonged QTc syndrome and intramyocardial tumors. Wide and frequently bizarre QRS complexes with a rapid rate are diagnostic; this ECG pattern may be simulated by SVT in patients with WPW syndrome, in whom there is antegrade conduction through the anomalous pathway (SVT with "aberration"). Ventricular tachycardia is a potentially unstable rhythm commonly with hemodynamic consequences. The underlying cause should be rapidly sought and treated. The hemodynamically stable patient should be treated with a lidocaine bolus, 1 to 2 mg/kg, followed by a lidocaine infusion, 20–50 mcg/kg/min. Direct current cardioversion (starting dose to 1 to 2 W-s/kg or 5 to 10 W-s) should be used if the patient is hemodynamically compromised, though will frequently be ineffective in the presence of acidosis. If a severe acidosis (pH <7.2) is present, it should be treated with hyperventilation and/or sodium bicarbonate prior to cardioversion. Phenytoin, 2 to 4 mg/kg, may be effective if the arrhythmia is due to digoxin toxicity (see VII.D).

b. Ventricular fibrillation in the neonate is almost always an agonal (preterminal) arrhythmia. There is a coarse irregular pattern on ECG with no identifiable QRS complexes. There are no peripheral pulses or heart sounds on examination. Cardiopulmonary resuscitation should be instituted and defibrillation (starting dose 1 to 2 W-s/kg or 5 to 10 W-s) performed. A bolus of lidocaine, 1 mg/kg, followed by a lidocaine infusion should be started. Once the infant has been resuscitated, the underlying problems should be evaluated and treated.

3. Bradycardia

a. Sinus bradycardia in the neonate is not uncommon especially during sleep or during vagal maneuvers, such as bowel movements. If the infant's perfusion and blood pressure are normal, transient bradycardia is not of major concern. Persistent sinus bradycardia may be secondary to hypoxemia, acidosis, and elevated intracranial pressure. Finally, a stable sinus bradycardia may occur with digoxin toxicity, hypothyroidism, or sinus node dysfunction (usually a complication of cardiac surgery).

b. Heart block

(1) First-degree atrioventricular block occurs when the PR interval is greater than 0.15 second. In the neonate, first-degree atrioventricular block may be due to a nonspecific conduction disturbance; medications (e.g., digoxin); myocarditis; hypothyroidism; or associated with certain types of congenital heart disease (e.g., complete atrioventricular canal or ventricular inversion). No specific treatment is generally indicated.

(2) Second-degree atrioventricular block. Second-degree atrioventricular block refers to **intermittent** failure of conduction of the atrial impulse to the ventricles. Two types have been described: (1) Mobitz I (Wenckebach phenomenon) and (2) Mobitz II (intermittent failure to conduct P waves, with a constant PR interval). Second-degree atrioventricular block may occur with SVT, digitalis toxicity, or a nonspecific conduction disturbance. No specific treatment is usually necessary other than diagnosis and treatment of the underlying cause.

(3) Complete heart block (CHB) refers to **complete** absence of conduction of any atrial activity to the ventricles. CHB typically has a slow, constant ventricular rate that is independent of the atrial rate. CHB is frequently detected in utero as fetal bradycardia. Although CHB may be secondary to surgical trauma, **congenital** CHB falls into two main categories. The most common causes include (1) anatomic defects (ventricular inversion and complete atrioventricular canal) and (2) fetal exposure to maternal antibodies related to systemic lupus erythematosus. The presence of CHB without structural heart disease should alert the clinician to investigate the mother for connective tissue disease.

Symptoms related to CHB are related both to the severity of the associated cardiac malformation (when present) and the degree of bradycardia. Fortunately, the fetus with CHB adapts well by increasing stroke volume, and will usually come to term without difficulty. Infants with isolated congenital CHB usually have a heart rate greater than 50 beats per minute, are asymptomatic, and grow normally.

4. Irregular rhythms

a. Premature atrial contractions (PACs, Fig. 25.19) are common in neonates, are usually benign, and do not require specific therapy. Most APBs result in a normal QRS morphology (Fig. 25.19A), distinguishing them from premature ventricular contractions. If the PAC occurs while the atrioventricular node is partially repolarized, an aberrantly conducted ventricular depolarization pattern may be observed on the surface ECG (Fig. 25.19B). If the premature beat occurs when the atrioventricular node is refractory (i.e., early in the cardiac cycle, occurring soon after the normal sinus beat), the impulse will not be conducted to the ventricle ("blocked") and may thus give the appearance of a marked sinus bradycardia (Fig. 25.19C).

b. Premature ventricular contractions (PVCs, Fig. 25.20) are "wide QRS complex" beats that occur when a ventricular focus stimulates a spontaneous beat prior to the normally conducted sinus beat. Isolated PVCs are not uncommon in the normal neonate and do not generally require treatment. Although PVCs frequently occur sporadically, they occasionally are grouped, such as every other beat (bigeminy, see Fig. 25.20A), every third beat (trigeminy), etc. These more frequent PVCs are typically no more worrisome than isolated PVCs, though their greater frequency usually prompts a more extensive diagnostic workup. PVCs may be caused by digoxin toxicity, hypoxemia, electrolyte disturbances, catecholamine, or xanthine toxicity. PVCs occurring in groups of two or more (i.e., couplets, triplets, etc; see Fig. 25.20B) are pathologic and "high grade"; they may be a marker for myocarditis or myocardial dysfunction and further evaluation should be strongly considered.

C. Emergency treatment in the hemodynamically compromised patient. With all therapies described in the following, it is important to have easily accessible resuscitation equipment available before proceeding with these antiarrhythmic interventions.

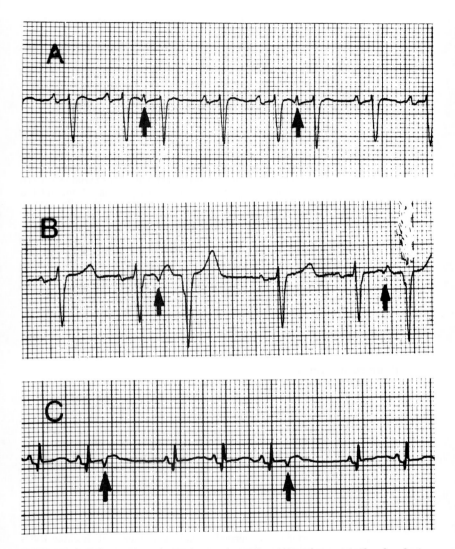

FIG. 25.19. Atrial premature beats (arrows) causing: (A) early ventricular depolarization with a normal QRS complex; (B) early ventricular depolarization with "aberration" of the QRS complex; (C) block at the atrioventricular node. (From Fyler D.C. *Nada Pediatric Cardiology*, with permission)

1. Tachycardias
    a. Adenosine. Adenosine has become the drug of choice for acute management. Adenosine transiently blocks AV node conduction, allowing termination of rapid reentrant rhythms involving the AV node. It must be given by very rapid intravenous push since its half-life is 10 seconds or less. Due to this short half-life, adenosine is a relatively safe medication; however, it has been reported to cause transient AV block severe enough to require pacing (albeit briefly) so it should be used with cau-

A.

B.

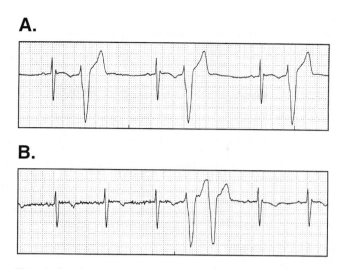

FIG. 25.20. Ventricular premature beats. (A) Ventricular premature beats alternating with normal sinus beats (ventricular bigeminy) are usually not indicative of significant pathology. (B) Paired ventricular premature beats ("couplet") are a potentially more serious rhythm and require further investigation.

tion and in consultation with a pediatric cardiologist. Adenosine, by virtue of its acute action on the AV node, is frequently **diagnostic** as well. Patients who respond with abrupt termination of the SVT have reentrant tachycardias involving the AV node; those with SVT due to atrial flutter will have acute AV block and easily visible flutter waves with reappearance of SVT in 10 to 15 seconds.

  b. **Cardioversion.** In the hemodynamically unstable patient, the **first** line of therapy is synchronized direct current cardioversion.The energy should start at 1 J/kg and be increased by a factor of 2 if unsuccessful. Care should be taken to avoid skin burns and arcing of the current outside the body by only using electrical transmission gel with the paddles. Paddle position should be anterior-posterior if possible.

  c. **Transesophageal pacing.** When available, esophageal overdrive pacing is a very effective maneuver for terminating tachyarrhythmias. The close proximity of the left atrium to the distal esophagus allows electrical impulses generated in the esophagus to be transmitted to atrial tissue; burst pacing may then terminate reentrant tachyarrhythmias.

2. **Bradycardias.** Therapeutic options for treating a symptomatic bradyarrhythmia are more limited. A transvenous pacemaker is a temporary measure in severely symptomatic neonates while preparing for placement of permanent epicardial pacemaker leads; however, transvenous pacing in a small neonate is technically difficult and frequently requires fluoroscopy. A number of transcutaneous pacemakers (Zoll) are available but long-term use must be avoided due to cutaneous burns. An isoproterenol infusion may temporarily increase the ventricular rate and cardiac output in an infant with congestive heart failure. The treatment of choice for sinus node dysfunction is transesophageal pacing at an appropriate rate, but this can only be accomplished with intact atrioventricular conduction and is not effective in patients with CHB. For the infant with transient bradycardia (due to increased vagal tone), intravenous atropine may be used.

References

1. Ainsworth S. B., et al. Prevalence and clinical significance of cardiac murmurs in neonates. *Arch Dis in Child Fetal Neonatal Ed* 1999;80(1): 43F–45F.
2. Allan L., et al. *Textbook of Fetal Cardiology.* 2000. London: Greenwich Medical Media Limited.
3. Allan L. D., et al. Prospective diagnosis of 1006 consecutive cases of congenital heart disease in the fetus. *J Am Coll Cardiol* 1994;23(6): 1452–1458.
4. Allen H. D., et al. *Moss and Adams' Heart Disease in Infants, Children and Adolescents Including the Fetus and Young Adult.* 2001. Philadelphia: Lippincott Williams & Wilkins.
5. Braudo M., Rowe R. D. Auscultation of the heart—early neonatal period. *Am J Dis Child* 1961;101: 67–78.
6. Burke R. P., et al. Video-assisted thoracoscopic surgery for congenital heart disease. *J Thorac Cardiovasc Surg* 1995;109(3): 499–507.
7. Castaneda A. R., et al. *Cardiac Surgery of the Neonate and Infant.* 1994. Philadelphia: W.B. Saunders.
8. Chang A. C., et al. Management and outcome of low birth weight neonates with congenital heart disease. *J Pediatr* 1994;124(3): 461–466.
9. Chang A. C., Wernovsky G., et al. Management of the neonate with transposition of the great arteries and persistent pulmonary hypertension. *Am J Cardiol* 1991;68(11): 1253–1255.
10. Colli A. M., et al. Balloon dilation of critical valvar pulmonary stenosis in the first month of life. *Catheterization Cardiovasc Diagn* 1995;34(1): 23–28.
11. Egito E., et al. Tranvascular balloon dilation for neonatal critical aortic stenosis: early and midterm results. *J Am Coll Cardiol* 1997;29(2): 442–447.
12. Ellison R. C., et al. Evaluation of the preterm infant for patent ductus arteriosus. *Pediatrics* 1983;71(3): 364–372.
13. Fyler D. C. Report of the New England Regional Infant Cardiac Program. *Pediatrics* 65(Suppl): 1980;377–461.
14. Fyler D. C. *Nadas' Pediatric Cardiology.* 1992. Philadelphia: Hanley & Belfus.
15. Garson A., et al. *The Science and Practice of Pediatric Cardiology.* 1998; Baltimore: Williams & Wilkins.
16. Gersony W. M., et al. Effects of indomethacin in premature infants with patent ductus arteriosus: results of a national collaborative study. *J Pediatr* 1983;102 (6): 895–906.
17. Goldmuntz E., et al. Frequency of 22q11 deletions in patients with conotruncal defects. *J Am Coll Cardiol* 1998;32(2): 492–498.
18. Hoffman J. I. E., Kaplan S. The incidence of congenital heart disease. *J Am Coll Cardiol* 2002;39(12'): 1890–1900.
19. Kirklin J. W., Barratt-Boyes B. G. *Cardiac Surgery.* 1993; New York: Churchill Livingstone.
20. Lawless S., et al. Amrinone pharmacokinetics in neonates and infants. *J Clin Pharmacol* 1988;28(3): 283–284.
21. Pihkala J., et al. Interventional cardiac catheterization. *Pediatr Clin North Am* 1999;46(2): 441–464.
22. Vitiello R., et al. Complications associated with pediatric cardiac catheterization. *J Am Coll Cardiol* 1998;32(5): 1433–1440.
23. Woolf A. D., et al. The use of digoxin-specific Fab fragments for severe digitalis intoxication in children. *N Engl J Med* 1992;326(26): 1739–1744.

26. HEMATOLOGIC PROBLEMS

Anemia

Helen A. Christou and David H. Rowitch

I. **Hematologic physiology of the newborn** (2,3,6,10,11). Significant changes occur in the red blood cell (RBC) mass of an infant during the neonatal period and ensuing months. The evaluation of anemia must take into account this developmental process, as well as the infant's physiologic needs.

   A. **Normal development: The physiologic anemia of infancy** (2)

   1. *In utero*, the fetal aortic oxygen saturation is 45%; erythropoietin levels are high, RBC production is rapid, and reticulocyte values are 3 to 7%.

   2. After birth, the oxygen saturation is 95%, and erythropoietin is undetectable. RBC production by day 7 is less than one-tenth the level in utero. Reticulocyte counts are low, and the hemoglobin level falls (Table 26.1).

   3. Despite dropping hemoglobin levels, the ratio of hemoglobin A to hemoglobin F increases, and the levels of 2,3-diphosphoglycerate (2,3-DPG) (which interacts with hemoglobin A to decrease its affinity for oxygen, thus enhancing oxygen release to the tissues) are high. As a result, oxygen delivery to the tissues actually increases. This physiologic "anemia" is not a functional anemia in that oxygen delivery to the tissues is adequate. Iron from degraded red blood cells is stored.

   4. At 8 to 12 weeks, hemoglobin levels reach their nadir (Table 26.2), oxygen delivery to the tissues is impaired, erythropoietin production is stimulated, and RBC production increases.

   5. Infants who have received transfusions in the neonatal period have lower nadirs than normal because of their higher percentage of hemoglobin A (2).

   6. During this period of active erythropoiesis, iron stores are rapidly utilized. The reticuloendothelial system has adequate iron for 15 to 20 weeks in term infants. After this time, the hemoglobin level decreases if iron is not supplied.

   B. **Anemia of prematurity** is an exaggeration of the normal physiologic anemia (see Tables 26.1 and 26.2).

   1. RBC mass is decreased at birth, although the hemoglobin level is the same as in the term infant.

   2. The hemoglobin nadir is reached earlier than in the term infant because of the following:

      a. RBC survival is decreased in comparison with the term infant.

      b. There is a relatively more rapid rate of growth in premature babies than in term infants. For example, a premature infant gaining 150 g/wk requires approximately a 12 mL/wk increase in total blood volume.

      c. Vitamin E deficiency is common in small premature infants, unless the vitamin is supplied exogenously.

   3. The hemoglobin nadir in premature babies is lower than in term infants because erythropoietin is produced by the term infant at a hemoglobin level of 10 to 11 g/dL but is produced by the premature infant at a hemoglobin level of 7 to 9 g/dL. This reflects the lower oxygen requirements in healthy preterm infants rather than a defect in erythropoietin production (2).

   4. Iron administration before the age of 10 to 14 weeks does not increase the nadir of the hemoglobin level or diminish its rate of reduction. However, this iron is stored for later use.

   5. Once the nadir is reached, RBC production is stimulated, and iron stores are rapidly depleted because less iron is stored in the premature infant than in the term infant.

461

TABLE 26.1. HEMOGLOBIN CHANGES IN BABIES IN THE FIRST YEAR OF LIFE

	Hemoglobin Level		
Week	Term Babies	Premature Babies (1200–2500 gm)	Small Premature Babies (< 1200 gm)
0	17.0	16.4	16.0
1	18.8	16.0	14.8
3	15.9	13.5	13.4
6	12.7	10.7	9.7
10	11.4	9.8	8.5
20	12.0	10.4	9.0
50	12.0	11.5	11.0

Source: From Glader B., Naiman J. L. Erythrocyte Disorders in Infancy. In: Taeusch H. W., Ballard R. A., Avery M. E. (Eds.), *Diseases of the Newborn.* 1991. Philadelphia: Saunders.

II. **Etiology of anemia in the neonate** (9)
   A. **Blood loss** is manifested by a decreased or normal hematocrit, increased or normal reticulocyte count, and a normal bilirubin level (unless the hemorrhage is retained) (10,11). If blood loss is recent (e.g., at delivery), the hematocrit and reticulocyte count may be normal and the infant may be in shock. The hematocrit will fall later as a result of hemodilution. If the bleeding is chronic, the hematocrit will be low, the reticulocyte count up, and the baby normovolemic.
      1. **Obstetric causes of blood loss,** including malformations of placenta and cord:
         a. Abruptio placentae.
         b. Placenta previa.
         c. Incision of placenta at cesarean section.
         d. Rupture of anomalous vessels (e.g., vasa previa, velamentous insertion of cord, or rupture of communicating vessels in a multilobed placenta).
         e. Hematoma of cord caused by varices or aneurysm.
         f. Rupture of cord (more common in short cords and in dysmature cords).
      2. **Occult blood loss**
         a. **Fetomaternal bleeding** may be chronic or acute. It occurs in 8% of all pregnancies, and in 1% of pregnancies the volume may be as large as 40 mL. The diagnosis of this problem is by Kleihauer-Betke stain of

TABLE 26.2. HEMOGLOBIN NADIR IN BABIES IN THE FIRST YEAR OF LIFE

Maturity of Baby at Birth	Hemoglobin Level at Nadir	Time of Nadir
Term babies	9.5–11.0	6–12 wk
Premature babies (1200–2500 gm)	8.0–10.0	5–10 wk
Small premature babies (< 1200 gm)	6.5–9.0	4–8 wk

Source: From Glader B., Naiman J. L. Erythrocyte disorders in infancy. In: Taeusch H. W., Ballard R. A., Avery, M. E. (Eds.), *Diseases of the Newborn.* 1991. Philadelphia: Saunders.

maternal smear for fetal cells (3). Many conditions may predispose to this type of bleeding:

(1) Placental malformations—chorioangioma or choriocarcinoma.

(2) Obstetric procedures—traumatic amniocentesis, external cephalic version, internal cephalic version, breech delivery.

(3) Spontaneous fetomaternal bleeding.

b. Fetoplacental bleeding:

(1) Chorioangioma or choriocarcinoma with placental hematoma.

(2) Cesarean section, with infant held above the placenta.

(3) Tight nuchal cord or occult cord prolapse.

c. Twin-to-twin transfusion.

3. Bleeding in the neonatal period may be due to the following causes:

a. Intracranial bleeding associated with:

(1) Prematurity.

(2) Second twin.

(3) Breech delivery.

(4) Rapid delivery.

(5) Hypoxia.

b. Massive cephalhematoma, subgaleal hemorrhage, or hemorrhagic caput succedaneum.

c. Retroperitoneal bleeding.

d. Ruptured liver or spleen.

e. Adrenal or renal hemorrhage.

f. Gastrointestinal bleeding:

(1) Peptic ulcer.

(2) Necrotizing enterocolitis.

(3) Nasogastric catheter.

(4) Maternal blood swallowed from delivery or breast should be ruled out by the Apt test (see Bleeding).

g. Bleeding from umbilicus.

4. **Iatrogenic causes.** Excessive blood loss may result from blood sampling with inadequate replacement.

B. Hemolysis is manifested by a decreased hematocrit, increased reticulocyte count, and an increased bilirubin level (2,3).

1. **Immune hemolysis** (see Chap. 18):

a. Rh incompatibility.

b. ABO incompatibility.

c. Minor blood group incompatibility (e.g., c, E, Kell, Duffy).

d. Maternal disease (e.g., lupus), autoimmune hemolytic disease, rheumatoid arthritis (positive direct Coombs' test in mother and newborn, no antibody to common red cell antigen Rh, AB, etc.), or drugs (e.g., penicillin antibodies in mother or infant, child on penicillin (4)).

2. **Hereditary RBC disorders:**

a. RBC membrane defects such as spherocytosis, elliptocytosis, or stomatocytosis.

b. Metabolic defects—glucose-6-phosphate dehydrogenase (G6PD) deficiency (significant neonatal hemolysis due to G6PD deficiency is usually seen only in Mediterranean or Asian G6PD-deficient males; blacks in the United States have a 10% incidence of G6PD deficiency but rarely have significant neonatal problems unless an infection or drug is operative), pyruvate-kinase deficiency, 5'-nucleotidase deficiency, and glucose-phosphate isomerase deficiency.

c. Hemoglobinopathies:

(1) Alpha- and gamma-thalassemia syndromes.

(2) Alpha- and gamma-chain structural abnormalities.

3. **Acquired hemolysis:**

a. Infection—bacterial or viral.

b. Disseminated intravascular coagulation.

c. Vitamin E deficiency and other nutritional anemias (2).

   d. Microangiopathic hemolytic anemia—cavernous hemangioma, renal artery stenosis, and severe coarctation of the aorta.
C. **Diminished RBC production** is manifested by a decreased hematocrit, decreased reticulocyte count, and normal bilirubin level.
   1. **Diamond-Blackfan syndrome.**
   2. **Congenital leukemia** or other tumor.
   3. **Infections,** especially rubella and parvovirus (see Chap. 23).
   4. **Osteopetrosis,** leading to inadequate erythropoiesis.
   5. **Drug-induced suppression of RBC production.**
   6. **Physiologic anemia or anemia of prematurity** (see I.A and B).
III. **Diagnostic approach to anemia in the newborn** (Table 26.3)
   A. The **family history** should include questions about anemia, jaundice, gallstones, and splenectomy.
   B. The **obstetric history** should be evaluated.
   C. The **physical examination** may reveal an associated abnormality and provide clues to the origin of the anemia.
      1. **Acute blood loss** leads to shock, with cyanosis, poor perfusion, and acidosis.
      2. **Chronic blood loss** produces pallor, but the infant may exhibit only mild symptoms of respiratory distress or irritability.
      3. **Chronic hemolysis** is associated with pallor, jaundice, and hepatosplenomegaly.
   D. **Complete blood cell count.** Capillary blood samples are 3.7 to 2.7% higher than venous hematocrits. Warming the foot reduced the difference from 3.9 to 1.9% (2,3).
   E. **Reticulocyte count** (elevated with chronic blood loss and hemolysis, depressed with infection and production defect).
   F. **Blood smear** (see Table 26.3).
   G. **Coombs' test and bilirubin level.**
   H. **Apt test** (see Bleeding) on gastrointestinal blood of uncertain origin.
   I. **Kleihauer-Betke preparation** of the mother's blood. A 50-mL loss of fetal blood into the maternal circulation will show up as 1% fetal cells in the maternal circulation (3).
   J. **Ultrasound of abdomen and head.**
   K. **Test on parents**—complete blood cell count, smear, RBC indices, RBC enzymes (G6PD, pyruvate kinase).
   L. Studies for infection [toxoplasmosis, other infections, rubella, cytomegalovirus infection, and herpes simplex (TORCH) infection; see Chap. 23].
   M. **Bone marrow** (rarely used except in cases of bone marrow failure from hypoplasia or tumor).
IV. **Therapy**
   A. **Transfusion** (see Blood Products Used in the Newborn)
      1. **Indications for transfusion.** The decision to transfuse must be made in consideration of the infant's condition and physiologic needs (13).
         a. Infants with significant respiratory disease or congenital heart disease (e.g., large left-to-right shunt) may need their hematocrit maintained above 40%. Transfusion with adult RBCs provides the added benefit of lowered oxygen affinity, which augments oxygen delivery to tissues. Blood should be fresh (3 to 7 days old) to ensure adequate 2,3-DPG levels.
         b. Healthy, asymptomatic newborns will self-correct a mild anemia, provided that iron intake is adequate.
         c. Infants with ABO incompatibility who do not have an exchange transfusion may have protracted hemolysis and may require a transfusion several weeks after birth. If they do not have enough hemolysis to require treatment with phototherapy, they will usually not become anemic enough to need a transfusion.
         d. Premature babies may be quite comfortable with hemoglobin levels of 6.5 to 7.0 mg/dL. The level itself is not an indication for transfusion. Sick infants (e.g., with sepsis, pneumonia, or bronchopulmonary dysplasia) may require increased oxygen-carrying capacities and therefore

TABLE 26.3. CLASSIFICATION OF ANEMIA IN THE NEWBORN

Reticulocytes	Bilirubin	Coombs' Test	RBC Morphology	Diagnostic Possibilities
Normal or ↓	Normal	Negative	Normal	Physiologic anemia of infancy or prematurity; congenital hypoplastic anemia; other causes of decreased production
Normal or ↑	Normal	Negative	Normal	Acute hemorrhage (fetomaternal, placental, umbilical cord, or internal hemorrhage)
			Hypochromic microcytes	Chronic fetomaternal hemorrhage
↑	↑	Positive	Spherocytes	Immune hemolysis (blood group incompatibility or maternal autoantibody)
Normal or ↑	↑	Negative	Spherocytes	Hereditary spherocytosis
			Elliptocytes	Hereditary elliptocytosis
			Hypochromic microcytes	Alpha- or gamma-thalassemia syndrome
			Spiculated RBCs	Pyruvate-kinase deficiency
			Schistocytes and RBC fragments	Disseminated intravascular coagulation; other microangiopathic processes
			Bite cells (Heinz bodies with supravital stain)	Glucose-6-phosphate dehydrogenase deficiency
			Normal	Infections; enclosed hemorrhage (cephalohematoma)

RBC = red blood cell; ↓ = decreased; ↑ = increased.
Source: Adapted from the work of Dr. Bertil Glader, Director of Division of Hematology-Oncology, Children's Hospital at Stanford, California.

need transfusion. Growing premature infants also may manifest a need for transfusion by exhibiting poor weight gain, apnea, tachypnea, or poor feeding (13). Transfusion guidelines are shown in Table 26.4. Desipite efforts to adopt uniform transfusion critera, significant variation in transfusion practices among neonatal intensive care units (NICUs) has been reported (17).

In our units when we instituted the practice of requiring parental permission for elective transfusion, the transfusion rate dropped markedly for premature infants.

2. **Blood products and methods of transfusion** [see Blood Products Used in the Newborn and (2)]

   a. **Packed RBCs.** The volume of transfusion may be calculated as follows:

   $$\frac{\text{Weight in kg} \times \text{blood volume per kilogram} \times (\text{hematocrit desired} - \text{hematocrit observed})}{\text{Hematocrit of blood to be given}} = \text{volume of transfusion}$$

   The average newborn blood volume is 80 mL/kg; the hematocrit of packed RBCs is 60 to 90% and should be checked prior to transfusion. We generally transfuse 15 to 20 mL/kg; larger volumes may need to be divided.

   b. **Whole blood** is indicated when there is acute blood loss.

   c. **Exchange transfusion** with packed RBCs may be required for severely anemic infants, when routine transfusion of the volume of packed RBCs necessary to correct the anemia would result in circulatory overload (see Chap. 18).

   d. **Irradiated** (5000 rads) (12) or frozen RBCs may be used if there is concern about the immunocompetence of the infant, and are recommended in premature infants weighing less than 1200 g. Premature infants may be unable to reject foreign lymphocytes in transfused blood. **We use irradiated blood for all neonatal transfusions. Leukocyte depletion** with third-generation transfusion filters has substan-

TABLE 26.4. TRANSFUSION GUIDELINES FOR PREMATURE INFANTS ASYMPTOMATIC INFANTS WITH HCT < 21% AND RETICULOCYTES <100,000/UL. (2%)

Infants with Hct< 31%	and	hood O2<36% or mean airway pressure < 6 cm H2O by CPAP or IMV
	or	>9 apneic and bradycardic episodes per 12 hours or 2/24 hours requiring bag and mask ventilation while on adequate methylxanthine therapy
	or	HR > 180/min or RR> 80/min sustained or 24 hours
	or	weight gain of < 10 grams/day for 4 days on 100 Kcal/k/d
	or	having surgery
Infants with Hct<36%	and	requiring > 35%O2 or mean airway pressure 6–8 cm H2O by CPAP or IMV

CPAP = continuous positive airway pressure by nasal or endotracheal route; HR = heart rate; IMV = intermittent mandatory ventilation; RR = respiratory rate.
Source: From the multicenter trial of recombinant human erythropoietin for preterm infants (14).

tially reduced the risk of exposure to foreign lymphocytes and cytomegalovirus (CMV) (1,10). Frozen RBCs probably reduce the incidence of transfusion-related infection. In the past we used only blood from CMV-negative donors for neonatal transfusion. We now use blood treated by prestorage leukodestruction as approved by the American Association of Blood Banks for prevention of CMV infection.

    e. Directed-donor transfusion is requested by many families. Irradiation of directed-donor cells is especially important, given the human leukocyte antigen (HLA) compatibility among first-degree relatives and the enhanced potential for foreign lymphocyte engraftment.

    f. Because of concern for multiple exposure risk associated with repeated transfusions in extremely low-birth-weight (ELBW) infants, **we recommend transfusing stored red blood cells from a single unit reserved for an infant** (18).

B. Prophylaxis

  1. Term infants should be sent home from the hospital on iron-fortified formula (2 mg/kg per day) if they are not breastfeeding (5).

  2. Premature infants (preventing or ameliorating the anemia of prematurity). The following is a description of our usual nutritional management of premature infants from the point of view of providing RBC substrates and preventing additional destruction:

    a. Iron supplementation in the preterm infant prevents late iron deficiency (7). We routinely supplement iron in premature infants at a dose of 2 to 4 mg of elemental iron per kilogram per day once full enteral feeding is achieved (see Chap. 10).

    b. Mother's milk or formulas similar to mother's milk in that they are low in linoleic acid are used to maintain a low content of polyunsaturated fatty acids in the RBCs (6).

    c. Vitamin E (15 to 25 IU of water-soluble form) is given daily until the baby is 38 to 40 weeks' postconceptional age (this is usually stopped at discharge from the hospital).

    d. These infants should be followed carefully, and additional iron supplementation may be required.

    e. Methods and hazards of transfusion are described in Blood Products Used in the Newborn.

    f. Recombinant human erythropoietin (REPO) offers promise in ameliorating the anemia of prematurity (8,13,14). Although studies in which we participated showed that recombinant human erythropoietin may decrease the frequency and volume of RBC transfusions administered to premature infants, we have not yet used it as a routine procedure (2,8,13–16). Though many studies have shown that the erythropoietin does not significantly reduce packed red blood cell (PRBC) transfusions once strict transfusion criteria are instituted, this therapy may have a role in individual babies. "A meta-analysis of the most scientifically rigorous studies on this topic indicate that administration of rEpo to VLBW infants reduces 'late' erythrocyte transfusions in a dose-dependant manner (20)."

    In conclusion, for infants in whom it is desirable to maintain a relatively high hematocrit, for example, babies with bronchopulmonary dysplasia or cyanotic congenital heart disease, initiation of erythropoietin may play a role in decreasing late transfusions.

    "It is still too early to endorse or to be become a nay-sayer when it comes to rEPO used in the nursery, it is hoped that a few more good studies properly designed will convincingly sway the debate (21)."

    Complementary strategies to reduce phlebotomy losses and the use of conservative standardized transfusion criteria are thought to contribute to significant reductions in transfusions. The utility of erythropoietin therapy is likely to depend on careful targeting to the population most likely to benefit (19).

References

1. Andreu G. Role of leucocyte depletion in the prevention of transfusion-induced cytomegalovirus infection. *Semin Hematol* 1991;28(Suppl. 5):26.
2. Bifano E. M., Ehrenkranz Z. (Eds.). Perinatal hematology. *Clin Perinatol* 1995;23(3).
3. Blanchette V., et al. Hematology. In: Avery G. B. (Ed.), *Neonatology,* 4th Ed. 1994; Philadelphia: Lippincott, 952.
4. Clayton E. M., et al. Penicillin antibody as a cause of positive direct antiglobulin tests. *Am J Clin Pathol* 1965;44:648.
5. Committee on Nutrition AAP. Iron-fortified infant formulas. *Pediatrics* 1989;84: 1114.
6. Glader B., Naiman J. L. Erythrocyte disorders in infancy. In: Taeusch H. W., Ballard R. A., Avery M. E. (Eds.), *Diseases of the Newborn.* 1991; Philadelphia: Saunders.
7. Hall R. T., et al. Feeding iron-fortified premature formula during initial hospitalization to infants less than 1800 grams birthweight. *Pediatrics* 1993;92:409.
8. Maier R. F., et al. The effect of epoietin beta (recombinant human erythropoietin) on the need for transfusion in very low-birth-weight infants. European Multicentre Erythropoietin Study Group. *N Engl J Med* 1994;330:1173.
9. Molteni R. A. Prenatal blood loss. *Pediatr Rev* 1990;12:47.
10. Nathan D. G., Oski F. A. *Hematology of Infancy and Childhood.* 1992; Philadelphia: Saunders.
11. Oski F. A., Naiman J. L. *Hematologic Problems in the Newborn,* 3rd Ed., 1982; Philadelphia: Saunders.
12. Parkman R., et al. Graft-versus-host disease after intrauterine and exchange transfusions for hemolytic disease of the newborn. *N Engl J Med* 1974;290:359.
13. Ross M. P., et al. A randomized trial to develop criteria for administering erythrocyte transfusions to anemic preterm infants 1 to 3 months of age. *J Perinatol* 1989;9:246.
14. Shannon K. M., et al. Recombinant human erythropoietin stimulates erythropoiesis and reduces erythrocyte transfusions in preterm infants. *Pediatrics* 1995;95:1.
15. Straus R. G. Erythropoietin and neonatal anemia (Editorial). *N Engl J Med* 1994;330:1227.
16. Willmas J. A. Erythropoietin—not yet a standard treatment for anemia of prematurity. *Pediatrics* 1995;95:9.
17. Ringer S. A., et al. Variations in transfusion practice in neonatal intensive care. *Pediatrics* 1998;101:194.
18. Strauss R. G. Blood banking issues pertaining to neontal red blood cell transfusions. *Transfus Sci* 1999;21(1):7.
19. Soubasi V., et al. In which neonates does early recombinant human erythropoietin treatment prevent anemia of prematurity? Results of a randomized, controlled study. *Pediatr Res* 1993;34(5):675.
20. Garcia M. G., et al. Effect of recombinant erythropoietin on "late" transfusions in the neonatal intensive care unit: A meta-anaysis. *J Perinatol* 2002;22:108.
21. Stockman J. A. Anemia of prematurity: Current concepts in the issue of when to transfuse. *Pediatr Clin North Am* 1986;22:111.

BLEEDING

Allen M. Goorin and Ellis Neufeld

The hemostatic mechanism in the neonate differs from that in the older child. In neonates there is decreased activity of certain clotting factors, impaired platelet function, and suboptimal defense against clot formation.References 1, 3, 6, 9, and 10 are reviews of this subject.

I. Etiology
A. Deficient clotting factors
1. **Transitory deficiencies** of the procoagulant vitamin K-dependent factors II, VII, IX, and X; and anticoagulant proteins C and S are characteristic of the newborn period and may be accentuated by the following:
   a. **The administration of total parenteral alimentation or antibiotics or the lack of administration of vitamin K** to premature infants.
   b. **Term infants may develop vitamin K deficiency** by day 2 or 3 if they are not supplemented with vitamin K parenterally, because of negligible stores and inadequate intake.
   c. **The mother may have received certain drugs during pregnancy that can cause bleeding in the first 24 hours of the infant's life.**
      (1) Phenytoin (Dilantin), phenobarbital, and salicylates interfere with the vitamin K effect on synthesis of clotting factors.
      (2) Coumadin compounds given to the mother interfere with the synthesis of vitamin K–dependent clotting factors by the livers of both the mother and the fetus, and the bleeding may not be immediately reversed by administration of vitamin K.
2. **Disturbances of clotting** may be related to associated diseases such as disseminated intravascular coagulation (DIC) due to infection, shock, anoxia, necrotizing enterocolitis (NEC), renal vein thrombosis (RVT), or the use of vascular catheters. Any significant liver disease may interfere with the production of clotting factors by the liver.
   a. Extracorporeal membrane oxygenation **(ECMO)** in neonates with critical cardiopulmonary disease is a special case of coagulopathy related to the bypass circuit and anticoagulation together.
3. **Inherited abnormalities of clotting factors**
   a. **Sex-linked recessive** (expressed predominantly in males):
      (1) Factor VIII clotting activity is decreased in the newborn with classic hemophilia A (1 in 5000 boys).
      (2) Hemophilia B, or Christmas disease is due to an inherited quantitative deficiency of factor IX (1 in 25,000 boys).
   b. **Autosomal dominant** (expressed in boys and girls with one parent affected):
      (1) Von Willebrand's disease, the most common inherited coagulation defect, involves decreased levels of von Willebrand factor, which is responsible for platelet adhesiveness, and serves as a carrier for factor VIII.
      (2) Dysfibrinogenemia (very rare) is due to fibrinogen functional mutations.
   c. **Autosomal recessive** (occurs in both boys and girls; the parents are carriers). Deficiencies of factors V, VII, X, and XIII. Factor XII deficiency, not a bleeding disorder, but a cause of long partial thromboplastin time (PTT), is recessive. Combined factor V and VIII deficiency is caused by defect in common protein processing (1).
      (1) Severe factor VII deficiency can present as intracranial hemorrhage in neonates.
      (2) Prothrombin (factor II) or fibrinogen (factor I) deficiency.
      (3) Factor XI deficiency is incompletely recessive and is often classified as autosomal dominant, since heterozygotes will have some minor bleeding problems.
      (4) von Willebrand's disease Type III (rare, complete absence of VW factor).

B. **Platelet problems** (see Thrombocytopenia)
   1. **Qualitative disorders** include hereditary conditions (e.g., Glanzmann's thrombasthenia) and disorders that result from the mother's use of aspirin.
   2. **Quantitative disorders** include immune thrombocytopenia (maternal idiopathic thombocytopenic purpura (ITP) or alloimmune), disseminated intravascular coagulation due to infection or asphyxia, congenital megakaryocytic hypoplasia, leukemia, inherited thrombocytopenia, giant congenital vascular malformations, hyperviscosity, RVT, and NEC.
C. **Other causes of bleeding** are **vascular** in etiology, and may include central nervous system hemorrhage, pulmonary hemorrhage, arterial-venous (A-V) malformations, and hemangiomas.
D. **Miscellaneous problems**
   1. **Trauma** (see Chap. 20):
      a. Rupture of spleen or liver associated with breech delivery.
      b. Retroperitoneal or intraperitoneal bleeding may present as scrotal ecchymosis.
      c. Subdural hematoma, cephalhematoma, or subgaleal hemorrhage (the latter may be associated with vacuum extraction).
   2. **Liver dysfunction.**
II. **Diagnostic workup of the bleeding infant**
   A. The **history** includes: (a) family history of excessive bleeding or clotting; (b) maternal medications (aspirin, phenytoin); (c) information about the pregnancy and the birth; (d) maternal history of a previous birth of an infant

TABLE 26.5. DIFFERENTIAL DIAGNOSIS OF BLEEDING IN THE NEONATE

Clinical Evaluation	Laboratory Studies			Likely Diagnosis
	Platelets	PT	PTT	
"Sick"	D−	I+	I+	DIC
	D−	N	N	Platelet consumption (infection, necrotizing enterocolitis, renal vein thrombosis)
	N	I+	I+	Liver disease
	N	N	N	Compromised vascular integrity (associated with hypoxia, prematurity, acidosis, hyperosmolality)
"Healthy"	D−	N	N	Immune thrombocytopenia, occult infection, thrombosis, bone marrow hypoplasia (rare) or bone marrow infiltrative disease
	N	I+	I+	Hemorrhagic disease of newborn (vitamin K deficiency)
	N	N	I+	Hereditary clotting factor deficiencies
	N	N	N	Bleeding due to local factors (trauma, anatomic abnormalities); qualitative platelet abnormalities (rare); factor XIII deficiency (rare)

PT = prothrombin time; PTT = partial thromboplastin time; D2 = decreased; I+ = increased; DIC = disseminated intravascular coagulation; N = normal.
Source: Modified from Glader B. E., Amylon M. D. Bleeding disorders in the newborn infant. In: Taeusch H. W., Ballard R. A., Avery M. E. (Eds.), *Diseases of the Newborn.* 1991. Philadelphia: Saunders.

with a bleeding disorder; and (e) any illness, medication, anomalies, or procedures done to the infant.

B. **Examination.** The crucial decision in diagnosing and managing the bleeding infant is determining whether the infant is sick or well (Table 26.5).

   1. **Sick infant.** Consider disseminated intravascular coagulation (DIC), infection, or liver disease (vascular injury induced by hypoxia may lead to DIC).

   2. **Well infant.** Consider vitamin K deficiency, isolated clotting factor deficiencies, or immune thrombocytopenia.

   3. **Petechiae, small superficial ecchymosis, or mucosal bleeding** suggest a platelet problem.

   4. **Large bruises** suggest deficiency of clotting factors, DIC, liver disease, or vitamin K deficiency.

   5. **Enlarged spleen** suggests congenital infection or erythroblastosis.

   6. **Jaundice** suggests infection, liver disease or resorption of a large hematoma.

   7. **Abnormal retinal findings** suggest infection (see Chap. 23).

C. **Laboratory tests** (Table 26.6)

   1. **The Apt test** is used to rule out maternal blood. If the child is well and only gastrointestinal bleeding is noted, an Apt test is performed on gastric aspirate or stool to rule out the presence of maternal blood swallowed during labor or delivery or from a bleeding breast. A breast pump can be used to collect milk to confirm the presence of blood in the milk, or the infant's stomach can be aspirated before and after breastfeeding.

      a. **Procedure.** Mix 1 part bloody stool or vomitus with 5 parts water; centrifuge it and separate the clear pink supernatant (hemolysate); add 1 mL of sodium hydroxide 1% to 4 mL of hemolysate.

TABLE 26.6. NORMAL VALUES FOR LABORATORY SCREENING TESTS IN THE NEONATE

Laboratory Test	Premature Infant Having Received Vitamin K	Term Infant Having Received Vitamin K	Child over 1 to 2 Months of Age
Platelet count/μl	150,000–400,000	150,000–400,000	150,000–400,000
PT (sec.)*	14–22	13–20	12–14
PTT (sec.)*	35–55	30–45	25–35
Fibrinogen (mg/dl)	150–300	150–300	150–300

PT = prothrombin time; PTT = partial thromboplastin time.
*Normal values may vary from laboratory to laboratory, depending on the particular reagent employed. In full-term infants who have received vitamin K, the PT and PTT values generally fall within the normal "adult" range by several days (PT) to several weeks (PTT) of age. Small premature infants (under 1500 gm) tend to have longer PT and PTT than larger babies. In infants with hematocrit levels greater than 60%, the ratio of blood to anticoagulant (sodium citrate 3.8%) in tubes should be 19:1 rather than the usual ratio of 9:1; otherwise, spurious results will be obtained, since the amount of anticoagulant solution is calculated for a specific volume of plasma. Blood drawn from heparinized catheters should not be used. The best results are obtained when blood from a clean venipuncture is allowed to drip directly into the tube from the needle or scalp vein set. Factor levels II, VII, IX, and X are decreased. Three-day-old full-term baby not receiving vitamin K has levels similar to a premature baby. Factor XI and XII levels are lower in preterm infants than in term infants and account for prolonged PTT. Fibrinogen, factor V, and factor VII are normal in premature and term infants. Factor XIII is variable.
Source: Data from normal laboratory values at the Hematology Laboratory, The Children's Hospital, Boston; Alpers J. B., Lafonet M. T. (Eds.), *Laboratory Handbook.* 1984. Boston: The Children's Hospital.

   b. Result. Hemoglobin A (HbA) changes from pink to yellow brown (maternal blood); hemoglobin F (HbF) stays pink (fetal blood).

2. **Blood smear** is used to determine the number, size, and kind of platelets and the presence of fragmented red blood cells as seen in DIC. Large platelets are young platelets and imply an immune cause of thrombocytopenia.

3. **Significant bleeding** from thrombocytopenia **is usually associated with platelet counts under 20,000 to 30,000/mL or less,** except in alloimmune thrombocytopenia due to antibodies against the platelet alloantigen, phospholipase A 1 (PLA1), which may cause bleeding up to 50,000 platelets (see Thrombocytopenia).

4. **Prothrombin time (PT)** is a test of the "extrinsic" clotting system. Factor VII and tissue factor activate factor X; Factor Xa activates prothromin (II) to thrombin, with factor Va as a cofactor. Thrombin cleaves fibrinogen to fibrin.

5. **Partial thromboplastin time (PTT)** is a test of the "intrinsic" clotting system and of the activation of factor X by factors XII, XI, IX, and VIII. PTT is also a test of the final coagulation pathway (factors V and II and fibrinogen).

6. **Fibrinogen** can be measured on the same sample used for PT. It may be decreased in liver disease and consumptive states.

7. ***d*-Dimer assays** have replaced Fibrin split products (FSP) assays to measure degradation products of fibrin found in the plasma of patients with DIC and in patients with liver disease who have problems clearing FSP. Improper collection of blood will result in increased FSP in the sample. *d*-Dimers are formed from the action of plasmin on the fibrin clot, generating derivatives of cross-linked fibrin containing *d*-dimer. Normal levels are less than 0.5 mg/mL. Levels are higher in DIC, deep vein thrombosis, and pulmonary embolism.

8. **Specific factor assays and Von Willerand panels** for patients with positive family history **can be measured in cord blood.** Age-specific norms must be consulted.

9. **Bleeding times are to be discouraged in all patients, but especially in neonates.** This test measures response to a standardized razor blade cut, and does not predict surgical bleeding, at least in adults. The apparatus is not well suited to infants.

III. **Treatment of neonates with abnormal bleeding parameters who have not had clinical bleeding.** In one study, preterm infants with respiratory distress syndrome (RDS) or term infants with asphyxia were treated for abnormal bleeding parameters (without DIC) to correct the hemostatic defect. Although the treatment was successful in correcting the defect, no change in mortality was seen in comparison with controls (11).

In general, we treat clinically ill infants or infants weighing less than 1500 g with fresh-frozen plasma (10 mL/kg) if the PT or PTT or both are greater than two times normal or with platelets (1 unit) (see IV.C) if the platelet count is under 20,000/ml (see Thrombocytopenia and Blood Products Used in the Newborn). This will vary with the clinical sutiations, trend of the laboratory values, impending surgery, and so forth. Some babies will receive platelets if their platelet count is under 50,000.

IV. **Treatment of bleeding**

A. **Vitamin K₁ oxide (Aquamephyton).** An intravenous or intramuscular dose of 1 mg is administered in case the infant was not given vitamin K at birth. Infants receiving total parenteral nutrition and infants receiving antibiotics for more than 2 weeks should be given 0.5 mg of vitamin K_1 (IM or IV) weekly to prevent vitamin K depletion. Ideally, Vitamin K rather than fresh frozen plasma (FFP) should be given for long PT and PTT due to vitamin K deficiency, rather than plasma, which should be reserved for bleeding or emergencies.

B. Fresh-frozen plasma (see Blood Products Used in the Newborn) (10 mL/kg) is given intravenously for active bleeding and is repeated every 8 to 12 hours as needed, or as a drip of 1 cc/kg per hour. This is used because it replaces the clotting factors immediately.

C. Platelets (see Thrombocytopenia). If there is no increased platelet destruction (as a result of DIC, immune platelet problem, or sepsis), 1 unit of platelets given to a 3-kg infant will raise the platelet count to 50,000 to 100,000/mL. If no new platelets are made or transfused, the platelet count will drop slowly over 3 to 5 days. If available, platelets from the mother or from a known platelet-compatible donor should be used if the infant has an alloimmune platelet disorder. The blood of the donor should be matched for Rh factor and type and washed, because red blood cells will be mixed in the platelet concentrates. Platelets are irradiated before transfusion.

D. Fresh whole blood (see Blood Products Used in the Newborn). The baby is given 10 mL/kg; more is given as needed.

E. Clotting factor concentrates (see Blood Products Used in the Newborn). When there is a known deficiency of factor VIII or IX, the plasma concentration should be raised to normal adult levels (50 to 100% of pooled normal control plasma, or 0.5 to1 unit/mL) to stop serious bleeding. Recombinant-DNA derived factor VIII and IX should be used if the diagnosis is clear. If severe von Willebrand's disease is considered, cryoprecipitate or a VW-containing factor VIII concentrate should be used. For other factor deficiencies, 10 mL/kg of fresh-frozen plasma will transiently raise the factor level approximately to 20% of adult control.

F. Disorders due to problems other than hemostatic proteins. Diagnosis and treatment should be aimed at the underlying cause (e.g., infection, liver rupture, catheter, or NEC).

G. Treatment of specific disorders

1. **Disseminated intravascular coagulation (DIC).** The baby usually appears sick and may have petechiae, gastrointestinal hemorrhage, oozing from venipunctures, infection, asphyxia, or hypoxia. The platelet count is decreased, and PT and PTT are increased. Fragmented red blood cells (RBCs) are seen on the blood smear. Fibrinogen is decreased, and d-dimers (or FSPs) are increased. Treatment involves the following steps:

   a. **The underlying cause should be treated** (e.g., sepsis, NEC, herpes).

   b. **Vitamin K$_1$, 1.0 mg IV, is given.**

   c. **Platelets and fresh-frozen plasma are given** as needed to keep the platelet count over 50,000/mL and to stop the bleeding.

   d. **If the bleeding persists,** one of the following steps should be taken, depending on the availability of blood, platelets, or fresh-frozen plasma:

      (1) Exchange transfusion with fresh citrated whole blood or packed red blood cells mixed with fresh-frozen plasma.

      (2) Continued transfusion with platelets and fresh-frozen plasma.

      (3) Administration of cryoprecipitate (10 mL/kg).

   e. If consumption coagulopathy is associated with thrombosis of large vessels and not with concurrent bleeding, **low-dose heparinination without a bolus may be considered** (for example, 10 to 15 units/kg per hour as a continuous infusion). Platelets and plasma are continued after the heparin has been started. Platelet counts should be kept at or above 50,000/mL. The aim of heparin treatment is to keep the PTT at 1.5 to 2 times normal. The plasma is essential to provide ATIII and other anticoagulant proteins. However, if bleeding accompanies DIC and thrombosis concurrently, heparin may be contraindicated, consult an expert. See Major Arterial and Venous Thrombosis Management for treatment of thrombosis.

2. **Hemorrhagic disease of the newborn** (HDN) occurs in 1 of every 200 to 400 neonates not given vitamin K prophylaxis.
   a. In the healthy infant, **hemorrhagic disease of the newborn may occur when the infant is not given vitamin K.** The infant may have been born in a busy delivery room, at home, or transferred from elsewhere. Bleeding and bruising may occur after the infant is 48 hours old. The platelet level is normal, and PT and PTT are prolonged. If there is active bleeding, 10 mL/kg of fresh-frozen plasma and an IV dose of 1 mg of vitamin K are given.
   b. **If the mother has been treated with phenytoin (Dilantin), primidone (Mysoline), methsuximide (Celontin), or phenobarbital, the infant may be vitamin K deficient and bleed during the first 24 hours.** The mother should be given vitamin K, 24 hours prior to delivery (10 mg of vitamin K_1 IM). The newborn should have PT, PTT, and platelet counts monitored if any signs of bleeding occur. The usual dose of vitamin K_1 (1 mg) should be given to the baby postpartum and repeated in 24 hours. Repeated infusions of fresh-frozen plasma are given if any bleeding occurs.
   c. **Delayed hemorrhagic disease** of the newborn can occur at 4 to 12 weeks of age. This may happen in breastfed infants who are not receiving supplementation. Infants who are undergoing treatment with broad-spectrum antibiotics or infants with malabsorption (liver disease, cystic fibrosis) are at greater risk of hemorrhagic disease. Vitamin K_1, 1 mg/week orally for the first 3 months of life, may prevent late hemologic disease of the newborn. An oral preparation as used in Europe has not yet been approved in the United States. Although blood tests show that breastfed infants are at potential risk for HDN, HDN has not been reported in infants who received intramuscular vitamin K at birth [see comments from Fanaroff (4)]. Concerns about an increased risk of childhood cancer after neonatal administration of vitamin K have proved unfounded (5,7,8).

References

1. Andrew M. The homeostatic system in the infant. In: Nathan, D. G. and Oski, F. A. (Eds.), *Hematology of Infancy and Childhood,* 5th ed. 1998. Philadelphia: Saunders.
2. Atkinson J. B., et al. Major surgical intervention during extracorporeal membrane oxygenation. *J Pediatr Surg* 1992;27(9):1197.
3. Christensen R. D. *Hematologic problems of the Neonate.* 2000. Philadelphia: Saunders.
4. Fanaroff A. A. *Yearbook of Neonatal and Perinatal Medicine.* St. Louis: Mosby, 1994; 330.
5. Green F. R. Vitamin K deficiency and hemorrhage in infancy. *Clin Perinatol* 1995;22: 759.
6. Hawiger J., et al. Hemostasis. In: Nathan D. G., Oski F. A. (Eds.), *Hematology of Infancy and Childhood,* 4th ed. 1993. Philadelphia: Saunders.
7. Klaus M. H. Editorial comment. In: *Yearbook of Neonatal and Perinatal Medicine.* 1994; St. Louis: C. V. Mosby, 380.
8. Klebanoff M. A., et al. The risk of childhood cancer after neonatal exposure to vitamin K. *N Engl J Med* 1993;329:905.
9. Oski F. A., et al. *Hematologic Problems in the Newborn,* 3rd ed. 1982. Philadelphia: Saunders.
10. Pramanik A. K. Bleeding disorders in neonates. *Pediatr Rev* 1992;13:163.
11. Turner T. Treatment of premature infants with abnormal clotting parameters. *Br J Hematol* 1981;47:65.
12. Wilson J. M., et al. Aminocaproic acid decreases the incidence of intracranial hemorrhage and other hemorrhagic complications in ECMO. *J Pediatr Surg* 1993;28: 536.

Polycythemia

Allen M. Goorin

As the central (venous) hematocrit rises, there is increased viscosity and decreased blood flow; when the hematocrit increases to more than 60%, there is a fall in oxygen transport (7) (Fig. 26.1). Newborns have erythrocytes that are less deformable than the erythrocytes of adults. As viscosity increases, there is impairment of tissue oxygenation and decreased glucose in plasma, and a tendency to form microthrombi. If these events occur in the cerebral cortex, kidneys, or adrenal glands, significant damage may result. Hypoxia and acidosis increase viscosity and deformity further. Poor perfusion increases the possibility of thrombosis.

I. **Definitions**
   A. **Polycythemia.** Venous hematocrit of over 65% (5), a venous hematocrit over 64% or more at 2 hours of age (16), an umbilical venous or arterial hematocrit over 63% or more (16). The mean venous hematocrit of term infants is 53 in cord blood, 60 at 2 hours of age, 57 at 6 hours of age, and 52 at 12 to 18 hours of age (16).
   B. **Hyperviscosity** is defined as greater than 14.6 centipoise at a shear rate of 11.5 s^{-1} as measured by a viscometer (15). The relationship of hematocrit and viscosity is nearly linear below a hematocrit of 60%, but viscosity increases exponentially at a hematocrit of 70% or greater (Fig. 26.1) (7,14).

   Other factors may alter viscosity. These include plasma proteins, especially fibrinogen, and local blood flow (16). The hyperviscosity syndrome is usually seen only in infants with venous hematocrits above 60.

II. **Incidence.** The incidence of polycythemia in newborns is increased in babies who are small for gestational age (SGA) and in post-term babies; on average it is 0.4 to 5% (11,16,17).

III. **Causes of polycythemia** (16)
   A. **Placental red cell transfusion**
      1. **Delayed cord clamping** may occur either intentionally or in unattended deliveries.

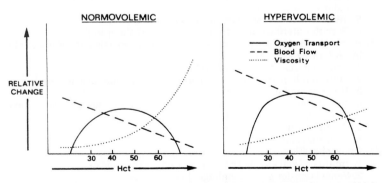

FIG. 26.1. Effect of hematocrit on viscosity, blood flow, and oxygen transport. (Adapted from Glader B., Naiman J. L. Erythrocyte disorders in infancy. In: Taeusch H. W., Ballard R. A., Avery M. E. (Eds.). *Diseases of the Newborn.* Philadelphia: Saunders, 1991, 823.

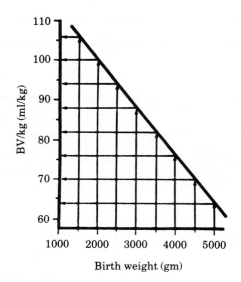

FIG. 26.2. Nomogram designed for clinical use, correlating blood volume per kilogram with birth weight in polycythemic neonates. BV, blood volume. (From Rawlings J. S. et al. Estimated blood volumes in polycythemic neonates as a function of birth weight. *J Pediatr* 1982;101:594.)

    a. When the cord is clamped within 1 minute after birth, the blood volume of the infant is 83.4 mL/kg.
    b. When the cord is clamped 2 minutes after delivery, the blood volume of the infant is 93 mL/kg.
    c. In newborns with polycythemia, blood volume per kilogram of body weight varies inversely in relation to birth weight (Fig. 26.2).
  2. Cord stripping (thus pushing more blood into the infant).
  3. Holding the baby below the mother at delivery.
  4. Maternal-to-fetal transfusion is diagnosed with the Kleihauer-Betke stain technique of acid elution to detect maternal cells in the newborn circulation (see Anemia).
  5. Twin-to-twin transfusion (see Chap. 7).
  6. Forceful uterine contractions before cord clamping.
 B. Placental insufficiency (increased fetal erythropoiesis secondary to chronic intrauterine hypoxia)
  1. Small-for-gestational-age (SGA) infants.
  2. Maternal hypertension syndromes (toxemia, renal disease, etc.).
  3. Postmature infants.
  4. Infants born to mothers with chronic hypoxia (heart disease, pulmonary disease).
  5. Pregnancy at high altitude.
  6. Maternal smoking.
 C. Other conditions
  1. Infants of diabetic mothers (increased erythropoiesis).
  2. Some large-for-gestational-age (LGA) babies.
  3. Infants with congenital adrenal hyperplasia, Beckwith-Wiedemann syndrome, neonatal thyrotoxicosis, congenital hypothyroidism, trisomy 21, trisomy 13, trisomy 18.

    4. Drugs (maternal use of propranolol).
    5. Dehydration of infant.
IV. Clinical findings. Most infants with polycythemia are asymptomatic. Clinical symptoms, syndromes, and laboratory abnormalities that have been described in association with polycythemia include the following:
    A. Central nervous system (CNS). Poor feeding, lethargy, hypotonia, apnea, tremors, jitteriness, seizures, cerebral venous thrombosis.
    B. Cardiorespiratory. Cyanosis, tachypnea, heart murmurs, congestive heart failure, cardiomegaly, elevated pulmonary vascular resistance, prominent vascular markings on chest X ray.
    C. Renal. Decreased glomerular filtration, decreased sodium excretion, renal vein thrombosis, hematuria, proteinuria.
    D. Other. Other thrombosis, thrombocytopenia, poor feeding, increased jaundice, persistent hypoglycemia, hypocalcemia, testicular infarcts, necrotizing enterocolitis, priapism, disseminated intravascular coagulation.
    All of these symptoms may be associated with polycythemia/hyperviscosity but may not be caused by it. They are common symptoms in many neonatal disorders.
V. Screening. The routine screening of all newborns for polycythemia/hyperviscosity is being advocated by some authors (6,18). The timing and site of blood sampling alter the hematocrit value (12,13). We do not routinely screen well term newborns for this syndrome, since there are few data showing that treatment of asymptomatic patients with partial exchange transfusion is beneficial in the long term (1,5,16).
VI. Diagnosis. The capillary blood or peripheral venous hematocrit level should be determined in any baby who appears plethoric, who has any predisposing cause of polycythemia, who has any of the symptoms mentioned in IV, or who is not well for any reason.
    A. Depending on local perfusion, the **capillary blood hematocrit** will be 5 to 20% higher than the central hematocrit (16). Warming the heel prior to drawing blood for a capillary hematocrit determination will give a better correlation with the peripheral venous or central hematocrit. If the capillary blood hematocrit is above 65%, the peripheral venous hematocrit should be determined. The hematocrit should be measured with an automated hematology analyzer. Most of the old studies of hematocrits were done with spun hematocrits, which may give falsely high levels (16).
    B. Few hospitals are equipped to measure blood viscosity. If the equipment is available, the test should be done, because some infants with venous hematocrits under 65% will have hyperviscous blood (17).
VII. Management
    A. Any child with symptoms that could be due to hyperviscosity should have a **partial exchange transfusion if the peripheral venous hematocrit is more than 65%.**
    B. Asymptomatic infants with a peripheral venous hematocrit between 60 and 70% **can usually be managed by increasing fluid intake and repeating the hematocrit in 4 to 6 hours.**
    C. Most neonatologists perform an **exchange transfusion when the peripheral venous hematocrit is more than 70% in the absence of symptoms, but this is controversial** (1,2,5,12,13).
    D. The following formula can be used to calculate the exchange with albumin 5% or normal saline that will bring the hematocrit to 50 to 60%. In infants with polycythemia, the blood volume varies inversely with the birth weight (see Fig. 26.2). **We usually take the blood from the umbilical vein and replace it with albumin 5% or normal saline in a peripheral vein.** Since randomized trials show no advantage to albumin, and there is less chance of infection, nonhuman products, such as saline, are preferred. There are many methods of exchange (see Chap. 18).

Volume of exchange (in mL)

$$= \frac{\text{blood volume} \times (\text{observed hematocrit} - \text{desired hematocrit})}{\text{observed hematocrit}}$$

Example: A 3-kg infant, hematocrit 75%, blood volume 80 mL/kg—to bring hematocrit to 50%:

$$\text{Volume of exchange (in mL)} = \frac{(80 \text{ mL} \times 3 \text{ kg}) \times (75-50)}{75}$$

$$= \frac{240 \text{ ml} \times 25}{75}$$

$$= 80\text{-mL exchange}$$

The total volume exchanged is usually 15 to 20 mL/kg of body weight. This will depend on the observed hematocrit. (Blood volume may be up to 100 mL/kg in polycythemic infants.)

VIII. Outcome

A. **Infants with polycythemia and hyperviscosity who have decreased cerebral blood flow velocity and increased vascular resistance develop normal cerebral blood flow following partial exchange transfusion** (12). They also have improvement in systemic blood flow and oxygen transport (1,13,15,16).

B. **The long-term neurologic outcome** in infants with asymptomatic polycythemia/hyperviscosity, whether treated or untreated, **remains controversial.**

   1. One trial with small numbers of randomized patients has shown decreased IQ scores in school-age children who had neonatal hyperviscosity syndrome, whether or not the newborns were treated (3,5).

   2. Another retrospective study, with small numbers of patients, showed no difference in the neurologic outcome of patients with asymptomatic neonatal polycythemia, whether they were treated or not (10).

   3. Some earlier preliminary prospective studies favored treatment (2,8).

   4. A small prospective study showed no difference at follow-up between control infants and those with hyperviscosity, between those with symptomatic and asymptomatic hyperviscosity, and no difference between asymptomatic infants treated with partial exchange transfusion and those who were observed. Analysis revealed that other perinatal risk factors and race, rather than polycythemia or partial exchange transfusion, significantly influenced the long-term outcome (1,16).

   5. An increased incidence of necrotizing enterocolitis (NEC) following partial exchange transfusions by umbilical vein has been reported (2,4). NEC was not seen in one retrospective analysis of 185 term polycythemic babies given partial exchange transfusions with removal of blood from the umbilical vein and reinfusion of a commercial plasma substitute through peripheral veins (9).

   6. A large prospective, randomized clinical trial comparing partial exchange transfusion with symptomatic care (increased fluid intake, etc.) equally balanced for risk factors and the etiologies of the polycythemia will be necessary to give guidelines for treatment of the asymptomatic newborn with polycythemia/hyperviscosity.

   7. Partial exchange transfusion will lower hematocrit, decrease viscosity, and reverse many of the physiologic abnormalities associated with polycythemia/hyperviscosity but has not been shown to significantly change the long-term outcome of these infants (16).

References

1. Bada H., et al. Asymptomatic syndrome of polycythemic hyperviscosity: Effect of partial plasma transfusion. *J Pediatr* 1992;120:578.

2. Black V. D., et al. Neonatal polycythemia and hyperviscosity. *Pediatr Clin North Am* 1982;5:1137.
3. Black V. D., et al. Developmental and neurologic sequelae in neonatal hyperviscosity syndrome. *Pediatrics* 1982;69:426.
4. Black V. D., et al. Gastrointestinal injury in polycythemic term infants. *Pediatrics* 1985;76:225.
5. Delaney-Black V. D., et al. Neonatal hyperviscosity: Association with lower achievement and IQ scores at school age. *Pediatrics* 1989;83:662.
6. Drew J.H., et al. Neonatal whole blood hyperviscosity: the important factor influencing later neurologic function is the viscocosity, and not the polycythemia. *Clin Hemorheol Microcirc* 1997;17:67.
7. Glader B. Erythrocyte Disorders in Infancy. In: Taeusch, H. W., Ballard R. A., Avery M. E. (Eds.). *Diseases of the Newborn*, 6th ed. 1991. Philadelphia: Saunders.
8. Goldberg K., et al. Neonatal hyperviscosity. II. Effect of partial plasma exchange transfusion. *Pediatrics* 1982;69:419.
9. Hein H. A., et al. Partial exchange transfusion in term, polycythemic neonates: Absence of association with severe gastrointestinal injury. *Pediatrics* 1987;80:75.
10. Host A., et al. Late prognosis in untreated neonatal polycythemia with minor or no symptoms. *Acta Paediatr Scand* 1982;71:629.
11. Lindermann R., et. al. Evaluation and treatment of polycythemia in the neonate. In: Christensen R. D. (Ed). *Hematologic Problems of the Neonate*. 2000. Philadelphia: Saunders.
12. Oski F. A., Naiman J. L. *Hematologic Problems in the Newborn*, 3rd ed. 1982. Philadelphia: Saunders, 87–96.
13. Phibbs R. H., et al. Hematologic problems. In: M. H. Klaus and A. A. Fanaroff (Eds.). *Care of the High Risk Neonate*. 1993. Philadelphia: Saunders, 421.
14. Ramamurthy R. S. J., et al. Postnatal alteration in hematocrit and viscosity in normal and polycythemic infants. *J Pediatr* 1987;110:929.
15. Swernam S. M., et al. Hemodynamic consequences of neonatal polycythemia. *J Pediatr* 1987;110:443.
16. Wexner E. J. Neonatal polycythemia and hyperviscosity. *Clin Perinatol* 1995;22:693.
17. Wirth F. H., et al. Neonatal hyperviscosity I. Incidence. *J Pediatr* 1979;63:833.
18. Wiswell T. E., et al. Neonatal polycythemia: Frequency of clinical manifestations and other associated findings. *Pediatrics* 1986;78:26.

Thrombocytopenia

Allen M. Goorin and John P. Cloherty

Neonatal thrombocytopenia is a platelet count of less than $150,000/mm^3$. The causes include increased consumption or decreased production (rare). Consumption may be caused by antibodies, mechanical problems, or intravascular coagulation. The incidence in the general neonatal population is small (approximately 0.1% of cord bloods had counts <50,000), and most neonates with thrombocytopenia have only a modest reduction in platelet counts (50,000 to 100,000). These are generally self-resolved (5). More serious reductions, under 20,000, or 50,000 with bleeding, warrant evaluation and intervention.

In contrast, thrombocytopenia in the neonatal intensive care unit is quite common. Indeed, in one prospective study, thrombocytopenia developed in 22% of 807 neonatal intensive care unit (NICU) admissions. The etiology in about 80% of cases is generally consumptive. This is particularly true for sick infants, in whom thrombocytopenia may represent just part of a spectrum of consumptive coagulopathy (18). The most severe sequelae of severe thrombocytopenia, such as intracranial hemorrhage, are associated with alloimmunization or are related to the degree of prematurity.

Thrombocytopenia may precede delivery. A recent retrospective review observed an incidence of approximately 5% of thrombocytopenia in fetal blood samplings. Congenital infections or chromosomal disorders accounted for almost half of these (reflecting the indications for the fetal blood sampling itself). Antibody-mediated causes included both maternal autoimmune and alloimmune conditions (11).

I. Diagnosis (Fig. 26.3)
   A. Maternal history. There may be a history of thrombocytopenia, bleeding before or during pregnancy, a previous splenectomy, drug use, or infection. A history of pre- or postnatal bleeding in a previous pregnancy is important.
   B. Infant. The baby may seem healthy or may appear sick. There may be petechiae or large bruises, hepatosplenomegaly, jaundice, limb enlargement, hemangioma, or bruits (3).
   C. Laboratory studies
      1. Mother. Needs to have a platelet count and platelet typing (if the maternal count is normal).
      2. Baby. Complete blood count (CBC), platelet count, prothrombin time (PT), and partial thromboplastin time (PTT).
II. Therapy
   A. Platelet transfusion
      1. Indications:
         a. When bleeding or platelets <20,000: There have been few prospective controlled trials of the best time to transfuse platelets in neonates. One attempt randomized sick preterm infants to conventional therapy (typically keeping platelets >50,000) versus maintaining platelets >150,000 with 1 to 3 transfusions) over the first week of life. There was no difference in the rate of intracranial hemorrhage in either group (2).
         b. This confirms that routine platelet transfusion does not help in severe prematurity, but it does not address the minimum number to which platelet counts should be allowed to fall.
      2. Source. Use a random donor, except for the infant with alloimmune thrombocytopenia. In this case, use the mother's platelets after appropriate testing (washed to remove the alloantibody) or platelets from a platelet antigen–compatible donor.

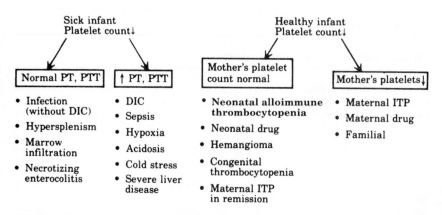

FIG. 26.3. Clinical status in neonatal thrombocytopenia with features that determine a quick differential diagnosis. PT = prothrombin time; PTT = partial thromboplastin time; DIC = disseminated intravascular coagulation; ITP = immune thrombocytopenic purpura; ↑, increase; ↓, decrease.

3. **Quantity.** One unit of platelets per 3 kg raises the platelet count by 50,000 to 100,000/mL, unless there is peripheral destruction of the platelets.
4. **Frequency.** The normal half-life of platelets is 4 to 5 days; it is shorter if there is increased platelet consumption.
5. **Route.** Give platelets intravenously through a peripheral vein. Never give platelets through an arterial line or into the liver (umbilical line) because thrombosis may occur.
6. **Irradiate all platelet transfusions for newborns.**
   B. **Steroid therapy** in bleeding infants. Prednisone 2 mg/kg per day (Prednisolone IV) may reduce bleeding.
   C. In an emergency, **whole blood may be used for exchange transfusion.**
III. **Thrombocytopenia with decreased platelet survival**
   A. **Immune.** In immune thrombocytopenias (ITP), maternal antibody crosses the placenta, resulting in destruction of neonatal platelets. Considerable amounts of antibody may cross, resulting in thrombocytopenias that persist for several weeks. It is called an **AUTOAntibody** when the antibody is directed against an antigen on the mother's own platelets shared in common with the baby's platelets. **ALLOAntibodies** are antibodies directed against antigens on the baby's platelets (and, perforce, paternal platelets) but not present on maternal platelets.
   1. **Auto-maternal ITP.** These include various autoimmune syndromes such as systemic lupus erythematosus (SLE).
      a. **Clinical picture.** The baby usually has mild to moderate thrombocytopenia (20,000 to 50,000) and is healthy, but has petechiae or bruising. There may be increased bruising at the vitamin K injection site or bleeding at circumcision or heel-stick sites. The mother usually has thrombocytopenia or a history of ITP.
      b. **Pathophysiology.** Maternal autoantibodies cross the placenta and bind to neonatal platelets. A normal maternal platelet count does not rule out this cause, as the maternal count may reflect compensated increased destruction. Although it is rare, one center had 11 mothers with normal platelet counts, in whom alloimmune differences were excluded, who delivered 17 infants with severe thrombocytopenia. In 10 of these 11, the center was able to identify a maternal autoanti– GP1b antibody and subsequently demonstrate compensated maternal thrombocytolysis or hypersplenism (20). This may be more common if the mother has had a splenectomy. Elicit a **maternal history** of thrombocytopenia or symptoms of autoimmune syndromes. Maternal thrombocytopenia at delivery is common (about 7% of women at delivery have platelet counts <150,000). Almost all infants born to women with thrombocytopenia are either unaffected or have mild to moderate reductions that are self-resolving. Only 1 of 756 of infants born to women with incidental thrombocytopenia, 5 of 1414 with hypertension, and 4 of 46 with ITP had cord blood platelet counts less than 50,000, and all of them were over 20,000 and without sequelae (5). Identification of autoantibody on maternal platelets is not sufficient to diagnose an autoimmune cause. There was elevated platelet-associated immunoglobulin G(IgG) (not directed against Gp1b) in the serum of about one-third of mothers of infants with documented anti–HPAa1 alloimmune thrombocytopenia (14).
      c. **Treatment of autoimmune thrombocytopenia**
         (1) **Prenatal management:** Even if the mother has true ITP, it appears that fetal hemorrhage in utero is very rare (compared with the small but definite risk of such hemorrhage in alloimmune thrombocytopenia (5,7). One uncontrolled study (10) showed a 3.6-fold increase in neonatal platelet counts following steroid administration to mothers with ITP and positive antiplatelet antibodies.
            Prednisone, 10 to 20 mg qd, was given for 10 to 14 days prior to delivery. A small prospective randomized trial of low-dose

betamethasone (1.5 mg orally per day from day 259 to day 273 and 1 mg until delivery) failed to prevent thrombocytopenia in newborns (9). These discrepant data need further study before steroid administration becomes routine practice. Intravenous gammaglobulin (IGG) given prenatally to the mother with ITP has not been clearly shown to affect the fetal platelet count. Percutaneous umbilical blood sampling (PUBS) is beginning to be used as a safe, accurate, and direct method of obtaining the fetal platelet counts. In experienced hands, the mortality from this procedure is less than 1% (7). This may still be too great a risk for cases of maternal ITP (see Chap. 1, Fetal Assessment and Prenatal Diagnosis). There may be little correlation between fetal and maternal platelet counts. Mothers who have had recent platelet counts under 80,000, who are on steroids, or who have had a splenectomy are at increased risk to have a child with significant thrombocytopenia. Since a cesarean section reduces trauma to the infant, it would decrease the risk of bleeding in the occasional infant who is severely thrombocytopenic. The issue of when to do cesarean sections in mothers known to have ITP is controversial. The maternal mortality from cesarean sections in most centers is the same as from vaginal deliveries. Our usual management of these cases is to allow vaginal delivery to progress until a fetal scalp platelet count can be done. If the fetal scalp platelet count is over 50,000 and labor is progressing normally, the infant is delivered vaginally. If these criteria are not met, then a cesarean section is done. One should remember that obstetricians would like a maternal platelet count of 50,000 to 100,000 before they are willing to operate, and anesthesiologists are often unwilling to give epidural anesthesia to mothers with platelet counts under 100,000. The use of steroids, IgG, PUBS, or cesarean sections in the prenatal management of maternal ITP is controversial and requires cooperation between the obstetrician, neonatalogist, hemotologist, and family. These therapies are not usually required in maternal ITP (3,13).

(2) **Postnatal treatment** of infants affected by maternal ITP may include platelet transfusion, steroids, IgG, or exchange transfusion (treatment is as in Bleeding, III,IV).

2. **Alloimmune thrombocytopenia.** Maternal serum that shows antibodies that react against the father's but not against the mother's own platelets demonstrates an alloantibody. Of 19 fetuses known to be at risk for alloimmune thrombocytopenia (typically because of severely affected siblings from a prior delivery), 6 had platelet counts under 20,000 and 3 suffered intracranial bleeding episodes, 2 of which were antenatal (5). Hence, alloimmune thrombocytopenia, although uncommon, when present, may result in severe hemorrhagic complications in utero. We have seen one mother who had recurrent episodes of severe fetal hemorrhage. A majority of cases are secondary to antiHPA1 (P1A-1) antibody; however, there are also numerous other antigens as targets (Table 26.7) (8).

a. **Clinical picture.** The baby appears healthy but has petechiae, bruising, bleeding, and a low platelet count (often < 20,000). The mother has a normal platelet count; it may be her first pregnancy, or she may have a history of a previously affected pregnancy. There may be a history of alloimmune thrombocytopenia in children born to the mother's sisters.

b. **Pathophysiology.** Approximately 97% of Caucasians are HPA-1a+ and, hence about 3% of pregnancies involve an HPA-1a negative mother carrying an HPA-1a positive fetus. Roughly 1 in 1000 to 5000 deliveries are affected; therefore, 3% of pregnancies at risk are actually affected (5,6). There is a link between maternal production of alloantibodies and HLA type DR-3; there may be other factors that also regulate maternal antibody formation (4). Virtually all identified platelet

TABLE 26.7. PLATELET-SPECIFIC ALLOANTIGEN SYSTEMS

New HPA Nomenclature	Original Designations	Caucasian Phenotype Frequency	Clinical Alloimmune Syndromes Described
HPA-1a	Zw^a, P1^{A1}	0.97	NAIT, PTP, PTR, PAT, TAT
HPA-1b	Zw^b, P1^{A2}	0.27	NAIT, PTP, PTR
HPA-2a	Ko^b	0.992	
HPA-2b	Ko^a, Sib^a	0.169	NAIT, PTR
HPA-3a	Bak^a, Lek^a	0.85	NAIT, PTP
HPA-3b	Bak^b, Lek^b	0.66	NAIT, PTP, PTR
HPA-4a	Pen^a, Yuk^b	>0.999	NAIT, PTP
HPA-4b	Pen^b, Yuk^a	<0.0001	NAIT
HPA-5a	Br^b, Zav^b	0.99	NAIT
HPA-5b	Br^a, Zav^a, Hc^a	0.21	NAIT, PTP, PTR, PAT
HPA-6b	Tu^a, Ca	<0.007	NAIT
HPA-7b	Mo^a	<0.002	NAIT
HPA-8b	Sr^a	<0.01	NAIT
	P1^{E1}	0.999	—
	P1^{E2}	0.05	NAIT
	Gov^a	0.81	NAIT, PTP
	Gov^b	0.74	
	Va^a	<0.004	NAIT
	Nak^a GPIV isoantibody	0.9966	PTR

NAIT = neonatal alloimmune thrombocytopenia; PTP = post-transfusion purpura; PTR = platelet transfusion refractoriness; PAT = passive alloimmune thrombocytopenia; TAT = transplant-associated thrombocytopenia; HPA = human platelet antigen.
From Burrows R. F., Kelton J. G. Prenatal thrombocytopenia. *Clin Perinatol* 1995;22:779.

antigens have been implicated in neonatal alloimmune thrombo-cytopenia (16). In one series of 295 patients with suspected neonatal alloimmune thrombocytopenia referred to a platelet serology reference laboratory, only 36% were found to have platelet-specific antibody. Two-thirds of them were anti-HPA-1a directed, and 4% anti-HPA-3a (19). Twenty-four percent revealed only HLA antibodies, although the presence of an anti-HLA antibody does not prove that the antibody resulted in the thrombocytopenia.

   c. **Diagnostic evaluation.** DNA techniques that define platelet-specific polymorphisms add to the diagnostic armamentarium but do not eliminate the usefulness of serological techniques (15). The identification of numerous polymorphisms, including those in Table 26.7, makes the role of a centralized platelet serology laboratory paramount (17). The Blood Center of Southeastern Wisconsin (1–800-245-3117), Tom

Kickler (Johns Hopkins, Baltimore, Maryland), and Scott Murphy (Temple University, Philadelphia, Pennsylvania) have excellent labs providing outside diagnostic services. Proper identification of the cause of the thrombocytopenia may be more important for the proper management of future pregnancies than for acute treatment of the thrombocytopenic infant. In cases of paternal heterozygosity, amniocentesis will identify the platelet antigen genotype of the fetus (8). Although controversial, the antenatal treatment of alloimmune thrombocytopenia with PUBS (percutaneous umbilical cord blood sampling) and administration of IVIG to the mother may affect the natural history of a disorder associated with intracranial hemorrhage during the third trimester (6,8,14).

Infusion of maternal compatible platelets at the time of cordocentesis may decrease the incidence of hemorrhage during the procedure.

DNA testing is performed on 1 to 5 mL of the mother's and the infant's (or, alternatively, the father's) blood. Serologic testing typically requires testing of both maternal and paternal platelets, as testing of the affected infant's platelets generally proves impossible because of thrombocytopenia. Again, not all infants of HPA-a1 (P1A1)-negative women with documented anti-HPA-a1 (P1A1) Ab are thrombocytopenic; use caution when interpreting treatment results of such "high-risk" women (4).

d. Treatment

(1) Prenatal treatment. Intravenous gammaglobulin, steroids, prenatal (by PUBS) platelet transfusion, fetal scalp platelet counts in labor, and elective cesarean section should be considered as management tools on a case-by-case basis with cooperation between the obstetrician, neonatologist, and hematologist. If the fetal platelet count is over 50,000/mL as measured by PUBS or fetal scalp platelet count, we allow **vaginal delivery** if presentation and labor are normal. If these criteria are not met, a **cesarean section** is done.

(2) Postnatal treatment (see II)

(a) Platelet transfusion. If the diagnosis is known to be alloimmune neonatal thrombocytopenia, the mother's platelets are collected 24 hours prior to delivery. If the baby has a platelet count of less than 20,000/mL, or if the baby shows any signs of bleeding, the mother's platelets (P1A1 negative) are transfused into the baby. The mother's serum will have P1A1 positive antibody, which potentially can react with the newborn's platelets. Using washed maternal platelets resuspended in plasma will avoid this complication. If there is an emergency secondary to bleeding in the newborn, and the mother's platelets have not been previously collected, either the mother's whole blood or platelets from a previously typed P1A1 negative platelet donor can be used. Random platelets should be used if there is serious bleeding and P1A1 negative platelets are not available. To avoid the possibility that the infant will develop **graft-versus-host (GVH) disease,** the blood products should be irradiated (see Blood Products Used in the Newborn).

Apheresis services are generally not necessary, as a single unit of antigen negative platelets should give a 50,000 to 100,000 boost. By collecting the platelet-rich plasma from the mother and reinfusing the red blood cells to the mother, there can be multiple collections over the ensuing several days. Although an apheresis unit could be obtained and aliquoted to achieve a platelet supply for up to 5 days of transfusions, it is unclear that this benefits the patient (13).

(b) Gamma-globulin (IgG). There has been successful postnatal use of intravenous IGG 0.4 g/kg per day for 2 to 5 days (1,7).

(c) Prednisone (Prednisolone IV). Usually, 2 mg/kg per day is given to newborns with continued low platelet counts or continued bleeding (7).

(3) Treatment of additional children. It is important to make the diagnosis for other children and to refer the family to a high-risk center for additional pregnancies. Sisters of P1A1-negative mothers should have platelet typing done to anticipate problems. If they are P1A1-negative and their husbands are P1A1-positive, anticipatory planning is indicated. Three platelet serology laboratories are The Blood Center of Southeastern Wisconsin (1-800-245-3117), Tom Kickler (Johns Hopkins, Baltimore, Maryland), and Scott Murphy's lab (Temple University, Philadelphia, Pennsylvania).

(4) Outcome. Roughly 20% of all infants with identified cases of neonatal alloimmune thrombocytopenia (NAIT) have intracranial hemorrhages. As many as half occur antenatally. We have seen two fetal deaths with bleeding associated with fetal alloimmune thrombocytopenia. Obtain a cranial ultrasound study after delivery to document any intracranial bleeding, since intracranial hemorrhages are sometimes clinically silent.

3. Drug-induced. Although a long list of drugs is associated with neonatal thrombocytopenia, it is unclear how many of them are the true cause. If the mother has an antibody that results in thrombocytopenia by immune mechanisms, the infant may become thrombocytopenic if given the same medication. (Treatment is as in Bleeding, III, IV.)

B. Peripheral consumption of platelets

1. Disseminated intravascular coagulation (DIC) (see Bleeding).

a. Clinical picture. The infant appears sick and has thrombocytopenia, a prolonged PT, and a prolonged PTT. There is a decrease in fibrinogen, and an increase in d-dimers.

b. Therapy

(1) Treat the underlying disorder (e.g., sepsis, acidosis, hypoxia, or hypothermia). Give vitamin K and replace clotting factors and platelets.

(2) Perform exchange transfusion with fresh whole blood for patients with active bleeding that does not respond to repeated plasma and platelet transfusions.

2. Giant hemangioma (Kasabach-Merritt syndrome) (3)

a. Clinical picture. The baby appears healthy, and has a large hemangioma and thrombocytopenia.

b. Therapy involves platelet transfusion, clotting factors, and prednisone. Most hemangiomas involute by 1 to 2 years of age, so attempt medical management. We and others have had good results treating some of these hemangiomas with alpha-interferon but an increase in cerebral palsy in children treated with alpha interferon has stopped us from using this therapy. Embolization or surgery is sometimes necessary.

3. Necrotizing enterocolitis (see Chap. 32)

a. Clinical picture. Thrombocytopenia with necrotizing enterocolitis.

b. Therapy. Treat the underlying disorder and give platelet transfusions as necessary.

4. Type IIB Von Willebrand's disease may present as thrombocytopenia secondary to platelet aggregation in newborns (10).

C. Direct toxic injury to platelets

1. Sepsis may be of bacterial or viral origin. Therapy involves treatment of the underlying disorder. Platelet transfusion is necessary if there is bleeding.

a. Thrombocytopenia as an early sign of sepsis in newborns is nonspecific, although high mean platelet volume and high platelet distribution widths correlated with late sepsis.

b. There is some evidence that an immune mechanism may be involved in the thrombocytopenia of neonatal sepsis.

2. **Drug injury.** Thiazides, tolbutamide, hydralazine, and aspirin have been implicated. Therapy involves the removal of the offending drug, and platelet transfusion if there is bleeding. Maternal ingestion of **aspirin** during pregnancy should be avoided. If ingestion occurs within 1 week of delivery, 90% of newborns will have bleeding tendencies. Maternal use of aspirin has been associated with a reduced mean birth weight of the offspring, prolongation of gestation and labor, increased blood loss at delivery, and increased perinatal mortality (3).

3. **Neonatal cold injury:** Massive pulmonary hemorrhage secondary to hyperaggregation of platelets has been associated with infants who die while being rewarmed.

D. **Hypersplenism**

1. **Clinical picture.** The baby has an enlarged spleen and thrombocytopenia; there may or may not be hemolytic anemia. The condition is associated with congenital hepatitis, congenital viral infection, and portal vein thrombosis.

2. **Therapy.** Treat the underlying disorder. Administer platelet transfusion if there is bleeding. Splenectomy is the last resort for uncontrollable bleeding.

E. **Familial shortened platelet survival** results from intrinsic problems with platelets. Production also may be abnormal.

1. **Wiskott-Aldrich syndrome** is manifested by the presence of abnormal, small platelets.

2. **May-Hegglin anomaly** is an autosomal dominant disorder in which the infant has giant, bizarre platelets with Döhle bodies, abnormal platelet survival, and impaired production of platelets.

3. **Bernard-Soulier syndrome** is demonstrated by large platelets with granules clumped to appear as a nucleus.

IV. **Thrombocytopenia with normal platelet survival and decreased platelet production**

A. **Toxic injury to megakaryocytes** due to bacterial or viral infections or drug-induced injury.

B. **Congenital thrombocytopenias** due to syndrome of thrombocytopenia with absent radii, Fanconi's anemia, familial thrombocytopenias, or marrow aplasia, which may be isolated or general.

C. **Marrow infiltration** due to neonatal leukemia, congenital neuroblastoma, or storage disease.

V. **Thrombocytopeni associated with erythroblastosis fetalis.** The mechanism may possibly involve platelet trapping in the liver and spleen, anoxia with secondary intravascular coagulation, or associated antiplatelet antibodies.

VI. **Thrombocytopenia after exchange or other transfusion.** Blood more than 24 hours old has few viable platelets.

VII. **The management of a high-risk fetus** requires orchestration of interventional obstetricians, reference lab, and comprehensive blood bank services. A review of platelet problems in the newborn is found in ref. 3.

References

1. Amato M., et al. Treatment of neonatal thrombocytopenia. *J Pediatr* 1985; 107: 650.
2. Andrew M., et al. A randomized, controlled trial of platelet transfusions in thrombocytopenic premature infants. *Pediatrics* 1993;123:285.
3. Beardsley D. S. Platelet abnormalities in infancy and childhood. In: Nathan D. G., Oski F. A. (Eds.). *Hematology of Infancy and Childhood,* 5th ed. 1992. Philadelphia: Saunders.
4. Blanchette V. S., et al. Alloimmunization to the P1A1 platelet antigen: Results of a prospective study. *Br J Haematol* 1990;74:209.
5. Burrows R. F. Fetal thrombocytopenia and its relation to maternal thrombocytopenia. *N Engl J Med* 1993;329:1463.

6. Burrows R. F., et al. Perinatal thrombocytopenia. *Clin Perinatol* 1995;22:779.
7. Bussel J. B., et al. Recommendations for the evaluation and treatment of neonatal autoimmune and alloimmune thrombocytopenia. *Thromb Haemost* 1991;65:631.
8. Bussel J. B., et al. Fetal alloimmune thrombocytopenia. *N Engl J Med* 1997;337:23.
9. Christiaens G. C., et al. Idiopathic thrombocytopenic purpura in pregnancy: A randomized trial on the effect of antenatal low dose corticosteroids on neonatal platelet counts. *Br J Obstet Gynaecol* 1990;97:893.
10. DeCarolis S., et al. Immune thrombocytopenic purpura and percutaneous umbilical blood sampling: An open question. *Fetal Diagn Ther* 1993;8:154.
11. Hohlfeld P., et al. Fetal thrombocytopenia: A retrospective survey of 5194 fetal blood samplings. *Blood* 1994;84:1851.
12. Karpatkin M. Platelet counts in infants of women with autoimmune thrombocytopenia: Effect of steroid administration to the mother. *N Engl J Med* 1981; 305: 936.
13. Kaplan C., et al. Fetal and neonatal alloimmune thrombocytopenia: Current trends in diagnosis and therapy. *Transfusion Med* 1992;2:265.
14. Kickler T. S. Elevated platelet-associated IgG in PLA1-negative mothers following sensitization to the PLA-1 antigen during pregnancy. *Vox Sang* 1992;63:210.
15. McFarland J. G., et al. Prenatal diagnosis of neonatal alloimmune thrombocytopenia using allele-specific oligonucleotide probes. *Blood* 1991;78:2276.
16. Menell J. S., et al. Antenatal management of the thrombocytopenias. *Clin Perinatol* 1994;21:591.
17. Pao M., et al. Importance of platelet serologic testing for defining the cause of neonatal thrombocytopenia. *Am J Pediatr Hematol Oncol* 1991;13:71.
18. Schmidt B. K. Coagulation screening in high risk neonates: A prospective cohort study. *Arch Dis Child* 1992;67:1196.
19. Schnell M., et al. Serologic investigation of 295 cases of suspected neonatal alloimmune thrombocytopenia. *Transfusion* 1994;34:16S(abstr):64.
20. Tchernia G., et al. Neonatal thrombocytopenia and hidden maternal autoimmunity. *Br J Haematol* 1993;84:457.

Blood Products Used in the Newborn

Steven R. Sloan

I. **Introduction.** Blood components consist of packed red blood cells (PRBCs), platelets, frozen plasma, fresh frozen plasma, cryoprecipitate (CRYO), and granulocytes (1). In addition, intravenous immunoglobulin (IVIG) is purified from blood. In some special cases, whole blood, usually in the form of reconstituted whole blood can be used. The indications for transfusions and types of transfusions are described earlier in this chapter (see Anemia).

II. **Packed red blood cells (PRBCs)**

    A. **Contents.** Several types of PRBCs units are available that vary in the preservatives added. Chemical additives delay storage damage to red blood cells allowing for extended storage times. The types of units that are currently available in the United States are:

        1. **Anticoagulant-preservative solution units.** These units contain approximately 250 ml of a concentrated solution of red blood cells. The average hematocrit of these units is 70 to 80%. In addition, these units contain 62 mg of sodium, 222 mg of citrate, and 46 mg of phosphate. Three types of units are currently approved for use in the United States. These are:

a. **CPD.** This contains 773 mg of dextrose and has a 21-day shelf-life.
b. **CP2D.** This contains 1546 mg of dextrose and has a 21-day shelf-life.
c. **CPDA-1.** This contains 965 mg of dextrose and 8.2 mg of adenine and has a 35-day shelf-life.
2. **Additive solution units.** Three additive solutions are currently approved for use in the United States. Each of these units contains approximately 350 mL, has an average hematocrit of 50 to 60%, and has a 42-day shelf-life. Contents of these units are as follows (2):

	AS-1	AS-3	AS-5
Dextrose (mg)	2973	2645	1673
Sodium (mg)	962	406	407
Citrate (mg)	222	711	222
Phosphate (mg)	46	233	46
Adenine (mg)	27	30	30
Mannitol (mg)	750	0	525

For simple transfusions of 5 to 20 cc/kg, additive units can be used. For larger transfusions such as exchange transfusions or transfusions for surgical procedures with substantial blood loss, mannitol may cause a dangerously rapid diuresis and adenine may be a nephrotoxin in the premature infant. Hence, for these transfusions, PRBCs may be washed or PRBCs stored in an anticoagulant-preservative solution can be used.
3. **Several changes occur in PRBCs during storage:**
   a. The pH decreases from 7.4 to 7.55 to pH 6.5–6.6 at the time of expiration.
   b. Potassium is released from the red blood cells. The initial plasma K+ concentration is ~4.2 mM and increases to 78.5 mM in CPDA-1 units at day 35 and 45 to 50 mM in additive solution units on day 42. CPDA-1 units contain about one-third the plasma volume as additive units so the total amount of extracellular potassium is similar in all units of the same age.
   c. 2,3-diphosphoglycerol (2,3-DPG) levels drop rapidly during the first 2 weeks of storage. This increases the affinity of the hemoglobin for oxygen and decreases its efficiency in delivering oxygen to tissue. The 2,3-DPG levels replenish over several hours after being transfused.

   None of these changes is significant for simple transfusions of 5 to 20 cc/kg. However, hyperkalemia and decreased oxygen delivery can be important in large transfusions such as exchange transfusions or transfusions for cardiac surgery. Ideally, fresher units can be provided for these transfusions. At Children's Hospital Boston, PRBCs less than 7 days old are transfused to children less than 4 months of age receiving a large transfusion (e.g., cardiac surgery).

   If fresh PRBCs are unavailable, washing blood will temporarily remove the plasma potassium. This is not ideal, since the cells will have low levels of 2,3-DPG, but this is an acceptable alternative.
B. Donor exposures can be minimized by reserving a fresh unit of PRBCs for a neonate at his or her first transfusion and transfusion of an aliquot of that unit for each transfusion (3). This is useful for patients receiving frequent simple transfusions.
III. **Frozen plasma** (see Bleeding). The two frozen plasma products that are available are fresh frozen plasma (FFP) and frozen plasma. FFP is frozen within 8 hours of collection and frozen plasma is frozen within 24 hours of collection.

A. Contents

1. Each component has approximately 1 unit/mL of each coagulation factor except that frozen plasma may have approximately two-thirds the levels of the unstable factors (V and VIII).
2. 160 to 170 mEq/L sodium and 3.5 to 5.5 mEq/L potassium.
3. All plasma proteins including albumin and antibodies.
4. 1440 g sodium citrate.

B. Indications. FFP and frozen plasma are indicated to correct coagulopathies due to factor deficiencies. Although plasma contains proteins and albumins, these components are not indicated for intravascular volume expansion or for antibody replacement since other components and safer and better for those indications.

C. Dosage. 10 to 20 mL/kg is usually an adequate dose, and this may need to be repeated every 8 to 12 hours depending on the clinical situation.

D. Citrate Toxicity. The amount of citrate is unlikely to cause transient hypocalcemia in most situations but this can happen with rapid infusions of large amounts of FFP.

IV. Platelets. (see Thrombocytopenia). Platelets can be prepared from whole blood donations or collected by apheresis. If they are collected by apheresis, an aliquot is obtained for a neonatal transfusion.

A. Contents. Each unit of whole blood derived platelets contains at least 5×10^{10} in 50 mL of anticoagulated plasma including proteins and electrolytes. Because platelets are stored at room temperature for up to 5 days, there may be low levels of unstable coagulation factors V and VIII.

B. Indications. No good studies exist, but NICU patients at increased risk for intracranial hemorrhage should probably be maintained at a platelet count of 50,000 to 100,000 platelets/mm^3.

C. Dose. 0.1 unit/kg should **raise** the platelet count by 30,000/mm^3.

D. Concentration of platelets. Platelets can be concentrated by centrifugation resulting in a volume of 15 to 20 mL. This may damage the platelets.

V. Granulocytes. Granulocyte transfusions are a controversial therapy that may benefit patients with severe neutropenia or dysfunctional neutrophils and a bacterial or fungal infection not responding to antimicrobial therapy. Granulocyte transfusions can only be used as a temporary therapy until the patient starts producing neutrophils or until another curative therapy can be instituted.

A. Adverse effects. Granulocyte transfusions can cause pulmonary symptoms and must be administered slowly to minimize the chances of severe reactions.

B. Dose. 10 to 15 mL/kg. This may need to be repeated every 12 to 24 hours.

C. Special considerations. Collections need to be specially scheduled and the granulocytes need to be transfused soon after collection.

VI. Whole blood (see Chap. 18). Few units are stored as whole blood.

A. Indications. Exchange transfusions. Also, may be used as a substitute for blood components in priming circuits for cardiopulmonary bypass or extracorporeal membrane oxygenation (ECMO). Whole blood may be useful for neonates immediately following disconnection from a cardiopulmonary bypass circuit for cardiac surgery.

B. Freshness. Whole blood is stored at 1 to 6°C and coagulation factors and platelet function decays at this temperature. If whole blood is transfused, it must be relatively fresh. When used just after cardiopulmonary bypass, the blood should be no more than 2 to 3 days old. When used in other situations, the whole blood should be no more than 5 to 7 days old.

C. Alternatives. If fresh blood is unavailable, then an acceptable alternative is to mix FFP and PRBCs for an exchange transfusion or to prime a circuit. Immediately following cardiopulmonary bypass, platelets should also be infused since bypass circuits damage platelets.

VII. Intravenous immunoglobulin (IVIG) (see Chap. 23). Several brands of IVIG are available. When administered, IVIG is a concentrated purified solution of immunoglobulins with some stabilizers such as sucrose. Most products contain over 90% IgG with small amounts of immunoglobulin M (IgM) and immunoglobulin A (IgA).

A. **Indications.** IVIG can have an immunosuppressive effect that may be useful for alloimmune disorders such as immune hemolytic anemia and neonatal alloimmune thrombocytopenia. Both of these disorders are due to maternal antibodies to antigens on the neonate's cells. Hemolytic anemia is not routinely treated with IVIG, but alloimmune thrombocytopenia is often treated with IVIG (4,6).

Some studies have attempted to determine whether IVIG is useful as a prophylaxis or treatment for neonatal sepsis. Results from these studies are mixed and not enough evidence exists for routine use of IVIG for general sepsis (7).

1. **Hyperimmune Immunoglobulins.** High titer disease-specific immunoglobulins are available for several infectious agents including varicella-zoster virus and respiratory syncytial virus (8, 9). These immunoglobulins may be useful for infants at high risk for these infections.

B. **Dose.** IVIG (nondisease-specific) is usually given at a dose of 500 to 900 mg/kg. Doses for the disease-specific immunoglobulins should follow manufactures recommendations.

C. **Adverse reactions.** Rare complications include transient tachycardia or hypertension. Also, several cases of renal damage in older patients receiving IVIG have been reported.

VIII. **Modifications of blood components and directed donations**
A. **Leukoreduction.** Current leukoreduction filters can remove approximately 99.9% of the white blood cells from PRBCs and platelets. In addition, most platelets collected by apheresis are often leukoreduced even without additional filtration. Benefits of leukoreduction include (10):

1. Decreased immunization to antigens on leukocytes such as human leukocyte antigen (HLA) antigens.
2. Decreased rate of febrile transfusion reactions.
3. Minimization of a possible (and contraversial) immunomodulatory effect of blood transfusions.
4. Decreased rate of cytomegalovirus transmission (CMV) (see Chap. 23).

Although the first three indications are not essential for neonates, neonates often receive leukoreduced blood components to decrease transmission of CMV. This is often a cheaper and easier approach than identifying blood components that test negative for CMV.

B. **Irradiation.** Irradiation prevents graft-versus-host disease (GVHD) from transfused leukocytes in cellular blood components. Among those at risk are premature infants and children with certain congenital immunodeficiencies. To ensure that nobody gets this fatal consequence of transfusion, we irradiate all PRBCs, platelets, and glanulocytes for all children less than 1 year old. (see Chap. 18)

C. **Directed donations.** Directed donations have, on average, a small increase in rate of infectious disease transmission. The difference is minimal and parents often want to donate for their children. This blood must be irradiated since it is at increased risk for causing GVHD if the blood donors are first-degree blood relatives of the patient.

IX. **Acute transfusion reactions.**
A. **Acute hemolytic transfusion reactions.** These reactions are usually due to incompatibility of donor red blood cells with antibodies in the patient's plasma. The antibodies usually responsible for acute hemolytic transfusion reactions are isohemagglutinins (anti-A, anti-B). These reactions are rare in neonates because they do not make isohemagglutinins until they are 4 to 6 months old. However, maternal isohemagglutinins can be present in the neonatal circulation.

Similar symptoms can also occur from transfusion of plasma that is incompatible with the patient's red blood cells. This is only likely to occur with platelet or FFP transfusions. These hemolytic reactions are milder than transfusion of incompatible erythrocytes.

1. **Symptoms.** Possible symptoms include hypotension, fever, tachycardia, and hematuria.

**TABLE 26.8. CURRENT INFECTIOUS DISEASE RISKS FROM
BLOOD TRANSFUSIONS**

Pathogen	Risk per Unit
HIV	1 in 1.4 $\times$ 10^6
Hepatitis C virus (HCV)	1 in 1.2 $\times$ 10^6
Hepatitis A virus	1 in 1 $\times$ 10^6
Hepatitis B virus (HBV)	1 in 150,000
Human T-cell leukemia (HTLV)	1 in 641,000
Parvovirus B19	1 in 10,000

    2. **Treatment.** Administer fluids, mannitol or furosemide to protect kidneys, and to treat hypotension and DIC if they develop. May need to transfuse compatible PRBCs.

B. **Allergic transfusion reactions.** These are also unusual in neonates. Allergic reactions are due to antibodies in the patient's plasma that react with proteins in donor plasma.

    1. **Symptoms.** Mild allergic reactions are characterized by hives and possibly wheezing. More severe reactions can present as anaphylaxis.

    2. **Treatment.** These reactions can be treated with antihistamines, brochodilators, and corticosteroids as needed. These reactions are usually specific to individual donors. If they are serious or reoccur, red blood cells and platelets can be washed.

C. **Volume overload.** Blood components have high oncotic pressure and rapid infusion can cause excessive intravascular volume. This can cause a sudden deterioration of vital signs.

D. **Hypocalcemia.** Rapid infusion of components, especially FFP, can cause transient hypocalcemia, usually manifested by hypotension.

E. **Hypothermia.** Cool blood can cause hypothermia. Transfusion through blood warmers can prevent this.

F. **Transfusion-associated acute lung injury (TRALI).** This is often due to antibodies in donor plasma that react with the patient's histocompatibility (HLA) antigens. These reactions present as respiratory compromise and are more likely to occur with blood components containing significant amounts of plasma such as frozen plasma or FFP.

X. **Infectious diseases.** A variety of infectious diseases can be transmitted by blood transfusion. The most serious ones are screened for but new pathogens can enter the blood supply (11) (Table 26.8) (see Chap. 23).

    CMV can also be transmitted by blood but this is extremely rare if the blood is leukoreduced. Other diseases known to be capable of being transmitted by blood transfusions include malaria, babesiosis, Chagas disease, syphilis, and West Nile virus. Of these, the one responsible for the most number of confirmed cases of transfusion transmitted infections in recent years is West Nile virus. Animal studies suggest that Variant Creutzfeldt-Jakob disease (vCJD) can also be transmitted by blood transfusion but no cases of transfusion transmitted vCJD have been reported to date.

References

1. Technical Manual Committee. *Technical Manual*, 13th ed. Bethesda, Md.: American Association of Blood Banks, 1999;798.
2. Luban N.L., Strauss R.G., Hume H.A. Commentary on the safety of red cells preserved in extended-storage media for neonatal transfusions. *Transfusion* 1991; 31:3, 229–235.

3. Strauss R.G., et al. AS-1 red cells for neonatal transfusions: A randomized trial assessing donor exposure and safety. *Transfusion* 1996;36:10, 873–878.
4. Alcock G.S., Liley H. *Immunoglobulin infusion for isoimmune haemolytic jaundice in neonates. Cochrane Database Syst Rev* 2002;3: CD003313.
5. Spencer J.A., Burrows R.F. Feto-maternal alloimmune thrombocytopenia: A literature review and statistical analysis. *Aust NZ J Obstet Gynaecol* 2001; 41:1, 45–55.
6. Kaplan C. Immune thrombocytopenia in the foetus and the newborn: Diagnosis and therapy. *Trans Clin Biol* 2001;8:3, 311–314.
7. Ohlsson A., Lacy J.B. Intravenous immunoglobulin for suspected or subsequently proven infection in neonates. *Cochrane Database Syst Rev* 2000;2: CD001239
8. Atkins J.T., et al. Prophylaxis for respiratory syncytial virus with respiratory syncytial virus-immunoglobulin intravenous among preterm infants of thirty-two weeks gestation and less: Reduction in incidence, severity of illness and cost. *Pediatr Infect Dis J* 2000;19:2, 138–143.
9. Huang Y.C., et al. Prophylaxis of intravenous immunoglobulin and acyclovir in perinatal varicella. *Eur J Pediatr* 2001;160:2, p. 91–94.
10. Dzik W.H. Leukoreduction of blood components. *Curr Opin Hematol* 2002;9:6, 521–526.
11. Strong D.M., Katz L. Blood-bank testing for infectious diseases: How safe is blood transfusion? *Trends Mol Med* 2002;8:7, 355–358.
12. Busch M.P., et al. Current and emerging infectious risks of blood transfusions. *JAMA* 2003;289:959–962.

Neonatal Thrombosis

Munish Gupta and Yao Sun

I. Physiology
A. Physiology of thrombosis
1. **Thrombin** is the primary procoagulant protein, converting fibrinogen into a fibrin clot. The intrinsic and extrinsic pathways of the coagulation cascade result in formation of active thrombin from prothrombin.
2. **Inhibitors of coagulation** include antithrombin, heparin cofactor I, protein C, protein S, and tissue factor pathway inhibitor (TFPI). Antithrombin activity is potentiated by heparin.
3. **Plasmin** is the primary fibrinolytic enzyme, degrading fibrin in a reaction that produces fibrin degradation products and *d*-dimers. Plasmin is formed from plasminogen by numerous enzymes, most important of which is tissue plasminogen activator (tPA).
4. In neonates, factors contributing to thrombus formation can affect blood flow, blood composition (leading to hypercoagulability), and vascular endothelial integrity.

B. Unique physiologic characteristics of hemostasis in neonates
1. *In utero,* coagulation proteins are synthesized by the fetus, and do not cross the placenta.
2. Both thrombogenic and fibrinolytic pathways are altered in the neonate compared with the older child and adult, resulting in increased vulnerability to both hemorrhage and pathologic thrombosis. However, under normal physiologic conditions, the hemostatic system in premature and

term newborns is in balance, and healthy neonates do not clinically demonstrate hypercoagulable or bleeding tendencies.

3. Concentrations of most procoagulant proteins are reduced in neonates compared with adult values, although fibrinogen levels are normal or even increased. Values for the prothrombin time (PT) and the activated partial thromboplastin time (PTT) are prolonged.

4. Concentrations of most antithrombotic and fibrinolytic proteins are also reduced, including protein C, protein S, plasminogen, and antithrombin. Thrombin inhibition by plasmin is diminished compared with adult plasma.

5. Platelet number and lifespan appear to be similar to that of adults. The bleeding time, an overall assessment of platelet function, and interaction with vascular endothelium is shorter in neonates than in adults, suggesting more rapid platelet adhesion and aggregation.

II. Epidemiology and risk factors

A. Epidemiology

1. Thrombosis occurs more frequently in the neonatal period than at any other age in childhood.

2. The presence of an **indwelling vascular catheter** is the single greatest risk factor for arterial or venous thrombosis. Indwelling catheters are responsible for more than 80% of venous and 90% of arterial thrombotic complications.

3. Autopsy studies show 20 to 65% of infants who expire with an umbilical venous catheter in place are found to have a thrombus associated with the catheter.

4. **Umbilical arterial catheterization (UAC) appears to result in clinically severe symptomatic vessel obstruction in approximately 1% of patients.** Asymptomatic catheter-associated thrombi have been found in 3 to 59% of cases by autopsy and 10 to 90% of cases by angiography.

5. Other risk factors include infection, increased blood viscosity, polycythemia, dehydration, hypoxia, hypotension, maternal diabetes, and intrauterine growth restriction (IUGR).

6. Infants undergoing surgery involving the vascular system, including repair of congenital heart disease, are at increased risk for thrombotic complications. Diagnostic or interventional catheterizations also increase the risk for thombosis.

7. **Renal vein thrombosis (RVT)** is the most common type of noncatheter related pathologic thrombosis.

8. In 1995, a Canadian and international registry published a review of 97 cases of neonatal thrombosis, excluding stroke, confirmed with imaging.

   a. Overall incidence of clinically apparent thrombosis was estimated at 2.4 per 1000 admissions to the neonatal intensive care unit.

   b. Twenty-one (22%) were spontaneous renal vein thrombosis; 39 (40%) were other venous; 33 (34%) were arterial; and 4 (4%) were mixed venous and arterial.

   c. Excluding renal vein thrombosis, 89% of cases were associated with indwelling vascular catheter.

   d. Twenty-five percent of all cases occurred in the context of a systemic infection.

   e. Management varied greatly for similar clinical conditions among participating centers.

   f. Eighty-two percent of all infants survived to discharge. Mortality rates were 5% for RVT, 18% for other venous thrombosis, 21% for arterial thrombosis, and 25% for mixed venous and arterial. Mortality was concentrated in extremely low-birth-weight and extremely premature infants. Among older and larger infants, mortality appears to be most concentrated in cases of thrombosis in the aorta or the right atrium and superior vena cava.

9. In 1997, a German registry published a review of 79 cases of neonatal thrombosis, confirmed with imaging.
   a. Overall incidence of clinically significant thrombosis was estimated to be 5.1 per 100,000 births.
   b. Thirty-five (44%) were renal vein thrombosis, 25 (32%) were other venous, and 19 (24%) were arterial. One patient had both venous and arterial thrombosis.
   c. Seventy percent of all cases, including renal vein thrombosis, were associated with identifiable risk factors. 32% were associated with indwelling central lines, which was the most common risk factor. Others included infection, asphyxia, and dehydration.
   d. Ninety-one percent of patients survived to discharge. Mortality rates were 3% for RVT, 12% for other venous, and 16% for arterial thrombosis.

B. **Inherited thrombophilias**
   1. **Congenital thrombophilias** are characterized by positive family history, early age of onset, recurrent disease, and unusual or multiple locations of thromboembolic events. It is estimated that a genetic risk factor can be identified in approximately 70% of patients with thrombophilia.
   2. Important **inherited thrombophilias** include:
      a. **Deficiencies of protein C, protein S, and antithrombin,** which appear to have the largest increase in relative risk for thromboembolic disease but are relatively rare.
      b. **Activated protein C resistance,** including the factor V Leiden mutation, and the prothrombin G20210A mutation, which have high incidence, particularly in certain populations, but appear to have low risk of thrombosis in neonates.
      c. Hyperhomocysteinemia, increased lipoprotein(a) levels, and mutation in the methylene tetrahydrofolate reductase (MTHFR) gene, whose significance in neonatal thrombosis is still poorly understood.
   3. Multiple other defects in the anticoagulation, fibrinolytic, and antifibrinolytic pathways have been identified, including abnormalities in thrombomodulin, tissue factor pathway inhibitor, fibrinogen, plasminogen, tissue plasminogen activator, and plasminogen-activator inhibitors. The frequency and importance of these defects in neonatal thrombosis is poorly understood.
   4. The incidence of thrombosis in patients heterozygous for most inherited thrombophilias is small; however, increasing evidence suggests that the presence of a second risk factor substantially increases the risk for thrombosis. This second risk factor can be an acquired clinical condition or illness, or another inherited defect. Patients with single defects for inherited prothrombotic disorders rarely present in neonatal period, unless another pathologic process or event occurs.
   5. Patients who are homozygous for a single defect or double heterozygotes for different defects can present in the neonatal period, often with significant illness due to thrombosis. The classic presentation of homozygous prothrombotic disorders is **purpura fulminans** with homozygous protein C or S deficiency, which presents within hours or days of birth, often with evidence of *in utero* cerebral damage.
   6. Overall, the importance of inherited thrombophilias as independent risk factors for neonatal thrombosis is still undetermined. It appears that the absolute risk of thrombosis in the neonatal period in all patients with inherited thrombophilia (nonhomozygous) is actually quite small; however, among neonates with thrombotic disease, the incidence of an inherited thrombophilia appears to be substantially increased compared with incidence in the general population.

C. **Acquired thrombophilias**
   1. Newborns can acquire significant coagulation factor deficiencies due to placental transfer of maternal antiphospholipid antibodies, including the lupus anticoagulant and anti-cardiolipin antibody. These neonates can present with significant thrombosis, including purpura fulminans.

III. Specific clinical conditions
  A. Venous thromboembolic disorders
  1. General considerations:
  a. Most venous thrombosis occurs secondary to **central venous catheters.** Spontaneous (i.e., noncatheter-related) venous thrombosis can occur in renal veins, adrenal veins, inferior vena cava, portal vein, hepatic veins, and the venous system of the brain.
  b. Spontaneous venous thrombi usually occur in the presence of another risk factor. Less than 1% of significant venous thromboembolic events in neonates are idiopathic.
  c. Thrombosis of the **sinovenous system of the brain** is an important cause of neonatal cerebral infarction.
  d. Short-term complications of venous catheter-associated thrombosis include loss of access, pulmonary embolism, superior vena cava syndrome, and specific organ impairment.
  e. It is likely that the frequency of pulmonary embolism in sick neonates is underestimated, as signs and symptoms would be similar to multiple other common pulmonary diseases.
  f. Long-term complications of venous thrombosis are poorly understood. Initial series suggest inferior vena cava thrombosis, if extensive, is associated with a high rate of persistent partial obstruction and symptoms such as leg edema, abdominal pain, lower extremity thrombophlebitis, varicose veins, and leg ulcers.
  2. Major venous thrombosis—signs and symptoms:
  a. Initial sign of catheter-related thrombosis is usually difficulty infusing through or withdrawing from the line.
  b. Signs of venous obstruction include swelling of the extremities, possibly including the head and neck, and distended superficial veins.
  c. The onset of **thrombocytopenia** in the presence of a central venous line also raises the suspicion of thrombosis.
  3. Major venous thrombosis—diagnosis:
  a. Ultrasound. Ultrasound is diagnostic in most cases of significant venous thrombosis. In smaller infants or low flow states, however, the ultrasound may not provide sufficient information about the size of the thrombus, and recent data suggests a significant false-negative rate for ultrasound diagnosis.
  b. Contrast studies. A radiographic line study can be helpful for diagnosis of catheter-associated thrombosis. Venography through peripheral vessels may be needed for diagnosis of thrombosis proximal to the catheter tip, for spontaneous thrombosis in the upper body, and for thrombosis not seen by other methods (see IV).
  4. Prevention of catheter-associated venous thrombosis:
  a. Heparin 0.5 units/mL is added to all infusions (compatability permitting) through central venous lines.
  b. Umbilical venous catheters should be removed as soon as clinically feasible. Our usual practice is to place a peripherally inserted central catheter (PICC) line if anticipated need for central access is greater than 7 days.
  5. Management of major venous thrombosis:
  a. Nonfunctioning central venous line (CVL):
  (1) If fluid can no longer be easily infused through the catheter, remove the catheter unless the CVL is absolutely necessary.
  (2) If continued central access through the catheter is judged to be clinically necessary, clearance of the blockage with thrombolytic agents or HCl can be considered (see V.F).
  b. Local obstruction. If a small occlusive catheter-related thrombosis is documented, a low-dose infusion of thrombolytic agents through the catheter can be considered for localized site-directed thrombolytic therapy (see V.E). If infusion through the catheter is not possible, the CVL should be removed and heparin therapy considered.

    c. Extensive venous thrombosis. Consider leaving the catheter in place and attempting systemic thrombolytic therapy. Otherwise, remove the catheter and begin heparin therapy. Systemic thrombolytic therapy should be considered for extensive noncatheter-related venous thrombosis and for venous thrombosis with significant clinical compromise.

B. Aortic or major arterial thrombosis

  1. General Considerations:

    a. Spontaneous arterial thrombi in absence of a catheter is unusual but does occur in ill neonates.

    b. Acute complications of catheter-related and spontaneous arterial thrombi depend on location, and can include renal hypertension, intestinal necrosis, peripheral gangrene, and other organ failure.

    c. Thrombosis of cerebral arteries is an important cause of neonatal cerebral infarction.

    d. Long-term effects of symptomatic and asymptomatic arterial thrombi are not well studied, but may include increased risk for atherosclerosis at the affected area and chronic renal hypertension.

  2. Aortic thrombosis—signs and symptoms:

    a. Initial sign is often isolated dysfunction of umbilical artery catheter (UAC).

    b. Mild clinical signs include: hematuria in absence of transfusions or hemolysis; hematuria with RBCs on microscopic analysis; hypertension; and intermittent lower extremity decreased perfusion or color change.

    c. Strong clinical signs include: persistent lower extremity color change or decreased perfusion; blood pressure differential between upper and lower extremities; decrease or loss of lower extremity pulses; signs of peripheral thrombosis; oliguria despite adequate intravascular volume; signs of necrotizing enterocolitis; and signs of congestive heart failure.

  3. Aortic thrombosis—diagnosis:

    a. Ultrasound. Ultrasound with Doppler flow imaging should generally be performed in all cases of suspected aortic thrombosis; if signs of thrombis are mild and resolve promptly after removal of the arterial catheter, an ultrasound may not be necessary. Ultrasound is diagnostic in most cases, although recent data suggest a significant false-negative rate.

    b. Contrast study. If ultrasound is negative or inconclusive, and major arterial thrombosis is suspected, a radiographic contrast study can be performed, via the arterial catheter.

  4. Prevention of catheter-associated arterial thrombosis:

    a. Heparin 0.5 to 1 unit/mL is added to all infusions (compatability permitting) through arterial catheters; heparin infusion through arterial catheters has been shown to prolong patency and to likely reduce incidence of local thrombus, without risk of significant complications.

    b. Review of the literature suggests **"high" umbilical arterial lines** (tip in descending aorta below left subclavian artery and above diaphragm) are preferable to "low" lines (tip below renal arteries and above aortic bifurcation), with fewer clinically evident ischemic complications, an apparent trend to reduced incidence of thrombi, and no difference in serious complications such as necrotizing enterocolitis and renal dysfunction.

    c. Consider placing **peripheral arterial line** rather than umbilical in infants weighing > 1500 g.

    d. Monitor carefully for clinical evidence of thrombus formation when an umbilical arterial catheter is present:

      (1) Monitor for evidence of UAC dysfunction, including waveform dampening and difficulty flushing or withdrawing blood.

      (2) Monitor lower extremity color and perfusion.

      (3) Check all urine for heme.

      (4) Check upper and lower extremity blood pressure three times daily.

      (5) Monitor for hypertension and decreased urine output.

e. Umbilical arterial catheters should be removed as soon as clinically feasible. Our general practice is to leave umbilical arterial catheters in place for no longer than 7 days, and to place a peripheral arterial line should continued arterial access be needed.

5. Management of aortic and major arterial thrombosis:

a. Minor aortic thrombi. Small aortic thrombi with limited mild symptoms can often be managed with prompt removal of the umbilical arterial catheter, with rapid resolution of symptoms.

b. Large but nonocclusive thrombus. For large thrombi that are nonocclusive to blood flow (as demonstrated by ultrasound or contrast study) and that are not accompanied by signs of significant clinical compromise, the arterial catheter should be removed and anticoagulation with heparin considered. Close follow-up with serial imaging studies is indicated.

c. Occlusive thrombus or significant clinical compromise. Large occlusive aortic thrombi or thrombi accompanied by signs of significant clinical compromise including renal failure, congestive heart failure, necrotizing enterocolitis, and signs of peripheral ischemia, should be managed aggressively:

(1) If catheter is still present and patent, consider local thrombolytic therapy through the catheter (see V.E).

(2) If catheter has already been removed or is obstructed, consider systemic thrombolytic therapy. The catheter should be removed if still in place and obstructed.

d. Surgical thrombectomy is not indicated, since the mortality and morbidity far exceed that of current medical management.

6. Peripheral arterial thrombosis

a. Congenital occlusions of large peripheral arteries are seen, although rare, and can present with symptoms ranging from a poorly perfused pulseless extremity to a black, necrotic limb, depending on duration and timing of occlusion.

(1) Common symptoms include decreased perfusion, decreased pulses, pallor, and embolic phenomena that may manifest as skin lesions or petechiae.

(2) Diagnosis can often be made by Doppler flow ultrasound.

b. Peripheral arterial catheters, including radial, posterior tibial, and dorsalis pedis catheters, are rarely associated with significant thrombosis.

(1) Poor perfusion to the distal extremity is frequently seen, and usually resolves with prompt removal of the arterial line.

(2) We infuse heparin 0.5 to 1 unit/mL at 1 to 2 mL/hr through all peripheral arterial lines.

(3) Treatment of significant thrombosis or persistently compromised extremity perfusion associated with a peripheral catheter should consist of heparin anticoagulation and consideration of systemic thrombolysis for extensive lesions. Close follow-up with serial imaging is indicated.

C. Renal vein thrombosis

1. Renal vein thrombosis occurs primarily in newborns and young infants, and most often presents in the first week of life. A significant proportion of cases appear to result from in utero thrombus formation.

2. Affected neonates are usually term and are **often** large for gestational age **(LGA).** There is an increased incidence among infants of diabetic mothers, and males are more often affected than females. Other associated conditions and risk factors include perinatal asphyxia, hypotension, polycythemia, increased blood viscosity, and cyanotic congenital heart disease.

3. Presenting symptoms in the neonatal period **include flank mass, hematuria, proteinuria, thrombocytopenia, and renal dysfunction.** Coagulation studies may be prolonged, and fibrin degration products are usually increased.

4. **Disease is often bilateral.**
5. Some physicians suggest all patients with renal vein thrombosis should be **screened for inherited pro-thrombotic disorders.**
6. **Diagnosis is usually by ultrasound.**
7. **Management is usually aggressive:**
   a. Unilateral renal vein thrombosis without significant renal dysfunction and without extension into the inferior vena cava is often managed with supportive care alone.
   b. Unilateral renal vein thrombosis with renal dysfunction or extension into the inferior vena cava and bilateral renal vein thrombosis should be considered for anticoagulation with heparin.
   c. Bilateral renal vein thrombosis with significant renal dysfunction should be considered for thrombolysis.

IV. **Diagnostic considerations**
   A. **Ultrasound.** Ultrasound with Doppler flow analysis is the most commonly used diagnostic modality.
      1. Advantages include relative ease of performance, noninvasiveness, and ability to perform sequential scans to assess progression of thrombosis or response to treatment.
      2. Sensitivity of ultrasound may be somewhat limited: several recent studies suggest that significant venous and arterial thrombi may be missed by ultrasonography. Ultrasound remains our test of first choice, but if ultrasound is inconclusive or negative in the context of significant clinical suspicion of thrombosis, a contrast study should be considered.
   B. **Radiographic line study.** Imaging after injection of contrast material through a central catheter often is diagnostic for catheter-associated thrombi, and has the advantage of relative ease of performance.
   C. **Venography.** Venography with injection of contrast through peripheral vessels may be necessary when other diagnostic methods fail to demonstrate the extent and severity of thrombosis.
      1. A contrast line study will not provide information on venous thrombosis proximal to catheter tip (i.e., along the length of the catheter).
      2. Upper extremity and upper chest venous thromboses, either catheter-related or spontaneous, are particularly difficult to visualize with ultrasound.

V. **Management**
   A. **Evaluation for thrombophilia**
      1. Consider evaluating for congenital or acquired thrombophilias those neonates with severe or unusual manifestations of thrombosis or with positive family histories of thrombosis.
      2. Initial evaluation should include consideration of deficiencies of protein C, protein S, or antithrombin; presence of activated protein C resistance and the Factor V Leiden mutation; presence of the prothrombin G20210A mutation; and passage of maternal antiphospholipid antibodies.
         a. **Protein C, protein S, and antithrombin deficiencies** can be evaluated by measurement of antigen or activity levels. Results of testing of neonates should be compared with standard gestational age-based reference ranges, as normal physiologic values can be as low as 15 to 20% of adult values. In addition, levels will be physiologically depressed in the presence of active thrombosis, and low results should be repeated in several weeks. We usually do not test the babies at birth, but do the tests 2 to 3 months later. Alternative to or in conjunction with testing of the neonate, parents can be tested for carrier status by measurement of protein C, protein S, and antithrombin levels.
         b. **Factor V Leiden and prothrombin G20210A mutations** can be assayed by specific genetic tests in the neonate. Alternatively, parents can be tested for carrier status.

   c. The mother can be tested for antinuclear antibodies, lupus anticoagulant, and anticardiolipin antibodies.

  3. If all of the above are negative, subsequent specialized laboratory evaluation includes consideration of abnormalities or deficiencies of homocysteine, lipoprotein(a), methylene tetrahydrofolate reductase, plasminogen, and fibrinogen. Very rarely seen are abnormalities or deficiencies of heparin cofactor II, thrombomodulin, plasminogen activator inhibitor-1, platelet aggregation, and tissue plasminogen activator.

B. General considerations

  1. Precautions

    a. Avoid IM injections and arterial punctures during anticoagulation or thrombolytic therapy.

    b. Avoid indocin or other antiplatelet drugs during therapy.

    c. Use minimal physical manipulation of patient (i.e., no physical therapy) during thrombolytic therapy.

    d. Thrombolytic therapy should not be initiated in the presence of active bleeding or significant risk for local bleeding, and should be carefully considered if there is a history of recent surgery of any type (particularly neurosurgery).

    e. Monitor clinical status carefully for signs of hemorrhage, including internal hemorrhage and intracranial hemorrhage.

    f. Consider giving **fresh frozen plasma (FFP) 10 mL/kg to any patient who needs anticoagulation.**

  2. Guidelines for choice of therapy

    a. Small asymptomatic nonocclusive arterial or venous thrombi related to catheters can often be treated with catheter removal and supportive care alone.

    b. Large or occlusive venous thrombi can be treated with anticoagulation with heparin or low-molecular-weight heparin; usually relatively short courses (7 to 14 days) of anticoagulation are sufficient, but occasionally long-term treatment may be necessary.

    c. Most arterial thrombi should be treated with anticoagulation with heparin or low-molecular weight heparin.

    d. In cases of massive venous thrombi or arterial thrombi with significant clinical compromise, treatment with local or systemic thrombolysis should be considered.

C. Heparin

  1. General considerations

    a. Term newborns generally have increased clearance of heparin compared with adults, and thus require relatively increased heparin dosage. This increased clearance is significantly diminished, however, in premature neonates.

    b. Heparin should be infused through a dedicated IV line that is not used for any other medications or fluids, if possible.

    c. Lab work. Prior to starting heparin therapy, obtain CBC, prothrombin time (PT), and partial thromboplastin time (PTT).

    d. Adjustment of heparin infusion rate is based on clinical response, serial evaluation of thrombus (usually by ultrasound), and monitoring of laboratory parameters.

    e. Significant patient-to-patient variability in heparin dosage requirements is seen.

    f. Use of partial thromboplastin time (PTT) to monitor heparin effect is problematic in neonates due to significant variability of coagulation factor concentrations and baseline prolongation of the PTT; **heparin activity level** is generally considered to be a more reliable marker.

    g. Therapeutic heparin activity for treatment of most thromboembolic events is considered to be an anti-factor Xa level of 0.3 to 0.7 U/mL or a heparin level by protamine titration of 0.2 to 0.4 U/mL. Most laboratories report heparin activity levels as an anti-factor Xa level.

  h. Follow CBC frequently while on heparin treatment to monitor for heparin-associated thrombocytopenia, which can be diagnosed by assay of heparin-associated antiplatelet antibodies.

  i. **Heparin activity is dependent on presence of antithrombin.** Consider administration of **fresh frozen plasma** (10 mL/kg) or antithrombin concentrate (one vial of 500 u) when effective anticoagulation with heparin is difficult to achieve.

   (1) Antithrombin levels can be measured directly to aid in therapy, although administration of exogenous antithrombin can increase sensitivity to heparin even in patients with near normal antithrombin levels.

   (2) Note that measurement of heparin activity levels, unlike measurement of PTT, is independent of presence of antithrombin. Therefore, measured heparin activity levels may be therapeutic even though effective anticoagulation is not seen due to antithrombin deficiency.

2. Dosing guidelines

  a. Heparin is given as an initial bolus of 75 units/kg, followed by a continuous infusion that is begun at 28 units/kg per hour. Slightly lower dosing can be used in premature infants under 36 weeks' gestation, with an initial bolus of 50 units/kg followed by a continuous infusion begun at 20 units/kg per hour.

  b. Heparin activity levels and/or PTT should be measured 4 hours after initial bolus and 4 hours after each change in infusion dose, and every 24 hours once a therapeutic infusion dose has been achieved.

DOSAGE MONITORING AND ADJUSTMENT

PTT (sec)*	Heparin Activity (U/mL)	Bolus (U/kg)	Hold	Rate	Recheck
<40	0–0.15	50	—	+20%	4 h
40–50	0.16–0.2	0	—	+20%	4 h
50–59	0.21–0.29	0	—	+10%	4 h
60–85	0.3–0.7	0	—	—	24 h
86–95	0.71–0.8	0	—	−10%	4 h
96–120	0.81–1.0	0	30 min	−10%	4 h
>120	>1	0	60 min	−15%	4 h

*PTT values may vary by laboratory depending on reagents used. Generally, PTT values of 1.5 to 2.5 × the baseline normal for a given laboratory correspond to heparin activity levels of 0.3 to 0.7 U/mL.
Source: Monagle P. et al. Antithrombotic therapy in children. *Chest* Jan. 2001;110: 344–370S.

3. Duration of therapy. Anticoagulation with heparin may continue 10 to 14 days. Oral anticoagulants are generally not recommended in neonates; if long-term anticoagulation is needed, consult hematology.

4. Reversal of anticoagulation

  a. Termination of heparin infusion will quickly reverse anticoagulation effects of heparin therapy, and is usually sufficient.

  b. If rapid reversal is necessary, protamine sulfate may be given IV. Protamine can be given in a concentration of 10 mg/mL at a rate not to exceed 5 mg/min. Hypersensitivity can occur in patients who have received protamine-containing insulin or previous protamine therapy.

c. Dosing. Based on total amount of heparin received in last 2 hours as follows:

PROTAMINE DOSAGE TO REVERSE HEPARIN THERAPY*
Based on total amount heparin received in prior 4 hours

Time since last heparin dose (min)	Protamine dose (mg/100 U heparin received)
<30	1.0
30–60	0.5–0.75
60–120	0.375–0.5
>120	0.25–0.375

*Maximum dosage is 50 mg. Maximum infusion rate is 5 mg/min of 10 mg/mL solution.
Source: Adapted from Monagle P. et al. Antithrombotic therapy in children. *Chest* Jan. 2001;110: 344–370S.

D. Low-molecular-weight heparin
  1. General considerations:
    a. Although data on low-molecular-weight (LMW) heparin usage in neonatal patients is limited, growing evidence of safety and efficacy in adult and pediatric patients has led to increased use in neonatal populations.
    b. Several **advantages of LMW heparins** over standard heparin exist: predictable pharmacokinetics; decreased need for laboratory monitoring; subcutaneous BID dosing; probable reduced risk of heparin-induced thrombocytopenia; and possible reduced risk of bleeding at recommended dosages.
    c. Therapeutic dosage of LMW heparins are extrapolated from adult/pediatric data, and are titrated to anti-factor Xa levels. **Target anti-factor Xa levels** for treatment of most thromboembolic events are 0.50 to 1.0 U/mL, measured 4 to 6 hours after a subcutaneous injection. When used for prophylaxis, target levels are 0.2 to 0.4 U/mL. After therapeutic levels have been achieved for 24 to 48 hours, levels should be followed at least weekly.
    d. Several different low-molecular-weight heparins are available, and the dosages are **not** interchangeable. **Enoxaparin (Lovenox)** has the most widespread pediatric usage and is generally preferred.
    e. Follow CBCs, as thrombocytopenia can occur.
  2. Dosing guidelines:

INITIAL DOSING OF ENOXAPRIN,
AGE-DEPENDENT (IN MG/KG/DOSE SQ)

Age	Initial Treatment Dose	Initial Prophylactic Dose
< 2 mo	1.5 q12h	0.75 q12h
>2 mo	1.0 q12h	0.5 q12h
Preterm infants*	1.0 q12h	0.75 q12h

Source: Adapted from Young T.E., Mangum B. *Neofax 2001.* 2001. Raleigh: Acorn; also Monagle P. et al. Antithrombotic therapy in children. *Chest* Jan. 2001;110: 344–370S.
*For preterm infants with significant risk of bleeding, see V.D.1.d.

MONITORING AND DOSAGE ADJUSTMENT OF ENOXAPARIN BASED ON ANTI-FACTOR Xa LEVEL MEASURED 4 HOURS AFTER DOSE OF ENOXAPARIN

Anti-factor Xa Level (U/mL)	Hold Dose	Dose Change	Repeat Anti-Xa Level
<0.35	—	+25%	4 h after next dose
0.35–0.49	—	+10%	4 h after next dose
0.5–1.0	—	—	24 h
1.1–1.5	—	–20%	Before next dose
1.6–2.0	3 h	–30%	Before next dose, then 4h after next dose
>2.0	Until level is 0.5 U/mL	–40%	Before next dose; if level not < 0.5 U/mL, repeat q12h

Adapted from Monagle P. et al. Antithrombotic therapy in children. *Chest* Jan. 2001;110: 344–370S.

3. **Reversal of anticoagulation:**
   a. Termination of subcutaneous injections usually is sufficient to reverse anticoagulation when clinically necessary.
   b. If rapid reversal is needed, protamine sulfate can be given within 3 to 4 hours of last injection, although protamine may not completely reverse anticoagulant effects. Administer 1 mg protamine sulfate per 1 mg LMW heparin given in last injection. See V.C.4 for administration guidelines.

E. **Thrombolysis**
   1. **General considerations:**
      a. Thrombolytic agents act by converting endogenous plasminogen to plasmin. Plasminogen levels in neonates are reduced compared with adult values, and thus effectiveness of thrombolytic agents may be diminished. Cotreatment with plasminogen can increase thrombolytic effect of these agents.
      b. **Indications include recent arterial thrombosis, massive thrombosis with evidence of organ dysfunction or compromised limb viability, and life-threatening thrombosis.** Thrombolytic agents can also be used to restore patency to thrombosed central catheters (see F), and local infusions of low-dose thrombolytic agents can be used for small to moderate occlusive thrombosis near a central catheter.
      c. **Minimal data exist in newborn populations regarding all aspects of thrombolytic therapy,** including appropriate indications, safety, efficacy, choice of agent, duration of therapy, use of heparin, and monitoring guidelines. Recommendations for use are generally based on small series and case reports, which overall suggest that thrombolytic therapy in neonates can be effective with limited significant complications.
      d. **Consider evaluating all patients for intraventricular hemorrhage** prior to initiating thrombolytic therapy.
   2. **Treatment guidelines:**
      a. **Preparation for thrombolytic therapy**
         (1) Place sign at head of bed indicating thrombolytic therapy.
         (2) Have topical thrombin available in unit refrigerator.
         (3) Notify blood bank to insure availability of cryoprecipitate.
         (4) Notify pharmacy to ensure availability of amino caproic acid (Amicar).

(5) Obtain good venous access; consider access to allow frequent blood draws to minimize need for phlebotomy.

(6) Consider hematology consult.

b. **Thrombolysis can be achieved by local, site-directed administration of thrombolytic agents in low doses** directly onto or near a thrombosis via a central catheter; or by **systemic** administration of thrombolytic agents in higher doses. Local therapy is generally limited to small or moderate-sized thromboses. Minimal data exist supporting one method over the other.

c. **Urokinase versus tissue-plasminogen activator (tPA) versus streptokinase.** Minimal data exist comparing safety, efficacy, and cost of different thrombolytic agents in children. **tPA has become the agent of choice,** although significantly more expensive, for several reasons:

(1) Streptokinase has the greatest potential for allergic reactions.

(2) Urokinase has limited availability due to manufacturing problems.

(3) tPA has the shortest half-life.

(4) tPA theoretically has less stimulation of a systemic prolytic state, due to its poor binding of circulating plasminogen and its maximal impact on fibrin-bound plasminogen.

d. **Obtain CBC, platelets, PT, PTT, and fibrinogen** prior to initiating therapy.

e. **Monitor PT, PTT, and fibrinogen** every 4 hours initially, and then at least every 12 to 24 hours. Monitor hematocrit and platelets every 12 to 24 hours. Monitor thrombosis by imaging every 6 to 24 hours.

f. **Expect fibrinogen to decrease by 20 to 50%.** If no decrease in fibrinogen is seen, obtain d-dimers or fibrinogen split products to show evidence that a thrombolytic state has been initiated.

g. **Maintain fibrinogen level above 100 mg/dL** and **platelets above 50,000 to 100,000/mm^3** to minimize the risks of clinical bleeding. Administer cryoprecipitate 10 mL/kg (or 1 unit per 5 kg) or platelets 10 mL/kg as needed. If fibrinogen level drops below 100, decrease the dose of thrombolytic agent by 25%.

h. If no improvement in clinical condition or thrombosis size is seen after initiating therapy, and if fibrinogen levels remain high, **consider giving fresh frozen plasma 10 mL/kg,** which may correct deficiencies of plasminogen and other thrombolytic factors.

i. **Duration of therapy.** Thrombolytic therapy is usually provided for a brief period, (i.e., 6 to 12 hours), but longer durations can be used for refractory thromboses with appropriate monitoring. Overall, therapy should balance resolution of the thrombus and improvement in clinical status against signs of clinical bleeding.

j. **Concomitant heparin therapy.** heparin therapy, usually without the loading bolus dose, should be initiated during or immediately after completion of thrombolytic therapy.

3. **Dosing**

SYSTEMIC THROMBOLYTIC THERAPY

Agent	Load	Infusion*	Notes
tPA	none	0.1–0.5 mg/kg/hr for 6 h	Duration usually 6 h; can continue for 12 h or repeat after 24 h, although lysis of clot will continue for hours after infusion stops
Streptokinase	2000–4000 U/kg over 10 min	1000–2000 U/kg/h for 6 h.	Only one course should be given Consider premed with Tylenol and benadryl

(continues)

(continued)

Agent	Load	Infusion*	Notes
Urokinase	4000 U/kg over 10 min	4000 U/kg/h for 6 h	Longer duration may be necessary based on clinical response

Consider concomitant heparin therapy at 20 U/kg per hour without bolus dose for all three agents; target PTT at 1.5 to 2.5 × control or heparin activity level of 0.3 to 0.7 U/mL.
*Optimal duration of therapy is uncertain, and can be individualized based on clinical response.

LOCAL SITE-DIRECTED THROMBOLYTIC THERAPY

Agent	Infusion	Notes*
tPA	0.03–0.05 mg/kg/h	Adjust infusion rate if no clinical effect to 0.1–0.5 mg/kg/h
Urokinase	150 U/kg/h	Increase infusion by 200 U/kg/h if no clinical effect

*Monitor laboratory studies as for systemic treatment.

4. **Treatment of bleeding during thrombolytic therapy:**
    a. Localized bleeding. Apply pressure, administer topical thrombin, and provide supportive care; thrombolytic therapy does not necessarily need to be stopped if bleeding is controlled.
    b. Severe bleeding. Stop infusion and administer cryoprecipitate (1 unit/ 5 kg).
    c. Life-threatening bleeding: stop infusion, give cryoprecipitate, and infuse amino caproic acid (Amicar) (at usual dose of 100 mg/kg IV every 6 hours); consult hematology prior to giving Amicar.
5. **Post-thrombolytic therapy.** Consider initiating heparin therapy, but without the initial loading dose. Consider discontinuing heparin if no reaccumulation of the thrombus occurs after 24 to 48 hours.
F. **Treatment of central catheter thrombosis**
    1. **Treatment guidelines:**
        a. Central catheters may become occluded because of thrombus or chemical precipitate, which is usually secondary to parenteral nutrition.
        b. Nonfunctioning central catheters should be removed whenever possible, unless continued access through that catheter is absolutely necessary.
        c. Thrombolytic agents may be used for thrombosis and hydrochloric acid (HCL) may be attempted for chemical blockage.
        d. General procedure:
            (1) Instill chosen agent at volume needed to fill catheter (up to 1 to 2 mL) with gentle pressure; agent should not be forced in if resistance is too high. If instillation is difficult, a three-way stopcock can be used to create a vacuum in the catheter: attach catheter, 10 mL empty syringe, and 1 mL syringe containing agent to the stopcock, and create vacuum by gently drawing back several mL in the 10-mL syringe while the stopcock is off to the 1-mL syringe. While holding pressure, turn stopcock off to the 10-cc syringe and allow vacuum in catheter to draw in infusate from the 1-mL syringe.
            (2) Use of HCL for catheter clearance in neonates is based on limited clinical data and experience, and should be performed with caution. Suggested volumes to use range from 0.1 mL to 1 mL of 0.1 molar solution. As severe tissue damage may result from peripheral

administration or extravasation of HCL, consultation with a surgeon prior to HCL use should be considered.

(3) Wait 1 to 2 hours for thrombolytic agents and 30 to 60 minutes for HCl and attempt to withdraw fluid through the catheter.

(4) If unsuccessful, above steps can be repeated once. Urokinase can also be left in place for 8 to 12 hours if shorter intervals are unsuccessful.

(5) If clearance of catheter is not successful after two attempts or longer urokinase infusion, catheter should be removed or contrast study performed to delineate extent of blockage.

e. Low-dose continuous infusion of thrombolytic agents can be considered for local thrombosis occluding catheter tip (see above).

2. Dosing guidelines

LOCAL INSTILLATION OF AGENTS FOR CATHETER BLOCKAGE

Agent	Dosing
tPA	0.5 mg per lumen diluted in NS to volume needed to fill line, to max 3 mL.
Urokinase	5000 U/mL, 1–2 mL per lumen. Comes in unit doses prepared expressly for catheter clearance.
HCL	0.1 M, 0.1–1 mL per lumen.

Suggested Readings

Andrew M. Developmental hemostasis: Relevance to newborns and infants. In: *Hematology of Infancy and Childhood*, eds. Nathan D.G., Orkin S.H. (Eds.). 1998. Philadelphia: Saunders.

Andrew M., Brooker L.A. Hemostatic disorders in newborns. In: *Fetal and Neonatal Physiology*. Polin R.A., Fox W.W. (Eds.). 1998. Philadelphia: Saunders.

Andrew M., et al. Thromboembolic disease and antithrombotic therapy in newborns. *Hematology* Jan. 2001;358–374.

Barrington K.J. Umbilical artery catheters in the newborn: Effects of position of the catheter tip. *Cochrane Database of Systematic Reviews*. 2001;Issue 3.

Chalmers E.A. Neonatal thrombosis. *J Clin Pathol* June 2000;53: 419–423.

Chalmers E.A., Gibson B.E.S. Thrombolytic therapy in children. *Br J Haematol* 1999;104:14–21.

deVeber G.A., et al. Cerebral thromboembolism in neonates: Clinical and radiographic features. *Thromb Haemost* 1997;78(suppl):725.

Dix D., et al. The use of low molecular weight heparin in pediatric patients: A prospective cohort study. *J Pediatr* Apr. 2000;136:439–345.

Duffy L.F., et al. Treatment of central venous catheter occlusions with hydrochloric acid. *J Pediatr* 1989;114:1002–1004.

Gunther G., et al. Symptomatic ischemic stroke in full-term neonates: Role of acquired and genetic prothrombotic risk factors. *Stroke* Oct. 2000;31:2437–2441.

Hartmann J., et al. Treatment of neonatal thrombus formation with recombinant tissue plasminogen activator: Six years experience and review of the literature. *Arch Dis Child Fetal Neonatal Ed* 2001;85:F18–22.

Hausler M., et al. Long-term complications of inferior vena cava thrombosis. *Arch Dis Child* 2001;85:228–233.

Heller C., et al. Abdominal venous thrombosis in neonates and infants: Role of prothrombotic risk factors—a multicenter case-control study. *Br J Hematol* 2000;111: 534–539.

Luchtman-Jones L., Schwartz A.L., Wilson D.B. Hematologic problems in the fetus and neonate. In: *Neonatal-Perinatal Medicine* Fanaroff A.A., Martin R.J. (Eds.). 2002. St. Louis: Mosby.

Manco-Johnson M.J., Nuss R. Neonatal thrombotic disorders. *NeoReviews* Oct 2000;1:e201–5.

Monagle P., et al. Antithrombotic therapy in children. *Chest* Jan. 2001;110:344–370S.

Nowak-Gottl U., et al. Neonatal symptomatic thromboembolism in Germany: Two year survey. *Arch Dis Child Fetal Neonatal Ed* 1997;76:F163N167.

Roy M., et al. Incidence and diagnosis of neonatal thrombosis associated with umbilical venous catheters. *Thromb Haemost* 1997;78(suppl):724.

Schmidt B., Andrew M. Neonatal thrombosis: Report of a prospective Canadian and international registry. *Pediatrics* 1995;96:939N943.

Werlin S.L., et al. Treatment of central venous catheter occlusions with ethanol and hydrochloric acid. *J Parent Ent Nutr* 1995;19:416–418.

Young T.E., Mangum B. *Neofax 2001*. 2001. Raleigh: Acorn Publishing.

27. NEUROLOGY

Neonatal Seizures

Adré J. du Plessis

I. **Introduction.** Seizures are the most distinctive manifestation of neurologic dysfunction in the newborn infant. Moreover, neonatal seizures often herald potentially devastating forms of brain injury. Recent advances in diagnostic technology have provided important insights into neonatal seizures. Techniques such as bedside video-electroencephalogram (EEG) monitoring and magnetic resonance imaging (MRI) have challenged earlier beliefs and raised fundamental questions regarding the diagnosis, etiology, and management of seizures in the newborn infant. It is well known that the vast majority of seizures in the newborn are symptomatic of a specific etiology; with these diagnostic advances, an etiology is increasingly identifiable. In addition, these advances have further highlighted the essential differences between seizures in newborn infants and older patients, including their response to conventional anticonvulsant agents. Such age-related differences in the manifestations and treatment response are due in large part to the immature developmental state of the newborn brain and the different etiologies involved. These are discussed in the following.

In earlier reports, seizures occurred in up to 3/1000 full-term infants and up to 60/1000 premature infants. However, the reported incidence of neonatal seizures varies widely across studies, a variability that is primarily the result of inconsistent diagnostic criteria, as well as the often subtle clinical manifestations of neonatal seizures, and their potential confusion with nonepileptic neonatal behaviors (discussed below). Regardless of their precise incidence, it is clear that seizures are more common in the newborn period than at any other time in life, and that the tendency toward recurrent seizures and status epilepticus is far greater in the newborn.

The **decreased seizure threshold in the newborn** reflects the developmental events active in the immature brain. In essence, the newborn brain has a transient over-development of excitatory systems compared to inhibitory systems. For example, the immature brain has a transient overexpression in the density of excitatory amino acid (primarily glutamate) receptors and a relative paucity of glutamate reuptake transporters. Together these features translate into more prolonged and intense contact of glutamate with postsynaptic receptors. Furthermore, these immature glutamate receptors are far more permissive for cationic influx, facilitating membrane depolarization and seizure activation. In contrast, inhibitory gamma-aminobutyric acid (GABA) ion channels are relatively underexpressed in the immature brain. In fact, in certain areas of the developing brain these immature GABA may be depolarizing (i.e., excitatory) rather than hyperpolarizing (i.e., inhibitory).

In addition to these cellular factors, differential development of neural systems may enhance the excitatory state of the immature brain and predispose to seizures. For example, the excitatory projections of the immature substantia nigra develop in advance of the inhibitory anticonvulsant pathways. By virtue of this relatively proconvulsant effect, the immature substantia nigra may actually function as an amplifier rather than inhibitor of epileptic discharges.

II. **Diagnosis of neonatal seizures.** The clinical manifestations of neonatal seizures differ in many ways from those in older patients. The behavioral features of seizures in the newborn may be very subtle, in some cases confined to autonomic and subtle motor phenomena. In addition, the motor manifestations are often disorganized, and an orderly homunculus-based progression of convulsive activity (i.e., "Jacksonian march") is very uncommon. Furthermore, continuous video-EEG monitoring has shown an often inconsistent temporal association between clinical and electrographic seizures.

The peculiar clinical characteristics of seizures in the newborn infant likely reflect the immature state of brain development. In late gestation and early postnatal life, active but incomplete developmental processes include cortical organization, axonal and dendritic branching, and the development of synaptic connections. Myelination commences around term but at this stage is largely confined to the deep subcortical regions of the brain. The relatively underdeveloped organization of the cortex and undermyelination of axons likely underlies the disorganized convulsive activity and lack of orderly seizure propagation in the newborn. For the same reasons, primary generalized seizures are very rare in the newborn. In accordance with the caudal-to-rostral gradient of brain development, the cortical development of the deep limbic system, including its connections to the diencephalic and brainstem structures, is relatively advanced compared to the more rostral neocortex. This fact may underlie the prevalence of behaviors referable to the limbic system, diencephalon, and brainstem, such as the sucking and chewing oromotor automatisms, excessive drooling, oculomotor activity, and respiratory irregularities seen in subtle seizures.

A. Clinical diagnosis of neonatal seizures

1. **Clinical seizure subtypes.** Broadly speaking, clinical seizures may be defined as paroxysmal alterations of neurologic function, including behavioral, motor, and/or autonomic changes. Continuous video EEG monitoring has demonstrated a number of important facts about seizures in the newborn. First, nonepileptic mimics of clinical seizures are common in the newborn. These seizurelike behavior patterns may occur in the normal newborn (e.g., non-nutritive sucking) and nonepileptic paroxysmal clinical changes are common in encephalopathic newborns.

   Given these diagnostic challenges, clinical seizure types may be categorized broadly into four groups: subtle seizures, clonic seizures, tonic seizures, and myoclonic seizures. In many cases, more than one type of seizure occurs in a newborn over time.

   a. **Subtle seizures** are the most common subtype, **comprising about half of all seizures in term and premature newborns.** Subtle seizures are rarely isolated and infants with subtle seizures will almost always have other seizure types as well. Subtle seizures include a broad spectrum of behavioral phenomena, occurring in isolation or in combination. Ocular phenomena are common and include tonic eye deviation, roving "nystagmoid" eye movements, and sudden sustained eye opening with apparent visual fixation. Tonic eye deviation is sometimes classified as a form of tonic seizure. Oro-bucco-lingual movements include chewing, sucking, or lip-smacking movements, and are often associated with a sudden increase in drooling. Various alternating limb movements ("progression movements") have been described, including pedaling, boxing, rowing, or swimming movements. Autonomic phenomena, including sudden changes in skin color and capillary size, may occur alone or in combination with various motor manifestations. Such autonomic paroxysms are usually associated with initial tachycardia, and if sustained, with later bradycardia and possibly apnea. Epileptic apnea is discussed in II.A.2.a. Uncommonly, and unlike clonic seizures, some cases of subtle seizures may be provoked or intensified by stimulation. Although the association between clinical and EEG events is variable, most subtle seizures are not associated with EEG seizures. Based on their inconsistent association with EEG seizures, as well as their poor response to conventional anticonvulsants, many consider these subtle seizures to be nonepileptic "brainstem release phenomena."

   b. **Clonic seizures** are stereotypic and repetitive biphasic movements with a fast contraction phase and a slower relaxation phase. The rhythm of clonic seizures tends to be slower in the newborn than in older patients. Clonic seizures may be unifocal, multifocal, or generalized. Clonic seizures that remain unifocal are usually not associated with loss of consciousness. **The most common cause for clonic seizures that remain unifocal is neonatal stroke** (see II.C.1.b). Other causes of unifocal seizures include focal traumatic contusions, subarachnoid hemorrhage, or metabolic disturbances. In the newborn, multifocal clonic seizures rarely follow a "Jacksonian march"; even when these multifocal seizures are sequential, they are rarely ordered in their progression. Each sequential seizure may appear independent with clinical and EEG features (e.g., rhythm and amplitude) that are different from the previous seizure. Primary generalized clonic seizures are extremely rare in the newborn, probably due to the inability of the immature brain to propagate highly synchronized discharges simultaneously to the entire brain. (One exception to this is benign familial neonatal seizures; see II.C.1.g.(1).(a).)

   c. Tonic seizures have a sustained period (seconds) of muscle contraction without repetitive features. Tonic seizures may be generalized or focal. Generalized tonic seizures, which may closely mimic decerebrate or decorticated posturing, are **most common in premature infants with diffuse neurologic dysfunction or major intraventricular hemorrhage.** Generalized tonic seizures are often associated with other motor automatisms or with clonic seizures, as well. Typically, infants are lethargic or obtunded between these seizures. Certain features suggest that these seizures may be nonepileptic in origin. Specifically, they may be precipitated by tactile or other stimuli, suggesting reflex discharges, and may be abolished by repositioning or light restraint. Finally, the clinical events are typically not associated with electrographic seizure patterns. The background EEG pattern tends to have multifocal or generalized voltage depression and undifferentiated frequencies, and, in some cases, a markedly abnormal burst suppression pattern. Overall, **the prognosis of tonic seizures is very poor,** except in some cases of postasphyxial seizures where an outcome may be less grim.

   d. Myoclonic seizures are distinguished from clonic seizures by their lightning-fast contractions and nonrhythmic character. These seizures may occur in a multifocal or generalized pattern. Even when repetitive, myoclonic seizures tend to be irregular or erratic in nature. In some cases, myoclonic seizures may be elicited by tactile or auditory stimulation or suppressed by restraint. The electro-clinical association of myoclonic seizures is variable, and when present, the myoclonic contraction is usually associated with a single high-voltage spike and followed by a slow wave complex. Conversely, myoclonic movements in stimulus-sensitive myoclonic seizures or in those with chaotic fragmentary movement patterns are usually not associated with electrographic seizure activity. The EEG background activity tends to be low-voltage, slow-wave activity or a burst suppression pattern with focal sharp waves. These patterns may later evolve to a high-voltage, chaotic hypsarrhythmic pattern. Typically, **myoclonic seizures are associated with diffuse and usually serious brain dysfunction** resulting from etiologies such as perinatal asphyxia, inborn errors of metabolism, cerebral dysgenesis, or major brain trauma. **Myoclonic seizures are usually associated with a poor long-term outcome.**

  2. Seizure mimics. In the newborn it may be difficult to distinguish between normal immature behaviors (e.g., non-nutritive sucking), abnormal but nonepileptic behaviors (e.g., "jitteriness"), and true epileptic manifestations. The following clinical guidelines may help distinguish true epileptic seizures from seizure mimics. These guidelines are most reliable with suspected clonic seizures but even then are not infallible.

First, **true epileptic seizures are rarely stimulus-sensitive. Second, epileptic seizures cannot be abolished by passive restraint or repositioning of the infant. Third, epileptic seizures are often associated with autonomic changes or ocular phenomena.** "Jitteriness" (tremor) may be distinguished from clonic seizures by the equal amplitude and faster equiphasic rhythm, compared to the slower, fast-and-slow components of clonic seizures. Generally, normal nonepileptic behaviors are associated with a normal interictal examination. Conversely, abnormal but nonepileptic repetitive behaviors often occur in encephalopathic infants with an abnormal interictal exam.

A temporal association between repetitive clinical events and simultaneous repetitive EEG changes is the strongest supportive evidence for true epileptic seizures. However, using electrographic monitoring to confirm the epileptic nature of suspicious clinical events is more complicated and controversial in the newborn. This is particularly true when clinical seizure events are not accompanied by EEG changes, a situation most often seen with subtle seizures and generalized tonic seizures. There are two opposing views regarding electrically silent clinical "seizures," based on different interpretations of the same fundamental assumptions. In both views, cerebral hemispheric dysfunction results in "disconnection" between higher cortical regions and deeper brainstem areas, thereby causing the electro-clinical dissociation in these "spells." On the one hand, these behavioral paroxysms are considered nonepileptic seizure mimics. In this model, the paroxysmal movements are considered to arise from "central pattern generators" in the brainstem. Normally, these brainstem centers are under tonic-descending inhibitory input from higher cortical centers. However, injury to the more rostral hemispheric regions disconnects the inhibitory input to the brainstem, "releasing" the primitive reflex movement patterns. These released movements may include relatively complex progression movements, or simple tonic posturing that originates from the brainstem reticulospinal nuclei. Several features support the theory that these spells are disinhibited reflex movements. First, they can often be elicited by external stimuli (spontaneous events may be the result of endogenous stimuli). Second, there is often a temporal and spatial summation of these movements to stimulation, with repeated stimuli eliciting movements that radiate or spread to sites distant from the point of stimulation.

In contrast to this "reflex release" concept of electrically silent clinical seizures, others consider these events to have a true epileptic origin. According to this model, seizure discharges originating in the inferomedial cortex are transmitted to deep brainstem centers where they elicit paroxysmal behavioral phenomena. However, these deep discharges cannot be transmitted through the injured and dysfunctional hemispheric pathways to higher cortical regions, and therefore remain undetected by conventional EEG montages. Support for this model includes the fact that these clinical events with no EEG changes may at other times be coupled to EEG discharges in the same patient. To date, these difficult issues remain unresolved.

a. **Epileptic apnea in the newborn.** Apnea is not uncommon during neonatal seizures, but is rarely the only manifestation. The vast majority of infants with epileptic apnea will at some point in their course develop other seizure manifestations. Epileptic apnea may be difficult to distinguish from apnea due to other causes, such as neurologic depression, prematurity, sedative medications, and respiratory illness. However, there are several helpful distinguishing features. Neonatal epileptic apnea rarely lasts longer than 10 to 20 seconds. Bradycardia is often an early accompaniment of nonepileptic apnea, whereas in epileptic apnea, an initial tachycardia is more common, only followed in more prolonged seizures by later bradycardia. The EEG discharges that accompany epileptic apnea are often monorhythmic (most commonly alpha frequency); in addition, they are usually focal over the temporal regions, suggesting an epileptogenic focus in the limbic system. Conversely, nonepileptic apnea is not accompanied by EEG changes except for amplitude suppression that may develop during prolonged apnea.

   b. **Benign neonatal sleep myoclonus** is a relatively common and sometimes dramatic nonepileptic form of myoclonus. This condition presents in the first week of life, and resolves spontaneously (i.e., without treatment) over weeks to months. The convulsive activity emerges during quiet [nonrapid eye movement (REM)] sleep and is rapidly abolished by arousal. Myoclonic activity often builds up dramatically in both intensity and distribution over a period of minutes. Unlike other nonepileptic behaviors, this form of myoclonus may be precipitated in some cases by gentle rhythmic rocking or tactile stimuli, and gentle restraint may actually increase rather than abolish the myoclonus. These events never occur during wakefulness and the neurologic examination is normal. Immediately prior to and during the episodes, the EEG shows features of quiet sleep (sometimes open-eye sleep) with no ictal changes. The interictal EEG is unremarkable. The mechanism is unclear but may be related to a transient dysmaturity of the brainstem reticular-activating system. Anticonvulsants are not indicated, and, in fact, benzodiazepines may exacerbate the myoclonic jerks. The long-term outcome is normal and later epilepsy does not develop.

B. EEG diagnosis of neonatal seizures. By definition, an electrographic seizure is a repetitive series of electrical discharges that evolves in frequency, amplitude and topographic field. As with the clinical manifestations, the electrographic features of neonatal seizures differ in a number of ways from those in more mature patients. Unlike older patients, focal-onset seizures are the rule in the newborn, and primary generalized seizures are exceptionally rare. In addition, there are rhythmic EEG patterns that are normal at specific gestational ages. Abnormal but nonepileptic rhythmic changes may occur on abnormal EEG background in encephalopathic infants. Somewhat arbitrarily, the threshold criterion for the diagnosis of an electrographic seizure has been set at 10 seconds or more of repetitive electrographic discharges. Gestational age has an important influence on the electrographic expression of seizures in the newborn. Such EEG seizures are rare before 34 weeks of gestation; with increasing maturation, the frequency and duration of electrographic seizures increase.

    Although the amplitude and frequency of an electrographic seizure tend to evolve as the focal seizure unfolds, the topographic field of seizure spread remains relatively circumscribed in the newborn. Even when several focal seizures develop in different brain regions at the same time, each seizure appears independent in frequency, amplitude, and morphology. Finally, unlike the interictal EEG in older patients with seizures, the neonatal EEG lacks interictal epileptiform patterns that reliably predict the risk for subsequent seizures; in fact, the development of electrographic seizures in the newborn has been described as an all-or-none phenomenon.

   1. The role and timing of EEG studies in the newborn with suspected seizures. Ideally an EEG study should be recorded as soon as a seizure is first suspected, and preferably no later than 24 hours after. If such an EEG is normal, particularly if a suspected clinical event is captured during the EEG recording, then subsequent EEGs are only indicated if the clinical spells keep recurring. Whenever possible, several suspect events should be captured on EEG to confirm the true epileptic nature of the events. The absence of EEG changes during several clinical events, especially when the interictal EEG background is normal, is suggestive of a nonepileptic process.

If the initial EEG captures the features of seizure activity and antiepileptic drugs are started, a period of continuous video-EEG monitoring is recommended because anticonvulsant medications may abolish only the clinical manifestations, allowing ongoing and undetected EEG seizures to persist. Ideally, EEG monitoring should continue for 24 to 48 hours after the last recorded electrographic seizure. A repeat EEG after 1 week may have particular prognostic value. The need for subsequent EEG studies as a guide to discontinuation of anticonvulsant medications is controversial.

C. Etiologic diagnosis of neonatal seizures. At the first suspicion of neonatal seizures, the immediate focus should be the exclusion of rapidly correctable and potentially injurious processes, including hypoglycemia, hypocalcemia, and hypomagnesemia, among others. After seizures are confirmed and management has commenced, the etiology should be pursued through a rational and orderly approach, with a stepwise interpretation of the facts, and refocusing of the diagnostic plan. The evaluation should start with a careful history of pregnancy, labor and delivery, and family, followed by a detailed clinical examination for signs of dysmorphism, trauma, skin lesions, and unusual odors. The neurologic examination should include a careful and accurate clinical description of the seizure features, the infant's mental status, and cranial nerve examination as well as interictal movements, muscle tone, and deep tendon and primitive reflexes. Certain clinical signs may suggest specific etiologies and may facilitate a more rapid etiologic diagnosis. Next, selected special diagnostic techniques may be necessary to pursue or confirm the etiology of seizures, including blood studies, cerebrospinal fluid (CSF) analysis, EEG recording, and neuroimaging studies. Using such an orderly and rational approach, the vast majority of neonatal seizure etiologies should be identifiable. A list of these seizure etiologies is given in Table 27.1.

1. Specific etiologies

a. Hypoxic ischemic encephalopathy (see also Chap. 27, Perinatal Asphyxia). The leading cause of neonatal seizures is cerebral hypoxia-ischemia, which may occur in the antenatal, intrapartum, or neonatal periods. Perinatal asphyxia is implicated in 25 to 40% of neonatal seizures. However, there is substantial variability in the reported incidence of this etiology, primarily due to the inconsistency of diagnostic cri-

TABLE 27.1. ETIOLOGIES OF NEONATAL SEIZURES

Etiology	Incidence (%)
1. Cerebral hypoxia-ischemia	
a. Global (e.g., perinatal asphyxia)	40
b. Focal infarction (arterial or venous)	15
2. Intracranial hemorrage	15
3. CNS infection	5
4. Metabolic disease	
a. Transient	5
b. Inborn errors of metabolism	1
5. Cerebral dysgenesis	5
6. Neonatal epileptic syndromes	1
7. Neonatal abstinence syndrome	1
8. Unknown	10

teria used in different reports. The advent of more sophisticated imaging techniques such as MRI and MR spectroscopy have allowed the more precise *in vivo* diagnosis and timing of hypoxic-ischemic lesions. With such imaging, earlier (i.e., antepartum) hypoxic-ischemic lesions are diagnosed, even in cases without significant neonatal encephalopathy.

Postasphyxial seizures occur in infants with moderate-to-severe grades of encephalopathy, that is, with obtundation, stupor, or coma. In addition, these infants tend to have muscle hypotonia, altered deep tendon reflexes and, in severe cases, brainstem abnormalities. **Intrapartum asphyxia should never be a diagnosis of exclusion,** and should satisfy certain criteria, including evidence of significant fetal distress, immediate postnatal "depression" at birth, and subsequent altered mental status. Significant fetal distress manifests with evidence of certain abnormal fetal heart rate patterns and/or evidence of "significant" fetal metabolic acidosis. Although the absolute criteria for significant metabolic acidosis remain controversial, most agree that an umbilical artery pH less than 7.0 with a base deficit of > 12 mEq reflects fetal asphyxia capable of causing neonatal encephalopathy and seizures. Commonly accepted criteria for immediate neonatal depression include an Apgar score of less than 5 at 5 minutes of life. In cases where there is a prolonged latency between a fetal asphyxial insult (e.g., an antepartum or early intrapartum insult) and delivery, the above criteria may not be satisfied. In these cases, specialized MRI studies have demonstrated characteristic features of hypoxic-ischemic brain injury despite the absence of significant acidosis or immediate neonatal depression.

The vast majority of postasphyxial seizures in the newborn occur within the first 24 hours after the insult, 50% or more occurring within 12 hours of birth. The seizure onset in each case is likely influenced by the severity, duration, and onset of the intrauterine asphyxial insult. It is likely that more severe insults are followed by earlier onset seizures, but this is not firmly established.

b. Focal ischemic injury:

   (1) Neonatal arterial stroke occurs in around 1/4000 live births. In a large proportion of cases, the etiology of neonatal strokes remains unknown; however, certain risk factors have been identified and are discussed elsewhere. **Seizures are the most common presentation of stroke in the newborn period, and stroke is the second most common cause of neonatal seizures,** accounting for 15 to 20% of cases. The onset of clinical seizures is variable and may be missed, since the majority of strokes occur in otherwise well term infants, without previously known risk factors. These infants usually appear normal immediately before and after seizures. In fact, in the absence of identified seizures, the diagnosis of neonatal stroke may be delayed until the onset of infant hand use around 4 to 5 months when motor asymmetries become evident. These seizures are typically unifocal, with minimal spread. Since neonatal arterial stroke most commonly involves the left middle cerebral artery, right-sided clonic seizures are the most common clinical presentation. The clonic activity is generally slower than that in older patients. Post-stroke seizures usually have a very good association between clinical and electrographic manifestations.

   (2) Cerebral vein thrombosis usually occurs in the large dural sinuses, particularly the posterior aspects of the superior sagittal sinus. Although the presentation of cerebral vein thrombosis may be subtle, with lethargy often the only feature, about 60% of cases develop neonatal seizures. Unlike the relatively normal mental status of infants with arterial stroke and seizures, infants with cerebral vein thrombosis and seizures are more encephalopathic, with depressed mental status before and between seizures.

   c. **Intracranial hemorrhage** (see also Intracranial Hemorrhage). Intra-
      cranial hemorrhage is implicated in approximately 10% of neonatal
      seizures. The location of hemorrhage and the clinical features of the
      seizures varies with gestational age. With term infants, posthemor-
      rhagic seizures are most commonly associated with **primary subarach-
      noid hemorrhage** and less often with subdural hemorrhage. Primary
      subarachnoid hemorrhage occurs more frequently after difficult pro-
      longed or traumatic labor, including forceps and vacuum deliveries.
      However, primary subarachnoid hemorrhage may occur after appar-
      ently uncomplicated labor (i.e., so-called parturitional hemorrhage).
      Such primary parturitional subarachnoid hemorrhage results in focal
      or multifocal seizures, usually starting on the second day of life, in in-
      fants who appear relatively well between seizures. These seizures often
      have good clinical and electrical association. **Infants with seizures
      associated with primary subarachnoid hemorrhage have a good
      long-term outcome in 90% of cases.**
      About half of all subdural hemorrhages (SDHs) diagnosed in the
      newborn are complicated by seizures, usually presenting in the first
      days of life. Neonatal SDH usually occurs in large babies, breech deliv-
      ery, or difficult instrumented delivery, as a result of sheering forces
      and tears of the tentorium, falx, or cortical bridging veins. Infratentor-
      ial SDHs in the limited posterior fossa space demand urgent evalua-
      tion since potentially fatal brainstem dysfunction may evolve rapidly.
      **Posthemorrhagic seizures in the preterm infant have different
      features and a more ominous prognosis.** These seizures are usually
      associated with **severe intraventricular hemorrhage (IVH),** or its paren-
      chymal complication, periventricular hemorrhagic infarction (PVHI)
      (see Chap. 27, Intracranial Hemorrhage) Seizures following severe IVH
      usually present within the first 3 days of life in sick, very premature
      infants. The seizures are usually generalized tonic seizures with poor
      electro-clinical association. They form part of a critical illness, which
      often evolves to coma and death in the acute phase. Seizures associ-
      ated with PVHI tend to occur after the third day of life.
   d. **Central nervous system infections** (see also Chap. 23). Central nervous
      system infections from a variety of agents, including viral, bacterial, or
      other organisms such as toxoplasmosis, may have neonatal seizures as a
      prominent part of their presentation. These infections may originate in
      the fetus, for example, congenital encephalitis due to cytomegalovirus
      (CMV) and toxoplasmosis. When CMV encephalitis occurs in earlier ges-
      tation it may cause cerebral dysgenetic lesions, which may further in-
      crease the risk of seizures. Intrauterine infections with toxoplasmosis or
      CMV that are severe enough to cause neonatal seizures usually do so
      within the first three days of life. Other viral infections of importance
      are herpes simplex virus infections that may become symptomatic in the
      first days of life after intrapartum infection [usually herpes simplex
      virus (HSV) type II] or have a more delayed presentation (usually post-
      natal acquisition of HSV type I). The development of bacterial menin-
      gitis, most commonly Group B streptococcal meningitis, may also have
      a biphasic appearance with early and late forms. The mechanism of
      seizures in central nervous system infections may be through direct
      cerebritis or vaso-occlusive injury with secondary seizures. The onset of
      infection-related seizures obviously depends on the various organisms
      and onset of infection. Of the bacterial infections, meningitis due to Group
      B streptococcus and *Escherichia coli* are the most common, and in these
      cases, seizures usually develop in the latter part of the first week or later.
   e. **Metabolic disturbances** (see also Chap. 29). Two types of metabolic
      disturbances may result in neonatal seizures: (1) transient and rapidly
      correctable disturbances, and (2) inherited and usually persistent
      causes.

(1) **Transient metabolic disturbances** include disturbances of blood glucose and electrolyte disturbances such as hypoglycemia, hypocalcemia and hypomagnesemia. These conditions frequently occur in conjunction with other potentially epileptogenic conditions such as perinatal asphyxia.

    (a) **Hypoglycemia** (see also Chap. 29, Hypoglycemia and Hyperglycemia) is especially common in infants with intrauterine growth retardation, diabetic mothers, or perinatal asphyxia. Less commonly, hypoglycemia may be a prominent feature of certain inborn errors of metabolism (e.g., galactosemia, glycogen storage diseases) or hyperinsulinemic conditions (e.g., Beckwith-Wiedeman syndrome, nesidioblastosis). Glucose transporter deficiency is a more recently described condition in which blood glucose levels are normal but CSF glucose levels are low. The timing of seizures in neonatal hypoglycemia is usually on the second day of life, but the primary link between hypoglycemia and seizures may be difficult to establish. Since seizures usually develop after sustained hypoglycemia, these infants often have a poor outcome.

    (b) **Hypocalcemia** (see also Chap. 29, Hypocalcemia, Hypercalcemia, and Hypermagnesemia) accounts for approximately 3% of neonatal seizures. Currently, hypocalcemic seizures are usually associated with perinatal asphyxia or endocrinopathies due to maternal neonatal hypoparathyroidism or deletion syndromes of chromosome 22, including the DeGeorge syndrome.

    (c) **Hyponatremic** seizures may develop in the setting of inappropriate antidiuretic hormone (ADH secretion), perinatal asphyxia, and inadvertent water intoxication (see also Chap. 9).

(2) **Inborn errors of metabolism** (see also Chap. 29, Inborn Error of Metabolism) are an uncommon cause of neonatal seizures; nevertheless, neonatal seizures have been described in a long list of such conditions (see partial list in Table 27.2). Certain of these conditions are more likely to be associated with seizures, including nonketotic hyperglycinemia, pyridoxine dependency, sulfate oxidase deficiency,

---

TABLE 27.2. SOME OF THE INBORN ERRORS OF METABOLISM PRESENTING WITH NEONATAL SEIZURES

Pyridoxine dependency

Nonketotic hyperglycinemia

Urea cycle defects

Sulfite oxidase deficiency

Glutaric aciduria type II

Maple syrup urine disease

Menkes disease

Molybdenum cofactor deficiency

Propionic aciduria

Methylmalonic aciduria

Mitochondrial diseases

Glucose transporter deficiency

glutaric aciduria type II, and urea cycle defects. The most common diagnostic abnormalities associated with these conditions include metabolic acidosis, hyperammonemia, hypoglycemia and ketosis. The clinical features and definitive diagnostic tests for these conditions are detailed in Chap. 29. Most of these conditions are due to permanent enzyme defects, and are largely incurable. However, their recognition is important for two reasons. First, some metabolic disturbances have transient forms that resolve over time (e.g., nonketotic hyperglycinemia). Second, some of these conditions are treatable (e.g., pyridoxine dependency). In both these situations, early diagnosis and treatment may prevent or limit brain injury.

(a) **Pyridoxine dependency results from impaired binding of the active form of pyridoxine to the enzyme glutamatic acid decarboxylase (GAD).** This enzyme is responsible for the conversion of the excitatory amino acid neurotransmitter, glutamate, to the inhibitory neurotransmitter, gamma-aminobutyric acid (GABA). Therefore, impaired GAD activity causes a marked increase in excitatory versus inhibitory neurotransmitter levels. Not only does this elevated excitatory state precipitate seizures, but high glutamate levels may be lethal to both neurons and oligodendroglia. Seizures in pyridoxine dependency often present early, that is, within the first hours of life or even in the fetus. The diagnosis is usually made by a therapeutic trial of intravenous pyridoxine with simultaneous EEG monitoring. In addition, affected infants have low GABA levels and high glutamate levels in the cerebrospinal fluid.

(b) **Glycine encephalopathy (nonketotic hyperglycinemia)** is an autosomal recessive condition in which a deficiency in the glycine cleavage system results in very high levels of glycine in the brain and CSF. Glycine is a coagonist at the excitatory cerebral N-methyl-D-aspartate (NMDA) glutamate receptor, but is inhibitory in the brainstem and spinal cord. The marked elevation of glycine levels results in refractory myoclonic seizures (due to excitation of cortical NMDA receptors), stupor, respiratory disturbances, and hypotonia (due to brainstem inhibition). **The diagnosis is made by demonstrating markedly elevated glycine levels in the CSF,** and may be missed if only serum or urine levels are measured since these may be normal or mildly elevated. The EEG background pattern typically shows burst-suppression. Most infants with nonketotic hyperglycinemia die by 1 year of age, but a transient and potentially benign form may present with seizures in early neonatal life. Consequently, aggressive support is indicated until such a transient form is excluded. Antenatal diagnosis is possible by chorionic villus sampling.

f. **Cerebral dysgenesis.** A number of dysgenetic cerebral lesions may be associated with neonatal seizures. In many, but not all, cases these lesions can be demonstrated *in vivo* by computed tomography (CT) or MRI scan. Conditions most commonly associated with neonatal seizures are disorders of neuronal migration (e.g., heterotopias, lissencephalies) or disorders of neuronal organization (e.g., polymicrogyria). These ectopic or disorganized collections of neurons are abnormally prone to hyperexcitability and bursts of discharges leading to seizures. The genetic lesions causing these disorders are being uncovered. Occasionally cerebral dysgenesis may be associated with and possibly caused by inborn metabolic disturbances, such as 7-dehydrocholesterol deficiency in certain holoprosencephalies, and carbohydrate-deficient glycoprotein syndrome and nonketotic hyperglycinemia in some cases of agenesis of the corpus callosum. Infants with cerebral dysgenesis and fluctuating consciousness, vomiting, and apparent regression, should be evaluated for metabolic conditions that may cause ongoing neuro-degeneration.

g. **Epileptic syndromes in the newborn infant**

(1) There are two benign and two malignant epileptic syndromes presenting with seizures in the newborn infant.

(a) **Benign familial neonatal seizures** is an autosomal dominant seizure disorder presenting in newborn infants without obvious risk factors for seizures. In this condition, seizures typically have their onset around the second to third day of life and may recur for days to weeks before gradually resolving. The interictal neurologic examination is normal, and **the vast majority of cases have a normal long-term neurodevelopmental outcome.** Less than 10% of cases develop later epilepsy, usually in adulthood. Neither the number of neonatal seizures, nor their treatment, appears related to the long-term outcome. These features have suggested that aggressive anticonvulsant therapy may not be indicated in this condition.

Benign familial neonatal seizures are a rare form of primary generalized seizures in the newborn. The clinical phenomena are variable but include a brief initial phase of apnea, tachycardia, and tonic posturing (with abduction or adduction of the arms, flexion of the hips, and extension of the knees) followed by a phase of clonic activity. As such, this condition is one of the rare instances in which tonic-clonic seizures occur in the newborn. These seizures tend to occur mainly during active sleep and may be preceded by brief arousal. The ictal EEG features consist of a sudden brief period of generalized voltage attenuation (during the apneic and tonic phase) followed by a longer generalized discharge of repetitive spike and/or sharp waves (during the clonic phase). Rarely do benign familial neonatal seizures have a consistent EEG focus or a postictal phase. The interictal EEG is either normal or has occasional bursts of alternating theta rhythmic activity (theta pointu alternant). All laboratory and imaging studies aimed at identifying an etiology are normal. Two separate genetic loci have been identified. The majority of families have a locus at chromosome 20q13.3, which encodes for a potassium channel, suggesting an impairment of potassium-dependent neuronal repolarization as the basis for the seizures. In other families, the locus is at chromosome 8q24.

(b) **Benign idiopathic neonatal seizures** make up about 5% of seizures in term infants. Certain diagnostic criteria have been proposed, including: (1) birth after 39 weeks' gestational age; (2) normal pregnancy and delivery; (3) Apgar scores > 8; (4) normal neonatal course prior to the seizures; (5) seizure onset between days 4 and 6 of life; (6) normal neurologic state before and between seizures; (7) clonic and/or apneic (never tonic) seizures; (8) normal diagnostic testing; (9) an ictal EEG showing brief (1–3 minute) seizures (never alpha frequency) in the rolandic regions; and (10) a normal interictal EEG except for theta pointu alternant pattern (in 60% cases). The cause for these seizures remains unknown, but may be related to a transient zinc deficiency, since CSF zinc levels may be decreased. Several features distinguish these idiopathic seizures from benign familial seizures; these include: (1) absence of a family history; (2) later seizure onset, around day 5 of life; (3) convulsions that are clonic and/or apneic, but never tonic; (4) multifocal clonic seizures that are never primary generalized; and (5) lack of the initial voltage attenuation on the ictal EEG. Instead, the ictal EEG shows lateralized or secondarily generalized rhythmic spikes and slow waves. The period of seizure activity is usually brief but intense, with frequent or serial seizures, and even status epilepticus. This phase is followed by gradual resolution, with seizures seldom persisting longer than 2 weeks. The long-term outcome is invariably favorable and later epilepsy does not occur.

(2) There are two early epileptic encephalopathies with an invariably poor prognosis.

(a) Neonatal myoclonic encephalopathy (NME) presents with erratic and fragmentary partial seizures and massive **myoclonus.** These seizures typically start as focal motor seizures, and later evolve into typical infantile spasms. The most common etiologies associated with this condition are metabolic disorders (especially nonketotic hyperglycinemia). The ictal EEG shows high-amplitude EEG bursts coinciding with the massive myoclonic seizures. The interictal pattern shows a burst suppression pattern with complex bursts and sharp waves alternating with periods of low-amplitude quiescence. **The long-term outcome is universally poor,** with a high mortality in the first year and severe retardation in all survivors.

(b) Ohtahara's syndrome usually presents within the first 10 days of life but may present as late as 3 months. The seizures are typically numerous brief **tonic** spasms (and not clonic or fragmentary myoclonic). In contrast to the metabolic causes of NME, the causes of Ohtahara's syndrome tend to be structural, with most being dysgenetic or, occasionally, destructive, such as hypoxic-ischemic injury. The interictal EEG is usually an invariant burst-suppression pattern, with no sleep-wake cycling. Unlike the ictal EEG of NME, the tonic spasms tend to occur with a period of EEG suppression and not with the bursts. As in NME, **the prognosis of Ohtahara's syndrome is universally grim,** with early death or, among survivors, severe handicap and frequently infantile spasms.

III. Treatment of neonatal seizures (Table 27.3). As a general rule, seizures in the newborn are less responsive to conventional anticonvulsants than are seizures in older patients. This is particularly true of seizures with electroclinical dissociation in which seizures may remain refractory to high doses and sometimes multiple anticonvulsants. The risk:benefit ratio of such high doses in the treatment of neonatal seizures has been questioned. Specifically, the potential for seizures to cause direct injury to the immature brain has to be weighed against the effect of high levels of anticonvulsants on the developing brain. These issues have triggered a vigorous but unresolved debate about the management of neonatal seizures.

A number of potentially deleterious effects on the systemic and cerebral systems support the treatment of neonatal seizures. First, seizures may cause significant hemodynamic and respiratory disturbances, which in the sick newborn, may complicate management and potentially extend brain injury. Seizures disrupt cerebral pressure autoregulation and cause wide fluctuations in blood pressure, a combination with potentially serious consequences for the immature brain. Second, massive amounts of cerebral energy are consumed during the repeated neuronal depolarization-repolarization associated with seizures. Neonatal seizures cause a rapid fall in cerebral glucose and rise in brain lactate, even with normal or elevated blood glucose levels. In the insulted brain, such energy depletion may seriously compromise recovery. Third, seizures release large amounts of glutamate, and, in conditions of cerebral energy failure, seizures inhibit the reuptake of glutamate. Together these mechanisms result

TABLE 27.3. ACUTE MANAGEMENT OF NEONATAL SEIZURES

After each step below, evaluate the infant for ongoing seizures. If seizures persist, advance to next step.

Step 1. Stabilize vital functions

Step 2. Correct transient metabolic disturbances
    a. Hypoglycemia (target blood sugar 70–120 mg/dL)
       10% dextrose water IV bolus dose 2 mL/kg
       +/−continuous infusion @ 8 mg/kg per minute
    b. Hypocalcemia 5% calcium gluconate IV @ 4 mL/kg (need cardiac monitoring)
    c. Hypomagnesemia 50% magnesium sulfate IM @ 0.2 mL/kg

Step 3. Phenobarbital 20 mg/kg IV load
    Cardiorespiratory monitoring
    5 mg/kg IV (may repeat to total dose of 40 mg/kg)
    Consider continuous EEG monitoring
    Consider intubation/ventilation

Step 4. Lorazepam   0.05 mg/kg IV (may repeat to total dose of 0.1 mg/kg)

Step 5. Phenytoin   20 mg/kg slow IV load
     (fosphenytoin)

                     5 mg/kg slow IV (may repeat to total dose of 30 mg/kg)

Step 6. Pyridoxine 50–100 mg/kg IV (with EEG monitoring)

Step 7. Other agents (see text)

---

in the accumulation of extracellular glutamate to toxic levels that are potentially lethal to postsynaptic neurons and immature oligodendrocytes.

In animal studies, the immature brain is remarkably resistant to even prolonged seizures induced by proconvulsant drugs. Conversely, in a model that mimics postasphyxial seizures in the human newborn, seizures preceded by an asphyxial insult cause extensive cellular loss in the immature brain. These studies suggest that seizures superimposed on insults that deplete or disrupt cerebral energetics are capable of causing or extending brain injury. Seizures may also disrupt protein and lipid metabolism of immature neurons, and activate genes that stimulate axonal growth and new synapse formation. These sublethal insults may result in aberrant neuronal pathways and a long-term reduction in seizure threshold. Together, these mechanisms likely contribute to the epilepsy, motor, and cognitive impairment seen in some survivors of neonatal seizures.

The lack of a single highly effective anticonvulsant regimen in the newborn has spawned many different approaches. However, the following protocol is used in many major centers, including our own (see Table 27.3). The initial steps in management consist of stabilization of the vital functions, exclusion or treatment of rapidly correctable conditions, and establishing the diagnosis of seizures by the clinical or EEG criteria detailed above. Specific therapies against other treatable conditions (e.g., meningitis, narcotic withdrawal) should commence but should not delay the initiation of anticonvulsant therapy.

A. Reversing rapidly correctable causes
    1. **Hypoglycemia** (see also Chap. 29 and Fig. 10.2). Even when other primary etiologies are identified for seizures, hypoglycemia should be excluded or corrected. In the newborn with seizures, the target goal for blood glucose should be 70 to 120 mg/dL. If the hypoglycemic infant is actively seizing, an IV loading dose of 10% dextrose at 2 mL/kg (0.2 g/kg)

should be given, followed by a continuous infusion of up to 8 mg/kg per minute to achieve the above target levels. In rare cases where these measures do not achieve normoglycemia, glucagon or hydrocortisone may be necessary. Experimental studies show that (1) brain tissue levels of glucose may fall during seizures even when blood glucose is normal, and (2) hyperglycemia may be neuroprotective. These data are interesting, but more data are required before supranormal blood glucose targets can be recommended.

2. **Hypocalcemia and hypomagnesemia** (see also Chap. 29). Even if hypocalcemic seizures respond to antiepileptic medications, the low calcium levels should be corrected. An IV dose of 5% calcium gluconate at 4 mL/kg (200 mg/kg) should be given under careful cardiac monitoring. Hypomagnesemia is best treated with an IM dose of 50% magnesium sulfate at 0.2 mL/kg. Infants treated for hypocalcemia should also receive magnesium because calcium administration increases renal magnesium excretion, and magnesium administration increases serum calcium levels. Of note, magnesium administration may result in transient weakness and hypotonia, even with normal serum levels.

B. **Specific anticonvulsant agents** (see also Appendix A).
1. **Acute management.** Once the diagnosis of seizures is strongly suspected or confirmed, anticonvulsant agents should be started. The administration of these agents should occur with careful cardiorespiratory monitoring.
   a. **Phenobarbital** should be started as an IV loading dose of 20 mg/kg given over 10 to 15 minutes. This usually achieves blood levels around 20 mg/dL, levels at which an anticonvulsant effect begins to be apparent in the newborn. If seizures persist, further bolus doses of 5 mg/kg should be given, up to a total dose of 40 mg/kg or control of seizures. At these levels, significant respiratory depression is usually not evident. However, in a recent randomized trial these levels achieved seizure control in less than half of infants. The use of higher levels has been advocated but remains controversial because additional therapeutic benefit may be outweighed by the risk of cardiorespiratory depression. In asphyxiated infants with hepatic dysfunction, the above doses may result in higher blood levels, with sedation that persists for days. For this reason, in the severely asphyxiated infant with hepatic dysfunction it may be advisable to add a second, less-sedating agent such as phenytoin if seizures persist after the first 20 mg/kg loading dose of phenobarbital.
   b. **Phenytoin,** the usual second-line agent, is given as an initial loading dose of 20 mg/kg which usually produces therapeutic blood levels around 15 to 20 mg/dL. Phenytoin is given into normal saline (it precipitates in dextrose solutions) and no faster than 1 mg/kg per minute to avoid cardiac arrhythmias. If seizures persist, an additional dose of 5 mg/kg may be used. **Fosphenytoin** is a more recently developed prodrug form that is rapidly converted into phenytoin. This agent has several advantages over phenytoin including greater solubility in standard intravenous solutions (including dextrose-containing solutions), safe faster rates of infusion, safe IM dosing, and no tissue injury with IV infiltration. Initial studies have supported the use of this agent in the newborn.
   c. **Benzodiazepines.** The combination of phenobarbital and phenytoin will control seizures in up to 85% of infants. For neonatal seizures that remain refractory to these measures, benzodiazepines may add further benefit. Lorazepam, diazepam, and midazolam have all demonstrated potent anticonvulsant effects in the newborn. Although all three agents gain rapid entry into the brain, important differences in their subsequent kinetics, efficacy, and adverse effect profile make lorazepam the preferred agent for neonatal seizures. Lorazepam has several advantages over diazepam. Specifically: (1) diazepam is rapidly redistributed

after an IV dose and cleared from the brain within minutes; (2) diazepam has greater respiratory and circulatory depressant effects (particularly when used with a barbiturate); (3) the anticonvulsant effect of diazepam lasts minutes, while its sedative effect exceeds 24 hours; and (4) sodium benzoate, the vehicle for IV diazepam, uncouples bilirubin from albumin, increasing the risk for kernicterus in jaundiced infants. **Lorazepam** at 0.05 mg/kg IV has an anticonvulsant onset within 2 to 3 minutes, which lasts between 6 and 24 hours (and much longer in infants with postasphyxial liver dysfunction). The dose may be repeated after several minutes to a total dose of 0.10 mg/kg. **Diazepam** is an effective anticonvulsant in the newborn and is given as an IV dose of 0.1 mg/kg increasing slowly up to 0.3 mg/kg given until the seizure stops. Because of their short anticonvulsant half-lives, both diazepam and **midazolam**, the newest benzodiazepine to be used as an anticonvulsant in the newborn, are most effective when given as a continuous infusion. Midazolam is given at an initial IV dose of 0.02 to 0.1 mg/kg, followed by a continuous infusion of 0.06 to 0.4 mg/kg per hour.

   d. Pyridoxine. When neonatal seizures prove refractory to the preceding regimen, pyridoxine dependency should be excluded. This condition is diagnosed by the rapid (within minutes) cessation of EEG seizures to an IV dose of 50 to 100 mg pyridoxine. Since pyridoxine administration increases the cerebral synthesis of the inhibitory transmitter GABA, apnea and hypotonia may occasionally develop, necessitating close respiratory monitoring. If the diagnosis is made, maintenance oral doses of pyridoxine should be given at 10 to 100 mg/day, depending on the response.

   e. Other agents. Although not commonly used in the United States, **lidocaine** has been used in Europe as an effective adjunctive anticonvulsant for neonatal seizures, usually after failure of phenobarbital and diazepam. The anticonvulsant effects are seen within 10 minutes after starting an IV infusion of 4 to 6 mg/kg per hour, with or without a preceding loading dose. Once seizures are controlled, the lidocaine infusion is tapered over several days. In spite of its potential cardiac toxicity, the only adverse effect described in these reports is recurrence of seizures during the weaning period.

  2. Maintenance and withdrawal of anticonvulsant drugs. Decisions regarding duration of therapy depend on the underlying etiology. Certain conditions, such as primary hypocalcemia, cause acute ("symptomatic") seizures with relatively low risk of later recurrent seizures, if the primary condition is appropriately managed. In these conditions discontinuation of anticonvulsant medications may be considered prior to intensive care unit (ICU) discharge. In conditions such as cerebral dysgenesis, the high risk for subsequent epilepsy warrants ongoing anticonvulsant treatment. Infants with postasphyxial seizures, have a 20 to 30% incidence of epilepsy, although subsequent seizures may present months to years later. If at the time of discharge from the neonatal intensive care unit (NICU) the infant's neurologic exam and EEG show good recovery towards normal, an early withdrawal of phenobarbital may be considered. Otherwise, the need for continued phenobarbital treatment should be reevaluated at 6- to 12-week intervals, maintaining interim blood levels around 20 mg/dL.

IV. Prognosis after neonatal seizures. The overall prognosis for survival in neonatal seizures is around 85%, a significant improvement from earlier decades. Unfortunately, the prognosis for long-term neurodevelopmental outcome remains largely unchanged. Specifically, an adverse outcome occurs in about 50% of cases, with sequelae such as mental retardation, motor dysfunction, and seizures. The range of outcomes after neonatal seizures varies widely, with the three major predictors of long-term outcome being (1) the underlying etiology, (2) the electro-

TABLE 27.4. PROGNOSIS OF NEONATAL SEIZURES BY ETIOLOGY

Etiology	Normal Outcome (%)
Hypoxia-ischemia	50
Meningitis	50
Hypoglycemia	50
Subarachnoid hemorrhage	90
Early hypocalcemia	50
Late hypocalcemia	100
Intraventricular hemorrhage	10
Dysgenesis	0
Unknown	75

graphic features, and (3) gestational age. Other useful predictors include the neonatal neurologic examination and neuroimaging findings.

A. Etiology as a prognostic factor (see Table 27.4). Neonatal seizures reflect significant brain dysfunction. The nature and severity of the insult causing these seizures might be expected to influence long-term brain function. Therefore, it is not surprising that in most studies the underlying etiology of neonatal seizures is the most powerful predictor of long-term outcome. Infants with hypoxic-ischemic encephalopathy, when accompanied by seizures, currently have an approximately 50% chance for normal development. Similarly, about half of infants with seizures due to bacterial meningitis have a favorable outcome. The overall outcome for infants with neonatal seizures after arterial or venous vaso-occlusive disease is relatively benign. However, there are certain features that predict a worse outcome. In arterial stroke, EEG and MRI studies may identify infants at risk for worse prognosis. Specifically, an abnormal interictal EEG background has a less favorable outcome. Likewise, an MRI study showing involvement of an entire vascular territory, e.g., in the middle cerebral artery (MCA) with injury to the hemispheres, the basal ganglia, and the internal capsule, is associated with significant hemiparesis in the long term. Although uncommon, involvement of multiple arteries, especially if bilateral, predicts worse outcome. About 75% of infants with cerebral vein thrombosis and seizures have a favorable outcome, and only 20% develop later epilepsy. Features that predict a worse outcome include the development of extensive hemorrhagic infarction, as well as venous occlusion that extends into the deep venous system. The outcome of intracranial hemorrhage depends on the degree of parenchymal injury and the gestational age. The vast majority of infants who develop seizures after primary subarachnoid (parturitional) hemorrhage have a good long-term outcome. Conversely, premature infants who develop seizures after intraventricular hemorrhage are usually critically ill and often have parenchymal hemorrhagic infarction; consequently, the outcome is significantly worse in these infants. Hypoglycemia severe and persistent enough to cause seizures is associated with a normal outcome in around 50% of cases. This prognosis is substantially worse when hypoglycemia complicates postasphyxial encephalopathy. The prognosis for infants with cerebral dysgenesis who develop seizures in the newborn period is universally dismal. If a thorough diagnostic evaluation fails to identify an etiology for neonatal seizures, the outcome is likely to be favorable.

B. **Both the interictal and ictal EEG features have prognostic value.** With severe interictal EEG background abnormalities, such as burst suppression, marked voltage suppression, and an isoelectric background, an adverse neurological outcome occurs in 90% or more of cases. Conversely, a normal EEG background at presentation is associated with a favorable outcome. Although somewhat less reliable, the ictal EEG features may also be useful predictors of outcome. A better outcome may be expected when the clinical and EEG seizures are consistently correlated, whereas electrically silent clinical seizures or clinically silent EEG seizures are associated with a worse outcome. The EEG seizure morphology may also be helpful, with alpha-frequency seizures, seizures associated with electrodecremental changes, or myoclonic seizures coupled with spike bursts, having a worse prognosis. Others have associated an increased number and duration of EEG seizures (particularly seizures lasting more than 30 minutes) with a worse outcome.

C. **Gestational age has prognostic significance,** with neonatal seizures in infants under 32 weeks' gestation having a high mortality up to 80% in some studies, and a significantly higher risk of adverse neurologic outcome in survivors, when compared to term infants.

Suggested Readings

Neonatal seizures. In: Volpe J. J. (Ed.) *Neurology of the Newborn,* 4th ed. Philadelphia: Saunders, 2001;178–216.

Mizrahi E., Kellaway P., *The Diagnosis and Management of Neonatal Seizures.* Philadelphia: Lippincott-Raven, 1997.

Intracranial Hemorrhage

Janet S. Soul

OVERVIEW

The incidence of intracranial hemorrhage (ICH) varies from 2 to >30% in newborns, depending on gestational age (GA) at birth and the type of ICH. Bleeding within the skull can occur: (1) external to the brain into the epidural, subdural, or subarachnoid spaces; (2) into the parenchyma of the cerebrum or cerebellum; or (3) into the ventricles from the subependymal germinal matrix or choroid plexus (Table 27.5). The incidence, pathogenesis, clinical presentation, diagnosis, management, and prognosis of these hemorrhages vary according to their location, severity, and the GA of the infant (1,2). There is often a combination of two or more types of ICH, as an ICH in one location often extends into an adjacent compartment—for example—extension of a parenchymal hemorrhage into the subarachnoid space or ventricles.

Diagnosis typically depends on clinical suspicion, when an infant presents with typical neurological signs, such as seizures, irritability, or depressed level of consciousness, and focal neurologic deficits referable either to the cerebrum or brainstem. Diagnosis is confirmed preferably with an appropriate neuroimaging study. Management varies according to the size and location of the ICH, and presenting neurological signs. In general, only very large hemorrhages require surgical intervention for removal of the ICH itself. With a large ICH, there may be a requirement for pressor support or volume replacement (with normal saline, albumin, or packed red blood cells) because of significant blood loss. More commonly, management is focused on treating complications such as seizures or the development of posthemorrhagic hydrocephalus. In general, although a larger ICH is more likely to result in greater morbidity or mortality, the presence and severity of parenchymal injury (whether due to hemorrhage or other neuropathology) is usually the best predictor of outcome.

TABLE 27.5. ILLUSTRATING NEONATAL ICH BY LOCATION, AND WHETHER EACH ICH TYPE IS PREDOMINANTLY PRIMARY (1°) OR SECONDARY (2°) SOURCE OF BLEEDING, AND THE RELATIVE INCIDENCE IN PRETERM (PT) OR TERM (T) NEWBORNS

Type (Location) of Hemorrhage	Principal Source of ICH	Relative Incidence in PT vs. T
1. Subdural and epidural hemorrhage	1° > 2°	T > PT
2. Subarachnoid hemorrhage (SAH)	2° > 1°*	?*
3. Intraparenchymal hemorrhage		
Cerebral	2° > 1°	PT > T
Cerebellar	2° > 1°	PT > T
4. Germinal matrix/intraventricular hemorrhage	1° > 2°	PT > T

*True incidence unknown, small 1° SAH may be more common than is recognized.

I. **Subdural hemorrhage (SDH) and epidural hemorrhage (EH)**

   A. **Etiology and pathogenesis.** The pathogenesis of SDH relates to rupture of the draining veins and sinuses of the brain that occupy the subdural space. Vertical molding, fronto-occipital elongation, and torsional forces acting on the head during delivery may provoke laceration of dural leaflets of either the tentorium cerebelli or the falx cerebri. This results in rupture of the vein of Galen, inferior sagittal sinus, straight sinus and/or transverse sinus, and a posterior fossa SDH. Breech presentation also predisposes to occipital osteodiastasis, a depressed fracture of the occipital bone or bones, which may lead to direct laceration of the cerebellum or rupture of the occipital sinus. Clinically significant SDH in the posterior fossa often results from trauma in the full-term infant, although small, inconsequential SDH may be fairly common in uncomplicated deliveries (the true incidence in apparently well newborns is unknown.). SDH in the supratentorial space usually results from rupture of the bridging, superficial veins over the cerebral convexity. Other risk factors for SDH include factors that increase the likelihood of significant forces on the infant's head, such as large head size, rigid pelvis (e.g., in a primiparous or older multiparous mother), nonvertex presentation (breech, face, etc.), or very rapid, or prolonged labor or delivery, difficult instrumented delivery, or rarely, a bleeding diathesis.

   B. **Clinical presentation.** When the accumulation of blood is rapid and large, as occurs with rupture of large veins or sinuses, the presentation follows shortly after birth and evolves rapidly. This is particularly true in infratentorial SDH, where compression of the brainstem may result in nuchal rigidity or opisthotonus; obtundation or coma; apnea; other abnormal respiratory patterns; or unreactive pupils and abnormal extraocular movements (i.e., compression of third or sixth cranial nerve by herniating cerebrum). With increased intracranial pressure (ICP), there may be a bulging fontanelle and/or widely split sutures. With large hemorrhages, there may be systemic signs of hypovolemia. When the sources of hemorrhage are small veins, there may be few symptoms or signs for up to a week, at which time either the hematoma attains a critical size, imposes on the brain parenchyma and produces neurological signs, or hydrocephalus develops. Seizures may occur in up to half of neonates with SDH, particularly with SDH over the cerebral convexity. With cerebral convexity SDH, there may also be subtle focal cerebral signs and mild disturbances of consciousness, such as irritability. Subarachnoid hemorrhage (SAH) probably coexists in the majority of cases of neonatal SDH, as demonstrated by a CSF exam (3). Finally, a chronic subdural effusion may gradually develop over months, presenting as abnormal head growth in the first weeks to months after birth.

C. **Diagnosis.** The diagnosis should be suspected on the basis of history and clinical signs, and confirmed with a computed tomography (CT) scan. Although ultrasound (US) may be valuable in evaluating the sick newborn at the bedside, **ultrasonic imaging of structures adjacent to bone (i.e., the subdural space) is often inadequate.** Magnetic resonance imaging (MRI) has recently proven to be quite sensitive to small hemorrhage, and can aid in the timing of a hemorrhage. MRI is also superior in detecting other lesions, such as contusion, thromboembolic infarction, or hypoxic-ischemic injury that may occur in some infants with severe hypovolemia or other risk factors for parenchymal abnormalities. However, a computed tomography (CT) scan is much quicker to obtain and usually adequate in an unstable infant with elevated ICP who may require neurosurgical intervention. **When there is clinical suspicion of a large SDH, a lumbar puncture (LP) should not be performed until after the CT is obtained,** and the LP may be contraindicated if there is a large hemorrhage within the posterior fossa or supratentorial compartment. With a smaller SDH, an LP should be performed to rule out infection in the newborn with signs such as seizures, depressed mental status, or other systemic signs of illness.

D. **Management and prognosis.** Most infants with SDH do not require surgical intervention, and can be managed with supportive care and treatment of any accompanying seizures. Infants with rapid evolution of a large infratentorial SDH require prompt stabilization with volume expansion, pressors, and respiratory support, as needed. An urgent head CT and neurosurgical consultation should be obtained in any infant with signs of progressive brainstem dysfunction (i.e., coma, apnea, cranial nerve dysfunction), opisthotonus, or tense, bulging fontanelle. Open surgical evacuation of the clot is the usual management for the minority of infants with large SDH in any location accompanied by such severe neurologic abnormalities or obstructive hydrocephalus. It has been suggested that when the clinical picture is stable and no deterioration in neurologic function or unmanageable increase in ICP exists, supportive care and serial CT examinations should be utilized in the management of posterior fossa SDH instead of surgical intervention (4). Laboratory testing to rule out sepsis or a bleeding diathesis should be considered with large SDH. The infant should be monitored for the development of hydrocephalus, which can occur in a delayed fashion following SDH. Finally, chronic subdural effusions may occur rarely, and can present weeks to months later with abnormally increased head growth. The outcome for infants with nonsurgical SDH is usually good, provided there is no other significant neurologic injury or disease. The prognosis for normal development is also good for cases in which prompt surgical evacuation of the hematoma is successful and there is no other parenchymal injury.

E. **Epidural hemorrhage (EH).** There are approximately 20 case reports of neonatal EH in the literature. EH appears to be correlated with trauma (e.g., difficult instrumented delivery), and a large cephalohematoma or skull fracture was found in about half the reported cases. Removal or aspiration of the hemorrhage was performed in the majority of cases, and the prognosis was quite good, except when other ICH or parenchymal pathology was present.

II. **Subarachnoid hemorrhage (SAH)**

A. **Etiology and pathogenesis.** Subarachnoid hemorrhage (SAH) is a common form of ICH among newborns. Primary SAH (i.e., SAH not due to extension from ICH in an adjacent compartment) is probably quite frequent but clinically insignificant. In these cases, the SAH may go unrecognized (the true incidence of small SAH remains unknown) because of a lack of clinical signs. Hemorrhagic or xanthochromic cerebrospinal fluid (CSF) may be the only indication of such a hemorrhage, for example, in infants who undergo a CSF exam to rule out sepsis. Small SAH probably results from the normal "trauma" associated with the birth process. The source of bleeding is usually ruptured bridging veins of the subarachnoid space or ruptured small leptomeningeal vessels (This is quite different from SAH in adults, where the source of bleeding is usually arterial and therefore produces a much more emergent clinical syndrome.) SAH should be distinguished from subarachnoid extension of blood from a germinal matrix hemorrhage/intraventricular hemorrhage (GMH/IVH), which occurs most commonly in the preterm infant. SAH may also result from extension of SDH (e.g., particularly in the posterior fossa) or a cerebral contusion (parenchymal hemorrhage). Finally, SAH may be subpial in origin, which often produces a more localized than diffuse hemorrhage.

B. Clinical presentation. As with other forms of ICH, clinical suspicion of SAH may result because of blood loss or neurologic dysfunction. Only rarely is the volume loss large enough to provoke catastrophic results. More often, neurologic signs manifest as seizures, irritability, or other mild alteration of mental status, particularly with SAH or subpial hemorrhage occurring over the cerebral convexities.

C. Diagnosis. Seizures, irritability, lethargy, or focal neurologic signs should prompt investigation to determine whether there is a SAH (or other ICH). Often, babies with small SAHs may have seizures but appear otherwise quite well. The diagnosis is best established with a CT or MRI scan, or by LP to confirm or diagnose a small SAH. CT scans are usually adequate to diagnose SAH, but an MRI may be useful to determine whether there is evidence of any other parenchymal pathology, since SAH may occur in the setting of hypoxia-ischemia or meningoencephalitis. Ultrasonography is not a sensitive technique for identifying a small SAH, and thus is less preferable to CT or MRI.

D. Management and prognosis. Management of SAH usually requires only symptomatic therapy, such as an anticonvulsant for seizures (see Neonatal Seizures) and nasogastric feeds or IV fluids if the infant is too lethargic to feed orally. The vast majority of infants with small SAH do well without recognized sequelae. In rare cases, a very large SAH will result in a catastrophic syndrome with profound depression of mental status, seizures, and/or brainstem signs. In such cases, blood transfusions and cardiovascular support should be provided as needed, and neurosurgical intervention may be required. It is most important to establish whether there is coexisting hypoxia-ischemia or other serious neuropathology that will be the crucial determinant of a poor outcome and thus make neurosurgical intervention unnecessary because such interventions will not improve outcome. Occasionally hydrocephalus will develop after a large SAH, and thus a repeat CT or US should be performed in infants with late-onset bulging fontanelle, lethargy, or abnormal extraocular movements.

III. Intraparenchymal hemorrhage (IPH)

A. Etiology and pathogenesis

1. Primary intracerebral IPH is uncommon in all newborns, while intracerebellar IPH is found in 5 to 10% of autopsy specimens in the premature infant. An intracerebral hemorrhage occurs rarely as a primary event related to rupture of an arteriovenous malformation or aneurysm, or from a coagulation disturbance (e.g., hemophilia, thrombocytopenia), or from an unknown cause. More commonly, cerebral IPH occurs as a secondary event, such as hemorrhage into a region of hypoxic-ischemic brain injury. For example, IPH can occur in a region of arterial distribution infarction [term (T) > preterm (PT)] or occasionally periventricular leukomalacia (PT > T). IPH may also occur as a result of (hemorrhagic) venous infarction, either in relation to a large GMH/IVH (PT > T, see IV), or as a result of sinus venous thrombosis (T > PT). IPH can also occur in infants undergoing extracorporeal membrane oxygenation (ECMO) therapy (as can GMH/IVH). Cerebral IPH can occur secondary to a large ICH in another compartment, such as large IVH, SAH, or SDH, as rarely occurs with significant trauma or coagulation disturbance.

2. **Intracerebellar hemorrhage** occurs more commonly in the PT newborn, and may be missed by routine cranial US (CUS), since the reported incidence is much higher in neuropathological than clinical studies. Intracerebellar IPH may be a primary hemorrhage or result from venous hemorrhagic infarction or from extension of GMH/IVH (PT >T). It is often difficult to distinguish the etiology of such hemorrhages by CUS. Cerebellar IPH rarely occurs as an extension of large SAH/SDH in the posterior fossa related to a trauma (T>PT) (see I).

B. **Clinical presentation.** The presentation of IPH is similar to that of SDH, where the clinical syndrome differs depending on whether the IPH is in the anterior or posterior fossa. In the PT infant, IPH is often clinically silent in either intracranial fossa, unless the hemorrhage is quite large.

   In the term infant, intracerebral hemorrhage typically presents with focal neurologic signs such as seizures, hemiparesis, or gaze preference, along with irritability or depressed level of consciousness. A large cerebellar hemorrhage (+/− SDH/SAH) presents as described in I, and should be managed as for a large posterior fossa SDH.

C. **Diagnosis.** CT or MRI scans provide the best visualization of an IPH, but CUS may be used in the PT infant, or when a rapid bedside imaging study is needed. MRI is superior in demonstrating the extent and age of the hemorrhage, and the presence of any other parenchymal abnormality. In addition, MR angiography may demonstrate a vascular anomaly, lack of flow distal to an arterial embolus, or sinus venous thrombosis. Thus MRI is more likely than CT or US to establish the etiology of the IPH and long-term outcome in the term infant. Finally, an LP should be performed to rule out infection, unless there is significant mass effect or herniation.

D. **Management and prognosis**

   1. The management of IPH is similar to that for SDH and SAH, where most small hemorrhages require symptomatic treatment and support, and only a large IPH with severe neurologic compromise should prompt neurosurgical intervention. It is important to diagnose and treat any coexisting pathology, such as infection or sinus venous thrombosis, as these are more likely to have a significant impact on long-term outcome. A large IPH, especially in association with IVH or SAH/SDH may cause hydrocephalus, and thus head growth and neurologic status should be monitored for days to weeks following IPH.

   2. The prognosis largely relates to location and size of the IPH and gestational age (GA) of the infant. A small IPH may have relatively few or no long-term neurological consequences. A large cerebral IPH may result in a life-long seizure disorder, hemiparesis, feeding difficulties, and cognitive impairments ranging from learning disabilities to occasionally mental retardation, depending on the location. Cerebellar hemorrhage in the term newborn often has a relatively good prognosis, although may result in cerebellar signs of ataxia, hypotonia, tremor, nystagmus, and mild cognitive deficits. A large cerebellar IPH in a preterm newborn may result in severe cognitive and motor impairments, for those infants who survive the newborn period (such infants often die of systemic illness rather than IPH).

IV. **Germinal matrix hemorrhage/intraventricular hemorrhage (GMH/IVH)**

   A. **Etiology and pathogenesis**

   1. **GMH/IVH is principally found in the PT infant,** where the incidence is currently 15 to 20% in infants born at <32 weeks' GA, but is infrequent in the term newborn. The etiology and pathogenesis are different for these two groups of infants. In the term newborn, primary IVH typically originates in the choroid plexus or in association with deep venous sinus thrombosis and thalamic infarction, although IVH may also occur in the small remnant of the subependymal germinal matrix. One study utilizing CT imaging suggested that IVH might occur secondary to venous hemorrhagic infarction in the thalamus in 63% of term infants with clinically significant IVH (5). The pathogenesis of IVH in the term infant is more

likely to be related to trauma or perinatal asphyxia. However, at least 25% of infants have no such identifiable risk factors.

2. **In the PT infant, GMH/IVH originates from the fragile involuting vessels of the subependymal germinal matrix, located in the caudo-thalamic groove.** The pathogenesis of GMH/IVH in the PT infant has been demonstrated to be related to numerous risk factors, which can be divided into intravascular, vascular, and extravascular factors. The intravascular risk factors are probably the most important, and are also the factors most amenable to preventive efforts.

   The intravascular risk factors predisposing to GMH/IVH include ischemia/reperfusion, increases in cerebral blood flow (CBF), fluctuating CBF, or increases in cerebral venous pressure. Ischemia/reperfusion occurs commonly when hypotension due to disease or to iatrogenic intervention is quickly corrected. This commonly occurs shortly after birth, when a premature infant may have hypovolemia or hypotension that is treated with infusion of colloid, normal saline, or hyperosmolar solutions such as sodium bicarbonate. In particular, rapid infusions of such solutions are thought to be particularly likely to contribute to GMH/IVH. Indeed, studies of the beagle puppy model showed that ischemia/reperfusion (hypotension precipitated by blood removal followed by volume infusion) reliably produces GMH/IVH. Other causes of sustained increases in CBF that may contribute to GMH/IVH include pneumothorax, seizures, hypercarbia, anemia, and perhaps hypoglycemia, all of which result in a compensatory increase in CBF. Fluctuating CBF has also been demonstrated to be associated with GMH/IVH in PT infants. In one study, infants with significant fluctuations in CBF velocity by Doppler US were much more likely to develop GMH/IVH than infants with stable patterns of CBF velocity (6). These fluctuations typically occurred in infants breathing out of synchrony with the ventilator, but such fluctuations have also been observed in infants with large patent ductus arteriosus or hypotension, for example. Increases in cerebral venous pressure are also thought to contribute to GMH/IVH. Sources of such increases include ventilatory strategies where intrathoracic pressure is high (e.g., high continuous positive airway pressure), pneumothorax, tracheal suctioning, and both labor and delivery, where fetal head compression likely results in significantly increased venous pressure. Indeed a higher incidence of GMH/IVH is found in PT infants delivered vaginally compared with those delivered via caesarean section, and in those with a longer duration of labor. In all of these intravascular factors related to changes in cerebral arterial and venous blood flow, the role of a **pressure-passive** cerebral circulation is likely to be important. Several studies have shown that PT infants, particularly asphyxiated newborns, have an impaired ability to regulate CBF in response to blood pressure changes (hence "pressure-passive") (7,8). Such impaired autoregulation puts the infant at increased risk of rupture of the fragile germinal matrix vessels in the face of significant increases in cerebral arterial or venous pressure, and particularly when ischemia precedes such increased pressure. Finally, impaired coagulation and platelet dysfunction are also intravascular factors that can contribute to the pathogenesis of GMH/IVH.

   Vascular factors that contribute to GMH/IVH include the fragile nature of the involuting vessels of the germinal matrix. There is no muscularis mucosa and little adventitia in this area of relatively large diameter, thin-walled vessels; all of these factors make the vessels particularly susceptible to rupture. Extravascular risk factors for GMH/IVH include deficient extravascular support and likely excessive fibrinolytic activity.

B. **Pathogenesis of complications of GMH/IVH.** There are two major complications of GMH/IVH, namely periventricular hemorrhagic infarction (PVHI) and posthemorrhagic hydrocephalus (PHH); the pathogenesis of these two complications are discussed here (Table 27.6).

TABLE 27.6.   FACTORS IN THE PATHOGENESIS OF GMH/IVH

Intravascular factors	Ischemia/Reperfusion (e.g., volume infusion after hypotension)
	Fluctuating CBF (e.g., with mechanical ventilation)
	Increase in CBF (e.g., with hypertension, anemia, hypercarbia)
	Increase in cerebral venous pressure (e.g., with high CPAP)
	Platelet dysfunction and coagulation disturbances
Vascular factors	Tenuous, involuting capillaries with large luminal diameter
Extravascular factors	Deficient vascular support
	Excessive fibrinolytic activity

1. The first, **PVHI,** has previously been considered an **extension** of a large IVH. However, careful neuropathological and US studies have shown that the finding of a large, often unilateral or asymmetric echogenic lesion dorsolateral to the lateral ventricle is **not** an extension of the original IVH. Rather, this lesion represents a hemorrhagic venous infarction, which results from obstruction of flow in the terminal vein by the large IVH. Evidence supporting this view includes the observation that PVHI occurs on the side of the larger IVH, and Doppler US studies show markedly decreased or absent flow in the terminal vein on the side of the large IVH (9). Neuropathological studies demonstrate the fan-shaped appearance of a typical hemorrhagic venous infarction in the distribution of the medullary veins that drain into the terminal vein. Furthermore, the ependymal lining of the lateral ventricle between the IVH and the PVHI is often intact, demonstrating that the IVH does not **extend** into the adjacent cerebral parenchyma, but that the **PVHI is a separate lesion.**

2. **Progressive ventricular dilation (PVD)** may occur days to weeks following the onset of GMH/IVH. The pathogenesis likely relates to obliterative arachnoiditis that prevents CSF resorption, and/or obstruction of the aqueduct or the foramina of Luschka or Magendie by particulate clot (10). The pathogenesis of the **brain injury** that results from PHH is probably related in large part to regional hypoxia-ischemia and mechanical distension of the periventricular white matter, based on animal and human studies (11–13). In addition, the presence of non-protein-bound iron in the CSF of infants with PHH may lead to the generation of reactive oxygen species that contribute to the injury of immature oligodendrocytes in the white matter (14). This results in a principally bilateral cerebral white matter injury that bears some similarities with periventricular leukomalacia (PVL) in its neuropathology and long-term outcome (15).

C. **Clinical presentation**
1. **GMH/IVH in the PT newborn is usually a clinically silent syndrome,** and thus recognized only when a routine CUS is performed. However, some infants present in hours to days with decreased levels of consciousness and spontaneous movements, hypotonia, abnormal eye movements, or skew deviation. Rarely, an infant will present with a rapid and severe neurologic deterioration with obtundation or coma, severe hypotonia and lack of spontaneous movements, and generalized tonic posturing that is often thought to be seizure [but does not have an electrographic correlate by electroencephalogram (13)].

2. **The term newborn with IVH typically presents with such signs as seizures, apnea, irritability or lethargy, and a full fontanelle.** It is rare to

find a catastrophic presentation, unless there is another ICH, such as a large SDH or parenchymal hemorrhage.

3. **PHH may develop over days to weeks following IVH,** and may present with increasing head growth (crossing percentiles on the growth chart), bulging fontanelle, splitting of sutures, decreased level of consciousness, impaired upgaze or sunsetting sign, apnea, worsening respiratory status, or feeding difficulties. However, PHH may be relatively asymptomatic in PT newborns, as ICP is often normal in this population, particularly with slowly progressive dilation. Thus serial CUS are critical for diagnosis of PHH in PT infants with known IVH. A recent study of infants with IVH showed that 50% of infants with a birth weight <1500 g will not show ventricular dilation, 25% will develop nonprogressive ventricular dilation (or stable ventriculomegaly), and the remaining 25% will develop PVD (16). The incidence of PVD increases with increasing severity of GMH/IVH; it is uncommon with grades I-II IVH (up to 5 to 12%), but occurs in up to 75% of infants with grade III IVH +/− PVHI. The incidence of PHH increases with younger GA at birth. The ventricular dilation may proceed rapidly (over a few days) or slowly (over weeks). About 40% of infants with PVD will have spontaneous resolution of PVD without any treatment. The remaining 60% will likely require medical and/or surgical therapy (and ~15% of these infants may not survive the newborn period).

D. **Diagnosis**
1. **The diagnosis of GMH/IVH is almost invariably made by real-time portable CUS in the premature infant.** Routine CUS should be performed in infants born at <32 weeks' GA. In addition, CUS may be considered in older infants born at >32 weeks' GA who have risk factors such as perinatal asphyxia or pneumothorax, or who present with abnormal neurological signs as described above. Given that >90% of GMH/IVH occurs in the first 72 hours after birth, the first routine CUS is often performed on the third day of postnatal life. However, in a very sick, very-low-birth-weight infant, consideration should be given to performing a CUS within 24 hours after birth, as a large IVH may be present. The finding of a severe IVH and/or other intracranial pathology (e.g., PVH1) might be an important factor in considering withdrawal of care, or may require early follow-up CUS to determine whether rapidly progressive ventricular dilation develops. We perform routine CUS on or around days 3, 7, 30, and 60 (or just prior to discharge) for infants born at <32 weeks GA (or birth weight <1500 g). Recently, in stable infants in whom the CUS will not change management, we have eliminated the day 3 CUS. Infants with a GMH/IVH may require more frequent CUS to monitor for complications of GMH/IVH such as PHH and PVH I, and for other lesions such as PVL. In addition, any infant who develops abnormal neurologic signs or a significant risk factor for IVH (such as pneumothorax, sepsis, sudden hypotension or volume loss for any reason) should undergo a CUS.

2. **Grading of GMH/IVH is important for determining management and prognosis.** While there is no universally accepted grading system, two grading systems are in wide usage, as outlined in Table 27.7. Grading of the GMH/IVH should be assigned based on the earliest CUS obtained when the IVH itself is of maximal size. Specifically, ventricular dilation that occurs days to weeks following GMH/IVH is not a grade III IVH; it represents either PHH or ventriculomegaly secondary to parenchymal volume loss. Given the variability in grading systems and in CUS interpretation, a detailed description of the CUS findings should be reported. Specifically, the description should include the following:

   a. Presence or absence of blood in the germinal matrix.
   b. Laterality (or bilaterality) of the hemorrhage.
   c. Presence or absence of blood in each ventricle, including volume of blood in relation to ventricle size.

TABLE 27.7. GRADING OF GMH/IVH

Grading System	Severity of GMH/IVH	Description of Findings
Papile (by CT)	I	Isolated GMH (no IVH)
	II	IVH without ventricular dilatation
	III	IVH with ventricular dilatation
	IV	IVH with parenchymal hemorrhage
Volpe (by CUS)	I	GMH with no or minimal IVH (<10% ventricular volume)
	II	IVH occupying 10–50% of ventricular area on parasagittal view
	III	IVH occupying >50% of ventricular area on parasagittal view, usually distends lateral ventricle *(at time of IVH diagnosis)*
	Separate notation	Periventricular echodensity (location and extent)

Source: From refs. 2, 17.

    d. Presence or absence of blood in cerebral parenchyma, with specification of location.
    e. Presence or absence of ventricular dilation, with measurements of ventricles when dilated.
    f. Presence or absence of other any other hemorrhage (e.g., SAH) or parenchymal abnormalities.
  3. In the term newborn, IVH is usually diagnosed when a head CT or CUS is performed because of seizures, apnea, or abnormal mental status. A brain MRI is superior for the demonstration of other lesions that may be associated with IVH in full-term newborns, such as thalamic hemorrhagic infarction, hypoxic-ischemic brain injury, or sinus venous thrombosis.
E. Management and prognosis
  1. Prevention of GMH/IVH should be the primary goal; the decreased incidence of GMH/IVH since the 1980s is likely related to numerous improvements in maternal and neonatal care. Although antenatal administration of **glucocorticoids** has clearly been shown to decrease the incidence of GMH/IVH, antenatal phenobarbital, vitamin K, and magnesium sulfate have not been conclusively demonstrated to lead to prevention of GMH/IVH. Postnatal prevention of GMH/IVH should be directed toward minimizing risk factors outlined above in IV.A and B. In particular, infusions of colloid or hyperosmolar solutions should be given slowly, and all efforts should be directed to avoiding hypotension and large fluctuations or sustained increases in arterial blood pressure or cerebral venous pressure. Elimination of CBF fluctuation related to mechanical ventilation may be achieved by administration of sedative or paralytic medication. This recommendation is based on the randomized study showed a marked reduction in the incidence of GMH/IVH in premature infants with fluctuating CBF who were paralyzed for the first 72 hours after birth (1 of 14 with IVH in the first 72 hours, 4 later onset, none severe), compared with infants who were not paralyzed (100% IVH) (18).
  2. Management of GMH/IVH in the premature newborn largely consists of supportive care of the infant, and monitoring for and treatment of complications of GMH/IVH. A GMH/IVH can increase in size, and thus appropriate early care may prevent enlargement of the IVH. Supportive care should be directed toward maintaining stable cerebral perfusion by main-

taining normal blood pressure and circulating volume. Transfusions of packed red blood cells may be required in cases of large IVH to restore normal blood volume and hematocrit. Thrombocytopenia or coagulation disturbances should be corrected when possible.

3. **Management of IVH in the term newborn is directed at supportive care of the infant and treatment of seizures during the acute phase.** However, as symptomatic IVH in this group of newborns is frequently large, PHH develops in many infants, and **may require serial LPs, and/or eventual ventriculoperitoneal (VP) shunt placement in up to 50% of such infants.** Outcome in this group of infants likely relates to factors other than IVH alone, as uncomplicated IVH has a good prognosis. Infants with a history of trauma or perinatal asphyxia, or with neuroimaging evidence of thalamic hemorrhagic infarction or hypoxic-ischemic brain injury are at much higher risk for significant cognitive and/or motor deficits.

4. **Management of PHH consists of careful monitoring of ventricle size by serial CUS, and appropriate intervention to reduce CSF accumulation, such as serial lumbar punctures (LPs), medications to reduce CSF production, and surgical interventions.** The goal of therapy is to alleviate abnormal neurologic signs and prevent secondary brain injury. There are significant animal data and some human data to suggest that earlier treatment of PHH improves neurologic outcome (19–22).

   a. In cases of **slowly progressive PHH** (over weeks), close monitoring of clinical status and ventricle size (by CUS) may be sufficient. Up to two-thirds of such cases will have spontaneous resolution of PHH without intervention or will prove to have stable ventriculomegaly. **It is critical to determine by serial CUS which infants have progressive dilation, versus those infants who have static ventriculomegaly due to other causes (such as atrophy due to PVL).**

   b. When serial CUS show persistent PVD, intervention is usually required, particularly if the infant is symptomatic. We typically begin therapy when progressive dilation persists for about 2 weeks, although the rate of ventricular dilation and size of ventricles will need to be assessed in each case to decide whether therapy should be initiated sooner or later. Therapy should begin with LPs performed every 1 to 3 days, depending on the rate of ventricular dilation and the effectiveness of CSF removal. The opening pressure should be measured whenever possible. A CUS performed before and after removal of 10–15 ml of CSF per kg body weight is often helpful in establishing the diagnosis of PHH and determining the effect of CSF removal in decreasing ventricle size. A recently published preliminary trial of continuous drainage, irrigation, and fibrinolytic therapy in 24 infants with PHH showed an apparent reduction in shunt surgery, mortality, and disability compared with historical controls. However, this very intensive high-risk therapy should be tested in larger trials before it is widely applied as a routine therapy for the care of the newborn with PHH (32)

   c. **Measurement of the resistive index (RI) can be helpful in guiding management of PHH.** The RI is a measure of resistance to blood flow, and may indicate when intracranial compliance is compromised sufficiently to diminish CBF and thus intervention is needed to prevent secondary brain injury. RI is measured by Doppler US, usually in the anterior cerebral artery.

$$RI = \frac{(\text{systolic} - \text{diastolic})}{\text{systolic blood flow velocity}}$$

A significant rise in RI from baseline RI values when gentle fontanelle compression is applied may indicate hemodynamic compromise and the need to remove CSF (we typically treat for a >30% increase in RI with compression compared to baseline RI, or a baseline RI >0.9) (23).

d. A combination of the infant's clinical status, ventricular size and shape by serial CUS, measurement of ICP by manometry, RI by Doppler US, and response to CSF removal should be used to determine **the need for and frequency of LPs** (or other interventions) to reduce CSF volume.

e. **Acetazolamide and furosemide** are carbonic anhydrase inhibitors **that can be used to decrease CSF production.** However, their combined use often produces nephrocalcinosis, and may be associated with a worse neurologic outcome (24,25). The use of acetazolamide alone may be considered, since it was shown to be effective in three of five infants in one small study (26). Acetazolamide could be used in cases where intermittent CSF removal is inadequate, or to reduce the frequency of intermittent CSF removal. It should be noted that the safety and efficacy of acetazolamide monotherapy for PHH has not been demonstrated in large studies.

Medications that decrease CSF production can also help to correct the imbalance between inflow and outflow. Such drugs include furosemide (Lasix), carbonic anhydrase inhibitors (e.g., acetazolamide [Diamox]), and osmotic agents (e.g., glycerol). Acetazolamide directly reduces CSF production, and its effects are augmented by the addition of furosemide. The combination of these diuretics can result in almost complete cessation of CSF production. Osmotic agents increase serum osmolality, which, in turn, decreases CSF production.

(1) Logistics. Pharmacologic therapy used as an adjunct to serial LPs may increase the interval necessary between spinal taps in the initial therapy of PHH. Pharmacotherapy by itself is usually ineffective in the most severe cases of PHH. Accepted diuretic therapy includes acetazolamide (25 to 150 mg/kg per day, given every 6 hours, administered intravenously or orally, starting dose of 25 mg/kg per day increased by 25 mg/kg per day to a maximum of 150 mg/kg per day); furosemide (1 to 3 mg/kg per day, given every 6 to 12 hours, administered intravenously or orally, starting dose of 1 mg/kg per day); or glycerol (4 to 8 mg/kg per day, given every 6 hours). Because of the dramatic osmotic changes caused by glycerol, it is currently only used in crises.

Use of these agents requires careful monitoring for resultant electrolyte imbalances, dehydration, and metabolic acidosis. When furosemide is administered, hypocloremia, hypercalciuria, and nephrocalcinosis must specifically be followed. Newborns and infants who receive long-term acetazolamide therapy often need replacement of sodium, potassium, and bicarbonate, most conveniently provided in the form of Polycitra (ALZA) (Na citrate, K citrate, and citric acid 2 mEq/mL based on the citrate). The starting dose is 1 to 3 mEq/kg per day divided into 3 or 4 doses. If K is not needed then Bicitra (ALZA) (Na citrate and citric acid 1 mEq Na and the equivalent of 1 mEq of bicarbonate (HCO_3)/ml) is used. The starting dose is 2 to 4 mEq/kg per day divided into 3 to 4 doses. The goal is to keep the serum HCO_3^- over 10 mEq/mL.

The lowest effective dose of acetazolamide and furosemide should be used because of concerns about potentially toxic effects of high doses of acetazolamide on developing myelin as well as the increased risk of nephrocalcinosis in the setting of combined acetazolamide and furosemide therapy. Currently, the combination of acetazolamide and furosemide provides the best combination of efficacy and safety and has gained favor as the agent of choice in the pharmacotherapy of PHH.

(2) Benefits. Pharmacotherapy is not invasive and therefore can generally be tolerated as a prolonged treatment course until the patient either recovers spontaneously or is large enough for a ventricularperitoneal (VP) shunt. Often, these patients have coexisting chronic lung disease; therefore, the use of diuretics can play an additional role in minimizing interstitial pulmonary fluid.

(3) Risks. Because of the effect of these diuretic agents on electrolyte balance, Na^+, K^+, HCO_3^-, and Ca^{++} need to be monitored carefully with serial blood tests. Replacement therapy is often needed. Other side effects include metabolic acidosis, dehydration, gastrointestinal upset, and hypercalciuria with a risk of nephrocalcinosis. Because phlebotomy is often difficult in these tiny patients and total blood volume is small with a tendency toward physiologic nadir of the hematocrit coinciding with progression of PHH, the monitoring of electrolytes in these newborns and infants is not a trivial consideration.

Newborns and infants receiving prolonged furosemide therapy must be monitored for nephrocalcinosis. Serial renal US scans should be performed to monitor for calcifications. The urine Ca^{++}: Cr ratios should be intermittently measured, with a ratio of greater than 0.21 suggesting a degree of hypercalciuria that might promote nephrocalcinosis. The diagnosis of hypercaliuria and nephrocalcinosis, made by either renal ultrasound scan or Ca^{++}: Cr ratio, requires discontinuation of diuretic therapy. Nephrocalcinosis is a reversible condition; therefore, diuretic therapy may possibly be reinstituted at a decreased dose (27).

f. If the foregoing medical therapy does not successfully reduce ventricle size, and/or PHH is rapidly progressive, surgical intervention is indicated. Surgical intervention will be required if LPs are unsuccessful (e.g., when there is a lack of communication between fourth ventricle and spinal fluid, hence little CSF can be drained). **A ventriculosubgaleal shunt (VSG), ventricular access device (reservoir), or external ventricular drain** should be placed. A VSG may be sufficient for adequate CSF drainage into the subgaleal space, although often only for a matter of days to weeks (28). Alternatively, CSF may be removed intermittently by a needle placed in the reservoir of the VSG or access device (e.g., every 1 to 3 days, as in the case of serial LPs). External ventricular drains are less favored because of the high incidence of infection, especially if the catheter is not tunneled subcutaneously.

g. If PHH has persisted for >4 weeks despite adequate therapy with intermittent CSF removal and/or medication, **a permanent shunt is usually required.** If the infant weighs <1500 grams, a VSG or ventricular access device may be preferable. A permanent ventriculo-peritoneal (VP) shunt can be placed in infants weighing >1500 to 2000 g.

h. Rarely (5%), PHH will recur weeks to months later despite apparent resolution in the neonatal period. Monitoring of head growth and fontanelle should continue after discharge home.

5. **The prognosis for infants with GMH/IVH varies considerably depending on the severity of IVH and the presence of complications and associated brain lesions, the birth weight/GA, and other significant illnesses.** PT infants with uncomplicated grade I to II IVH usually have a similar prognosis to infants of the same GA without IVH. These infants may still have school difficulties that are found in up to 25 to 50% of very-low-birth-weight infants. These subtle cognitive impairments may relate more to coexisting cerebral white matter injury (i.e., PVL), which has many of the same risk factors as GMH/IVH. Infants with GMH/IVH and stable ventriculomegaly are at increased risk of long-term neurologic impairments, likely because ventriculomegaly is a result of white matter injury. Infants with PVH I and PHH are at much higher risk of neurologic impairments. Infants with PHH may manifest spastic diparesis and cognitive impairments due to bilateral periventricular white matter injury. Infants with a localized, unilateral PVHI may develop a spastic hemiparesis affecting the arm and leg with minimal or mild cognitive impairments. Quadriparesis and significant cognitive deficits (including mental

retardation) are more likely if the PVHI is very extensive or bilateral, or if there is also co-existing PVL (29). Recent studies show that MRI is superior to CUS in improving detection, classification and hence prognosis of GMH/ IVH, PVHI, PVL and the periventricular white matter injury associated with PHH (30–32).

References

1. Volpe J.J. Intracranial hemorrhage: Subdural, primary subarachnoid, intracerebellar, intraventricular (term infant), and miscellaneous. In: *Neurology of the Newborn.* 2001. Philadelphia: Saunders, p. 397.
2. Volpe J.J. Intracranial hemorrhage: Germinal matrix-intraventricular hemorrhage of the premature infant. In: *Neurology of the Newborn.* 2001. Philadelphia: Saunders, p. 428.
3. Chamnanvanakij S., et al. Subdural hematoma in term infants. *Pediatr Neurol* 2002;26:301.
4. Perrin R.G., et al. Management and outcomes of posterior fossa subdural hematomas in neonates. *Neurosurgery* 1997;40:1190; discussion 1199.
5. Roland E.H., et al. Thalamic hemorrhage with intraventricular hemorrhage in the full-term newborn. *Pediatrics* 1990;85:737.
6. Perlman J.M., et al. Fluctuating cerebral blood-flow velocity in respiratory-distress syndrome. Relation to the development of intraventricular hemorrhage. *N Engl J Med* 1983;309:204.
7. Lou H., et al. Impaired autoregulation of cerebral blood flow in the distressed newborn infant. *J Pediatr* 1979;94:118.
8. Pryds O., et al. Heterogeneity of cerebral vasoreactivity in preterm infants supported by mechanical ventilation. *J Pediatr* 1989;115:638.
9. Taylor G.A. Effect of germinal matrix hemorrhage on terminal vein position and patency. *Pediatr Radiol* 1996;25 Suppl 1:S37.
10. Larroche J.C. Post-haemorrhagic hydrocephalus in infancy. Anatomical study. *Biol Neonate* 1972;20:287.
11. da Silva M., et al. High-energy phosphate metabolism in a neonatal model of hydrocephalus before and after shunting. *J Neurosurg* 1994;81:544.
12. da Silva, M.C., et al. Reduced local cerebral blood flow in periventricular white matter in experimental neonatal hydrocephalus-restoration with CSF shunting. *J Cereb Blood Flow Metab* 1995;15:1057.
13. Del Bigio M.R., et al. Cell death, axonal damage, and cell birth in the immature rat brain following induction of hydrocephalus. *Exp Neurol* 1998;154:157.
14. Savman K., et al. Non-protein-bound iron is elevated in cerebrospinal fluid from preterm infants with posthemorrhagic ventricular dilatation. *Pediatr Res* 2001;49:208.
15. Fukumizu M., et al. Neonatal posthemorrhagic hydrocephalus: Neuropathologic and immunohistochemical studies. *Pediatr Neurol* 1995;13:230.
16. Murphy B.P., et al. Posthaemorrhagic ventricular dilatation in the premature infant: natural history and predictors of outcome. *Arch Dis Child Fetal Neonatal.* 2002;Ed 87:F37.
17. Papile L.A., et al. Incidence and evolution of subependymal and intraventricular hemorrhage: a study of infants with birth weights less than 1500 gm. *J Pediatr* 1978;92:529.
18. Perlman J.M., et al. Reduction in intraventricular hemorrhage by elimination of fluctuating cerebral blood-flow velocity in preterm infants with respiratory distress syndrome. *N Engl J Med* 1985;312:1353.
19. Del Bigio M.R., et al. Myelination delay in the cerebral white matter of immature rats with kaolin-induced hydrocephalus is reversible. *J Neuropathol Exp Neurol* 1997;56:1053.
20. del Bigio M.R., et al. Magnetic resonance imaging and behavioral analysis of immature rats with kaolin-induced hydrocephalus: Pre- and postshunting observations. *Exp Neurol* 1997;148:256.
21. Ehle A., et al. Visual evoked potentials in infants with hydrocephalus. *Neurology* 1979;29:1541.

22. de Vries L.S., et al. Early versus late treatment of posthaemorrhagic ventricular dilatation: results of a retrospective study from five neonatal intensive care units in The Netherlands. *Acta Paediatr* 2002;91:212.
23. Whitelaw A., Pople I., Cherian S., et al. 2003 Phase 1 trial of prevention of hydrocephalus after intraventricular hemorrhage in newborn infants by drainage, irrigation, and fibrinolytic therapy. *Pediatrics* 111:759–765.
24. Taylor G.A., et al. Neonatal hydrocephalus: Hemodynamic response to fontanelle compression—correlation with intracranial pressure and need for shunt placement. *Radiology* 1996;201:685.
25. International PHVD Drug Trial Group 1998 International randomised controlled trial of acetazolamide and furosemide in posthaemorrhagic ventricular dilatation in infancy. *Lancet* 1998;352:433.
26. Kennedy C.R., et al. Randomized, controlled trial of acetazolamide and furosemide in posthemorrhagic ventricular dilation in infancy: follow-up at 1 year. *Pediatrics* 2001;108:597.
27. Mercuri E., et al. Acetazolamide without frusemide in the treatment of posthaemorrhagic hydrocephalus. *Acta Paediatr* 1994;83:1319.
28. Hansen A.R., et al. Medical management of neonatal post-hemorrhagic hydrocephalus. *Neurosurg Clin North Am* 1998;9:85
29. Rahman S., et al. Ventriculosubgaleal shunt: a treatment option for progressive posthemorrhagic hydrocephalus. *Child's Nerv Syst* 1995;11: 650. [see comments]
30. Guzzetta F., et al. Periventricular intraparenchymal echodensities in the premature newborn: critical determinant of neurologic outcome. *Pediatrics* 1986;78:995.
31. De Vries L.S., et al. Asymmetrical myelination of the posterior limb of the internal capsule in infants with periventricular haemorrhagic infarction: An early predictor of hemiplegia. *Neuropediatrics* 1999;30:314.
32. Valkama A.M., et al. Magnetic resonance imaging at term and neuromotor outcome in preterm infants. *Acta Paediatr* 2000;89:348. [see comments]
33. de Vries L.S., et al. Unilateral parenchymal haemorrhagic infarction in the preterm infant. *Eur J Paediatr Neurol* 2001;5:139.

PERINATAL ASPHYXIA

Sanjay Aurora and Evan Y. Snyder

I. **Definition.** Perinatal asphyxia is an insult to the fetus or newborn due to a lack of oxygen (hypoxia) and/or a lack of perfusion (ischemia) to various organs of sufficient magnitude and duration to produce more than fleeting functional and/or biochemical changes. It is associated with tissue lactic acidosis. If accompanied by hypoventilation, it also may be associated with hypercapnia. The effects of hypoxia and ischemia may not be identical, but they are difficult to separate clinically. Both factors probably contribute to asphyxial injury. Normal blood gas values in term newborns are shown in Table 27.8.

A. Assessment and medical record documentation of infants with potential perinatally acquired brain injury is necessary. Precise documentation is critical when caring for an infant whose perinatal circumstances place the infant at risk for brain injury.

Definitions of specific terms:

1. **Perinatal hypoxia, ischemia, asphyxia.** These terms describe, respectively, lack of oxygen, blood flow, and gas exchange to the fetus or newborn. This term should be reserved for circumstances when there is rigorous pre-, peri-, and postnatal data to support its use.

2. **Neonatal depression.** This is a general term that describes the condition of the infant in the immediate postnatal period (interpreted to be approximately the first hour after birth) without making an association with

TABLE 27.8. NORMAL BLOOD GAS VALUES IN TERM NEWBORNS

	At Birth			At Age		
	Maternal Artery	Umbilical Vein	Umbilical Artery	10 Minutes	30 to 60 Minutes (Umbilical Artery)	5 Hours
PO_2	95	27.5	16	50	54	74
CO_2	32	39	49	46	38	35
pH*	7.4	7.32	7.24	7.21	7.29	7.34

PO_2 = partial pressure of oxygen; PCO_2 = partial pressure of carbon dioxide.
*A scalp pH in labor of 7.25 or above is considered normal (see Chaps. 1, 4).

prenatal condition or postnatal physical exam, laboratory tests, imaging studies, or EEGs. This is the preferred term unless or until there is objective scientific evidence to support the use of other diagnoses.

3. **Encephalopathy.** This is a clinical—not an etiologic—term that describes an altered level of consciousness at the time of the exam. It includes such reversible conditions as hypoglycemia and exposure to maternal medications.

4. **Hypoxic ischemic encephalopathy (HIE).** This term describes encephalopathy as defined earlier with objective data to support a hypoxic/ischemic mechanism.

5. **Hypoxic ischemic brain injury.** This describes brain injury due to exposure to hypoxia and/or ischemia as evidenced by biochemical [creatine kinase brain fraction (CK-BB)], electrophysiologic (EEG), by neuroimaging (MRI, CT scan), or pathologic (postmortem examination) means.

II. **Incidence.** The incidence of perinatal asphyxia is about 1.0 to 1.5% of live births in most centers and is inversely related to gestational age and birth weight, lowering considerably in later gestation (1,3,20). It occurs in 0.5% of live born infants more than 36 weeks' gestational age and accounts for 20% of perinatal deaths (or as high as 50% of deaths if stillborns are included). The incidence is higher in term infants of diabetic or toxemic mothers; these factors correlate less well in preterm infants. In both preterm and term infants, intrauterine growth retardation (IUGR) and breech presentation are associated with an increased incidence of asphyxia. Postmature infants are also at risk.

III. **Pathophysiology and etiology of asphyxia.** In term neonates, 90% of asphyxial insults occur in the antepartum or intrapartum periods as a result of placental insufficiency, resulting in an inability to provide oxygen (O_2) to and remove carbon dioxide (CO_2) and H^+ from the fetus. The remainder are postpartum, usually secondary to pulmonary, cardiovascular, or neurologic abnormalities. The proportion of postpartum events is higher in premature neonates, especially the extremely low-birth-weight infant (25,27).

During **normal labor,** uterine contractions and some degree of cord compression result in reduced blood flow to the placenta, and hence decreased O_2 delivery to the fetus. Because there is a concomitant increase in O_2 consumption by both mother and fetus, fetal O_2 saturation falls. Maternal dehydration and maternal alkalosis from hyperventilation may further reduce placental blood flow; maternal hypoventilation may also contribute to decreased maternal and fetal O_2 saturation. These normal events cause most babies to be born with little O_2 reserve. Newborns, however, including their central nervous systems (CNS), are fairly resistant to asphyxic damage. Late decelerations are uncommon until the partial pressure of O_2 (PO_2) is less than 20 mm Hg (2). Furthermore, partial asphyxia under an hour is unlikely to result in an **encephalopathy,** defined simply as an altered level of consciousness without etiological implications (3,25).

In addition to the normal factors mentioned, any process that (1) impairs maternal oxygenation, (2) decreases blood flow from the mother to the placenta or from the placenta to the fetus, (3) impairs gas exchange across the placenta or at the fetal tissue, or (4) increases fetal O_2 requirement will exacerbate perinatal asphyxia. Such factors include: maternal hypertension (either chronic or preeclampsic); maternal vascular disease; maternal diabetes; maternal drug use; maternal hypoxia from pulmonary, cardiac, or neurologic disease; maternal hypotension; maternal infection; placental infarction or fibrosis; placental abruption; cord accidents (prolapse, entanglement, true knot, compression); abnormalities of umbilical vessels; fetal anemia; fetal or placental hydrops; fetal infection; intrauterine growth retardation; and postmaturity. In the presence of a hypoxic-ischemic challenge to the fetus, reflexes are initiated, causing shunting of blood to the brain, heart, and adrenals and away from the lungs, gut, liver, kidneys, spleen, bone, skeletal muscle, and skin ("diving reflex"). In mild hypoxia, there is a decreased heart rate, slight increase in blood pressure (BP) to maintain cerebral perfusion, increased central venous pressure (CVP), and little change in cardiac output. As asphyxia progresses with severe hypoxia and acidosis, there is a decreased heart rate, decreased cardiac output, and initially increased then falling BP as oxidative phosphorylation fails and energy reserves become depleted. During asphyxia, anaerobic metabolism produces lactic acid, which, because of poor perfusion, remains in local tissues. Systemic acidosis may actually be mild until perfusion is restored and these local acid stores are mobilized.

A. **Perinatal assessment of risk** includes awareness of preexisting maternal or fetal problems and assessment of changing placental and fetal conditions by ultrasound, biophysical profile (BPP), nonstress tests (NSTs), and urinary estriol measurements (see Chap. 1, Fetal Assessment and Prenatal Diagnosis).

B. **Perinatal management of high-risk pregnancies** consists of fetal heart monitoring, evaluation of fetal scalp pH, when indicated, and awareness of the progress of labor and the presence of meconium. While the value of any one of these parameters is uncertain, and even controversial (4), the presence of a constellation of abnormal findings may alert and allow proactive mobilization of the perinatal team for a newborn that may potentially require immediate intervention. The pH is considered a better determinant of fetal oxygenation than PO_2; if a hypoxic-ischemic insult occurs intermittently, the PO_2 may improve transiently, whereas pH will fall progressively; pH less than 7.0 and a base deficit more than 12 (5) is good evidence of substantial and prolonged intrauterine asphyxia. (It should be remembered, however, that scalp and cord pH values may be profoundly affected by maternal acid–base status.). Fetal scalp blood lactate has been found to be technically easier and more reliable than the pH by some, but has not gained widespread acceptance (6). Abnormalities of fetal heart rate (FHR) and rhythm plus heavy meconium staining may provide possible supporting evidence of asphyxia but provide no information concerning the severity or duration of the asphyxia. The decision to perform a cesarean section, to augment a vaginal delivery, or to allow labor to progress is the most difficult obstetric decision. Each medical center should have guidelines for intervention in cases of suspected fetal distress (see Chap. 1, Fetal Assessment and Prenatal Diagnosis).

IV. **Delivery room management** (see Chaps 4, 17, and 24). Asphyxiated infants usually present in the delivery room as having depressed cardiovascular-respiratory responsiveness, diminished neurological reaction to stimuli, and decreased muscle tone, all items tallied in and contributing to the Apgar score. This type of clinical presentation is designated nonspecifically as "Neonatal Depression" pending a more definitive assessment of etiology and diagnosis. An Apgar score of 3 or less prolonged for more than 5 minutes is generally regarded as consistent with asphyxia. However, a low Apgar score may not indicate asphyxia in preterm or small-for-gestational-age (SGA) infants (see Chap. 4), who are more likely to be hypotonic, have cyanotic extremities, and have diminished responsiveness; a score of 6 to 7 may be maximal for a "normal" preterm infant. Infants below 30 weeks' gestation often have an Apgar score of 2 to

3 without asphyxia. Low Apgar scores may be present in *non*asphyxiated infants with (1) depression from maternal anesthesia or analgesics; (2) trauma; (3) metabolic or infectious insults; (4) neuromuscular disorders; or (5) CNS, cardiac, or pulmonary malformations. Further, a low Apgar score, even when a marker of a depressed infant, does not indicate the mechanism for the depression, duration, or severity of the specific insult, or the adaptive response of the fetus. A high Apgar score (>6 by 5 minutes), however, speaks compellingly against substantial peripartum asphyxia.

V. Postnatal management of asphyxia

    A. The **differential diagnosis of acute asphyxia** in a newborn includes: the effect of maternal drugs or anesthesia; acute blood loss; acute intracranial bleeding; CNS malformation; neuromuscular disease; cardiopulmonary disease; mechanical impediments to ventilation (airway obstruction, pneumothorax, hydrops, pleural effusion, ascites, diaphragmatic hernia); and infection (including septic shock and hypotension). These problems may be the cause of asphyxia or merely coincident with it. A common presentation is the postmature infant with asphyxia, meconium aspiration, persistent pulmonary hypertension, pneumothorax, and birth trauma. Another common presentation is the premature infant with asphyxia, hyaline membrane disease, and an intracranial bleed. Intrauterine ischemia, early in gestation, may present in the newborn as a hypoplastic organ (e.g., lung, gut) or extremity (e.g., sirenomelia), as hydranencephaly, or as a more subtle congenital abnormality of neurocytoarchitecture.

    B. Target organs of perinatal asphyxia are the brain, heart, lungs, kidneys, liver, bowel, and bone marrow. In a study of asphyxiated newborns (7), 34% had no evidence of organ injury, 23% had an abnormality confined to one organ, 34% involved two organs, and 9% had three affected organs. The most frequent abnormalities involved the kidney (50%), followed by the CNS (28%), cardiovascular system (25%), and pulmonary (23%) system. Often, asphyxiated infants will succumb to dysfunctions of organs other than the CNS [e.g., persistent fetal circulation or persistent pulmonary hypertension of the newborn (PPHN)] while showing minimal evidence of hypoxic-ischemic brain injury. In such instances, the brain is spared at the expense of cardiac output to the affected organ. The degree of asphyxia required to cause severe permanent neurologic impairment is close to that which causes death from multisystem failure. However other studies looking at higher cutoffs of scalp pH (< 7.2) and Apgar scores (<7 at 5 minutes) to identify asphyxiated newborns, have reported isolated mild cerebral involvement in 20% of their neonates, with minimal motor deficit at 1 year (8).

      1. Hypoxic-ischemic brain injury

        a. Pathophysiology. Hypoxic-ischemic brain injury (7,8,25) is the most important consequence of perinatal asphyxia. Brief **hypoxia** impairs cerebral oxidative metabolism leading to an increase in lactate, a fall in pH, and given the inefficiency of anaerobic glycolysis to generate adenosine triphosphate (ATP), a decrease in glycogen, high-energy phosphate compounds (first phosphocreatine, then ATP) (9). The hypoxic brain, therefore, increases its glucose utilization. Vascular dilation, caused by hypoxia, increases glucose availability for anaerobic glycolysis, but this leads to increased local lactic acid production. The worsening acidosis is ultimately associated with decreased glycolysis, loss of cerebrovascular autoregulation, and diminished cardiac function, which causes local **ischemia** and decreased glucose delivery to the very tissue that has increased its substrate utilization. Local glucose stores therefore become depleted, energy reserves fall further, and accumulated lactic acid remains unremoved. During prolonged hypoxia, cardiac output falls, cerebral blood flow (CBF) is compromised, and a combined **hypoxic-ischemic insult** produces a secondary failure of oxidative phosphorylation and ATP production, that occurs in the first 48 hours after the initiating insult (9). Such energy failure impairs ion pumps with accumulation of Na^+, Cl^-, H_2O, and Ca^{2+} intracellularly and K^+ and excitatory amino acid neurotransmitters (e.g., glutamate, aspartate) extracellularly. The nature of asphyxial damage at the cellular level is presently the subject of intense investigation. Current theories implicate both an apoptotic and a necrotic cell death, dependent upon the nature of injury (chronic vs. acute) and both the location and developmental stage of the affected parenchyma (10,25). **Excitotoxic amino acids,** through action at ionotropic glutamate receptors [like the N-methyl-D-aspartate (NMDA) receptor], open ion channels allowing Na+ and Ca^{2+} to enter a cell, inducing **immediate** neuronal death from the osmolar load. Furthermore, these excitotoxins, by means of direct activation of the NMDA channel (mediated by the phosphoinositol second messenger system) and/or activation of voltage-dependent Ca^{2+} channels, provoke excessive Ca^{2+} influx. This, in turn, leads to a **delayed** form of neuronal death by: (1) activation of undesirable enzyme and second messenger systems (e.g., Ca^{2+}-dependent lipases and proteases); (2) perturbation of mitochondrial respiratory electron chain transport; (3) generation of free radicals and leukotrienes; (4) generation of NO via NO synthase; and (5) depletion of energy stores. Reperfusion of previously ischemic tissue may also promote the formation of excess oxygen-free radicals (e.g., superoxide ion, hydrogen peroxide, hydroxyl radical, singlet oxygen), which, when they overwhelm endogenous scavenger mechanisms, may damage cellular lipids, proteins, and nucleic acids and the blood-brain barrier. Reperfusion also brings with it neutrophils, which along with activated microglia release injurious cytokines [like interleukin 1 (IL-1 β) and tumor necrosis factor-α (TNF-α)]. Grossly, the following lesions may be seen after moderate or severe asphyxia:

(1) **Focal or multifocal cortical necrosis** (occasionally with cerebral edema) with resultant **cystic encephalomalacia** and/or **ulegyria** (attenuation of depths of sulci), due to loss of perfusion in one or several vascular beds (usually left middle cerebral artery) and affecting all cellular elements.

(2) **Watershed infarcts** in boundary zones between cerebral arteries (particularly following severe hypotension). Examples of this include **periventricular leukomalacia [PVL]** in the preterm infant, which reflects poor perfusion of the vulnerable periventricular border zones in the centrum semiovale and produces predominantly white matter injury; bilateral parasagittal cortical and subcortical white matter injury of the term infant; and injury to parietooccipital cortex.

(3) **Selective neuronal necrosis** is the most common type of injury. This injury occurs at specific sites to specific cell types (neurons > glia) [e.g., CA1 region of the hippocampus, Purkinje cells of the cerebellum (term neonates), internal granule cells of the cerebellum (premature neonates) and brain stem nuclei].

(4) **Necrosis of thalamic nuclei and basal ganglia (status marmoratus**), a subtype of selective neuronal necrosis.

The precise pathologic pattern seen in any case is not predictable. However, the longer the asphyxia, the more extensive is the pathology. Insults due to **prolonged partial episodes of asphyxia** (e.g., from placental abruption) seem to cause diffuse cerebral (especially cortical) necrosis, while **acute total asphyxia** (e.g., from cord prolapse) seems to spare the cortex and affect primarily the brainstem, thalamus, and basal ganglia. In the former instance, seizures and paresis might be expected. In the latter instance, one might see disturbances of consciousness, respiration, heart rate, BP, and temperature control; disorders of tone and reflexes; and cranial nerve palsies. Most cases, however, represent a combination of the two patterns: partial prolonged asphyxia followed by a terminal acute asphyxial event. If diffuse cerebral necrosis and subsequent swelling is severe, increased intracranial pressure (ICP) could theoretically compromise CBF with further damage to the thalamus and brainstem. Recent data, however, indicate that swelling is an effect from prior, rather than a cause of subsequent, neural damage (12) [see V.B.1.c.(7)].

b. The **syndrome of hypoxic-ischemic encephalopathy (HIE)** (7,8,11,25) has **a spectrum of clinical manifestations** from mild to severe. In its most dramatic form, the initial phase lasts about 12 hours after the insult and consists of signs of cerebral dysfunction. The infants are stuporous or comatose, have periodic breathing or irregular respiratory effort (a reflection of bihemispheric dysfunction), are hypotonic, and have lost most complex reflexes (Moro, suck, etc.). They may have roving eye movements while the papillary responses are intact. Subtle, tonic, or multifocal-clonic seizures occur 6 to 24 hours after the insult in 50% of moderately-to-severely asphyxiated infants. Between 12 and 24 hours there may be apnea requiring respiratory support, reflecting brainstem dysfunction. Severely affected infants have a progressive deterioration in CNS function over 24 to 72 hours following the insult, with coma, prolonged apnea, and further brainstem dysfunction (e.g., abnormalities of papillary reactivity, loss of oculomotor and caloric responses, loss of bulbar function). "Brain death" (see d) may ensue between 24 and 72 hours later. In the most severely affected infants, for whom the incidence of death or significant permanent neurologic sequelae is greatest, other organ systems inevitably also display evidence of asphyxial damage. The most striking reduction in blood flow, due to shunting of cardiac output to vital organs, involves the kidneys, particularly the proximal tubule, resulting in acute tubular necrosis (ATN) (see Chap. 31). In fact, persistent oliguria (<1 mL/kg per hour for the first 36 hours) is significantly associated with severe HIE and a poor outcome (90% of cases). This suggests that when the asphyxic insult is severe enough to manifest as persistent oliguria, it is likely the brain also has suffered ischemic injury. As previously noted, **the degree of asphyxia required to cause permanent neurologic impairment is close to that which causes death from multisystem failure.** We also use the **Sarnat clinical stages** to estimate the severity of asphyxial insult to infants more than 36 weeks' gestational age on an individual basis at the bedside (Table 27.9). The sequential appearance and resolution of various transitory clinical signs and their duration over the first 2 postnatal weeks not only suggest the extent and permanence of neurologic impairment but also define clinical categories that have proved fairly accurate for early assessment of prognosis in neonates with HIE (11) (e.g., prognosis is good if a neonate does not progress to and/or remain in stage 3 and if total duration of stage 2 is less than 5 days) (see VI). Electrodiagnostic tests such as **electroencephalography (EEG)** and **evoked potentials**, in conjunction with these clinical signs, may assist in evaluating and classifying the severity of the damage (e.g., seizure foci, or even more significantly, interictal and/or background activity—suppressed?, normal?) [see V.B.1.c.(7) and VI.C].). **Ultrasonic examination** of the brain may reveal hemorrhage or periventricular changes (useful in preterm infants) and, less well, the extent of edema (midline shift, ventricular compression). **Cranial computed tomography (CT)** is more useful in assessing the degree of edema, when performed early (2 to 4 days after the insult). CT may not be as useful in predicting sequelae in premature infants because the excess water and lower myelin content of the premature brain obscures gray-white differentiation. (In this case, serial ultrasound studies may suffice for localizing, for example, periventricular echoes suggestive of PVL.) CT is useful for demonstrating focal ischemic le-

TABLE 27.9. SARNAT AND SARNAT STAGES OF HYPOXIC-ISCHEMIC ENCEPHALOPATHY*

Stage	Stage 1 (Mild)	Stage 2 (Moderate)	Stage 3 (Severe)
Level of consciousness	Hyperalert; irritable	Lethargic or obtunded	Stuporous, comatose
Neuromuscular control:	Uninhibited, overreactive	Diminished spontaneous movement	Diminished or absent spontaneous movement
Muscle tone	Normal	Mild hypotonia	Flaccid
Posture	Mild distal flexion	Strong distal flexion	Intermittent decerebration
Stretch reflexes	Overactive	Overactive, disinhibited	Decreased or absent
Segmental myoclonus	Present or absent	Present	Absent
Complex reflexes:	Normal	Suppressed	Absent
Suck	Weak	Weak or absent	Absent
Moro	Strong, low threshold	Weak, incomplete high threshold	Absent
Oculovestibular	Normal	Overactive	Weak or absent
Tonic neck	Slight	Strong	Absent
Autonomic function:	Generalized sympathetic	Generalized parasympathetic	Both systems depressed
Pupils	Mydriasis	Miosis	Midposition, often unequal; poor light reflex
Respirations	Spontaneous	Spontaneous; occasional apnea	Periodic; apnea
Heart rate	Tachycardia	Bradycardia	Variable
Bronchial and salivary secretions	Sparse	Profuse	Variable
Gastrointestinal motility	Normal or decreased	Increased diarrhea	Variable
Seizures	None	Common focal or multifocal (6 to 24 hours of age)	Uncommon (excluding decerebration)

Electroencephalographic findings	Normal (awake)	Early: generalized low-voltage, slowing (continuous delta and theta) Later: periodic pattern (awake); seizures focal or multifocal; 1.0 to 1.5 Hz spike and wave	Early: periodic pattern with isopotential phases Later: totally isopotential
Duration of symptoms	<24 hours	2 to 14 days	Hours to weeks
Outcome	About 100% normal	80% normal; abnormal if symptoms more than 5 to 7 days	About 50% die; remainder with severe sequelae

*The stages in this table are a continuum reflecting the spectrum of clinical states of infants over 36 weeks' gestational age.
Source: From Sarnat H. B., Sarnat M. S. Neonatal encephalopathy following fetal distress: A clinical and electroencephalographic study. *Arch Neurol* 1976;33:696.

sions (commonly seen in the left middle cerebral-artery distribution area). **Magnetic resonance imaging (MRI)** particularly when accompanied by diffusion-weighted images (DWI) becomes the diagnostic modality of choice. DWI often can show abnormalities within the first few hours after the insult (13), and is prognostically useful (see VI C.). **DWI** reveals restricted water diffusion not apparent on conventional MRI, by detecting differences in the rates of diffusion of water protons. **Brain scans with isotopes** may reveal areas without blood flow (9), but have generally not been widely used clinically. Several studies documented significant increases (>5 IU) in the serum **creatine kinase brain fraction (CK-BB)** at 4 and 10 hours of life (peaking between 6 and 10 days) in asphyxiated infants who ultimately died or developed neurologic sequelae; however, CK-BB also may rise after intraventricular hemorrhage (IVH). This isoenzyme is also expressed in the placenta, lungs, gastrointestinal (GI) tract, and kidneys, all of which may be involved in the sequelae of asphyxia. A combination of protein S-100 (> 8.5 µg/L) and CK-BB or, CK-BB and cord blood arterial pH have been found to have a sensitivity of 71 % each and specificity of 95% and 91%, respectively, in predicting moderate to severe encephalopathy (16). Measures of **neuron-specific enolase (NSE)** have not proven sufficiently useful.

It should be emphasized that HIE is just one (and not the most common) of a number of etiologies in the differential diagnosis of neurologic dysfunction or depression in the neonate, which also includes: genetic and structural abnormalities; drugs and toxins; infection; inherited metabolic diseases; trauma; intracranial hemorrhage (ICH); and transient homeostatic derangements, such as hypoglycemia, hypocalcemia, hypermagnesemia, hypomagnesemia, hypernatremia, and hypothermia. Asphyxia may be suspected and HIE reasonably included in the differential diagnosis of neonatal depression, coma, or neurologic dysfunction if the following have been documented: (1) 5- to 10-minute Apgar score (or more reliably, 15- to 20-minute Apgar score) less than 3; (2) fetal heart rate (FHR) of less than 60; (3) prolonged (1 hour) antenatal acidosis; (4) neonatal seizure within the first 24 to 48 hours (though 50% of seizures are not asphyxial in etiology); (5) burst-suppression pattern on electroencephalogram (EEG); and (6) need for positive-pressure resuscitation for more than 1 minute or more than 5 minutes until the first cry. Whether permanent neurologic sequelae can be **attributed** to HIE is a completely different question and is addressed in VI.

   c. **Management of hypoxic-ischemic brain injury.** The initial management of hypoxic-ischemic damage in the delivery room is described in Chap. 4. Other specific management consists of supportive care to maintain temperature, perfusion, ventilation, and a normal metabolic state, including glucose, Ca^{2+}, and acid–base balance. Control of seizures is important. It is important to emphasize that the most significant portion of neuronal death occurs after the initiating insult. Hence in cases of birthing-related insult, the initial management is quite important.

   (1) **O_2 levels should be kept in the normal range** by monitoring arterial PO_2 or transcutaneous PO_2 or percent O_2 saturation by pulse oximeter (recognizing that the latter two may be rendered inaccurate by diminished peripheral perfusion). Hypoxia should be treated with O_2 and/or ventilation. Hyperoxia also may cause a decrease in CBF or exacerbate free-radical damage. Aminophylline may decrease CBF and should not be used in the initial management of apnea due to asphyxia.

   (2) **CO_2 should be kept in the normal range** because hypercapnia causes cerebral acidosis and may cause cerebral vasodilation,

which may cause more flow to uninjured areas with relative ischemia to damaged areas ("steal phenomenon") and extension of infarct size. The excess flow to uninjured areas may furthermore be associated with ICH because of loss of autoregulation of CBF (see Intracranial Hemorrhage). Excessive hypocapnia (CO_2 < 25 mm Hg) may decrease CBF. Hyperventilation is not recommended.

(3) **Perfusion.** Cardiovascular stability and adequate mean systemic arterial blood pressure are key to the management of HIE. It is important to maintain cerebral perfusion pressure (CPP) within a normal range. Too little can cause ischemic injury; too much can cause hemorrhage in the areas of damaged blood vessels, with germinal matrix hemorrhage and IVH in premature infants. Excessive reperfusion of infarcted tissue may cause the infarct to become hemorrhagic because of loss of vascular integrity. Abrupt changes in perfusion and rapid infusions of volume expanders or sodium bicarbonate may be associated with IVH (25). Because cerebrovascular autoregulation is lost, cerebral perfusion entirely reflects systemic BP in a pressure-passive fashion. To maintain cerebral perfusion, a **systemic mean arterial BP of at least 45 to 50 mm Hg is usually desirable for term infants, 35 to 40 mm Hg for infants weighing 1000 to 2000 g, and 30 to 35 mm Hg for infants weighing less than 1000 g (12,25).** Conversely, if hypertension develops and persists despite the discontinuation of pressors and the institution of adequate sedation, the systemic BP should not be lowered further, since it may be needed to maintain adequate CPP in the face of increased ICP. The following recommendations should be adhered to:

(a) Continuously monitor arterial BP. Continuously monitor CVP, if possible, to ensure there is adequate preload—that is—the infant is not hypovolemic due to vasodilatation or third spacing.

(b) Keep systemic mean arterial BP at no lower than 45 to 50 mm Hg in term infants, 35 to 40 mm Hg in 1000- to 2000-g infants, and 30 to 35 mm Hg in infants weighing less than 1000 g. Keep CVP 5 to 8 mm Hg in term infants and 3 to 5 mm Hg in preterm infants.

(c) Minimize acute, abrupt pushes of colloid or sodium bicarbonate, but regularly replace intravascular volume losses as needed to avoid lactic acidosis and insure vascular tone.

(d) Give volume replacement slowly.

(e) Minimize administered free H_2O (insensible losses plus urine output); however, if urine output is low, first ensure that intravascular volume is adequate (i.e., rule out prerenal etiology) before fluid restriction (see Chaps. 9, 31).

(f) Judicious use of pressors may help minimize the need for colloid in maintaining BP and perfusion (see Chap. 17).

(g) Monitor ICP if possible.

(h) Avoid hyperviscosity from a hematocrit over 65 as it may exacerbate the preexisting hypoxia and ischemia.

(4) **Glucose** (see Chap. 27, Neonatal Seizures, and Chap. 29). **Blood glucose level should be kept at 75 to 100 mg/dL** to provide adequate substrate for the brain. Higher levels may lead to elevation of brain lactate, damage to cellular integrity, increased edema, and further disturbances in vascular autoregulation (17,25). Lower levels may potentiate excitotoxic amino acids and extend the infarct size. **Hypoglycemia,** due both to glycogen depletion secondary to catecholamine release and to an unexplained hyperinsulinemic state, is often seen in asphyxiated infants. An initial phase of hyperglycemia and hypoinsulinemia (5 to 10 minutes following an acute event due to a catecholamine surge which inhibits insulin release

and stimulates glucagons release) may be followed within 2 to 3 hours by profound hypoglycemia. Normal glucose infusion rates of 5 to 8 mg/kg per minute may not be sufficient to maintain normoglycemia; rates as high as 9 to 15 mg/kg per minute may be required for short periods. Because hypoglycemia may be difficult to control without causing fluid overload, concentrated glucose infusions may be necessary by means of a central line (e.g., a "high" umbilical venous line with its tip at the inferior vena cava-right atrial junction). Since rapid glucose boluses should be avoided, serum glucose level should be monitored frequently and adjustments anticipated. Glucose infusions should be discontinued slowly to avoid rebound hypoglycemia. Seizures may result from hypoglycemia; therefore, if seizures do occur, the possibility of hypoglycemia should be ruled out or treated appropriately before reflexly instituting anticonvulsant therapy. Seizures in such an instance would not be used for Sarnat clinical staging.

(5) Temperature should be kept in a normal range. Initial results of selective head cooling, which acts through multiple pathways (decreasing energy depletion, inhibiting glutamate release, and inhibiting apoptosis) in asphyxiated newborns have shown promising results at 6 and 12-month follow-up (18); however, the results of multicenter studies presently under way to evaluate safety and efficacy will be needed before this modality can be recommended for routine treatment.

(6) Calcium level should be kept in a normal range. Hypocalcemia is a common metabolic alteration in the neonatal postasphyxial syndrome. A subnormal serum Ca^{2+} level will not forestall neuronal damage and may only serve to compromise cardiac contractility or cause seizures (see Chap. 29, Hypocalcemia, Hypercalcemia, and Hypermagnesemia).

(7) Seizures. Seizures should be controlled as described in Neonatal Seizures. In neonatal HIE, they are typically focal or multifocal (myelinization and synaptogenesis not having developed sufficiently for generalization of seizures). Seizures occur in about 20 to 50% of infants with HIE in most series (7,8,11), characteristically on the first or second day, usually in stage 2, only rarely in stage 3, and almost never in stage 1 (see Sarnat and Sarnat stages, Table 27.9). They may be associated with an increased cerebral metabolic rate, which in the absence of adequate O_2 and perfusion may lead to a fall in blood glucose level, an increase in brain lactate level, and a fall in high-energy phosphate compounds. In infants not mechanically ventilated, seizures may be associated with hypoxemia and/or hypercapnia. Abrupt elevations in BP associated with seizures may contribute to ICH in preterm infants. When seizures are clinically apparent and of typical morphology, an EEG is not necessary to confirm the diagnosis (though data regarding interictal background activity may be useful for assessing the overall "well-being" of the brain). **In infants paralyzed with pancuronium for mechanical ventilation, seizures may be manifested by abrupt changes in BP, heart rate, and oxygenation.** An EEG should be obtained in these circumstances. Whether seizures alone, in the absence of metabolic or cardiopulmonary abnormalities, lead to brain injury is controversial. Although one should have a low threshold for diagnosing seizures in the setting of HIE, there is inadequate evidence, despite initial trial showing some long-term benefits (19), of prophylactic use of anticonvulsants in the absence of clinical seizures or electrical seizures on EEG. There is actually very little change in ICP during most electrographic seizures (12). The clinical distinction between multifocal seizures and the "jitteriness" (actually a rhythmic segmental myoclonus) seen frequently in stage 1 and even stage 2 HIE is often difficult to make by observation alone. Taking hold of the clonic extremity and changing the tension on the muscle stretch receptor by slightly flexing or extending the joint immediately arrests clonus but does not alter true seizure activity, during which rhythmic convulsive movements continue to be felt in the examiner's hand. When seizures are diagnosed, **phenobarbital** should be given slowly, 20 mg/kg intravenously to be followed by a maintenance dose of 3 to 5 mg/kg per day. One should always be vigilant for respiratory depression and/or cardiovascular compromise with hypotension. If the infant is already mechanically ventilated, respiratory depression is not a concern. In nonintensive care unit (ICU) settings, one may divide the loading dose of phenobarbital or use phenytoin (or fosphenytoin). Phenobarbital, especially at high levels, itself can cause lethargy, stupor, and occasionally brain stem signs. If seizures persist, **phenytoin** may be administered slowly as a second drug (20 mg/kg intravenously as a loading dose followed by 4 to 8 mg/kg per day as a maintenance dose). The dose of **fosphenytoin** is the same as phenytoin, calculated and written in terms of phenytoin equivalents (PE), to avoid medication errors. One should, of course, ascertain that metabolic derangements that may complicate asphyxia and cause seizures have been addressed (e.g., hypoglycemia, hypocalcemia, and hyponatremia) (see Chap. 29). **Pyridoxine-dependency seizures** and local anesthetic toxicity may mimic postasphyxic seizures and should be considered in the differential diagnosis. If seizures nevertheless persist, a **benzodiazepam** (e.g., lorazepam 0.05 to 0.10 mg/kg per dose intravenously) may be given transiently as a third drug. If vascular access cannot be achieved in the non-ICU setting, rectal diazepam, valproate, or paraldehyde (in that order) may provide a stopgap. (Intramuscular phenobarbital is absorbed too slowly and, because it may confound subsequent management, its use is discouraged.) Seizures in HIE are notoriously difficult to control and often resistant to even aggressive anticonvulsant therapy in the early stages (first 72 hours) of the syndrome. Once levels of conventional anticonvulsants are maximized (phenobarbital level to 40 mg/dL, phenytoin level to 20 mg/dL), unless there is cardiopulmonary compromise from the seizures, there is often little utility in eliminating every "twitch" or electrographic seizure. For unexplained reasons, even refractory seizures in HIE ultimately "burn themselves out" and cease after approximately 48 hours. **When the infant's condition has been stable for 3 to 4 days, all anticonvulsants are weaned except phenobarbital** (the level of which may be allowed to drop to 15 to 20 mg/dL if possible). If seizures have resolved, if neurologic findings are normal, and if the EEG is normal, anticonvulsants are stopped in the neonatal period (14 days of life). If this is not the case, anticonvulsants are continued for 1 to 3 months. If the neurologic findings are then normal with no recurrent seizures and a nonepileptiform EEG, phenobarbital is tapered over 4 weeks. If the neurologic results are not normal, the advisability of continued anticonvulsant therapy requires consideration of the initial cause of the seizures. The risk of subsequent epilepsy is 100% with seizures secondary to cerebral cortical dysgeneses but only 20 to 30% after seizures secondary to perinatal asphyxia and essentially nil after seizures secondary to transient metabolic disturbances. Infants with a higher risk of subsequent seizures are those with a persistent neurologic deficit (50% risk) and those with an abnormal EEG between seizures (40% risk). If the result of neurologic examination is not normal, an EEG is obtained; if there is no electrographic seizure activity, phenobarbital is tapered and discontinued over 4 weeks, even if the infant has abnormal neurologic signs.

(8) Cerebral edema. Devices applied to the anterior fontanel provide noninvasive methods for measuring ICP (12). Cerebral edema may be minimized by avoiding fluid overload, although initial resuscitation of an asphyxiated infant and maintenance of cardiovascular stability and CPP (CPP = systemic mean arterial BP minus ICP) should always take priority. Two processes may predispose to fluid overload in asphyxiated infants: (1) syndrome of inappropriate secretion of antidiuretic hormone (SIADH) (see Chap. 9) and (2) ATN (see Chap. 31). SIADH, often seen for 3 to 4 days after the insult, is manifested by hyponatremia and hypoosmolarity with excretion of an inappropriately concentrated and Na^+-containing urine (elevated urine-specific gravity, osmolarity, and Na^+). SIADH should be monitored by daily determinations of serum and urinary Na^+ and osmolarity. Urine output may further be compromised by ATN resulting from shunting of cardiac output away from the kidneys. Persistent oliguria (<1 mL/kg per hour for the first 36 hours of life) can provide an index of the severity of asphyxia and risk for neurologic sequelae. **To avoid fluid overload and the exacerbation of cerebral edema, both SIADH and ATN should be managed by limitation of free H_2O administration only to replacement of insensible losses and urine output (usually, 60 mL/kg per day)** (see Chap. 9). Before attributing oliguria to SIADH or ATN, rule out prerenal etiologies (hypovolemia, vasodilation) with a 10 to 20 mL/kg fluid challenge followed by a loop diuretic (e.g., furosemide) if there is no urine output. Cerebral edema and increased ICP (>10 mm Hg) are actually fairly uncommon concomitants of perinatal asphyxia (12). When present, they more often reflect extensive prior cerebral necrosis rather than swelling of intact cells, and because they bespeak such extensive cell death, they have a uniformly bad prognosis. They peak 36 to 72 hours after the insult. They are more properly regarded as an effect rather than a cause of brain damage. For this reason, efforts specifically to reduce cerebral edema or ICP do not affect outcome; neither do ICP elevations reduce cerebral perfusion or introduce any acute functional neurologic disturbances (12,25). Therefore, such interventions previously explored in the literature as antiedema agents (e.g., high-dose phenobarbital, steroids, mannitol, and other hypertonic solutions) are not employed at our institution. The infant's patent sutures and open fontanel are protective of any acute increases in ICP that might occur. **Our major efforts are devoted to ensuring an adequate CPP through maintaining an adequate systemic mean arterial BP,** shown in recent studies to be a more important variable than ICP in ensuring adequate CBF. A simple estimate of ICP can be made in infants (assuming no elevations of CVP such as occurs with pneumothorax or during treatment with continuous positive airway pressure [CPAP]) by measuring the vertical distance between the anterior fontanel and the heart, measured at the point that the midportion of the fontanel flattens as the baby is tilted up. Normal will be 50 mm H_2O or lower.

(9) Many **brain-sparing, cerebroprotective, and/or infarct-limiting interventions** have been proposed in recent years, many based on the postulated mechanisms of asphyxial damage described earlier (V.B.1.a) (reviewed in (20). Administration of naloxone (for endogenous opioid blockade) has proved ineffective in humans despite its initial promise in animal models. Newer possibilities such as (1) antagonists of excitotoxic neurotransmitter receptors (e.g.,

NMDA receptor blockers); (2) free-radical scavengers (e.g., allopurinol, superoxide dismutase, vitamin E); (3) Ca^{2+} channel blockers (e.g., nimodipine, nicardipine); (4) cyclooxygenase inhibitors (e.g., indomethacin); (5) hypothermia; (6) benzodiazepine receptor stimulation (e.g., midazolam); (7) enhancers of protein synthesis (e.g., dexamethasone); and (8) vasodilators (e.g., prostacyclin) all have a theoretical basis (see V.B.1.a) but most have not yet undergone large systemic neonatal trials (13). At this point, **selective head hypothermia** seems the most promising based on initial results (see V.C.5), (but still requires multicenter validation before becoming a routine part of management.

d. **Brain death in the neonate.** In 1987, recommendations for determination of brain death in children and infants older than 7 days were proposed by an ad hoc task force committee (14). The guidelines avoided specific recommendations in infants less than 7 days old, citing lack of published data. Though controversial, Ashwal et al. (15) argued that the current task force guidelines might be extended to include the term infant and the preterm infant more than 32 weeks' gestational age. The clinical diagnosis of brain death might, in their opinion, be made on the basis of (1) coma, manifested by lack of response to pain, light, or auditory stimulation; (2) apnea, confirmed by documentation of failure to breathe when partial pressure of carbon dioxide (PCO_2) is higher than 60 mm Hg (tested by 3 minutes without ventilator support while continuing 100% O_2 supplementation or for shorter periods if hypotension or bradycardia intervene); (3) absent bulbar movements and brain stem reflexes (including midposition or fully dilated pupils with no response to light or pain and with absent oculocephalic, caloric, corneal, gag, cough, rooting, and sucking reflexes), all normally elicitable by 33 weeks' gestation; and (4) flaccid tone and absence of spontaneous or induced movements (excluding activity mediated at the spinal cord level). If these clinical findings remain unchanged for 24 hours, there is electrocerebral silence in the absence of a barbiturate level over 25 mg/mL, hypothermia (<24°C), or cerebral malformations (e.g., hydranencephaly, hydrocephalus), it is confirmatory of brain death. Further, if the initial EEG (done after 24 hours of life) shows electrocerebral silence and the infant remains brain-dead for 24 hours, a repeat study is not necessary. Absence of radionuclide uptake (a reliable estimate of CBF) contemporaneous with initial electrocerebral silence is also associated with brain death. Alternatively, if no radionuclide uptake is demonstrated initially (signifying CBF <2 mL/min/100 g) and the infant remains clinically brain-dead for 24 hours, a diagnosis of brain death also can be made, even if some EEG activity persists. Sensitivity is increased in this regard by repeating the scan in 24 hours and reconfirming no uptake. Term infants clinically brain-dead for 2 days and preterm infants brain-dead for 3 days do not survive regardless of the EEG or CBF status, indicating that determination of brain death in the newborn might be made solely by using clinical criteria over this prolonged period of observation. Therefore, confirmatory neurodiagnostic studies are of value in potentially shortening the period of observation to 24 hours. Phenobarbital levels higher than 25 mg/mL may suppress EEG activity in this age group. The diagnosis of brain death must also be made in the appropriate clinical setting, wherein the cause of coma has been determined and all remediable or reversible conditions eliminated. In isolation, neither EEG alone nor radionuclide flow studies alone are sufficiently sensitive to diagnose brain death. Persistent EEG activity and/or prognostically small variations in radionuclide uptake do **not** obviate the diagnosis of brain death in the newborn. (Unlike in adults or older children, minimal radionuclide uptake may persist in brain-dead neonates, perhaps due to patent sutures, which may moderate acute increases in ICP, which would otherwise diminish CPP to a no-flow state.) Clinical correlation and/or coupled neurodiagnostic studies are necessary. These recommendations, Ashwal et al. contend (15), take into account all reported cases to date of possible misdiagnosis of brain death. Based on these, the combination of neurologic assessment, an EEG showing electrocerebral silence, and isotope estimation of CBF followed by 24 hours of observation seems valid, they suggest, in deciding that irreversible cessation of brain function has occurred in the preterm and term infant. At present, insufficient information is available to warrant the use of brainstem-evoked response testing for confirmation of brain death in the newborn. In neonates, an additional clinical clue to brain death is a fixed heart rate without decelerations or accelerations. (See Chap. 22 and Table 22.1.)

2. **Cardiac effects of asphyxia** (see Chap. 25)
   a. **Diagnosis.** Infants with perinatal asphyxia may have **transient myocardial ischemia** and the electrocardiogram (ECG) may show ST depression in the midprecordium and T-wave inversion in the left precordium. A serum creatine kinase plasma MB isoenzyme fraction higher than 5 to 10% may be present in myocardial damage. More recently troponin T (which is found to be superior in older patients as an indicator of myocardial ischemia) levels of ≥ 0.1 ng/mL have been associated with neonatal ischemia (21). The echocardiogram/Doppler study will show normal cardiac structures but decreased left ventricular contractions, especially of the posterior wall, and perhaps persistent pulmonary hypertension. It is important to rule out Epstein's disease of the tricuspid valve, pulmonary stenosis, and pulmonary atresia with intact ventricular septum. The ventricular end-diastolic pressures are usually elevated because of poor ventricular function. Some infants will show **tricuspid regurgitation** with right-to-left shunting at the atrial level. In a study of moderately to severely asphyxiated newborns (7), left ventricular dysfunction occurred in less than 10% of infants, while right ventricular dysfunction was found in 30% of infants. Many of these infants will have meconium aspiration syndrome with persistent pulmonary hypertension (see Chap. 24). Of significance, the presence of a **fixed heart rate without variation** may raise suspicion of clinical brain death.
   b. **Management of the cardiac effects of asphyxia.** The treatment is adequate ventilation with correction of hypoxemia, acidosis, and hypoglycemia. Volume overload must be avoided. (Diuretics may be ineffective if there is concomitant renal failure.) These infants will require continuous monitoring of systemic mean arterial BP, CVP, and urine output. Infants with cardiac collapse will require inotropic drugs such as **dopamine** and/or **dobutamine** (see Chap. 17). Some infants in great distress may require afterload reduction with a peripheral beta-agonist (e.g., isoproterenol), a peripheral alpha blocker (e.g., phentolamine or tolazoline), or nitroprusside (see Chap. 25). The prognosis for the heart is good, with most surviving infants having normal cardiac findings in 3 weeks and a normal ECG in 3 months. If there is severe cardiogenic shock, the infant usually dies or has a severe insult to the brain or other vital organ.

3. **Renal effects of asphyxia.** The asphyxiated infant is at risk for **ATN** and for **syndrome of inappropriate antidiuretic hormone (SIADH). Urine output, urinalysis, urine-specific gravity, and urine and serum osmolarity and electrolytes should be monitored. Measurement of serum and urine creatinine together with serum and urine Na$^+$** allows calculation of the **fractional excretion of Na$^+$ (Fe-Na** and the **renal index** to help confirm a renal insult (see Chap. 31 for diagnosis and management of ATN). Mea-

surement of urinary levels of **beta-2-microglobulin,** a low-molecular-weight protein freely filtered through the glomerulus and reabsorbed almost completely in the proximal tubule of even immature kidneys, may provide a sensitive indicator of subtle proximal tubular dysfunction. Renal size should be monitored by ultrasound. Dopamine infusion at 1.25 to 2.50 mg/kg per hour intravenously may aid renal perfusion. **Oliguria should not be attributed to SIADH or ATN until prerenal etiologies such as hypovolemia or vasodilation have been ruled out since one does not want to compromise system blood pressure inappropriately** (see Chaps. 9, 31).

4. **Gastrointestinal effects of asphyxia.** The asphyxiated infant is at risk for bowel ischemia and **necrotizing enterocolitis (NEC).** We usually do not feed **severely asphyxiated** infants for 5 to 7 days after the insult or until good bowel sounds are heard and stools are negative for blood and/or reducing substance (see Chap. 32).

5. **Hematologic effects of asphyxia.** Disseminated intravascular coagulation (DIC) may be seen in asphyxiated infants because of damage to blood vessels. The liver may fail to make clotting factors, and the bone marrow may not produce platelets. Clotting factors [partial thromboplastin time (PTT) and prothrombin time (PT)], fibrinogen, and platelets should be monitored and replaced as needed (see Chap. 26).

6. **Liver.** The liver may be so damaged ("shock liver") that it cannot provide its basic functions. Liver function [transaminases (ALT, AST), clotting factors (PT, PTT, fibrinogen), albumin, and bilirubin] should be monitored, and serum ammonia level should be measured. Clotting factors should be provided as indicated. Serum glucose level should be kept at 75 to 100 mg/dL; glycogen stores have usually been depleted. Drugs that are detoxified by the liver must have their levels monitored closely. Total liver failure is usually a bad prognostic sign.

7. **Lung.** The pulmonary effects of asphyxia include **increased pulmonary vascular resistance, pulmonary hemorrhage, pulmonary edema** secondary to cardiac failure, and possibly failure of surfactant production with secondary hyaline membrane disease (acute respiratory distress syndrome). Meconium aspiration may be present. Treatment consists of oxygenation and ventilation (and possibly mild alkalinization). The method of ventilation may be different if the primary problem is hyaline membrane disease, persistent pulmonary hypertension, or meconium aspiration (see Chap. 24). High-frequency ventilation may play a role in some of these strategies (see Chap. 24). Nitric oxide (NO) may also be indicated for severe pulmonary hypertension. Extracorporeal membrane oxygenation (ECMO) may also provide a therapeutic modality in an asphyxiated infant whose CNS appears otherwise intact (see Chap. 24).

VI. **Prognosis of perinatal asphyxia** (16,22–27). The degree of asphyxia necessary to cause severe permanent brain damage in experimental animals is quite close to that which causes death (25 minutes of acute, total asphyxia). Survival with brain damage due to asphyxia is actually uncommon in this model, the extremes of death or intact survival being the most likely outcomes. Likewise, in humans, birth asphyxia severe enough to damage the fetal brain irreversibly usually kills before or soon after birth. Approximately one-fourth of asphyxiated term newborns die. The remainder, however, even those with seizures, will overwhelmingly be normal. The only group of neonates with significant neurologic impairment are those who were severely asphyxiated, yet narrowly escape death, a relatively small few. Except in extreme cases where an infant is asphyxiated to near-lethal proportions, if an infant does not die from the asphyxia, the prognosis is quite favorable for normal neurologic status (including absence of mental retardation and epilepsy).

Thus a diagnosis of asphyxia severe enough to offer a poor prognosis must hinge on assessment of other systems in addition to the CNS. A corollary of this

statement is that **no significant neurologic abnormality diagnosed later in childhood (e.g., cerebral palsy) can be ascribed to perinatal asphyxia in the absence of evidence in the perinatal period of severe, multisystemic asphyxial insult.**
A. **Outcome** (9,22–27). Overall, full-term asphyxiated infants have a mortality of 10 to 20%. The incidence of neurologic sequelae in survivors is 20 to 45% (approximately 40% of these are minimal; 60% severe); i.e., the majority will be normal. Analyzed according to **Sarnat's stages** of severity (11) (see Table 27.9), virtually 100% of newborns with evidence of mild encephalopathy (stage 1) have normal neurologic outcome; 80% of those with moderate encephalopathy (stage 2) are normal neurologically (those who are abnormal exhibiting stage 2 signs over 7 days); and virtually all the children with severe encephalopathy (stage 3) die (one-half) or develop major neurologic sequelae (the other half) [e.g., cerebral palsy (CP), retardation, epilepsy, microcephaly]. (Preterm infants may have a higher morbidity and mortality at less severe stages because of the high frequency of ICH and problems with other systems.) While the **risk** of CP in the asphyxiated newborn is elevated—5 to 10% versus 2 per 1000 in the general population of live births—the actual number is quite small in absolute terms. Regarding the existence of school problems among the "neurologically and mentally normal" survivors of HIE, the data are controversial. In one study (26), at 8 years of age, all unimpaired children from the Sarnat mild HIE group and a majority (65 to 82%) of unimpaired children from the Sarnat moderate HIE group were performing at expected grade level, indistinguishable from a matched peer group. In another study, however, in which children with evidence of neonatal encephalopathy following an Apgar score under 4 were followed to 8 to 13 years, there was a 3.3 times risk of problems with mathematics, a 4.6 times risk of problems with reading, a 7 times risk of epilepsy, 13 times risk of minor motor problems, and 14 times risk of attention deficit-hyperactivity disorder (ADHD) compared to controls with normal Apgar scores and no neonatal evidence of encephalopathy (22).

The cardiac, renal, gastrointestinal, pulmonary, hepatic, and hematologic problems usually resolve if the infant survives.
B. **Risk of CP** (1,25,27). Data from the National Collaborative Perinatal Project (NCPP) and the British National Child Development Study (BNCDS) suggest that **perinatal factors of labor and delivery contribute little to the incidence of mental retardation and seizure. Only 3 to 13% of infants with CP had evidence of actual intrapartum asphyxia.** In support of this assessment is the observation that despite improvements in perinatal care, the incidence of long-term neurologic sequelae has not decreased. The following previously implicated obstetric events **do not correlate with CP: oxytocin administration, nuchal cord, midforceps use, and duration of labor. Factors found to be statistically associated with an increased risk for the development of CP were gestational age less than 32 weeks, fetal heart rate less than 60 beats per minute, breech presentation (although not breech delivery), chorioamnionitis, low placental weight, placental complications, and birth weight less than 2000 g.** Most of these factors, however, reflect preexistent, unpreventable sources of neurologic dysfunction that occur independent of asphyxia but that might also predispose to concomitant asphyxia at birth. An abnormal CNS may cause otherwise unexplained premature onset of labor. Conversely, a fetus with CNS abnormalities might not possess appropriate reflex cardiovascular responses to stress during labor and delivery to ensure proper fetal and placental perfusion or a smooth transition to extra-uterine physiology (4). **No constant relationship between measures of fetal distress and subsequent long-term neurologic outcome has been demonstrated;** that is, most infants with only one of the following predictors do not develop CP: meconium staining (98% do not develop CP), fetal heart rate less than 60 beats per minute (98% do not develop CP), pH less than 7.1 (no correlation with CP), more than 5 minutes to the first cry (98% do not develop CP), and 10-minute Apgar score less than 3 (83% do not develop CP). These

clearly better reflect clinical status during the perinatal period than they do ultimate long-term outcome. Clustering perinatal events improves prediction of CP. For example, seizures alone were associated with CP in only 0.13%, but low Apgar score, signs of HIE, and seizures identified a small subgroup in whom the risk for CP was 55%. Most CP, however, is not related to birth asphyxia, and most birth asphyxia does not cause CP.

C. **Indicators of poor outcome.** Although permanent brain damage from perinatal asphyxia is actually uncommon, are there reliable prognostic indicators of the small subgroup in which this does occur? Within the first 2 weeks of life it is very difficult to offer a prognosis for an individual infant because the present methods of prognostication are so unreliable. Unfavorable signs are: (1) **severe, prolonged asphyxia;** (2) **Sarnat stage 3 encephalopathy;** (3) **seizures of early onset (<12 hours)** that are difficult to control when accompanied by other signs of asphyxia in multiple systems; (4) **elevated ICP** (>10 mm Hg); (5) persistence of **abnormal neurologic signs** at discharge (usually for more than 1 to 2 weeks), especially absence of the **Moro reflex;** (6) **MRI** findings showing an abnormal signal in DWI correlate with poor outcomes in both premature and term neonates (13,23); (7) abnormalities on **brain scan** (24); (8) **an elevated CK-BB level** when combined with a cord arterial base deficit > 17 mM/L (16); and (9) **persistent oliguria** (<1 mL/kg per hour for the first 36 hours of life). Although a single early Apgar score correlates poorly with acid–base status, which itself correlates poorly with outcome, the **extended Apgar score** may help predict outcome. Term infants with Apgar scores of 0 to 3 at 10, 15, and 20 minutes have mortality rates of 18, 48, and 59%, respectively; in survivors, the CP rates are 5, 9, and 57%, respectively (27). It should be noted that many features of the Apgar score relate to **cardiovascular integrity** and **not** neurologic function. (Clearly, if an infant responds in the delivery room by 15 to 20 minutes, it has an excellent chance of being normal; conversely, only a small percentage of infants have a score less than 3 at 20 minutes and survive.) By electrodiagnostic criteria, the neonate with seizures was 50 to 70 times more likely to develop CP than one without seizures; however, more important, 70 to 80% of infants with neonatal seizures who survived had no CP. Of neonates, however, who required resuscitation (not merely intubation) after 5 minutes of life and subsequently developed seizures, one-half died and almost half the survivors had CP. Simply stated, **seizure without depression is not ominous, and depression without seizure is not ominous. Background EEG activity** is actually a better indicator of prognosis than ictal patterns per se. Term infants with normal or maturationally delayed interictal EEGs after seizures have an almost 86% probability of normal development at the age of 4 years. However, interictal background abnormalities, such as burst-suppression (not pharmacologically induced), low-voltage, or electrocerebral inactivity are associated with poor outcome (30 to 75% likelihood). When EEG records are categorized as mild, moderate, or marked severity, only markedly abnormal records predict subsequent morbidity or mortality. For example, 93% of neonates with **extreme burst-suppression activity** have a poor outcome. It should be noted that not all neonates who have seizures and later neurologic deficits have those seizures because of asphyxia; often there is concurrent evidence of a metabolic disorder, infection, or malformation that might predispose to both asphyxia and neurologic deficit. Evoked potentials have not yet proved to be reliable prognosticators. Monitoring CPP by Doppler in the asphyxiated infant may prove of benefit in prognostication. While still an experimental modality, in the future **near-infrared spectroscopy (NIRS)** (which detects the concentrations of various chromophores within biologic tissue whose light-absorbing properties in the near-infrared region of the spectrum vary with oxygenation) may provide noninvasive quantification of indices of cerebral oxygenation and hemodynamics. For example, in preliminary studies (24), elevated cerebral blood volume, assessed noninvasively by NIRS in asphyxiated full-term infants within the first 24 hours after birth, appeared to correlate with the clinical severity of the encephalopathy and with adverse outcome.

In perinatal cardiac arrest, several studies indicated that if the heartbeat is back within 5 minutes and if the baby is breathing regularly and spontaneously within 30 minutes, the prognosis is good. If this is not the case, the outcome is poor (28).

D. **Clinical manifestations of neurologic sequelae.** The precise neurologic sequelae one will see following a severe asphyxic insult will reflect the location, identity, and extent of the neural cellular population affected. **CP** is a nonprogressive motor and/or postural deficit of early onset. The specific types—**pyramidal,** that is, **spastic quadriplegia** commonly associated with **mental retardation** and **epilepsy; spastic diplegia** (more common in "preemies") or **hemiplegia;** and **extrapyramidal** (including **dystonic** and **choreoathetoid** types)—are determined by the topography of brain injury. Mixed varieties exist. Focal or multifocal **cortical necrosis,** especially in the distribution of the middle cerebral artery, usually at the depths of sulci, may lead to **pyramidal CP** (unilateral or bilateral spastic hemiplegia or quadriplegia), **focal seizures,** and **mental retardation,** depending on the extent of the damage. A **boundary zone infarct** in a term newborn involving predominantly the parasagittal cortical regions (a watershed between the anterior, middle, and posterior cerebral arteries) may be recognized as weakness of the shoulder girdle and proximal upper extremities. **Auditory, visual-spatial,** or **language** difficulties probably reflect more extensive **parasagittal injury** more laterally and posteriorly in the border zones of the parieto-occipital lobe. In the initially preterm infant, **spastic diplegia** probably represents an ischemic cystic lesion in watershed zones of the periventricular white matter at the angles of the ventricle superior to the germinal matrix **(PVL)**; concomitant **visual impairment** suggests involvement of the optic radiations as well. **Extrapyramidal CP** is probably the long-term clinical correlate of necrosis of the basal ganglia and thalamus **(status marmoratus).** There are also indications in experimental animals that oligodendrocytes (especially in preterm mammals) may be particularly vulnerable to asphyxial insult and hence impact the functional myelinated pathways (25).

References

1. Grether J.K. et al. Prenatal and perinatal factors and cerebral palsy in very-low-birth-weight infants. *J Pediatr* 1996;128(3):407.
2. Aarnoudse J.G. et al. Fetal subcutaneous scalp PO_2 and abnormal heart rate during labor. *Am J Obstet Gynecol* 1985;153(5):565.
3. Low J.A., et al. Predictive value of electronic fetal monitoring for intrapartum fetal asphyxia with metabolic acidosis. *Obstet Gynecol* 1999;93(2):285.
4. Painter M.J. Fetal heart rate patterns, Perinatal asphyxia, and brain injury [Review]. *Pediatr Neurol* 1989;5:137.
5. Low J.A., et al. Threshold of metabolic acidosis associated with newborn complications. *Am J Obstet Gynecol* 1997;177:391.
6. Kruger K., et al. Predictive value of fetal scalp blood lactate concentration and pH as markers of neurologic disability. *Am J Obstet Gynecol* 1999;181:1072.
7. Perlman J.M., et al. Acute systemic organ injury in term infants after asphyxia. *Am J Dis Child* 1989;143:617.
8. Martin-Ancel A., et al. Multiple organ involvement in perinatal asphyxia. *J Pediatr* 1995;127:786.
9. Martin E., et al. Diagnostic and prognostic value of cerebral ^{31}P magnetic resonance spectroscopy study in neonates with perinatal asphyxia. *Pediatr Res* 1996;40:749.
10. Edwards A.D., et al. Apoptosis in the brain of infants suffering intrauterine cerebral injury. *Pediatr Res* 1997;42:684.
11. Sarnat H.B., et al. Neonatal encephalopathy following fetal distress: A clinical and electroencephalographic study. *Arch Neurol* 1976;33:696.

12. Clancy R., et al. Continuous intracranial pressure monitoring and serial electroencephalographic recordings in severely asphyxiated term neonates. *Am J Dis Child* 1988;142:740.

13. Cowan F.M., et al. Early detection of cerebral infarction and hypoxic ischemic encephalopathy in neonates using diffusion weighted magnetic resonance imaging. *Neuropediatrics* 1994;25:172.

14. Ad Hoc Task Force. Guidelines for the determination of brain death in children. American Academy of Pediatrics Task Force on Brain Death in Children. *Pediatrics* 1987;80:298.

15. Ashwal S., et al. Brain death in the newborn [see comments]. *Pediatrics* 1989; 84:429.

16. Nagdyman N., et al. Early biochemical indicators of hypoxic-ischemic encephalopathy after birth asphyxia. *Pediatr Res* 2001;49:502.

17. Vannucci R.C., et al. Cerebral carbohydrate and energy metabolism in perinatal hypoxic-ischemic brain damage. *Brain Pathol* 1992;2:229.

18. Gunn A.J., et al. Selective head cooling in newborn infants after perinatal asphyxia: A safety study. *Pediatrics* 1998;102:885.

19. Hall R.T., et al. High-dose phenobarbital therapy in term newborn infants with severe perinatal asphyxia: A randomized, prospective study with three-year follow up. *J Pediatr* 1998;132:345.

20. Gluckman P.D., et al Hypoxic-ischemic brain injury in the newborn: Pathophysiology and potential strategies for intervention. [Review]. *Semin Neonatol* 2001;6:109.

21. Makikallio K., et al. Association of severe placental insufficiency and systemic venous pressure rise in the fetus with increased neonatal cardiac troponin T levels. *Am J Obstet Gynecol* 2000;183:726.

22. Moster D., et al. Joint association of Apgar scores and early neonatal symptoms with minor disabilities at school age. *Arch Dis Child Fetal Neonatol Ed* 2002; 86: F16.

23. Johnson A.J., et al. Echoplanar diffusion-weighted imaging in neonates and infants with suspected hypoxic-ischemic injury: correlation with patient outcome. *Am J Roentgenol* 1999;172:219.

24. Meek J.H., et al. Abnormal cerebral haemodynamics in perinatally asphyxiated neonates related to outcome *Arch Dis Child Fetal Neonatol Ed* 1999;81: F110.

25. Volpe J. J. Hypoxic-Ischemic Encephalopathy. In: Volpe J. J. (Ed.), *Neurology of the Newborn,* 3rd ed. Philadelphia: Saunders, 2001;217, 277, 296, 331.

26. Robertson C.M., et al. School performance of survivors of neonatal encephalopathy associated with birth asphyxia at term. *J Pediatr* 1989;114:753.

27. Goldenberg R.L., and Nelson K.B. Cerebral palsy. In Cresey R. K., Resnik R. (Eds.), *Maternal-Fetal Medicine* (4th ed.). 1999. Philadelphia: Saunders, 1194.

28. Steiner H., et al. Perinatal cardiac arrest. Quality of the survivors. *Arch Dis Child* 1975;50:696.

NEURAL TUBE DEFECTS

Revised by John A. F. Zupancic*

I. **Definitions and pathology.** Neural tube defects constitute one of the most common congenital malformations in newborns. The term refers to a group of disorders that is heterogeneous with respect to embryologic timing, involvement of specific elements of the neural tube and its derivatives, clinical presentation, and prognosis.

---

*This is a revision of the chapter by Lawrence C. Kaplan in the 4th edition.

A. **Types of neural tube defects**
1. **Primary neural tube defects.** These constitute approximately 95% of all neural tube defects. They are due to primary failure of closure of the neural tube or possibly disruption of an already closed neural tube between 18 and 28 days' gestation. The resulting abnormality usually consists of two anatomic lesions: an exposed (open or operta) neural placode along the midline of the back caudally, and rostrally, the Arnold-Chiari II malformation (malformation of pons and medulla, with downward displacement of cerebellum, medulla, and fourth ventricle into the upper cervical region), with associated aqueductal stenosis and hydrocephalus (2).
   a. **Myelomeningocele.** This is the most common primary neural tube defect. It involves a saccular outpouching of neural elements (neural placode), typically through a defect in the bone and the soft tissues of the posterior thoracic, sacral, or lumbar regions, the latter comprising 80% of lesions. Dura and arachnoid are typically included in the sac (meningo-), which contains visible neural structures (myelo-), and the skin is usually discontinuous over the sac (4). Hydrocephalus occurs in 84% of these children; Arnold-Chiari II malformation occurs in approximately 90%. Various associated anomalies of the central nervous system are noted, most important, cerebral cortical dysplasia in up to 92% of cases.
   b. **Encephalocele.** This defect of anterior neural tube closure is an outpouching of dura with or without brain, noted in the occipital region in 80% of cases, and less commonly in the frontal or temporal regions. It may vary in size from a few millimeters to many centimeters.
   c. **Anencephaly.** In the most severe form of this defect, the cranial vault and posterior occipital bone are defective, and derivatives of the neural tube are exposed, including both brain and bony tissue. The defect usually extends through the foramen magnum and involves the brainstem. It is not compatible with long-term survival.
2. **Secondary neural tube defects.** Five percent of all neural tube defects result from abnormal development of the lower sacral or coccygeal segments during secondary neurulation. This leads to defects primarily in the lumbosacral spinal region. These heterogeneous lesions rarely are associated with hydrocephalus or the Arnold-Chiari II malformation, and the skin is typically intact over the defect (4).
   a. **Meningocele.** This is an outpouching of skin and dura without obvious involvement of the neural elements. These may be bone and contiguous soft-tissue abnormalities.
   b. **Lipomeningocele.** A lipomeningocele is a lipomatous mass usually in the lumbar or sacral region, occasionally off the midline, typically covered with full-thickness skin. Adipose tissue frequently extends through the defect into the spine and dura and adheres extensively to a distorted spinal cord or nerve roots.
   c. **Sacral agenesis/dysgenesis, diastematomyelia, myelocystocele.** These and others all may have varying degrees of bony involvement. Although rarely as extensive as with primary neural tube defects, neurologic manifestations may be present representing distortion or abnormal development of peripheral nerve structures. These lesions may be inapparent on physical examination of the child, resulting in the use of the term "occulta" to describe them (See Chap. 2, Diabetes Mellitus).
B. **Etiologies** proposed for both primary and secondary neural tube defects are heterogeneous. They include such **known** factors as maternal alcohol, aminopterin, or thalidomide ingestion; maternal diabetes; prenatal x-irradiation; and amniotic band disruption. **Suspected** factors and associations are maternal hyperthermia; hallucinogen, trimethadione, or valproate ingestion; and prenatal exposure to rubella. Both dominant and recessive mendelian inheritance have been documented, and neural tube defects can occur with trisomies 13 and 18, triploidy, and Meckel syndrome (autosomal recessive syndrome of encephalocele, polydactyly, polycystic kidneys, cleft lip and palate), as well as

other chromosome disorders. There is concordance for neural tube defect in monozygotic twins and an increased incidence with consanguinity. Both zinc and folic acid deficiencies have been proposed as possible etiologies.

C. Epidemiology and recurrence risk. In the United States, the overall frequency of neural tube defects is 1 in 2000 live births, and this appears to be decreasing. A well-established increased incidence is known among individuals living in parts of Ireland and Wales (4.2 to 12.5 per 1000), and carries over to descendants of these individuals who live elsewhere in the world. This also may be true for other ethnic groups, including Sikh Indians and certain groups in Egypt. The exact cause of failed neural tube closure remains unknown. Over 95% of all neural tube defects occur to couples with no known family history. Primary neural tube defects carry an increased empiric recurrence risk of approximately 2 to 3% for couples with one affected pregnancy. Similarly, affected individuals have a 3% risk of having one offspring with a primary neural tube defect. Recurrence risk is strongly affected by the level of the lesion in the index case, with risks as high as 7.8% for lesions above T11. In 5% of cases, neural tube defects may be associated with uncommon disorders; some, like Meckel syndrome, are inherited in an autosomal recessive manner, resulting in a 25% recurrence risk. Secondary neural tube defects are generally sporadic and carry no increased recurrence risk. In counseling families for recurrence, however, it is critical to obtain a careful history of drug exposure and/or family history (3).

D. Prevention. Controlled, randomized clinical studies of prenatal multivitamin administration both for secondary prevention in mothers with prior affected offspring (6) and for primary prevention in those without a prior history (7) suggest a much lower recurrence risk than in control groups. The Centers for Disease Control of the U.S. Public Health Service recommends that women of childbearing age who are capable of becoming pregnant should consume 0.4 mg of folic acid per day to reduce their risks of having a fetus affected with spina bifida or other neural tube defects (1). Higher doses are recommended for women with prior affected offspring. In addition, folate supplementation of enriched cereal-grain products has been mandated by the Food and Drug Administration in the United States; however, the level of folate intake from this source is not high enough to forgo additional supplementation in the large majority of women (1).

II. Diagnosis

A. Prenatal diagnosis. The combination of maternal serum alpha-fetoprotein (AFP) determinations and prenatal ultrasound, along with AFP and acetylcholinesterase determinations on amniotic fluid where indicated, greatly improves the ability to make a prenatal diagnosis. Maternal serum AFP measurements of 2.5 multiples of the median (MoM) in the second trimester (16 to 18 weeks) have a sensitivity of 80 to 90% for myelomeningocele. The exact timing of this measurement is critical as AFP levels change throughout pregnancy. Ultrasound diagnosis through direct visualization of the spinal defect or through indirect signs related to Arnold Chiari malformation has a sensitivity of greater than 90%. Determining the prognosis based on prenatal ultrasound remains difficult, except in obvious cases of encephalocele or anencephaly (see Chap. 1).

B. Postnatal diagnosis. Except for some secondary neural tube defects, most neural tube defects, especially meningomyelocele, are immediately obvious at birth. Occasionally some saccular masses, including sacrococcygeal teratomas, are confused with these. These are usually in the low sacrum.

III. Evaluation

A. History. Obtain a detailed family history. Ask about the occurrence of neural tube defects, and other congenital anomalies or malformation syndromes. Note should be made of any maternal medication use in the first trimester.

B. Physical examination. It is important to do a thorough physical examination, including a neurologic examination. The following are portions of the examination likely to reveal abnormal conditions:

1. **General newborn assessment.** Without exception, evaluate all newborns with neural tube defects for the presence of congenital heart disease, renal malformation, and structural defects of the airway, gastrointestinal tract, ribs, and hips. Although uncommon in primary neural tube defects, these can be encountered and should be considered before beginning surgical treatment or before discharge from the hospital. In addition, plan an ophthalmologic examination and hearing evaluation during the hospitalization or following discharge.

2. **Back.** Inspect the defect and note if it is leaking cerebrospinal fluid (CSF). Use a sterile nonlatex rubber glove when touching a leaking sac (in most circumstances, only the neurosurgeon needs to touch the back). Note the location, shape, and size of the defect, and observe the size of the cutaneous defect or thin "parchment-like" skin, although it has little relation to the size of the sac. Often the sac is deflated and has a wrinkled appearance. It is important to note the curvature of the spine and the presence of a bony gibbus underlying the defect. Occasionally, there is more than one meningomyelocele.

3. **Head.** Record the head circumference and plot daily throughout the first hospitalization. At birth, some infants will have macrocephaly due to hydrocephalus, and still more will develop hydrocephalus after closure of the defect on the back.

4. **Intracranial pressure (ICP).** Assess the ICP by palpating the anterior fontanel and tilting the head and torso forward until the midportion of the anterior fontanel is flat. The fontanels may be quite large and the calvarial bones widely separated. (See Intracranial Hemorrhage.)

5. **Eyes.** Abnormalities in conjugate movement of the eyes are common and include esotropias, esophorias, and abducens paresis.

6. **Lower extremities.** Look for deformities and evidence of muscle weakness. Abnormalities in the lower extremities, some representing deformations, are common. Look at thigh positions and skinfolds for evidence of congenital dislocation of the hips. Dislocation of the hips can be diagnosed clinically and by ultrasound (see Chap. 28).

7. **Neurologic examination.** Observe the child's spontaneous activity and response to sensory stimuli in all extremities. Predicting ambulation and muscle strength based on the "level" of the neurologic deficit can be misleading, and very often the anal reflex, or "wink," will be present at birth and absent postoperatively, owing to spinal shock and edema. Repeating neurologic examinations at periodic intervals is more helpful in predicting functional outcome than a single newborn examination. Similarly, sensory examination of the newborn can be misleading because of the potential absence of a motor response to pinprick. Carefully examine deep tendon reflexes (Table 27.10).

8. **Bladder and kidneys.** Observe bladder function, particularly for the possibility of inadequate emptying. Palpate the abdomen for evidence of kidney enlargement. Observe the pattern of urination, and check the child's response to Credé's maneuver by monitoring residual urine in the bladder.

IV. **Consultation.** The care of infants with neural tube defects requires the coordinated efforts of a number of medical and surgical specialists as well as specialists in nursing, physical therapy, and social service. If follow-up is by a myelodysplasia team, follow their protocols. If not, the following specialties represent the areas needing careful assessment:

A. **Specialty consultations**

1. **Neurosurgery.** The initial care of the child with a neural tube defect is predominantly neurosurgical. The neurosurgeon is responsible for assessment and surgical closure of the defect, and for control and treatment of elevated ICP.

2. **Pediatrics.** A thorough evaluation before surgical procedures is important, particularly for detecting other abnormalities that might influence surgical risk.

TABLE 27.10. CORRELATION BETWEEN SEGMENTAL INNERVATION; MOTOR, SENSORY, AND SPHINCTER FUNCTION; REFLEXES; AND AMBULATION POTENTIAL

Lesion	Segmental Innervation	Cutaneous Sensation	Motor Function	Working Muscles	Sphincter Function	Reflex	Potential for Ambulation
Cervical/thoracic	Variable	Variable	None	None	—	—	Poor, even in full braces
Thoracolumbar	T12	Lower abdomen	None	None	—	—	Full braces, long-term ambulation unlikely
	L1	Groin	Weak hip flexion	Iliopsoas	—	—	
	L2	Anterior upper thigh	Strong hip flexion	Iliopsoas and sartorius	—	—	
Lumbar	L3	Anterior distal thigh and knee	Knee extension	Quadriceps	—	Knee jerk	May ambulate with braces and crutches
	L4	Medial leg	Knee flexion and hip abduction	Medial hamstrings	—	Knee jerk	
Lumbosacral	L5	Lateral leg and medial knee	Foot dorsiflexion and eversion	Anterior tibial and peroneals	—	Ankle jerk	Ambulate with or without short leg braces
	S1	Sole of foot	Foot plantar flexion	Gastrocnemius, soleus, and posterior tibial	—	Ankle jerk	
Sacral	S2	Posterior leg and thigh	Toe flexion	Flexor hallucis	Bladder and rectum	Anal wink	Ambulate without braces
	S3	Middle of buttock	—	—	Bladder and rectum	Anal wink	
	S4	Medial buttock	—	—	Bladder and rectum	Anal wink	

Source: From Noetzel M. J. Myelomeningocele: Current concepts of management. *Clin Perinatol* 1984;6:318.

3. **Clinical genetics.** Begin a complete dysmorphology evaluation and genetic counseling during the first hospitalization and follow up during outpatient visits.

4. **Urology.** Consult a urologist on the day of birth because of the risk of obstructive uropathy.

5. **Orthopedics.** The pediatric orthopedic surgeon is responsible for the initial assessment of musculoskeletal abnormalities and long-term management of ambulation, seating, and spine stability. Clubfeet, frequently encountered in these newborns, should be assessed and may be managed during this hospitalization.

6. **Physical therapy.** Perform a thorough muscle examination as early as possible and involve physical therapists in planning for outpatient physical therapy programs.

7. **Social service.** Arrange for a social worker familiar with the special needs of children with neural tube defects to meet the parents as early as possible. Children with meningomyelocele may require a considerable amount of parents' time and resources, thereby placing considerable strain on parents and siblings.

B. **Diagnostic tests.** During the first hospitalization, the following tests should be done on most children with meningomyelocele. Scheduling these tests will vary depending on each situation.

1. **Radiographs:**

   a. **Chest.** Rib deformities are common; cardiac malformations also may be identified.

   b. **Spine.** Abnormalities in vertebral bodies, absent or defective posterior arches, and evidence of kyphosis are common.

   c. **Hips.** Evidence of dysplasia of hips is common, and some children with neural tube defects are born with dislocated hips. As noted, ultrasound examination of the hips can be very helpful to the orthopedic surgeon (see Chap. 28).

2. **Serum creatinine** level should be measured if voiding patterns appear initially abnormal. Occasionally, potassium levels may be elevated in the nonvoiding newborn.

3. **Ultrasound of the urinary tract** is useful to assess possible hydronephrosis and/or structural abnormalities of the upper urinary tract.

4. **Urodynamic study** should be done early in the hospitalization or shortly after discharge to document the status of the bladder and urinary sphincter function and innervation and to serve as a basis for comparison later in life.

5. Consider a **voiding cystourethrogram** if there is an abnormality seen on ultrasound or urodynamic study or in the setting of a rising serum creatinine level.

6. **Computed tomography (CT) of the head** is usually not necessary before repair of the defect on the back, but generally should be done soon thereafter, even if there is no clinical evidence of hydrocephalus. If ultrasonography is available and can accurately evaluate the presence of hydrocephalus, this may be a useful alternative to an initial CT. **Magnetic resonance imaging (MRI)** is particularly valuable in assessment of the posterior fossa and syringomyelia but should not necessarily replace CT or ultrasound in the initial assessment period.

V. **Selection of an approach to caring for children with neural tube defects**

A. **Initial general approach and ethical Issues.** There has long been debate regarding whether universal, aggressive treatment or selective treatment is most appropriate for infants with spina bifida. Early surgery permits survival of increased numbers of patients with neural tube defects, with outcomes similar to those previously published even for selected patients. It is our practice to identify risk factors that will likely contribute to poor outcome; these include major cerebral anomalies, hemorrhage, established infection, severe hydrocephalus, or high cord lesions. Although the prognosis for infants with these conditions is definitely worse, we do not base management decisions on any set protocol or scoring system. Prognostic criteria, if considered, should guide discussion, not replace the dialogue that is necessary between parents and care providers. Consult a hospital ethics committee to guide decision-making and to help establish a forum to discuss various opinions and treatment options.

Regardless of the management plan ultimately undertaken, every child with neural tube defects should receive well-planned and consistent care that respects his or her need for nutrition, comfort, and dignity and that honors the right of parents to participate in all decisions regarding care.

B. Specific selection of care

1. **Supportive care.** This implies no surgical repair of the back or placement of a ventriculoperitoneal (VP) shunt but includes nurturing, feeding on demand, and consideration of the child's comfort. The child may die of infection of the open lesion not treated with antibiotics or of complications from hydrocephalus or other congenital malformations. If death appears inevitable, exercise care not to prolong undue suffering with such interventions as ventilator support and pressors. Survival without surgery may occur for months or even years. In children who stabilize (e.g., complete epithelialization of the spinal defect), periodic reassessment of treatment options and discussion with the family become critical. Acceptable options to consider may include placement of a VP shunt to arrest progressive hydrocephalus, referral for foster and adoptive care, and alternative feeding techniques.

2. **Aggressive care.** The goal here is rehabilitation and planning intervention as completely as possible to prevent any further injury to the central nervous system or to prevent morbidity secondary to complications of bladder and bowel dysfunction and progressive orthopedic deformity.

VI. Management

A. Fetal surgery. Animal evidence suggests that in utero closure of myelomeningocele leads to improved peripheral function and prevention of Arnold-Chiari malformation. A multicenter randomized controlled trial of in utero surgical correction with standard management is currently in progress (8).

B. Perinatal. Consideration should be given to cesarean section given evidence of improved neuromotor outcomes with operative delivery. At birth, the very thin sac is often leaking. Keep the newborn in the prone position, with a sterile saline-moistened gauze sponge placed over the defect. This reduces bacterial contamination and damage related to dehydration. Administer intravenous antibiotics (ampicillin and gentamicin) to diminish the risk of meningitis, particularly that due to group B streptococci. Children with an open spinal defect can receive a massive inoculation of bacteria directly into the nervous system at the time of vaginal delivery or even in utero if the placental membranes rupture early. Meningitis is a particularly devastating complication. Because of the potential for allergy to latex rubber and possible anaphylaxis, no latex equipment should be used.

C. Surgical treatment. The initial neurosurgical treatment of an open meningomyelocele consists of (1) closing the defect to prevent infection and (2) reducing the elevated ICP. The back should be closed on the first day of life or as soon thereafter as safely possible to minimize bacterial contamination and the risk of infection. Techniques are available to close rapidly even very large cutaneous defects without skin grafting. Intracranial hypertension can be initially controlled by continuous ventricular drainage. Typically, once the back is sealed, a VP shunt catheter can be placed. Some neurosurgeons may elect to insert the catheter at the time of back closure. If a shunt is to be placed as a second procedure after back closure, careful monitoring of head circumference should be done because ICP often increases following closure of the back in unshunted patients.

Children whose defect is covered with skin and whose nervous system is therefore not at risk of bacterial contamination can undergo elective repair. This may be done at the age of 1 month or later.

D. Parents. Keep parents accurately informed of their child's condition. The involvement of multiple specialists heightens the importance of the identification of a primary care provider to coordinate the flow of information.

VII. Prognosis

A. Survival. Nearly all children with neural tube defects, even those severely affected, can survive for many years. The overall 1-year survival rate for children with myelomeningocele exceeds 96%, and the 10-year survival rate is 90%. It should be noted that survival rates are significantly influenced by decisions to intervene or to withhold aggressive medical and surgical care in the early neonatal period. Most deaths occur in the most severely affected children and are likely related to brainstem dysfunction, which is present in 1/3 (1).

B. Motor and intellectual outcome

1. **Motor outcome.** This depends more on the level of paralysis and surgical intervention than it does on congenital hydrocephalus. There is a likelihood that there will be a delay in motor progress in most children with neural tube defects, but appropriate bracing, physical therapy interventions, and monitoring and treatment of kyphosis and scoliosis can mitigate this. Also, such factors as obesity, frequent hospitalizations, tethering of the spinal cord, and decubitus ulcers can contribute to motor delays (3). Table 27.10 is a rough guide to motor, sensory, and sphincter function and ambulation potential.

2. **Intellectual outcome.** Three identifiable subgroups are at risk for mental retardation: those with severe hydrocephalus at birth, those who develop infection in the central nervous system early in life, and those whose intracranial hypertension is not properly controlled. True mental retardation is encountered most commonly in children who have high thoracic level lesions, a history of central nervous system infection, and hydrocephalus with less than 1 cm of cortical mantle. Formal developmental testing is critical, since visual/perceptual deficits and fine motor difficulties may interfere with intellectual functioning. In addition, complex partial seizures can contribute to impaired intellectual function and should be considered in children, especially school-age children who have lost cognitive milestones. Eighty-five percent of children whose spinal lesions are at L3 or lower usually complete twelfth grade or beyond.

C. Morbidity. The numbers of hospitalizations, of days in the hospital, and of operations required are much lower for children with sacral level lesions and much higher for those with thoracic lesions. Of 132 children consecutively admitted to the Children's Hospital of Boston for whom outcome is known beyond the age of 2 years, 12% have a "normal" gait, 7% have an abnormal gait but require no braces, 38% require braces, and 16% are only able to sit. Eighty-six percent live at home with the parents, and 4.6% live in a skilled nursing facility. Of children over 4 years old, 18% have "normal" bladder function, 21% receive intermittent catheterization, 42% void by Credé's maneuver, and 19% have an ileal conduit. Parents of 45% of the children over 4 years old report bowel function to be acceptable, and 49% report chronic bowel dysfunction, including encopresis. Of children over 5 years old, 45% attend regular public schools, and 89% of these are believed to be at grade level. Approximately 5% of newborns with open neural tube defects develop symptoms related to the Arnold-Chiari II malformation. These pontomedullary symptoms include stridor, ophthalmoplegia, apnea, abnormal gag, and vomiting (often confused with gastroesophageal reflex). These symptoms may indicate shunt malfunction but frequently disappear without treatment. If they persist, especially in association with cyanosis, the prognosis is poor, with the risk of respiratory failure and death. Posterior fossa decompression and cervical laminectomy are surgical options but are often not successful.

References

1. American Academy of Pediatrics, Committee on Genetics. Folic Acid for the Prevention of Neural Tube Defects. *Pediatrics* 1999;104:325–327.
2. Dias M. S., et al. Spinal dysraphism. In Weinstein, S. L. (Ed.), *The Pediatric Spine: Principles and Practice*. 1994. New York: Raven.
3. Kaplan L. C. Evaluation of the child with congenital anomalies. In: Rubin I. L., Crocker A. C. (Eds.), *Developmental Disabilities: Medical Care for Children and Adults*. 1989. Philadelphia: Lea & Febiger.
4. McLaughlin D. G., et al. Early neural development and the embryogenesis of dysraphism. In Chadduck W. (Ed.), *Pediatric Neurosurgery* (3rd ed.). 1994. Philadelphia: Saunders.
5. Volpe J. J. Human brain development. In: Volpe J. J. (Ed.), *Neurology of the Newborn* (4th ed.). 2001. Philadelphia: Saunders, p. 3.
6. MRC Vitamin Study Research Group. Prevention of neural tube defects: Results of the Medical Research Council Vitamin Study. *Lancet* 1991;338:131.
7. Czeizel A. E., Duds I. Prevention of the first occurrence of neural tube defects by periconceptual vitamin supplementation. *N Engl J Med* 1992;327:1832.
8. Jobe A. H. Fetal surgery for myelomeningocele. *N Engl J Med* 2002;347:4–6.

28. ORTHOPEDIC PROBLEMS

James R. Kasser

This chapter considers common musculoskeletal abnormalities that may be detected in the neonatal period. Consultation with an orthopedic surgeon is often required to provide definitive treatment after the initial evaluation.

I. **Torticollis**
   A. **Torticollis** is a disorder characterized by limited motion of the neck, asymmetry of the face and skull, and a tilted position of the head. It is usually caused by shortening of the **sternocleidomastoid (SCM) muscle** but may be secondary to muscle adaptation from an abnormal in utero position of the head and neck.
      1. The **etiology** of the shortened SCM muscle is unclear; in many infants it is due to an abnormal in utero position, and in some it may be due to stretching of the muscle at delivery. The result of the latter is a contracture of the muscle associated with fibrosis. One hypothesis is that the SCM abnormality is secondary to a compartment syndrome occurring at the time of delivery.
      2. **Clinical course.** The limitation of motion is minimum at birth, but increases over the first few weeks. At 10 to 20 days, in torticollis related to stretching, a mass is frequently found in the SCM muscle. This mass gradually disappears, and the muscle fibers are partially replaced by fibrous tissue, which contracts and limits head motion. Because of the limited rotation of the head, the infant rests on the ipsilateral side of the face in the prone position and on the contralateral side when supine. The pressure from resting on one side of the face and the opposite occipital bone contributes to the facial and skull asymmetry. The ipsilateral zygoma is depressed and the contralateral occiput flattened.
      3. **Treatment.** Most infants will respond favorably to positioning the head in the direction opposite to that produced by the tight muscle. Padded bricks or sandbags can be used to help maintain the position of the head until the child is able to move actively to free the head. Passive stretching by rotating the head to the ipsilateral side and tilting it toward the contralateral side also may help. The torticollis in most infants resolves by the age of 1 year. Patients who have asymmetry of the face and head and limited motion after 1 year should be considered for surgical release of the SCM muscle.
   B. **Torticollis with limited motion of the neck** may be due to a congenital abnormality of the cervical region of the spine. Some infants with this disorder also have a tight SCM muscle. These infants are likely to have significant limitation of motion at birth. Radiologic evaluation of the cervical region is necessary to make this diagnosis.
   C. A **third type of torticollis** is associated with congenital asymmetric contractures of the hip abductor and unilateral metatarsal adduction. The torticollis always subsides spontaneously. Since some infants with this type of torticollis have unilateral hip dysplasia, ultrasonography of the hips should be performed if examination reveals tightness in the hip abductors sufficient to cause a pelvic obliquity.
II. **Polydactyly**
   A. **Duplication of a digit** may range from a small cutaneous bulb to an almost perfectly formed digit. Treatment of this problem is variable. Syndromes associated with polydactyly include Laurence-Moon-Biedl syndrome, chondroectodermal dysplasia, Ellis-van Creveld syndrome, and trisomy 13. Polydactyly is

generally thought to be inherited in an autosomal dominant fashion with variable penetrance.

B. Treatment

1. The small functionless skin bulb without bone or cartilage at the ulnar border of the hand or lateral border of the foot can be ligated and allowed to develop necrosis for 24 hours. The part distal to the suture should be removed. The residual stump should have an antiseptic applied twice a day to prevent infection. Do not tie off digits on the radial side of the hand (thumb) or the medial border of the foot.

2. When duplicated digits contain bony parts, the decision about treatment is more difficult and should be delayed until the patient is evaluated by an orthopedist or hand surgeon. In general, polydactyly is managed surgically in the first year of life. X rays can be delayed until necessary for definitive management.

III. Fractured clavicle (see Chap. 20, Birth Trauma)

A. The **clavicle** is the site of the most common fracture associated with delivery.

B. Diagnosis is usually made soon after birth, when the infant does not move the arm on the affected side or cries when that arm is moved. There may be tenderness, swelling, or crepitance at the site. Occasionally, the bone is angulated. Diagnosis can be confirmed by radiographic examination. A "painless" fracture discovered by radiography of the chest is more likely a congenital pseudarthrosis (nonunion). Nearly all pseudarthroses occur on the right side.

C. The **clinical course** is such that clavicle fractures heal without difficulty. **Treatment** consists of providing comfort for the infant. If the arm and shoulder are left unprotected, motion occurs at the fracture site when the baby is handled. We usually pin the infant's sleeve to the shirt and put a sign on the baby to remind personnel to decrease motion of the clavicle. No reduction is necessary. If the fracture appears painful, a wrap to decrease motion of the arm is useful.

IV. Congenital and infantile scoliosis

A. Congenital scoliosis is a lateral curvature of the spine secondary to a failure either of formation of a vertebra or of segmentation. Scoliosis in the newborn may be difficult to detect; by bending the trunk laterally in the prone position, however, a difference in motion can usually be observed. Congenital scoliosis must be differentiated from **infantile scoliosis**, in which no vertebral anomaly is present. Infantile scoliosis often improves spontaneously, although the condition may be progressive in infants who have a spinal curvature of more than 20 degrees. If the scoliosis is progressive, treatment is indicated.

B. Clinical course. Congenital scoliosis will increase in many patients. Bracing of congenital curves is usually not helpful. Surgical correction and fusion are frequently indicated before the curve becomes severe. Since many patients with congenital curves have renal or other visceral abnormalities, studies should be done to detect these abnormalities.

V. Congenital dislocation of the hip. Most (but not all) hips that are dislocated at birth can be diagnosed by a careful physical examination (see Chap. 3). Ultrasound examination of the hip is useful for diagnosis in high-risk cases. In general, ultrasound is delayed as a screening technique until 1 month of age to avoid a high incidence of false-positive examinations. X-ray examination will not lead to a diagnosis in the newborn because the femoral head is not calcified but will reveal an abnormal acetabular fossa seen with hip dysplasia. There are three types of congenital dislocations.

A. The **classic congenitally dislocated hip** is diagnosed by the presence of Ortolani's sign. The hip is unstable and dislocates on adduction and also on extension of the femur but readily relocates when the femur is abducted in flexion. No asymmetry of the pelvis is seen. This type of dislocation is more common in females and is usually unilateral, but it may be bilateral. Hips that are unstable at birth often become stable after a few days. The infant with hips that are unstable after 5 days of life should be treated with a splint that keeps the hips flexed and abducted. The **Pavlik harness** has been used effectively to treat this group of patients. Ultrasound is used to monitor the hip during treatment as well as to confirm the initial diagnosis.

B. The **teratologic type of dislocation** occurs very early in pregnancy. The **femoral head does not relocate on flexion and abduction**; that is, Ortolani's sign is not present. If the dislocation is unilateral, there may be asymmetry of the gluteal folds and asymmetric motion with limited abduction. In bilateral dislocation, the perineum is wide and the thighs give the appearance of being shorter than normal. This may be easily overlooked, however, and requires an extremely careful physical examination. Treatment of the teratologic hip dislocation is by open reduction. Exercise to decrease contracture is indicated but use of the pavlik harness is generally not beneficial.

C. The **third type of dislocation** occurs late, is unilateral, and is associated with a **congenital abduction contracture** of the contralateral hip. The abduction contracture causes a pelvic obliquity. The pelvis is lower on the side of the contracture, which is unfavorable for the contralateral hip, and the acetabulum may not develop well. After the age of 6 weeks, infants with this type of dislocation develop an apparent short leg and have asymmetric gluteal folds. Some infants will develop a dysplastic acetabulum, which may eventually allow the hip to subluxate. Treatment of the dysplasia is with the Pavlik harness, but after the age of 8 months, other methods of treatment may be necessary.

VI. **Genu recurvatum,** or hyperextension of the knee, is not a serious abnormality and is easily recognized and treated. It must be differentiated, however, from subluxation or dislocation of the knee, which also may present with hyperextension of the knee. The latter two abnormalities are more serious and require more extensive treatment.

A. **Congenital genu recurvatum** is secondary to in utero position with hyperextension of the knee. This can be treated successfully by repeated cast changes, with progressive flexion of the knee until it reaches 90 degrees of flexion. Minor degrees of recurvatum can be treated with passive stretching exercises.

B. All infants with **hyperextension of the knee** should have a radiographic examination to differentiate genu recurvatum **from true dislocation of the knee**. In congenital genu recurvatum, the tibial and femoral epiphyses are in proper alignment except for the hyperextension. In the subluxed knee with dislocation, the tibia is completely anterior or anterolateral to the femur. The tibia is shifted forward in relation to the femur and is frequently lateral as well. Congenital fibrosis of the quadriceps is frequently associated with the subluxed and dislocated knee, and open reduction is essential, for attempted treatment of the dislocated knee by stretching or by repeated cast changes is hazardous and may result in epiphyseal plate damage.

VII. **Deformities of the feet**

A. **Metatarsus adductus** is a condition in which the metatarsals rest in an adducted position, but the appearance does not always reveal the severity of the condition. Whether or not treatment is necessary is determined by the difference in the degree of structural change in the metatarsals and tarsometatarsal joint.

1. Most infants with metatarsus adductus have **positional deformities** that are probably caused by in utero position. The positional type of metatarsus adductus is flexible and the metatarsals can be passively corrected into abduction with little difficulty. **This condition does not need treatment.**

2. The **structural metatarsus adductus** has a relatively fixed adduction deformity of the forefoot and the metatarsals cannot be abducted passively. The etiology has not been definitely identified but is probably related to in utero position. This is seen more commonly in the firstborn infant and

in pregnancies with oligohydramnios. Most infants with the structural types of metatarsus adductus have a valgus deformity of the hindfoot. **The structural deformity needs to be treated with manipulation and cast immobilization** until correction occurs. Although there is no urgency to treat this condition, it is more easily corrected earlier than later and should be done before the child is of walking age.

B. **Calcaneovalgus deformities** result from an in utero position of the foot that holds the ankle dorsiflexed and abducted. At birth, the top of the foot lies up against the anterior surface of the leg. Structural changes in the bones do not seem to be present. The sequela to this deformity appears to be a valgus or pronated foot that is more severe than the typical pronated foot seen in toddlers. Whether this disorder is treated or not is variable, and no study supports either course. **Treatment consists of either exercise or application of a short-leg cast** that will keep the foot plantar flexed and inverted. If the foot cannot be plantar flexed to a neutral position, casts are indicated. Casts are changed appropriately for growth and maintained until plantar flexion and inversion are equal to those of the opposite foot. Generally, the foot is held in plaster for about 6 to 8 weeks. Feet that remain in the calcaneovalgus position for several months may be more likely to have significant residual pes valgus; a fixed or rigid calcaneovalgus deformity probably represents a congenital vertical talus.

C. **Congenital clubfoot** is a congenital deformity with a multifactorial etiology. A first-degree relative of a patient with this deformity has 20 times the risk of having a clubfoot than does the normal population. The risk in subsequent siblings is 3 to 5%. The more frequent occurrence in the firstborn and the association with oligohydramnios suggest an influence of in utero pressure as well. Sometimes clubfoot is part of a syndrome. Infants with neurologic dysfunction of the feet (spina bifida) often have clubfoot.

1. **There are three and sometimes four components to the deformity.** The foot is in equinus, cavus, and varus position, with a forefoot adduction; thus the clubfoot is a talipes equinocavovarus with metatarsal adduction. Each of these deformities is sufficiently rigid to prevent passive correction to a neutral position by the examiner. The degree of rigidity is variable in each patient.

2. **Treatment** should be started early, within a few days of birth. An effective method of treatment **consists of manipulation and application of either tapes, or plaster or fiberglass casts that are changed every few days.** If conservative treatment does not successfully correct the deformities, surgical correction will be necessary.

Suggested Readings

Cooperman D.R., Thompson G.H. Neonatal Orthopaedics. In: Fanatoff A.A., Martin R.J. (Eds.), *Neonatal Perinatal Medicine,* 6th ed. 1997. St. Louis: Mosby, 1709.

Jones K.L. *Smith's Recognizable Patterns of Human Malformation,* 5th ed. 2002. Philadelphia: W.B. Saunders.

29. METABOLIC PROBLEMS

Hypoglycemia and Hyperglycemia

Richard E. Wilker

Hypoglycemia is one of the most common metabolic problems seen in both the newborn nursery and neonatal intensive care unit (NICU). However, its definition, clinical significance, and management remain controversial. Blood glucose levels are frequently lower in newborn babies than in older children or adults, but confirming a diagnosis of clinically significant hypoglycemia requires that one interpret the blood glucose level within the clinical context. Most cases of neonatal hypoglycemia are transient, respond readily to treatment, and are associated with an excellent prognosis. Persistent hypoglycemia, however, is more likely to be associated with abnormal endocrine conditions and possible neurologic sequelae.

Hyperglycemia is very rarely seen in the newborn nursery, but frequently occurs in very-low-birth-weight (VLBW) babies in the NICU.

I. **Hypoglycemia.** Glucose provides the fetus with approximately 60 to 70% of its energy needs. Almost all fetal glucose derives from the maternal circulation by the process of transplacental-facilitated diffusion that maintains fetal glucose levels at approximately two-thirds of maternal levels. The severing of the umbilical cord at birth abruptly interrupts the source of glucose, and to maintain adequate glucose levels, the newborn must rapidly respond by glycogenolysis of hepatic stores, inducing gluconeogenesis, and utilizing exogenous nutrients from feeding. During this transition, newborn glucose levels fall to a low point in the first 1 to 2 hours of life, and then increase and stabilize at mean levels of 65 to 70 mg/dL by the age of 3 to 4 hours.

A. **Incidence.** The reported incidence of hypoglycemia varies with its definition, but it has been estimated to occur in 8% of large-for-gestational-age (LGA) infants and 15% of small-for-gestational-age (SGA) babies.

B. **Definition.** Discussion of the incidence, effects, and treatment of hypoglycemia has been hampered by lack of agreement on its definition.

1. **Epidemiologic definition:**

a. Early definitions of normal neonatal glucose levels were derived by measuring glucose levels in populations of infants, some of whom were not being fed or given other sources of glucose. The statistical definition of normal, values that are within 2 standard deviations of the mean, resulted in the acceptance of glucose levels in the range of 20 to 30 mg/dL.

This definition was affected by clinical practice at the time, and did not define "optimal" glucose level in newborns.

2. Clinical definition (**Whipple's triad**):

a. Requires reliable measurement of a low glucose level.

b. Signs and symptoms consistent with hypoglycemia. **Development of clinical signs or symptoms may be a late sign of hypoglycemia.**

c. Resolution of signs and symptoms after blood glucose level is restored to normal range.

3. More recently, Cornblath recommended use of an "**Operational Threshold**" for blood-sugar management in newborn infants. The Operational Threshold is an indication for action, not diagnostic of disease.

a. Defines glucose level at which intervention should be considered based on current knowledge.

b. Differs from therapeutic goal.

c. Is dependent on clinical state.

d. Does not define normal or abnormal.

e. Provides margin of safety.

f. Operational thresholds as suggested by Cornblath et al.

(1) Healthy full-term infant:

(a) <24 hours of age—30 to 35 mg/dL may be acceptable once, but raised to 45 mg/dL if it persists after feeding or recurs in first 24 hours.

(b) After 24 hours, threshold should be increased to 45 to 50 mg/dL.

(2) Infant with abnormal signs or symptoms—45 mg/dL.

(3) Asymptomatic infants with risk factors for low blood sugar—36 mg/dL. Close surveillance is required and intervention is needed if plasma glucose remains below this level, it does not increase after feeding, or if abnormal clinical signs are seen.

(4) For any baby, if glucose levels are <20 to 25 mg/dL, IV glucose is needed to raise the plasma glucose to >45 mg/dL.

4. The significance of a given glucose level depends on the method of measurement, the infant's gestational age, chronological age, and other risk factors.

5. The absence of overt symptoms at low glucose levels does not rule out central nervous system (CNS) injury. There is no evidence indicating that the premature or young infant is protected from the effects of inadequate glucose delivery to the CNS.

6. There is no single value below which brain injury definitely occurs.

7. A glucose level less than 40 mg/dL at any time in any newborn requires follow-up glucose measurements to document a normal value.

8. Within the first hours of life, a normal asymptomatic baby may have a transient glucose level in the 30s (mg/dL) that will increase either spontaneously or in response to feeding. These babies have an excellent prognosis.

9. On the basis of recent developmental, neuroanatomic, metabolic, and clinical studies, our goal is to maintain the glucose value above 45 mg/dL in the first day, and more than 50 mg/dL thereafter.

C. Etiology

1. Increased utilization of glucose: hyperinsulinism

a. Diabetic mothers (see Chap. 2, Maternal Conditions That Affect the Fetus).

b. Large for gestational age (LGA) infants.

c. Erythroblastosis (hyperplastic islets of Langerhans) (see Chaps. 18 and 26).

d. Islet-cell hyperplasia, hyperfunction, focal hyperinsulinism, or diffuse hyperinsulinism (mutations of *SUR1* [high-affinity sulfonylurea receptor] or $K_{IR}6.2$ [potassium-channel gene]).

e. Beckwith-Weidemann syndrome (macrosomia, mild microcephaly, omphalocele, macroglossia, hypoglycemia, and visceromegaly).

f. Insulin-producing tumors (nesidioblastosis, islet-cell adenoma, or islet-cell dysmaturity).

g. Maternal tocolytic therapy with beta-sympathomimetic agents (terbutaline).

h. Maternal chlorpropamide therapy (Diabinese); possibly maternal thiazide diuretics (chlorothiazide).

i. Malpositioned umbilical artery catheter used to infuse glucose in high concentration into the celiac and superior mesenteric arteries T11 to 12, stimulating insulin release from the pancreas.

j. Abrupt cessation of high-glucose infusion.

k. After exchange transfusion with blood containing high-glucose concentration.

l. Exaggerated response to neonatal transition.

2. Decreased production/stores

a. Prematurity.

b. Intrauterine growth restriction (IUGR).

c. Inadequate caloric intake.

d. Delayed onset of feeding.

3. **Increased utilization and/or decreased production.** Any baby with one of the following conditions should be evaluated for hypoglycemia; parenteral glucose may be necessary for the management of these infants.

 a. **Perinatal stress**

 (1) Sepsis.

 (2) Shock.

 (3) Asphyxia.

 (4) Hypothermia (increased utilization).

 (5) Respiratory distress.

 b. **Exchange transfusion** with heparinized blood that has a low glucose level in the absence of a glucose infusion; reactive hypoglycemia after exchange with relatively hyperglycemic citrate-phosphate-dextrose (CPD) blood.

 c. **Defects in carbohydrate metabolism** (see Chap. 29)

 (1) Glycogen storage disease.

 (2) Fructose intolerance.

 (3) Galactosemia.

 d. **Endocrine deficiency**

 (1) Adrenal insufficiency.

 (2) Hypothalamic deficiency.

 (3) Congenital hypopituitarism.

 (4) Glucagon deficiency.

 (5) Epinephrine deficiency.

 e. **Defects in amino acid metabolism** (see Chap. 29)

 (1) Maple syrup urine disease.

 (2) Propionic acidemia.

 (3) Methylmalonic acidemia.

 (4) Tyrosinemia.

 (5) Glutaric acidemia type II.

 (6) Ethylmalonic adipic aciduria.

 (7) Glutaricidemia.

 f. **Polycythemia.** Hypoglycemia may be due to higher glucose utilization by the increased mass of red blood cells. The decreased amount of serum per drop of blood may cause a reading consistent with hypoglycemia on whole blood measurements, but may yield a normal glucose level on laboratory analysis of serum.

 g. **Maternal therapy with beta-blockers (e.g., labetalol or propranolol).** Possible mechanisms include the following:

 (1) Prevention of sympathetic stimulation of glycogenolysis.

 (2) Prevention of recovery from insulin-induced decreases in free fatty acids and glycerol.

 (3) Inhibition of epinephrine-induced increases in free fatty acids and lactate after exercise.

D. **Diagnosis**

 1. **Symptoms attributed to hypoglycemia are nonspecific.**

 a. Lethargy, apathy, and limpness.

 b. Apnea.

 c. Cyanosis.

 d. Weak or high-pitched cry.

 e. Seizures, coma.

 f. Poor feeding, vomiting.

 g. Tremors, jitteriness, or irritability.

 h. Seizures.

 i. Some infants may have no symptoms.

 2. **Screening.** Serial blood-glucose levels should be routinely measured in infants who have risk factors for hypoglycemia and in infants who have symptoms that could be due to hypoglycemia (see I.C and I.D.1).

   a. Babies with risk factors should have their glucose levels measured within the first 1 to 2 hours after birth. The length of time to continue screening depends on the glucose levels measured and the etiology of hypoglycemia. (See I.)

   (1) Infants of diabetic mothers usually develop hypoglycemia in the first hours of life and should have frequent early measurements of blood-glucose level (see Chap. 2, Maternal Conditions That Affect the Fetus).

   (2) Preterm and SGA infants should have blood-glucose measurements followed during the first 3 to 4 postnatal days.

   (3) Infants with erythroblastosis fetalis should have blood-glucose levels measured after exchange transfusions with CPD blood.

   (4) Infants with symptoms should be evaluated for hypoglycemia when the symptoms are present.

3. Reagent strips with reflectance meter. Although in widespread use as a screening tool, reagent strips are of unproven reliability in documenting hypoglycemia in neonates.

   a. Reagent strips measure whole blood glucose, which is 15% lower than plasma levels.

   b. Reagent strips are subject to false-positive and false-negative results, even when used with a reflectance meter.

   c. A confirmatory laboratory glucose determination is required before one can diagnose hypoglycemia.

   d. If a reagent strip reveals a concentration less than 45 mg/dL, treatment should not be delayed while one is awaiting confirmation of hypoglycemia by laboratory analysis. If an infant has either symptoms that could be due to hypoglycemia and/or a low glucose level as measured by reagent strip, treatment should be initiated immediately after the confirmatory blood sample is obtained.

4. Laboratory diagnosis

   a. The laboratory sample must be obtained and analyzed promptly to avoid the measurement being falsely lowered by glycolysis. The glucose level can fall 18 mg/dL per hour in a blood sample that awaits analysis.

5. Clinical confirmation of the diagnosis of symptomatic hypoglycemia requires both of the following:

   a. A laboratory-determined serum glucose level of less than 40 mg/dL at the time symptoms are present.

   b. Prompt resolution of the symptoms with the administration of intravenous glucose and correction of the hypoglycemia.

6. Additional testing. When the hypoglycemia or need for large glucose infusions lasts over 1 week, evaluation of some of the rare causes of hypoglycemia should be considered [See I.C.1]. At that time an endocrine consultation may be helpful and measurements of the following should be considered:

   a. Insulin.

   b. Growth hormone.

   c. Cortisol.

   d. Adrenocorticotropic hormone (ACTH).

   e. Thyroxine (T4).

   f. Glucagon.

   g. Plasma amino acids.

   h. Urine ketones.

   i. Urine-reducing substance.

   j. Urine amino acids.

   k. Urine organic acids.

7. Differential diagnosis. The symptoms mentioned in I.D can be due to many other causes with or without associated hypoglycemia. If symptoms

persist after the glucose concentration is in the normal range, other etiologies should be considered. Some of these are as follows:
  a. Adrenal insufficiency.
  b. Maternal drug use.
  c. Heart failure.
  d. Renal failure.
  e. Liver failure.
  f. CNS disease.
  g. Metabolic abnormalities
    (1) Hypocalcemia.
    (2) Hyponatremia or hypernatremia.
    (3) Hypomagnesemia.
    (4) Pyridoxine deficiency.
  h. Sepsis.
  i. Asphyxia.
E. **Management.** Anticipation and prevention, when possible, are key to the management of hypoglycemia.
  1. Well infants who are at risk for hypoglycemia (see I.C) should have serial blood-glucose levels measured. **Infants of diabetic mothers** should have glucose measured, and be treated, according to the protocol in Chap. 2.
  2. Other **asymptomatic** infants who are at risk for hypoglycemia should have blood glucose measured in the first 1 to 2 hours of life. As soon after birth as their condition allows they should be nursed or given formula. This feeding should be repeated every 2 to 3 hours.
  3. **The interval between measurement of glucose levels requires clinical judgment.** If the glucose concentration is as low as 20 to 25 mg/dL, the baby should be treated with intravenous glucose with a goal of maintaining the glucose greater than 45 mg/dL in the first 24 hours, and > 50 mg/dL thereafter.
  4. **Feeding.** Some infants with early glucose levels in the 30s (mg/dL) will respond to feeding (breast or bottle). A follow-up blood glucose should be measured within 1 hour of the feeding. If the glucose level does not rise or falls again, more aggressive therapy may be needed. While early feeding of glucose water will transiently raise the serum glucose level, there is often an associated rebound hypoglycemia, within 1 to 2 hours of the glucose water feeding. The early introduction of milk feeding will often result in raising glucose levels to normal, maintaining normal stable levels, and avoiding problems with rebound hypoglycemia. We sometimes find it useful to add Polycose (4 Kcal/oz) to feedings in infants who feed well but have marginal glucose levels.
  5. **Breastfeeding.** Babies who are breastfed have lower glucose levels but higher ketone body levels than those who are formula-fed. The use of alternate fuels may be an adaptive mechanism during the first days of life as breastfeeding is developing. Early breastfeeding enhances gluconeogenesis and increases the production of gluconeogenic precursors. Some infants will have difficulty in adapting to breastfeeding, and symptomatic hypoglycemia has been reported to develop in breastfed babies after hospital discharge. It is important to document that breastfed babies are latching on and appear to be sucking milk, but there is no need to routinely monitor glucose levels in healthy full-term breastfed babies.
  6. **IV therapy**
    a. **Indications:**
      (1) Unable to tolerate oral feeding.
      (2) Symptomatic.
      (3) Oral feedings do not maintain normal glucose levels.
      (4) Glucose levels less than 25 mg/dL.
    b. **Urgent treatment:**
      (1) 200 mg/kg of glucose over 1 minute; to be followed by continuing therapy below

This is equivalent to 2 mL/kg of dextrose 10% in water (10% D/W) infused intravenously over 1 minute

$$10\% \text{ D/W} = \frac{10 \text{ g glucose}}{100 \text{ mL}} = \frac{1 \text{ g glu}}{10 \text{ mL}} = 100 \text{ mg/mL}$$

200 mg dextrose is present in 2 ml 10% DW
Dose of 200 mg/kg = 2 mL/kg

c. Continuing therapy:
(1) Infusion of glucose at a rate of 6 to 8 mg of glucose/kg per minute.
(2) 10% D/W at a rate of 86.4 mL/kg per day or 3.6 mL/kg per hour gives 6 mg/kg per minute of glucose (Fig. 29.1, glucose rate calculation).
(3) Recheck glucose level after 20 to 30 minutes and hourly until stable, to determine if additional therapy is needed.
(4) Additional bolus infusions of 2 mL/kg of 10% D/W may be needed.
(5) If glucose is stable and in acceptable range feedings may be continued and the glucose infusion tapered as permitted by glucose measurements prior to feeding.

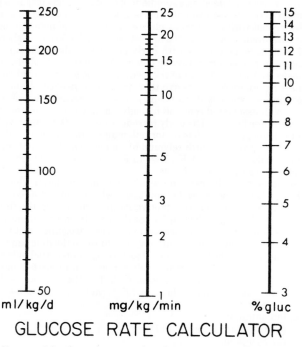

GLUCOSE RATE CALCULATOR

Use a straight edge to determine the volume required per 24 hours.

FIG. 29.1. Interconversion of glucose infusion units. (From Klaus M. H. Faranoff A. A. (Eds.), *Care of the High-risk Neonate,* 2nd ed. Philadelphia: Saunders, 1979, p. 430.)

d. For most infants, intravenous 10% D/W at daily maintenance rates will provide adequate glucose. The concentration of the dextrose in fluids will depend on the daily water requirement. It is suggested that calculation of both glucose intake (i.e., milligrams of glucose per kilogram per minute) and water requirements be done each day. For example, on the first day the fluid requirement is 80 mL/kg per day, or 0.055 mL/kg per minute; therefore, 10% D/W provides 5.5 mg of glucose per kilogram per minute, and 15% D/W provides 8.25 mg of glucose per kilogram per minute.

e. Some infants with hyperinsulinism and infants with IUGR will require 12 to 15 mg of dextrose per kilogram per minute (often as 15% or 20% D/W).

f. The concentration of glucose and the rate of infusion are increased as necessary to maintain a normal blood glucose level. A central venous catheter may be necessary to give adequate glucose (15% to 20% D/W) in an acceptable fluid volume. Taper glucose to 4 to 6 mg/kg per minute, monitoring glucose levels; then wean slowly while oral feedings are advanced.

7. Consider adding **hydrocortisone,** 10 mg/kg per day intravenously in two divided doses, if the infant requires more than 12 mg of glucose per kilogram per minute to maintain an adequate serum level. Hydrocortisone reduces peripheral glucose utilization, increases gluconeogenesis, and increases the effects of glucagons. The hydrocortisone will usually result in stable and adequate glucose levels, and it can then be rapidly tapered over the course of a few days. Before administering hydrocortisone, obtain a blood sample for measurements of glucose, insulin, and cortisol levels. Cortisol levels can be used to screen for the integrity of the hypothalamic-pituitary-adrenal axis.

8. Unless there is a suspicion of a metabolic defect, feedings of mothers milk or formula can be started and advanced as the clinical situation allows. As the feedings are advanced and the intravenous glucose infusion is tapered, it is important to continue to monitor glucose levels.

9. Glucagon 0.025–0.3 mg/kg intramuscularly (maximum 1.0 mg) may be given to hypoglycemic infants with good glycogen stores but it is only a temporizing measure to mobilize glucose for 2 to 3 hours in an emergency until intravenous glucose can be given. The glucose level will often fall after the effects of glucagon have worn off, and it remains important to obtain intravenous access to adequately treat these babies. For infants of diabetic mothers, the dose is 0.3 mg/kg (maximum dose is 1.0 mg) (see Chap. 2, Diabetes Mellitus).

10. Diazoxide (2 to 5 mg/kg per dose orally given q8h) may be given for infants who are persistently hyperinsulinemic. It inhibits insulin release by acting as a specific adenosine triphosphate (ATP)-sensitive potassium channel agonist in normal pancreatic beta cells decreasing insulin release. A positive response is usually seen in 48 to 72 hours if it is going to occur.

11. Other. Epinephrine and growth hormone are used rarely and only in treatment of persistent hypoglycemia. Surgical subtotal pancreatectomy may be necessary for insulin-secreting tumors.

12. Additional evaluation. Most hypoglycemia will resolve in 2 to 3 days. A requirement of more than 8 mg of glucose per kilogram per minute suggests increased utilization due to hyperinsulinism. This is usually transient as in infants of diabetic mothers. If it lasts more than 7 days, endocrine evaluation may be necessary to rule out excess insulin secretion from an insulin-secreting tumor or other cause as listed in I.B.

a. A sample drawn to determine insulin level at the same time as low blood glucose will document an inappropriate secretion of insulin.

b. If the insulin level is normal for the blood glucose level, other causes of persistent hypoglycemia such as defects in carbohydrate metabolism (see I.C.3.c), endocrine deficiency (see I.C.3.d), and defects in amino acid metabolism (see I.C.3.e) should be considered.

c. Evaluation will often require allowing the blood glucose level to reach a level as low as (20 mg/dL) and then drawing blood for insulin, cortisol, and amino acids. Many evaluations are not productive because they are done too early in the course of a transient hypoglycemic state or the samples to determine hormone levels are drawn when the glucose level is normal.

d. Genetic testing is available for *SUR1* and $K_{ir}6.2$ mutations.

II. **Hyperglycemia** is usually defined as a whole-blood glucose level higher than 125 mg/dL or plasma glucose values higher than 145 mg/dL. This problem is commonly encountered in low-birth-weight premature infants receiving parenteral glucose but is also seen in other infants who are sick. There are usually not any specific symptoms associated with neonatal hyperglycemia, but the major clinical problems associated with hyperglycemia are hyperosmolarity and osmotic diuresis. Osmolarity of more than 300 mOsm/L usually leads to osmotic diuresis (each 18 mg/dL rise in blood-glucose concentration increases serum osmolarity 1 mOsm/L). Subsequent dehydration may occur rapidly in small premature infants with large insensible fluid losses.

The hyperosmolar state, an increase of 25 to 40 mOsm or a glucose level of more than 450 to 720 mg/dL, can cause water to move from the intracellular compartment to the extracellular compartment. The resultant contraction of the intracellular volume of the brain may be a cause of intracranial hemorrhage.

A. **Etiology**

1. **Exogenous parenteral glucose** administration of more than 6.0 mg of glucose per kilogram per minute in normal term infants or of more than 6.6 mg of glucose per kilogram per minute in preterm infants weighing less than 1000 g may be associated with hyperglycemia.

2. **Drugs.** The most common association is with steroids used for treatment of hypotension. Other drugs associated with hyperglycemia are caffeine, theophylline, phenytoin, and diazoxide.

3. **Very-low-birth-weight infants** (<1000 g), possibly due to variable insulin response, to persistent endogenous hepatic glucose production despite significant elevations in plasma insulin, or to insulin resistance that may in part be due to immature glycogenolysis enzyme systems. Very-low-birth-weight infants will often have fluid requirements exceeding 200 mL/kg per day. A minimum glucose concentration of dextrose 5% must be used to avoid infusing a hypotonic solution and when this fluid is administered the infant may be presented with an excessive glucose load.

4. **Lipid infusion.** Free fatty acids are associated with increased glucose levels.

5. **Sepsis,** possibly due to depressed insulin release, cytokines, or endotoxin, resulting in decreased glucose utilization. Stress hormones such as cortisol and catecholamines are elevated in sepsis. In an infant who has normal glucose levels and then becomes hyperglycemic without an excess glucose load, sepsis should be the prime consideration.

6. **"Stressed" premature infants** requiring mechanical ventilation or other painful procedures, from persistent endogenous glucose production due to catecholamines and other "stress hormones." Insulin levels are usually appropriate for the glucose level.

7. **Hypoxia,** possibly due to increased glucose production in the absence of a change in peripheral utilization.

8. **Surgical procedures.** Hyperglycemia in this setting is possibly due to the secretion of epinephrine, glucocorticoids, and glucagon as well as excess administration of glucose-containing intravenous fluids.

9. **Transient neonatal diabetes mellitus**. In this rare disorder, infants present with hyperglycemia usually before the age of 15 days (range 2 days to 6 weeks). They characteristically are small for gestational age (SGA)

term infants, they have no gender predilection, and a third have a family history of diabetes mellitus. They present with marked glycosuria, hyperglycemia (240 to 2300 mg/dL), polyuria, severe dehydration, acidosis, mild or absent ketonuria, reduced subcutaneous fat, and failure to thrive. Insulin values are either absolutely or relatively low for the corresponding blood-glucose elevation. **Treatment** consists of rehydration, and the majority require insulin (regular 0.5 to 3.0 units/kg per day subcutaneously divided q6h or 0.01 to 0.10 unit/kg per hour by constant infusion). Start with the intravenous dose, and then switch to the subcutaneous dose. Monitor serum electrolytes, glucose, and acid–base balance. Repeated plasma insulin values are necessary to distinguish transient from permanent diabetes mellitus. The average length for insulin treatment is 65 days (range, 3 days to 18 months). Fifty percent of the cases are transient. Some transient cases will have a later recurrence. Some cases are permanent. Cases presenting after 3 weeks and in infants with HLA-DR3+DR4 haplotypes have a higher incidence of permanent diabetes. The transient nature of this disorder may be due to delayed or abnormal maturation of the B cell, transiently deficient or delayed insulin secretion, or secretion of an abnormal insulin molecule.

10. **Diabetes due to pancreatic lesions** such as pancreatic aplasia, or hypoplastic or absent pancreatic beta cells is usually seen in SGA infants who may have other congenital defects. They usually present soon after birth and rarely survive.

11. **Transient hyperglycemia associated with ingestion of hyperosmolar formula.** Clinical presentation may mimic transient neonatal diabetes with glycosuria, hyperglycemia, and dehydration. A history of inappropriate formula dilution is key. Treatment consists of rehydration, discontinuation of the hyperosmolar formula, and appropriate instructions for mixing concentrated or powder formula. Insulin has been used briefly but cautiously.

12. **Hepatic glucose production** can persist despite normal or elevated glucose levels.

13. **Immature development of glucose transport proteins,** such as GLUT-4.

B. **Treatment.** The primary goal is prevention and early detection of hyperglycemia by carefully adjusting glucose-infusion rates, and frequent monitoring of blood-glucose levels and urine for glycosuria. If present, evaluation and possible intervention are indicated.

1. Measure glucose levels in premature infants or infants with abnormal symptoms.

2. Extremely low-birth-weight premature infants (<1000 g) should start with an intravenous glucose concentration no higher than 5%. If hyperglycemia is documented, parenteral glucose intake is reduced to 4.0 to 6.0 mg of glucose per kilogram per minute by adjusting the concentration or the rate (or both) of glucose infusion and monitoring the falling blood-glucose level. Hypotonic fluids (solutions < dextrose 5%) should be avoided.

3. If appropriate, decrease the glucose infusion by 2 mg/kg per minute every 4 to 6 hours (see Fig. 29.1).

4. Begin parenteral nutrition as soon as possible in low-birth-weight infants. Some amino acids promote insulin secretion.

5. Feed if condition allows; feeding can promote the secretion of hormones that promote insulin secretion.

6. Many small infants will initially be unable to tolerate a certain glucose load (e.g., 6 mg/kg per minute) but will eventually develop tolerance if they are presented with just enough glucose to keep their glucose level high yet not enough to cause glycosuria.

7. Exogenous insulin therapy has been used when glucose values exceed 250 mg/dL despite efforts to lower the amount of glucose delivered or when prolonged restriction of parenterally administered glucose would

substantially decrease the required total caloric intake. Neonates may be extremely sensitive to the effects of insulin. It is desirable to decrease the glucose level gradually to avoid rapid fluid shifts. Very small doses of insulin are used and the actual amount delivered may be difficult to determine because some of the insulin is adsorbed on the glass or plastic surfaces of the intravenous tubing.

a. Continuous insulin infusion

(1) The standard dilution is 10 units regular insulin/100 mL D5 or D10.

(2) Flush the IV tubing with 50 to 100 mL of this insulin solution to saturate binding sites.

(3) Rate of infusion is 0.01 to 0.2 unit/kg per hour.

(4) Check glucose levels every 30 minutes until stable to adjust the infusion rate.

(5) Monitor potassium level.

(6) Monitor for rebound hyperglycemia.

b. Subcutaneous insulin

(1) (This is rarely used except in neonatal diabetes. Dose is 0.10 to 0.20 unit/kg every 6 hours Monitor glucose level at 1, 2, and 4 hours.

(2) Monitor potassium level every 6 hours initially.

Suggested Readings

Cornblath M., Ichord, R. Hypoglycemia in the neonate. *Semin Perinatology* 2000; 24:136.

Cornblath M., et al. Controversies regarding definition of neonatal hypoglycemia: Suggested operational thresholds. *Pediatrics* 2000;105:1141.

Cowett R.M. Neonatal hypoglycemia: A little goes a long way. *J Pediatr* 1999; 134:389.

deLonlay-Debeney P., et al. Clinical features of 52 neonates with hyperinsulinism. *N Engl J Med* 1999; 340:1169.

Duvanel C.B., et al. Long-term effects of neonatal hypoglycemia on brain growth and psychomotor development in small-for-gestational-age preterm infants. *J Pediatr* 1999;134:492.

Eidelman A. Hypoglycemia and the breastfed neonate. *Pediatr Clin North Am* 2001;48:377.

Farrag H.M., Cosett R.M. Glucose homeostasis in the micropremie. *Clin Perinatol* 2000; 27:1.

Hemachandra A.H., Cosett R.M. Neonatal hyperglycemia. *NeoReviews* July 1999. Available: www.neoreviews.org.

Kalhan S., Peter-Wohl S. Hypoglycemia: What is it for the neonate? *Am J Perinatol* 2000;17:11.

Kinnala A., et al. Cerebral magnetic resonance imaging and ultrasonographic findings after neonatal hypoglycemia. *Pediatrics* 1999;103:724.

McGwan J.E. Neonatal hypoglycemia. *NeoReviews* July 1999. Available: www.neo reviews.org.

Menni F., et al. Neurologic outcomes of 90 neonates with persistent hyperinsulinemic hypoglycemia. *Pediatrics* 2001;107:476.

Moore A.M., Perlman M. Symptomatic hypoglycemia in otherwise healthy, breastfed newborns. *Pediatrics* 1999;103:837.

Srinivasan G., et al. Plasma glucose values in normal neonates: A new look. *J Pediatr* 1986;109:114.

HYPOCALCEMIA, HYPERCALCEMIA, AND HYPERMAGNESEMIA

Kenneth M. Huttner

Calcium is physiologically important in two general ways. First, **calcium salts in bone** provide structural integrity. Decreased skeletal calcium is a hallmark of neonatal metabolic bone disease (see Metabolic Bone Disease of Prematurity). Second, **calcium ions (Ca^{2+}) in cellular and extracellular fluid (ECF)** are essential for many biochemical processes. Significant aberrations of serum calcium concentrations are observed frequently in the neonatal period. One must evaluate these alterations in light of the normal dynamic changes in serum calcium level that take place during the first week of life. Consequently, a given serum calcium level cannot be interpreted without knowing the newborn's postnatal age.

I. **Principles of mineral metabolism**
    A. **Laboratory measurement of serum calcium**
        1. There are **three definable fractions of calcium** in serum: (a) **ionized calcium** (about 50% of serum total calcium); (b) **calcium bound to serum proteins,** principally albumin (about 40%); and (c) **calcium complexed to serum anions,** mostly phosphates, citrate, and sulfates (about 10%). **Ionized calcium is the only biologically available form of calcium.**
        2. For routine clinical purposes, measurement of serum total calcium level usually is adequate. Some clinical laboratories can measure the ionized calcium level in microspecimens of anticoagulated blood collected anaerobically. Algorithms for correcting serum total calcium level for alterations in serum albumin concentration and/or pH or for calculating "free" calcium concentrations are not reliable compared with actual measurements of ionized calcium.
        3. Calcium concentration reported as milligrams per deciliter can be converted to molar units by dividing by 4 (e.g., 10 mg/dL converts to 2.5 mmol/L).
    B. **Hormonal regulation of calcium homeostasis** (Fig. 29.2). Regulation of serum and ECF-ionized calcium concentration within a narrow range is critical for blood coagulation, neuromuscular excitability, cell membrane integrity and function, and cellular enzymatic and secretory activity. The principal calcitropic or calcium-regulating hormones are **parathyroid hormone (PTH)** and **1,25-dihydroxyvitamin D ($1,25(OH)_2D_3$).**
        1. **PTH.** When ECF-ionized calcium level declines, parathyroid cells secrete PTH. PTH mobilizes calcium from bone, increases calcium resorption in the renal tubule, and stimulates renal production of $1,25(OH)_2D_3$. PTH also mobilizes phosphate from bone and produces significant phosphaturia. Therefore, **PTH secretion causes the serum calcium level to rise and the serum phosphorus level to be maintained or fall.** Newborns in the first 2 days of life may exhibit decreased renal responsiveness to PTH.
        2. **$1,25(OH)_2D_3$ (calcitriol).** Inactive vitamin D is synthesized in skin exposed to sunlight and is also ingested in the diet. The liver then synthesizes **$25(OH)D_3$ (the major storage form of the hormone)** and the kidney synthesizes the **biologically active hormone, $1,25(OH)_2D_3$.** $1,25(OH)_2D_3$ increases intestinal calcium and phosphate absorption and mobilizes calcium and phosphate from bone.

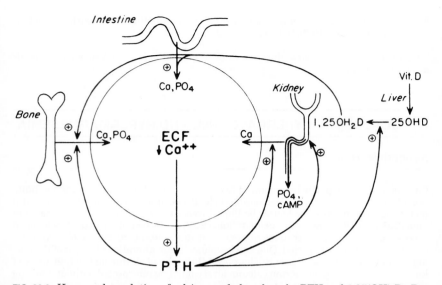

FIG. 29.2. Hormonal regulation of calcium and phosphate by PTH and $1,25(OH)_2D_3$. Decreased Ca^{2+} stimulates PTH and $1,25 (OH)_2D$ secretion. Renal, gastrointestinal, and skeletal mechanisms will increase Ca^{2+}, inhibiting PTH secretion and closing the negative-feedback loop. (PTH = parathyroid hormone; $1,25(OH)_2D$ = 1,25-dihydroxyvitamin D; 25(OH)D = 25-hydroxyvitamin D; Ca^{2+} = ionized calcium; PO_4 = inorganic phosphate; ECF = extracellular fluid; cAMP = cyclic adenosine monophosphate.) (From Brown E. M. Regulation of synthesis, metabolism, and actions of parathyroid hormone. *Contemp Iss Nephrol* 1983;151.)

    3. Calcitonin. Calcitonin, secreted by thyroid C cells, **inhibits bone resorption and has an antihypercalcemic effect.** Its significance for calcium regulation in the human adult is controversial. Calcitonin may play a more important calcitropic role during fetal and/or neonatal development.

  C. Postnatal changes in serum calcium concentrations. The flow of calcium ions from mother to fetus during the third trimester of gestation is associated with **fetal chronic hypercalcemia.** At birth, the umbilical serum calcium level is elevated (10 to 11 mg/dL). In healthy term babies, calcium concentrations decline for the first 24 to 48 hours; the nadir is usually 7.5 to 8.5 mg/dL. Thereafter, calcium concentrations progressively rise to the mean values observed in older children and adults.

    Serum calcium concentrations in the first 3 days of life are also positively correlated with gestational age.

II. Hypocalcemia. Neonatal **hypocalcemia** usually is defined as a total serum calcium concentration of less than 7.0 mg/dL and an ionized calcium concentration of less than 4.0 mg/dL (1.0 mmol/L).

  A. Etiology

    1. Early-onset hypocalcemia (during the first 3 days)

      a. Preterm newborns are born amid the third-trimester growth spurt. They are poorly adapted to the cessation of maternal calcium flow and at birth face a calcium crisis. About 50% of low-birth-weight infants and **nearly all** very-low-birth-weight (VLBW) infants exhibit total serum calcium levels of less than 7.0 mg/dL by day 2. This hypocalcemia appears to be an exaggeration of the normal term pattern; the nadir occurs by 12 to 24 hours, with little change until 72 hours. The pathogenesis is probably multifactorial. Preterm newborns do mount a PTH response, but target-organ responsiveness to PTH may be diminished. Even VLBW newborns can synthesize $1,25(OH)_2D_3$ if vitamin D stores are adequate. Hypercalcitoninemia may be important. High renal sodium excretion in preterm newborns may aggravate calciuric losses.

   b. Infants of diabetic mothers (IDMs) (see Chap. 2) have a 25 to 50% incidence of hypocalcemia during the first 24 to 48 hours. The natural history may be similar to that of early neonatal hypocalcemia in preterm infants, or hypocalcemia may persist for several days. Hypercalcitoninemia, hypoparathyroidism, abnormal vitamin D metabolism, and hyperphosphatemia have been implicated, but none has been found consistently. The lower mean maternal and umbilical calcium and magnesium levels associated with diabetes may be important. Strict metabolic control during pregnancy reduces this neonatal complication.

   c. Severe neonatal birth depression is associated frequently with hypocalcemia and hyperphosphatemia, (see Chap. 27, Perinatal Asphyxia). Decreased calcium intake, increased endogenous phosphate load, and increased calcitonin concentrations may contribute.

2. **Late-onset hypocalcemia** usually presents at the end of the first week, but onset ranges from the first days to several weeks after birth. The classical syndrome was described in term infants fed **high-phosphate diets.** Contributing factors probably include neonatal immaturity of renal tubular phosphate excretion, hypoparathyroidism, hypomagnesemia, and vitamin D deficiency. Specific etiologies include the following:

   a. Hypoparathyroidism (most common)
      (1) Idiopathic, transient.
      (2) Congenital. Parathyroids may be absent in **DiGeorge's sequence** (hypoplasia or absence of the third and fourth branchial pouch structures) as an isolated defect in the development of the parathyroid glands, or as part of the Kenny-Coffey syndrome.
      (3) Pseudohypoparathyroidism.
      (4) Maternal hyperparathyroidism induces transient neonatal hypoparathyroidism.
      (5) Magnesium deficiency (including inborn error of intestinal magnesium transport) impairs PTH secretion.

   b. Vitamin D deficiency
      (1) Secondary to **maternal vitamin D deficiency.**
      (2) Malabsorption.
      (3) Maternal anticonvulsant therapy during pregnancy increases catabolism of vitamin D.
      (4) Renal insufficiency may impair $1,25(OH)_2D_3$ production.
      (5) Nephrosis and **impaired enterohepatic circulation** accelerate losses of $25(OH)D_3$.
      (6) Hepatobiliary disease may decrease production of $25(OH)D_3$.

   c. Miscellaneous
      (1) Rapid or excessive skeletal mineral deposition **("hungry bones" syndrome)** may occur in small-for-gestational-age (SGA) infants or in infants with rickets or hypoparathyroidism who receive aggressive vitamin D therapy.
      (2) Hyperphosphatemia is associated with phosphate-rich diets, excessive phosphate administration, renal insufficiency, asphyxia, hypervitaminosis D, hypoparathyroidism, and rhabdomyolysis.
      (3) Hypoalbuminemia. Ionized calcium level is unchanged.
      (4) Alkalosis and **bicarbonate therapy.**
      (5) Rapid infusion of **citrate-buffered blood** (exchange transfusion) chelates ionized calcium.

     (6) Lipid infusions may lower the ionized calcium level by enhancing calcium-albumin binding.

     (7) Furosemide produces marked hypercalciuria.

     (8) Shock or **sepsis.**

     (9) Hypothyroidism infrequently is associated with hypocalcemia in patients with pseudohypoparathyroidism.

    (10) Rapid **albumin infusion** may lead to a transient increase in protein-bound and a decrease in ionized calcium.

    (11) Phototherapy may be associated with hypocalcemia by decreasing melatonin secretion and increasing bone uptake of calcium.

B. Evaluation

  1. Clinical manifestations

    a. Hypocalcemia increases cellular permeability to sodium ions and increases cell membrane excitability. The signs are usually nonspecific: apnea, seizures, jitteriness, increased extensor tone, clonus, hyperreflexia, and stridor (laryngospasm). Carpopedal spasm and Chvostek's sign are present less frequently.

    b. Early-onset hypocalcemia in preterm newborns is usually asymptomatic or clinically mild.

    c. Late-onset syndromes, in contrast, may present as hypocalcemic seizures.

  2. Laboratory evaluation

    a. Suggested schedule for monitoring calcium levels in infants at risk for developing hypocalcemia:

     (1) Preterm infants (>1000 g): at 24 and 48 hours of life.

     (2) Preterm infants (<1000 g): at 12, 24, and 48 hours.

     (3) Sick or stressed infants: at 12, 24, and 48 hours, and then as indicated.

     (4) Healthy preterm infants (>1500 g) and healthy IDMs who begin milk feedings on the first day do not need to be monitored in the absence of signs or symptoms.

    b. An electrocardiographic Q–T_c interval longer than 0.4 second (due to prolonged systole), when present, is a useful indicator of hypocalcemia and helpful in monitoring therapy (0.44 sec is the ninety-seventh percentile for infants 3–4 days old).

$$Q\text{–}T_c = \text{corrected QT interval} = \frac{\text{measured QT (sec)}}{\sqrt{R\text{—}R \text{ interval (sec)}}}$$

    c. For other than straightforward early-onset hypocalcemia, measure calcium, ionized calcium, phosphorus, and magnesium levels. Assessment of albumin, urinary calcium, PTH, vitamin D_3 metabolite levels and renal function also may be helpful.

     (1) Elevated serum phosphorus level suggests phosphate loading, renal insufficiency, or hypoparathyroidism.

     (2) Magnesium level of 0.8 mg/dL or less strongly suggests primary **hypomagnesemia.**

     (3) Normal to moderately elevated $1,25(OH)_2D_3$ levels are consistent with hypoparathyroidism.

     (4) Absence of a thymic shadow on a chest radiograph and the presence of conotruncal cardiac abnormalities may suggest a diagnosis of 22q11 syndrome also known as CATCH22 or DiGeorge sequence.

     (5) Urinary calcium excretion of more than 4 mg/kg per day or a 24-hour urine calcium:creatinine ratio of more than 0.2 (mg/ mg) is indicative of hypercalciuria in individuals with mature renal function. Hypercalciuria associated with hypocalcemia suggests a deficiency of PTH. In the premature infant, especially one receiving large amounts of supplemental calcium, these values may not be applicable.

C. Management

1. **Treatment of hypocalcemia is associated with certain risks,** which are minimized by attention to details.

   a. Rapid intravenous infusion of calcium can cause sudden elevation of serum calcium level, leading to bradycardia or other dysrhythmias. Intravenous calcium should only be "pushed" for treatment of hypocalcemic crisis (e.g., with seizures).

   b. Infusion by means of the umbilical vein may result in hepatic necrosis if the catheter is lodged in a branch of the portal vein.

   c. Rapid infusion by means of the umbilical artery can cause arterial spasms and, at least experimentally, intestinal necrosis.

   d. Intravenous calcium solutions are incompatible with sodium bicarbonate, since calcium carbonate will precipitate.

   e. Intravenous infusion of calcium chloride may produce chloride loading and hyperchloremic acidosis in neonates.

   f. **Extravasation of calcium solutions** into subcutaneous tissues can cause severe necrosis and subcutaneous calcifications.

      (1) Scrupulous attention to the peripheral intravenous site is indicated when calcium-containing solutions are infused.

      (2) Extravasations have been treated successfully with **hyaluronidase** injection. Subcutaneous injection around the periphery of the extravasation is reported most commonly, although injection through the peripheral intravenous line has theoretical advantages in that it would deliver the hyaluronidase to the same tissue plane as the calcium. The small gauge needles used for subcutaneous injection dull with repeated use and are changed frequently during this procedure.

      (3) The dose of injected hyaluronidase is 150 units/ml solution in normal saline, injected in 0.2 ml amounts subcutaneously in five separate sites around leading edge of infiltrate. Treatment of extravasation within the first hour is preferable.

2. **Calcium preparations.** We prefer calcium gluconate 10% solution for intravenous (and occasionally oral) use (Table 29.1). Calcium glubionate syrup (Neo-Calglucon) is a convenient oral preparation. However, the high sugar content and osmolality may cause gastrointestinal irritation or diarrhea.

3. **Treatment of early-onset hypocalcemia**

   a. Hypocalcemic preterm infants who have no symptoms and are not ill from any other cause do not require specific treatment. The hypocalcemia should resolve spontaneously by day 3. We avoid the use of peripheral calcium infusion in asymptomatic, well newborns.

   b. If the serum calcium level drops to 6.5 mg/dL or less (usually VLBW newborns), we recommend beginning a continuous calcium infusion with the goal of producing a sustained serum calcium level (7 to 8

TABLE 29.1. COMMON CALCIUM PREPARATIONS

Preparation	Elemental Calcium Content (mg/mL)
Calcium gluconate (10% injection)	9.0
Calcium chloride (10% injection)	27.2
Calcium glubionate syrup	23.6

mg/dL). A convenient starting dose is 45 mg/kg per day (5 mL/kg per day of calcium gluconate 10%). Bolus infusions are ineffective and hazardous. Prophylaxis or treatment with pharmacologic doses of vitamin D is **not recommended.**

   c. It may be desirable to prevent the onset of hypocalcemia for newborns who exhibit cardiovascular compromise (e.g., severe respiratory distress syndrome, asphyxia, septic shock, persistent pulmonary hypertension of the newborn) and require cardiotonic drugs or blood pressure support. Use a continuous calcium infusion, preferably by means of a central catheter, to maintain a total calcium level higher than 7.0 mg/dL and an ionized calcium level higher than 4.0 mg/dL (1.0 mmol/L).

4. Treatment of hypocalcemic crisis with seizures, apnea, or tetany. Serum calcium level is usually less than 5.0 mg/dL.

   a. Emergency calcium therapy consists of 1 to 2 mL of calcium gluconate 10% per kilogram (9 to 18 mg of elemental calcium per kilogram) by intravenous infusion over 5 minutes.

      (1) Monitor heart rate and the infusion site.

      (2) Repeat the dose in 10 minutes if there is no clinical response.

      (3) Following the initial dose(s), maintenance calcium should be given parenterally or orally (see II.C.3.b). Patients in acute hypocalcemic crisis as a consequence of the hypoparathyroidism associated with the 22q11/CATCH22/DiGeorge sequence may require both calcium therapy and vitamin D to maintain normocalcemia. Dihydrotachysterol (DHT) is the vitamin D analog of choice based on its rapid onset of activity and its enhanced effect on calcium mobilization from bone.

   b. Symptomatic hypocalcemia unresponsive to calcium therapy may be due to **hypomagnesemia.**

      (1) The preferred preparation for treatment is magnesium sulfate. The 50% solution contains 500 mg, or 4 mEq/mL.

      (2) Correct severe hypomagnesemia (<1.2 mg/dL) with 0.1 to 0.2 mL of magnesium sulfate 50% per kilogram intravenously or intramuscularly. When administering intravenously, infuse slowly and monitor heart rate; intramuscular administration may cause local tissue necrosis. The dose may be repeated every 6 to 12 hours. Obtain serum magnesium levels before each dose.

      (3) Maintenance magnesium therapy consists of oral administration of magnesium sulfate 50%, 100 mg or 0.2 mL/kg per day. If there is significant malabsorption, the dose may be increased twofold to fivefold.

5. Treatment of specific hypocalcemic syndromes

   a. Hypocalcemia associated with hyperphosphatemia

      (1) Classic late-onset neonatal hypocalcemia is preventable in most cases by ensuring adequacy of maternal vitamin D stores during pregnancy and avoiding nonformula, high-phosphate diets in infants.

      (2) The goal of therapy is to **reduce renal phosphate load.** Reduce phosphate intake by feeding the infant human milk or a low-phosphorus formula (Similac PM 60/40). Mineral contents of some infant diets are shown in Table 29.2.

      (3) Increase the calcium-phosphate ratio of the milk to 4:1 with oral calcium supplements (e.g., 0.5 ml of Neo-Calglucon per 30 ml of PM 60/40). This will inhibit intestinal absorption of phosphorus. Phosphate binders are generally not necessary.

      (4) Gradually wean calcium supplements over 2 to 4 weeks. Monitor serum calcium and phosphorus levels one to two times weekly.

   b. Hypoparathyroid infants are hypocalcemic and hyperphosphatemic. Use a low-phosphate diet, for example, Sim PM60/40, with calcium sup-

TABLE 29.2. MINERAL CONTENTS OF COMMON INFANT DIETS

Type of Milk	Approximate Mineral Content	
	Calcium (mg/L)	Phosphorus (mg/L)
Human milk	280	140
Similac PM 60/40	380	190
Similac	527	284
Enfamil	527	358
Isomil	710	510
ProSobee	710	561
Human milk/HMF 24 cal*	1450	810
Similac Special Care 24	1452	806
Enfamil Premature 24	1330	669
Similac Lactofree	554	372
Carnation Good Start	432	240
Similac Neosure	784	463
Enfacare	902	496
Pregestimil	777	507
Nutramigen	635	426
Alimentum	709	507

*Human milk with fortifier to 24 kcal/oz.

plementation [see II.C.5.a.(1)–(4)], and correct vitamin D deficiency if present.

  c. Vitamin D disorders

    (1) Vitamin D deficiency in neonates is usually treatable with initial doses up to 5000 units per day of oral vitamin D_2 (Drisdol, 8000 units/mL), although occasionally higher doses may be required. We recommend the involvement of a pediatric endocrinologist. Wean slowly as the deficiency resolves. Frequent assay of serum calcium level is necessary to avoid rebound hypervitaminosis D.

    (2) Defects in vitamin D metabolism are treated with vitamin D analogues, for example, dihydrotachysterol (Hytakerol) and calcitriol (Rocaltrol). The rapid onset of action and short half-life of these drugs lessen the risk of rebound hypercalcemia.

III. Hypercalcemia. Neonatal hypercalcemia (serum total calcium level >11.0 mg/dL, serum ionized calcium level >5.0 mg/dL) may be asymptomatic and discovered incidentally during routine screening. Alternatively, the presentation of severe hypercalcemia (>14.0 mg/dL) can be dramatic and life-threatening, requiring immediate medical intervention.

  A. Etiology. The physiologic mechanisms that prevent hypercalcemia are inhibition of PTH and $1,25(OH)_2D_3$ synthesis, which **reduces calcium mobilization from bone, absorption from intestine, and reclamation from kidney.** (The potential pathophysiologic role for calcitonin is unclear.) Elevated serum calcium concentration, therefore, implies inappropriately increased calcium efflux from one of these pools into the extracellular fluid (ECF).

1. **Increased bone resorption**
   a. **Hyperparathyroidism**
      (1) **Congenital hyperparathyroidism associated with maternal hypoparathyroidism** usually resolves over several weeks. Decreased availability of maternal calcium for the fetus stimulates the fetal parathyroids.
      (2) **Neonatal severe primary hyperparathyroidism (NSPHP).** The parathyroids are refractory to regulation by calcium, producing marked hypercalcemia (frequently 15 to 30 mg/dL) and lack of response to subtotal parathyroidectomy. Milder forms of the disorder probably occur also. NSPHP occurs frequently in **familial hypocalciuric hypercalcemia** kindreds (see III.A.3.b) as the consequence of homozygosity for a gene encoding a mutated calcium sensor.
      (3) Self-limited secondary **hyperparathyroidism** associated with neonatal renal tubular acidosis.
   b. **Hyperthyroidism.** Thyroid hormone stimulates bone resorption and bone turnover.
   c. **Hypervitaminosis A** accelerates bone resorption.
   d. **Phosphate depletion** can cause hypercalcemia in preterm infants fed phosphate-poor diets, usually human milk, or undergoing parenteral nutrition. Low phosphate intake stimulates $1,25(OH)_2D_3$ production, which mobilizes phosphate and calcium from bone into the ECF.
   e. **Hypophosphatasia,** an autosomal recessive bone dysplasia, produces severe bone demineralization and fractures.

2. **Increased intestinal absorption of calcium**
   a. **Hypervitaminosis D** may result from excessive vitamin D ingestion by the mother (during pregnancy) or the neonate. Since vitamin D is extensively stored in fat, intoxication may persist for weeks to months (see Chap. 10 for nutritional requirements for vitamin D).
   b. Variation in vitamin D content of **human milk fortifier** may lead to excessive vitamin D intake in premature infants fed breast milk supplemented to 24 kcal/oz.

3. **Decreased renal calcium clearance**
   a. **Thiazide diuretics** can induce or exacerbate hypercalcemia, largely by hypocalciuric effects.
   b. **Familial hypocalciuric hypercalcemia,** a clinically benign autosomal dominant disorder, can present in the neonatal period. The gene mutation is on chromosome 3q21–24. Mutations in the calcium sensor lead to a dual defect in parathyroid cells (causing parathyroid hyperplasia) and renal tubules (causing hypocalciuria).

4. **Uncertain mechanisms**
   a. **Idiopathic neonatal/infantile hypercalcemia** occurs in the constellation of **Williams syndrome** (hypercalcemia, supravalvular aortic stenosis or other cardiac anomalies, "elfin" facies, psychomotor retardation) and in a familial pattern lacking the Williams phenotype. Increased calcium absorption has been demonstrated; increased vitamin D sensitivity and impaired calcitonin secretion are proposed as possible mechanisms.
   b. **Subcutaneous fat necrosis** is a sequela of trauma or asphyxia. Only the more generalized necrosis seen in asphyxia is associated with significant hypercalcemia. Granulomatous (macrophage) inflammation of the necrotic lesions may be a source of unregulated $1,25(OH)_2D_3$ synthesis. The accompanying hypercalcemia may present several weeks postnatally.
   c. **Acute renal failure,** usually during the diuretic or recovery phase
   d. **Acute adrenal insufficiency,** which may be transient in preterm infants. Diagnosis may be made by an ACTH-stimulation test.

e. Blue diaper syndrome, a defect in intestinal transport of tryptophan, causes excretion of water-insoluble blue tryptophan metabolites (indacanuria). The pathogenesis of the hypercalcemia is uncertain.

B. Evaluation

1. The **clinical manifestations** of severe hypercalcemia (usually hyperparathyroidism) include hypotonia, encephalopathy (lethargy or irritability, occasionally seizures), hypertension, respiratory distress (due to hypotonia and demineralization and deformation of the rib cage), poor feeding, vomiting, constipation, polyuria, hepatosplenomegaly, anemia, and extraskeletal calcifications, including nephrocalcinosis. Mortality is high for untreated infants. Milder hypercalcemia may present as feeding difficulties or poor linear growth.

2. **History**

   a. Maternal/family history of hypercalcemia or hypocalcemia, parathyroid disorders, nephrocalcinosis, and unexplained fetal losses.

   b. Maternal dietary and drug history (e.g., excessive vitamin A or D, thiazides).

   c. Family history of hypercalcemia or familial hypocalciuric hypercalcemia.

   d. Medications (e.g., vitamin A or D, thiazides, antacids).

   e. Low-phosphate diet in preterm infants or excessive dietary calcium.

3. **Physical examination**

   a. Small for dates (hyperparathyroidism, Williams syndrome).

   b. Craniotabes, fractures (hyperparathyroidism), or characteristic bone dysplasia (hypophosphatasia).

   c. "Elfin" facies (Williams syndrome).

   d. Cardiac murmur (supravalvular aortic stenosis and peripheral pulmonic stenosis associated with Williams syndrome).

   e. Indurated, bluish-red lesions (subcutaneous fat necrosis).

   f. Evidence of hyperthyroidism.

   g. Blue discoloration of diaper.

4. **Laboratory evaluation**

   a. The clinical history and **serum and urine mineral levels** [e.g., calcium, ionized calcium (if available), phosphorus, and urinary calcium:creatinine ratio (U_{Ca}/U_{Cr})] should suggest a likely diagnosis.

   (1) Very elevated serum calcium level (>15 mg/dL) usually indicates primary hyperparathyroidism or in VLBW infants, phosphate depletion.

   (2) Low phosphorus level indicates phosphate depletion, hyperparathyroidism, or familial hypocalciuric hypercalcemia.

   (3) Very low U_{Ca}/U_{Cr} suggests familial hypocalciuric hypercalcemia.

   b. Specific serum hormone levels (immunoreactive PTH, $25(OH)D_3$, $1,25(OH)_2D_3$) will confirm the diagnostic impression.

   c. Serum alkaline phosphatase level increases with increased bone resorption. Very low activity suggests hypophosphatasia (confirmed by increased urinary phosphoethanolamine level).

   d. Radiographs of hand/wrist may suggest hyperparathyroidism (demineralization, subperiosteal resorption) or hypervitaminosis D (submetaphyseal rarefaction).

C. Treatment

1. **Emergency medical treatment** (symptomatic or calcium >14 mg/dL)

   a. Volume expansion with isotonic saline solution. Hydration and sodium promote urinary calcium excretion. If cardiac function is normal, infuse normal saline solution (10 to 20 mL/kg) over 15 to 30 minutes (monitoring blood glucose level), then about one to three times "maintenance" fluids using, for example, dextrose 5% in water (5% D/W) with 40 to 60 mEq/L sodium chloride and 20 mEq/L potassium chloride.

   b. Furosemide (1 mg/kg q6–8h intravenously) induces calciuria. Since potassium and magnesium may become depleted, monitor and supplement as necessary.

   c. Inorganic phosphate may lower serum calcium levels in **hypophosphatemic patients** by inhibiting bone resorption and promoting bone mineral accretion. Parenteral phosphate should be avoided in severely hypercalcemic patients (serum total calcium level >12 mg/dL) unless hypophosphatemia is severe (<1.5 mg/dL). **Extraskeletal calcification** may occur. Oral phosphate (e.g., Neutra-phos, 200 mg of phosphate per milliliter) is preferred. Initial dosage (orally, or in parenteral nutrition) is 3.0 to 5.0 mg/dL.

   d. Glucocorticoids are effective in hypervitaminosis A and D and subcutaneous fat necrosis by inhibiting both bone resorption and in testinal calcium absorption; they are ineffective in hyperparathyroidism. Administer hydrocortisone, 10 mg/kg per day, or methylprednisolone, 2 mg/kg per day.

  2. Other therapies

   a. Low-calcium, low-vitamin D diets are an effective adjunctive therapy for hypervitaminosis A or D, subcutaneous fat necrosis, and Williams syndrome. Prolonged use may induce rickets.

   b. Calcitonin is a potent inhibitor of bone resorption. The antihypercalcemic effect is transient but may be prolonged if glucocorticoids are used concomitantly. There is little reported experience in neonates.

   c. Parathyroidectomy with autologous reimplantation may be indicated for severe persistent neonatal hyperparathyroidism.

IV. Hypermagnesemia

  A. Etiology. Usually an exogenous magnesium load exceeding renal excretion capacity produces hypermagnesemia.

   1. Magnesium sulfate therapy for maternal preeclampsia or preterm labor.

   2. Administration of magnesium-containing antacids to the newborn.

   3. Excessive magnesium in parenteral nutrition.

   4. Magnesium sulfate enemas (contraindicated in newborns).

  B. Diagnosis

   1. Elevated serum magnesium level (normal newborn range, 1.6 to 2.8 mg/dL).

   2. Hypermagnesemic signs are unusual in term infants if the serum magnesium level is less than 6.0 mg/dL. The common curariform effects include apnea, respiratory depression, lethargy, hypotonia, hyporeflexia, poor suck, decreased intestinal motility, and delayed passage of meconium.

   3. Administration of aminoglycosides to a hypermagnesemic infant can lead to an additive inhibition of cholinergic function and an increased risk of respiratory compromise. An alternative antibiotic should be considered in this setting (see Chap. 23, Bacterial and Fungal Infections).

  C. Treatment

   1. Often the only intervention necessary is removal of the source of exogenous magnesium.

   2. When hypermagnesemic symptoms are severe, an intravenous calcium infusion may reverse them. (Calcium acts as a magnesium antagonist.)

   3. Exchange transfusion, peritoneal dialysis, and hemodialysis are usually not necessary.

   4. Begin feedings only after suck and intestinal motility are established.

   5. Saline enemas or glycerin suppositories may be used to initiate bowel movements.

Suggested Readings

De Marini S., et al. Disorders of calcium, phosphorus, and magnesium metabolism. In: Fanaroff A. A., Mouton R. J. (Eds.), *Neonatal–Perinatal Medicine,* 6th ed. St. Louis: Mosby, 1997.

Tsang R. C. Calcium, phosphorus, and magnesium metabolism. In: Polin R. A., Fox W. W. (Eds.), *Fetal and Neonatal Physiology.* Philadelphia: Saunders, 1992.

METABOLIC BONE DISEASE OF PREMATURITY

Kenneth M. Huttner

Metabolic bone disease occurs in more than 30% of infants weighing 1500 g or less at birth and 50% of those weighing less than 1000 g. **Osteopenia** ("washed out" or undermineralized bones) develops during the first postnatal weeks. Signs of **rickets** (epiphyseal dysplasia and skeletal deformities) usually become evident in 2 to 4 months or by term-corrected gestational age. The risk of bone disease is greatest for the sickest, most premature infants.

I. Etiology

A. **Deficiency of calcium and phosphorus is the principal cause.** Demands for rapid growth in the third trimester are met by intrauterine mineral accretion rates of 120 to 150 mg of calcium and 60 to 120 mg of phosphorus per kilogram per day. Poor mineral intake and absorption after birth result in undermineralized new and remodeled bone.

1. **Diets** low in mineral content predispose preterm newborns to metabolic bone disease.

   a. Unsupplemented human milk.

   b. Parenteral nutrition.

   c. Formulas not designed for use in preterm infants (e.g., soy-based).

2. **Furosemide** therapy causes renal calcium wasting. However, in animal studies calcium homeostasis is maintained via increased gastrointestinal absorption. Data from preterm infants demonstrates that the use of alternative day enteral furosemide improves pulmonary function without associated renal calcium loss.

3. **Renal phosphorus wasting**

   a. Acquired tubular acidosis.

   b. The Fanconi syndromes.

   c. X-linked hypophosphatemic rickets may present in late infancy.

   d. Tumor osteomalacia. Many mesenchymal tumors, including **sclerosing hemangiomas,** produce humoral phosphaturic factors.

B. **Vitamin D deficiency.** Human milk has a total antirachitic sterol content of only 25 to 50 IU/L, insufficient for maintaining normal 25-hydroxyvitamin D $(25(OH)D_3)$ levels in preterm infants (400 to 1000 IU per day required). However, when vitamin D intake is adequate, even very-low-birth-weight newborns can synthesize 1,25-dihydroxyvitamin D $(1,25(OH)_2D_3)$.

1. **Maternal vitamin D deficiency** can cause **congenital rickets**.

2. Inadequate vitamin D intake or absorption produces **nutritional rickets**.

3. **Hepatobiliary rickets** results largely from vitamin D malabsorption.

4. **Chronic renal failure** (renal osteodystrophy).

5. Chronic use of phenytoin or phenobarbital increases 25(OH)D metabolism.

6. Hereditary pseudo–vitamin D deficiency: type I (abnormality or absence of 1-alpha-hydroxylase activity) or type II (tissue resistance to $1,25(OH)_2D_3$).

II. Diagnosis

A. **Clinical signs** include respiratory insufficiency or failure to wean from a ventilator, hypotonia, pain on handling due to pathologic fractures, decreased linear growth with sustained head growth, frontal bossing, enlarged anterior fontanel and widened cranial sutures, craniotabes (posterior flattening of the skull), "rachitic rosary" (swelling of costochondral junctions),

Harrison's grooves (indentation of the ribs at the diaphragmatic insertions), and enlargement of wrists, knees, and ankles.

B. Radiographic signs include widening of epiphyseal growth plates; cupping, fraying, and rarefaction of the metaphyses; subperiosteal new-bone formation; osteopenia, particularly of the skull, spine, scapula, and ribs; and occasionally osteoporosis or pathologic fractures.

C. Laboratory evaluation

1. **Serum calcium level** (low, normal, or slightly elevated) **and phosphorus level** (low to normal) generally are **not** good indicators of the presence or severity of metabolic bone disease.

2. **Serum alkaline phosphatase level** (an indicator of osteoclast activity) is often but not invariantly correlated with disease severity (>1000 U/L in severe rickets). Note the following:

   a. Normal neonatal range may be up to four times the adult upper limit.

   b. Hepatobiliary disease also elevates alkaline phosphatase level.

   c. Solitary elevated alkaline phosphatase level rarely occurs in the absence of bone or liver disease (transient hyperphosphatasemia of infancy).

3. **25(OH)D$_3$** levels are usually low to normal. Measures of 25(OH)D$_3$ are useful for establishing the sufficiency of vitamin D stores; levels are less than 6 ng/mL in severe vitamin D deficiency.

4. **Radiographs.** A loss of up to 40% of bone mineralization can occur without radiographic changes. Chest films may show osteopenia and sometimes rachitic changes. Wrist or knee films and a skeletal series (pathologic fractures) can be useful.

5. Measurement of **bone mineral content** by photon densitometry remains investigational.

6. Reserve measurement of 1,25(OH)$_2$D$_3$ or PTH for complicated or refractory cases.

III. Prevention and treatment

A. Dietary management (see Chap. 10)

1. In LBW infants, early enteral feeding significantly enhances the establishment of full-volume enteral intake, leading to increased calcium accumulation and decreased osteopenia. Mineral-fortified human milk or "premature" formulas are the appropriate diets for preterm infants; their use can prevent and treat metabolic bone disease of prematurity (see Table 29.2). Calcium retention is dependent on phosphorus availability, hence calcium supplementation alone may not prevent rickets. In addition, the dietary carbohydrate composition, especially the inclusion of glucose polymers, has been shown to be a significant contributor to calcium absorption in preterm infants.

2. Use of other diets and specific supplementation with calcium gluconate or glubionate (see Table 29.1, to a total of 200 mg of elemental calcium per kilogram per day) and/or potassium phosphate (93 mg phosphate per milliliter, to a total of 100 mg/kg per day) is less desirable because of concern over medication error. The addition of both calcium and phosphorus supplements directly to standard formulas should be avoided, as it will lead to the formation of a precipitate.

B. Ensure adequate vitamin D stores by an intake of 150 to 400 IU per day (see Chap. 10).

1. Vitamin D deficiency rickets has been treated with initial doses of up to 5000 IU of vitamin D per day. However, early prophylactic administration of vitamin D$_2$ doses of 2000 IU/day produced no consistent improvement in the incidence of neonatal rickets. Oral calcium supplements may be necessary during high-dose vitamin D therapy, since serum calcium levels may drop precipitously as bone mineralizes rapidly.

2. Defects in vitamin D metabolism may respond better to dihydrotachysterol (DHT) or calcitriol (see Chap. 29, Hypocalcemia, Hypercalcemia, and Hypermagnesemia).

C. Furosemide-induced renal calcium wasting can be lessened by adding a thiazide diuretic or by alternate-day administration.

D. Avoid nonessential handling and vigorous chest physiotherapy in preterm infants with severely undermineralized bones. Recent data suggests that daily passive physical activity (range of motion, 5 to 10 minutes) may enhance both growth and bone mineralization.

E. Infants receiving mineral-modified human milk as "premature" formula or extra vitamin D should have calcium, PO_4, and alkaline phosphate levels monitored periodically. (See Chap. 10, Nutrition.)

F. Former LBW infants discharged to home on unsupplemented mother's milk are at risk for hypophosphatemia and should be started on vitamin D supplementation. This patient population may be candidates for a repeat rickets screen at 4 to 8 weeks post-discharge.

Suggested Readings

Koo W.W.K., et al. Calcium, magnesium, phosphorus, and Vitamin D. In: Tsang R.C., et al., (Eds.), *Nutritional Needs of the Preterm Infant: Scientific Basis and Practical Guidelines*. Baltimore: Williams & Wilkins, 1993;135.

Rigo J., et al. Bone mineral metabolism in the micropremie. *Clin Perinatol* 2000; 27:147–170.

Tsang R.C. Calcium, phosphorus and magnesium metabolism. Section XXV. In: Polin R.A., Fox W.W. (Eds.), *Fetal and Neonatal Physiology*. Philadelphia: Saunders, 1995.

Ziegler E.E., et al. Body composition of the reference fetus. *Growth* 1976;40:329.

INBORN ERRORS OF METABOLISM

Sule U. Cataltepe and Harvey L. Levy

Infants with inborn errors of metabolism (IEM) are usually normal at birth. In those disorders that present in the neonatal period, the signs and symptoms often develop in hours to days after birth. Since the newborn infant has a limited repertoire of responses to acute illness, the manifestations of IEM are common to several other neonatal conditions, such as infections and cardiopulmonary dysfunction. Thus, in the face of such nonspecific features, it is important to maintain a high index of suspicion of IEM in sick neonates since most of these disorders are lethal unless diagnosed and treated immediately. Even if the disorder is untreatable, establishing the diagnosis in the index case is crucial for prenatal diagnosis in subsequent pregnancies.

I. **Incidence.** Although IEM are individually rare, their overall incidence is as high as 1 in 2000. About 100 different IEM may present clinically in the neonatal period.

II. **Inheritance.** Most IEM are transmitted as autosomal recessive genetic traits. A history of parental consanguinity, unexplained neonatal deaths, or severe illness in the immediate family should alert the clinician to the possibility of an IEM. Some IEM, such as ornithine transcarbamylase (OTC) deficiency, are X-linked. As in any X-linked disorder, the affected family member can be a maternal uncle, a brother, or a mildly affected mother.

III. **Clinical presentation**

A. **Pregnancy.** Women carrying fetuses with long chain 3-hydroxyacyl-coenzyme A (CoA) dehydrogenase deficiency (LCHADD) as well as one or two other disorders of fatty acid oxidation are predisposed to developing acute fatty liver of pregnancy and the syndrome of hemolysis, elevated liver enzymes, and low platelet counts (the HELLP syndrome). In most IEM, however, the pregnancy is normal.

B. Time and pattern of onset. IEM can be divided into two groups based on the timing and pattern of presentation in the newborn infant. In the **intoxication type,** the typical course is that of a newborn infant who is born healthy and deteriorates clinically after an initial symptom-free period. The first signs are usually poor feeding and vomiting followed by neurological deterioration with lethargy, apnea, seizures, and coma. The organic acidemias and urea cycle defects classically present in this manner. In **energy deficiencies,** the most common presentation is an overwhelming neurologic illness with apnea, seizures, and coma without an apparent symptom-free period. The diseases in this group include mitochondrial and peroxisomal disorders, nonketotic hyperglycinemia, molybdenum cofactor deficiency, and primary lactic acidosis.

C. Patterns of presentation. Newborns with IEM present with one or more of the following manifestations:
1. **Neurological abnormalities. Encephalopathy, seizures, and tone abnormalities.** Encephalopathy and seizures are commonly seen in organic acidemias, urea cycle defects, maple-syrup urine disease, fatty-acid oxidation defects and congenital lactic acidosis. Seizures may be the presenting symptom in pyridoxine-dependent seizures, folinic-acid-responsive seizures, nonketotic hyperglycinemia, sulfite oxidase deficiency, and peroxisomal disorders. A few IEM present as predominant hypotonia in the neonatal period. These disorders include nonketotic hyperglycinemia, sulfite oxidase deficiency, peroxisomal disorders, and respiratory chain disorders.
2. **Disorders of acid-base status.** Metabolic acidosis with a raised anion gap is an important laboratory feature of many IEM. A flowchart for the investigation of metabolic acidosis with anion gap in patients with suspected IEM is presented in Fig. 29.3. The organic acidemias, fatty-acid oxidation defects, and primary lactic acidemias (defects of gluconeogenesis, glucogenolysis, pyruvate metabolism, Krebs cycle, and respiratory chain) cause metabolic acidosis with an increased anion gap. Measurement of

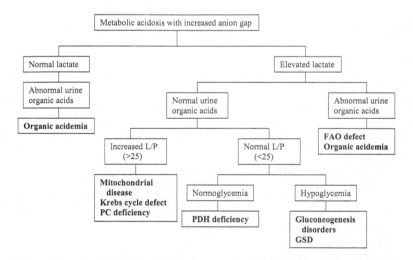

FIG. 29.3. Approach to the investigation of neonatal metabolic acidosis. (L/P = lactate/pyruvate ratio; FAO = fatty acid oxidation; PC = pyruvate carboxylase; PDH = pyruvate dehydrogenase; GSD = glycogen storage disease.)

lactate/pyruvate ratio can be helpful to differentiate various causes of primary lactic acidosis (Fig. 29.3). Respiratory alkalosis can be associated with hyperammonemia syndromes.

3. **Hypoglycemia.** Hypoglycemia, a frequent finding in neonates, should raise a suspicion of IEM if it is severe and persistent without any other etiology. Hypoglycemia associated with metabolic acidosis suggests an organic acidemia or a defect of gluconeogenesis, such as glycogen storage disease type I or fructose 1,6-diphosphatase deficiency. Nonketotic hypoglycemia is the hallmark of defects of fatty acid oxidation.

  A flowchart for the evaluation of persistent hypoglycemia is presented in Fig. 29.4.

4. **Liver dysfunction.** Galactosemia is the most common metabolic cause of liver disease in the neonate. Hepatomegaly with hypoglycemia and seizures suggest glycogenosis type I or III, gluconeogenesis defects, or hyperinsulinism. Hereditary fructose intolerance (in the case of fructose-containing diet), tyrosinemia type I, neonatal hemochromatosis and mitochondrial diseases can also present predominantly with liver dysfunction in the neonate. Cholestatic jaundice with failure to thrive is observed primarily in α_1- antitrypsin deficiency, Byler Disease, and Niemann-Pick Disease Type C.

5. **Dysmorphic features.** Several IEM can present with facial dysmorphism (Table 29.3). Congenital disorders of glycosylation and some lysosomal storage diseases can present with hydrops fetalis (Table 29.4).

6. **Cardiac disease.** Long-chain fatty-acid oxidation defects and mitochondrial respiratory-chain defects present with cardiomyopathy, arrhythmias and hypotonia in neonates (Table 29.5). Neonatal form of Pompe disease, a glycogen storage disorder, presents with generalized hypotonia, failure to thrive, and cardiomyopathy.

7. **Abnormal urine odor.** Abnormal urine odors can best be detected on a drying filter paper or by opening a container that has been closed at room temperature for a few minutes. Table 29.6 lists IEM associated with characteristic odors.

IV. **Initial evaluation of a neonate with suspected IEM.** Initial screening of a sick newborn infant with a suspected underlying metabolic disease should include the investigations listed on Table 29.7. The first line laboratory studies can be

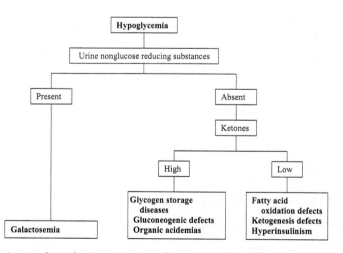

FIG. 29.4. Approach to the investigation of persistent hypoglycemia in the newborn with suspected IEM.

TABLE 29.3. INBORN ERRORS OF METABOLISM ASSOCIATED WITH
DYSMORPHIC FEATURES

Disorder	Dysmorphic features
Peroxisomal disorders Zellweger syndrome	Large fontanelle, prominent forehead, flat nasal bridge, epicanthal folds, hypoplastic supraorbital ridges
Pyruvate dehydrogenase deficiency	Epicanthal folds, flat nasal bridge, small nose with anteverted flared alae nasi, long philtrum
Glutaric aciduria type II	Macrocephaly, high forehead, flat nasal bridge, short anteverted nose, ear anomalies, hyposbadias, rocker-bottom feet
Cholesterol biosynthetic defects Smith-Lemli-Opitz syndrome	Epicanthal folds, flat nasal bridge, toe 2/3 syndactyly, genital abnormalities, cataracts
Congenital disorders of glycosylation	Inverted nipples, lipodystrophy
Lysosomal storage disorders I-cell disease	Hurler-like phenotype

performed by any clinical laboratory and should be obtained immediately once
IEM is suspected. The results of these simple tests can provide important information about the underlying disease and help to narrow down the specialized
tests required for definitive diagnosis.

A. Initial evaluation
   1. **The complete blood cell count** should include examination of cell morphol-
      ogy as well as differential cell count. Neutropenia and thrombocytopenia

TABLE 29.4. INBORN ERRORS OF METABOLISM ASSOCIATED WITH
HYDROPS FETALIS

Lysosomal disorders
   Mucopolysaccharidosis types I, IVA, and VII
   GM1 gangliosidosis
   Gaucher disease
   Niemann-Pick disease type C
   Sialidosis
   Galactosialidosis
   Farber disease

Hematologic disorders
   Glucose-6-phosphate dehydrogenase deficiency
   Pyruvate kinase deficiency
   Glucosphosphate isomerase deficiency
Others
   Congenital disorders of glycosylation
   Neonatal hemochromatosis
   Respiratory chain disorders
   Glycogen storage disease type IV

TABLE 29.5. INBORN ERRORS OF METABOLISM ASSOCIATED WITH NEONATAL CARDIOMYOPATHY

Disorders of fatty acid oxidation
Carnitine uptake deficiency
Carnitine-acylcarnitine translocase (CAT) deficiency
Carnitine palmitoyltransferase II (CPT II) deficiency
Long-chain 3-hydroxyacyl-CoA dehydrogenase deficiency (LCHADD)
Trifunctional protein deficiency
Very-long-chain acyl-CoA dehydrogenase deficiency (VLCADD)

Mitochondrial respiratory chain disorders

Tricarboxylic acid cycle defects
Alpha-ketoglutarate dehydrogenase deficiency

Glycogen storage disorders
Pompe disease (GSD type II)
Phosphorylase b kinase deficiency

Lysosomal storage disorders
I-cell disease

---

may be associated with a number of organic acidemias (isovaleric acidemia, methylmalonic acidemia, and propionic acidemia). Neutropenia may also be found with glycogen storage disease type 1b and respiratory chain defects, such as Barth syndrome and Pearson syndrome.

2. **Electrolytes and blood gases** are required to determine whether an acidosis or alkalosis is present and, if so, whether the abnormality is associated with an increased anion gap. The organic acidemias and the primary lactic acidosis cause metabolic acidosis with a raised anion gap in early stages. Most metabolic conditions result in acidosis in late stages as encephalopathy and circulatory disturbances progress. A persistent metabolic acidosis with normal tissue perfusion may suggest an organic acidemia or a congenital lactic acidosis. A mild respiratory alkalosis in nonventilated babies almost certainly suggests hyperammonemia. However, in late stages of hyperammonemia, vasomotor instability and collapse can cause metabolic acidosis, as well.

3. **Glucose.** Hypoglycemia is a critical finding in some IEM. Ketones are useful in developing a differential diagnosis for newborns with hypoglycemia (Fig. 29.4). Nonketotic hypoglycemia is the hallmark of defects

---

TABLE 29.6. INBORN ERRORS OF METABOLISM ASSOCIATED WITH ABNORMAL URINE ODOR IN NEWBORNS

Inborn Error of Metabolism	Odor
Glutaric acidemia (type II)	Sweaty feet
Isovaleric acidemia	Sweaty feet
Maple syrup urine disease	Maple syrup
Hypermethioninemia	Boiled cabbage
Multiple carboxylase deficiency	Tomcat urine

TABLE 29.7. LABORATORY STUDIES FOR A NEWBORN SUSPECTED OF HAVING AN INBORN ERROR OF METABOLISM

First line laboratory studies
Complete blood count with differential
Serum electrolytes, calcium, magnesium
Blood glucose
Blood gases
Plasma ammonia
Plasma lactate, pyruvate
Liver function tests
Urine-reducing substances
Urine ketones if acidosis or hypoglycemia present

Second line laboratory studies
Plasma amino acids, quantitative
Urine organic acids
Plasma carnitine and acylcarnitine profile
Plasma uric acid
CSF amino acids
Peroxisomal function tests
Plasma and urine for storage at $-20°C$

of fatty acid oxidation. Hypoglycemia associated with metabolic acidosis and ketones suggests an organic acidemia or defect of gluconeogenesis (glycogen storage disease type 1 or fructose 1,6-biphosphatase deficiency).

4. **Plasma ammonia level** should be determined in all neonates with unexplained lethargy and neurologic intoxication. Early recognition of severe neonatal hyperammonemia is crucial since irreversible damage can occur within hours.

5. **Plasma lactate level.** A high plasma lactate can be secondary to hypoxia, cardiac disease, infection, or seizures, whereas primary lactic acidosis may be caused by disorders of pyruvate metabolism and respiratory chain defects. Some IEM (fatty-acid oxidation disorders, organic acidemias, and urea cycle defects) may also be associated with a secondary lactic acidosis. Persistent increase of plasma lactate above 3 mmol/L in a neonate who did not suffer asphyxia and who has no evidence of other organ failure should lead to further investigation for an IEM (see Fig. 29.3). Specimens for lactate measurement should be obtained from a central line or via an arterial stick since use of tourniquet during venous sampling may result in a spurious increase in lactate.

6. **Liver function tests (LFTs).** Galactosemia is the most common metabolic cause of liver dysfunction in the newborn period. Other causes of abnormal LFTs in the newborn include tyrosinemia, alpha1-antitrypsin deficiency, neonatal hemochromatosis, mitochondrial respiratory chain disorders and Niemann-Pick disease type C.

7. **Urine ketones.** The presence of ketonuria is abnormal in neonates. Excessive urinary excretion of ketones (acetone and acetoacetate) can be investigated with the Acetest or Ketostix reactions. The dinitrophenylhydrazine (DNPH) test screens for the presence of alpha keto acids, such as are seen in maple syrup urine disease (MSUD).

8. **Urine-reducing substances.** Urine specimens should be tested for reducing substances. The Clinitest reaction detects excess excretion of galactose and glucose, but not fructose. A positive reaction with the Clinitest should be investigated further with the Clinistix reaction (glucose oxidase) which is specific for glucose.

B. Second line evaluations
   1. **Plasma amino acid analysis.** Plasma amino acid analysis is indicated for any infant suspected of having IEM. A biochemical geneticist who is informed of the patient's clinical presentation and nutritional status should evaluate the results.
   2. **Urine organic acid analysis** is indicated for patients with unexplained acidosis, seizures, hyperammonemia, hypoglycemia, and/or ketonuria.
   3. **Plasma carnitine and acylcarnitine profile.** Carnitine transports long-chain fatty acids across the inner mitochondrial membrane. An elevation of carnitine esters may be seen in fatty-acid oxidation defects, organic acidemias, and ketosis. In addition to patients with inherited disorders of carnitine biosynthesis, low carnitine levels are common in preterm infants and neonates receiving total parenteral nutrition without adequate carnitine supplementation. Several metabolic diseases may cause secondary carnitine deficiency.
   4. **Plasma uric acid** test is a convenient screen for the few inborn errors of metabolism that are associated with either hyperuricemia (type I glycogen storage disease) or hypouricemia (xanthine dehydrogenase deficiency).
   5. **CSF amino acids.** Nonketotic hyperglycinemia is diagnosed by finding of an elevated CSF to plasma glycine ratio.
   6. **Peroxisomal function tests** include plasma very-long-chain fatty acids, phytanic acid, and erythrocyte plasmalogen levels.
V. Inborn errors of metabolism that are potentially lethal in the newborn
   A. Galactosemia
   1. **Inheritance and enzyme deficiency.** Galactosemia is inherited as an autosomal recessive trait and develops as a result of the deficiency of galactose-1-phosphate uridyl transferase (GALT).
   2. **Clinical manifestations.** Typical symptoms of galactosemia in the newborn develop after ingestion of lactose (a disaccharide of glucose and galactose) through a standard formula or breast milk. Clinical manifestations include jaundice, hepatosplenomegaly, feeding difficulties and vomiting, hypoglycemia, lethargy, irritability, seizures, cataracts, and increased risk of *Escherichia coli* neonatal sepsis. Delayed diagnosis results in cirrhosis and mental retardation.
   3. **Laboratory findings.** The preliminary diagnosis is made by demonstrating nonglucose-reducing substance in urine while the patient is receiving lactose-containing formula or breast milk. The reducing substance is found in urine by Clinitest and can be specifically identified by chromatography or by specific enzymatic test for galactose. The Clinistix urine test result is negative because this test is based on the action of glucose oxidase, therefore specific for glucose and is nonreactive with galactose. Semiquantitative assay of blood for GALT, known as the Beutler test, can be performed on a newborn screening blood specimen by the newborn screening program. Most newborn screening programs screen for galactosemia. Newborns with galactosemia who have received a lactose-free formula from birth, however, may be missed on screening programs that test only for galactose but do not measure the GALT enzyme. Conversely, the GALT assay result will be normal if the infant has received a blood transfusion.
   4. **Management** consists of substituting a lactose-free formula for breast-feeding or a standard formula, and, later, a full galactose-free diet.
   B. Hereditary fructose intolerance
   1. **Inheritance and enzyme deficiency.** Autosomal recessive inheritance, deficiency of fructose 1,6-biphosphate aldolase (aldolase B).
   2. **Clinical manifestations** develop when the infant is exposed to fructose (the fruit sugar) or sucrose (in soy-based formulas) in the diet. Early manifestations include hypoglycemia, jaundice, hepatomegaly, vomiting, lethargy, irritability, seizures, and abnormal liver function tests (LFTs).
   3. **Laboratory findings.** Diagnosis is suspected on the basis of hypoglycemia and clinical manifestations that may suggest galactosemia. However, the

diagnosis of galactosemia is eliminated when reducing substance is absent in urine and blood GALT activity is normal. Definitive diagnosis is made by assay of fructaldolase activity in the liver or by DNA analysis of point mutations in the aldolase B gene.

4. **Management** is elimination of sucrose, fructose, and sorbitol from the diet.

C. Maple syrup urine disease (MSUD)

1. **Inheritance and enzyme deficiency.** Autosomal recessive, deficiency of branched-chain α-ketoacid dehydrogenase.

2. **Manifestations.** Poor feeding and vomiting during the first week of life; lethargy, seizures and coma, hypertonicity and muscular rigidity with severe opisthotonus, maple syrup odor in body fluids.

3. **Laboratory findings.** High plasma and urine levels of leucine, isoleucine, valine, and their respective ketoacids. These ketoacids may be qualitatively detected in urine by adding a few drops of 2,4-dinitrophenylhydrazine reagent (0.1% in 0.1N HCl) to the urine; a yellow precipitate of 2–4 dinitrophenylhydrazone is formed in a positive test. Many newborn screening programs include MSUD.

4. **Management** is aimed at quick removal of the branched-chain amino acids and their metabolites from the tissues and body fluids. Hemodialysis is the most effective means of therapy and should be promptly instituted. Treatment after recovery from the acute state requires a low branched-chain amino acid diet. Patients with MSUD should remain on the diet for the rest of their lives.

D. Organic acidemias. Branched-chain organic acidemias are a group of disorders that result from a deficiency of any of the degradative enzymes involving the catabolism of branched-chain amino acids valine, leucine, and isoleucine. Collectively, isovaleric acidemia (IVA), propionic acidemia (PPA), and methylmalonic acidemia (MMA) are the most commonly encountered organic acidemias in the neonatal period. These disorders have similar clinical and biochemical findings.

1. **Isovaleric acidemia (IVA)**

   a. **Inheritance and enzyme deficiency.** Autosomal recessive, deficiency of isovaleryl-CoA dehydrogenase.

   b. **Manifestations.** Vomiting (sometimes severe enough to suggest pyloric stenosis) and severe acidosis in the first few days of life, followed by lethargy, convulsions, coma, and death if proper therapy is not initiated. The characteristic odor of "sweaty feet" may be present.

   c. **Laboratory findings.** Laboratory findings are severe ketoacidosis, neutropenia, thrombocytopenia, and occasionally pancytopenia, hyperammonemia, and hypocalcemia. **Diagnosis** is established by demonstrating elevations of isovalerylcarnitine in blood and isovalerylglycine in urine. Measuring the enzyme in cultured skin fibroblasts confirms the diagnosis. Newborn screening programs that have expanded metabolic screening include IVA. Antenatal diagnosis has been accomplished by measuring isovalerylglycine in amniotic fluid or by enzyme assay in cultured amniocytes.

   d. **Management** of the acute attack is aimed at hydration, sodium bicarbonate infusion, and removal of the excess isovaleric acid. Glycine (250 mg/kg per 24 h) and carnitine (100 mg/kg per 24 h) administration is recommended to enhance excretion of isovaleric acid in urine. Exchange transfusion and peritoneal dialysis may be needed if above measures fail.

2. **Propionic acidemia (PPA)**

   a. **Inheritance and enzyme defect.** Autosomal recessive deficiency of propionyl-CoA carboxylase.

   b. **Manifestations.** Poor feeding, vomiting, hypotonia, lethargy, dehydration, and clinical signs of acidosis progress rapidly to coma and death.

   c. **Laboratory findings.** Laboratory findings are severe metabolic acidosis with a large anion gap, ketosis, neutropenia, thrombocytopenia, hypoglycemia, hyperglycinemia (ketotic hyperglycinemia due to inhibition of glycine cleavage enzyme by the high levels of accumulated organic acid) and hyperammonemia, elevated plasma propionylcarnitine, and plasma and urine concentrations of propionic acid and methylcitric acid. Newborn screening programs that have expanded metabolic screening include propionic acidemia.

    d. Management of acute attacks include rehydration, correction of acidosis, and prevention of catabolic state by provision of adequate calories through parenteral hyperalimentation. To control the possible production of propionic acid by intestinal bacteria, sterilization of the intestinal tract flora by antibiotics (e.g., oral neomycin, metronidazole) should be promptly initiated. In patients with concomitant hyperammonemia, measures to reduce blood ammonia should be employed.

3. Methylmalonic acidemia (MMA)

    a. Inheritance and enzyme deficiency. Autosomal recessive deficiency of methylmalonyl-CoA mutase or its B_{12} coenzyme adenosylcobalamin.

    b. Manifestations. Fulminant neonatal form is more common in patients with methylmalonic acidemia than in patients with propionic acidemia. Some infants have characteristic facial features with a triangular mouth and high forehead.

    c. Laboratory findings. Large quantities of methylmalonic acid is detected in body fluids. Propionic acid and its metabolites 3-hydroxypropionate and methylcitrate are also found in urine. Newborn screening programs that have expanded metabolic screening include methylmalonic acidemia.

    d. Management is similar to propionic acidemia, except that large doses of vitamin B_{12} are used.

E. Hyperammonemia syndromes. Figure 29.5 summarizes approach to neonatal hyperammonemia.

    1. Transient hyperammonemia is manifested in premature babies by respiratory distress during the first 24 hours of life and may progress to seizures and coma within 48 hours. Ammonia levels may exceed 1000 µmol/L and require vigorous treatment. Asymptomatic transient hyperammonemia (range 40 to 72 µmol/L), on the other hand, is not associated with any short-term or long-term neurologic deficits.

    2. Urea cycle defects (UCD)

        a. Inheritance. Aside from the x-linked ornithine transcarbamylase deficiency, UCD are inherited as autosomal recessive traits.

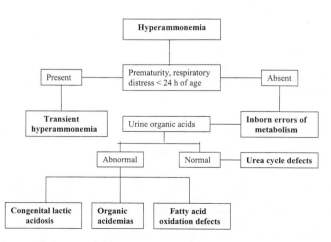

FIG. 29.5. Approach to neonatal hyperammonemia.

b. Manifestations. Infants with complete urea cycle enzyme deficiencies present with poor feeding, vomiting, lethargy, hypotonia, and hyperventilation between 1 to 5 days of age. These patients may develop seizures, apnea, coma, and increased intracranial pressure unless hyperammonemia is diagnosed and treated promptly. Since almost all neonates with UCD are initially thought to be septic, the plasma ammonia level should be measured in septic-appearing patients without microbiologic evidence of infection.

c. Laboratory findings. In neonatal-onset UCD, ammonia levels are usually higher than 300 μmol/L and are often in the range of 500 to 1500 μmol/L. Respiratory alkalosis secondary to hyperventilation is an important initial clue for the diagnosis of a UCD. Other laboratory abnormalities may include mild serum liver enzyme elevations and coagulopathy. Prior to initiation of therapy, samples should be sent for plasma amino acid analysis and for urinary amino acid, organic acid, and orotic acid determination. Plasma and urine should be frozen for future testing. These tests will help identify the cause of hyperammonemia (Figs. 29.5 and 29.6). Newborn screening programs that have expanded metabolic screening include some of the UCD.

d. Management. All neonates with symptomatic hyperammonemia should be transferred to a level III neonatal unit with hemodialysis facilities. Dialysis is the only means of rapid removal of ammonia from blood in acute neonatal hyperammonemia, and hemodialysis is preferred over peritoneal dialysis because it is much more effective. All feedings containing protein should be discontinued and administration of intra-

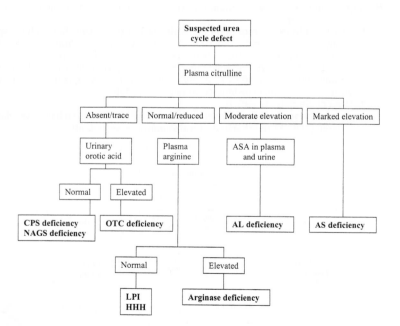

FIG. 29.6. Approach to differential diagnosis of suspected urea cycle defect. (ASA = argininosuccinic acid; CPS = carbamyl phosphate synthetase I; NAGS = N-acetyl glutamate synthase; OTC = ornithine transcarbamylase; AL = argininosuccinic acid lyase; AS = argininosuccinic acid synthetase; LPI = lysinuric protein intolerance; HHH = hyperornithinemia, hyperammonemia, homocitrullinuria.)

venous glucose and fluids should be started before transport. Calories should be provided as intravenous glucose and lipids. Intravenous therapy with ammonia-scavenging drugs should be started when ammonia elevation causes any central nervous system symptoms. For acute neonatal hyperammonemic coma, a loading dose of 600 mg/kg L-arginine-HCL and 250 mg/kg each of sodium benzoate and sodium phenylacetate in 25 to 35 mL/kg of 10% dextrose solution given over a 90-minute period is recommended. This is followed by a sustained infusion of 250 mg/kg L-arginine-HCL and 250 mg/kg each of sodium benzoate and sodium phenylacetate over a 24-hour period for carbamyl phosphate synthetase I and ornithine transcarbamylase deficiency; 600 mg/kg L-arginine-HCL and 250 mg/kg each of sodium benzoate and sodium phenylacetate over a 24-hour period for citrullinemia and argininosuccinic acidemia. For argininosuccinic aciduria, arginine therapy alone may suffice. Intravenous therapy with ammonia-scavenging drugs should be continued while dialysis is being performed. A repeat loading dose of ammonia-scavenging drugs should be given only in neonates with severe disorders who are receiving dialysis. Toxicity is associated with high drug doses (750 mg/kg/d and higher).

F. **Nonketotic hyperglycinemia (NKH)**
   1. **Inheritance and enzyme deficiency.** Autosomal recessive disorder characterized by defective glycine degradation and glycine accumulation in tissues.
   2. **Clinical manifestations.** Patients with neonatal form of NKH present with lethargy, hypotonia, and poor feeding within a few days of birth. Seizures, hiccups, and apneic episodes are common. EEG shows the characteristic burst-suppression pattern. The majority of these infants die within a few weeks of life; survivors develop severe psychomotor retardation. In transient NKH, which is secondary to the immaturity of glycine cleavage enzymes, laboratory and clinical abnormalities return to normal by 2 to 8 weeks of age.
   3. **Laboratory findings.** Diagnosis is established by the findings of elevated glycine levels in body fluids and an elevated CSF/plasma glycine ratio. Measurement of glycine cleavage system activity in hepatocytes confirms the diagnosis.
   4. **Management.** There is no known effective treatment for NKH.

G. **Holocarboxylase synthetase deficiency (HCS) (Multiple carboxylase deficiency—infantile or early form)**
   1. **Inheritance and enzyme deficiency.** Holocarboxylase synthetase (HCS) is inherited as an autosomal recessive trait. HCS catalyzes the binding of biotin with the inactive apocarboxylases, leading to carboxylase activation. Deficiency of this enzyme causes malfunction of all carboxylases and is fatal unless diagnosed and treated rapidly.
   2. **Clinical manifestations.** Affected infants become symptomatic in the first few weeks of life with respiratory distress, hypotonia, seizures, vomiting and failure to thrive. The urine may have a peculiar odor (tomcat urine). Skin manifestations include generalized erythematous rash with exfoliation and alopecia totalis. These infants may also have an immunodeficiency manifested by a decrease in the number of T-cells.
   3. **Laboratory findings** include metabolic acidosis, ketosis, organic aciduria, and hyperammonemia. Diagnosis is confirmed by measuring the enzyme activity in lymphocytes or cultured fibroblasts. Prenatal diagnosis is available.
   4. **Management.** Almost all patients respond to treatment with biotin (10 to 20 mg/day), although some may require higher doses (40 to 80 mg/day) and may have a partial response.

H. **Mitochondrial disorders.** The principal function of mitochondria is to produce ATP from the oxidation of fatty acids and sugars via the electron transport chain. Thus, tissues that are more dependent on aerobic metabolism, such as brain, muscle, and heart, are more likely to be affected in these disorders. Relatively common mitochondrial disorders with potentially lethal presentations in the neonate fall into three main subgroups:

1. **Defects in the carnitine cycle**
   a. Carnitine is required for the transfer of long-chain fatty acids to the mitochondrial matrix for their oxidation. Defects in the carnitine–acylcarnitine translocase cause neonatal onset of seizures, cardiac arrhythmias, and apnea. Laboratory studies show nonketotic hypoglycemia, hyperammonemia, and low carnitine levels.

2. **Defects of fatty acid oxidation**
   a. Very-long-chain acyl-CoA dehydrogenase deficiency (VLCADD) and long-chain 3-hydroxyacyl-CoA dehydrogenase deficiency (LCHADD) can present in the neonatal period with hypotonia, cardiomyopathy, and hypoketotic hypoglycemia.

3. **Defects of pyruvate metabolism**
   a. Pyruvate dehydrogenase complex deficiency (PDHC) can present with severe lactic acidosis, hypotonia, feeding and breathing abnormalities, seizures, dysmorphic facial features (see Table 29.4), agenesis of corpus callosum, and white matter abnormalities. Diagnosis is confirmed by measuring PDH activity in cultured fibroblasts.
   b. Pyruvate carboxylase deficiency can present with lactic acidosis, profound hypotonia, and seizures in the neonatal period.

I. Peroxysomal disorders

Zellweger syndrome, neonatal adrenoleukodystrophy (ALD), and infantile Refsum disease represent a continuum, with the Zellweger syndrome the most severe. In all three disorders, the basic defect is the failure to import one or more proteins into the peroxisome. Newborn infants with Zellweger syndrome have dysmorphic facies (see Table 29.4), severe weakness and hypotonia, neonatal seizures, and eye abnormalities. Patients with neonatal ALD show fewer dysmorphic features. Neonatal seizures are common. The diagnosis is established by measurement of very-long-chain fatty acids (VLCFA) and other metabolites that are elevated secondary to the defect in peroxisome structure.

VI. Management of infant with a suspected metabolic disorder[1]

A. When a sibling has had symptoms consistent with a metabolic disorder, or has died of a metabolic disorder, the following steps should be taken:

1. **Preliminary considerations**
   a. Old hospital charts and postmortem material should be reviewed.
   b. There should be a prenatal discussion of possible diagnoses, and the parents and relatives should be screened for possible clues to diagnosis.
   c. When a diagnosis is known, intrauterine diagnosis by measurement of abnormal metabolites in the amniotic fluid or by enzyme assay of amniocytes obtained by amniocentesis should be considered.
   d. The baby should be delivered in a facility equipped to handle potential metabolic or other complications, preferably closely associated with a laboratory capable of performing or arranging the necessary diagnostic tests.

2. **Initial evaluation** includes a careful physical examination, seeking any of the signs described in III. All nonmetabolic causes of symptoms such as infection or asphyxia should be excluded. Careful examination of the eyes, skin, and liver should also be performed. Tests should be targeted toward the hereditary anomaly, if it is known. Blood and urine tests should be obtained as summarized in Table 29.7. It is important to obtain

[1]Adapted from protocol of Mark Korson, M.D., New England Medical Center, Tufts University, Boston, MA.

these specimens at the time of presentation before starting treatment for metabolic disease. The specimens can be frozen (plasma, urine) and analysis performed later. Enzyme assay or DNA analysis of red blood cells, white blood cells, fibroblasts, or liver tissue may be done for confirmation of diagnosis.

3. **Initial feedings for the asymptomatic infant at risk for metabolic disease** will vary with the diagnosis; for example, in disorders of protein metabolism the infant may be given IV glucose or fed 10% glucose or dextrose polymer (Polycose, Ross Laboratories, Columbus, OH) as tolerated. This may be followed by fat in the form of medium-chain triglycerides (e.g., Product 80056, Mead Johnson Laboratories, Evansville, IN). If the results of tests performed at 48 hours are all negative, protein may be introduced in the form of breast milk or any low-protein milk.

The tests are repeated after 48 hours of protein intake. If no abnormalities are found , the child may be cautiously fed. If metabolic abnormalities are found, the specific problem should be identified and the appropriate diet or treatment started.

The initial feeding will vary with the type of suspected disorder. Many special products are available for various metabolic diseases. More information about these products are available through the following companies' Web sites:

http://www.meadjohnson.com/metabolics/metabolicsforhcp.html (Mead Johnson)

http://www.ross.com/productHandbook/metabolic.asp (Ross Products)
http://www.shsna.com/html/metabolic.htm (SHS North America)
http://www.medicalfood.com (Applied Nutrition Corp.)

B. When an infant has signs or symptoms of an acute metabolic disease, the condition should be managed as follows:

1. Other causes of the symptoms should be ruled out, for example, asphyxia, infection, or intracranial hemorrhage. Even when one of these is the likely cause, if an inborn error cannot be ruled out, obtain acute specimens and keep frozen.

2. Tests as in IV should be performed. Note: Organic acids and ammonia are toxic to the brain, and accumulation of these substances may result in cerebral edema. Caution should be exercised when the need for lumbar puncture is considered in a situation where sepsis should be ruled out.

3. The therapy for acute metabolic decompensation in these disorders includes
   a. Hydration.
   b. Correction of the biochemical abnormalities (metabolic acidosis, hyperammonemia, hypoglycemia).
   c. Reversal of catabolism/promotion of anabolism.
   d. Elimination of toxic metabolites, for example, by hemodialysis.
   e. Treatment of the precipitating factor when possible (e.g., infection, excess protein ingestion).
   f. Cofactor supplementation.

4. The infant should be adequately hydrated, and provided with glucose (and in some cases lipids) to prevent catabolism and with alkali to treat acidosis.
   a. The patient should be kept NPO (nothing by mouth) for 1 to 2 days with intravenous glucose in high doses. Added insulin should be considered if metabolic stability cannot be achieved (see Hypoglycemia and Hyperglycemia, above). If a diagnosis is not available, a protein source at 0.5 g/kg per day by parenteral nutrition (PN) or enteral formula is given with other non-nitrogenous caloric supplements (carbohydrates and fats).

   In galactosemia the infant can be fed a lactose-free formula immediately. Ringer's lactate should not be used for fluid or electrolyte therapy in a child with a known or suspected metabolic disorder.

b. In undiagnosed cases of acidosis, when the lactate and pyruvate are markedly elevated, the possibility of a **disorder of pyruvate metabolism** must be considered. In pyruvate dehydrogenase deficiency, specifically, excess glucose will make the acidosis worse. Glucose and lactate levels should be monitored. In this disorder, lipids are given to prevent catabolism. Small amounts of glucose are given only to keep the blood glucose normal.

5. If the infant is acidotic (pH <7.22) or the bicarbonate level is <14 mEq/L, give $NaHCO_3$ (1 mEq/kg) as a bolus followed by a continuous infusion of bicarbonate. If hypernatremia is a problem, use potassium acetate as part of the solution.

6. Correct hypoglycemia (see Hypoglycemia and Hyperglycemia).

7. Lipids. Intralipid may be given to supply extra calories. Intralipid is composed of even-chain fatty acids, so it is not contraindicated in propionic and methylmalonic acidemia.

8. Calories. Caloric consumption during a period of decompensation, in order to support anabolism, should be about 20% greater than that needed for ordinary maintenance. One must remember that withholding natural protein from the diet also eliminates this source of calories, which should be replaced using other dietary or nutritional (non-nitrogenous) sources.

9. Insulin. Insulin is a potent anabolic hormone, promoting protein and lipid synthesis. It will allow extra glucose to be metabolized and prevent hyperglycemia (see Hypoglycemia and Hyperglycemia).

10. Protein. All natural protein (containing amino acids) should be withheld for 48 to 72 hours while the patient is acutely ill. Afterward, amino acid therapy may be very beneficial in facilitating clinical improvement, but it should be implemented only under the supervision of a physician/nutritionist with expertise in metabolic management. Special parenteral amino acid solutions and specialized formulas are available for many disorders.

11. Elimination of toxic metabolites. Correction of acute metabolic perturbations (acidosis, hypoglycemia, dehydration) may help clear some of the factors contributing to the encephalopathy associated with acute metabolic crisis. However, large quantities of toxic intermediate metabolites, believed to be toxic to the brain as well, are not cleared with glucose or bicarbonate. Hydration promotes renal excretion of toxins. Consideration should be given to providing the means to facilitate the excretion of these compounds.

a. L-Carnitine. Free carnitine levels are low in the organic acidemias because of increased esterification with organic acid metabolites. While the benefit of carnitine supplementation is controversial, there is evidence that carnitine facilitates excretion of these metabolites. If administered, it should be mixed in 10% glucose and given as an infusion to provide 25–100 mg/kg per 24-hour period. When oral fluids are tolerated, carnitine may be administered PO at a dose of 100 to 400 mg/kg/day. Diarrhea is the primary adverse effect of oral carnitine.

b. Antibiotics. For certain organic acidemias (e.g., propionic acidemia, methylmalonic acidemia), gut bacteria are a significant source of organic acid synthesis (e.g., propionic acid). Eradicating the gut flora with a short course of a broad-spectrum antibiotic (e.g., neomycin, metronidazole) orally or intravenously may speed the recovery of a patient in acute crisis. In a newborn with galactosemia there is a significant risk of sepsis. Acute propionic acidemia and methylmalonic acidemia are often associated with neutropenia as well as thrombocytopenia.

c. In hyperammonemia due to a urea cycle disorder, a mixture of sodium benzoate and sodium phenyllactate may be used in addition to glucose, lipids, and electrolytes to facilitate the removal of ammonia (see V.E.2d). Arginine is given in all the urea cycle defects except arginase deficiency to prevent arginine deficiency and to stimulate further excretion of waste nitrogen by stimulating the activity of ornithine transcarboxylase. When ammonia levels exceed 500 to 600 mg/dL, hemodialysis is far more effective in reducing them.

d. Hemodialysis is indicated in cases of intractable metabolic acidosis, unresponsive hyperammonemia (>500 to 600 mg/dL), coma, or severe (usually iatrogenic) electrolyte disturbances.

12. **Treatment of precipitating factors.** Infection should be treated vigorously when possible. Neutropenia (and thrombocytopenia) frequently accompany metabolic decomposition. Bone marrow recovery can be expected once the levels of toxic metabolites have diminished significantly.

13. **Cofactor supplementation.** Pharmacologic doses of appropriate cofactors may be useful in cases of vitamin-responsive enzyme deficiencies.

14. **Monitoring the patient.** The patient should be monitored closely for any mental status changes, overall fluid balance, evidence of bleeding (if thrombocytopenic) and symptoms of infection (if neutropenic). Biochemical parameters including electrolytes, measured CO_2, glucose, ammonia, blood gases, CBC with differential, platelets, urine for ketones and urine-specific gravity at every voiding should be followed.

15. **Recovery.** The patient should be kept NPO until his or her mental status is more stable. Anorexia, nausea, and vomiting during the acute crisis period make significant oral intake unlikely. If the patient is not significantly neurologically compromised, consideration should be given to providing the patient (PO or by NG tube) with a modified formula preparation containing all but the offending amino acids. When the infant is able to take oral feedings, a specific diet must be used. The diet will be individualized for each child and his or her metabolic defect.

VII. **Postmortem diagnosis.** If an infant is dying or has died of what may be a metabolic disease, it is very important to make a specific diagnosis in order to help the parents with genetic counseling for future reproductive planning. Sometimes families that will not permit a full autopsy will allow the collection of some premortem or immediately postmortem specimens that may help in diagnosis. Specimens that should be collected include the following:

A. **Blood,** both clotted and heparinized. The specimen should be centrifuged and the plasma frozen. Lymphocytes may be saved for culture.

B. **Urine,** refrigerated.

C. **Spinal fluid,** refrigerated.

D. **Skin biopsy** for fibroblast culture to be used for chromosomal analysis or enzyme assay. Two samples should be taken from a well-perfused area in the torso. The skin should be well cleaned, but any residual cleaning solution should be washed off with sterile water. The skin can be placed briefly in sterile saline until special media are available.

E. **Liver biopsy samples,** both premortem samples and generous-size postmortem samples, should be flash-frozen to preserve enzyme integrity as well as tissue histology.

F. **Other.** Depending on the nature of the disease, other tissues such as skeletal muscle, cardiac muscle, brain, and kidney should be preserved.

Photographs should be taken and a full skeletal radiologic screening done of any infant with dysmorphic features. A full autopsy should be done if permitted. Information on the proper handling of the tissue should be obtained from one of the regional information centers (see VIII).

VIII. **Regional information centers.** Metabolic problems in the newborn are complicated and require sophisticated diagnosis and treatment. There are regional centers for assistance with these problems. More information about regional centers can be found at the following web addresses:

http://www.meadjohnson.com/metabolics/metabolicdirectory.html
http.//www.geneclinics.org

IX. **Routine newborn screening.** Each state in the United States mandates its own newborn screening program. Recent advances have enabled automated tandem mass spectrometry to be applied to the newborn screening specimen.

This technique is currently being used in several states to offer screening for many treatable IEM. Routine newborn screening always includes phenylketonuria and congenital hypothyroidism, almost always includes maple syrup urine disease, galactosemia, and sickle cell disease, and very often includes congenital adrenal hyperplasia, and biotinidase deficiency. Newborn screening coverage among states in the United States can be found on the following Web site: http://genes-r-us.uthscsa.edu/resources/newborn/screenstatus.htm.

Suggested Readings

Behrman E.R., et al. (Eds.). Metabolic diseases. In: *Nelson Textbook of Pediatrics,* 16th ed. Philadelphia: Saunders, 2000.

Burton B.K. Inborn errors of metabolism in infancy: A guide to diagnosis. *Pediatrics* 1998;102:e69.

Chakrapani A., et al. Detection of inborn errors of metabolism in the newborn. *Arch Dis Child Neonatal Ed* 2001;84:205.

Enns G.M., et al. Diagnosing inborn errors of metabolism in the newborn: Clinical features. *NeoReviews* 2001;2:183.

Enns G.M., et al. Diagnosing inborn errors of metabolism in the newborn: Laboratory investigations. *NeoReviews* 2001;2:192.

Leonard J.V., et al. Inborn errors of metabolism around time of birth. *Lancet* 2000;356:583.

Scaglia F., Longo N. Primary and secondary alterations of neonatal carnitine metabolism. *Semin Perinatol* 1999;23:152.

Scriver C.R., et al. (Eds.). *The Metabolic and Molecular Bases of Inherited Disease,* Vols. I–III. New York: McGraw-Hill, 2001.

Sue C.M., et al. Neonatal presentations of mitochondrial metabolic disorders. *Semin Perinatol* 1999;23:113.

Summar M., et al. Proceedings of a consensus conference for the management of patients with urea cycle disorders. *J Pediatr* 2001;138:S6.

The Urea Cycle Disorders Conference Group. Consensus statement from a conference for the management of patients with urea cycle disorders. *J Pediatr* 2001; 138:S1.

Zinn A.B. Inborn errors of metabolism. In: Fanaroff A.A., Martin R.J. (Eds.). *Neonatal-Perinatal Medicine,* 6th ed. St. Louis: Mosby, 1997.

30. AMBIGUOUS GENITALIA

Norman P. Spack and Mary Deming Scott

I. **Definition.** The normal full-term male infant has a phallus length of at least 2.5 cm measured stretched from the pubic ramus to the tip of the glans. (Fig. 30.1). Testes usually migrate into the scrotum during the last 6 weeks of gestation. The normal full-term female infant has a clitoris less than 1 cm in length. The term ambiguous genitalia applies to any confusing appearance of the external genitalia. This includes any infant with:
   1. A phallus and bilaterally nonpalpable testes.
   2. Unilateral cryptorchidism and hypospadias.
   3. Penoscrotal or perineoscrotal hypospadias, with or without microphallus, even if the testes are descended.
      The internal genital anatomy, karyotype, and sex for rearing cannot be determined from the baby's external appearance; a thorough evaluation is required. The evaluation must be expedited because of conditions such as salt-losing congenital adrenal hyperplasia that could be life-threatening in the first 2 weeks of life.

II. **Assignment of a sex for rearing.** Rapidity in the determination of sex assignment is essential for the parents' peace of mind. Most causes can be clarified in 1 to 2 days, although some cases may take 1 to 2 weeks. Sex assignment depends on anatomy, functional prenatal and postnatal endocrinology, and the potential for sexual functioning and fertility, which may be independent of chromosomal sex. Until a gender assignment is made, gender-specific names or references should be withheld. Premature inappropriate statements may have profound psychosocial consequences for families. After their infant's genitalia are examined in their presence, the parents should be told about the process of genital differentiation; that their child's genitalia are incompletely formed; and that further tests will clarify the problem and provide the necessary information to be able to assign the gender. If future hormonal therapy is necessary, parents should be reassured that it will enable their child to live a normal life. Options for surgery on the internal and/or external genitalia should be discussed in the context of a team approach consisting of a pediatric endocrinologist, pediatric surgeon, geneticist, and counselor experienced in dealing with these issues. No guarantees should be made about fertility.

III. **Normal sexual development.** The process of gonadal and genital differentiation is described in Fig. 30.2. Sex determination progresses in stages. At fertilization, **genetic sex** is determined. Under the influence of specific genes such as SRY (testis-determining factor) located on the short arm of the Y chromosome, **gonadal sex** is determined by the seventh week of gestation. Specific ovarian-determining genes have also been identified. 46,XX males and 46,XY females result from aberrant X-Y interchange during paternal meiosis.
   The testis secretes two hormones critical for genital formation: Antimüllerian hormone (AMH) from the Sertoli cells, which causes regression of the Müllerian ducts (which would otherwise become uterus, fallopian tubes, and upper vagina), and testosterone from the Leydig cells, which promotes development of the Wolffian ducts into the vas deferens, seminal vesicles, and epididymis. Müllerian duct regression and Wolffian duct development require high **local** concentrations of AMH and testosterone, respectively. Failure of a testis to develop on one side may result in retained Müllerian structures and undeveloped Wolffian structures on that side. The enzyme 5α-reductase converts testosterone to dihydrotestosterone, which is responsible for masculinizing of the genital tubercle and labioscrotal folds to form the penis and scrotum, respectively. Formation of normal male internal and external genitalia requires that the target tissues contain functional androgen receptors.

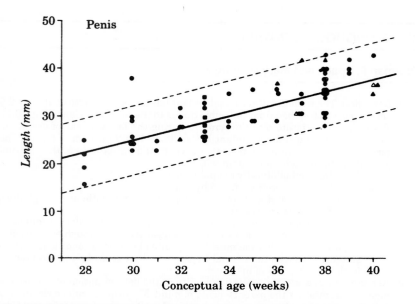

FIG. 30.1. Stretched phallic length of normal premature and full-term babies (closed circles), showing lines of mean 2 standard deviations. Correlation coefficient is 0.80. Superimposed are data for two small-for-gestational-age infants (open triangles), seven large-for-gestational-age infants (closed triangles), and four twins (closed boxes), all of whom are in the normal range. (From Feldman K.W., Smith D.W. Fetal phallic growth and penile standards for newborn male infants. *J Pediatr* 1975;86:395.)

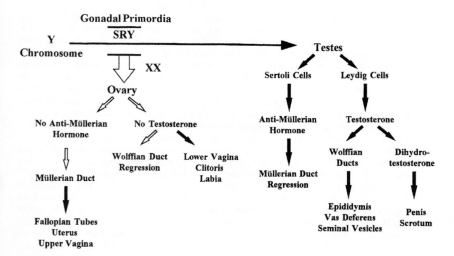

FIG. 30.2. The process of gonadal, internal, and genital differentiation. (From Holm I.A. Ambiguous genitalia in the newborn. In: Emans S.J. et al. (Eds.), *Pediatric and Adolescent Gynecology*. Philadelphia: Lippincott-Raven, 1998:53.)

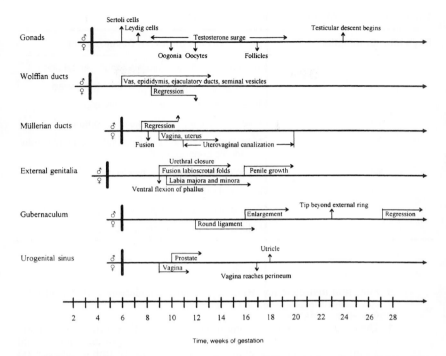

FIG. 30.3. Timelines for five aspects of sexual differentiation. (From White P.C., Speiser P.W. Congenital adrenal hyperplasia due to 21-hydroxylase deficiency. *Endocrine Rev.* 21(3), 2000:245–291. Adapted from Barthold J.S., Gonzalez R. Intersex states. In: Gonzalez E.T., Bauer S.B. (Eds.), *Pediatric Urology Practice*. Philadelphia: Lippincott Williams & Wilkins, 1999;547–578.)

The time course of fetal sexual differentiation is depicted in Fig. 30.3 and Table 30.1. **Phenotypic sex** is established at the end of the first trimester. If a female infant is exposed to excessive androgens during the first trimester, her clitoris and labioscrotal folds will virilize and may appear indistinguishable from a normal male phallus and scrotum, although the latter will be empty. In the second and third trimesters, male phallic growth and scrotal maturation is dependent on testicular androgens stimulated by gonadotrophins from the fetal pituitary. Endogenous growth hormone also contributes to penile growth. A female fetus only exposed to increased androgen concentrations during the second and third trimesters will manifest clitoromegaly but not labial fusion. High intrauterine concentrations of testosterone can influence the brain in terms of later behavior and **gender identity** formation.

IV. **Nursery evaluation of a newborn with ambiguous genitalia**
  A. **History**
  1. **Family history** of hypospadias, congenital adrenal hyperplasia, cryptorchidism, infertility, consanguinity.
  2. **Maternal drug exposure** in pregnancy (progestins, danazol, testosterone, aminoglutethimide, finasteride).
  3. **Maternal virilization** in pregnancy (maternal adrenal hyperplasia; virilizing adrenal or ovarian tumor).
  4. **Neonatal deaths.** Death from vomiting/dehydration of a male sibling in early infancy, possibly from undiagnosed congenital adrenal hyperplasia (CAH). Genital manifestations of CAH in a male are subtle.

TABLE 30.1. TIMETABLE OF SEXUAL DEVELOPMENT

Days after Conception	Events of Sexual Development
19	Primordial germ cells migrate to the genital ridge
40	Genital ridge forms an undifferentiated gonad
44	Müllerian ducts appear; testes develop
62	Müllerian inhibitor (from testes) becomes active
71	Testosterone synthesis begins (induced by placental chorionic gonadotropin)
72	Fusion of the labioscrotal swellings
73	Closure of the median raphe
74	Closure of the urethral groove
77	Müllerian regression is complete

5. Placental insufficiency. Human chorionic gonadotropin (HCG) initiates synthesis of testosterone in the fetal testis.

B. Physical examination

1. The examiner should note phallic stretched length, width of the corpora, presence of chordee, position of the urethral orifice, presence of a vaginal opening, and pigmentation and symmetry of the scrotum or labioscrotal folds. Posterior fusion of the labioscrotal folds is defined as an increased "anogenital ratio," which is determined by measuring the distance between the anus and posterior fourchette divided by the distance between the anus and base of the clitoris. An anogenital ratio >0.5 is indicative of early intrauterine androgen exposure.

2. Gonadal size, position, and descent should be carefully noted. A gonad below the inguinal ligament is usually a testis, but an ovotestis and a uterus are capable of presenting as a hernia. Genital ambiguity with clitoromegaly or an apparently well-formed phallus, with or without hypospadias or chordee, and an empty scrotum should raise immediate concern that the infant is a female virilized by CAH.

3. Bimanual rectal examination may reveal Müllerian structures: a palpable cervix or uterus in the midline.

4. Associated anomalies: Dysmorphic features suggest a more generalized disorder. Denys-Drash syndrome (Wilms' tumor and nephropathy) or WAGR syndrome (Wilms' tumor, aniridia, genitourinary anomalies, and mental retardation) can affect both 46,XY and 46,XX infants and are due to mutations of the WT1 gene on 11p13. Other syndromes associated with genital ambiguity include Smith-Lemli-Opitz, Robinow, Goldenhar syndromes, and Trisomy 13.

5. Circumcision is contraindicated until a determination is made concerning the need for surgical reconstruction.

C. Diagnostic tests

1. **Pelvic ultrasound** can determine whether a uterus is present. Ovaries and testes can often be visualized. Magnetic resonance imaging (MRI) may be needed to locate intra-abdominal testes.

2. **The voiding orifice should be injected with radiopaque contrast.** This procedure may reveal a vagina with cervix at its apex or a utricle.

3. **Chromosome analysis** on peripheral blood can be performed using standard techniques within 72 hours and more rapidly via fluorescent *in situ*

hybridization (FISH). A standard karyotype may reveal 46,XX, but portions of the Y chromosome containing the SRY region may be translocated to an X chromosome requiring FISH techniques to locate the Y material.

V. 46,XX females with genital ambiguity/virilization. The infant has no Wolffian structures, normally developed Müllerian structures, and evidence of external genital virilization.

    A. The most common form of genital ambiguity is a female infant with 21-hydroxylase (21-OH in Fig. 30.4 or CYP21) deficiency. Virilization may occur in other adrenogenital syndromes: 11β-hydroxylase (11-OH in Fig. 30.4 or CYP11B1) deficiency, or 3β-hydroxysteroid dehydrogenase (3βHSD3) deficiency (see Fig. 30.4).

        1. Determinations of **17-hydroxyprogesterone (17-OHP)**, 11-deoxycortisol, dehydroepiandrosterone level (DHEA), and testosterone concentrations should be performed on the second or third day of life. Newborn screening

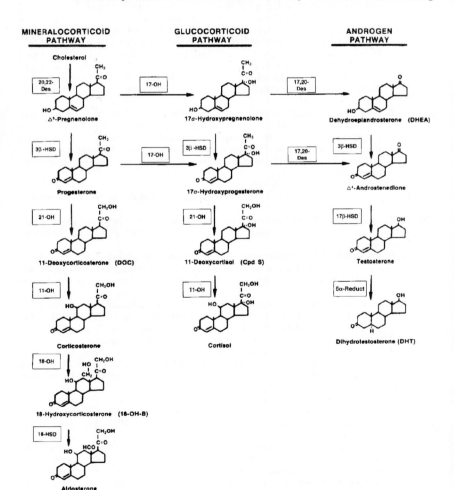

FIG. 30.4. Pathways of steroid biosynthesis. (From Esoterix, 4301 Lost Hills Road, Calabasas Hills, CA 91301.)

programs screen for 21-hydroxylase (21-OH or CYP21) deficiency by measuring 17-OHP concentrations, which should exceed 5000 ng/dl (50 ng/ml) 24 hours after birth in affected full-term infants. In 90% of girls with adrenogenital syndrome, the 17-OHP will be elevated. Worldwide newborn filter-paper screening programs for 17-OHP show an incidence of 1:14,554 births; the incidence varies markedly by country. Salt-losers outnumber non-salt-losers by 3:1. The male:female sex ratio is 1:1. False-positive results occur in sick, premature, and low-birth-weight infants. The false positive rate is as high as 0.19% and the recall rate is 0.2%. Normal values must be determined for each individual program, since they depend on the filter-paper thickness and the radioimmunoassay used. Rapid turnaround of results is critical to avert salt-wasting crises.

2. Virilized females suspected of 21-hydroxylase deficiency should be started on hydrocortisone 20 mg/m² per day (divided into q8h dosing) after the above laboratory tests have been obtained. Salt-wasting crises usually do not develop until the fifth to fourteenth day of life and may occur in affected infants whose virilization is not severe. Weight and fluid balance must be monitored closely with blood samples every 2 days to detect hyponatremia or hyperkalemia during the first 2 weeks of life. If salt-wasting occurs, salt loss should be replaced with intravenous normal saline with glucose added. Once the infant is stabilized, 2 to 3 g of salt per day should be added to the formula and 0.05 to 0.2 mg per day of fludrocortisone acetate (Florinef) is given for mineralocorticoid replacement.

3. In a virilized 46,XX female suspected of having a form of CAH, who has normal 17-OHP levels, an ACTH (Cortrosyn) stimulation test may be necessary to demonstrate the adrenal enzyme defect (see Fig. 30.4). The second most common form of virilizing adrenal hyperplasia, 11β-hydroxylase (11-OH or CYP11B1) deficiency, may present with fluid retention, hypertension, and hypokalemia.

B. Placental aromatase deficiency.

C. Maternal masculinizing CAH or virilizing tumors of the maternal adrenal or ovary.

VI. 46,XY karyotype. The undervirilized male. Even if the chromosomes contain Y material, the parents should not be hastily told that the child should be raised as a male.

A. Environmental disorders: maternal drug ingestion (finasteride, phenytoin).

B. Hereditary disorders. Usually at least one gonad is palpable and there are no Müllerian structures because of anti-Müllerian hormone secreted from the testes.

1. Enzyme defects in testosterone synthesis: deficiencies of 17-ketosteroid reductase (17β-HSD3), 3β-hydroxysteroid dehydrogenase (3βHSD3), 17α-hydroxylase (labeled 17-OH or CYP17), and 17-lyase ("17,20 Des" in Fig. 30.4).

2. Defects in testosterone metabolism (5α-reductase deficiency).

3. Partial end-organ resistance to testosterone (X-linked recessive).

C. Laboratory evaluation of the infant with 46,XY and no Müllerian structures will determine the ability to synthesize testosterone and convert testosterone to dihydrotestosterone.

1. Obtain blood samples for measurement of follicle-stimulating hormone (FSH), luteinizing hormone (LH), dehydroepiandrosterone (DHEA), androstenedione, testosterone, and dihydrotestosterone (DHT). HCG, 500 IU, is given intramuscularly every other day for a total of three doses. Measurements of DHEA, androstenedione, testosterone, and DHT concentrations are repeated 24 hours after the final dose. Inability to increase the testosterone level in response to HCG is characteristic of a biosynthetic defect in testosterone synthesis or gestational loss of testicular tissue ("vanishing testes"). An elevated testosterone:DHT (>20:1) ratio after HCG stimulation suggests 5 α-reductase deficiency.

2. An ACTH stimulation test may be necessary to define earlier enzyme defects in testosterone synthesis such as salt-losing (3βHSD) or salt-retaining (17-OH or 17α-hydroxylase) enzyme deficiencies, which also produce cortisol insufficiency and congenital adrenal hyperplasia (Fig. 30.4)

3. If the initial laboratory tests show high levels of testosterone that do not increase when HCG is given and the ratios of testosterone:androstenedione and testosterone:dihydrotestosterone are normal, the infant probably has a **partial** form of androgen resistance (AR). This can be further evaluated by the administration of 25 to 50 mg of intramuscular depot testosterone monthly for 3 months. Failure of the phallus stretched length to increase by 2.0 ± 0.6 cm in stretch length supports the suspicion of AR. At the time of puberty, these patients will not achieve normal adult phallic size. In the past, infants with partial AR were given a female gender assignment, and underwent gonadectomy and feminizing genitoplasty. This policy has recently become controversial. When a testis is retained, these patients will virilize to a variable degree during puberty, but will develop gynecomastia.

Newborns with the **complete** form of androgen resistance have normal-appearing female genitalia. They may be identified by an antepartum 46,XY karyotype (amniocentesis) or the presence of an apparent inguinal hernia that proves to be a testis. Infants with complete androgen resistance should be raised female. Their gender identities are invariably female.

D. **Other causes of microphallus** (<2.5 cm in a full-term infant) with or without cryptorchidism include: hypothalamo-pituitary disorders of fetal gonadotrophin production such as septo-optic dysplasia or Kallman's Syndrome. Infants with panhypopituitarism often have neonatal hypoglycemia and hyperbilirubinemia. Other syndromes that may be associated with microphallus include: Prader-Willi, Robinow, Klinefelter, Carpenter, Meckel-Gruber, Noonan, de Lange, trisomy 21, Fanconi, and fetal hydantoin. Treatment with testosterone enanthate, 25 mg given intramuscularly monthly for 3 months, may produce substantial increase in penile length.

E. **Bilateral cryptorchidism.** Bilateral cryptorchidism at birth occurs in 3:1000 infants, most of whom are premature. By 1 month of life, the testes are still undescended in 1:1000. Fewer than 1:1000 term infants have bilaterally non-palpable undescended testes. Ultrasound or MRI may reveal a testis in an intra-abdominal location. If testicular tissue cannot be found, serum FSH, LH, and testosterone levels should be measured. Thereafter, three doses of 500 IU of HCG should be given intramuscularly every other day, and serum testosterone remeasured 24 hours after the final dose to determine the presence and responsiveness of testicular tissue. Elevated serum gonadotropins and a low basal testosterone concentration that fails to rise suggest absent or nonfunctioning testes. A surgeon should be consulted and early orchidopexy performed by 1 year of life. If abdominal testes cannot be brought into the scrotum, they should be removed because of the three- to tenfold risk of germ cell cancer in cryptorchid testes. Cryptorchidism occurs in congenital ichthyosis, anencephaly, neural tube defects, Prader-Willi, Laurence-Moon-Biedl, Aarskog, Cockayne, Fanconi, Noonan's, Trisomy 21, and Klinefelter's syndromes.

VII. **Gonadal Differentiation Disorders**

A. **True hermaphroditism.** Less than 10% are 46,XY, 50% are 46,XX, and the remainder show mosaicism (45,X/46,XY or 46,XY/47,XXY) or are chimeric for 46,XX/46,XY. Laparotomy, gonadal biopsy, or both, may be required to diagnose the rare true hermaphrodite. Diagnosis is based on the histology of the gonads, which, by definition, contain both testicular and follicle-containing ovarian tissue. Whether or not the internal structures contain Wolffian or Müllerian elements depend on the presence of testosterone and anti-Müllerian hormone on that side. Sex assignment should be based on the external and internal genitalia and the degree of intrauterine androgen exposure. An HCG stimulation test that produces a rise in serum testosterone concentration indicates the presence of testicular tissue. Dysgenetic

TABLE 30.2. CAUSES OF AMBIGUOUS GENITAL DEVELOPMENT (INTERSEX)

Disorder	Phenotype			Karyotype
	External Genitalia	Gonads		
Disorders of gonadal differentiation				
True hermaphroditism	Ambiguous	Ovarian and testicular tissue		46,XX; 46,XY; 46,XX/46,XY chimerism or mosaic
"Pure" gonadal dysgenesis	Female	Streak gonads or hypoplastic ovaries		46,XX
	Female or ambiguous	Dysgenetic testes or dysgenetic testes and streak gonads		46,XY
Mixed gonadal dysgenesis	Ambiguous	Streak gonad and dysgenetic testis		45,X/46,XY;46,XYp⁻
Female pseudohermaphroditism (masculinization of the genetic female)				
Congenital adrenal hyperplasia				
21α-hydroxylase deficiency	Ambiguous	Ovaries		46,XX
11β-hydroxylase deficiency	Ambiguous	Ovaries		46,XX
3β-OH steroid dehydrogenase deficiency	Ambiguous	Ovaries		46,XX
Transplacental synthetic progestogens	Ambiguous	Ovaries		46,XX
Maternal androgen excess	Ambiguous	Ovaries		46,XX
Male pseudohermaphroditism (incomplete masculinization of the genetic male)				
Testicular unresponsiveness to HCG and LH (Leydig cell hypoplasia or agenesis)	Ambiguous	Testes		46,XY

614

Disorder	Phenotype	Gonads	Karyotype
Disorders of testosterone synthesis	Ambiguous	Testes	46,XY
Side chain cleavage enzyme deficiency			
17α-hydroxylase deficiency			
3β-OH steroid dehydrogenase deficiency			
17-lyase deficiency			
17-ketosteroid reductase deficiency			
End-organ resistance to testosterone			
Complete testicular feminization	Female	Testes	46,XY
Incomplete testicular feminization	Ambiguous	Testes	46,XY
Disorder of testosterone metabolism			
5α-reductase deficiency	Ambiguous	Testes	46,XY
Vanishing testes syndrome	Variable	Absent gonads	46,XY
Lack of Müllerian inhibiting substance	Male	Testes, uterus, fallopian tubes	46,XY

Source: From Wolfsdorf J.I., Muglia L., Endocrine Disorders. In: Graef J.W. (Ed.), *Manual of Pediatric Therapeutics.* Philadelphia: Lippincott-Raven, 1997:381–413.
HCG = human chorionic gonadotropin; LH = luteinizing hormone.

Y chromosome-containing gonads should be removed. If a male sex assignment is made, Müllerian structures should be removed.

B. **Mixed gonadal dysgenesis.** This disorder has a 45,X/46,XY chromosomal complement. The genitalia range from completely male to completely female, and a uterus and a fallopian tube are frequently present. Gender assignment is discretionary because of the marked phenotypic and hormonal variability. The external genitalia are usually asymmetric, with a gonad palpable in one labioscrotal fold and a streak gonad intra-abdominally. If an HCG stimulation test causes a significant rise in serum testostosterone concentration indicative of testicular tissue, the testis should be removed or brought into the scrotum for close observation if a male sex assignment is made. Gonadal neoplasia (gonadoblastoma) may arise in the first 20 years of life in up to 20% of these children. Therefore, streak gonads should be removed in infancy. Other features of the disorder may be more typical of Turner's syndrome: webbed neck, lymphedema, short stature, and occasional cardiac defects, specifically coarctation of the aorta.

C. **"Complete" gonadal dysgenesis.** Karyotype may be 46,XX or 46,XY and most do not usually have genital ambiguity at birth. Infants with 46,XY gonadal dysgenesis fail to masculinize, owing to incomplete testicular differentiation as a result of abnormal functioning of the SRY gene or of transcription factors that regulate the gene's activity. The external genitalia usually appear female, but clitoromegaly may occur, and streak gonads are present. Up to 30% of patients with 46,XY gonadal dysgenesis will develop gonadoblastoma or dysgerminoma. These gonads should be removed in infancy.

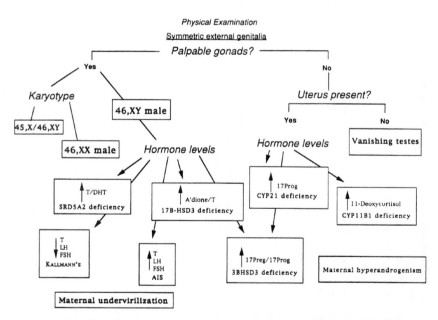

FIG. 30.5. Algorithm for the evaluation of symmetrical genital ambiguity. A'dione = androstenedione; AIS = androgen insensitivity syndrome; DHT = dihydrotestosterone; FSH = follicle stimulating hormone; LH = luteinizing hormone; 17 Preg = 17-hydroxypregnenolone; 17 Prog = 17-hydroxyprogesterone; T = testosterone. (From Witchel S.S., Lee P.A., Ambiguous genitalia. In: Sperling M.A. (Ed.), *Pediatric Endocrinology.* Philadelphia: Saunders, 1996:31–49.)

A uterus is often present due to inadequate production of anti-Müllerian hormone from the undifferentiated gonads. These patients are usually raised female and may not be diagnosed until they fail to initiate puberty and exhibit high gonadotrophins consistent with gonadal failure. With gonads retained, these patients may virilize at puberty.

VIII. Table 30.2 summarizes causes and Figs. 30.5 and 30.6 describe an approach to patients with ambiguous genitalia.

IX. **Issues of Gender Assignment**

In the past, a primary criterion for male gender assignment was phallic size adequate for sexual function. This issue is currently being debated. 46,XY infants born with little or no penile tissue have usually been given female sex assignment and surgically and hormonally feminized by means of genitoplasty early in life and estrogen treatment at the age of puberty. The decision to assign gender is, however, complicated by our current understanding that the prenatal hormonal environment influences gender identity formation and behavior. During the second trimester, the normal fetal testis produces levels of testosterone approaching concentrations seen in the adult male. The 46,XY neonate born with minimal penile tissue, who is not androgen resistant and who has been exposed to normal intrauterine testosterone concentrations, may retain a male gender identity regardless of gender assignment. Fueling the debate are the new techniques such as intracytoplasmic sperm injection (ICSI) which makes fertilization possible without penetration or ejaculation.

Likewise, the issue of gender assignment in the case of the most severely virilized 46,XX newborns with congenital adrenal hyperplasia who have completely fused labioscrotal folds and a phallic urethra is also under debate. A minority

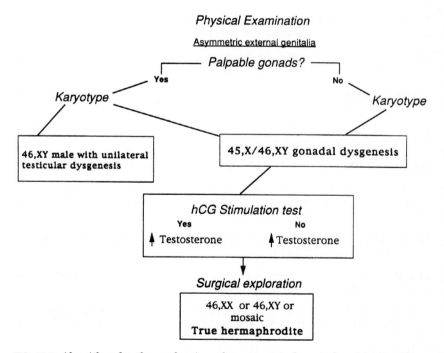

FIG. 30.6. Algorithm for the evaluation of asymmetrical genital ambiguity. (From Witchel S.S., Lee P.A. Ambiguous genitalia. In: Sperling M.A. (Ed.), *Pediatric Endocrinology*. Philadelphia: Saunders, 1996:31–49.)

opinion recommends male assignment and gonadectomy, thereby eliminating the need for feminizing genitoplasty. Nevertheless, most geneticists and endocrinologists continue to recommend female assignment to preserve fertility.

Whether and when to perform genital surgery, particularly clitoral reduction in virilized females, is now also the subject of controversy. Whereas some intersexual adults view their genital surgery as mutilation, most parents prefer surgery so that their child's genitalia appear consistent with the gender of rearing. One-stage surgical procedures that preserve the neurovascular bundle can be done in infancy and are much improved compared to the ablative procedures and clitorectomies that were routinely performed several decades ago.

Parents require a thorough explanation of their child's condition as the laboratory and imaging data become available so that they can participate in the decision-making as the various options for medical and surgical therapy and future prospects for sexual functioning, fertility, and gender identity are evaluated. Long-term studies of gender identity and sexual functioning in individuals born with various forms of genital ambiguity are underway. The results will enhance our understanding of the complex and subtle issues and will contribute to the difficult task of assigning the most appropriate gender for a specific infant.

Suggested Readings

American Academy of Pediatrics. Committee on Genetics. Evaluation of the newborn with developmental anomalies of the external genitalia. *Pediatrics* 2000;106:138.

Anhalt H., et al. Ambiguous genitalia. *Pediatr Rev* 1996;17: 213.

Berenbaum S.A. Effects of early androgens on sex-typed activities and interests in adolescents with congenital adrenal hyperplasia. *Horm Behav* 1999;35:102.

Creighton S.M., et al. Objective cosmetic and anatomical outcomes at adolescence of feminising surgery for ambiguous genitalia done in childhood. *Lancet* 2001;358:124.

Diamond M., Sigmundson H.K. Management of intersexuality: Guidelines for dealing with persons with ambiguous genitalia. *Arch Pediatr Adolesc Med* 1997;151:1046.

Drummond-Borg M., et al. Nonfluorescent dicentric Y in males with hypospadias. *J Pediatr* 1988;113:469.

Federman D.D., Donahoe P.K. Ambiguous genitalia—etiology, diagnosis and therapy. *Adv Endocrinol Metab* 1995;6:91.

Hawkins J.R. The SRY gene. *Trend Endocrinol Metab* 1993;4:328.

Hawkins J.R., et al. Evidence for increased prevalence of SRY mutations in XY females with complete rather than partial gonadal dysgenesis. *Am J Hum Genet* 1992;51:979.

Lee P.A. Fertility in cryptorchidism: Does treatment make a difference? *Endocrinol Metab Clin North Am* 1993;22:479.

Page D.C, et al. Exchange of terminal portions of X- and Y- chromosomal short arms in human XX males. *Nature* 1987;328:437.

Pang S., et al. Congenital adrenal hyperplasia due to 21 hydroxylase deficiency: Newborn screening and its relationship to the diagnosis and treatment of the disorder. *Screening* 1993;2:105.

Pritchard-Jones K., et al. The candidate Wilms' tumour gene is involved in genitourinary development. *Nature* 1990;346:194.

Reiner W.G. Assignment of sex in neonates with ambiguous genitalia. *Curr Opin Pediatr* 1999;11:363.

Saenger P. Male pseudohermaphroditism. *Pediatr Ann* 1981;10:15.

Savage M.O., Lowe D.G. Gonadal neoplasia and abnormal sexual differentiation. *Clin Endocrinol* 1990;32:519.

Schnitzer J.J., Donahoe P.K. Surgical treatment of congenital adrenal hyperplasia. *Endocrinol Metab Clin North Am* 2001;30:137.

Styne D.M. The testes: Disorders of sexual differentiation and puberty. In: Sperling M.A. (Ed.), *Pediatric Endocrinology.* Philadelphia: Saunders, 1996;424.

Therell B.L. Newborn screening for congenital adrenal hyperplasia. *Endocrinol Metab Clin North Am* 2001;30:15.

Vainio S., et al. Female development in mammals is regulated by Wnt-4 signalling. *Nature* 1999;397:405.

Warne G.L., Zajac J.D. Disorders of sexual differentiation. *Endocrinol Metab Clin North Am* 1998;27:945.

Witchel S.S., Lee P.A. Ambiguous genitalia. In: Sperling M.A. (Ed.), *Pediatric Endocrinology.* Philadelphia: Saunders, 1996;32.

31. RENAL CONDITIONS

Melanie S. Kim and John T. Herrin

I. **Renal embryogenesis and functional development**
   A. **Embryology**
      1. Three paired renal systems develop from the nephrogenic ridge of the mesoderm.
      2. The first two systems, the **pronephros** and the **mesonephros,** have limited function in the human being and are transient. The mesonephric tubules and duct form the efferent ductules of the epididymis, the vas deferens, the ejaculatory ducts, and the seminal vesicles in the male. In the female they result in the vestigial epoophoron and the paroophoron.
      3. The **metanephros** is the third and final excretory system and appears in the fifth week of gestation. The metanephros is made up of two different cell types. These differentiate into the **pelvicalyceal** system, which is well delineated by the thirteenth or fourteenth week, and the **nephrons,** which continue to form up to the thirty-fifth week of gestation to a final complement of one million nephrons per kidney. Urine is produced by the twelfth week.
      4. Parallel development of the lower urinary tract occurs with opening of the mesonephric duct to the allantois and cloaca at 5 weeks' gestation. Shortly thereafter at 6 weeks, the urorectal fold forms as a septum dividing the gastrointestinal (GI) tract (posterior compartment) from the anterior genitourinary (GU) compartment—the urogenital sinus. At 7 weeks separate vesicoureteral openings form and the allantois degenerates to a cord that becomes the urachus and the upper bladder, while the trigone develops from the Wolffian duct remnant. Müllerian system development produces a uretero-vaginal cord, which in the female becomes the vaginal vestibule, vagina, and uterine cervix. In the male, Müllerian system regression leads to the prostatic urethra.
      5. Disruption of normal renal development may lead to renal malformations such as renal agenesis, renal hypoplasia, renal ectopy, renal dysplasia, and cystic disease.
   B. **Functional development.** At birth, the kidney replaces the placenta as the major homeostatic organ, maintaining fluid and electrolyte balance and removing harmful waste products. This transition occurs with changes in renal blood flow, glomerular filtration rate and tubular functions. The level of renal function relates more closely to the postnatal age than to the gestational age at birth.
      1. **Renal blood flow (RBF)** remains low in the fetus, accounting for only 2 to 3% of cardiac output. At birth, RBF rapidly increases to 15 to 18% of cardiac output because of (1) a decrease in renal vascular resistance, which is proportionally greater in the kidney compared to other organs,; (2) an increase in systemic blood pressure,; (3) increase in inner to outer cortical blood flow.
      2. **Glomerular filtration** begins soon after the first nephrons are formed and glomerular filtration rate (GFR) increases in parallel with body and kidney growth (approximately 1 mL/min per kilogram of body weight). Once all the glomeruli are formed by 34 weeks' gestation, the GFR continues to increase until birth because of decreases in renal vascular resistance. After birth, the GFR rises quickly, doubling by 2 weeks of age and reaching adult levels by 1 year of age. The rate of GFR maturation is not altered by premature birth and increases in response to solute load. GFR is less well autoregulated in the neonate. It is controlled by maintenance of glomerular capillary pressure by the greater vasoconstrictive effect of

angiotension II at the efferent then afferent arteriole where the effect is attenuated by concurrent prostglandin induced vasodilatation.

3. **Tubular function:**

a. **Sodium (Na+) handling:** The capacity to reabsorb Na+ is developed by 24 weeks' gestation. However, tubular resorption of Na+ is low until 34 weeks' gestation, with fractional excretion of sodium (FeNa; see Table 31.1) ranging from 5 to 10%. In severely ill infants, urinary Na losses can be very high, with FeNa reaching 15%. Very premature infants cannot conserve Na+ even when Na+ balance is negative. Hence premature infants below 34 weeks' gestation receiving formula or breast milk without Na+ supplementation can develop hyponatremia. After 34 weeks' gestation, Na+ reabsorption becomes more efficient, so that 99% of filtered Na+ can be reabsorbed, resulting in a FeNa of less than 1%. Full-term neonates can retain Na+ when in negative Na+ balance but, like premature infants, are also limited in their ability to excrete a Na+ load because of their low GFR.

b. **Water handling:** The newborn infant has a limited ability to concentrate urine. The maximal urine osmolality is 500 mOsm/L in premature infants and 800 mOsm/L in term infants. Although this is of little consequence in infants receiving appropriate amounts of water with hypotonic feeding, it can become clinically relevant in infants receiving high osmotic loads. In contrast, both premature and full-term infants can dilute their urine with a minimal urine osmolality of 25 to 35 mOsm/L. Their low GFR, however, limits their ability to handle water loads.

c. **Potassium (K+) handling:** The limited ability of premature infants to excrete large K+ loads is related to decreased distal tubular K+ secretion, a result of decreased aldosterone sensitivity, low Na-K+ adenosine triphosphatase (ATPase) activity, and low GFR.

d. **Acid and bicarbonate handling** are limited by (1) a low serum bicarbonate threshold in the proximal tubule (14 to 16 mEq/L in premature infants, 18 to 21 mEq/L in full-term infants) which improves as matu-

TABLE 31.1. COMMONLY USED EQUATIONS AND FORMULAS

$$CrCl \ (ml/min/1.73 \ m^2) = K \times \frac{Length \ (cm)}{P_{Cr}}$$

$K = 0.34$ in premature infants <34 wks and 0.44 in infants from 35 wks to term

$$CrCl \ (ml/min/1.73 \ m^2) = \frac{U_{Cr} \times U_{vol} \times 1.73}{P_{Cr} \times BSA}$$

$$FeNa = 100 \times \left(\frac{U_{Na^+} \times P_{Cr}}{P_{Na^+} \times U_{Cr}} \right)$$

$$TRP = 100 \times \left(1 - \frac{U_P \times P_{Cr}}{P_P \times U_{Cr}} \right)$$

Calculated $P_{osm} \geqslant 2 \times$ plasma $[Na^+] + \frac{[glucose]}{18} + \frac{BUN}{2.8}$

Plasma anion gap $= [Na^+] - [Cl^-] - [HCO^-_3]$

CrCl = creatinine clearance, U_{Cr} = urinary creatinine, U_{vol} = urinary volume per minute, P_{Cr} = plasma creatinine, P_{Na} = plasma sodium, BSA = body surface area, FeNa = fractional excretion of sodium, TRP = tubular reabsorption of phosphorus, P_{osm} = plasma osmolarity.

ration of Na^+-K^+ ATPase and Na^+-H transporter occurs. In addition, the production of ammonia in the distal tubule and proximal tubular glutamine synthesis are decreased. The lower rate of phosphate excretion limits the generation of titratable acid, further limiting their ability to eliminate an acid load. Very-low-birth-weight infants can develop mild metabolic acidosis during the second to fourth week after birth that may require administration of additional sodium bicarbonate.

   e. Calcium and phosphorous handling in the neonate is characterized by a pattern of increased phosphate retention associated with growth. The intake and filtered load of phosphate, parathyroid hormone (PTH), and growth factors modulate phosphate transport. The higher phosphate level and higher rate of phosphate reabsorption are not explained by a low GFR or tubular unresponsiveness to extrarenal factors (PTH, vitamin D). More likely, there is a developmental mechanism that favors renal conservation of phosphate in part due to growth hormone effects, as well as a growth-related Na^+-dependent phosphate transporter, so that a positive phosphate balance for growth is maintained. Tubular reabsorption of phosphate is also altered by gestational age, increasing from 85% at 28 weeks to 93% at 34 weeks and 98% by 40 weeks.

   Calcium levels in the fetus and cord blood are higher than those in the neonate. Calcium levels fall in the first 24 hours, but low levels of PTH persist. This relative hypoparathyroidism in the first few days after birth may be the result of this physiologic response to hypercalcemia in the normal fetus. Although plasma Ca^+ values less than 8 mg% in premature infants are common, they are usually asymptomatic, because the ionized calcium level is usually normal. Factors that favor this normal ionized Ca^+ fraction include lower serum albumin and the relative metabolic acidosis in the neonate.

   Urinary calcium excretion is lower in premature infants and correlates with gestational age. At term, calcium excretion rises and persists until approximately 12 months of age. The urine calcium excretion in the premature infants varies directly with Na^+ intake, urinary Na^+ excretion, and inversely with plasma Ca^{2+}. Neonatal stress and therapies such as aggressive fluid use or furosemide administration increase Ca^{2+} excretion, aggravating the tendency to hypocalcemia.

   f. Fetal urine contribution to amniotic fluid volume is minimal in the first half of gestation but increases significantly to an average of 50 mL/hr and is a necessary contribution to pulmonary development. Oligohydramnios will follow decreased renal function.

II. Clinical assessment of renal function
   Assessment of renal function is based on the patient's history, physical examination, and appropriate laboratory and radiologic tests.
   A. History
   1. Prenatal history includes any maternal illness, drug use, or exposure to known and potential teratogens.
      a. Maternal use of captopril or indomethacin decrease glomerular capillary pressure and GFR and has been associated with neonatal renal failure.
      b. Oligohydramnios may indicate a decrease in fetal urine production. It is often associated with renal agenesis, renal dysplasia, polycystic kidney disease, or severe obstruction of the urinary-tract system. Polyhydramnios may be a result of renal tubular dysfunction with inability to fully concentrate urine.
      c. Elevated serum and amniotic fluid alpha-fetoprotein have been associated with congenital nephrotic syndrome.
   2. Family history. The risk of renal disease is increased if there is a family history of urinary-tract anomalies, polycystic kidney disease, consanguinity, or inherited renal tubular disorders.

3. **Delivery history.** Fetal distress, perinatal asphyxia, or shock due to volume loss may lead to ischemic or anoxic injury, resulting in acute tubular necrosis.

4. **Micturition.** 17% of newborns void in the delivery room, 93% void by 24 hours, and 98% void by 48 hours. The rate of urine formation ranges from 0.5 to 5.0 mL/kg per hour at all gestational ages. The most common cause of delayed or decreased urine production is inadequate perfusion of the kidneys; however, delay in micturition may be due to intrinsic renal abnormalities or obstruction of the urinary tract.

B. **Physical examination.** Careful examination will detect abdominal masses in 0.8% of neonates. The majority of these masses are either renal in origin or related to the GU system. It is important to consider in the differential diagnosis whether the mass is unilateral or bilateral (Table 31.2). Edema may be present in infants with congenital nephrotic syndrome, renal failure, or fluid overload. Concentrating defects or tubular defects with salt wasting may cause dehydration.

Other congenital anomalies detected by physical examination which are associated with renal abnormalities include low-set ears, ambiguous genitalia, anal atresia, abdominal wall defect, vertebral anomalies, aniridia, meningomyelocele or tethered cord, pneumothorax, hemihypertrophy, persistent urachus, hypospadias, and cryptorchidism (Table 31.3). Spontaneous pneumothorax is associated with an increased risk of renal abnormalities.

C. **Laboratory evaluation.** Renal function tests must be interpreted in relationship to gestational and postnatal age (Tables 31.4 and 31.5).

1. Urinalysis reflects the developmental stages of renal physiology.

   a. **Specific gravity.** Full-term infants have a limited concentrating ability with a maximum specific gravity of 1.021 to 1.025.

   b. **Protein excretion** varies with gestational age. Urinary protein excretion is higher in premature infants and decreases progressively with postnatal age. In normal full-term infants, protein excretion is minimal after the second week of life.

   c. **Glycosuria** is commonly present in premature infants of less than 34 weeks' gestation. The tubular resorption of glucose is less than 93% in infants born before 34 weeks' gestation compared with 99% in infants born after 34 weeks' gestation. Glucose excretion rates are highest in infants born before 28 weeks' gestation.

TABLE 31.2. ABDOMINAL MASSES IN THE NEONATE

Type of Mass	% Total
I. Renal	55
Hydronephrosis	
Multicystic Dysplastic Kidney	
Polycystic Kidney Disease	
Mesoblastic Nephroma	
Renal Ectopia	
Renal Vein Thrombosis	
Nephrobastomatosis	
Wilms' Tumor	
II. Genital	15
Hydrometrocolpos	
Ovarian Cyst	
III. Gastrointestinal	20

From Pinto E., Guignard J.P. Renal masses in the neonate. *Biol Neonate* 1995;68:175–184.

TABLE 31.3. CONGENITAL SYNDROMES WITH RENAL COMPONENTS

Dysmorphic Disorders, Sequences, and Associations	General Features	Renal Abnormalities
Oligohydramnios sequence (Potter syndrome)	Altered facies, pulmonary hypoplasia, abnormal limb and head position	Renal agenesis, severe bilateral obstruction, severe bilateral dysplasia, autosomal recessive polycystic kidney disease
VATER and VACTERL syndrome	Vertebral anomalies, anal atresia, tracheo-esophageal fistula, radial dysplasia, cardiac and limb defects	Renal agenesis, renal dysplasia, renal ectopia
MURCS association and Rokitansky sequence	Failure of paramesonephric ducts, vaginal and uterus hypoplasia/atresia, cervicothoracic somite dysplasia	Renal hypoplasia/agenesis, renal ectopia, double uterers
Prune belly	Hypoplasia of abdominal muscle, cryptorchidism	Megaureters, hydronephrosis, dysplastic kidneys, atonic bladder
Spina bifida	Meningomyelocele	Neurogenic bladder, vesicoureteral reflux, hydronephrosis, double ureter, horseshoe kidney
Caudal dysplasia sequence (caudal regression syndrome)	Sacral (and lumbar) hypoplasia, disruption of the distal spinal cord	Neurogenic bladder, vesicoureteral reflux, hydronephrosis, renal agenesis
Anal atresia (high imperforate anus)	Rectovaginal, rectovesical, or rectourethral fistula tethered to the spinal cord	Renal agenesis, renal dysplasia
Hemihypertrophy	Hemihypertrophy	Wilms' tumor, hypospadias
Aniridia	Aniridia, cryptorchidism	Wilms' tumor
Drash syndrome	Ambiguous genitalia	Mesangial sclerosis, Wilms' tumor
Small deformed or low-set ears		Renal agenesis/dysplasia

(continues)

TABLE 31.3. *(continued)*

Hereditary Disorders	General Features	Renal Abnormalities
Autosomal recessive		
Cerebrohepatorenal syndrome (Zellweger syndrome)	Hepatomegaly, glaucoma, brain anomalies, chondrodystrophy	Cortical renal cysts
Jeune syndrome (thoracic asphyxiating dystrophy)	Small thoracic cage, short ribs, abnormal costochondral junctions, pulmonary hypoplasia	Cystic tubular dysplasia, glomerulosclerosis, hydronephrosis, horseshoe kidneys
Meckel-Gruber syndrome (dysencephalia splanchnocystica)	Encephalocele, microcephaly, polydactyly, cryptorchidism, cardiac anomalies, liver disease	Polycystic/dysplastic kidneys
Johanson-Blizzard syndrome	Hypoplastic alae nasi, hypothyroidism, deafness, imperforate anus, cryptorchidism	Hydronephrosis, caliectasis
Schinzel-Giedon syndrome	Short limbs, abnormal facies, bone abnormalities, hypospadias	Hydronephrosis, megaureter
Short rib–polydactyly syndrome	Short horizontal ribs, pulmonary hypoplasia, polysyndactyly, bone and cardiac defects, ambiguous genitalia	Glomerular and tubular cysts
Bardet-Biedl syndrome	Obesity, retinal pigmentation, polydactyly	Interstitial nephritis
Autosomal dominant		
Tuberous sclerosis	Fibrous-angiomatous lesions, hypopigmented macules, intracranial calcifications, seizures, bone lesions	Polycystic kidneys, renal angiomyolipomata
Melnick-Fraser syndrome (branchio-otorenal [BOR] syndrome)	Preauricular pits, branchial clefts, deafness	Renal dysplasia, duplicated ureters
Nail-patella syndrome (hereditary osteoonychodysplasia)	Hypoplastic nails, hypoplastic or absent patella, other bone anomalies	Proteinuria, nephrotic syndrome
Townes syndrome	Thumb, auricular and anal anomalies	Various renal abnormalities
X-Linked		
Oculocerebrorenal syndrome (Lowe's syndrome)	Cataracts, rickets, mental retardation	Fanconi syndrome
Oral-facial-digital (OFD) syndrome, type I	Oral clefts, hypoplastic alae nasi, digital asymmetry (X-linked, lethal in male)	Renal microcysts

(continues)

TABLE 31.3. *(continued)*

Chromosomal Abnormalities	General Features	Renal Abnormalities
Trisomy 21 (Down syndrome)	Abnormal facies, brachy-cephaly, congenital heart disease	Cystic dysplastic kidney and other renal abnormalities
X0 syndrome (Turner syndrome)	Small stature, congenital heart disease, amenorrhea	Horseshoe kidney, duplications and malrotations of the urinary col-lecting system
Trisomy 13 (Patau syndrome)	Abnormal facies, cleft lip and palate, congenital heart disease	Cystic dysplastic kidneys and other renal anomalies
Trisomy 18 (Edwards syndrome)	Abnormal facies, abnormal ears, overlapping digits, congenital heart disease	Cystic dysplastic kidneys, horse-shoe kidney, or duplication
XXY, XXX syndrome (Triploidy syndrome)	Abnormal facies, cardiac defects, hypospadias and cryptorchidism in male, syndactyly	Various renal abnormalities
Partial trisomy 10q	Abnormal facies, micro-cephaly, limb and cardiac abnormalities	Various renal abnormalities

  d. Hematuria is abnormal and may indicate intrinsic renal damage or re-sult from a bleeding or clotting abnormality (see III.G).
  e. The sediment exam will usually demonstrate multiple epithelial cells (thought to be urethral mucosal cells) for the first 24 to 48 hours. In in-fants with asphyxia, there is an increase in epithelial cells and transient microscopic hematuria with leukocytes is common. Further investigation is necessary if these sediment findings persist. Hyaline and fine granular casts are common in dehydration or hypotension. Uric acid crystals are common in deyhdration states and concentrated urine samples. They may be seen as pink or reddish brown diaper staining (particularly with the newer absorptive diapers).
2. Method of collection
  a. Suprapubic aspiration is the most reliable method of detecting urinary-tract infection.
  b. Bladder catheterization is used if an infant has failed to pass urine by 36 to 48 hours and is not apparently hypovolemic (see III.B), or if urine volume, flow, or sedimentary exam is important.
  c. Bag collections are adequate for most studies such as determinations of specific gravity, pH, electrolytes, protein, glucose, and sediment but not urine culture. It is the preferred method for detecting red blood cells in the urine.
  d. Diaper urine specimens are reliable for estimation of pH and qualita-tive determination of the presence of glucose, protein, and blood.
3. Evaluation of renal function
  a. Serum creatinine at birth reflects maternal renal function. In infants, serum creatinine levels after a transient rise over the first 24 to 36

TABLE 31.4. NORMAL URINARY AND RENAL VALUES IN TERM AND PRETERM INFANTS

	Preterm Infants <34 wks	Term Infants at Birth	Term Infants 2 wks	Term Infants 8 wks
GFR (ml/min/1.73 m^2)	13–58	15–60		63–80
FeNa (%) (oliguric patient)	>1%	<1%	<1%	<1%
Bicarbonate threshold (mEq/L)	14–18	21	21.5	
TRP (%)	>85%	>95%		
Protein excretion (mg/m^2/24h) (mean ± 1 SD)	60 ± 96	31 ± 44		
Maximal concentration ability (mOsmol/L)	500	800	900	1200
Maximal diluting ability (mOsmol/L)	25–30	25–30	25–30	25–30
Specific gravity	1.002–1.015	1.002–1.020	1.002–1.025	
Dipstick				
pH	5.0–8.0	4.5–8.0	4.5–8.0	4.5–8.0
Proteins	Neg to ++	Neg to +	Neg	Neg
Glucose	Neg to ++	Neg	Neg	Neg
Blood	Neg	Neg	Neg	Neg
Leukocytes	Neg	Neg	Neg	Neg

TABLE 31.5. NORMAL SERUM CREATININE VALUES IN TERM AND PRETERM INFANTS (MEAN ±SD)

Age (days)	<28 weeks	28–32 weeks	32–37 weeks	>37 weeks
3	1.05 ± 0.27	0.88 ± 0.25	0.78 ± 0.22	0.75 ± 0.2
7	0.95 ± 0.36	0.94 ± 0.37	0.77 ± 0.48	0.56 ± 0.4
14	0.81 ± 0.26	0.78 ± 0.36	0.62 ± 0.4	0.43 ± 0.25
28	0.66 ± 0.28	0.59 ± 0.38	0.40 ± 0.28	0.34 ± 0.2

From: (1) Rudd P.T., et al. Reference ranges for plasma creatinine during the first month of life. *Arch Dis Child* 1983;58:212. (2) Van den Anker J.N., et al. Assessment of glomerular filtration rate in preterm infants by serum creatinine: comparison with insulin clearance. *Pediatrics* 1995;96:1156–8.

hours (particularly in premature infants) fall quickly from 0.8 mg/dL at birth to 0.5 mg/dL at 5 to 7 days and reach a stable level of 0.3 to 0.4 mg/dL by 9 days. The rate of decrease in serum creatinine in the first few weeks is slower in younger gestational age infants with lower GFR (see Table 31.5).

  b. Serum urea nitrogen (BUN) is a useful indicator of renal function. However, BUN can be elevated as a result of increased production of urea nitrogen in hypercatabolic states, sequestered blood, tissue breakdown, hemoconcentration, or increased protein intake. Renal insufficiency is suspected if BUN is greater than 20 mg/dL or rises at a rate of 5 mg/dL per day or higher.

  c. Glomerular filtration rate can be measured by clearance studies of either exogenous substances (insulin, Cr-EDTA [chromium ethylene diamene tetra-acetic acid], sodium iothalamate) or endogenous substances such as creatinine. Practical considerations such as frequent blood sampling, urine collection, or infusion of an exogenous substance limit their use. GFR can be estimated from serum creatinine and body length (see Table 31.1).

  d. Measurement of serum and urine electrolytes is used to guide fluid and electrolyte management and in assessing renal tubular function.

D. Radiological studies

  1. Ultrasound is the initial imaging study to delineate renal parenchymal architecture. Color flow Doppler techniques can estimate renal blood flow. The length of the kidneys in millimeters is approximately the gestational age in weeks. The renal cortex has echogenicity similar to that of the liver or spleen in the neonate, in contrast to the hypoechoic renal cortex seen in adults and older children. In addition, the medullary pyramids in the neonate are much more hypoechoic than the cortex and hence are more prominent in appearance.

  2. Intravenous pyelography (IVP) is rarely used in the newborn period, since the neonate has a limited concentrating ability and difficulty in excreting a highly osmolar load.

  3. Voiding cystourethography (VCUG), with fluoroscopy, is indicated in infants with urinary-tract infections or with renal anomalies on ultrasound to rule out vesicoureteral reflux (VUR) and in neonates with obstructive uropathy to define associated reflux and define lower-tract anatomy more specifically. Radionuclide cystography is often used to evaluate VUR because of its lower radiation dose. However, VCUG produces better static imaging for anatomical defects and is preferred for the initial evaluation of obstructive uropathy.

  4. Radionuclide scintography is useful in demonstrating the position and relative function of the kidneys. Isotopes such as technetium-99m-diethylene triamine pentacetic acid (DTPA) or mercaptoacetyltriglycine

(MAG 3) are handled by glomerular filtration and can be used to assess renal blood flow and renal function. In conjunction with intravenously administered furosemide, it can help differentiate obstructive from nonobstructive hydronephrosis. Isotopes that bind to the renal tubules, such as technetium-99m-dimercaptosuccinic acid (DMSA), produce static images of the renal cortex. This may be helpful for assessing acute pyelonephritis and renal scarring from renal artery emboli, or renal vascular disorders and to quantify the amount of renal cortex in patients with renal dysplasia and hypoplasia.

III. Common clinical renal problems

A. **Prenatal ultrasound:** Routine maternal ultrasound screening detects an incidence of fetal genitourinary abnormalities of 0.3 to 0.5%.

1. The most common finding is **hydronephrosis,** reported in over 80% of the cases. Approximately 75% of these are confirmed postnatally.

a. Initial management of a newborn with prenatally identified hydronephrosis depends on the clinical condition of the patient and the suspected nature of the lesion.

b. Unilateral hydronephrosis is more common and is not associated with systemic or pulmonary complications if the contralateral kidney is normal. Postnatal ultrasound confirmation may be carried out electively at about 1 month, depending on severity. It is important to not perform the ultrasound examination in the first few days after birth, when hydronephrosis may not be detected because of physiologic dehydration.

c. Bilateral hydronephrosis is more worrisome, especially if oligohydramnios or pulmonary disease is present. In the male infant, postnatal evaluation (VCUG and ultrasound) should be performed within the first day to rule out the possibility of posterior urethral valves (PUV). With post-bladder obstruction such as PUV, ultrasound will often demonstrate a trabeculated and thickened bladder wall.

d. Prophylactic antibiotics (amoxicillin 20 mg/kg orally every day) is recommended before VCUG is performed, as hydronephrosis may be due to vesicoureteral reflux.

2. Routine prenatal ultrasound has increased the diagnosis of multicystic dysplastic kidney (MCDK) especially with unilateral involvement. Infants with unilateral MCDK are usually asymptomatic, and the affected kidney has no renal function as demonstrated by dimercapto succinic acid (DMSA) renal scan. There is general agreement that surgical removal is indicated in cases with associated hypertension or infection, or with respiratory compromise secondary to abdominal compression by the abnormal kidney. In asymptomatic patients, the relative merits of conservative observation versus surgical removal remain controversial.

3. Renal abnormalities may be associated with other congenital anomalies including neural tube defects, congenital heart lesions, intestinal obstructive lesions, abdominal wall defects, central nervous system (CNS) or spinal abnormailites, and urological abnormalities of the lower urinary tract.

B. **Acute renal failure** may be secondary to prerenal, intrinsic, or postrenal disorders (Table 31.6). **Prerenal failure** is due to hypoperfusion to the kidneys. This is the most common cause of renal failure in the neonate, and if not corrected it may lead to intrinsic renal damage. **Intrinsic renal failure** implies direct damage to the kidneys from an insult or congenital anomaly. **Postrenal failure** results from obstruction to urinary flow in both kidneys. In boys, the most common lesion occurs in the posterior urethral valves. Renal function may be abnormal even after correction of the obstruction.

1. **Diagnosis and management** should proceed simultaneously to correct the defect as quickly as possible, so that compromise of the kidney will be limited.

a. Suspect renal failure if oliguria is present (urine flow less than 0.5 mL/kg per hour) and/or if serum creatinine is elevated 2 standard devi-

TABLE 31.6. CAUSES OF RENAL FAILURE IN THE NEONATAL PERIOD

I. Prerenal

  A. Reduced effective circulatory volume
    Hemorrhage
    Dehydration
    Sepsis
    Necrotizing enterocolitis
    Congenital heart disease
    Hypoalbuminemia

  B. Increased renal vascular resistance
    Polycythemia
    Indomethacin
    Adrenergic drugs (e.g., tolazoline)

  C. Hypoxia/asphyxia

II. Intrinsic or renal parenchymal

  A. Sustained hypoperfusion leading to acute tubular necrosis

  B. Congenital anomalies
    Agenesis
    Hypoplasia/dysplasia
    Polycystic kidney disease

  C. Thromboembolic disease
    Bilateral renal vein thrombosis
    Bilateral renal arterial thrombosis

  D. Nephrotoxins
    Aminoglycosides
    Radiographic contrast media
    Maternal use of captopril or indomethacin

III. Obstructive

  A. Urethral obstruction
    Posterior urethral valves
    Stricture

  B. Ureterocele

  C. Ureteropelvic/ureterovesical obstruction

  D. Extrinsic tumors

  E. Neurogenic bladder

  F. Megacystis or megaureter syndrome

---

ations above the mean value for gestational age (see Table 31.5) or rising (0.3 mg/dL per day).
  b. Evaluate history for oligohydramnios, perinatal asphyxia, bleeding disorders, polycythemia, thrombocytsis, thrombocytopenia, or maternal drug use.
  c. Identify abdominal mass or congenital anomaly.
  d. Perform ultrasound exam of genitourinary system.
  e. Catheterize the bladder to rule out lower urinary-tract obstruction, measure residual urine volume, collect urine for analysis, and monitor subsequent urinary flow rate.

   f. To rule out prerenal failure, give a fluid challenge of normal saline 10 to 20 mL/kg over 1 hour if there is no evidence of heart failure or volume overload, administer a diuretic (furosemide, 1 mg/kg). No response suggests intrinsic or postrenal failure. Infuse low-dose dopamine to improve renal blood flow and urine output.

   g. Table 31.7 lists laboratory tests that are helpful in differentiating prerenal from intrinsic renal failure in the oliguric patient.

2. **Management of renal failure** (see Chap. 9)

   a. Discontinue or minimize potassium (K^+) intake. Low-K^+ formula such as Similac PM 60/40 or K^+-free IV solution is used. Treatment of hyperkalemia ($K^+ > 6$ mEq/L) is as follows:

   (1) **Sodium polystyrene sulfonate (Kayexalate)** is administered rectally in a dose of 1.0 to 1.5 g/kg (dissolved in normal saline at 0.5 g/ML saline) or orally in a dose of 1.0 g/kg (dissolved in dextrose 10% in water) every 4 to 6 hours. The enema tube, a thin Silastic feeding tube, is inserted 1 to 3 cm. If possible, we avoid using Kayexalate in low-birth-weight infants. 1 g/kg of resin removes 1 mEq/L of potassium.

   (2) **Calcium** is given as 1 to 2 mL/kg of calcium gluconate 10% over 2 to 4 minutes while the electrocardiogram (ECG) is monitored.

   (3) **Sodium bicarbonate.** 1 mEq/kg given intravenously over 5 to 10 minutes, will decrease serum potassium by 1 mEq/L.

   (4) **Glucose and insulin.** Begin with a bolus of regular human insulin (0.05 units/kg) and dextrose 10% in water (2 mL/kg) followed by a continuous infusion of dextrose 10% in water at 2 to 4 mL/kg per hour and human regular insulin (10 units/100 mL) at 1 mL/kg per hour. Monitor blood glucose level frequently. Maintain a ratio of 1 or 2 units of insulin to 4 g glucose.

   (5) **Furosemide.** 1 mg/kg is given when renal function is adequate or as a trial to establish urine flow as kaliuresis as well as natriuresis occurs with this diuretic.

   (6) **Dialysis** is considered when hyperkalemia cannot be controlled or if anuria is present. All modes of dialysis—hemodialysis (HD), peritoneal dialsyis (PD), continuous veno-venous hemoperfusion (CVVH)—can be used, however, special expertise is needed in this age group (see j).

   b. Fluid management is based on the patient's fluid status and should be limited to replacement of insensible losses and urine output (see Chap. 9).

   c. Sodium (Na^+) is restricted and Na^+ concentration is monitored, accounting for fluid balance. Hyponatremia is usually secondary to excess free water. Close monitoring of electrolytes especially sodium is needed during diuretic therapy or with dialysis.

TABLE 31.7. RENAL FAILURE INDICES IN THE OLIGURIC NEONATE

Indices	Prerenal Failure	Intrinsic Renal Failure
Urine sodium (mEq/L)	10–50	30–90
Urine/plasma creatinine	29.2 ± 1.6	9.7 ± 3.6
FeNa[1]	0.9 ± 0.6	4.3 ± 2.2

[1]Fractional excretion of sodium defined in Chap. 9.
Modified from Mathew O. P., et al. Neonatal renal failure: Usefulness of diagnostic indices. *Pediatrics* 1980;65:57.

d. Phosphorus is restricted by using a low-phosphorus formula (e.g., Similac PM 60/40). Oral calcium carbonate can be used as a phosphate-binding agent.

e. Calcium supplementation is given if ionized calcium is decreased or the patient is symptomatic. In infants with chronic renal failure, 1,25-dihydroxyvitamin D or its analog is given to maximize Ca^{+2} absorption and prevent renal osteodystrophy (see Chap. 29).

f. Metabolic acidosis is usually mild unless there is (1) significant tubular dysfunction with decreased ability to reabsorb bicarbonate, or (2) increased lactate production due to decreased perfusion due to heart failure or volume loss from hemorrhage (see III.B). Use sodium bicarbonate or sodium citrate to correct severe metabolic acidosis.

g. Nutrition is limited by severe fluid restriction. Infants who can take oral feedings are given a low-phosphate formula with a low renal solute load (e.g., Similac PM 60/40). Caloric density is increased to a maximum of 50 kcal/oz with glucose polymers (Polycose) and corn oil. Parenteral nutrition is given when oral feeding is not tolerated. Protein is limited to 0.5 g/kg per day and is increased as tolerated.

h. Hypertension (see III. D)

i. Drugs that are renally excreted must have their dosing schedule adjusted in accordance with the patient's renal function. Potential nephrotoxic drugs such as indomethacin and aminoglycosides should be avoided.

j. Dialysis is indicated when conservative management has been unsuccessful in correcting severe fluid overload, hyperkalemia, acidosis, and uremia. Inadequate nutrition because of severe fluid restriction in the anuric infant is a relative indication. Since the technical aspects and the supportive care is specialized and demanding, this procedure must be performed in centers where the staff have experience with dialysis in infants and neonates.

C. Congenital anomalies may be defined by prenatal or postnatal ultrasound. The common lesions are hydronephrosis and multicystic dysplastic kidney (MCDK). Differential diagnosis includes other renal masses (see Table 31.2). Search for other renal symptoms such as poor urinary stream or dribbling, urinary-tract infection, hematuria, and fever.

D. **Blood pressure** in the newborn is related to weight and gestational age. Blood pressure rises with postnatal age, 1 to 2 mm Hg per day during the first week and 1 mm Hg per week during the next 6 weeks in both the preterm and full-term infant.

1. Normative values of blood pressure are shown for full-term infants and premature infants in Tables 31.8, 31.9, and 31.10.

2. **Hypertension** is defined as persistent blood pressure greater than 2 standard deviations above the mean. Premature infants with bronchopulmonary dysplasia or who have undergone umbilical artery catheterization are at increased risk for hypertension. The clinical signs and symptoms, which may be absent or nonspecific, include cardiorespiratory abnormalities such as tachypnea, cardiomegaly, or heart failure; neurologic findings such as irritability, lethargy, or seizure; failure to thrive; or gastrointestinal difficulties.

3. Neonatal hypertension has many causes (Table 31.11), which may be determined by history and physical examination and a review of fluid status, medications, use and location of umbilical arterial catheter, maternal history, and other clinical findings such as intracranial hemorrhage and chronic lung disease. If a particular cause is suspected, proceed with appropriate laboratory evaluation. Otherwise, focus initial evaluation on renovascular and renal causes, which are most commonly responsible for neonatal hypertension. Obtain urinalysis, renal function studies, serum electrolyte levels, and renal ultrasound examination. Color Doppler flow studies may detect aortic or renal vascular thrombosis. A DMSA renal

TABLE 31.8. NORMAL LONGITUDINAL BLOOD PRESSURE IN FULL-TERM INFANTS (MM HG)

	Boys		Girls	
Age	Systolic	Diastolic	Systolic	Diastolic
1st day	67 ± 7	37 ± 7	68 ± 8	38 ± 7
4th day	76 ± 8	44 ± 9	75 ± 8	45 ± 8
1 month	84 ± 10	46 ± 9	82 ± 9	46 ± 10
3 months	92 ± 11	55 ± 10	89 ± 11	54 ± 10
6 months	96 ± 9	58 ± 10	92 ± 10	56 ± 10

From Gemeilli M., Managanaro R., Mami C., et al. Longitudinal study of blood pressure during the 1st year of life. *Eur J Pediatr* 1990;149:318.

TABLE 31.9. SYSTOLIC AND DIASTOLIC BLOOD PRESSURE RANGES IN INFANTS OF 500–2000 GRAMS BIRTH WEIGHT AT 3–6 HOURS OF LIFE

Birth Weight (g)	Systolic (mm Hg)	Diastolic (mm Hg)
501–750	50–62	26–36
751–1000	48–59	23–36
1001–1250	49–61	26–35
1251–1500	46–56	23–33
1501–1750	46–58	23–33
1751–2000	48–61	24–35

From Hegyi T., et al. Blood pressure ranges in premature infants. 1. The first hours of life. *J Pediatr* 1994;124:627–633.

TABLE 31.10. MEAN ARTERIAL BLOOD PRESSURE (MAP) IN INFANTS OF 500–1500 GRAMS BIRTH WEIGHT

	MAP ± SD (mm Hg)		
Birth Weight (g)	Day 3	Day 17	Day 31
501–750	38 ± 8	44 ± 8	46 ± 11
751–1000	43 ± 9	45 ± 7	47 ± 9
1001–1250	43 ± 8	46 ± 9	48 ± 8
1251–1500	45 ± 8	47 ± 8	47 ± 9

From Klaus M. H., Fanaroff A. A. (eds.). *Care of the High-risk Neonate.* Philadelphia: Saunders, 1993; 497.

TABLE 31.11.   CAUSES OF HYPERTENSION IN THE NEONATE

Vascular
  Renal artery thrombosis
  Renal vein thrombosis
  Coarctation of the aorta
  Renal artery stenosis
  Idiopathic arterial calcification

Renal
  Obstructive uropathy
  Polycystic kidney disease
  Renal insufficiency
  Renal tumor
    Wilms' tumor
  Glomerulonephritis
  Pyelonephritis

Endocrine
  Congenital adrenal hypoplasia
  Primary hyperaldosteronism
  Hyperthyroidism

Neurologic
  Increased intracranial pressure
  Cushing's disease
  Neural crest tumor
  Cerebral angioma
  Drug withdrawal

Pulmonary
  Bronchopulmonary dysplasia

Drugs
  Corticosteroids
  Theophylline
  Adrenergic agents
  Phenylephrine

Other
  Fluid/electrolyte overload
  Abdominal surgery
  Associated with extracorporeal membrane oxygenation (ECMO)

scan may detect segmental renal arterial infarctions. Plasma renin levels are difficult to interpret in newborns.

4. Management is directed at correcting the underlying cause whenever possible. Antihypertensive therapy (Table 31.12) is administered for sustained hypertension not related to volume overload or medications.

E. **Renal vascular thrombosis** (see Chap. 26)

1. **Renal artery thrombosis (RAT)** is often related to the use of indwelling umbilical artery catheters. Management is controversial. The options include surgical thrombectomy, thrombolytic agents, and conservative medical care including antihypertensive therapy. The surgical renal salvage rate is no better than medical management, and carries a considerable mortality rate of 33%. Patients with unilateral RAT who received conservative medical treatment are usually normotensive by 2 years of age, no longer receiving antihypertensive medications, and have normal

TABLE 31.12. ANTIHYPERTENSIVE AGENTS FOR THE NEWBORN (SEE APPENDIX A FOR SPECIFIC DOSING RECOMMENDATIONS)

	Dose	Comment
Diuretics		
Furosemide	0.5–1.0 mg/kg/dose IV, IM, PO	May cause hyponatremia, hypokalemia, hypercalciuria
Chlorothiazide	20–40 mg/kg/day PO; divided Q12h 2–8 mg/kg/day IV divided Q12h	May cause hyponatremia, hypokalemia, hypochloremia
Vasodilators		
Hydralazine	1–8 mg/kg/day; divided q 6–8 hr	May cause tachycardia
Nitroprusside	0.2–6 µg/kg/min continuous IV infusion	Monitor isothiocyanate levels
Calcium channel blockers		
Nifedipine	0.2 mg/kg/dose SL, PO	Limited use in neonates; may cause tachycardia
Beta receptor antagonist		
Propranolol	0.5–5.0 mg/kg/day PO; divided q 6–8 hr	May cause bronchospasm
Alpha/beta receptor antagonist		
Labetalol	0.5–1.0 mg/kg/dose IV, q 4–6 hr	Limited use in neonates
ACE inhibitor		
Captopril	0.15–2.0 mg/kg/day PO, divided q 8–12 hr	May cause oliguria, hyperkalemia, renal failure
Enalapril	5–10 µg/kg/dose IV, q 8–24 hr	May cause oliguria, hyperkalemia, renal failure

IV = intravenously; IM = intramuscularly; PO = per os; SL = sublingual; ACE = angiotensin-converting enzyme.

creatinine clearance, although some have unilateral renal atrophy with compensatory contralateral hypertrophy. There have been reports of long-term complications with hypertension and/or proteinuria and progression to renal failure in adolescence.

2. **Renal vein thrombosis (RVT)** has the predisposing conditions of hyperosmolarity, polycythemia, hypovolemia, and hypercoagulable states and is thus commonly associated with infant of diabetic mother, or use of umbilical venous catheters. Cases of interuterine renal venous thrombosis have been described and present with calcification of the clot in the inferior vena cava (IVC). The clinical findings include gross hematuria often with clots, enlarged kidneys, hypertension, and thrombocytopenia. Other symptoms include vomiting, shock, lower extremity edema, and abdominal distention. The diagnosis of RVT is confirmed by ultrasound, which typically shows an enlarged kidney with diffuse homogenous hyperechogenicity; Doppler-flow studies may detect thrombi in the IVC or renal vein. Differential diagnosis include renal masses or hemolytic uremic syndrome.

   The management of RVT also is controversial. Initial therapy should focus on the maintenance of circulation, fluid, and electrolyte balance while examining for underlying predisposing clinical conditions. Assessment of the coagulation status includes platelet count, prothrombin time (PT), partial thromboplastin time (PTT), fibrinogen, and fibrin split products and, if suggested by maternal history, lupus antiphospholipid antibodies.

   No consensus exists on the use of heparin. Our approach depends on the patient's clinical status. If there is unilateral involvement without evidence of disseminated intravascular coagulation (DIC), we use conservative management. If there is bilateral involvement and evidence of DIC, we initiate heparin therapy with an initial bolus of 50 to 100 units/kg followed by continuous infusion at 25 to 50 units/kg to maintain PTT of 1.5 times normal. Anti-thrombin III (AT III) activity should be reassessed before heparin therapy is instituted as AT III is required for the anticoagulant action of heparin. Heparin-induced hyperkalemia is a risk, hence monitoring K^+ is necessary. Recently, low-molecular-weight heparin has been used both as initial treatment for thrombosis and as prophylactic therapy after recannulization of the occluded vessel. In the treatment of patients with thrombosis, dosages of 200 to 300 anti-Fxa U/kg are reported to reach a therapeutic level of 0.5–1.0 anti-Fxa U/ml. Reported dosages range from 45 to 100 anti-Fxa units/kg to reach prophylactic levels of 0.2 to 0.4 anti-Fxa U/mL.

   Thrombolytic therapy with streptokinase and urokinase have been used in both RAT and RVT, with variable success (see Chap. 26) but are no longer commercially available. There is limited experience with the use of thromboplastin activator (TPA). This is used in low dose (0.02 to 0.03 mg/kg) if there is evidence of bleeding, and titrated to PTT value of 1.5 times normal. Plasma infusion may be necessary to provide thromboplastin activation. Protamine and e-caproic acid should be present at the bedside since significant bleeding can occur. Surgical intervention should be considered if there has been an indwelling umbilical vein catheter, the thrombosis is bilateral, and involves the main renal renal veins leading to renal failure. This type of thrombosis is likely to have started in the IVC rather than intrarenal and hence is more likely amenable to surgical attention.

F. **Proteinuria** in newborns is frequently normal. After the first week, persistent proteinuria greater than 250 mg/m^2 per 24 hours should be investigated (see Table 31.4).

   1. In general, **mild proteinuria** reflects a vascular or tubular injury to the kidney. Administration of large amounts of colloid can exceed the reabsorptive capacity of the neonatal renal tubules and may result in mild proteinuria.

2. **Massive proteinuria** (>1.5 g/m² per 24 hours), hypoalbuminemia with serum albumin levels less than 2.5 g/dL, and edema are all components of congenital nephrotic syndrome. A renal biopsy is often required for final diagnosis. Prenatal diagnosis of Finnish-type nephrotic syndrome is possible before the 20th week of gestation by detection of elevated maternal and amniotic alpha-fetoprotein levels.

3. No specific treatment is required for mild proteinuria. Treat the underlying disease and monitor the proteinuria until resolved.

4. Glomerular disease is rare and usually associated with congenital nephrotic syndrome if presentation is in the nursery.

G. **Hematuria** is defined as greater than 5 red blood cells per high-power field. It is uncommon in newborns and should always be investigated.

1. Hematuria has many causes (Table 31.13) including hemorrhagic disease of the newborn if vitamin K supplementation has not been given. The differential diagnosis for hematuria includes urate staining of the diaper, myoglobinuria, or hemoglobinuria. A negative dipstick with benign sediment suggests urates, while a positive dipstick with negative sediment for red blood cells (RBCs) indicates the present of globin pigments. Vaginal bleeding ("pseudo-menses") in girls or a severe diaper rash is also a possible cause of blood in the diaper or positive dipstick for heme.

2. Evaluation of neonatal hematuria depends on the clinical situation. In most cases, the initial investigation includes the following tests: urinalysis with examination of the sediment, urine culture, ultrasound of the upper and lower urinary tract, evaluation of renal function [serum creatinine and blood urea nitrogen (BUN)], and coagulation studies.

H. **Urinary-tract infection (UTI)** (see Chap. 23)

1. Infections of the urinary tract in newborns can result in asymptomatic bacteriuria or can lead to pyelonephritis and/or sepsis. A urine culture

TABLE 31.13. ETIOLOGY OF HEMATURIA IN THE NEWBORN

Acute tubular necrosis

Cortical necrosis

Vascular diseases
  Renal vein thrombosis
  Renal artery thrombosis

Bleeding and clotting disorders
  Disseminated intravascular coagulation
  Severe thrombocytopenia
  Clotting factors deficiency

Urological anomalies

Urinary-tract infection

Glomerular diseases (see proteinuria)

Tumors
  Wilms' tumor
  Neuroblastoma
  Angiomas

Nephrocalcinosis

Trauma
  Suprapubic bladder aspiration
  Urethral catheterization

should be obtained from every infant with fever, poor weight gain, poor feeding, unexplained prolonged jaundice, or any clinical signs of sepsis.

2. The diagnosis is confirmed by positive urine culture obtained by suprapubic bladder aspiration or catheterized specimen with a colony count exceeding 1000 colonies per millimeter. A blood culture should also be obtained, even from asymptomatic infants. Although most newborns with UTIs have leukocytes in the urine, an infection can be present in the absence of leukocyturia.

3. *Escherichia coli* accounts for approximately 75% of the infections. The remainder are caused by other gram-negative bacilli (Klebsiella, Enterobacter, Proteus) and by gram-positive cocci (enterococci, *Staphylococcus epidermidis, Staphylococcus aureus*).

4. Evaluation of the urinary tract by ultrasound is required emergently to rule out obstructive uropathy or neurogenic bladder with inability to empty the bladder. Adequate drainage or relief of obstruction is necessary for antibiobic control of the infection. VCUG is needed to detect reflux and define lower tract abnormalities. Vesicoureteral reflex occurs in 40% of neonates with UTIs and predominates slightly in boys. If renal abnormality is detected, a renal scan is done to assess renal cortex and function. Inadequate therapy, particularly in the presence of urological abnormalities, could lead to renal scarring with potential development of hypertension and loss of renal function.

5. The initial treatment is antibiotics, usually a combination of ampicillin and gentamicin, given parenterally. The final choice of antibiotic is based on the sensitivity of the cultured organism. Treatment is continued for 10 to 14 days, and amoxicillin prophylaxis (20 mg/kg/day) is administered until a VCUG is performed. If VUR is present, prophylactic treatment should continue until the reflux has resolved.

I. Tubular disorders

1. **Fanconi syndrome** is a group of disorders with generalized dysfunction of the proximal tubule resulting in excessive urinary losses of amino acids, glucose, phosphate, and bicarbonate. The glomerular function is usually normal.

   a. **Clinical and laboratory findings** include:

      (1) Hypophosphatemia due to the excessive urinary loss of phosphate. In these patients the tubular reabsorption of phosphate (TRP) is abnormally low. Rickets and osteoporosis are secondary to hypophosphatemia and can appear in the neonatal period.

      (2) Metabolic acidosis is secondary to bicarbonate wasting (proximal renal tubular acidosis).

      (3) Aminoaciduria and glycosuria do not result in significant clinical signs or symptoms.

      (4) These infants are often polyuric and therefore at risk for dehydration.

      (5) Hypokalemia, due to increased excretion by the distal tubule to compensate for the increased sodium reabsorption, is also frequent and sometimes profound.

   b. **Etiology.** The primary form of Fanconi syndrome is rare in the neonatal period and is a diagnosis of exclusion. Although familial cases (mainly autosomal dominant) have been reported, it is generally sporadic. Most secondary forms of the syndrome in the neonatal period are related to inborn errors of metabolism, including cystinosis, hereditary tyrosinemia, hereditary fructose intolerance, galactosemia, glycogenosis, Lowe syndrome (oculocerebro-renal syndrome), and mitochondrial disorders. Cases associated with heavy metal toxicity have also been described.

2. **Renal tubular acidosis (RTA)** is defined as metabolic acidosis resulting from the inability of the kidney to excrete hydrogen ions or to reabsorb bicarbonate. Poor growth may result from RTA.

a. **Distal RTA (type I)** is caused by a defect in the secretion of hydrogen ions by the distal tubule. The urine cannot be acidified below a pH of 6. It is frequently associated with hypokalemia and hypercalciuria. Nephrocalcinosis is common later in life. In the neonatal period, distal RTA may be primary, due to a genetic defect, or secondary to several disorders including nephrocalcinosis, obstructive uropathies, drugs such as amphotericin B, heavy metals, and hereditary elliptocytosis.

b. **Proximal RTA (type II)** is a defect in the proximal tubule with reduced bicarbonate reabsorption leading to bicarbonate wasting. Serum bicarbonate concentration falls until the abnormally low threshold for bicarbonate reabsorption is reached in the proximal tubule (generally below 16 mEq/L). Once this threshold has been reached, no significant amount of bicarbonate reaches the distal tubule, and the urine can be acidified at that level. Proximal RTA can occur as an isolated defect or in association with Fanconi syndrome (see III.I).

c. **Hyperkalemic RTA (type IV)** is a result of a combined impaired ability of the distal tubule to excrete hydrogen ions and potassium. In the neonatal period, this disorder is seen in infants with aldosterone deficiency, adrenogenital syndrome, reduced tubular responsiveness to aldosterone, or associated obstructive uropathies. It can also be induced by treatment with angiotensin-converting enzyme (ACE) inhibitors or spironolactone.

d. **The treatment of RTA** is based on correction of the acidosis with alkaline therapy. Bicitra or sodium bicarbonate, 2 to 3 mEq/kg per day in divided doses, is usually sufficient to treat type I and type IV RTA. The treatment of proximal RTA requires larger doses sometimes as high as 10 mEq/kg/day bicarbonate. In secondary forms of RTA, the treatment of the primary cause often results in the resolution of the RTA.

J. **Nephrocalcinosis (NC)** is detected by renal ultrasound examinations (see Chap. 29).

1. NC is generally associated with a hypercalciuric state. Drugs that are associated with NC and increased urinary calcium excretion include loop diuretics such as furosemide, methylxanthines, glucocorticoids, and vitamin D in pharmacological doses. In addition, hyperoxaluria, often associated with parenteral nutrition, and hyperphosphaturia facilitate the deposition of calcium crystals in the kidney.

2. Renal stones and NC secondary to primary hyperoxaluria/oxalosis, renal tubular acidosis, or urinary-tract infections are rare in newborns.

3. Few follow-up studies of NC in premature infants are available. In general, renal function is not significantly impaired, and most cases resolve spontaneously within the first year of life as demonstrated by ultrasound. However, significant tubular dysfunction at 1 to 2 years of age has been reported.

4. It is unclear whether NC requires a specific treatment. If possible, drugs that cause hypercalciuria should be discontinued. Change to or addition of thiazide diuretics and supplemental magnesium in patients with bronchopulmonary dysplasia with a need for long-term diuretic therapy may be helpful. Monitoring of urinary calcium excretion (urine calcium:creatinine ratio) help in determining response to therapy.

K. **Cystic disease of the kidney** may result from abnormalities in development, such as multicystic dysplasia, or from genetically induced diseases. The principal differential diagnosis of bilateral cystic kidney disease in the newborn includes **autosomal recessive polycystic kidney disease (ARPKD)**, the infantile form of autosomal dominant polycystic kidney disease **(ADPKD)**, and glomerulocystic kidney disease (which in some affected families represents a variant of ADPKD).

1. In ARPKD, the kidneys appear markedly enlarged and hyperechogenic by ultrasound, with a typical "snowstorm" appearance with concurrent liver fibrosis and/or dilated bile ducts. In contrast, macroscopic cysts are usually detected in cases of ADPKD and glomerulocystic disease and the

liver is spared. The clinical findings of ARPKD are variable and include bilateral smooth enlarged kidneys, varying degrees of renal insufficiency, which usually progresses to renal failure over time and severe renin-mediated hypertension. Infants with more severe involvement may have oligohydramnios with pulmonary hypoplasia and Potter's syndrome but those patients who survive the neonatal period can be carried to renal transplantation in later childhood or adolesence. ARPKD is always associated with liver involvement, which may progress to liver failure requiring transplantation in adolesence. The diagnosis is confirmed by renal and liver biopsy, unless the family history is certain.

2. In ADPKD, an abnormal gene PKD1 has been identified and located on the short arm of chromosome 16, and a second gene PKD2 located on the long arm of chromosome 4. These two genes account for the large majority of ADPKD patients. Clinical manifestations include bilateral renal masses that are usually less symetrical than in ARPKD. Hypertension is also less common than ARPKD.

3. Other hereditary syndromes that can manifest as renal cystic disease include tuberous sclerosis; von Hippel-Landau disease; Jeune's asphyxiating thoracic dysplasia; oral-facial-digital syndrome, type 1; brachymesomelia-renal syndrome; and Trisomy 9, 13, and 18.

L. The decision for circumcision is based primarily on cultural or ethnic background. Medical indications for circumcision include urinary retention due to adhesions of the foreskin or to tight phimosis. Circumcision should be avoided in cases of hypospadias, ambiguous genitalia, and bleeding disorders (see Chap. 5).

M. Renal tumors are rare in the neonatal period. These include mesoblastic nephroma and nephroblastomatosis. The differential diagnosis includes other causes of renal masses (see Table 31.2).

Suggested Readings

Bailie M.D., (Ed.). Renal function and disease. *Clin Perinatol* 1992;19(1) (entire issue).

Guignard J.P., Drukker A. Clinical neonatal nephrology. In: Barratt T.M., Avner E.D., Harmon W.E., (Eds.), *Pediatric Nephrology*. Philadelphia: Lippincott, Williams and Williams, 1999.

32. NECROTIZING ENTEROCOLITIS

Karen R. McAlmon

I. **Background.** **Necrotizing enterocolitis (NEC)** is an acute intestinal necrosis syndrome of unknown etiology. Its pathogenesis is complex and multifactorial. Our understanding of the pathophysiology is increasing as we learn more about the crucial role of inflammatory mediators. Current clinical practice is directed toward prompt, early diagnosis and rapid institution of proper intensive-care management.

   A. **Epidemiology.** NEC is the most common serious surgical disorder among infants in a neonatal intensive care unit (NICU) and is a significant cause of neonatal morbidity and mortality.

      1. The **incidence** of NEC varies from center to center and from year to year within centers. There are endemic and epidemic occurrences. An estimated 0.3 to 2.4 cases occur in every 1000 live births. In most centers, NEC occurs in 2 to 5% of all NICU admissions and 5 to 10% of VLBW infants. If infants who die early are excluded and only infants who have been fed included, the incidence is approximately 15%.

      2. Sex, race, geography, climate, and season do not appear to play any determining role in the incidence or course of NEC.

      3. **Prematurity** is the single greatest risk factor. Decreasing gestational age is associated with an increased risk for NEC. The mean gestational age of infants with NEC is 30 to 32 weeks, and the infants are generally appropriate for gestational age. Approximately 10% of infants are full-term. The postnatal age at onset is inversely related to birth weight and gestational age. The mean age at onset is 12 days, and the mode is 3 days. More than 90% of infants have been fed prior to the onset of this disease.

      4. Infants exposed to cocaine have a 2.5 times increased risk of developing NEC. The vasoconstrictive and hemodynamic properties of cocaine may promote intestinal ischemia (see Chap. 19, Drug Abuse and Withdrawal).

      5. The overall **mortality** is 9 to 28% regardless of surgical or medical intervention. The mortality for infants weighing less than 1500 g is up to 45%; for those weighing less than 750 g, it may be much higher. The introduction of standardized therapeutic protocols with criteria for medical management and surgical intervention, a high index of suspicion for the disease, and general improvements in neonatal intensive care, have decreased the mortality rate. Infants exposed to cocaine who develop NEC have a significantly higher incidence of massive gangrene, perforation, and mortality than do infants not exposed.

      6. Case-controlled epidemiologic studies have revealed that almost all previously described risk factors for NEC, including maternal disorders (e.g., toxemia), the infant's course [e.g., asphyxia, patent ductus arteriosus (PDA)], and the type of management [e.g., umbilical artery catheterization (UAC)], simply describe a population of high-risk neonates. Excluding cocaine exposure, no maternal or neonatal factors other than prematurity are known to increase the risk of NEC. This suggests that immaturity of the gastrointestinal tract is the greatest risk factor.

   B. **Pathogenesis**

      1. The **causes** of NEC are not well defined. NEC is likely a heterogeneous disease resulting from complex interactions between mucosal injury secondary to a variety of factors (including ischemia, luminal substrate, and infection) and poor host protective mechanism(s) in response to injury.

      2. The concept of a **hypoxic or hemodynamic insult,** resulting in splanchnic vasoconstriction and reduced mesenteric flow, inducing bowel mucosal

hypoxia and rendering the intestine susceptible to injury, has long been considered a probable cause of NEC. The pathologic findings resemble those seen in older individuals with vascular compromise. However, in a significant number of cases no hypoxic or ischemic problems could be identified, and the temporal sequence of events does not support an ischemic event alone. Indomethacin use, both antenatal for tocolysis and postnatal for treatment of patent ductus arteriosus, has been associated with an increased incidence of NEC (see Chap. 25, Cardiac Disorders).

3. **Enteral feedings** have been implicated in the pathogenesis of NEC. Factors that have been considered include osmolality of formula, the lack of immunoprotective factors in formula, and the timing, volume, and rate of feeding. Breast milk has been shown to have protective factors; however, breast milk alone does not prevent development of NEC. Some studies have shown that very slow introduction of feedings and avoidance of large day-to-day volume increases may lower the incidence of NEC. However, the exact rate of feeding increment that predisposes infants to NEC has not been identified, and the mechanism by which excessive volumes predispose to the development of NEC is not known.

4. The **microbiologic flora** involved in NEC are not unique but represent the predominant bowel organisms present in the infant at the time of onset. Various bacterial and viral agents have been included in the microbial picture that is sometimes associated with NEC, especially with epidemic NEC, but none has yet been proved to be causal. Release of endotoxin and cytokines by proliferation of colonizing bacteria, and bacterial fermentation with gaseous distention, may play a role.

5. Increasing evidence supports a critical role for **platelet activating factor (PAF)** and other inflammatory mediators in the pathophysiology of NEC. Animal studies show that exogenous administration or endogenous increased production of PAF causes ischemic bowel necrosis pathologically similar to NEC. Several factors may promote (e.g., leukotrienes, oxygen radicals, tumor necrosis factor) or inhibit (e.g., acetylhydrolase, steroids, nitric oxide, prostacyclin) PAF-induced intestinal injury. PAF antagonists, including dexamethasone and PAF acetylhydrolase, prevent this histologic necrosis. All the NEC risk factors—prematurity, hypoxia, feeding, and bacteria—tend to increase the concentration of circulating or local PAF. Intestinal tissue's high biosynthetic activity for inflammatory mediators (especially PAF), make it particularly susceptible to necrosis.

6. **Histopathologic examination** of tissue after surgery or autopsy indicates that the terminal ileum and ascending colon are the most frequently involved areas, but in the most severe cases the entire bowel may be involved. This localization has implications for long-term sequelae (see IV). The pathologic lesions consist of coagulation necrosis, bacterial overgrowth, inflammation, and reparative changes. These suggest that the disease is initiated by subtotal ischemia and gradual tissue compromise that results in bacterial invasion and inflammation.

II. **Diagnosis.** Early diagnosis of NEC is the most important factor in determining outcome. This is accomplished by careful clinical observation for nonspecific signs in infants at risk.

A. **Clinical characteristics.** There is a broad spectrum of disease manifestations. The clinical features of NEC can be divided into systemic and abdominal signs. Most infants have a combination of both.

1. **Systemic signs.** Respiratory distress, apnea or bradycardia (or both), lethargy, temperature instability, irritability, poor feeding, hypotension (shock), decreased peripheral perfusion, acidosis, oliguria, bleeding diathesis.

2. **Abdominal (enteric) signs.** Bloody stools, abdominal distention or tenderness, gastric aspirates (feeding residuals), vomiting (of bile, blood, or both), ileus (decreased or absent bowel sounds), abdominal wall erythema or induration, persistent localized abdominal mass, ascites.

3. The **course of the disease** varies among infants. Most frequently, it will appear (1) as a fulminant, rapidly progressive presentation of signs consistent with intestinal necrosis and sepsis or (2) as a slow, paroxysmal presentation of abdominal distention, ileus, and possible infection. The latter course will vary with the rapidity of therapeutic intervention and require consistent monitoring and anticipatory evaluation (see III).

B. **Laboratory features.** The diagnosis is suspected from clinical presentation but must be confirmed by diagnostic radiographs, surgery, or autopsy. No laboratory tests are specific for NEC; nevertheless, some tests are valuable in confirming diagnostic impressions.

1. **Roentgenograms.** The abdominal roentgenogram will often reveal an abnormal gas pattern consistent with ileus. Both anteroposterior (AP) and cross-table lateral or left lateral decubitus views should be included. These films may reveal bowel wall edema, a fixed-position loop on serial studies, the appearance of a mass, pneumatosis intestinalis (the radiologic hallmark used to confirm the diagnosis), portal or hepatic venous air, pneumobilia, or pneumoperitoneum.

2. **Blood studies.** Thrombocytopenia, persistent metabolic acidosis, and severe refractory hyponatremia constitute the most common triad of signs and help to confirm the diagnosis.

3. **Analysis of stool** for blood and carbohydrate has been used to detect infants with NEC based on changes in intestinal integrity. Although grossly bloody stools may be an indication of NEC, occult hematochezia does not correlate well with NEC. Carbohydrate malabsorption, as reflected in a positive stool Clinitest result, can be a frequent and early indicator of NEC within the setting of signs noted in A.

C. **Bell staging criteria** with the Walsh and Kleigman modification allow uniformity of diagnosis and treatment based on severity of illness.

1. **Stage I** (suspect) clinical signs and symptoms, nondiagnostic radiographs.

2. **Stage II** (definite) clinical signs and symptoms, pneumatosis intestinalis on radiograph.
   a. Mildly ill.
   b. Moderately ill with systemic toxicity.

3. **Stage III** (advanced) clinical signs and symptoms, pneumatosis intestinalis on radiograph, and critically ill.
   a. Impending intestinal perforation.
   b. Proven intestinal perforation.

D. **Differential diagnosis**

1. **Pneumonia and sepsis** are common and frequently are associated with an abdominal ileus. The abdominal distention and tenderness characteristic of NEC will be absent, however.

2. **Surgical abdominal catastrophes** include malrotation with obstruction (complete or intermittent), malrotation with midgut volvulus, intussusception, ulcer, gastric perforation, and mesenteric vessel thrombosis (see Chap. 26, Hematologic Problems). The clinical presentation of these disorders may overlap with that of NEC. Occasionally, the diagnosis is made only at the time of exploratory laparotomy.

3. **Infectious enterocolitis** is rare in this population but must be considered if diarrhea is present. Campylobacter species have been associated with bloody diarrhea in the newborn. These infants lack any other systemic or enteric signs of NEC.

4. Severe forms of **inherited metabolic disease** (e.g., galactosemia with *Escherichia coli* sepsis) may lead to profound acidosis, shock, and vomiting and may initially overlap with some signs of NEC.

5. Severe **allergic colitis** can present with abdominal distension and bloody stools. Usually these infants are well appearing, and have normal abdominal radiographs and laboratory studies.

6. **Feeding intolerance** is a common but ill-defined problem in premature infants. Despite adequate gastrointestinal function in utero, some prema-

ture infants will have periods of gastric residuals and abdominal distention associated with advancing feedings. The differentiation of this problem from NEC can be difficult. Cautious evaluation by withholding enteral
feedings and administering intravenous fluids and antibiotics for 48 to 72
hours may be indicated until this benign disorder can be distinguished
from NEC.

E. Additional diagnostic considerations

1. Since the early features are often nonspecific, **a high index of suspicion**
   is the most reliable approach to early diagnosis. The entire picture of history, physical examination, and laboratory features must be considered in
   the context of the particular infant's course. Isolated signs or laboratory
   values often indicate the need for a careful differential diagnosis, despite
   the obvious concern over NEC.

2. **Diarrhea** is an uncommon presentation of NEC in the absence of bloody
   stools. This sign should point away from NEC.

3. **Roentgenographic findings** can often be subtle and confusing. For example, perforation of an abdominal viscus will not always cause pneumoperitoneum, and conversely, pneumoperitoneum does not necessarily
   indicate abdominal perforation from NEC. Careful serial review of the
   roentgenograms with a pediatric radiologist is indicated to assist in interpretation and to plan for further appropriate studies.

III. Management

A. Immediate medical management
(Table 32.1). Treatment should begin
promptly when signs suggestive of NEC are present. Therapy is based on
intensive-care measures and the anticipation of potential problems.

1. **Respiratory function.** Rapid assessment of ventilatory status (physical
   examination, arterial blood gases) should be made, and supplemental
   oxygen and mechanical ventilatory support should be provided as needed.

2. **Cardiovascular function.** Rapid assessment of circulatory status (physical examination, blood pressure) should be made, and circulatory support
   should be provided as needed. Volume in the form of normal saline or
   fresh frozen plasma (dose 10 mL/kg) may be used. Pharmacologic support
   may be necessary; in this case, we use low doses of dopamine (3 to 5 μg/kg
   per minute) to optimize the effect on splanchnic and renal blood flow. Impending circulatory collapse will often be reflected by poor perfusion and
   oxygenation, even though arterial blood pressure may be maintained. In-
   traarterial blood pressure monitoring is often necessary, but the proximity of the umbilical arteries to the mesenteric circulation precludes the
   use of these vessels. In fact, any umbilical artery catheter should be
   promptly removed and peripheral artery catheters used. Further monitoring of central venous pressure (CVP) may become necessary if additional pharmacologic support of the circulation or failing myocardium is
   needed (see Chap. 17, Shock).

3. **Metabolic function.** Severe metabolic acidosis will generally respond to
   volume expansion but may require treatment with sodium bicarbonate
   (2 mEq/kg). The blood pH should be carefully monitored; in addition,
   serum electrolyte levels and liver function should be measured. Blood
   glucose levels should be monitored as well.

4. **Nutrition.** All gastrointestinal feedings are discontinued, and the bowel is
   decompressed by suctioning through a nasogastric tube. Parenteral nutrition (PN) is given through a peripheral vein as soon as possible, with the
   aim of providing 90 to 110 cal/kg per day once amino acid solutions and
   intralipid are both tolerated. A central venous catheter is almost always
   necessary to provide adequate calories in the very-low-birth-weight infant.
   We wait to place a central catheter for this purpose until the blood cultures are negative for 2 to 5 days, during which time adaptation to peripheral PN can take place.

5. **Infectious disease.** Blood, urine, stool, and cerebrospinal fluid (CSF)
   specimens are obtained, examined carefully for indications of infection,

TABLE 32.1. MANAGEMENT OF NECROTIZING ENTEROCOLITIS

Bell Staging Criteria	Diagnosis	Management (Usual attention to respiratory, cardiovascular and hematologic resuscitation presumed)
Stage I (Suspect)	Clinical signs and symptoms Nondiagnostic radiograph	NPO with IV fluids Nasogastric drainage CBC, lytes, KUB q6–8 h × 48 h Blood culture Stool heme test and Clinitest Ampicillin and gentamicin × 48 hours
Stage II (Definite)	Clinical signs and symptoms Pneumatosis intestinalis on radiograph	NPO with parenteral nutrition (by CVL once sepsis ruled out) Nasogastric drainage CBC, lytes, KUB (AP and lateral) q6–8 h × 48–72 h then prn Blood culture Stool heme test and Clinitest Ampicillin, gentamicin and clindamycin × 14 days Surgical consultation
Stage III (Advanced)	Clinical signs and symptoms Critically ill Pneumatosis intestinalis or pneumoperitoneum on radiograph	NPO with parenteral nutrition (by CVL once sepsis ruled out) Nasogastric drainage CBC, lytes, KUB (AP and lateral) q6–8 h × 48–72 h then prn Stool heme test and Clinitest Ampicillin, gentamicin, and clindamycin × 14 days Surgical consultation with intervention, if indicated: Resection with enterostomy or primary anastomosis In selected cases (usually <1000 g and unstable), bedside drainage under local anesthesia

AP = anteroposterior; CBC = complete blood count; CVL = central venous line; KUB = kidney, urethra, bladder X ray; NPO = nothing by mouth.

and sent for culture and sensitivity. We routinely begin broad-spectrum antibiotics as soon as possible, utilizing ampicillin, gentamicin, and clindamycin to cover most enteric flora. Zosyn has recently been used due to its broad spectrum and the ability to use as a single agent. With changing antibiotic sensitivities, one must be aware of the predominant NICU flora, the organisms associated with NEC, and their resistance patterns and adjust antibiotic coverage accordingly. Stool should be tested for aminoglycoside-resistant organisms. Antibiotic therapy is adjusted on the basis of culture results, but only 10 to 40% of blood cultures will be positive, necessitating continued broad coverage in most cases. Treatment is generally maintained for 14 days. There is no evidence to support the use of enteral antibiotics.

6. **Hematologic aspects.** Analysis of the complete blood count and differential, with examination of the blood smear, is always indicated. We use platelet transfusions to correct severe thrombocytopenia and packed red blood cells (PRCs) to maintain the hematocrit above 35%. The prothrombin time, partial thromboplastin time, fibrinogen, and platelet count should be evaluated for evidence of disseminated intravascular coagulation. Fresh-frozen plasma is used to treat coagulation problems.

7. **Renal function.** Oliguria often accompanies the initial hypotension and hypoperfusion of NEC; careful evaluation of urine output is essential. In addition, serum blood urea nitrogen (BUN), creatinine, and serum electrolyte levels should be monitored. Impending renal failure from acute tubular necrosis, coagulative necrosis, or vascular accident must be anticipated, and fluid therapy must be adjusted accordingly (see Chap. 31, Renal Conditions).

8. **Neurologic function.** Evaluation of the infant's condition is difficult given the degree of illness, but one must be alert to the problems of associated meningitis and intraventricular hemorrhage. Seizures may occur secondary to either of these problems or from the metabolic perturbations associated with NEC. These complications must be anticipated and promptly recognized and treated.

9. **Gastrointestinal function.** Physical examination and serial (every 6 to 8 hours during the first 2 to 3 days) roentgenograms are used to assess ongoing gastrointestinal damage. Unless perforation occurs or full-thickness necrosis precipitates severe peritonitis, the management of this system will be medical. The evaluation for surgical intervention, however, is an important and complex management issue (see III.B).

10. **Family support.** Any family of an infant in the NICU may be overwhelmed by the crisis. Infants with NEC present a particular challenge because the disease often causes sudden deterioration for "no apparent reason." Furthermore, the impending possibility of surgical intervention and the high mortality and uncertain prognosis make this situation most difficult for parents. Careful anticipatory sharing of information must be utilized by the staff to establish a trusting alliance with the family.

B. **Surgical intervention**

1. **Prompt consultation** should be obtained with a pediatric surgeon. This will allow the surgeon to become familiar with the case and will provide an additional evaluation by another skilled individual. If a pediatric surgeon is not available, the infant should be transferred to a site where one is.

2. **Gastrointestinal perforation** is generally agreed on as an indication for intervention. Unfortunately, there is no reliable or absolute indicator of imminent perforation; therefore, careful monitoring is necessary. Perforation occurs in 20 to 30% of patients, usually 12 to 48 hours after the onset of NEC, although it can occur later. In some cases, the absence of pneumoperitoneum on the abdominal radiograph can delay the diagnosis, and paracentesis may aid in establishing the diagnosis. In general, an infant with increasing abdominal distention, an abdominal mass, a worsening clinical picture despite medical management, or a persistent fixed loop on

serial roentgenographic studies may have a perforation and may require operative intervention.

3. **Full-thickness necrosis of the gastrointestinal tract** may require surgical intervention, although this diagnosis is difficult to establish in the absence of perforation. In most cases, the infant with bowel necrosis will have signs of peritonitis, such as ascites, abdominal mass, abdominal wall erythema, induration, persistent thrombocytopenia, progressive shock from third-space losses, or refractory metabolic acidosis. Paracentesis may help to identify these patients before perforation occurs.

4. The mainstay of **surgical treatment** is resection with enterostomy although resection with primary anastomosis is useful in selected cases. At surgery, the goal is to excise necrotic bowel while preserving as much bowel length as possible. Peritoneal fluid is examined for signs of infection and sent for culture, necrotic bowel is resected and sent for pathologic confirmation, and viable bowel ends are exteriorized as stomas. All sites of diseased bowel are noted, whether or not removal is indicated. If there is extensive involvement, a "second look" operation may be done within 24 to 48 hours to determine whether any areas that appeared necrotic are actually viable. The length and areas of removed bowel are recorded. If large areas are resected, the length and position of the remaining bowel are noted, since this will affect the long-term outcome. In approximately 14% of infants with this condition, NEC totalis (bowel necrosis from duodenum to rectum) is found. In these cases mortality is almost certain.

5. More recently, **peritoneal drainage** has been considered in a select group of infants. In ELBW infants (<1000 g) and extremely unstable infants, peritoneal drainage under local anesthesia may be a management option. In many cases this temporizes laparotomy until the infant is more stable and in some cases no further operative procedure is required. Unlike for infants <1000 g, there is no increase in survival rate with drainage compared with laparotomy for infants > 1000 g.

C. **Long-term management.** Once the infant has been stabilized and effectively treated, feedings can be reintroduced. We generally begin this process after 2 weeks of treatment by stopping nasogastric decompression. If infants can tolerate their own secretions, feedings are begun very slowly while parenteral alimentation is gradually tapered. No conclusive data are available on the best method or type of feeding, but breast milk may be better tolerated and is preferred. The occurrence of strictures may complicate feeding plans. The incidence of recurrent NEC is 4% and appears to be independent of type of management. Recurrent disease should be treated as before and will generally respond similarly. If surgical intervention was required and an ileostomy or colostomy was created, intestinal reanastomosis can be electively undertaken after an adequate period of healing. Before reanastomosis, a contrast study of the distal bowel is obtained to establish the presence of a stricture that can be resected at the time of ostomy closure.

IV. **Prognosis.** Few detailed and accurate studies are available on prognosis. In uncomplicated cases of NEC, the long-term prognosis may be comparable with that of other low-birth-weight infants; however, those with Stage IIB and Stage III NEC have a higher incidence of growth delay (delay in growth of head circumference is of most concern). NEC requiring surgical intervention may have more serious sequelae, including increased morbidity and mortality secondary to infection, respiratory failure, parenteral nutrition–associated hepatic disease, rickets, and significant developmental delay.

A. **Sequelae** of NEC can be directly related to the disease process or to the long-term NICU management often necessary to treat it. Gastrointestinal sequelae include strictures, enteric fistulas, short bowel syndrome, malabsorption and chronic diarrhea, dumping syndromes related to loss of terminal ileum and ileocecal valve, fluid and electrolyte losses with rapid dehydration, and hepatitis or cholestasis related to long-term PN. Strictures occur in 25 to 35% of patients with or without surgery and are most common in the large bowel. Not all strictures are clinically significant. Short bowel syndrome occurs in approximately 10 to 20% following surgical treatment. Metabolic sequelae include failure to thrive, metabolic bone disease, and problems related to CNS function in the very-low-birth-weight infant.

B. **Prevention of NEC is the ultimate goal.** Unfortunately, this can best be accomplished only by preventing premature birth. If prematurity cannot be avoided, several preventive strategies may be of benefit:

1. **Induction of gastrointestinal maturation.** The incidence of NEC is significantly reduced after prenatal steroid therapy.

2. **Alteration of the immunologic status of the intestine.** Oral immunoglobulins may have potential benefit, and in one study immunoglobulin A (IgA) and immunoglobulin G (IgG) supplementation of feedings reduced the incidence of NEC. Breast milk contains many immunoprotective factors; however, no study has convincingly demonstrated that breast milk alone can prevent NEC.

3. **Optimization of enteral feedings** (see Chap. 10, Nutrition). Very slow introduction of feedings may be useful, but more data are required. Feeds with polyunsaturated fatty acids have been shown to be protective in animal models.

4. **Reduction or antagonism of inflammatory mediators.** Since many of the factors associated with NEC promote increased PAF concentrations and the subsequent inflammatory cascade resulting in bowel injury, trials of oral PAF antagonists may reduce the incidence and severity of NEC.

Suggested Readings

Azarow K.S., et al. Laparotomy or drain for perforated necrotizing enterocolitis: Who gets what and why? *Pediatr Surg Int* 1997;12 (2–3):137.

Muguruma K., et al. The central role of PAF in necrotizing enterocolitis development. *Adv Exp Med Biol* 1997;407:379.

Stoll B. J., Kliegman R. M., (Eds.) Necrotizing enterocolitis. *Clin Perinatol* Philadelphia: Saunders, 1994;21(2).

33. SURGICAL EMERGENCIES IN THE NEWBORN

Steven A. Ringer and Anne R. Hansen

I. **Fetal Surgical Disorders**
   A. **Polyhydramnios** (amniotic fluid volume > 2L) occurs in 1 in 1000 births.
      1. **Gastrointestinal** (GI) obstruction (including esophageal atresia) is the most frequent surgical cause of polyhydramnios.
      2. **Other causes** of polyhydramnios include abdominal wall defects (omphalocele and gastroschisis), anencephaly, diaphragmatic hernia, tight nuchal cord, inability of the fetus to concentrate urine, maternal diabetes, anything causing an inability of the fetus to swallow, and fetal death.
      3. All women in whom polyhydramnios is suspected should have an ultrasonographic examination. In experienced hands, these studies are the method of choice for the diagnosis of intestinal obstruction, abdominal wall defects, and diaphragmatic hernia, as well as abnormalities leading to an inability of the fetus to swallow.
      4. If an obstructing intestinal lesion is diagnosed antenatally and there is no evidence of dystocia, vaginal delivery is acceptable. Pediatric surgical consultation should be obtained prior to delivery.
   B. **Oligohydramnios** is usually associated with intrauterine growth retardation (IUGR), postmaturity, or fetal distress, but it may indicate renal dysgenesis or agenesis (Potter's syndrome; see Chap. 31) or amniotic fluid leak. It is important to anticipate respiratory compromise in these infants as adequate amniotic fluid volume is generally necessary for normal pulmonary development, particularly during the second trimester of gestation. Severity of pulmonary hypoplasia correlates with degree and duration of oligohydramnios.
   C. **Meconium peritonitis**
      1. Diagnosed prenatally by ultrasonography, which may reveal areas of calcification scattered throughout the abdomen. Postnatal confirmation of these calcifictions is by **plain film of the abdomen.**
      2. **Meconium peritonitis** is usually due to antenatal perforation of the intestinal tract. Therefore it is most commonly seen in association with a congenital lesion causing intestinal obstruction, either anatomic or functional. (see IV). Fifty percent of these infants will have cystic fibrosis.
   D. **Fetal ascites** is usually associated with urinary-tract anomalies (e.g., lower urinary tract obstruction due to posterior urethral valves). Other causes include hemolytic disease of the newborn, any severe anemia (e.g., alphathalassemia), peritonitis, thoracic duct obstruction, cardiac disease, hepatic or portal vein obstruction, hepatitis, and congenital infection [e.g., toxoplasmosis, rubella, cytomegalovirus, herpes simplex (TORCH) infections; see Chap. 23)] as well as other causes of hydrops fetalis (see Chap. 18). After birth, ascites may be seen in congenital nephrotic syndrome. Accurate prenatal ultrasonography is important in light of the potential for fetal surgery, which might allow decompression of either the bladder or a hydronephrotic kidney and to minimize renal parenchymal injury (see Chaps. 1, 31).
   E. **Dystocia** may result from fetal intestinal obstruction, abdominal wall defect, genitourinary anomalies, or fetal ascites.
   F. **Fetal surgery.** The potential for surgical intervention during fetal life continues to develop. It depends heavily on the availability of precise prenatal diagnostic techniques and experience in accurately characterizing disorders including the use of ultrasound and fast magnetic resonance imaging (MRI).
      Advances in obstetric and anesthesia management have also contributed to the feasibility of performing in utero procedures. The mother must be carefully managed through what is often a long and unpredictable anesthesia

course. Medications that reduce uterine irritability have been developed that maximally ensure that the uterus can be maintained without contractions during and after the procedure. The criteria for consideration of a procedure are in flux, but have included:

1. **Technical feasibility.** Ethical considerations are important, including balancing the risk to the fetus versus potential pain or harm to the mother, and the impact on the family as a whole.
2. Initially most cases dealt with conditions that are **life-threatening** and may cause either fetal death, or the inability to survive delivery without repair. More cases are now considered where the condition is not life-threatening, but may benefit from early repair.
3. **The surgery should positively alter the infant's course.** Either the condition itself is progressive (such as the growth of a large tumor partially obstructing the fetal airway), or the consequences of the condition are progressively worsening (such as worsening hydrops due to a large teratoma).
4. The **necessary resources** for the care of the fetus and potential baby during surgery, in the immediate postoperative period, and after birth are available in the institution where the surgery is to be performed.

   Fetal surgery has been successfully used for removal of an enlarging chest mass, such as an adenomatoid malformation of the lung or a bronchopulmonary sequestration. Other mass lesions such as sacrococcygeal teratoma, when diagnosed in utero, have been treated with excision or by fetoscopically guided laser ablation of the feeder vessels, resulting in involution. Progressive fetal urethral obstruction has been ameliorated by the use of shunts or fulgaration of posterior urethral valves. Similar fetoscopic laser ablation of connecting vessels has been used successfully in the treatment of twin–twin transfusion syndrome or twin-reversed arterial perfusion Fetal surgical correction of meningomyelocele is a rapidly evolving area of endeavor. Fetal intervention has been also been used for forms of congenital heart disease that progress in severity during fetal life. It is likely that indications for fetal intervention will continue to evolve and change.

II. **Postnatal surgical disorders.** Brief review of differential diagnoses and initial stabilization, ordered by presenting symptoms.
   A. **Respiratory distress** (see III and Chaps. 4, 24). Though most etiologies of respiratory distress are treated medically, some respiratory disorders do require surgical therapies:
      1. **Choanal atresia.** If bilateral, the baby is unable to breathe nasally, but will stabilize upon placement of an oral airway. (see III.C.1).
      2. **Laryngotracheal clefts** (see III.C.3).
      3. **Tracheal agenesis.**
      4. **Esophageal atresia** with or without tracheoesophageal fistula (TEF) (see III.A).
      5. **Congenital lobar emphysema.**
      6. **Cystic adenomatoid malformation of the lung.**
      7. **Biliary tracheobronchial communication** (extremely rare).
      8. **Diaphragmatic hernia** (see III.B). Stabilization generally consists of intubation, gastric decompression, initiation of intravenous fluids (IVF) and antibiotics, and consultation with a pediatric surgeon.
   B. **Scaphoid abdomen**
      1. Diaphragmatic hernia (see III.B).
      2. Esophageal atresia without TEF (see III.A).
   C. **Excessive mucus and salivation.** Esophageal atresia with or without TEF (see III.A).
   D. **Abominal distention.** Can be due to pneumoperitoneum or intestinal obstruction (mechanical or functional).
      1. **Pneumoperitoneum**
         a. Any perforation of the bowel may cause pneumoperitoneum (Chap. 32).

   b. Perforated stomach is associated with large amounts of free intraabdominal air. At times it is necessary to aspirate air from the abdominal cavity to relieve respiratory distress prior to definitive surgical repair. The lesion can be due to instrumentation (nasogastric tube) or localized ischemia of the stomach (associated with some medications such as indomethacin). It requires simple closure.

   c. Air from a pulmonary air leak may dissect into the peritoneal cavity of infants receiving mechanical ventilation.

2. Intestinal obstruction

   a. Obstruction of proximal bowel (e.g., complete duodenal atresia) causes rapid distention of the left upper quadrant. Obstruction of distal bowel causes more generalized distention, varying with location of obstruction. Esophageal atresia with TEF (see III.A) can also present as abdominal distention.

   b. The normal progression of the air column seen on an x-ray film of the abdomen is as follows: 1 hour after birth the air is past the stomach into the upper jejunum; 3 hours after birth it is at the cecum; by 8 to 12 hours after birth it is at the rectosigmoid. The movement of air through the bowel is slower in the premature infant.

E. Vomiting. The causes of vomiting can be differentiated by the presence or absence of bile.

1. Bilious emesis. The presence of bile-stained vomit in the newborn should be treated as a life-threatening emergency, with at least 20% of such infants requiring surgical intervention immediately after evaluation. Surgical consultation should be obtained immediately. Unless the infant is clinically unstable, a contrast study of the upper gastrointestianl tract should be obtained as quickly as possible.

   Intestinal obstruction may result from malrotation with or without volvulus; duodenal, jejunal, ileal, or colonic atresias; annular pancreas; Hirschsprung's disease; aberrant superior mesenteric artery; preduodenal portal vein; peritoneal bands; persistent omphalomesenteric duct; or duodenal duplication. Bile-stained emesis is occasionally seen in infants without intestinal obstruction, especially in setting of decreased motility (see IIE2c below). In these cases the bile-stained vomiting will only occur one or two times and will present without abdominal distention. However, a nonsurgical condition is a diagnosis of exclusion: Bileous emesis is malrotation until proven otherwise.

2. Nonbile-stained emesis

   a. Overfeeding (feeding excessive volume).

   b. Milk or formula intolerance.

   c. Decreased motility (e.g., prematurity, antenatal exposure to $MgSO_4$, narcotic exposure).

   d. Sepsis with ileus.

   e. Central nervous system (CNS) lesion.

   f. Lesion above ampulla of VATER.

      (1) Pyloric stenosis.

      (2) Upper duodenal stenosis.

      (3) Annular pancreas (rare).

F. Failure to pass meconium. Can occur in sick and/or premature babies with decreased bowel motility. It also may be the result of the following disorders:

1. Imperforate anus.

2. Functional intestinal obstruction, including meconium ileus (see IV.D.3).

G. Failure to develop transitional fecal stools after the passage of meconium:

1. Volvulus.

2. Malrotation.

H. Hematemesis and bloody stools:

1. Many patients with hematemesis, and the majority of patients with bloody stools, have a nonsurgical condition. Differential diagonisis includes:

   a. Formula intolerance/allergy (usually cow's milk protein allergy).

    b. Instrumentation (e.g., nasogastric tube).

    c. Swallowed maternal blood

        (1) Maternal blood is sometimes swallowed by the newborn during labor and delivery. This can be diagnosed by an Apt test performed on blood aspirated from the infant's stomach (see XIc and Chap. 26, Anemia).

        (2) In breastfed infants, if blood obtained from the infant's stomach is adult blood, inspection of the mother's breasts or her expressed milk may reveal the source of blood. Aspirating the contents of the baby's stomach after a feeding is most likely to yield milk for testing.

  2. Surgical conditions resulting in hematemesis and bloody stool:

    a. Necrotizing enterocolitis (most frequent cause of hematemesis and bloody stool in premature infants; see Chap. 32).

    b. Gastric or duodenal ulcers (due to stress).

    c. Coagulation disorders including disseminated intravascular coagulation (DIC) (see Chap. 26, Bleeding).

    d. Duodenal stenosis.

    e. Meckel's diverticulum.

    f. Duplications of the small intestine.

    g. Volvulus.

    h. Intussusception.

    i. Polyps, hemangiomas.

    j. Cirsoid aneurysm.

I. Abdominal masses (see VIII)

  1. Genitourinary anomalies including distended bladder (see VI and Chap. 31).

  2. Tumors (see VII).

J. Birth trauma (see Chap. 20)

  1. Fractured clavicle/humerus (see Chap. 28).

  2. Intracranial hemorrhage (see Chap. 27).

  3. Lacerated solid organs—liver, spleen.

  4. Spinal cord transection with quadriplegia.

III. Lesions causing respiratory distress

A. Esophageal atresia (EA) with or without tracheoesophageal fustula (TEF). At least 85% of infants with EA also have TEF. Diagnosis may be suspected on prenatal ultrasonography by the absence of a stomach bubble.

  1. Presentation

    a. Infants often present with excessive salivation and vomiting soon after feedings. They may develop respiratory distress due to:

        (1) Airway obstruction by excess secretions.

        (2) Compromised pulmonary capacity due to diaphragmatic elevation secondary to abdominal distention.

        (3) Reflux of gastric contents up the distal esophagus into the lungs via the fistula.

    b. If the fistula connects the trachea to the esophagus proximal to the atresia, no gastrointestinal (GI) gas will be seen on x-ray examination, and the abdomen will be scaphoid. Respiratory difficulties are less acute.

    c. TEF without esophageal atresia (H-type fistula) is extremely rare and usually presents after the neonatal period. The diagnosis is suggested by a history of frequent pneumonias or respiratory distress temporally related to meals.

  2. Diagnosis

    a. Esophageal atresia itself is diagnosed by the inability to pass a catheter into the stomach. To test whether the esophagus is patent, a catheter is passed into it until resistance is met. Air is then injected into the catheter while listening (for lack of air) over the stomach. The diagnosis is confirmed by x-ray studies showing the catheter coiled in the upper esophageal pouch. Plain x-ray films may demonstrate a distended blind upper esophageal pouch filled with air that is unable to progress into the stomach. (The plain films may also show associated vertebral anomalies of the cervical or upper thoracic region of the spine.) Pushing 50 mL of air into the catheter under fluoroscopic examination may show dilatation and relaxation of the upper pouch, thus avoiding the need for contrast studies.

b. H-type fistula. This disorder can often be demonstrated with administration of nonionic water-soluble contrast medium (Omnipaque) during cinefluoroscopy. The definitive examination is combined fiberoptic bronchoscopy and esophagoscopy with passage of a fine balloon catheter from the trachea into the esophagus. The H-type fistula is usually high in the trachea (cervical area).

3. Associated issues and anomalies. Babies with esophageal atresia with or without TEF are often of low birth weight. Approximately 20% of these babies are premature (five times the normal incidence), and another 20% are small for gestational age (eight times the normal incidence). Other anomalies may be present, including the chromosomal abnormlities and the VATER association: vertebral defects, imperforate anus, TEF with esophageal atresia, and renal dysplasia or defects.

4. Management. Preoperative management focuses on minimizing the risk of aspiration and avoiding gaseous distention of the GI tract with positive pressure crossing from the trachea into the esophagus.

a. A multiple end-hole suction catheter (Replogle) should be placed in the proximal pouch and put under intermittent suction at the time the diagnosis is made.

b. The head of the bed should be elevated to 45 degrees to diminish reflux of gastric contents into the fistula.

c. If possible, mechanical ventilation of these babies should be avoided until the fistula is controlled because the abdomen may become very distended, compromising ventilation. If intubation is required, the case should be considered an emergency. Guidelines for intubation are the same as for other types of respiratory distress (see Chap. 36). The endotracheal tube should be advanced to just above the carina in the hopes of obstructing airflow through the fistula. Most commonly, the fistula connects to the trachea near the carina. Care must be taken to avoid accidental intubation of the fistula. Optimally, if mechanical ventilation is required, it should be done using a relatively high rate and low pressure to prevent gastric and intestinal distention. Heavy sedation should be avoided since the patient's spontaneous respiratory effort generates negative intrathoracic pressure, minimizing passage of air through the fistula into the esophagus.

d. Surgical therapy usually involves immediate placement of a gastrostomy tube. As soon as the infant can tolerate further surgery, the fistula is divided, and if possible, primary repair of the esophagus is performed.

e. Many infants with esophageal atresia are premature or have other defects that make it advisable to delay primary repair. Mechanical ventilation and nutritional management may be difficult in these infants because of the TEF. These babies need careful nursing care to prevent aspiration, and total parenteral nutrition to allow growth until repair is possible. In some cases, the fistula can be divided, with deferral of definitive repair.

f. If the infant has cardiac disease that requires surgery, it is usually best to repair the fistula first. If not, the postoperative ventilatory management will be very difficult.

B. Diaphragmatic hernia (DH)

1. The most common site is the left hemithorax, with the defect in the diaphragm being posterior (foramen of Bochdalek) in 70% of infants. It can also occur on the right, with either an anterior or a posterior defect.

2. **The incidence is between 1 in 2000 and 5000.** Fifty percent of these hernias are associated with other malformations, especially neural tube defects, cardiac defects, and intestinal malrotation. In some cases diaphragmatic hernia is familial. Diaphragmatic hernia has been associated with trisomies 13 and 18, and 45 XO, and has been reported as part of Goldenhar, Beckwith-Wiedemann, Pierre Robin, Goltz-Gorlin, and the Rubella syndromes.

3. **Symptoms.** Infants with large diaphragmatic hernias usually present at birth with cyanosis, respiratory distress, a scaphoid abdomen, decreased or absent breath sounds on the side of the hernia, and heart sounds displaced to the side opposite the hernia. Small hernias, right-sided hernias, and substernal hernias of Morgagni may have a more subtle presentation, manifested as feeding problems and mild respiratory distress.

4. **Diagnosis**
   a. **Prenatal Dx.** DHs often occur after the routine 16-week prenatal ultrasound, therefor many of these cases are not diagnosed until after birth. The development of polyhydramnios can prompt a later fetal ultrasound that will detect DH. Symptoms early in gestation may correlate with a poorer prognosis due to severity of the condition. This prenatal diagnosis should also lead to delivery in a center equipped to optimize chances for survival. If delivery before term is likely, fetal lung maturity should be assessed to evaluate the need for maternal betamethasone therapy (see Chap. 24). Increased severity and poorer prognosis also correlate with whether the liver is present in the thorax. This may also guide initial therapy.
   b. **Postnatal Dx.** The diagnosis is made or confirmed by radiograph. Because of the posssiblity of marked mediastinal shift, a radiopaque marker should be placed on one side of the chest to aid interpretation of the x-ray film.

5. **Treatment**
   a. Severe cases that have been diagnosed before birth may be best managed by delivery by the ex utero intrapartum treatment (EXIT) procedure, with immediate institution of extracorporeal membrane oxygenation (ECMO) (See Chap. 24). EXIT was developed for the intrapartum management of airway obstruction of giant fetal neck masses. It requires a multidisciplinary team consisting of surgeons, obstetricians, neonatologists, specialized anesthesiologists, nurses, respiratory therapists, and ECMO technicians to be assembled at a specialized center. Deep general anesthesia is established in the mother, ensuring fetal anesthesia. Maternal laparotomy is performed, with exposure of the uterus. The uterus, which should be extremely hypotonic because of the anesthesia, is then opened using a special device that cuts a full thickness uterine incision and simultaneously places haemostatic clips along the incision, minimizing bleeding.

   The fetus is then partially delivered through the uterine opening, and a pulse oximeter probe is placed on the fetal hand to permit direct monitoring of heart rate and oxygen saturation, so that the percent of oxygen saturation can be maintained at fetal levels (approximately the 60% range). If the saturation gets too high, the umbilical vessels will constrict and umbilical blood supply will diminish. Monitoring may be augmented by palpation of the umbilical pulse.

   Intervention on the fetus is begun coincident with establishing monitoring. The fetus should be intubated, and then assessed. A decision is then made whether delivery should be completed at that point, and further care continued as noted in 5.b. If the fetal condition does not improve upon intubation or if the diaphragmatic hernia is known to be severe, the EXIT procedure may be used as a bridge to immediate initiation of ECMO. Once the fetus is partially delivered, the surgeons can expose the major vessels of the neck and insert the ECMO catheters. Portable ECMO equipment brought to the operating room is then used during transport to the intensive-care unit or during subsequent surgery on the delivered newborn.

   b. Intubation. All infants should be intubated immediately after delivery if the diagnosis has been made antenatally, or at the time of postnatal diagnosis. Bag and mask ventilation is contraindicated. Immediately after intubation, a large sump nasogastric tube should be inserted and attached to continuous suction. Care must be taken with assisted ventilation to keep inspiratory pressures low to avoid damage or rupture of the contralateral lung. Peripheral venous and arterial lines are preferable, as umbilical lines may need to be removed during surgery. However, if umbilical lines are the only practical access, these should be placed initially. Heavy sedation should be avoided as spontaneous respiratory effort enables the use of the assist-control mode of ventilation, which we have found to induce the least barotrauma.

   c. Preoperative management is focused on avoiding barotrauma and minimizing pulmonary hypertension. The use of high-frequency ventilation is controversial in this patient population. Avoidance of hypoxia and acidosis will aid in minimizing pulmonary hypertension.

6. **Surgical repair is through** either the **abdomen or** the **chest,** with reduction of intestine into the abdominal cavity.

7. **Mortality and prognosis**
   a. While improved with modern therapy, mortality from diaphragmatic hernias is as high as 40%. Repair of the defect itself is relatively straightforward; the underlying pulmonary hypoplasia and pulmonary hypertension are largely responsible for overall mortality (see Chap. 24, Persistent Pulmonary Hypertension of the Newborn).

   b. **Prognosis.** Initial oxygen tension (PO_2) and carbon dioxide tension (PCO_2) are predictive of prognosis. In addition, the later the onset of postnatal symptoms, the higher the survival rate. Extracorporeal membrane oxygenation and nitric oxide inhalation therapy offer the hope of improved survival (see Chap. 24, Extracorporeal Membrane Oxygenation).

C. **Other mechanical causes for respiratory distress**
   1. **Choanal atresia.** Bilateral atresia presents in the delivery room as respiratory distress that resolves with crying. Infants are obligate nasal breathers until approximately 4 months of age. An oral airway is effective initial treatment. Definitive therapy includes opening a hole through the bony plate, which can be accomplished with a laser in some settings.

   2. **Robin anomaly** (Pierre Robin syndrome) consists of a hypoplastic mandible associated with a secondary U-shaped midline cleft palate. Often the tongue occludes the airway causing obstruction. Prone positioning or forcibly pulling the tongue forward will relieve the obstruction. These infants often improve after placement of a nasopharyngeal or endotracheal tube. If the infant can be supported for a few days, he or she will sometimes adapt, and aggressive procedures can be avoided. In some cases, a procedure to adhere the tongue to the lip is done, which avoids the need for tracheostomy. A specialized feeder (Breck) facilitates PO feeding the infant, but sometimes a gastrostomy will be necessary. Severely affected babies will require tracheostomy and gastrostomy.

   3. **Laryngotracheal clefts.** The length of the cleft determines the symptoms. The diagnosis is made by instillation of contrast material into the esophagus and is confirmed by bronchoscopy. Very ill newborns should undergo immediate bronchoscopy without contrast studies.

   4. **Laryngeal web occluding the larynx.** Perforation of the web by a stiff endotracheal tube or bronchoscopy instrument may be lifesaving.

   5. **Tracheal agenesis.** This rare lesion is suspected when a tube cannot be passed down the trachea. The infant ventilates by way of bronchi coming

off the esophagus. Diagnosis is by use of contrast material in the esophagus and by endoscopy. Prognosis is poor as tracheal reconstruction is difficult.

6. **Congenital lobar emphysema** may be due to a malformation, a cyst in the bronchus, or a mucous or meconium plug in the bronchus. These lesions cause air trapping, compression of surrounding structures, and respiratory distress. There may be a primary malformation of the lobe (polyalveolar lobe). Overdistention from mechanical ventilation may cause lobar emphysema. Extrinsic pressure on a bronchus also can cause obstruction. Lower lobes are generally relatively spared. Diagnosis is by chest x-ray studies.

   a. **High-frequency ventilation** may resolve the lobar emphysema.

   b. **Elective intubation** of the opposite bronchus may decompress the lobe if overinflation is thought to be the cause and if the infant can tolerate it. After a maximum of 8 to 12 hours, the tube should be withdrawn to the trachea. The lobar emphysema may not recur. Occasionally, selective suctioning of the bronchus on the side of the lesion may remove obstructing mucus or meconium. Treatment of acquired lobar emphysema (from inflammation of a bronchus) has included dexamethasone, 0.5 mg/kg per day for 3 days. If the baby is symptomatic and conservative measures fail, surgical intervention should be considered. Bronchoscopy should be performed to remove any obstructing material or rupture a bronchogenic cyst; if this procedure fails, the involved lobe should be resected.

7. **Cystic adenomatoid malformation** of the lung may be confused with a diaphragmatic hernia. Respiratory distress is related to the effect of the mass on the uninvolved lung. This malformation can cause shifting of the mediastinal structures.

8. **Vascular rings.** The symptomatology of vascular rings is related to the architecture of the ring. Both respiratory (stridor) and GI symptoms (vomiting, difficulty swallowing) may occur, depending on the anatomy of the ring. Barium swallow radiography is diagnostic.

IV. **Lesions causing mechanical intestinal obstruction.** The most critical lesion to rule out is malrotation with midgut volvulus. All patients with suspected intestinal obstruction should have a nasogastric sump catheter placed to continuous suction without delay.

A. **Congenital mechanical obstruction**

   1. **Intrinsic types** include atresia; stenosis; hypertrophic pyloric stenosis; meconium ileus (associated with cystic fibrosis or a rare form that is not associated with cystic fibrosis); small left colon syndrome; cysts within the lumen of the bowel; and imperforate anus.

   2. **Extrinsic forms** include malrotation with or without midgut volvulus; volvulus without malrotation; congenital peritoneal bands with or without malrotation; incarcerated hernia (common in premature infants); annular pancreas; duplications of the intestine; aberrant vessels (usually the mesenteric artery or preduodenal portal vein); hydrometrocolpos; and obstructing bands (persistent omphalomesenteric duct).

B. **Acquired mechanical obstruction**

   1. Malrotation with volvulus.

   2. Intussusception.

   3. Peritoneal adhesions

      a. After meconium peritonitis.

      b. After abdominal surgery.

      c. Idiopathic.

   4. Mesenteric thrombosis.

   5. Meconium and mucous plugs.

   6. Strictures secondary to necrotizing enterocolitis.

   7. Formation of abnormal intestinal concretions not associated with cystic fibrosis.

C. Functional intestinal obstruction constitutes the major cause of intestinal obstruction seen in the neonatal unit.
   1. Immaturity bowel motility.
   2. Defective innervation (Hirschsprung's disease).
   3. Paralytic ileus
      a. Induced by medications
         (1) Narcotics (pre- or postnatal exposure).
         (2) Hypermagnesemia due to prenatal exposure to magnesium sulfate.
      b. Sepsis.
      c. Pseudomonas enteritis.
   4. Meconium plug syndrome.
   5. Endocrine disorders
      a. Hypothyroidism.
      b. Adrenal insufficiency.
   6. Intrinsic defects in the bowel wall.
D. Other disorders associated with intestinal obstruction
   1. **Duodenal atresia.** 70% of cases associated with other malformations, including Down syndrome, cardiovascular anomalies, and such other GI anomalies as annular pancreas, esophageal atresia, malrotation of the small intestine, small-bowel atresias, and imperforate anus.
      a. There may be a history of polyhydramnios.
      b. Commonly diagnosed prenatally by ultrasound.
      c. Vomiting of bile-stained material usually begins a few hours after birth.
      d. Abdominal distention is limited to the upper abdomen.
      e. The infant may pass meconium in the first 24 hours of life; then bowel movements cease.
      f. Diagnosis suggested if aspiration of the stomach yields more than 30 mL of gastric contents prior to feeding.
      g. A plain radiograph of the abdomen will show air in the stomach and upper part of the abdomen ("double bubble") with no air in the small or large bowel.
      h. The neonate may be jaundiced due to increased enterohepatic circulation.
      i. Preoperative management includes decompression with nasogastric suction. Contrast radiographs of the upper intestine are not mandatory.
   2. **Pyloric stenosis** typically presents with nonbilious vomiting after the age of 2 to 3 weeks, but it has been seen in the first week of life. Radiographic examination will show a large stomach with little or no gas below the duodenum. Often the pyloric mass, or "olive," cannot be felt in the newborn. The infant may have associated jaundice and hematemesis. Diagnosis often starts with an ultrasound. An upper GI series confirms the diagnosis.
   3. **Meconium ileus** is a frequent cause of meconium peritonitis. Unlike most other etiologies of obstruction in which flat and upright x-ray films will demonstrate fluid levels, in cases of nonperforated meconium ileus, the distended bowel may be granular in appearance or may show tiny bubbles mixed with meconium.
      a. No meconium will pass through the rectum, even after digital stimulation.
      b. Rare cases (both familial and nonfamilial) of meconium ileus are not associated with cystic fibrosis.
      c. Cheek brushing for DNA analysis is becoming the standard initial screening for cystic fibrosis. If the results are negative or equivocal, a sweat test should be performed. Some couples will have received prenatal CF genetic testing, and some states now include CF in the newborn screen. A family history can provide rapid information regarding expected risk.

d. As with all types of complete obstruction, results of tests of stool trypsin activity will be negative (see XI E).

e. Contrast enemas can be both diagnostic and therapeutic. Meglumine diatrizoate (Gastrografin) can be used in an adequately hydrated infant. Diatrizoate sodium (Hypaque) also can be used. Both of these contrast agents are hypertonic. Therefore, the baby should start the procedure well hydrated, and fluids should be run at two to three times the maintenance level. Meglumine diatrizoate is often diluted 1:4 before use.

If the diagnosis is certain and the neonate stable, repeat enemas may be administered to relieve the impaction.

f. Surgical therapy is required if the contrast enema fails to relieve the obstruction.

g. Decompression with nasogastric suction should be used to prevent further distention.

h. Microcolon distal to the atresia will generally dilate spontaneously with use. Atresias distal to the obstruction require surgery.

4. **Imperforate anus.** Often associated with other anomalies such as those in the VATER association. Infants with imperforate anus may pass meconium if a rectovaginal or rectourinary fistula exists; in these infants, the diagnosis may be delayed. There are two types of imperforate anus: low and high.

a. Low imperforate anus. Eighty percent of females and 50% of males have the low type. The rectum has descended through the puborectalis sling and exists on the perineum as a fistula.

   (1) Meconium may be visualized on the perineum. It may be found in the rugal folds or scrotum in boys, and in the vagina in girls.

   (2) Perineal fistulas may be dilated to allow passage of meconium to temporarily relieve intestinal obstruction.

b. High imperforate anus. The rectum ends above the puborectalis sling. No perineal fistula is present. The fistula may enter the urinary tract or vagina.

   (1) The presence of meconium particles in the urine is diagnostic of a rectovesical fistula. Vaginal examination with a nasal speculum or cystoscope may reveal a fistula.

   (2) A cystogram may show a fistula and the level of rectal descent. Injection of dye into the most distal portion of the pouch may also show the level of rectal descent.

   (3) Ultrasound is often helpful in defining the distal level of the rectum.

   (4) Temporary colostomy is necessary in all neonates with a high imperforate anus with or without fistula.

5. **Volvulus with or without malrotation of the bowel**

a. Malrotation may be associated with other GI abnormalities such as diaphragmatic hernia, annular pancreas, and bowel atresias, and is always seen with omphalocele.

b. If this condition develops during fetal life, it may cause the appearance of a large midabdominal calcific shadow on x-ray examination; this results from calcification of meconium in the segment of necrotic bowel.

c. After birth there is a sudden onset of bilious vomiting in an infant who has had some normal stools. If the level of obstruction is high, there may not be much abdominal distention.

d. Signs of shock and sepsis are often present.

e. Plain X rays will show a dilated small bowel. A normal X ray does not rule out malrotation, which can be intermittent.

f. If a malrotation is present, barium enema may show failure of barium to pass beyond the transverse colon or may show the cecum in an abnormal position.

g. An upper GI series should be to obtained, specifically looking for an absent or abnormal position of the ligament of Treitz that confirms the diagnosis of malrotation.

    h. Malrotation as the cause of intestinal obstruction is a surgical emergency because intestinal viability is at stake. Bileous emesis is malrotation until proven otherwise.

6. Annular pancreas may be nonobstructing but associated with duodenal atresia or stenosis. It presents as a high intestinal obstruction.

7. Hydrometrocolpos

    a. The hymen bulges.

    b. Accumulated secretions in the uterus may cause intestinal obstruction by bowel compression.

    c. Meconium peritonitis or hydronephrosis may occur.

    d. Edema and cyanosis of the legs may be observed.

    e. If hydrometrocolpos is not diagnosed at birth, the secretions will decrease, the bulging will disappear, and the diagnosis will be delayed until puberty.

8. Meconium and mucous plug syndrome. Seen in premature babies, infants of diabetic mothers, and sick babies; it also can be caused by functional immaturity of the bowel with a small left colon, as seen in infants of diabetic mothers or Hirschsprung's disease (see IV.D.9), which should always be considered when a newborn has difficulty passing stools. Cystic fibrosis should also be ruled out. Treatment consists of glycerin suppository, warm half-normal saline enemas (5 to 10 mL/kg), and rectal stimulation with soft rubber catheter. If these maneuvers fail, a contrast enema with a hyperosmolar contrast material may be both diagnostic and therapeutic. A normal stooling pattern should follow evacuation of a plug.

9. Hirschsprung's disease. Should be suspected in any newborn who fails to pass meconium spontaneously by 24 to 48 hours after birth and who develops distention relieved by rectal stimulation. This is especially so if the infant is neither premature nor born to a diabetic mother. The diagnosis should be considered until future development shows sustained normal bowel function.

    a. When the diagnosis is suspected, every effort should be made to rule the condition in or out. If the diagnosis is considerd but seems very unlikely, parents taking the newborn home must specifially understand the importance of immediately reporting any obstipation, diarrhea, poor feeding, distention, lethargy, or fever. Development of a toxic megacolon may be fatal.

    b. Barium enema frequently does not show the characteristic transition zone in the newborn.

    c. Rectal biopsy is obtained to confirm the diagnosis. If suspicion is relatively low, a suction biopsy is useful, as presence of ganglion cells in the submucosal zone rules out the diagnosis. If the index of suspicion is high, or the suction biopsy is positive, formal full-thickness rectal biopsy is the definitive method for diagnosis. Absence of ganglion cells and hypertrophic nonmyelinated axons is diagnostic. Histochemical tests of biopsy specimens show an increase in acetylcholine.

    d. Obstipation can be relieved by gentle rectal irrigations with warm saline solution. If the patient has had a barium enema, gentle rectal saline washes are helpful in removing trapped air and barium.

    e. Neonates require surgical intervention when the diagnosis is made. A primary pull-through procedure is possible in some cases. Otherwise, a colostomy is made and definitive repair is postponed until the infant is of adequate size and stability.

V. Other surgical problems

    A. Appendicitis is extremely rare in newborns. Its presentation may be that of pneumoperitoneum. The appendix usually perforates prior to the diagnosis; therefore, the baby may present with intestinal obstruction, sepsis, or even DIC related to the intraabdominal infection. Rule out Hirschsprung's disease.

B. Omphalocele. The sac may be intact or ruptured. The diagnosis is often made by prenatal ultrasound. Cesarean section may prevent rupture of the sac, but is not specifically indicated unless the defect is large (>5 cm) or contains liver.

    1. Intact sac. Emergency treatment includes the following:

        a. Use latex-free products, including gloves.

        b. Provide continuous nasogastric sump suction.

        c. It is preferable to encase intestinal contents in a bowel bag (e.g., Vi Drape Isolation Bag) as it is the least abrasive. Otherwise, cover the sac with warm saline-soaked gauze, then wrap the sac on abdomen with Kling gauze and cover with plastic wrap so as to support the intestinal viscera on the abdominal wall.

        d. Keep the baby warm, including thoroughly wrapping in warm blankets to prevent heat loss.

        e. Do not attempt to reduce the sac because this can rupture it, interfere with venous return from the sac, and cause respiratory distress.

        f. Place a reliable intravenous line in an upper extremity.

        g. Monitor temperature and pH.

        h. Start broad-spectrum antibiotics (ampicillin and gentamicin).

        i. Obtain a surgical consultation; definitive surgical therapy should be delayed until the baby is stabilized. In the presence of other more serious abnormalities (respiratory or cardiac), definitive care can be postponed as long as the sac remains intact.

    2. Ruptured sac. As above for intact sac except, surgery is more emergent. Also, bowel viability may be compromised with a small abdominal wall defect and an obstructed segment of eviscerated intestine. In these circumstances, prior to transfer, the defect must be enlarged by incising the abdomen cephalad or caudad to relieve the strangulated viscera.

    3. A careful search must be made for associated abnormalities, such as chromosomal defects, malrotation of the colon, congenital heart disease, or extrophy of the cloaca. The Beckwith-Wiedemann syndrome includes omphalocele, macroglossia, hypoglycemia, and hemihypertrophy.

C. Gastroschisis, by definition, contains no sac and the intestine is eviscerated.

    1. Preoperative management as per omphalocele with ruptured sac (V.B.2).

    2. Obtain immediate surgical evaluation.

    3. Ten percent of infants with gastroschisis have intestial atresia.

    4. Unlike omphalocele, gastroschesis is not commonly associated with anomalies unrealted to the GI tract.

VI. Renal disorders (see Chap. 31)

A. Genitourinary abnormalities should be suspected in babies with abdominal distention, ascites, flank masses, persistently distended bladder, bactiuria, pyuria, or poor growth. First void should be noted in all infants. Approximately 90% of babies void in the first 24 hours of life, and 99% within the first 48 hours of life. Male infants exhibiting the listed symptoms should be observed for the normal forceful voiding pattern.

    1. Posterior urethral valves may cause obstruction.

    2. Renal vein thrombosis should be considered in the setting of hematuria with a flank mass.

        a. Renal ultrasound will initially show a large kidney on the side of the thrombosis. Kidney will return to normal size over ensuing weeks to months.

        b. Doppler ultrasound will show diminished or absent blood flow to involved kidney.

        c. Current treatment in most centers starts with medical support in the hope of avoiding surgery. Heparin is generally not indicated, but its use has been advocated by some (see Chaps. 31, 26).

    3. Extrophy of the bladder. Ranges from an epispadias to complete extrusion of the bladder onto the abdominal wall. Currently, most centers are attempting bladder turn-in within the first 48 hours of life.

a. Preoperative Management

(1) Use moist, fine-mesh gauze or petroleum jelly–impregnated gauze to cover the exposed bladder.

(2) Transport the infant to a facility for definitive care as soon as possible.

(3) Obtain renal ultrasound. Intravenous pyelography (IVP) is generally not required preoperatively.

b. Intraoperative management. Surgical management of an extrophied bladder includes turn-in of the bladder to preserve bladder function. The symphysis pubis is approximated. The penis is lengthened. Iliac osteotomies are not necessary if repair is accomplished within 48 hours. No attempt is made to make the bladder continent at this initial procedure.

4. Cloacal extrophy is a complex GI and genitourinary anomaly that includes vesico-intestinal fissure, omphalocele, extrophied bladder, hypoplastic colon, imperforate anus, absence of vagina in females, and microphallus in males.

a. Preoperative management

(1) Gender assignment. It is surgically easier to create a phenotypic female, regardless of genotype. Understanding of the long-term psychological effects of this practice has made this decision controversial (see Chap. 30).

(2) Nasogastric suction relieves partial intestinal obstruction. The baby excretes stool through a vesicointestinal fissure that is often partially obstructed.

(3) A series of complex operations is required in stages to achieve the most satisfactory results.

b. Surgical management

(1) The initial procedure includes division of the vesicointestinal fissure and establishment of fecal and urinary stomas.

(2) The bladder can be closed during the initial procedure if the baby is stable.

(3) Subsequent procedures are designed to reduce the number of stomas and create genitalia.

VII. Tumors

A. Teratomas are the most common tumor in the neonatal period. Though they are most commonly found in the sacrococcygeal area, they can arise anywhere, including the retroperitoneal area or the ovaries. Approximately 10% contain malignant elements. Prenatal diagnosis is often made by ultrasound. After delivery, rectal examination, ultrasound, computed tomography (CT), magnetic resonance imaging (MRI), as well as serum alpha-fetoprotein and beta-human chorionic gonadotropin measurements are used in evaluation. Calcifications are often seen on x-ray films. Excessive heat loss, platelet trapping, and dystocia are possible complications. Masses compromising the airway have been successfully managed by the EXIT procedure (see III. B.5.a), and establishment of an airway before complete delivery of the baby.

B. Neuroblastoma is the most common malignant neonatal tumor, accounting for about 50%. It is irregular, stony hard, and ranges in size from minute to massive. There are many sites of origin; the adrenal-retroperitoneal area is the most common. On rare occasions this tumor can cause diarrhea or hypertension by the release of tumor by-products, especially catecholamines or vasointestinal peptides. Tests should be performed to determine levels of catecholamines and their metabolites. Calcifications can often be seen on plain radiographs. Ultrasound is the most useful diagnostic test. Prenatal diagnosis by ultrasound is associated with improved prognosis. Of note, many neuroblastomas diagnosed prenatally resolve spontaneously prior to birth.

C. Wilms' tumor is the second most common malignant tumor in the newborn. It presents as a smooth flat mass and may be bilateral. One should palpate gently to avoid rupture. Ultrasound is the most useful diagnostic test.

D. Sarcoma botryoides. This grapelike tumor arises from the edge of the vulva or vagina. It may be small and thus be confused with a normal posterior vaginal tag. Intravenous pylogram (IVP) is an important test preoperatively, especially to avoid confusing the lesion with an obstructing ureterocele.

E. **Other tumors** include hemangiomas, lymphangiomas, hepatoblastomas, hepatomas, hamartomas, and nephromas.

VIII. Abdominal masses

A. **Renal masses** (see VI and Chap. 31) are the most common etiology: polycystic kidneys, multicystic dysplastic kidney, hydronephrosis, renal vein thrombosis.

B. **Other causes of abdominal masses** include tumors (see VII), adrenal hemorrhage, ovarian tumor or cysts, pancreatic cyst, choledochal cyst, hydrometrocolpos, mesenteric or omental cyst, and intestinal duplications.

IX. Inguinal hernia is found in 5% of premature infants weighing under 1500 g, and as many as 30% of infants weighing less than 1000 g at birth. It is more common in small-for-gestational-age (SGA) infants and male infants. In females the ovary is often in the sac.

A. **Surgical repair.** Inguinal hernia repair is the most common operation performed on premature infants. In general, hernias in this patient population can be repaired shortly before discharge home if they are easily reducible and cause no other problems.

1. **Repair prior to discharge.** The operation may be difficult and should be performed by an experienced pediatric surgeon. The use of spinal anesthesia has simplified the care of the infants with respiratory problems. As these infants often develop postoperative apnea, they should be monitored for at least 24 hours, and not be sent home on the day of surgery.

2. **Repair after discharge.** Infants with significant pulmonary disease, such as bronchopulmonary dysplasia, are often best repaired at a later time when their respiratory status has improved. We have occasionally had well-instructed parents bring their babies home, and then have them readmitted later for repair. The risks and benefits of this option must be weighed carefully as there is a real risk of the hernia incarcerating at home. In a term infant, repair should be scheduled when the diagnosis is made. An incarcerated hernia can usually be reduced with sedation, steady firm pressure, and elevation of the feet. If a hernia has been incarcerated, it should be repaired as soon as the edema is gone.

X. Testicular Torsion

A. **About 70% of the cases** of testicular torsion that are diagnosed in the newborn period **occur prenatally.** In the newborn, testicular torsion is generally extravaginal (the twist occurs outside the tunica vaginalis) and is caused by an incomplete attachment of the gubernaculum to the testis, allowing torsion and infarction.

B. **Diagnosis is made be physical examination.** The testicle is generally nontender, firm, indurated, and swollen with a slightly bluish or dusky cast on the affected side of the scrotum. If the torsion is acute, rather than congenital, it will be extremely tender to palpation. The testicle can have a transverse lie or be high riding and the overlying skin may be erythematous or edematous, limited to the scrotum itself. Transillumination is negative and the cremasteric reflex is absent. Ultrasonography employing Doppler flow studies can be helpful if available, but testing should not delay referral for surgery if there is a possibility that the torsion is recent.

C. **Differential diagnosis of acute scrotal swelling** in the newborn includes:

1. **Trauma/scrotal hematoma.** Most commonly secondary to breech delivery. This is generally bilateral, and may present with hematocele, scrotal swelling, and ecchymoses. Rarely transilluminates. Resolution is usually spontaneous but severe cases may require surgical exploration, evacuation of the hematocele, and repair of the testes.

2. **Torsion of the testicular appendage.** Swelling is usually less marked, and may present on palpation or as a blue dot on the scrotum. The cremasteric reflexes are preserved, and Doppler flow ultrasonography may be helpful in ruling out testicular torsion. No treatment is needed.

3. **Incarcerated hernia.**
4. **Spontaneous idiopathic scrotal hemorrhage.** Most common in large for gestational (LGA) infants. Distinguishable from torsion by the appearance of a small but distinct ecchymosis over the superficial inguinal ring.
5. **Tumor.** These are usually nontender, solid, and firm. Transillumination is negative.
6. **Meconium peritonitis.**
D. **Treatment.** In the vast majority of cases the torsed testicle is already necrotic at birth, and surgical intervention will not salvage the testicle. However, if there is *any possibility* that the torsion occurred recently and the infant is otherwise healthy, emergency surgical exploration and detorsion should be performed within 4 to 6 hours. This may result in salvage of the torsed testicle. Because there have been reports of bilateral testicular torsion, surgical exploration should include contralateral orchiopexy. Even if emergency exploration is not indicated because of definitive evidence of chronicity of torsion, exploration should be performed on a nonemergent basis to rule out a tumor with clinical and imaging findings identical to testicular torsion. Testicular protheses are available.
E. **Oligospermia** has been reported after unilateral testicular torsion.
XI. **Common tests** used in the diagnosis of surgical conditions
   A. **Abdominal X ray examinations.** A flat plate radiograph of the abdomen is sufficient for assessing intraluminal gas patterns and mucosal thickness. A left lateral decubitus radiograph is obtained to ascertain the presence of free air in the abdomen.
      1. **Barium enema** may be diagnostic in suspected cases of Hirschsprung's disease. It may reveal microcolon in the infant with complete obstruction of the small intestine and may show a narrow segment in the sigmoid in the infant with meconium plug syndrome due to functional immaturity.
      2. **Barium swallow** with meglumine diatrizoate may be used to demonstrate H-type TEF without esophageal atresia.
      3. In patients with suspected malrotation, a combination of **contrast studies** may be necessary, starting with a contrast swallow/ upper GI. In combination with air or contrast media, an upper GI series will determine the presence or absence of the normally placed ligament of Treitz. A barium enema may show malposition of the cecum but will not always rule out malrotation. Neonates with intestinal obstruction presumed secondary to malrotation require urgent surgery to relieve possible volvulus of the midgut.
   B. **Ultrasonography** is the preferred method of evaluating abdominal masses in the newborn. It is useful for defining the presence of masses, together with their size, shape, and consistency.
   C. **The Apt test** differentiates maternal from fetal blood. A small amount of bloody material is mixed with 5 ml of water and centrifuged. One part 0.25N sodium hydroxide is added to five parts of pink supernatant. The fluid remains pink in the presence of fetal blood but rapidly becomes brown if maternal blood is present. The test is useful only if the sample is not contaminated by pigmented material (e.g., meconium/stool).
   D. **Cheek brush sampling** for DNA analysis is the initial test for cystic fibrosis, and will detect the majority of cases. When the test result is negative but clinical suspicion remains high, a sweat test should be done. This test can yield a false-positive result due to the relatively high chloride content of infants' sweat. The test can yield a false-negative or be uninterpretable if less than 100 mg of sweat is collected. It may be necessary to repeat the test when the infant is 3 to 4 weeks old if inadequate volume of sweat is collected.
   E. **Test for stool trypsin activity.** Lack of trypsin activity is not diagnostic of cystic fibrosis, since stool will have no enzyme activity with any type of complete bowel obstruction. The method involves making 1:5 and 1:10 dilutions of meconium or stool and placing them on the gelatin side of undeveloped

x-ray films. They should be incubated at 37°C for 1 hour. If trypsin activity is present, the gelatin will dissolve.

F. Computed tomography (CT) is an excellent modality to evaluate abdominal masses as well as their relationship to other organs. Contrast enhancement can outline the intestine, blood vessels, kidneys, ureter, and bladder.

G. IVP use should be restricted to evaluating genitourinary anatomy if other modalities (ultrasound and contrast CT) are not available. The IVP dye is poorly concentrated in the newborn.

H. Radionuclide scan of the kidneys can aid in determining function. This is especially useful in assessing complex genitourinary anomalies and in evaluating the contribution of each kidney to renal function.

I. MRI is useful to better define the anatomy and location of masses.

XII. Preoperative management by presenting symptom

A. Bilious vomiting and abdominal distention (important to concurrently proceed aggressively with diagnositic evaluation to rule out malrotation with midgut volvulous).

  1. Enteral feedings should be discontinued. Continuous gastric decompression with a sump catheter is mandatory if intestinal obstruction is suspected. All babies with presumed intestinal obstruction should be transported with a nasogastric suction catheter in place, attached to a catheter-tip syringe (Becton-Dickinson catheter-tip 60-mL syringe no. 5664) for continuous aspiration of gastric contents. Failure to decompress the stomach could lead to gastric rupture, aspiration, or respiratory compromise secondary to diaphragmatic compression. This is especially important in infants who are to be transported by air, since loss of cabin pressure may be associated with rupture of an inadequately drained viscus.

  2. Shock, dehydration, and electrolyte imbalance should be prevented, or treated if present (see Chap. 9).

  3. Broad-spectrum antibiotics (ampicillin and gentamicin) should be initiated if there is suspicion of volvulus or any question about bowel integrity. Clindamycin should be added in the setting of documented or high risk of perforation.

  4. Studies that should be performed include the following:
    a. Complete blood count with differential.
    b. Electrolytes.
    c. Blood gases and Ph.
    d. Clotting studies (e.g., prothrombin time, partial thromboplastin time).
    e. Monitoring of oxygen saturation, blood pressure, and urine output.

B. Nonbilious vomiting with distention. Many babies with nonbilious vomiting and distention respond to glycerin suppositories, half-strength saline enemas (5 mL/kg body weight), rectal stimulation with a soft rubber catheter, or a combination of these measures. It is important to rule out other nonfunctional causes of distention. Limited feedings, stimulation to the rectum, and care for the general condition of the baby will solve most of these problems. Plain x-ray studies are helpful. Barium enema should be undertaken with caution because it may be difficult to evacuate the barium.

C. Vomiting without distention

  1. If the baby's general condition is good, feedings of dextrose water should be attempted. If this is tolerated, milk should be tried again. If vomiting recurs, the baby should be given a trial of non-cow's-milk-based formula (e.g., soy-based, or elemental). If this is successful, a trial of a cow's milk formula should be undertaken in 2 weeks.

  2. The mechanics of feeding the baby should be observed. Rapid feeding, intake of excessive volume, and lack of burping, and are all causes of nonbilious vomiting without distention.

  3. Functional and mechanical causes must be ruled out.

D. Masses. The following steps may be taken to determine the etiology of abdominal masses:

1. Complete blood cell count and urinalysis.
2. Determination of the level of catecholamines and their metabolites.
3. X-ray examination of the chest and abdomen with the infant supine and upright.
4. Abdominal ultrasonography.
5. Contrast-enhanced CT.
6. MRI.
7. Angiography—venous and arterial.
8. Surgical consultation.

XIII. General intraoperative management
A. Monitoring devices
1. Temperature probe.
2. Electrocardiogram (ECG).
3. Pulse oximetry responds rapidly to changes in patient condition, but is subject to artifacts.
4. Arterial cannula to monitor blood gases and pressure. Transcutaneous partial pressure of oxygen (pO_2) (see Chap. 24, Blood Gas and Pulmonary Graphics Monitoring) is helpful if pulse oximetry is unavailable, but can be inaccurate in the setting of anesthetic agents that dilate skin vessels.
B. Well-functioning intravenous line. Babies with omphalocele or gastroschesis must have the intravenous line in the upper extremity or neck.
C. Maintenance of body temperature
1. Warmed operating room.
2. Humidified, warmed anesthetic agents.
3. Cover exposed parts of the baby, especially the head (with a hat).
4. Warmed blood and other fluids used intraoperatively.
D. Fluid replacement
1. Replace loss of more than 15% of total blood volume with warmed packed red blood cells (PRBCs).
2. Replace ascites loss with normal salinemilliliter per milliliter to maintain normal blood pressure.
3. The neonate loses approximately 5 mL of fluid per kilogram for each hour that the intestine is exposed. This should be replaced by Ringer's lactate or fresh-frozen plasma.
E. Anesthetic management of the neonate is reviewed in Chap. 37.
F. Postoperative pain management is discussed in Chap. 37.
G. Postoperatively, the newborn fluid requirement is approximately two-thirds the standard maintenance level for the first 24 to 48 hours, plus continuing losses that must be replaced.

Suggested Readings

Adzick N. S., Nance M. L.. Medical progress:pediatric surgery (second of two parts). *N Engl J Med* 2000;342:1726.

Altman R. P., et al. Pediatric surgery. *Pediatr Clin North Am* 1993;40:1121.

American Academy of Pediatrics, Committee on Bioethics: Fetal therapy: Ethical considerations. *Pediatrics* 1999;103:1061.

Brodeur A. E., et al. Abnormal masses in children: Neuroblastoma, Wilms tumor, and other considerations. *Pediatr Rev* 1991;12:196.

Dillon P. W., Cilley R. E. Newborn surgical emergencies. *Pediatr Clin North Am* 1993;40:1289.

Grosfeld J. Neuroblastoma: A 1990 review. *Pediatr Surg Int* 1991;6:9.

Guzzetta P. C., et al. General surgery. In: Avery G. B. (Ed.), *Neonatology.* Philadelphia: Lippincott, 1994.

Hansen A., Puder M. *Manual of Surgical Neonatal Intensive Care.* Hamilton, Ontario: B.C. Decker, 2003.

Johnson M. P., et al. In utero surgical treatment of fetal obstructive uropathy: A new comprehensive approach to identify appropriate candidates for vesicoamniotic shunt therapy. *Am J Obstet Gynecol* 1994;170:1770.

Liechty K. W., et al. Intrapartum airway management for giant fetal neck masses: The EXIT (ex utero intrapartum treatment) procedure. *Am J Obstet Gynecol* 1997;177:870.

Nakayama D., Bose C., Chescheir N., Valley R. *Critical Care of the Surgical Newborn.* Armonk, NY: Futura, 1997.

Nakayama D. K., et al. Inguinal hernia and the acute scrotum in infants and children. *Pediatr Rev* 1989;11:87.

Ringer S. A., Stark A. S. Management of neonatal emergencies in the delivery room. *Clin Perinatol* 1989;16:23.

Ross A. J. Intestinal obstruction in the newborn. *Pediatr Rev* 1994;15:338.

Sherer L. R. III, et al. Inguinal hernias and umbilical anomalies. *J Pediatr Surg* 1993;40:1121.

West K. N., et al. Delayed surgical repair and ECMO improves survival in congenital diaphragmatic hernia. *Ann Surg* 1992;216:454.

34. SKIN CARE

Stephanie Packard and Caryn Douma

I. **Introduction.** The skin is the largest organ of the human body. Its functions include protecting the internal organs, facilitating thermoregulation, barrier properties, and fluid and electrolyte balance. In addition, the skin is a sensory organ capable of receiving tactile input from the environment including touch, temperature, pain, and pressure.

   A. **Examination.** The skin is easily examined by direct observation and touch for color, temperature, hydration, and turgor.

   B. **Maturation** affects the resilience of the skin and wound healing. The epidermal layer of the skin in newborns is thin and functionally immature. The functionality of the skin decreases with gestational age, increasing the risk of infection, exposure to chemical and environmental toxins, electrolyte imbalance, and traumatic injury.

II. **Routine skin care practices** promote skin integrity and minimize complications.

   A. **Bathing**

      1. Newborns should be given an initial bath after temperature and physiologic condition are stable. This minimizes the risk of transmission of human immunodeficiency virus (HIV), hepatitis B virus (HBV), and other infectious agents. A mild, low-alkaline soap (Dove or Basis) should be used so the acid mantle of the skin is not disrupted.

      2. Soaps and shampoos containing perfumes and dyes are not recommended for newborns during the first 2 to 3 weeks of age as they may increase the risk of skin irritation. Low-alkaline soap may be added after the first week for term infants and 2 to 3 weeks for preterm infants.

      3. Warm sterile water should be used for infants with nonkeratinized skin or skin breakdown of any kind.

      4. The diaper area should be cleaned with warm water and a thin protective layer of petroleum jelly (Vaseline) applied to prevent irritant contact diaper dermatitis.

      5. Preterm infants less than 2 months of age should be bathed infrequently, generally not more than 2 or 3 times a week.

      6. Preterm infants may require additional heat during bathing. Radiant heat lamps may be used for this purpose.

      7. Creams and emollients should be avoided except in cases of extreme dryness with cracking and fissures.

      8. Generalized prophylactic application of the emollient Aquaphor in extremely low-birth-weight infants does not reduce the combined outcome of death or sepsis and may increase nosocomial infection. We do not use Aquaphor in preterm infants until after the first week.

   B. **Umbilical cord care.** The cord and surrounding area should be cleaned with mild soap during the initial bath. The cord should be kept clean and dry. If soiled, it should be cleaned with sterile water. The use of alcohol should be avoided. The umbilical cord typically falls off 7 to 10 days after birth.

   C. **Latex products should be avoided.** Latex is present in a variety of products throughout the hospital environment. Exposure should be avoided in infants at risk for developing serious skin sensitivities or allergy, such as those with neural tube defects, frequent surgery, or genitourinary abnormalities requiring frequent catheterizations.

   D. **Minimal use of adhesives.** Adhesives are a potential skin irritant and may cause trauma if applied or removed incorrectly. The use of adhesive tape should be minimized.

      1. Use nonadhesive products when available (gel electrodes, Velcro ties, and cloth wraps).

2. Use transparent dressings to secure IV catheters and tubes that allow direct visualization of underlying skin and minimize adhesive irritation.
3. Consider a thin pectin or hydrocolloid "anchor" to protect the skin when repeated tape removal is necessary. A pectin barrier may also be used when securing catheters, endotracheal tubes, feeding tubes, nasal cannulas, and urine bags.
4. Warm sterile water and patience should be used when removing adhesives from the skin. Adhesive removers or solvents containing hydrocarbon derivatives or petroleum distillates should be avoided in the preterm infant during the first 2 weeks after birth due to potential toxicity. If an adhesive remover is necessary, the skin should be rinsed thoroughly.
5. Avoid the use of adhesive bonding agents as they may cause irritation or be absorbed systemically. In preterm infants, the bond created by these agents is often stronger than the bond between the dermis and the epidermis and removal may cause epidermal stripping.

E. **Invasive procedures.** Antiseptic agents used to prepare the site for invasive procedures should be used sparingly. Remaining solution should be removed from the skin with sterile water to limit possible systemic absorption.

F. **Pressure necrosis** can result from any firm object that comes in contact with the infant's skin. The skin should be inspected frequently. Potential sources of injury in the environment should be identified. Interventions to help maintain skin integrity include changing the infant's position, alternating sites of monitoring devices at regular intervals, padding pressure points, and adherence to manufacturer's guidelines for use of medical devices. Alterations in skin integrity resulting from pressure injuries are more common in infants with multisystem disease, generalized edema, inadequate tissue perfusion, poor nutrition, and immobility.

G. **Thermal injury** should be avoided from heat sources such as water filled gloves, heated transcutaneous monitor electrodes, heating mattresses, and disposable heel warmers. The temperature of any products should not exceed 41°C/105°F. Warming mattresses should always be covered with a blanket. Monitoring electrodes should be used at the lowest possible temperature setting and the site should be changed at least every 4 hours. Heel warmers and mattresses should be used with caution on infants who weigh < 1000 g. Skin temperature probes on servo-controlled radiant warmers and incubators should be affixed securely to the infant and checked frequently for dislodgement and accuracy.

III. **Wound care.** Effective wound management is essential to optimize healing.
   A. **Wound healing occurs in three phases:**
      1. **Inflammatory phase** is characterized by erythema, warmth, edema, and pain.
      2. **Proliferative phase,** which overlaps with the inflammatory phase and continues until the wound is healed, is characterized by beefy, red granulation tissue surrounded by a thin silvery epithelial layer and wound shrinkage.
      3. **Maturation phase,** which begins three weeks after the wound and may continue for several years, is characterized by paling of the scar.
   B. **The elements of wound management** are: Identification of the etiology of the wound, wound assessment, appropriate dressing selection, and systematic documentation.
      1. **Description.** The wound location should be described using anatomical landmarks. Wounds should be measured accurately and include length, width, and depth. The presence or absence of drainage should be noted including amount, color, and odor of exudates, if present. The character of wound tissue should be assessed, including the presence of granulation tissue, slough (nonviable tissue), or eschar.
      2. **Management** for optimal wound healing is achieved through proper cleansing, treatment of infection, debridement if indicated, a moist wound base, and selection of the appropriate dressing. Routine cleansing of the

wound is essential to remove exudates and debris, assess the wound bed, and determine the appropriate dressing. Creating a moist environment improves collagen synthesis and granulation tissue formation. Cell migration and epithelial resurfacing occur more rapidly and scabs, crusts, and eschars do not form.

C. **Wound types**

1. **Primary intention wounds** are closed by sutures, tape, or staples. They are usually dressed with gauze and a transparent film dressing that can be removed in 2 to 3 days. The suture line is kept clean and protected. Once staples and sutures are removed, the wound is left open to air but protected from trauma. If steristrips are used to close the incision, they are left undisturbed until they peel off. Incisions that include a Penrose drain may require frequent dressing changes and absorbent foam or gauze to absorb exudate. The use of Montgomery straps (Johnson & Johnson Medical Inc., Arlington, TX) or pectin wafers as tape "anchors" to hold the dressing in place may be helpful to decrease contact dermatitis and epidermal stripping that may occur with frequent dressing changes and adhesive tape removal.

2. **Draining wounds** such as open abdominal wounds, heal by secondary intention. They are left open and allowed to heal by formation of new blood vessels and production of connective (scar) tissue. Open draining wounds require diligent effort to prevent cross-contamination from other wound sites and maintain surrounding intact skin. If wounds have excessive drainage and cannot be managed with exudate absorbers, a closed drainage and suction system may be necessary.

D. **Wound dressings** are used to create an optimal environment for tissue healing. Dressings are either primary or secondary. A primary dressing is placed in direct contact with the wound bed. A secondary dressing is applied over a primary dressing. Dressing changes should be made as frequently as demanded by the accumulation of fluid and debris in the wound. Before a new dressing is applied, the old dressing should be removed and analyzed.

1. **Gauze dressings** (dry or fine mesh) help to debride necrotic tissue or for packing and undermining the wound. They absorb exudates, protect the wound, and may be used to deliver topical solutions if kept moist. If gauze dressings are left to dry in the wound, they may remove viable tissue.

2. **Moisture vapor-permeable membranes** (MVP films) are used to help maintain a physiologic environment on the skin. They provide a transparent barrier to bacteria and water and conform to the wound margins. They may be used over a layer of gauze to absorb leakage. Care should be taken when removing this type of dressing as epithelial damage may occur.

3. **Hydrocolloid dressings** create a moist wound-healing environment by interacting with wound fluid. They provide a barrier to external bacteria, protect the wound from reinjury, foster autolytic debridement, and may reduce pain. In addition, they are waterproof, absorbent, and nonadherent to healing tissue. This type of dressing should be changed as needed, depending on the amount of exudate absorbed. They should be avoided in wounds with infection.

4. **Hydrogel dressings** maintain a physiologic wound-healing environment. They relieve pain and are nonadherent. They require some type of cover dressing to keep them securely in place. Because the dressing is 90% water, it may macerate surrounding skin. These dressings should be avoided in infected wounds and not allowed to dry out.

5. **Foam dressings, polymeric, and composite polymeric dressings** are used for highly exudative chronic wounds such as tracheostomy and gastrostomy drain sites. They maintain a physiologic environment, may reduce pain, permit some autolytic debridement, provide some padding, and do not adhere to the wound. One layer usually absorbs or wicks exudates away from the wound while another layer maintains a moist wound-heal-

ing environment. They should be changed every 24 hours or when leaking occurs.

6. **Wound exudate absorbers** are hydrophilic compounds that attract bacteria, exudates, and debris through osmotic forces in the wound. They are used for draining chronic wounds. They can cause pain when applied and require a cover dressing. They are difficult to remove from deep tracts and pockets in the wound.

IV. **Infiltration of intravenous solutions** containing vasoconstrictive agents or hyperosmolar or extremely alkaline solutions may cause tissue necrosis and sloughing. When an IV infiltrate occurs, the infusion should be stopped immediately and the site or affected extremity should be elevated. Heat or cold should not be applied, as this may further damage already compromised tissue. When pharmacologic intervention is needed, it should be administered as soon as possible but no later than 12 to 24 hours.

A. **Phentolomine** (Regitine, CIBA-GEIGY, Summit, NJ 07901) is used to treat dermal necrosis caused by extravasation of **vasoconstrictive** agents such as dopamine, dobutamine, or epinephrine. It is administered as a 1 mg/mL solution of phentolamine in normal saline using a 27- to 30-gauge needle, injecting 0.2 mL subcutaneously at five separate sites around the edge of the infiltration. The needle should be changed after each skin entry. This can be repeated as needed.

B. **Hyaluronidase** (Wydase, Wyeth-Ayerst Laboratories, Philadelphia, PA 19101) is used to minimize tissue injury caused by IV extravasation of hyperosmolar or extremely alkaline solutions. It is administered as a 150 U/mL solution in normal saline, injecting 0.2 mL subcutaneously in five separate sites around the leading edge of the infiltrate, using a 25- or 27-gauge needle. The needle should be changed after each injection.

C. **Infiltration** may require the use of bacitracin ointment and xeroform dressing for wound care. For severe lesions, we usually consult a plastic surgeon for both acute wound care and the need for future skin grafting.

V. **Transient cutaneous lesions** are common in the neonatal period.

A. **Milia** are multiple pearly white or pale yellow papules or cysts that are scattered about on the face of many infants, especially those born at term. They are mainly on the nose, chin, and forehead. Milia consist of epidermal cysts (up to 1 mm in diameter) that develop in connection with the pilosebaceous follicle. They will exfoliate and disappear within the first few weeks after birth. No treatment is necessary.

B. **Sebaceous gland hyperplasia** is similar to milia, but the lesions are smaller, more numerous, and usually confined to the nose, upper lip, and chin. They are related to maternal androgen stimulation. They present mainly in full-term babies and disappear within a few weeks after birth.

C. **Erythema toxicum** is a scattering of macules, papules, and even some vesicles, that usually occur on the trunk but frequently also appear on the extremities and face. It affects 50 to 70% of term infants. The cause is not known. The rash usually appears on the first or second day after birth and is self-limited without any treatment. It is not serious, but it may cause alarm when papules and vesicles are numerous, especially when the lesions are thought to be pustular.

1. If the vesicles are opened and the contents smeared and stained with Wright stain and examined microscopically, they are found to contain almost exclusively eosinophils. Cultures are sterile except for an occasional contaminant such as *Staphylococcus epidermidis*.

2. The incidence of erythema toxicum decreases with gestational age. It is rarely seen in infants less than 1500 g or 30 weeks' gestation.

D. **Transient neonatal pustular melanosis** is a benign, self-limited disorder seen at birth in 2 to 5% of term black infants and <1% of term white infants. The lesions consist of small papules, vesicles, pustular lesions, and hyperpigmented spots that occur most commonly on the forehead, neck, lower back, and shins. The lesions rupture easily, revealing white scales surrounding a hyperpigmented macule. Staining the contents of an open lesion with Wright stain will reveal neutrophils, few to no eosinophils, and cellular debris with no organisms. Transient neonatal pustular melanosis should be differentiated from pustules caused by staphylococci, candida, or herpes. The lesions resolve in 1 to 2 days, leaving a hyperpigmented macule that slowly disappears.

VI. **Abnormalities of pigmentation** occur frequently and may be cutaneous clues to underlying disease.

   A. **Flat lesions**
      1. **Mongolian spots** are benign pigmented lesions often found at birth. They are seen in over 90% of blacks and Native Americans, 81% of Asians, 70% of Hispanics, and 10% of white infants. The lumbosacral region is most commonly involved, but the upper part of the back, shoulders, arms, buttocks, legs, and face are occasionally included. The lesions may be small or large, grayish blue or bluish black, and irregularly round; they are never elevated or palpable. Mongolian spots result from an infiltration of melanocytes deep in the dermis. Although they frequently fade as the child gets older, this is probably due to decreasing transparency of the overlying skin rather than a true disappearance of the lesions.
      2. **Café au lait spots** are flat, brown, round or oval lesions with smooth edges. They are found anywhere on the body and occur in 10% of normal individuals. These lesions appear somewhat darker in black than in white infants. Many appear after birth. As the infant grows older, they do not resolve. A few small spots are of little or no significance, but larger ones or increasing numbers may indicate neurofibromatosis.
      3. **Albright syndrome** is characterized in the newborn by the presence of a large, very irregular, ragged pigmented area, as large as 9 to 12 cm. Other features, appearing later, are bony lesions and endocrine disorders.
      4. **Junctional nevi** are brown or black and flat to slightly raised lesions that are present at birth. They are composed of nests of cuboidal cells with melanocytes and occur at the border of the dermis and epidermis. They are benign lesions, needing no treatment unless excision is desired for cosmetic reasons.
      5. **Peutz-Jeghers syndrome** is characterized at birth by multiple scattered hyperpigmented macules, especially around the nose and mouth, but also on the hands and fingers, and frequently on the mucous membranes of the mouth. The more serious part of the syndrome appears later, with the development of polyposis of the small bowel and episodes of intussusception.

   B. **Raised lesions**
      1. **Giant hairy nevi** (bathing trunk nevi) are present at birth and may be huge, involving 20 to 30% of the body surface; they are leathery and hard and brown to black, with a large amount of hair. Other pigmentary abnormalities are frequently present on the remaining skin. Occasionally, deeper structures, such as the central nervous system, may be involved. Although it is sometimes difficult, surgical removal is indicated for cosmetic reasons and because at least 10% of these progress to malignant melanoma.
      2. **Compound nevi** are similar to junctional nevi in that they are composed of melanocytes. However, compound nevi tend to be larger, and are often hairy; they involve the dermis as well as the epidermis. Treatment involves surgical removal, if technically feasible, at age 5 or 6 years because of the possibility of later malignant change.
      3. **Other raised lesions.** Epidermal nevi, blue nevi, and juvenile melanoma are other forms of raised lesions rarely seen in the newborn; they require no treatment except occasional diagnostic excision.

   C. **Diffuse hyperpigmentation** occurs in a variety of conditions, such as:
      1. Melanism.
      2. Progressive familial hyperpigmentation.
      3. Congenital Addison's disease.
      4. Fanconi's syndrome.

     5. Generalized hereditary lentiginosis.

     6. Androgen excess.

D. Hypopigmentation

  1. Albinism is an autosomal recessive condition that leads to a deficiency in pigment production. The defect is most noticeable in the skin, hair, and eyes (iris). No treatment is effective; the infant must be protected from light.

  2. Piebaldism, also known as partial albinism, is inherited as an autosomal dominant disorder with decreased penetrance. The skin and hair are involved in a patchy way, with both hypomelanotic and normal areas. A white "forelock" of hair, as in Waardenburg's syndrome, is a feature of this disorder.

  3. Vitiligo is characterized by patchy areas of decreased or absent pigmentation. The lesions are occasionally present at birth, but may develop in later infancy or childhood. The characteristic microscopic appearance is few or no melanocytes in the junctional layer.

  4. Hypopigmented macules (white spots) may occur in tuberous sclerosis. The typical white spot seen in tuberous sclerosis is small (2 to 3 cm) with an irregular border and usually occurs on the trunk and buttocks. The number of spots is variable. The lesion differs from vitiligo in that many melanocytes are present, but the melanosomes are poorly pigmented. In fair-skinned infants, it may be difficult to demonstrate the white macule without the use of a Wood's lamp. Many infants with tuberous sclerosis also have at least one café au lait spot.

  5. Waardenburg syndrome and Chediak-Higashi syndrome are examples of other inherited conditions that include pigmentary deficits.

VII. Vascular abnormalities occur in up to 40% of newborns.

  A. A salmon patch, nevus simplex, or macular hemangioma is a flat, pink macular lesion found on the forehead, upper eyelid, nasolabial area, glabella, or nape of the neck (stork bite). It is the most common vascular lesion of the newborn, occurring in 30 to 40% of infants. The nevus consists of distended dermal capillaries representing persistence of the fetal pattern. Except for those on the neck, most resolve by 1 year of age.

  B. A port-wine stain, or **nevus flammeus,** is a flat or mildly elevated reddish purple lesion most commonly found on the face. It is often unilateral. The lesion is a vascular malformation of dilated capillarylike vessels. Port-wine stains do not involute. They are often associated with hemangiomas of the underlying structures. The association of nevus flammeus (port-wine stain) in the region of the first branch of the trigeminal nerve with cortical lesions in the brain is known as the Sturge-Weber syndrome. Ocular involvement may result in glaucoma. The skin lesions can be treated with pulsed dye laser.

  C. Strawberry hemangiomas may not be present at birth or may present as a pale macule with irregular margins. There are often a few blood vessels in the center of the macule. They are more common in the head, neck, and trunk but can occur anywhere. They are more common in premature infants and are not usually noticed until the infant is 1 to 2 weeks old. Strawberry hemangiomas grow rapidly during the first 6 months and continue to grow until 1 year. The majority involute completely with no scar by age 4 to 5 years. A strawberry hemangioma involving the eyelid may need treatment to prevent amblyopia.

  D. A cavernous hemangioma is a deep strawberry hemangioma composed of large, mature vascular elements. It is often present at birth. The lesion grows during the first year after birth, but regression is often less complete. Most regress but some do not. Cavernous hemangiomas may be associated with significant complications such as hemorrhage due to platelet trapping (Kasabach-Merritt syndrome), hypertrophy of involved structures (Klippel-Trénaunay syndrome), heart failure due to arteriovenous anastomoses, and infection in infants with large venous lakes. Treatment may involve surgery, occlusion, laser therapy, steroids, and alpha interferon.

E. Disorders of lymphatic vessels include
1. Lymphangiomas (simple, lymphangioma circumscriptum, and cavernous lymphangioma).
2. Cystic hygroma.
3. Lymphedema.
4. Milroy's disease (congenital hereditary lymphedema).

F. Purpura can result from one of the following conditions:
1. Infectious disorders such as TORCH or bacterial infections (see Chap. 23).
2. Giant hemangioma with thrombocytopenia.
3. Congenital leukemia.
4. Langerhans cell histiocytosis.
5. Immune thrombocytopenia (see Chap. 26).
6. Maternal drug ingestion.
7. Congenital megakaryocytic hypoplasia (see Chap. 26).
8. Inherited thrombocytopenias (see Chap. 26).
9. Coagulation defects (see Chap. 26).

VIII. Trauma. Various forms of contusions, abrasions, and ecchymoses occur as the result of forces associated with delivery. (see Chap. 20).

IX. Developmental abnormalities of skin
A. Skin dimples and sinuses can occur on any part of the body, but they are most common over bony prominences such as the scapula, knee joint, and hip. They may be simple depressions in the skin of no pathologic significance or actual sinus tracts connecting to deeper structures.
1. A pilonidal dimple or sinus may occur in the sacral area. A sinus that is deep but does not communicate to underlying structures usually does not cause problems. If the bottom of the dimple can be seen, it is usually of no significance. At puberty, if hair grows in the depths of the sinus, a cyst may form. The cyst occasionally gets infected and needs excision.
2. If the sinus connects to the central nervous system (CNS), serious infection can occur, but this is rare. Occasionally, a dimple, sometimes accompanied by a nevus or hemangioma, may signify an underlying spinal disorder such as diastematomyelia. Diagnosis of these connections usually requires ultrasound, computed tomography (CT), or magnetic resonance imaging (MRI).
3. Dermal sinuses or cysts along the cheek or jawline, or extending into the neck, may represent remnants of the branchial cleft structures of the early embryo. Sinuses or cysts in the sides of the neck usually arise from the second branchial cleft. They may or may not open into the mouth or pharynx.
4. The most common dermal sinus is the **preauricular sinus,** which is a leftover from the first branchial cleft. It appears in the most anterior upper portion of the tragus of the external ear. Preauricular sinuses may be unilateral or bilateral; they usually require no treatment unless secondary infection develops, in which case surgical excision is recommended. They rarely cause problems in the newborn period.

B. Small skin tags can occur on the chest wall near the breast. They usually have a narrow base and are of no significance.

C. Redundant skin usually occurs as loose folds of excess skin in the posterior part of the neck. It is common in some chromosomal disorders, such as trisomy 18, Down syndrome, trisomy 13, and especially Turner syndrome.

D. Hemihypertrophy is a condition in which one side of the body is larger than the other. The asymmetry is often apparent at birth, but it becomes more obvious with growth. The skin, which is thicker on the hypertrophied side, is one of many systems involved. Some affected patients have mental retardation and seizures. They are at increased risk for the development of embryonal tumors of the kidney, adrenal glands, and liver.

E. Aplasia cutis (congenital absence of skin) occurs most frequently in the midline of the posterior part of the scalp. It is usually a round, punched-out lesion 1 or 2 cm in diameter that is present at birth. The area is devoid of hair; it is sometimes covered with a thin membrane and is sometimes crusted and weeping. Rarely, other parts of the body may be involved. Treatment involves protection from trauma and infection; healing is usually slow. Plastic surgical repair may be considered for rare cases when the scar cannot be adequately covered by growing hair. Cutis aplasia of the scalp can occur in trisomy 13 and trisomy 18.

X. Scaling disorders include a variety of conditions, some of which are listed.
  A. **Harlequin fetus (ichthyosis).**
  B. **Ichthyosis vulgaris.**
  C. **Sex-linked ichthyosis.**
  D. **Nonbullous congenital ichthyosiform erythroderma.**
  E. **Bullous congenital ichthyosiform erythroderma.**
  F. **Ichthyosis linearis circumflexa.**
  G. **Erythrokeratodermia variabilis.**
  H. **Acrodermatitis enteropathica** is caused by zinc deficiency. The skin lesions may be dry or moist; they are scaling and impetiginous and appear primarily around the nose, mouth, and perineum, as well as around ostomy wounds. They frequently spread to adjacent areas and especially to the fingers and toes. The condition is often accompanied by severe diarrhea, irritability, and failure to thrive. Response to zinc therapy is prompt and dramatic.
  I. **Neonatal lupus erythematosus** can occur in infants born to mothers with systemic lupus erythematosus. Skin lesions are typically dry, scaly, and reddened areas that may appear on the face, trunk, or extremities or may be present at birth. Congenital heart block occurs in about half the affected infants.

XI. Vesicobullous eruptions
  A. **Hereditary causes (nonscarring)**
    1. Epidermolysis bullosa simplex.
    2. Epidermolysis bullosa lethalis.
    3. Bullous eruption of hands and feet (Cockayne-Weber syndrome).
  B. **Hereditary causes (scarring)**
    1. Epidermolysis bullosa dystrophica (dominant).
    2. Epidermolysis bullosa dystrophica (recessive).
  C. **Congenital porphyria.**
  D. **Incontinentia pigmenti.**
  E. **Juvenile dermatitis herpetiformis.**
  F. **Infiltrative diseases**
    1. Mast cell diseases
      a. Mastocytosis.
      b. Urticaria pigmentosa.
    2. Langerhans cell histiocytosis.
  G. **Infections caused by bacterial** (especially staphylococcal, **pseudomonas,** or listeria), **viral, fungal** (e.g., candida), or other **organisms.**

Suggested Reading
Curley M.A.Q., Maloney-Harmon P.A. Critical care of nursing infants and children (2nd Ed.). Philadelphia: Saunders, 2001: Chapter 16.

Lund C. et al. Neonatal skin care: The scientific basis for practice. *Neonatal Netw* 1999; 18:15.

35. AUDITORY AND OPHTHALMOLOGIC PROBLEMS

Retinopathy of Prematurity

John A.F. Zupancic and Jane E. Stewart

I. **Background.** **Retinopathy of prematurity (ROP)** is a multifactorial vasoproliferative retinal disorder that increases in incidence with decreasing gestational age. Approximately 65% of infants with a birth weight less than 1250 g and 80% of those with a birth weight less than 1000 g will develop some degree of ROP. In Massachusetts, ROP is the second most common cause of blindness for children under 6 years old.

II. **Pathogenesis**

A. **Normal development.** After the sclera and choroid have developed, retinal elements, including nerve fibers, ganglion cells, and photoreceptors, migrate from the optic disk at the posterior pole of the eye and move toward the periphery. The photoreceptors have progressed 80% of the distance to their resting place at the ora serrata by 28 weeks' gestation. Before the retinal vessels develop, the avascular retina receives its oxygen supply by diffusion across the retina from the choroid vessels. The retinal vessels, which arise from the spindle cells of the adventitia of the hyaloid vessels at the optic disk, begin to migrate outward at 16 weeks' gestation. Migration is complete by 36 weeks on the nasal side and by 40 weeks on the temporal side.

B. **Possible mechanisms of injury.** Clinical observations suggest that the onset of ROP consists of two stages.

1. The **primary stage** involves an initial insult or insults, such as hyperoxia, hypoxia, or hypotension, at a critical point in retinal vascularization that results in vasoconstriction and decreased blood flow to the developing retina with a subsequent arrest in vascular development. The relative hyperoxia after birth is hypothesized to down-regulate the production of growth factors such as vascular endothelial growth factor that are essential for the normal development of the retinal vessels.

2. During the **second stage,** neovascularization occurs. This aberrant retinal vessel growth is thought to be driven by excess angiogenic factors (such as vascular endothelial growth factor) released by the ischemic relatively hypoxic avascular retina. New vessels grow through the retina into the vitreous. These vessels are permeable and hemorrhage and edema can occur. Extensive and severe extraretinal fibrovascular proliferation can lead to retinal detachment and abnormal retinal function. In the majority of affected infants, however, the disease process regresses and the retinopathy gradually resolves.

C. **Risk factors.** Many factors have been associated with ROP. The most consistent association has been with low gestational age, low birth weight, and duration of mechanical ventilation. Other factors implicated in the pathogenesis include vitamin E deficiency, multiple red blood cell transfusions, intraventricular hemorrhage, bronchopulmonary dysplasia, oxygen exposure, fluctuation in blood gas tensions, and sepsis.

III. **Screening and diagnosis.** Because no early clinical signs or symptoms indicate developing ROP, early and regular retinal examination is necessary. The timing of the occurrence of ROP is related to the maturity of retinal vessels and thus postnatal age. The median postnatal ages at the onset of stage 1 ROP, prethreshold disease, and threshold disease (see IV.B) are 34, 36, and 37 weeks, respectively. Preterm infants who are discharged from level III facilities before they reach the postnatal age of highest incidence for severe ROP must continue to have ophthalmologic examinations until their retinal vessels have reached maturity.

ROP is diagnosed by retinal examination with indirect ophthalmoscopy; this should be performed by an ophthalmologist with expertise in neonatal disorders when the infant is 4 to 6 weeks old. We screen all infants with a birth weight less than 1500 g or gestational age less than 32 weeks. Infants who are born between 32 and 34 weeks' gestational age are examined if they have been ill (e.g., those who have had severe respiratory distress syndrome, hypotension requiring pressor support, or surgery in the first several weeks of life). Because the timing of ROP is related to postnatal age, infants who are born at 24 to 26 weeks' gestation are examined at the postnatal age of 6 weeks and those of more advanced gestational age are examined at the postnatal age of 4 weeks. Patients are examined every 2 weeks until their vessels have grown out to the ora serrata and the retina is considered mature. If ROP is diagnosed, the frequency of examination depends on the severity and rapidity of progression of the disease (see Table 35.1). Infants are examined more frequently until their retinopathy regresses and full maturity of vessels is noted or until they reach a threshold for treatment. (see IV.B).

IV. **Classification and definitions**

A. **Classification.** The International Classification of Retinopathy of Prematurity (ICROP) is used to classify ROP. This classification system consists of four components (Fig. 35.1).

1. **Location** refers to how far the developing retinal blood vessels have progressed. The retina is divided into three concentric circles or zones:

   a. **Zone 1** consists of an imaginary circle with the optic nerve at the center and a radius of twice the distance from the optic nerve to the macula.

   b. **Zone 2** extends from the edge of zone 1 to the equator on the nasal side of the eye and about half the distance to the ora serrata on the temporal side.

   c. **Zone 3** consists of the outer crescent-shaped area extending from zone 2 out to the ora serrata temporally.

2. Severity refers to the **stage** of disease.

TABLE 35.1. FREQUENCY OF SCREENING EXAMINATION FOR RETINOPATHY OF PREMATURITY

Findings on Most Recent Examination*

Zone	Stage	Next Examination
I	0	1–2 wk
I	1–2–3	1–7 days[†]
II	0	2–3 wks
II	1–2	2 wks
II	2 (with plus disease)	1 wk
II	3 (no plus disease)	1 wk
II	3 (with plus disease)	1 wk
III	0 (immature)	2–3 wks
III	0 (mature)	8 months

*These recommendations apply only if threshold criteria have not been met.
†Depending on severity and ophthalmologists discretion.
Source: Section on Ophthalmology, American Academy of Pediatrics. Screening examination of premature infants for retinopathy of prematurity. *Pediatrics* 2001;108:809–811.

Children's Hospital
300 Longwood Ave., Boston, Massachusetts

**OPHTHALMOLOGIC CONSULTATION FOR
RETINOPATHY OF PREMATURITY (ROP)**

Gestational Age (wks) _____ Birth Weight _____ g

Date of Exam _____ Age (wks) _____

Ophthalmologist _____ MD

USE PLATE OR PRINT

M.R. NO. _____ DATE _____

PT. NAME _____

DATE OF BIRTH _____

EXAMINATION:

Right Eye   Left Eye
(O.D.)   (O.S.)

ORA SERRATA

COMMENTS

_____
_____
_____
_____
_____
_____
_____

O.D.	**Other Findings** *(mark with an "X")*	O.S.
_____	Dilatation/Tortuosity	_____
_____	Iris Vessel Dilatation	_____
_____	Pupil Rigidity	_____
_____	Vitreous Haze	_____
_____	Hemorrhages	_____

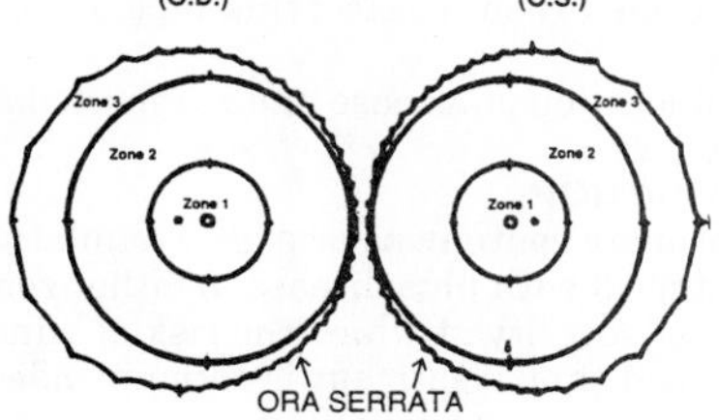

KEY

Stage 1 - line of demarcation

Stage 2 - ridge, elevated

Stage 3- ridge with ERVP

Stage 4 - partial detachment

Stage 5 - total detachment

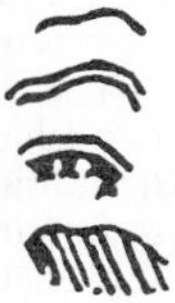

SUMMARY DIAGNOSIS

O.D.   O.S.

_____ Mature Retina _____

_____ Immature, No ROP _____
   Zone   Zone

ROP

Stage _____   Stage _____

Zone _____   Zone _____

clock hrs _____   # clock hrs _____

Other: _____
_____
_____
_____

Plan: Repeat Exam in : _____

Discussed with: _____ MD/NNP

Examined by: _____ MD

03241 10/96 25/PKG

FIG. 35.1. Sample of form for ophthalmologic consultation.

a. **Stage 1.** A demarcation line appears as a thin white line that separates the normal retina from the undeveloped avascular retina.
b. **Stage 2.** A ridge of scar tissue with height and width replaces the line of stage 1. It extends inward from the plane of the retina.
c. **Stage 3.** The ridge has extraretinal fibrovascular proliferation. Abnormal blood vessels and fibrous tissue develop on the edge of the ridge and extend into the vitreous.

    d. Stage 4. Partial retinal detachment may result when scar tissue pulls on the retina. Stage 4A is partial detachment outside the macula, so that the chance for vision is good if the retina reattaches. Stage 4B is partial detachment that involves the macula, thus limiting the likelihood of usable vision in that eye.

    e. Stage 5. Complete retinal detachment occurs. The retina assumes a funnel-shaped appearance and is described as open or narrow in the anterior and posterior regions.

  3. Plus disease is an additional designation that refers to the presence of vascular dilatation and tortuosity of the posterior retinal vessels. This indicates a more severe degree of ROP and may be associated with iris vascular engorgement, pupillary rigidity, and vitreous haze. Plus disease that is associated with zone 1 ROP is termed rush disease; this type of ROP tends to progress extremely rapidly.

  4. Extent refers to the circumferential location of disease and is reported as clock hours in the appropriate zone.

B. Definition of threshold and prethreshold ROP

  1. Threshold ROP is present if five or more contiguous or eight cumulative clock hours (30-degree sectors) of stage 3 with plus disease in either zone 1 or 2 are present. This is the level of severity at which the risk of blindness is predicted to approach 50% and thus treatment is recommended.

  2. Prethreshold ROP is any of the following: zone 1 ROP of any stage less than threshold; zone 2 ROP with stage 2 and plus disease; zone 2 ROP with stage 3 without plus disease; or zone 2 ROP at stage 3 with plus disease with fewer than the threshold number of sectors of stage 3. Infants with prethreshold ROP have a 1 in 3 chance of needing surgical treatment and a 1 in 6 chance of extreme loss of vision if treatment is not done promptly when threshold is reached. With therapy, they have a 1 in 12 chance of extreme visual loss.

V. Prognosis

A. Short-term prognosis. Factors that increase the risk of reaching threshold ROP include posterior location of the ROP in zone 1 or posterior zone 2, increased severity of stage, circumferential involvement, the presence of plus disease, and rapid progression of disease. Most infants with stage 1 or 2 ROP will have regression. In a large study of infants weighing less than 1250 g at birth, the overall incidence of ROP was 66%; stage 1 was the highest stage reached in 25% and stage 2 was the highest stage in 22%. Prethreshold ROP was reached in 18% and threshold in 6.0%. Zone 3 disease has a good prognosis for complete recovery. Tables 35.2 and 35.3 show the risk of progression and poor visual outcome according to severity of ROP and postnatal age.

B. Long-term prognosis. Infants with ROP have an increased risk of myopia, high myopia, anisometropia and other refractive errors, strabismus, amblyopia, astigmatism, late retinal detachment, glaucoma, and vitreal hemorrhage. **Cicatricial disease** refers to residual scarring in the retina and may be associated with much later retinal detachment. The prognosis for stage 4 ROP depends on the involvement of the macula; the chance for functional vision is greater when the macula is not involved. Once the retina has detached, the prognosis is poor even with surgical reattachment attempts. All premature infants who meet screening criteria regardless of the diagnosis of ROP are at risk for long-term ophthalmologic problems. We therefore recommend a follow-up evaluation by an ophthalmologist with neonatal expertise at approximately 8 months of age.

VI. Management

A. Prevention. Currently no proven methods are available to prevent ROP. Multiple large clinical trials to prevent retinopathy of prematurity have been performed evaluating the use of prophylactic vitamin E therapy, reducing the exposure to bright light, and administration of penicillamine. A meta-analysis of the vitamin E trials revealed some reduction in the num-

TABLE 35.2. PROBABILITY OF REACHING CRYOTHERAPY CRITERIA

	Postnatal Age (wks)					
	≤32	33–34	35–36	37–38	39–40	41–42
Zone 1a						
Incomplete	33%	37%	7%	36%	—†	—†
Stage 1 −	18%	33%	—†	—†	—†	—†
All others	—†	—†	—†	—†	—†	—†
Zone 2*						
Incomplete	9%	6%	3%	1%	2%	0%
Stage 1 −	8%	6%	4%	2%	1%	1%
Stage 2 −	4%	6%	4%	2%	1%	1%
Stage 3 −	—†	16%	13%	8%	2%	0%
Stage 1 +	—†	83%	42%	—†	—†	—†
Stage 2 +	—†	44%	34%	25%	17%	0%
Stage 3 +	—†	77%	61%	34%	31%	14%

*"+" means with plus disease; "2" means without plus disease.
†Too few to calculate risk.
Source: Modified from Schaffer D. B., et al. Prognostic factors in the natural course of retinopathy of prematurity. The Cryotherapy for Retinopathy of Prematurity Group. *Ophthalmology* 1993;100:230.

ber of infants developing more severe ROP. However, one trial revealed an increased incidence of adverse events including necrotizing enterocolitis and late onset sepsis, making the risks of treatment questionable. The trials that evaluated the reduction of retinal exposure to light showed no benefit. Some preliminary trials have demonstrated a potential benefit from the use of the anti-oxidant pennicillamine. However, long-term outcomes on these patients are still pending.

TABLE 35.3. PROBABILITY OF POOR VISUAL OUTCOME (WITHOUT CRYOTHERAPY)

	Postnatal Age (wks)					
Zone 2a	≤32	33–34	35–36	37–38	39–40	41–42
Incomplete	7%	4%	1%	2%	2%	3%
Stage 1 −	6%	3%	2%	<1%	1%	0%
Stage 2 −	0%	3%	2%	1%	0%	2%
Stage 3 −	—†	3%	2%	5%	4%	1%
Stage 1 +	—†	—†	—†	—†	—†	—†
Stage 2 +	—†	27%	29%	20%	12%	33%
Stage 3 +	—†	62%	48%	35%	30%	32%

*"+" means with plus disease; "2" means without plus disease.
†Not calculated due to small number.
Source: Modified from Schaffer D. B., et al. Prognostic factors in the natural course of retinopathy of prematurity. The Cryotherapy for Retinopathy of Prematurity Group. *Ophthalmology* 1993;100:230.

B. Treatment

1. **Cryotherapy.** A multicenter trial designed to evaluate the benefit of cryotherapy for threshold ROP demonstrated a reduction in unfavorable outcome from 51.4% in control eyes to 31.1% in treated eyes. That is, cryotherapy reduces the risk of extreme loss of vision by half, although these infants may not have normal vision. The cryoprobe is applied to the external surface of the sclera and areas beyond the region of the ridge of the ROP are frozen until the entire anterior avascular retina has been treated. Approximately 20 to 70 applications are made in each eye. The procedure is usually done under general anesthesia. In infants with bronchopulmonary dysplasia, this may result in a temporary pulmonary exacerbation.

   Close follow-up is required to detect continued progression and requirement of further cryotherapy.

2. **Laser therapy.** Laser photocoagulation therapy for ROP is the preferred initial treatment in many centers. Laser therapy is technically difficult if there is vitreal hemorrhage obscuring the view of the retinal vessels or if there is a significant remnant of the tunica vasculosa lentis (the vascular layer enveloping the lens of the fetal eye) with remnants of hyaloid vessels obscuring the view through the lens. When these situations occur, cryotherapy is preferred. Laser treatment is delivered through an indirect ophthalmoscope and is applied to the avascular retina anterior to the ridge of extraretinal fibrovascular proliferation for 360 degrees. Approximately 400 to 2000 spots are placed in each eye. Both argon and diode laser photocoagulation have been successfully used in infants with severe ROP. The advantage of this technique is that the equipment is portable and therefore the procedure can be performed in the newborn intensive care unit. In addition, the procedure can be performed with local anesthesia and sedation, avoiding some of the adverse effects of general anesthesia. Clinical observations suggest that it is as at least as effective as cryotherapy in achieving favorable visual outcomes. The development of cataracts following laser surgery has been reported. Further long-term follow-up studies are still needed for both modalities.

3. **Retinal reattachment.** Buckling procedures have proved to be of limited value. The anatomic success rate is 53.3% in the early postoperative phase, but later decreases to 33.3%, with a functional success rate of 20% at follow-up (with perception of large forms). Lensectomy–vitrectomy has an anatomic success rate of 29.8% at 5.5 years of age. Only 15% of patients had any functional vision at that time (light perception or low vision) and the rest were blind. Although these techniques are limited, the achievement of even minimal vision can result in a large difference in a child's overall quality of life.

4. **Supplemental oxygen.** A large clinical trial was performed to determine whether supplemental oxygen given to infants with prethreshold ROP would limit the progression from prethreshold to threshold ROP. This showed no significant reduction in the number of infants that progressed to threshold ROP. In a subgroup analysis, however, it appeared that supplemental oxygen therapy may be beneficial for infants with prethreshold ROP without plus disease.

Suggested Readings

Cryotherapy for Retinopathy of Prematurity Cooperative Group. Multicenter trial of cryotherapy for retinopathy at prematurity. *Arch Ophthalmol* 1990;108:195–209.

Page J. M., et al. Ocular sequelae in premature infants. *Pediatrics* 1993;92:787–790.

Palmer E., et al. Incidence and early course of retinopathy of prematurity. *Ophthalmology* 1991;98:1628–1640.

Phelps D. L. Retinopathy of prematurity. *Pediatr Clin North Am* 1993;40:705–714.

Pierce E.A., Foley E.D., Smith LE. Regulation of vascular endothelial growth factor by oxygen in a model of retinopathy of prematurity. *Arch Ophthalmol* 1996;114: 1219–1228.

Quinn G. E., et al. Visual acuity of eyes after vitrectomy for retinopathy of prematurity. *Ophthalmology* 1996;103:595–600.

Screening Examination of Premature Infants for Retinopathy of Prematurity. Policy Statement American Academy of Pediatrics. *Pediatrics* 2001;108:809–811.

Supplemental Therapeutic Oxygen for Prethreshold Retinopathy of Prematurity (STOP-ROP), a randomized, controlled trial. I: Primary outcomes. *Pediatrics* 2000;105: 295–310.

Tonse N.K., et al. Viatmin E prophylaxis to reduce retinopathy of prematurity: A reappraisal of published trials. *J Pediatr* 1997;131:844–850.

HEARING LOSS IN NEONATAL INTENSIVE CARE UNIT GRADUATES

Jane E. Stewart and Jeffrey W. Stolz

I. **Definition.** Neonatal intensive care unit (NICU) graduates are at high risk of developing hearing loss. When undetected, hearing loss can result in delays in language, communication, and cognitive development. Hearing loss falls into two major categories:
   A. **Sensorineural loss** is the result of abnormal development or damage to the cochlear hair cells (sensory end organ) or auditory nerve.
   B. **Conductive loss** is the result of interference in the transmission of sound from the external auditory canal to the inner ear. The most common cause for conductive hearing loss is fluid in the middle ear or middle ear effusion. Less common are anatomic causes such as microtia, canal stenosis, or stapes fixation that often occur in infants with craniofacial malformations.
II. **Incidence.** The overall incidence of severe congenital hearing loss is 1–3 in 1000 live births. However, 2 to 4 per 100 infants surviving neonatal intensive care have some degree of sensorineural hearing loss.
III. **Etiology**
   A. **Genetic.** Approximately 50% of congenital hearing loss is thought to be of genetic origin. The most common genetic cause of hearing loss is a mutation in the connexin 26(Cx26) gene, located on chromosome 13q11–12. The carrier rate for this mutation is 3% and it causes approximately 20 to 30% of congenital hearing loss. Approximately 30% of infants with hearing loss have other associated medical problems that are part of a syndrome. More than 200 syndromes are known to include hearing loss (e.g., Alport, Pierre Robin, Usher, Waardenburg Syndrome, Trisomy 21).
   B. **Nongenetic.** The remaining 50% of congenital hearing loss is secondary to injury to the developing auditory system in the intrapartum or perinatal period. This injury may be due to infection, hypoxia, ischemia, metabolic disease, ototoxic medication, or hyperbilirubinemia. Preterm infants and term infants who require newborn intensive care are often exposed to these factors.
   C. **Risk factors.** The Joint Committee on Infant Hearing listed the following risk indicators for progressive or delayed-onset sensorineural and/or conductive hearing loss.

1. Parental or caregiver concern regarding hearing, speech, language, or developmental delay.
2. Family history of permanent childhood hearing loss.
3. Stigmata or other findings associated with a syndrome known to include a sensorineural or conductive hearing loss or eustacian tube dysfunction.
4. Postnatal infections associated with sensorineural hearing loss, including bacterial meningitis.
5. In utero infections such as cytomegalovirus, herpes, rubella, syphilis, human immunodeficiency virus (HIV), and toxoplasmosis.
6. Neonatal indicators: specifically, hyperbilirubinemia at a serum level requiring exchange transfusion (some centers use a level of ≥20 mg/dL as a general guideline), persistent pulmonary hypertension of the newborn associated with mechanical ventilation, and conditions requiring the use of extracorporeal membrane oxygenation (ECMO).
7. Syndromes associated with progressive hearing loss such as neurofibromatosis, osteopetrosis, and Usher syndrome.
8. Neurodegenerative disorders, such as Hunter syndrome, or sensory motor neuropathies, such as Friedreich's ataxia and Charcot-Marie-Tooth syndrome.
9. Head trauma.
10. Recurrent or persistent otitis media with effusion for at least 3 months. However, a substantial proportion of infants with congenital hearing loss have no identified risk factors.

D. Detection. Universal newborn hearing screening is recommended to detect hearing loss as early as possible. The Joint Committee on Infant Hearing and the American Academy of Pediatrics endorse a goal that 100% of infants be tested during their hospital birth admission. The implementation of this recommendation is underway; many states have passed legislation to ensure this goal is achieved promptly.

IV. Screening tests. The currently acceptable methods for physiologic hearing screening in newborns are auditory brain-stem response and evoked otoacoustic emissions. A threshold of ≥35 dB has been established as a cutoff for an abnormal screen, which prompts further testing.

A. Auditory brain-stem responses (ABR). ABR measures the electroencephalographic waves generated by the auditory system in response to clicks via three electrodes placed on the infant's scalp. The characteristic waveform recorded from the electrodes becomes more well defined with increasing postnatal age. ABR is reliable after 34 weeks postnatal age. The automated version of ABR allows this test to be performed quickly and easily by trained hospital staff. Because it can detect injury to the auditory pathway beyond the cochlea (auditory nerve) and can be performed with moderate conductive hearing loss (e.g., due to vernix in the external ear canal), ABR is the preferred screening method to evaluate hearing loss in the NICU graduate.

B. Evoked otoacoustic emissions (EOAEs). EOAE records acoustic "feedback" from the cochlea through the ossicles to the tympanic membrane and ear canal following a click stimulus. EOAE is even quicker to perform than ABR. However, EOAE is more likely to be affected by debris or fluid in the external and middle ear, resulting in higher referral rates. Furthermore, EOAE is unable to detect some forms of sensorineural hearing loss. EOAE is often combined with automated ABR in a two-step screening system.

V. Follow-up testing. Infants with abnormal screening ABRs should have follow-up testing. Infants who are abnormal in both ears should have a diagnostic auditory brain-stem response performed within two weeks after their initial test. Infants with unilateral abnormal results should have follow-up testing within 3 months.

Testing should include a full diagnostic frequency-specific ABR to measure hearing threshold. Evaluation of middle ear function, observation of the infant's behavioral response to sound, and parental report of emerging communication and auditory behaviors should also be included.

A. Definitions of the degree and severity of hearing loss are:

Mild	15–30 dB HL
Moderate	30–50 dB HL
Severe	50–70 dB HL
Profound	70+ dB HL

B. Infants who have risk factors for progressive or delayed-onset sensorineural and/or conductive hearing loss require continued surveillance, even if the initial newborn screening results are normal. They should have audiologic testing performed at least every 6 months for the first 3 years of age.

VI. Medical evaluation. An infant diagnosed with true hearing loss should have the following additional evaluations:

   A. Complete evaluation should be performed by an otolaryngologist or otologist who has experience with infants.

   B. Genetic evaluation and counseling should be provided for infants without a definite etiology for their hearing loss.

   C. Examination should be performed by a pediatric ophthalmologist to detect eye abnormalities that may be associated with hearing loss.

VII. Habilitation/treatment: Infants with true hearing loss should be referred for early intervention services to enhance the child's acquisition of developmentally appropriate language skills. Infants who are appropriate candidates and whose parents have chosen to utilize personal amplification systems should be fitted with hearing aids as soon as possible. Early intervention resources and information for parents to make decisions regarding communication choices should also be provided as promptly as possible.

VIII. Prognosis. The prognosis depends largely on the extent of hearing loss, as well as on the time of diagnosis and treatment. The earlier habilitation starts, the better the child's chance of achieving age-appropriate language and communication skills. Fitting of hearing aids by the age of 6 months has been associated with improved speech outcome. Initiation of early intervention services before 3 months of age has been associated with improved cognitive developmental outcome at 3 years.

Suggested Readings

AAP Task Force on Newborn Hearing and Infant Screening. Newborn and Infant Hearing Loss: Detection and Intervention. *Pediatrics* 1999;103:527–530. www.aap.org/policy/re9846.html

Hereditary Hearing Loss homepage. http://www.uia.ac.be/dnalab/hhh.

Hone S.W., Smith R.J. Genetics of hearing impairment. *Semin Neonatol* 2001;6:531–41.

National Institute on Deafness and Other Communicative disorders. http://www.babyhearing.org.

NIH Joint Committee on Infant Hearing. Year 2000 Position Statement: Principles and Guidelines for Early Hearing Detection and Intervention Programs. *Pediatrics* 2000;106:798–817.

Utah State University National Center for Hearing Assessment and Management. http://www.infanthearing.org.

36. COMMON NEONATAL PROCEDURES

James E. Gray and Steven A. Ringer

Invasive procedures are a necessary but potentially risk-laden part of newborn intensive care. To provide maximum benefit, these techniques must be performed in a manner that both accomplishes the task at hand and maintains the patient's general well-being.

I. **General principles**
   A. **Consideration of alternatives.** For each procedure, all alternatives should be considered and risk-benefit ratios evaluated. Many procedures involve the placement of indwelling devices made of plastic. Polyvinylchloride-based devices leach a plasticizer, Di (2-ethylhexyl)-phthalate (DEHP) which may be toxic over long-term exposure. Whenever possible, devices that are DEHP-free should be used for procedures on neonates.
   B. **Monitoring and homeostasis.** Care providers should always maintain their primary focus on the patient, rather than on the procedure being performed. They must assess cardiorespiratory and thermoregulatory stability throughout the procedure, and apply interventions when needed. Continuous monitoring can be accomplished through a combination of invasive (e.g., arterial blood pressure monitoring) or noninvasive (e.g., oximeter) techniques. Whenever possible, the operator should delegate the responsibility for monitoring and managing the patient to another care provider during the procedure.
   C. **Pain control.** Treatment of procedure-associated discomfort can be accomplished with pharmacologic or nonpharmacologic approaches (see Chap. 37). The potential negative impact of any medication on the patient's cardiorespiratory status should be considered. Oral sucrose (0.2 to 0.4 mL/kg) is very effective in reducing pain of minor procedures and blood drawing. It can also be used as adjunctive therapy for more painful procedures when the patient can tolerate oral medication. Morphine or fentanyl are commonly administered prior to beginning potentially painful procedures. The use of pain scales to assess the need for medication is recommended.
   D. **Informing the family.** Other than during true emergencies, we notify parents of the need for invasive procedures in their child's care before we perform them. We discuss the indications for and possible complications of each procedure. In addition, alternative procedures, where available, are also discussed.
   E. **Precautions.** The operator should use universal precautions, including use of gloves, impermeable gowns, barriers, and eye protection to prevent exposure to blood and bodily fluids that may be contaminated with infectious agents.
   F. **Education and supervision.** Individuals should be trained in the conduct of procedures prior to performing the procedure on patients. This training should include a discussion of indications, possible complications and their treatment, alternatives, and the techniques to be used. Experienced operators should be available at all times to provide further guidance and needed assistance.
   G. **Documentation.** Careful documentation of procedures enhances patient care. For example, noting difficulties encountered at intubation or the size and positioning of an endotracheal tube used provides important information if the procedure must be repeated. We routinely write notes after all procedures, including unsuccessful attempts. We document the date and time, indications, techniques used, difficulties encountered, complications (if any), and results of any laboratory tests performed.
II. **Blood drawing.** The preparations for withdrawing blood depend somewhat on the blood studies that are required.

A. **Capillary blood** is drawn when there is no need for many serial studies in close succession.

1. **Applicable blood studies** include hematocrit, blood glucose (using glucometers or other point-of-care testing methods), and electrolyte determinations, and occasionally blood gas studies.

2. **Techniques**

   a. **The extremity to be used should be warmed** to increase peripheral blood flow.

   b. **Spring-loaded lancets minimize pain** while ensuring a puncture adequate for obtaining blood. The blood should flow freely, with minimal or no squeezing. This will ensure the most accurate determination of laboratory values.

   c. **Capillary punctures of the foot should be performed on the lateral side of the sole of the heel,** avoiding previous sites if possible.

   d. **The skin should be cleaned carefully** with povidone-iodine and alcohol before puncture to avoid infection of soft tissue or underlying bone.

B. **Catheter blood samples**

1. **Umbilical artery or radial artery catheters** are often used for repetitive blood samples, especially for blood gas studies.

2. **Techniques**

   a. **A needleless system for blood sampling** from arterial catheters **should be used.** Specific techniques for use vary with the product and the manufacturer's guidelines should be followed.

   b. For **blood gas studies,** a 1-mL preheparinized syringe, or a standard 1-mL syringe rinsed with 0.5 mL of heparin is used to withdraw the sample.

   c. **The catheter must be adequately cleared of infusate** prior to withdrawing samples, **to avoid false readings.** After the sample is drawn, blood should be cleared with a small volume of heparinized saline-flushing solution.

C. **Venous blood** for blood chemistry studies, blood cultures, and other laboratory studies **is usually obtained from either the antecubital vein, the external jugular vein, or the saphenous vein.** For blood cultures, the area should be cleaned with an iodine-containing solution; if the position of the needle is directed by using a sterile gloved finger, the finger should be cleaned in the same way. A new sterile needle should be used to insert the blood into the culture bottles.

III. **Bladder tap**

A. Since bladder taps are most often used to obtain urine for culture, **a sterile technique is crucial.** Careful cleaning with iodine and alcohol solution over the prepubic region is essential.

B. **Technique.** Bladder taps are done with a 5- to 10-mL syringe attached to a 22- or 23-gauge needle or to a 23-gauge butterfly needle. Before the tap, one should try to determine that the baby has not recently urinated. Ultrasound guidance is useful. One technique is as follows:

1. The pubic bone is located by touch.

2. The needle is placed in the midline, just superior to the pubic bone.

3. The needle is slid in, aimed at the infant's coccyx.

4. If the needle goes in more than 3 cm and no urine is obtained, one should assume that the bladder is empty and wait before attempting again.

IV. **Intravenous therapy.** The insertion and management of intravenous catheters require great care. As in older infants, hand veins are used most often, but veins in the scalp, foot, and ankle can be used. Transillumination of an extremity can help identify a vein.

V. **Arterial punctures** are usually carried out by using the radial artery or posterior tibial artery. Rarely, the brachial artery is used. Radial artery punctures are most easily done using 25- to 23-gauge butterfly needle, and transillumination often aids in locating the vessel. The radial artery is visualized and entered with the bevel of the needle facing up and at a 15-degree angle against the direction of flow. The artery is transfixed, and then the needle is slowly withdrawn and the syringe filled.

VI. Lumbar puncture

A. Technique

1. The infant should be placed in the lateral decubitus position or in the sitting position with legs straightened. The assistant should hold the infant firmly at the shoulders and buttocks so that the lower part of the spine is curved. Neck flexion should be avoided so as not to compromise the airway.

2. A sterile field is prepared and draped with towels.

3. A 22- to 24-gauge spinal needle with a stylet should be used. Use of a No. 25 butterfly needle may introduce skin into the subarachnoid space and is to be avoided.

4. The needle is inserted in the midline into the space between the fourth and fifth lumbar spinous processes. The needle is advanced gradually in the direction of the umbilicus, and the stylet is withdrawn frequently to detect the presence of spinal fluid. Usually a slight "pop" is felt as the needle enters the subarachnoid space.

5. The **cerebrospinal fluid (CSF)** is collected into three or four tubes, each with a volume of 0.5 to 1.0 mL.

B. Examination of the spinal fluid. CSF should be inspected immediately for turbidity and color. In many newborns normal CSF may be mildly xanthochromic, but it should always be clear.

1. **Tube 1.** Cell count and differential should be determined from the unspun fluid in a counting chamber. The unspun fluid should be stained with methylene blue; it should be treated with concentrated acetic acid if there are numerous red blood cells (RBCs). The centrifuged sediment should be stained with Gram stain and Wright stain.

2. **Tube 2.** Culture and sensitivity studies should be obtained.

3. **Tube 3.** Glucose and protein determinations should be obtained.

4. **Tube 4.** The cells in this tube also should be counted if the fluid is bloody. The fluid can be sent for latex fixation tests for infectious agents.

C. Information obtainable

1. When the CSF is collected in three or four separate containers, an **RBC count** can be done on the first and last tubes to see if there is a difference in the number of RBCs/mm^3 between these specimens. In fluid obtained from a traumatic tap, the final tube will have fewer RBCs than the first; more equal numbers suggest the possibility of an intracranial hemorrhage. CSF in the newborn may normally contain up to 600 to 800 RBCs/mm^3.

2. **White blood cell (WBC) count.** The normal number of WBCs/mm^3 in newborns is a matter of controversy. We accept up to 5 to 8 lymphocytes or monocytes as normal if there are no polymorphonuclear WBCs. Others accept as normal up to 25 WBCs/mm^3, including several polymorphonuclear cells. Data obtained from high-risk newborns without meningitis (Table 36.1) show 0 to 32 WBCs/mm^3 in term infants and 0 to 29 WBCs/mm^3 in preterm infants with about 60% polymorphonuclear cells to be within the normal range. Higher WBC counts are generally seen with gram-negative meningitis than with group B streptococcal disease; as high as 50% of the latter group will have 100 WBCs/mm^3 or less. Because of the overlap between normal infants and those with meningitis, the presence of polymorphonuclear leukocytes in CSF deserves careful attention. Ultimately, the diagnosis depends on culture results and clinical course.

3. Data on **glucose and protein levels** in CSF from high-risk newborns are shown in Table 36.1. The CSF glucose level is normally about 80% of the blood glucose level for term infants and 75% for preterm infants. If the blood glucose level is high or low, there is a 4- to 6-hour equilibration period with the CSF glucose.

TABLE 36.1.   CEREBROSPINAL FLUID EXAMINATION IN HIGH-RISK NEONATES WITHOUT MENINGITIS

Determination	Term	Preterm
White blood cell count (cells/μL)		
No. of infants	87	30
Mean	8.2	9.0
Median	5	6
Standard deviation	7.1	8.2
Range	0–32	0–29
± 2 Standard deviations	0–22.4	0–25.4
Percentage of polymorphonuclear cells	61.3%	57.2%
Protein (mg/dL)		
No. of infants	35	17
Mean	90	115
Range	20–170	65–150
Glucose (mg/dL)		
No. of infants	51	23
Mean	52	50
Range	34–119	24–63
Glucose in cerebrospinal fluid divided by blood glucose (%)		
No. of infants	51	23
Mean	81	74
Range	44–248	55–105

Source: From Sarff L. D., Platt L. H., McCracken G. H. Cerebrospinal fluid evaluation in neonates: Comparison of high-risk neonates with and without meningitis. *J Pediatrics* 1976;88:473.

The normal level of CSF protein in newborns may vary over a wide range. In full-term infants, levels below 100 mg/dL are acceptable. In premature infants, the acceptable level can be as high as 180 mg/dL. Values for high-risk infants are shown in Table 36.1. The level of CSF protein in the premature infant appears to be related to the degree of prematurity.

VII. Intubation

    A. Endotracheal intubation. In most cases an infant can be adequately ventilated by bag and mask so that endotracheal intubation can be done as a controlled procedure.

        1. Tube size and length. The correct tube size (see Chap. 4) and length (Fig. 36.1) can be estimated from the infant's weight.

        2. Route. Contradictory data exist over the preferred route for endotracheal intubation (i.e., oral versus nasal). In most circumstances local practice should guide this selection with two exceptions. First, oral intubation should be performed in all emergent situations, as it is generally easier and quicker than nasal intubation. Second, a functioning endotracheal tube should never be electively changed simply to provide an alternate route.

        3. Technique

            a. The patient should be preoxygenated with 100% oxygen. When possible, oxygen saturations higher than 98% should be achieved prior to laryngoscopy. Laryngoscopy and intubation of an active, unmedicated patient is more difficult for the operator, more uncomfortable for the patient, and the risk of complications may be increased. Whenever possible, the patient should be premedicated with a narcotic or short-acting benzodiazepine, unless the patient's condition is a contraindication (see Chap. 37).

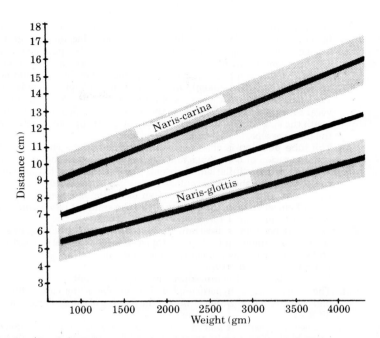

FIG. 36.1. The relationship of naris–carina and naris–glottis distance with body weight. The middle line represents the distance from naris to midtrachea. (Modified from Coldiron J. Estimation of nasotracheal tube length in neonate. *Pediatrics* 1968;41: 823, American Academy of Pediatrics.)

   b. Throughout the intubation procedure, **observation of the patient and monitoring of the heart rate are mandatory.** Pulse oximetry should also be used when available. Electronic monitoring with an audible pulse rate frees personnel to attend to other tasks. If bradycardia is observed, especially if accompanied by hypoxia, the procedure should be stopped and the baby ventilated with bag and mask. An anesthesia bag attached to the tube adapter can deliver oxygen to the pharynx during the procedure or free-flow oxygen at 5 L/min can be given from a tube placed ½ in. from the infant's mouth.
   c. **The baby's head should be slightly lifted anteriorly** (the "sniffing" position) with the baby's body aligned straight. The operator should stand looking down the midline of the body.
   d. The **laryngoscope** is held between the thumb and first finger of the left hand, with the second and third fingers holding the baby's chin and stabilizing the head.
   e. The **laryngoscope blade** is passed into the right side of the mouth and then to the midline, sweeping the tongue up and out of the way. The blade tip should be advanced into the vallecula, and the handle of the laryngoscope raised to an angle of about 60 degrees. The blade should then be lifted parallel to the handle with care being taken not to rock or lever the laryngoscope blade. Visualization of the vocal cords may be improved by pushing down on the larynx with the fourth or fifth finger of the left hand (or having an assistant do it) in order to displace the trachea posteriorly.
   f. The **endotracheal tube** is held with the right hand and inserted between the vocal cords to about 2 cm below the glottis (less in extremely

small infants). During nasotracheal intubation, the tube can be guided by moving the baby's head slightly, or with small Macgill-type forceps. If a finger is pressing on the trachea, the tube can be felt passing through.

g. The anatomic structures of the larynx and pharynx have different appearances. The esophagus is a horizontal muscular slit; it should never be accidentally or mistakenly intubated if this is kept clearly in mind. The glottis, in contrast, consists of a triangular opening formed by the vocal cords meeting anteriorly at the apex. This orifice lies directly beneath the epiglottis, which is lifted away by gentle upward traction with the laryngoscope.

h. The **tube position** is checked by auscultation of the chest to ensure equal aeration of both lungs and observation of chest movement with positive-pressure inflation. If air entry is poor over the left side of the chest, the tube should be pulled back until it becomes equal to the right side. The insertion length of an oral tube is generally between 6 and 7 cm when measured at the lip for the smallest babies, and 8 and 9 cm for term or near-term babies (Fig. 36.1).

4. Once correct position is ascertained, the tube should be held against the palate with one finger, until it can be taped securely in place; the position of the tube is confirmed by radiograph when possible.

5. Commonly observed errors

   a. Focus is placed on the procedure and not the patient.

   b. The baby's neck is hyperextended. This displaces the cords anteriorly and obscures visualization or makes the passing of the endotracheal tube difficult.

   c. Excessive pressure is placed on the infant's upper gum by the laryngoscope blade. This results from the tip of the laryngoscope blade being tilted or rocked upward instead of traction being exerted parallel to the handle.

   d. The tube is inserted too far and the position not assessed, resulting in continued intubation of the right mainstem bronchus.

B. Nasal continuous positive airway pressure (CPAP). Continuous distending pressure can be applied using nasal prongs as part of the ventilator circuit. These are simple to insert and are held on by a Velcro-fastened headset. In unusual circumstances, CPAP can be delivered via an appropriately sized endotracheal tube passed nasally and advanced to a pharangeal position just inferior to the uvula. This tube is then connected to the ventilator circuit as above.

VIII. Thoracentesis and chest tube placement (see Chap. 24, Pulmonary Air Leak)

IX. Vascular catheterization (see Figs. 36.2 and 36.3 for diagrams of the newborn venous and arterial systems).

A. Types of catheters

   1. Umbilical artery catheters (UAL) are used (1) for frequent monitoring of arterial blood gases, (2) as a stable route for infusion of parenteral fluids, and (3) for continuous monitoring of arterial blood pressure.

   2. Peripheral artery catheters are used when frequent blood gas monitoring is still required and an umbilical artery catheter is contraindicated, cannot be placed, or is removed because of complications. Peripheral artery catheters must not be used to infuse alimentation solution or medications. They require that motion of the infant's arm be kept restricted.

   3. Umbilical vein catheters (UVC) are used for exchange transfusions, monitoring of central venous pressure, infusion of fluids (when passed through the ductus venous and near the right atrium), and emergency vascular access for infusion of fluid, blood, or medications.

   4. Central venous catheters, used largely for prolonged parenteral nutrition and occasionally to monitor central venous pressure, also can be placed percutaneously through the external jugular, subclavian, basilic, or saphenous vein.

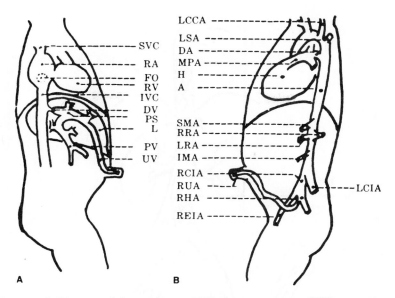

FIG. 36.2. A. Diagram of the newborn umbilical venous system (SVC = superior vena cava; RA = right atrium; FO = foramen ovale; RV = right ventricle; IVC = inferior vena cava; DV = ductus venosus; PS = portal sinus; L = liver; PV = portal vein; UV = umbilical vein). **B.** Diagram of the newborn arterial system, including the umbilical artery (LCCA = left common carotid artery; LSA = left subclavian artery; DA = ductus arteriosus; MPA = main pulmonary artery; H = heart; A = aorta; SMA = superior mesenteric artery; RRA = right renal artery; LRA = left renal artery; IMA = inferior mesenteric artery; LCIA = left common iliac artery). (From Kitterman J.A., Phibbs R.H., Tooley W.H. Catheterization of umbilical vessels in newborn infants. *Pediatr Clin North Am* 1970; 17:898.)

B. Umbilical artery catheterization
1. **Guidelines.** In general, only seriously ill infants should have an umbilical artery catheter placed. If only a few blood gas measurements are anticipated, peripheral arterial punctures should be performed together with noninvasive oxygen monitoring, and a peripheral intravenous route should be used for fluids and medications.
2. **Technique**
    a. **Sterile technique is used.** Before preparing cord and skin, make external measurements to determine how far the catheter will be inserted (Figs. 36.3–36.5). For a high UAC, the distance is usually (umbilicus-to-shoulder) +2 cm , plus the length of the stump. In a high setting, the catheter tip is placed between the eighth and tenth thoracic vertebrae; in a low setting, the tip is between the third and fourth lumbar vertebrae.
    b. **The cord stump is suspended with a clamp.** It and the surrounding area are washed carefully with an antiseptic solution. In infants older than 2 months of age chlorhexidine is recommended and iodine solutions are acceptable. In younger infants the referred choice of agent is not clear. It is important to avoid chemical burns caused by iodine solution by carefully cleaning the skin (including the back and trunk) with sterile water after the solution has dried. Following this, the abdomen is draped with sterile towels.

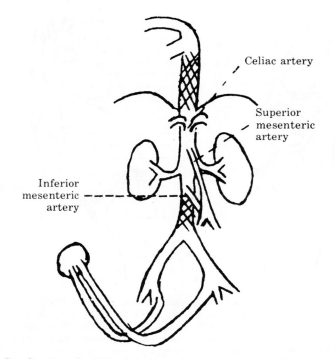

FIG. 36.3. Localization of umbilical artery catheters. The cross-hatched areas represent sites in which complications are least likely. Either site may be used for placement of the catheter tip.

c. **Umbilical tape** should be placed around the base of the cord itself. If it is necessary to place the tape on the skin, it must be loosened after the procedure. The tape is used to gently constrict the cord to prevent bleeding. The cord is then cut cleanly with a scalpel to a length of 1.0 to 1.5 cm.

d. **The cord is stabilized** with a forceps or hemostat, and the two arteries are identified.

e. The open tip of an iris forceps is inserted into the artery lumen and gently used to **dilate the vessel;** and then the closed tip is inserted into the lumen of an artery to a depth of 0.5 cm. Tension on the forceps tip is released, and the forceps is left in place to dilate the vessel for about 1 minute. This pause may be the most useful step in insertion of the catheter.

f. **The forceps is withdrawn,** and a sterile saline-filled 3.5F or 5F umbilical vessel catheter with an end hole is threaded into the artery. The smaller catheter is generally used for infants weighing less than 1500 g. A slightly increased resistance will be felt as the catheter passes through the base of the cord and as it navigates the umbilical artery–femoral artery junction. In about 5 to 10% of attempted umbilical artery catheterizations, one of the following problems may occur.

(1) **The catheter will not pass into the abdominal aorta.** Sometimes a double-catheter technique will allow successful cannulation in this situation.

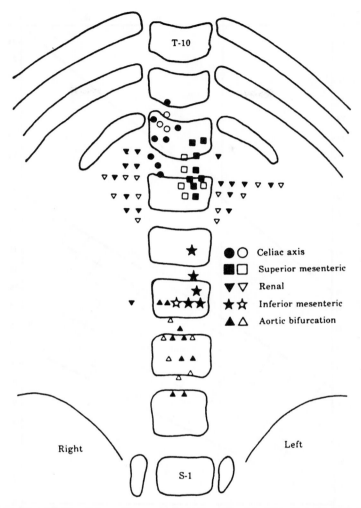

FIG. 36.4. Distribution of the major aortic branches found in 15 infants by aortography as correlated with the vertebral bodies. Filled symbols represent infants with cardiac or renal anomalies (or both); open symbols represent those without either disorder. Major landmarks appear at the following vertebral levels: diaphragm, T12 interspace; celiac artery, T12; superior mesenteric artery, L1 interspace; renal artery, L1; inferior mesenteric artery, L3; aortic bifurcation, L4. (From Phelps D.L. et al. The radiologic localization of the major aorta tributaries in the newborn. *J Pediatr* 1972; 81:336.)

(2) **The catheter may pass into the aorta but then loop caudad back down the contralateral iliac artery** or out one of the arteries to the buttocks. There may be difficulty advancing the catheter and cyanosis or blanching of the leg or buttocks may occur. This happens more frequently when a small catheter (3.5F) is placed in a large baby. Sometimes using a larger, stiffer catheter (5.0F) will

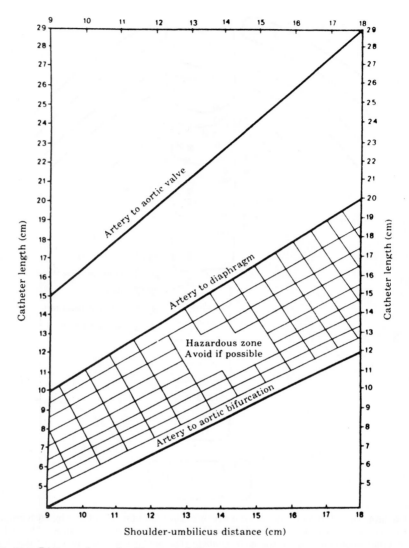

FIG. 36.5. Distance from shoulder to umbilicus measured from above the lateral end of the clavicle to the umbilicus, as compared with the length of umbilical artery catheter needed to reach the designated level. (From Dunn P.M. Localization of the umbilical catheter by postmortem measurement. *Arch Dis Child* 1969; 41:69.)

allow the catheter to advance up the aorta. Alternatively, retracting the catheter into the umbilical artery, rotating it, and reinserting it into the aorta will result in aoric placement. If this fails, the catheter should be removed and placement attempted via the other umbilical artery. Sometimes the catheter goes up the aorta and then loops back on itself. This also happens more frequently in a large baby when a small catheter is used. The catheter may also enter any of the vessels coming off the aorta. If the catheter cannot be advanced to the desired position, the tip should be pulled to a low position or the catheter removed.

(3) There is persistent cyanosis, blanching, or poor distal extremity perfusion. This may be improved by warming the contralateral leg, but if there is no improvement the catheter should be removed. Hematuria is an indication for catheter removal.

g. When the catheter is advanced the appropriate distance, placement should be confirmed by x-ray examination.

h. The catheter should be fixed in place with a purse-string suture using silk thread, and a tape bridge added for further stability (see Chap. 34).

3. **Catheter removal**

a. The umbilical artery catheter should be removed when either of the following criteria are met:

(1) The infant improves so that continuous monitoring and frequent blood drawings are no longer necessary.

(2) A maximum dwell time of 5 days is recommended to reduce infectious and thrombotic complications.

(3) Complications are noted.

b. **Method of catheter removal.** The catheter is removed slowly over a period of 30 to 60 seconds, allowing the umbilical artery to constrict at its proximal end while the catheter is still occluding the distal end. This usually prevents profuse bleeding. Old sutures should be removed.

4. **Complications associated with umbilical artery catheterization.** Significant morbidity can be associated with complications of umbilical artery catheterization. These complications are mainly due to vascular accidents, including thromboembolic phenomena to the kidney, bowel, legs, or rarely the spinal cord. These may manifest as hematuria, hypertension, signs of necrotizing enterocolitis or bowel infarction, and cyanosis or blanching of the skin of the back, buttocks, or legs. Other complications seen are infection, disseminated intravascular coagulation, and vessel perforation. All these complications are indications for catheter removal. Close observation of the skin, monitoring of the urine for hematuria, measuring blood pressure, and following the platelet count may give clues to complications.

a. We perform ultrasound examination of the aorta and renal vessels in infants in whom we are concerned about complications. If thrombi are observed, the catheter is removed.

b. If there are small thrombi without symptoms or with increased blood pressure alone, we usually remove the catheter, follow resolution of the thrombi by ultrasound examination, and treat hypertension if necessary (see Chap. 31). If there are signs of emboli or loss of pulses, or coagulopathy, and no intracranial hemorrhage is present, we consider heparinization, maintaining the partial thromboplastin time (PTT) at double the control value. Published data to guide practice are limited. If there is a large clot with impairment of perfusion, we consider the use of fibrinolytic agents (see Chap. 26). Surgical treatment of thrombosis is not generally effective.

c. **Blanching of a leg** following catheter placement is the most common complication noted clinically. Although this often occurs transiently, it deserves careful attention. One technique that may reverse this finding is to warm the opposite leg. If the vasospasm resolves, the catheter may be left in place. If there is no improvement, the catheter should be removed.

5. **Other considerations**

a. **Use of heparin for anticoagulation to prevent clotting.** Whether the use of heparin in the infusate decreases the incidence of thrombotic complications is not known. We use dilute heparin 0.5 to 1.0 unit/mL of infusate, depending on the rate of infusion.

b. Positioning of the catheter tip. Little helpful information convincingly supports the choice between high and low placement of umbilical artery catheters. A higher complication rate has been reported in infants with the catheter tip at L3 to L4, compared with T7 to T8, owing to more episodes of blanching and cyanosis of one or both legs. No difference between the high- and low-position groups was seen in the rate of complications requiring catheter removal. Renal complications and emboli to the bowel may be more common with catheter tips placed at T7 to T8 while catheters placed low (L3 to L4) are associated with complications such as cyanosis and blanching of the leg, which are easier to observe.

c. Indwelling time. The incidence of complications associated with umbilical artery catheterization appears to be directly related to the length of time the catheter is left in place.

6. Infection and use of antibiotics. We do not use prophylactic antibiotics for placement of umbilical artery catheters. In infants with umbilical artery catheters, we use antibiotics whenever infection is suspected and after appropriate cultures have been obtained.

C. Umbilical vein catheterization (see Figs. 36.2 and 36.6).

1. Indications. We use umbilical vein catheterization for emergency vascular access and exchange transfusions; in these cases, the venous catheter is replaced by a peripheral intravenous catheter or other access as soon as possible. In critically ill and extremely premature infants, we also use an umbilical vein catheter to infuse vasopressors and as the initial venous access.

2. Technique

a. The site is prepared as for umbilical artery catheterization after determining the appropriate length of catheter to be inserted (see Fig. 36.6).

b. Any clots seen are removed with a forceps, and the umbilical vein is gently dilated as with the umbilical artery in IX. C.

c. The catheter (3.5F or 5F), is prepared by filling the lumen with heparinized saline solution, 1 unit/mL of saline solution via an attached syringe. The catheter should never be left open to the atmosphere because negative intrathoracic pressure could cause an air embolism.

d. The catheter is inserted while gentle traction is exerted on the cord. Once the catheter is in the vein, one should try to slide the catheter cephalad just under the skin, where the vein runs very superficially. If the catheter is being placed for an exchange transfusion, it should be advanced only as far as is necessary to establish good blood flow (usually 2 to 5 cm). If the catheter is being used to monitor central venous pressure, it should be advanced through the ductus venosus into the inferior vena cava and its position verified by X ray.

e. Only isotonic solutions should be infused until the position of the catheter is verified by x-ray studies. If the catheter tip is in the inferior vena cava, hypertonic solutions may be infused.

f. Catheters may be left in place for up to 14 days, after which the increased risk of infectious or other complications increases. In very-low-birth-weight infants, our practice is to change access to a peripherally placed central venous catheter by 7 to 8 days if possible.

D. Multiple-lumen catheters for umbilical venous catheterization

1. Indications. Placement of a double- or triple-lumen catheter into the umbilical vein provides additional venous access for administration of incompatible solutions (e.g., those containing vasopressor agents, sodium bicarbonate, or calcium). The use of a multilumen catheter significantly reduces the need for multiple peripheral intravenous catheters and skin punctures, and is preferred in very-low-birth-weight infants.

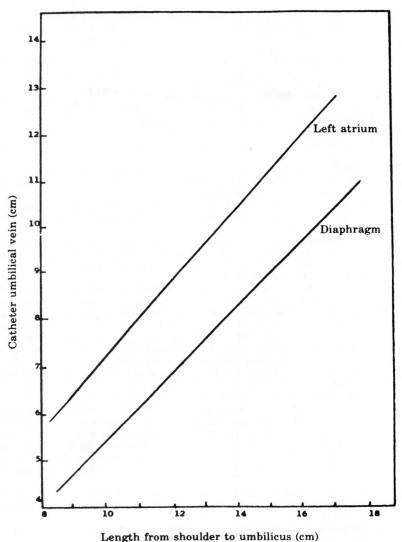

FIG. 36.6. Catheter length for umbilical vein catheterization. The catheter tip should be placed between the diaphragm and the left atrium. (From Dunn P.M. Localization of the umbilical catheter by postmortem measurements. *Arch Dis Child* 1966; 41:69.)

2. **Technique**
   a. **Modified Seldinger technique.** In patients with an indwelling single-lumen catheter, a wire exchange technique may be used to place a multiple-lumen catheter. Although this method decreases the probability of catheter loss during exchange, it entails the risks of wire passage including cardiac dysrhythmias and perforation, and should be attempted only by those familiar with the Seldinger technique.

    b. Direct placement. Multiple-lumen catheters can be placed directly following the outline provided for single-lumen catheters. The increased pliability of many of the multiple-lumen catheters makes passage into the hepatic veins more likely.

   3. Usage. Where possible, infusions that should not be interrupted (e.g., vasopressors) are placed in the proximal lumen to allow measurement of central venous pressure from the distal port.

E. Percutaneous radial artery catheterization. Placement of an indwelling radial artery catheter is a useful alternative to umbilical artery catheterization for monitoring blood gas levels and blood pressure.

   1. Advantages

    a. Accessibility (when the umbilical artery is inaccessible or has been used for a long period).

    b. Reflection of preductal flow (if the right radial artery is used).

    c. Avoidance of thrombosis of major vessels, which is sometimes associated with umbilical vessel catheterization.

   2. Risks are usually small if the procedure is performed carefully, but infection, air embolus, inadvertent injection of incorrect solution, and arterial occlusion may occur.

   3. Equipment required includes a 22- or 24-gauge intravenous cannula with stylet, a T-connector, heparinized saline flushing solution (0.5 to 1.0 unit of heparin per milliliter of solution), and an infusion pump.

   4. Method of catheterization

    a. The adequacy of the ulnar collateral flow to the hand must be assessed. The radial and ulnar arteries should be simultaneously compressed, and the ulnar artery should then be released. The degree of flushing of the blanched hand should be noted. If the entire hand becomes flushed while the radial artery is occluded, the ulnar circulation is adequate.

    b. The hand may be secured on an arm board with the wrist extended, leaving all fingertips exposed, to observe color changes.

    c. The wrist is prepared with an iodine-containing solution, and the site of maximum arterial pulsation is palpated.

    d. The intravenous cannula is inserted through the skin at an angle less than 30 degrees to horizontal and is slowly advanced into the artery. Transillumination may help delineate the vessel and its course. If the artery is entered as the catheter is advanced, the stylet is removed and the catheter is advanced in the artery. If there is no blood return, the artery may be transfixed. The stylet is then removed, and the catheter is slowly withdrawn until blood flow occurs; then it is advanced into the vessel.

   5. Caution. Only heparinized saline solution (0.45 to 0.9%) is infused into the catheter. The minimum infusion rate is 0.8 mL/h; the maximum is 2 mL/h.

F. Percutaneous central venous catheterization is useful for long-term venous access for intravenous fluids, particularly parenteral nutrition.

   1. Subclavian vein catheterization is useful in infants weighing more than 1200 g.

    a. The equipment required includes a 3.0F catheter with introducer needle and guidewire. Double-lumen 4.0F catheters may be used in larger infants (>2.5 kg).

    b. Technique. The infant is sedated and placed supine with a roll between the scapulae. Generally, the patient should be ventilated and muscle relaxed to afford maximum chance of success. The head is turned away from the side of insertion. The shoulders should drop posteriorly. The skin is prepared with an iodine-containing solution and infiltrated with local anesthetic. The introducer needle is inserted through the skin and immediately beneath the clavicle, a third of the way from the shoulder to the midline. The needle should be almost parallel to the chest wall and aimed at the sternal notch. When blood flow is established, the guidewire is passed and the catheter is placed over the wire. Catheter position is determined radiographically. The catheter tip should lie at the junction of the superior vena cava and right atrium.

    c. **Complications** include pneumothorax, hemothorax, and inadvertent subclavian artery puncture. The potential severity of these complications dictates that only those thoroughly familiar with this technique should attempt this form of venous cannulation.

  2. **Peripheral** or **external jugular vein catheterization** is useful in infants weighing less than 1500 g.

    a. **The equipment** required includes a 1.9F to 2.1F silicone catheter cut to the appropriate length, a splittable introducer needle, and iris forceps.

    b. **Technique.** An appropriate vein of entry is selected. This may be a basilic, greater saphenous, or external jugular vein. The cephalic vein should be avoided, as central placement is more difficult. The site is prepared with an antiseptic solution, and the introducer needle is inserted into the vein until blood flows freely. The silicone catheter is inserted through the needle with forceps and is slowly advanced the predetermined distance for central venous positioning. The introducer needle is removed, the extra catheter length is coiled on the skin near the insertion site, and the site is covered with transparent surgical covering. The catheter tip is positioned at the junction of the vena cava and right atrium, as confirmed by radiography. Some physicians inject a small amount of isotonic contrast material to make visualization easier.

    c. **Complications** are rare but include infection, thrombosis, and thrombophlebitis.

X. Abdominal paracentesis for removal of ascitic fluid

  A. Indications

    1. Therapeutic indications include respiratory distress resulting from abdominal distention (e.g., hydropic infants, infants with urinary ascites) for which removal of ascitic fluid will ameliorate respiratory symptoms. In addition, interference with urine production or lower extremity perfusion resulting from increased intraabdominal pressure may be improved by paracentesis.

    2. Diagnostic indications include the evaluation of suspected peritonitis.

  B. Technique

    1. The equipment needed includes an 18- to 22-gauge intravenous catheter, three-way stopcock, and a 10- to 50-mL syringe.

    2. The lower abdomen is prepared with povidone-iodine solution and the area is draped. If the bladder is distended, it is drained with manual pressure or a urinary catheter. A local anesthetic such as 1% lidocaine (Xylocaine) is infiltrated into the subcutaneous tissues when possible. The catheter is inserted just lateral to the rectus sheath one-third of the distance between the umbilicus and the symphysis pubis. Alternatively the catheter can be inserted in the midline, during aspiration with the syringe. The catheter is advanced approximately 1 cm until the resistance of passing through the abdominal wall diminishes or fluid is obtained. Five to 10 mL of fluid is removed for diagnostic paracentesis while 10 to 20 mL/kg should be removed for therapeutic effects. The catheter is removed and the site bandaged.

  C. Potential complications

    1. Cardiovascular effects, including tachycardia, hypotension, and decreased cardiac output, may result from rapid redistribution of intravascular fluid to the peritoneal space following removal of large amounts of ascites.

    2. Bladder or intestinal aspiration may occur more frequently in the presence of a dilated bladder or bowel. These puncture sites usually heal spontaneously and without significant clinical findings.

Suggested Readings

Fletcher M.A., McDonald M.G., Avery G.B. (Eds.), *Atlas of Procedures in Neonatology.* Philadelphia: Lippincott, 1994.

Garland J.S., Henrickson K., Maki D.G. The 2002 Hospital Infection Control Practices Advisory Committee Centers for Disease Control and Prevention Guideline for Prevention of Intravascular Device-Related Infection. *Pediatrics* 2002;110: 1009–1013.

Latini G. Potential hazards of exposure to Di-(2-Ethylhexyl)-phthalate in babies. *Biol Neonate* 2000;78: 269–276.

37. MANAGEMENT OF PAIN AND STRESS IN THE NICU

Linda J. Van Marter and Corinne Cyr Pryor

I. **Background.** The recognition that premature and full-term infants experience pain has led to increasing appreciation that the stress and pain of infants in the neonatal intensive care unit (NICU) probably is undertreated. Laboratory studies and clinical observations suggest that uncontrolled neonatal pain might result in adverse effects on neonatal health and long-term neurodevelopmental outcomes. Thus, both scientific and human considerations favor improved management strategies to prevent and treat infant pain and discomfort.

A. **Fetal and neonatal physiologic responses to pain.** Because sensory nerve terminals exist on all body surfaces by 22 to 29 weeks of gestation, the fetus is capable of experiencing pain. Early in development, overlapping nerve terminals create local hyperexcitable networks, enabling even low-threshold stimuli to produce an exaggerated pain response. Fetal wounds heal more quickly and with less scarring than those of infants, children, or adults. The process, in part, involves sprouting of sensory nerve endings in and near the wound. Although it seems to enhance wound healing, hyperinnervation results in hypersensitivity to painful stimuli that persists long after wound healing has occurred. Repeated noxious stimuli lower the pain threshold, slow recovery, and adversely effect long-term outcomes.

The fetus is capable of mounting a stress response beginning at approximately 23 weeks of gestation. Physiological responses to painful or stressful stimuli include increases in circulating catecholamines, increased heart rate and blood pressure, and elevated intracranial pressure. However, the stress response of the immature fetus or preterm infant is less competent than that of the more mature infant or child. Therefore, in immature infants, the classical vital signs of stress (e.g, tachycardia, hypertension, agitation) are not reliable indicators of painful stimuli. Even when the infant's stress response is intact, persistence of painful stimuli for hours or days fatigues or deactivates the sympathetic nervous system response, obscuring signs of pain or discomfort.

B. **Medical and developmental outcomes**
   1. **Medical and surgical outcomes.** Neonatal responses to pain contribute to hypoxia, hypercarbia, acidosis, hyperglycemia, respiratory dysynchrony, and pneumothoraces. Intraoperative courses are more stable and postoperative recoveries are improved among infants who receive adequate intraoperative analgesia and anesthesia. Increases in intrathoracic pressure due to diaphragmatic splinting and vagal responses produced in response to pain following invasive procedures precipitate hypoxemic events and alterations in oxygen delivery and cerebral blood volume.
   2. **Neurodevelopmental outcomes.** Behavioral and neurological studies suggest that preterm infants who experience numerous painful procedures and noxious stimuli are less responsive to painful stimuli at 18 months' corrected age. However, unlike their normal birth weight peers, at 8 to 10 years of age, infants born at or below 1000 g birth weight rate medical pain intensity greater than measures of psychosocial pain. These data provide evidence that neonatal pain and stress influence development and later perceptions of painful stimuli.

II. **Principles of prevention and management of neonatal pain and stress.** A policy statement by the Committee on the Fetus and Newborn of the American Academy of Pediatrics (AAP) identified a number of key principles pertaining to newborn pain and stress. These include the following concepts:
   - Neuroanatomical components and neuroendocrine systems of the neonate are sufficiently developed to allow transmission of painful stimuli.
   - Exposure to prolonged or severe pain may increase neonatal morbidity.

703

- Infants who have experienced pain during the neonatal period respond differently to subsequent painful events.
- Severity of pain and effects of analgesia can be assessed in the neonate using validated instruments.
- Newborn infants usually are not easily comforted when analgesia is needed.
- A lack of behavioral responses (including crying and movement) does not necessarily indicate the absence of pain.

A. AAP recommendations

1. To evaluate and reduce the stress and pain experienced by neonates, validated measures and assessment tools must be applied in a consistent manner. The assessments should continue as long as the neonate requires treatment for stress or pain.

2. Health-care professionals should use appropriate environmental, nonpharmacological (behavioral), and pharmacological interventions to prevent, reduce, or eliminate the stress and pain of neonates.

3. Pharmacological agents with known pharmacokinetic and pharmacodynamic properties and demonstrated efficacy in neonates should be used. Agents that might cause cardiorespiratory compromise should be administered only in settings with the capacity for continuous monitoring by persons experienced in neonatal airway management.

4. Health-care institutions should develop and implement patient-care policies to assess, prevent, and manage pain in neonates, including those receiving palliative care.

5. Educational programs to increase the skills of health-care professionals in the assessment and management of stress and pain in neonates should be provided.

6. There is a need for development and validation of neonatal pain assessment tools that are easily applicable in the clinical setting.

7. For research purposes, a minimal set of well-defined outcome measures, including short- and long-term effects of interventions aimed at reducing stress and pain in the neonate, should be identified to permit statistical synthesis of data (meta-analysis) and more accurate estimates of effect size.

III. Evaluating neonatal pain and stress. Several validated and reliable scales are available for pain assessment. Behavioral indicators (e.g., facial expression, crying, body/extremity movement) as well as physiological indicators (e.g., tachycardia or bradycardia, hypertension, tachypnea or apnea, oxygen desaturation, palmar sweating, changes in vagal tone, plasma cortisol, or catecholamine levels) can be useful in assessing the infant's level of comfort or discomfort.

Physiological responses to painful stimuli include release of circulating catecholamines, heart rate acceleration, blood pressure increase, and a rise in intracranial pressure. The stress response of the immature fetus or preterm infant is less competent than that of the more mature infant or child. Gestational age must be considered in evaluating the pain response among preterm infants experiencing pain, the vital signs associated with the stress response and agitation are not consistently evident. Even among infants with an intact response to pain, a painful stimulus that persists for hours or days exhausts sympathetic nervous system output, suppresses behavioral expression of pain, and obscures the clinician's ability to objectively assess the infant's level of discomfort.

A. Recommended assessment tools. Selecting the most appropriate tool for assessment of neonatal pain assessment must take into consideration the infant's gestational age and other clinical factors, such as severity of illness.

1. **Infants in intensive care.** Pain responses are influenced by gestational age. The Premature Infant Pain Profile (PIPP), a method that incorporates assessment of facial expression and physiological measures in the context of gestational age and neonatal state is the only method that has been validated for assessment of pain in preterm infants (Table 37.1).

2. **Infants intermediate care or well nursery.** Several pain assessment scales are available for full-term or growing former preterm infants. We recom-

TABLE 37.1. PREMATURE INFANT PAIN PROFILE FOR PRETERM AND TERM INFANTS IN THE NICU

Process	Indicator	0	1	2	3	Score*
Medical record review	Gestational age	36 weeks and more	32–35 6/7 weeks	28–31 6/7 weeks	< 28 weeks	—
Observe infant behavior (for 15 seconds)	Behavioral state	Active/awake, eyes open, facial movements	Quiet/awake, eyes open, no facial movements	Active/sleep, eyes closed, facial movements	Quiet/sleep, eyes closed, facial movements	—
Observe baseline	Heart rate ____ O₂ saturation ____					
Observe infant changes (for 30 seconds)	Heart rate Maximum ____	0–4 beats/min increase	5–14 beats/min increase	15–24 beats/min increase	25 beats/min or more increase	—
	O₂ saturation Minimum ____	0–2.4% decrease	2.5–4.9% decrease	5.0–7.4% decrease	7.5% or more decrease	—
	Brow bulge	None 0–9% of time	Minimum 10–39% of time	Moderate 40–69% of time	Maximum 70% of time or more	—
	Eye squeeze	None 0–9% of time	Minimum 10–39% of time	Moderate 40–69% of time	Maximum 70% of time or more	—
	Nasolabial furrow	None 0–9% of time	Minimum 10–39% of time	Moderate 40–69% of time	Maximum 70% of time or more	—
					Total score:	—

NICU = neonatal intensive care unit.
*A score of ≤ 6 indicates minimal or no pain.
A score of >12 indicates moderate to severe pain.
Source: Adapted from Stevens B. *Clin J Pain* 1990;12:13–22.

mend the Behavioral Pain Score (BPS), a method that assesses motor activity, cry, consolability, and sleep (Table 37.2). An alternative is the Neonatal Infant Pain Scale (NIPS), a research tool that has been used to assess pain pre- and postinterventions (Table 37.3).

IV. **Pain prevention and treatment**
　A. **Environmental and behavioral approaches.** Painful or stressful procedures should be minimized and coordinated with other aspects of the newborn's care.
　　1. During the procedure, the following environmental and developmentally supportive measures might prove useful to reduce infant pain and stress:
　　　a. Clustering painful interventions prior to a comforting event (e.g., feeding or holding).
　　　b. Swaddling during the procedure.
　　　c. Non-nutritive sucking; pacifier.
　　　d. Use of mechanical lancets for heel-stick blood draws.
　　2. Following the procedure, other measures are helpful:
　　　a. Reducing noise and light.
　　　b. Touch or massage.
　　　c. Parent–infant skin-to-skin contact (kangaroo care).
　　　d. Holding the baby following the procedure.
　　　e. Positional "nesting" or containment using blanket rolls.
　B. **Physiological interventions.** There are two primary approaches to physiological pain management. These are sucrose analgesia and competitive stimulation.
　　1. **Sucrose analgesia** (0.25 to 0.5 g) is given orally approximately 2 minutes prior to the painful procedure
　　2. **Competitive stimulation** consists of gently rubbing, tapping, or vibrating one extremity before and/or during painful stimulus to another extremity.
　C. **Pharmacological management.** A number of scientific principles guide the pharmacological management of neonatal pain.
　　1. **Complementary therapies.** Environmental and behavioral interventions should be used to comfort infant experiencing painful stimuli. These measures and sucrose analgesia often are useful in conjunction with pharmacological treatments.
　　2. **Prophylaxis versus pain treatment.** Narcotic analgesia given prophylactically on a scheduled basis results in a lower total dose and improved pain control compared with "as needed" dosing.
　　3. **Gestational maturity.** A prophylactic approach might be especially useful in the preterm acutely ill infant who is assumed to be incapable of mounting a stress response to signal his/her pain. The inability of the infant to mount an appropriate response is especially relevant when the infant is extremely immature or the painful stimulus is severe and/or prolonged.
　　4. **No long-term adverse effects of the use of morphine sedation among ventilated infants have been reported.** These include long-term studies assessing intelligence, motor function, and behavior.

V. **Pharmacological treatment of procedure-related pain** (Table 37.4)
　A. **Analgesia for minimally invasive procedures** (Table 37.5). In a full-term infant, sucrose analgesia is recommended for once or twice-daily blood draws, at a dose of: **sucrose** 0.25 to 0.5 g total dose (1.5 to 3 mL of 20% sucrose solution) approximately 2 minutes prior to the procedure. Studies of sucrose analgesia are largely limited to full-term infants. Data are scarce on the use of sucrose analgesia among premature infants. However, some Harvard NICUs use single doses of sucrose solution to treat moderately preterm infants (30 to 36 weeks' gestational age) who were undergoing minimally invasive procedures. For preterm infants, we recommend lower doses: 0.5 to 1.5 mL of sucrose 20% solution.
　B. **Analgesia for invasive procedures** (Table 37.6). **Narcotics** (e.g., morphine or Fentanyl) and **sedatives** (e.g., midazolam, phenobarbital) are useful in treating

TABLE 37.2. BEHAVIORAL PAIN SCORE FOR FULL-TERM INFANTS UNDERGOING INTERVENTIONS OR POST-OP CARE

Behavior	0 (Satisfactory)	1 (Mediocre)	2 (Poor)	Score*
Sleep (during preeding hour)	Longer naps (>10 minutes)	Short naps (5–10 minutes)	None	——
Facial expression of pain	Calm, relaxed	Less marked, intermittent	Marked, constant	——
Quality of cry	No cry	Modulated (distracted by normal sound)	Screaming, painful, high pitched	——
Spontaneous motor activity	Normal	Moderate agitation	Thrashing, incessant agitation	——
Spontaneous excitability and responsiveness to ambient stimulation	Quiet	Excessive reactivity (to any stimulation)	Tremulous, clonic movements, spontaneous Moro reflexes	——
Flexion of fingers and toes	Absent	Less marked, intermittent	Very pronounced, marked and constant	——
Sucking	Normal for age	Intermittent (three or four) stops with crying	Absent or disorganized sucking	——
Global evaluation of tone	Normal for age	Moderate tonicity	Strong hypertonicity	——
Consolability	Calm before 1 minute	Quiet after 1 minute of effort	None after 2 minutes	——
Sociability (eye contact), response to voice, smile; real interest in face	Easy and prolonged	Difficult to obtain	Absent	——
			Total:	——

*A score of 0–5 indicates adequate postoperative analgesia.
Source: Adapted from Attia J., et al. Post-operative pain score. *Anesthesiology* 1987;67:A532.

TABLE 37.3. NEONATAL INFANT PAIN SCALE (NIPS)

	0	1	2	Score*
Facial expression	Relaxed muscles	Tight facial muscles		____
Cry	No cry	Moaning	Continuous cry	____
Breathing patterns	Relaxed	Change in breathing pattern		____
Arms	Relaxed/restrained	Flexed/extended (tense, rigid or rapid extension)		____
Legs	Relaxed/restrained	Flexed/extended (tense, rigid, or rapid extension)		____
State of arousal	Sleeping/awake	Fussy		____
			Total score:	____

*A score of 0–3 indicates adequate analgesia.
Source: Adapted from Lawrence J., *Neonatal Network* 1993;12:59.

TABLE 37.4. COMMONLY USED ANESTHETIC, ANALGESIC, AND SEDATIVE AGENTS

Local anesthetics	Use	Maximum dose
Lidocaine 0.5%*		5 mg/kg SQ (1.0 mL/kg of 0.5% solution, 0.5 mL/kg of 1% solution)
EMLA 5% cream†	33–37 weeks GA and >1.8 kg	0.5 g for 1–2 hours (then remove excess)
	>37 weeks GA and >2.5 kg	1.0 g for 1–2 hours (then remove excess)

Analgesics	Single dose‡	Infusion§
Morphine sulfate‖	Intubated: 0.05–0.15 mg/kg IV or SQ	0.01–0.03 mg/kg/hour
	Nonintubated: 0.025–0.05 mg/kg IV or SQ	Not recommended
Fentanyl¶	Intubated: 2–5 μg/kg (over 5 minutes) IV	0.2–0.5 μg/kg/hour
	Nonintubated: 0.25–0.5 μg/kg (over 5 minutes) IV	Not recommended
Acetaminophen	10–15 mg/kg PO/PG/PR every 6 hours prn, maximum dose 40 mg/kg/24 hours	

Sedatives	Dose
Short-term	
Midazolam**	0.05–0.1 mg/kg IV or intranasal
Chloral hydrate††	20–30 mg/kg PO or PG
Long-term	
Phenobarbital	Loading dose: 5–10 mg/kg PO, PG, or IV
	Maintenance dose: 3–4 mg/kg PO, PG, or IV

EMLA = eutectic mixture of local anesthetic; IV = intravenous; PG = per gastric tube; GA = gestational age; PO = by mouth; PR = per rectum; prn = as needed; SQ = subcutaneous.

*Lidocaine toxicity may cause cardiac arrhythmia or seizure. 0.5% solution can be made by 1:1 dilution of 1% lidocaine with normal saline.

†EMLA should be limited to a *single dose* per day and it must be removed within 2 hours. It takes 40–60 minutes following application to achieve the maximum effect of EMLA. Prilocaine (in EMLA) may cause methemoglobinemia. Swelling associated with the use of EMLA might distort anatomical structures.

‡May repeat dosing at 10–15-minute intervals until initial therapeutic effect is achieved.

§May titrate above this dosing range to achieve a therapeutic effect.

‖Morphine may cause hypotension.

¶Rapid infusion of fentanyl may cause chest-wall rigidity. Fentanyl infusion often must be increased due to tachyphylaxis.

**Midazolam is recommended for use only in full-term infants. Abnormal movements have been described in premies treated with midazolam.

††Chloral hydrate is metabolized to trichloroethanol, which competes for glucuronidation and may exacerbate hyperbilirubinemia.

TABLE 37.5. ANALGESIA FOR MINIMALLY INVASIVE PROCEDURES*

	Intubated and ventilated infants	Nonintubated infants
Arterial puncture	20% sucrose 1.5–3 cc/kg PO/PG	20% sucrose 1.5–3 cc/kg/PO/PG
Venipuncture	20% sucrose 1.5–3 cc/kg PO/PG	20% sucrose 1.5–3 cc/kg PO/PG
Heel-stick blood draw	20% sucrose 1.5–3 cc/kg PO/PG	20% sucrose 1.5–3 cc/kg PO/PG
Intravenous placement	20% sucrose 1.5–3 cc/kg PO/PG	20% sucrose 1.5–3 cc/kg PO/PG
Lumbar puncture	20% sucrose 1.5–3 cc/kg PO/PG and morphine sulfate 0.05–0.15 mg/kg IV or SQ or fentanyl† 2–3 µg/kg IV and/or If ≥ 34 weeks: EMLA‡ or buffered lidocaine 0.5% (max: 0.5 cc/kg) SQ, skin only	20% sucrose 1.5–3 cc/kg PO/PG and If ≥ 34 weeks: EMLA‡ or buffered lidocaine 0.5% (max: 0.5 cc/kg) SQ, skin only
Dressing change	20% sucrose 1.5–3 cc/kg PO/PG and morphine sulfate 0.05–0.1 mg/kg IV or fentanyl† 2–3 µg/kg IV	20% sucrose 1.5–3 cc/kg PO/PG and/or morphine sulfate 0.025–0.05 mg/kg IV or SQ or fentanyl† 0.25–1 µg/kg IV
Endotracheal suctioning (mechanically ventilated)	morphine sulfate 0.05–0.15 mg/kg or fentanyl† 2–3 µg/kg IV	N/A
Immunization injection	N/A	20% sucrose 1.5–3 cc/kg PO/PG and/or EMLA* (if ≥ 34 weeks)

EMLA = eutectic mixture of local anesthetic; IV = intravenous; PG = per gastric tube; PO = by mouth; SQ = subcutaneous.
*Competitive stimulation may be used for any of these procedures, except suctioning.
†Fentanyl should be infused at ≤1 µg/kg minute (e.g., 3 µg/kg infused over ≥ 3 minutes).
‡Only one application per day of EMLA should be used. It takes 40–60 minutes to reach peak effect and should be removed within 2 hours of application.

TABLE 37.6. ANALGESIA FOR INVASIVE PROCEDURES: PRETERM AND TERM* INFANTS

Invasive procedures	Intubated and ventilated infants	Nonintubated infants
Intubation (emergency)	None	None
Intubation	N/A	Fentanyl[†] 0.25–1 µg/kg IV (infused over 2 minutes) IV or morphine 0.025–0.05 mg/kg IV or SQ
Mechanical ventilation		
First 24 hours (unless imminent extubation is anticipated)	Fentanyl[†] 2–3 µg/kg Q4 h and prn or morphine 0.05–0.15 mg/kg Q4 h and prn or fentanyl infusion 0.2–2 µg/kg/h (start at low rate and increase prn)	N/A
>24 hours	Fentanyl[†] 2–3 µg/kg Q4 h and prn or morphine 0.05–0.15 mg/kg Q4 h and prn or fentanyl infusion 0.2–2 µg/kg/h (start at low rate and increase prn)	N/A
Chest tube		
Insertion	Lidocaine 0.5% (max: 1 cc/kg) SQ and fentanyl[†] 2–5 µg/kg µg/kg × 1 or morphine 0.1–0.2 µg/kg IV (titrate prn)	Lidocaine 0.5% (max: 0.5 cc/kg) SQ and fentanyl[†] 0.5–2 µg/kg IV or morphine 0.05–0.1 µg/kg IV (titrate prn)
In place	Morphine 0.05–0.15 mg/kg Q 2–4 h prn or fentanyl[†] 2–4 µg/kg Q 2–4 h prn	Morphine 0.025–0.05 mg/kg IV or SQ or fentanyl[†] 0.25–1 µg/kg IV
Removal	Morphine 0.05–0.15 mg/kg or fentanyl[†] 2 µg/kg	Morphine 0.025–0.05 mg/kg IV or SQ or fentanyl[†] 0.25–1 µg/kg IV
Umbilical catheter placement	Morphine 0.05–0.1 mg/kg prn Fentanyl[†] 2–3 µg/kg prn	Morphine 0.025–0.05 mg/kg IV or SQ or fentanyl[†] 0.25–0.5 µg/kg IV

(continues)

TABLE 37.6. *(continued)*

Invasive procedures	Intubated and ventilated infants	Nonintubated infants
Peripheral arterial catheter placement	Morphine sulfate 0.05–0.1 mg/kg Q 2–4 hrs or fentanyl[†] 2–3 µg/kg Q 2–4 h or EMLA (if ≥ 34 weeks)	Morphine 0.025–0.05 mg/kg IV or SQ or fentanyl[†] 0.25–1 µg/kg IV or EMLA (if ≥ 34 weeks)
Percutaneously inserted central catheter	Morphine 0.05–0.1 mg/kg Q 2–4 h fentanyl[†] 2–3 µg/kg Q 2–4 h or EMLA (if ≥ 34 weeks)	Morphine EMLA (if ≥ 34 weeks) or fentanyl[†] 0.25–1 µg/kg IV or EMLA (if ≥ 34 weeks)
Laser surgery	*2 hrs before the procedure:* acetaminophen 15 mg/kg and *During the procedure:* Morphine sulfate 0.05–0.1 mg/kg Q 1–2 h or fentanyl[†] 2–4 µg/kg Q 1–2 h prn and, if ≥ 34 weeks: Midazolam 0.1 mg/kg Q 1–2 h prn	N/A
Circumcision	N/A	20% sucrose 1.5–3 cc/kg PO/PG and acetaminophen 10–15 mg/kg 2 h before and Q6 h after the procedure (×24 h) and Ring block (lidocaine 0.5%) (max.: 0.5 cc/kg) or dorsal penile block (lidocaine 0.5%) or *If ≥34 weeks GA and >1.8 kg:* EMLA
Preoperative (i.e., intubated infants undergoing general anesthesia)	Consider fentanyl[†] 1–3 µg/kg (infused over 5 minutes) 1 hour before transfer for the procedure	N/A

EMLA = eutectic mixture of local anesthetic; IV = intravenous; N/A = not applicable; PG = per gastric tube; GA = gestational age; prn = as required; SQ = subcutaneous.
*Full-term infants *only* also may receive midazolam 0.05–0.1 mg/kg for anxiety.
[†]Fentanyl should be infused at ≤1 µg/kg/minute (e.g., 3 µg/kg infused over ≥ 3 minutes).

TABLE 37.7. POSTOPERATIVE ANALGESIA

	Intubated and ventilated infants	Nonintubated infants
Herniorraphy	acetaminophen 10–15 mg/kg PO/PG/PR Q 4–6 h or fentanyl* 2–3 μg/kg Q 2–4 h prn or morphine 0.05–0.1 mg/kg Q 2–4 h prn	acetaminophen 10–15 mg/kg PO/PG/PR Q 6 h or fentanyl* 0.25–0.5 μg/kg Q 4 h prn or morphine 0.025–0.05 mg/kg IV or SQ Q 4 h prn
Laparotomy	1st 24 hours: fentanyl* 1–3 μg/kg Q 4–6 h or morphine 0.1 mg/kg Q 4–6 h Then: Morphine 0.05–0.1 Q 2–4 h prn or fentanyl* 1–3 μg/kg Q 2–4 h prn	Fentanyl* 0.25–0.5 μg/kg Q 4 h prn or morphine 0.025–0.05 mg/kg IV or SQ Q 4 h prn
Thoracotomy	1st 24 hours: fentanyl* 1–3 μg/kg Q 4 h or morphine 0.05–0.1 mg/kg Q4 h Then: Morphine 0.05–0.1 mg/kg Q 2–4 h prn or fentanyl* 1–3 μg/kg Q 2–4 h prn	acetaminophen 10–15 mg/kg Q6 h Q 6 h prn or fentanyl*0.25–0.5 μg/kg Q 4 h prn prn or morphine 0.025–0.05 mg/kg IV or SQ Q 4 h prn
Laser surgery	acetaminophen 15 mg/kg 2 h before and tylenol 10 mg/kg Q 6 h after the procedure (×24 hours); then Q6 h prn	acetaminophen 10 mg/kg Q6 h after the procedure (×24 h); then Q6 h prn
Neurosurgical (cranial)	Fentanyl* 1–3 μg/kg Q 2–4 h prn or morphine 0.05–0.1 mg/kg Q 2–4 h prn	acetaminophen 10–15 mg/kg Q6 h prn or fentanyl* 0.25–0.5 μg/kg Q 4 h prn or morphine 0.025–0.05 mg/kg IV or SQ Q 4 h prn
Neurosurgical (lumbar)	Fentanyl* 1–3 μg/kg Q 2–4 h prn or morphine 0.05–0.1 mg/kg Q 2–4 h prn	acetaminophen 10–15 mg/kg Q 6 h Q 4 h prn or fentanyl* 0.25–0.5 μg/kg (over 2 minutes) or morphine 0.025–0.05 mg/kg IV or SQ Q 4 h prn

IV = intravenous; PG = per gastric tube; PO = by mouth; PR = by rectum; prn = as needed; SQ = subcutaneous.
*Fentanyl should be infused at ≤ 1 μg/kg/minute (e.g., 3 μg/kg infused over ≥3 minutes).

critically ill newborns undergoing invasive or very painful procedures. Alleviating pain is the most important goal. Therefore, treatment with analgesics is preferred over sedation without analgesia. For term newborns, a sedative agent may be added, as needed.

1. For most invasive procedures, **pharmacological premedication** is recommended. Except in instances of emergency intubation, newborns should be premedicated for invasive procedures. Examples of procedures for which premedication is indicated include: elective intubation, mechanical ventilation, chest tube insertion or removal, arterial catheter placement, laser surgery, and circumcision.

2. **For intubation and the first few days of mechanical ventilation,** we recommend **around-the-clock medication with fentanyl 2 to 3 µg/kg or morphine sulfate 0.05 to 0.15 mg/kg IV every four hours.** Thereafter, we recommend dosing these medications on an 'as needed' basis. In nonintubated newborns, we recommend morphine sulfate 0.025 to 0.05 mg/kg or fentanyl 0.25 to 1 µg/kg with repeated administration "as needed." Fentanyl must be infused slowly (over 5 to 10 minutes) to avoid the complications of chest wall rigidity and impaired ventilation. In infants at or near term gestation undergoing an isolated procedure such as intubation, midazolam 0.1 mg/kg may be used in addition to narcotic analgesia.

3. **For circumcision,** we recommend treatment with oral 20% sucrose analgesia and acetaminophen 15 mg/kg preoperatively and, for the procedure, ring or dorsal penile block with a maximum dose of lidocaine 0.5% 0.5 mL. Following the procedure, we recommend acetaminophen 10 mg/kg every 6 hours for 24 hours (total dose not to exceed 40 mg/kg).

4. **Sedatives and narcotics cause respiratory depression.** They should be used in newborns only in settings in which respiratory depression can be promptly treated by medical staff with expertise in airway management.

C. **Perioperative analgesia.** We recommend premedicating intubated infants undergoing surgery with fentanyl 1 to 3 µg/kg 1 hour before transfer to the operating suite. Infants who are not intubated receive perioperative analgesia and sedation in the operating room just prior to intubation. The approach to management of postoperative pain depends on the surgical procedure (Table 37.7).

D. **Naloxone for reversal of opioid side effects.** Naloxone (Narcan) is used to treat the side effects of excessive opioid, most commonly respiratory depression. In neonatal resuscitation, a relatively large dose (0.1 mg/kg or more) is used. This is appropriate in the infant with profound respiratory depression. However, in an infant receiving narcotic analgesia, the optimal goal is to block the adverse effects without exacerbating pain. If the baby's clinical status permits, a preferable approach is to titrate administration of naloxone, giving it in increments of 0.05 mg/kg until the side effects are reversed.

Suggested Readings

Alkalay A.L., Sola A. Analgesia and local anesthesia for nonritual circumcision in stable healthy newborns. *Neonatal Intensive Care* 2000; 13:19–21.

Anand K.J.S., Hickey P.R. Pain and its effects in the human neonate and fetus *N Engl J Med* 1987; 317:1321–1329.

Belleini C. et al. Effect of multisensory stimulation on analgesia in term neonates: A randomized clinical trial. *Pediatr Res* 2002; 51:460–463.

Berde C., Sethna N. Analgesics for the treatment of pain in children. *N Engl J Med* 2002; 347:1094–1103.

Bhutta A., Anand K.J.S. Vulnerability of the developing brain: neuronal mechanisms. *Clin Perinatol* 2002; 29:357–372.

Committee on the Fetus and Newborn, American Academy of Pediatrics. Prevention and management of pain and stress in the neonate. *Pediatrics* 2000; 105:454–460.

Johnston C.C., Stevens B.J. Experience in a neonatal intensive care unit affects pain response. *Pediatrics* 1996; 98:925–930.

APPENDIX A. COMMON NICU MEDICATION GUIDELINES

Tola Dawodu, Caryn Douma, and Rita Patnode

ACETAZOLAMIDE

Classification: Diuretic, carbonic anhydrase inhibitor. **Indication:** To slow the progression of hydrocephalus. **Dosage/administration:** 5 mg/kg/dose orally or intravenously every 6 hours. If desired may increase by 25 mg/kg/day up to a maximum of 100 mg/kg/day if tolerated. Usual concentration for infusion is 25 mg/mL up to a maximum of 100 mg/mL. Maximum infusion rate is 500 mg/min. **Precautions:** Adjust dose for renal impairment. Intramuscular administration painful because of alkaline pH. Tolerance to diuretic effect occurs with long-term administration. **Monitoring:** Acid–base status, daily intake/output, weight, and weekly head circumference. **Adverse reactions:** Hyperchloremic metabolic acidosis, hypokalemia, and bone marrow suppression.

ACYCLOVIR

Classification: Antiviral agent. **Indications:** Treatment of herpes simplex infections, varicella zoster infections with central nervous system and pulmonary involvement, and herpes simplex encephalitis.
Dosage/administration:

TABLE A.1

Indication	Dosage
Localized HSV infection	20 mg/kg/dose IV Q8h for 14 days Infusion concentration must be ≤ 7 mg/mL, usual infusion concentration = 5 mg/mL
Disseminated or CNS infections	20 mg/kg/dose IV Q8h for 21 days
Varicella	20 mg/kg/dose PO Q6h for 5 days Initiate therapy within the first 24 h of disease onset

CNS = central nervous system; HSV = herpes simplex virus; IV = intravenously; PO = orally; Q6h = every 6 hours; Q8h = every 8 hours.

Do not refrigerate because it can cause precipitation of the drug. Infuse by syringe pump over 1 hour. **Precautions:** Reduce dosage for impaired renal function. **Monitoring:** Renal and hepatic function. **Adverse reactions:** Nephrotoxicity, bone marrow suppression, fever, thrombocytosis, and transitory increase of serum creatinine and liver enzymes. Rare encephalopathy associated with rapid intravenous administration (lethargy, obtundation, agitation, tremor, seizure, and coma).

ALPROSTADIL

Classification: Prostaglandin. **Indications:** Temporary maintenance of patent ductas arteriosis (PDA), in neonates with ductal-dependent congenital heart disease. **Dosage/administration:** *Initial:* 0.05 to 0.1 µg/kg/min; titrate to lowest effective dosage with therapeutic response. *Maintenance:* 0.01 to 0.4 µg/kg/min. Alprostadil is usually given at an infusion rate of 0.05 µg/kg/min as a continuous intravenous infusion on a syringe pump (central venous access preferred). Dilute with dextrose or normal saline (NS). Recommended concentration is 10 µg/mL. **Precautions:** Use cautiously in neonates with bleeding tendencies. If hypotension or pyrexia occurs, reduce infusion until symptoms subside. Severe hypotension, apnea, or bradycardia require drug discontinuation with cautious reinstitution at a lower dose. Apnea occurs in about 10% of neonates with congenital heart defects (especially in those weighing less than 2 kg at birth) and usually appears during the first hour of drug infusion. *Be prepared to intubate and resuscitate.* **Contraindications:** Respiratory distress syndrome, persistent pulmonary hypertension, coagulation abnormalities. **Adverse reactions:** apnea, respiratory depression, flushing, bradycardia, fever, seizurelike activity, systemic hypotension, hypocalcemia, hypoglycemia, and cortical proliferation of long bones has been seen with long-term infusions; diarrhea, gastric-outlet obstruction secondary to antral hyperplasia (occurrence related to duration of therapy and cumulative dose), inhibition of platelet aggregation.

AMINOPHYLLINE

Classification: Respiratory stimulant, bronchodilator.
Dosage/administration:

TABLE A.2

Indications	Dosage/Administration*
Apnea of prematurity	*Load:* 5 mg/kg/dose, IV (infuse for 30 min) or PO *Maintenance:* 6 mg/kg/day, IV, PO, divided Q6–8h. Start maintenance dose 6 to 8 h after loading dose
Bronchodilator	*IV load:* 6 mg/kg/dose, IV (infuse for 30 min). Each 1 mg/kg raises the serum theophylline concentration 2 mg/L *Maintenance:* 8 mg/kg/day IV or PO divided Q6h

IV = intravenously; PO = orally; Q6h = every 6 hours; Q8h = every 8 hours.
*When switching from intravenous to **oral aminophylline**, consider increasing dose by 20%. No dosage change is required when switching from intravenous **aminophylline** to **oral theophylline** (see Theophylline).

Precautions: Intramuscular administration causes intense local pain and sloughing. **Monitoring:** Heart rate, blood glucose periodically during loading-dose therapy, agitation, feeding intolerance. Withhold dose for heart rate greater than 180 beats per minute. Monitor serum trough levels before the fifth dose. Consider checking earlier if toxicity is suspected or spells increase in number or severity. If level is low, give a partial bolus of 1.0 mg/kg for each desired 2 mcg/mL in serum theophylline concentration. **Therapeutic ranges:** Apnea of prematurity: 7 to 10 µg/mL; bronchospasm: 10 to 20 µg/mL. **Adverse reactions:** Gastrointenstinal upset, arrhythmias, seizures, tachycardia (heart rate greater than 180 beats per minute) warrants determination of serum levels to detect excessive aminophylline levels.

AMPHOTERICIN-B LIPOSOME (AMBISOME)

Classification: Systemic antifungal agent. **Indication:** Treatment of suspected or proven systemic fungal infections.
Dosage/administration: 5 mg/kg IV q 24h infused over 2 h. Max concentration for infusion is 2mg/mL. Average duration of therapy is 2 to 4 weeks. **Precautions:** Concurrent use with other nephrotoxic medications may lead to additive nephrotoxicity. Corticosteroids may increase the potassium depletion caused by amphotericin. May intensify toxicity to neuromuscular blocking agents (e.g., pancuronium) secondary to hypokalemia. Use with caution in patients with electrolyte instabilities. **Do not confuse with conventional amphotericin-B or other lipid–based forms of amphotericin. Contraindications:** Do not dilute with normal saline (NS) or mix with any other medication that is diluted in NS. Do not mix with any other medication or electrolytes to avoid precipitation. **Adverse reactions:** Hypokalemia, nephrotoxicity, liver function test (LFT) abnormalities, thrombocytopenia and tachycardia. **Monitoring:** Blood urea nitrogen (BUN), serum creatinine, LFTs, serum electrolytes, complete blood count (CBC), vitals, I's & O's, monitor EKG changes for signs of hypokalemia.

TABLE A.3

Dosage	Administration	Comments
Initial dose: 0.25–0.5 mg/kg IV, Q24h	Dilute in dextrose to concentration of 0.1 mg/mL for peripheral lines or 0.5 mg/mL for central lines Infuse over 2 h	
Maintenance dose: Daily dose increased by 0.125 to 0.25 mg/kg/day Q24–48h until maximum daily dose of 0.5–1 mg/kg IV Q24h		Average duration of therapy is 2 to 4 weeks

IV = intravenously; Q24h = every 24 hours; Q48h = every 48 hours.

AMPICILLIN

Classification: Semisynthetic penicillinase-sensitive penicillin. **Indications:** Combined with either an aminoglycoside or cephalosporin for the prevention and treatment of infections with group B streptococci and Listeria monocytogenes. **Dosage/administration:**

TABLE A.4

Age	Weight	Dose
≤ 7 days	—	150 mg/kg/dose IV Q12h
>7 days	<1.2 kg	50–150 mg/kg/dose IV Q12h
>7 days	1.2 kg–2 kg	25–50 mg/kg/dose IV Q8h
>7 days	>2 kg	25–50 mg/kg/dose IV Q6h

IV = intravenously; Q12h = every 12 hours; Q8h = every 8 hours; Q6h = every 6 hours.

Infused over 15 minutes on syringe pump. Maximum final concentration for administration is 100 mg/mL in normal saline (NS). Intramuscular administration associated with sterile abscess formation. **Precautions:** Dosage adjustment for renal impairment. **Drug interactions:** Blunting of peak aminoglycoside concentration if administered simultaneously with ampicillin. Administer after aminoglycoside level is drawn. **Adverse reactions:** Diarrhea, hypersensitivity reaction (rubellalike rash and fever), nephritis (typically preceded by eosinophilia), elevated transaminases, and penicillin encephalopathy (central nervous system excitation and seizure activity associated with large or rapidly administered doses).

ATROPINE SULFATE

Classification: Anticholinergic agent. **Indications:** Prolonged cardiopulmonary resuscitation unresponsive to epinephrine. **Dosage/administration:** Intravenous: 0.01 to 0.03 mg/kg/dose, every 10 to 15 minutes, for two to three doses as needed. Endotracheal tube: 0.01 to 0.03 mg/kg/dose. Administer undiluted form for intravenous and endotracheal tube administration. **Clinical considerations:** Effective oxygenation and ventilation must precede atropine treatment of bradycardia. Low doses (< 0.1 mg) may cause paradoxical bradycardia secondary to central action. Monitor heart rate. **Contraindications:** Tachycardia, narrow-angle glaucoma, thyrotoxicosis, gastrointestinal or genitourinary obstruction. **Precautions:** Spastic paralysis or central nervous system damage.

Adverse reactions: Tachycardia, mydriasis, cycloplegia, abdominal distention/ileus, urinary retention, arrhythmias, esophageal reflux. **Antidote:** Physostigmine.

CAFFEINE CITRATE

Classification: Respiratory stimulant. **Indications:** Apnea of prematurity. **Dosage/ administration:** *Loading dose:* 20 mg/kg intravenously. Infuse over 30 minutes on syringe pump. *Maintenance dose:* 5 to 12 mg/kg intravenously or orally daily, starting 24 hours after loading dose. May increase maintenance dose by 1 mg/kg/day every 72 hours up to a maximum of 12 mg/kg/day. Minibolus = 5 mg/kg/dose. Infuse intravenous maintenance dose over 10 minutes on a syringe pump. A small loading dose of caffeine citrate (10 mg/kg) is required when switching from aminophylline/theophylline to caffeine citrate. This is because it takes about a week for caffeine citrate to reach steady-state levels because of its long half-life. *Do not push intravenous doses of caffeine citrate.* **Precautions:** Do not use caffeine-base formulations because of different dosage requirements. Do not use caffeine preparations that contain sodium benzoate. **Adverse reactions:** Cardiac arrhythmias, tachycardia (withhold dose for heart rate greater than 180), insomnia, restlessness, irritability, nausea, vomiting, diarrhea. Consider a decrease in dose to treat the central nervous system or/and gastrointestinal side effects. **Monitoring parameters:** Monitor heart rate, number and severity of apnea spells.

CAPTOPRIL

Classification: Angiotensin-converting enzyme inhibitor. **Indication:** Antihypertensive agent, treatment of congestive heart failure. **Dosage/administration:** 0.05 to 0.5 mg/kg/dose orally every 8 to 12 hours. May increase to maximum dose of 1 mg/kg orally every 8 to 12 hours. Administer on an empty stomach 1 hour before or 2 hours after feedings if possible. Food decreases absorption by approximately 50%. Administration times need to be consistent. **Precautions:** Use with caution and modify dosage in patients with renal impairment. **Contraindications:** Angioedema, bilateral renal artery stenosis, hyperkalemia, renal failure. **Adverse reactions:** Hypotension, rash, fever, eosinophilia, neutropenia, gastrointestinal disturbances, cough, dyspnea, acute renal failure, hyperkalemia. Development of jaundice or elevated hepatic enzymes is reason for immediate drug withdrawal. **Monitoring parameters:** Monitor blood pressure for hypotension within 1 hour after first dose or after a new higher dose, blood urea nitrogen, serum creatinine, renal function, urine dipstick for protein, complete blood count with differential, serum potassium.

CEFOTAXIME SODIUM

Classification: Third-generation cephalosporin. **Indications:** Reserved for suspected or documented gram-negative meningitis or sepsis. Combine with ampicillin or aqueous penicillin G for empiric therapy.
Dosage/administration:

Table A.5

Age	Dosage
≤ 7 days old	50 mg/kg/dose IV/IM Q12h
> 7 days old	50 mg/kg/dose IV/IM Q8h

IM = intramuscularly; IV = intravenously; Q8h = every 8 hours; Q12h = every 12 hours.

Maximum concentration for infusion is 100 mg/mL in dextrose 5% water (D5W), dextrose 10% water (D10W), or normal saline (NS). Infuse over 30 minutes on syringe pump. Maximum concentration for intramuscular dose is 300 mg/mL. **Precautions:** Dosage modification for impaired renal function. **Monitoring:** Complete blood count, blood urea nitrogen, creatinine, liver function tests (LFTs). **Drug interactions:** Blunting of peak aminoglycoside concentration if administered less than 2 hours before/after cefotaxime. **Adverse reactions:** Leukopenia, granulocytopenia, pseudomembranous colitis, positive direct Coombs' test, serum-sicknesslike reaction, and transient elevation of blood urea nitrogen, creatinine, eosinophils, and liver enzymes.

CEFTAZIDIME

Classification: Third-generation cephalosporin. **Indications:** Broad-spectrum cephalosporin and the only antipseudomonal cephalosporin. Treatment of gram-negative meningitis.
Dosage/administration:

TABLE A.6

Indication	Age	Dosage
Systemic infections	≤ 7 days old	50 mg/kg/dose IV/IM Q12h
Systemic infections	> 7 days old	50 mg/kg/dose IV/IM Q8h
Meningitis	All	50 mg/kg/dose IV/IM Q8h

IM = intramuscularly; IV = intravenously; Q8h = every 8 hours; Q12h = every 12 hours.

Final concentration for infusion is 100 mg/mL in dextrose 5% water (D5W) or normal saline (NS). Infuse over 30 minutes on syringe pump. **Clinical considerations:** Treat serious pseudomonal infections with ceftazidime in combination with an aminoglycoside. **Precautions:** Modify dosage for renal impairment. **Drug interaction:** Blunting of peak aminoglycoside concentration if administered simultaneously with ceftazidime. **Monitoring:** Complete blood count, renal and liver function tests (LFTs). **Adverse reactions:** Transient leukopenia and bone marrow suppression, positive direct Coombs' test, candidiasis, hemolytic anemia, pseudomembranous colitis, and transient elevation of eosinophils, platelets, renal, and LFTs.

CEFTRIAXONE SODIUM

Classification: Third-generation cephalosporin. **Indications:** Good activity against both gram-negative and gram-positive organisms except for *Pseudomonas spp.*, enterococci, methicillin-resistant staphylococci, and Listeria monocytogenes. Indicated for treatment of gonococcal meningitis and conjunctivitis. Not recommended for use in neonates with hyperbilirubinemia. Use cefotaxime instead.
Dosage/administration:

TABLE A.7

Indication	Dosage
Systemic infections	50 mg/kg/dose IV/IM Q24h
Meningitis	100 mg/kg IV/IM Q24h
Uncomplicated gonococcal ophthalmia	50 mg/kg IV/IM (max = 125 mg) single dose

IM = intramuscularly; IV = intravenously; Q24h = every 24 hours.

Maximum concentration for intravenous administration is 100 mg/mL in dextrose or saline. Infused over 30 minutes on syringe pump. Reconstitute intramuscular doses with 1% lidocaine without epinephrine to reduce pain at injection site. Maximum concentration for intramuscular administration is 350 mg/mL. **Precautions:** Do not use in gallbladder, biliary tract, liver, or pancreatic disease. Consider cefotaxime or ceftazidime instead. **Clinical considerations:** Do not use as sole therapy for staphylococcal or pseudomonal infections. Combine with ampicillin for initial empiric therapy of meningitis. Ceftriaxone displaces bilirubin from albumin binding sites, leading to increased free-serum bilirubin levels. *Routine or frequent use of cephalosporins in the neonatal intensive care unit will quickly result in the emergence of resistant enteric organisms.* Clinicians are advised to use aminoglycosides combined with ampicillin or penicillin for initial empiric therapy of suspected or proven neonatal sepsis. **Monitoring:** Complete blood count, electrolytes, and renal/liver function tests (LFTs). **Adverse reactions:** Leukopenia, anemia, gastrointestinal intolerance, and rash. Transient increase in eosinophils, platelets, bleeding time, free serum bilirubin concentration, and renal/LFTs. Transient formation of gallbladder precipitates characterized by vomiting and cholelithiasis. Gastrointestinal tract bacterial or fungal overgrowth.

CHLORAL HYDRATE

Classification: Sedative, hypnotic. **Indications:** Sedative/hypnotic. **Dosage/administration:** 25 to 50 mg/kg/dose orally (PO) or rectally (PR), every 6 to 8 hours as needed. *Maximum dose:* 50 mg/kg/dose. To reduce gastric irritation, dilute in feedings or administer after feedings. **Precautions:** Rectal suppositories are not recommended because of unreliable release characteristics. Use caution with concurrent administration of furosemide and anticoagulants. **Clinical considerations:** No analgesic properties. Excitation may occur instead of sedation in infants with pain. Assess level of sedation. Accumulation of the toxic metabolite (trichloroethanol) and direct hyperbilirubinemia occur with repeated doses. **Contraindications:** Hepatic or renal impairment. **Adverse reactions:** Paradoxical excitation, gastrointestinal intolerance, allergic manifestations, leukopenia, eosinophilia, vasodilation, cardiopulmonary depression (especially when coadministered with barbiturates and opiates), cardiac arrhythmias.

CHLOROTHIAZIDE

Classification: Thiazide diuretic, loop diuretic. **Indications:** Fluid overload, pulmonary edema, bronchopulmonary dysplasia (BPD), congestive heart failure, and hypertension. **Dosage/administration:** 20 to 40 mg/kg/day orally, divided every 12 hours. Intravenously 2 to 8 mg/kg/day, divided every 12 hours. When converting from oral to intravenous dose, use one-half of the oral dose. Intramuscular and subcutaneous (SC) administration not recommended because of local pain and irritation. **Contraindications:** Anuria or hepatic dysfunction. **Drug interactions:** Reduced antihypertensive effect with concurrent nonsteroidal anti-inflammatory drug use. **Monitoring:** Serum electrolytes, calcium, blood glucose, urine output, blood pressure, and daily weight. **Adverse reactions:** Hypochloremic alkalosis, prerenal azotemia, volume depletion, blood dyscrasias, decreased serum potassium and magnesium levels, and increased levels of glucose, uric acid, lipids, bilirubin, and calcium.

CITRATE MIXTURES, ORAL

Classification: Electrolyte supplement. **Indications:** Metabolic acidosis. **Dosage/administration:** 0.5 to 1 mEq/kg/dose, orally 3 or 4 times per day. Give with feedings. Adjust dose to maintain desired urine pH. One mEq citrate equivalent to 1 mEq HCO_3. **Content (mEq) in each mL of citrate mixture:**

TABLE A.8

Citrate mixtures	Na+	K+	Citrate
Polycitra	1	1	2
Polycitra-K	0	2	2
Bicitra	1	0	1
Oracit	1	0	1

Precautions: Use with caution in infants receiving potassium supplements. **Adverse reactions:** Laxative effect.

CLINDAMYCIN

Classification: Anaerobic antibiotic. **Indications:** Treatment of *B. fragilis* septicemia, peritonitis, necrotizing enterocolitis. Not indicated for meningitis. **Dosage/administration:**

TABLE A.9

Age	Dosage
Corrected gestational age ≤ 29 weeks	7.5 mg/kg/dose IV Q12h
Corrected gestational age > 29 weeks	7.5 mg/kg/dose IV Q8h

IV = intravenously; Q8h = every 8 hours; Q12h = every 12 hours.

Final concentration of 10 mg/mL in dextrose 5% water (D5W) or normal saline (NS). Infuse over 30 minutes on syringe pump. Maximum concentration for infusion is 18 mg/mL. Intramuscular administration associated with sterile abscess formation. **Contraindications:** Hepatic impairment. **Warnings:** Can cause severe and possibly fatal pseudomembranous colitis characterized by severe persistent diarrhea and possibly the passage of blood and mucus. **Drug interactions:** Potentiates neuromuscular blockade of tubocurarine, pancuronium. **Adverse reactions:** Pseudomembranous colitis, Stevens-Johnson syndrome, glossitis, pruritus, granulocytopenia, thrombocytopenia, hypotension, and increased liver function tests (LFTs).

DIAZOXIDE

Classification: Antihypoglycemic agent. **Indications:** Hyperinsulinemic hypoglycemia. **Dosage/administration:** 8 to 15 mg/kg/day, orally, divided every 8 to 12 hours. **Clinical considerations:** Used only for glucose-refractory hypoglycemia. **Contraindications:** Compensatory hypertension associated with aortic coarctation or arteriovenous (AV) shunts. **Precautions:** Diabetes mellitus, renal or liver disease. May displace bilirubin from albumin. **Monitoring:** Blood pressure, complete blood count, serum uric acid levels. **Drug interactions:** Phenytoin. **Adverse reactions:** Hyperglycemia (insulin reverses diazoxide-induced hyperglycemia), ketoacidosis, sodium and water retention, hypotension, hyponatremia, extrapyramidal symptoms, seizures, arrhythmias, leukopenia, thrombocytopenia, and hyperosmolar coma.

DIGOXIN

Classification: Antiarrhythmic agent, inotrope. **Indications:** Heart failure, paroxysmal atrioventricular nodal tachycardia, atrial fibrillation/flutter. **Dosage/administration:** Reserve total digitalizing dose (TDD) for treatment of arrhythmias and acute congestive heart failure. Administer TDD over 24 hours in 3 divided doses: first dose is one-half TDD, second dose is one-fourth TDD administered 8 hours after first dose, and third dose is one-fourth TDD administered 8 hours after second dose.
Administer intravenous doses over 10 minutes on syringe pump. Utilize maintenance dose schedule for nonacute arrhythmia and congestive heart failure conditions. Do not administer intramuscularly. The pediatric intravenous formulation (100 μg/mL) may be given undiluted. The pediatric oral elixir is 50 μg/mL. **Precautions:** Reduce dose for renal and hepatic impairment. Cardioversion or calcium infusion may precipitate ventricular fibrillation in the digoxin-treated neonate (may be prevented by lidocaine pretreatment). **Monitoring:** Heart rate/rhythm for desired effects and signs of toxicity,

TABLE A.10

	Total Digitalizing Dose		Maintenance Dose	
Age	PO	IV	PO	IV
< 37 weeks	20–30 µg/kg/day	15–25 µg/kg/day	5–7.5 µg/kg/day	4–6 µg/kg/day
≥ 37 weeks	25–35 µg/kg/day	20–30 µg/kg/day	6–10 µg/kg/day	5–8 µg/kg/day

IV = intravenously; PO = orally.

serum calcium, magnesium (especially in neonates receiving diuretics and amphotericin B, both of which predispose to digoxin toxicity). **Therapeutic levels:** 0.8 to 2 mg/mL. Neonates may have falsely elevated digoxin levels as a result of maternal digoxinlike substances. **Contraindications:** Atrioventricular block, idiopathic hypertrophic subaortic stenosis, ventricular dysrhythmias, atrial fibrillation/flutter with slow ventricular rates, or constrictive pericarditis. **Drug interactions:** Amiodarone, erythromycin, cholestyramine, indomethacin, spironolactone, quinidine, verapamil, and metoclopramide. **Adverse reactions:** Persistent vomiting, feeding intolerance, diarrhea, and lethargy, shortening of QT_c interval, sagging ST segment, diminished T-wave amplitude, bradycardia, prolongation of PR interval, sinus bradycardia or S-A block, atrial or nodal ectopic beats, ventricular arrhythmias. Toxicity enhanced by hypokalemia. Treat life-threatening digoxin toxicity with Digoxin Immune Fab.

DOBUTAMINE

Classification: Sympathomimetic, adrenergic agonist agent. **Indications:** Treatment of hypoperfusion, hypotension, short-term management of cardiac decompensation. **Dosage/administration:** 5 to 25 µg/kg/min continuous intravenous infusion on intravenous pump. Begin at a low dose and titrate to obtain desired mean arterial pressure. Central *venous* access is preferred. ***Do not administer via* umbilical arterial catheter (UAC).** Maximum concentration is 90 mg/100 mL = 900 µg/mL in normal saline (NS) or dextrose. **Precautions:** Hypovolemia should be corrected before use. Infiltration causes local inflammatory changes. Extravasation may cause dermal necrosis. Use phentolamine to treat extravasation. **Contraindications:** Idiopathic hypertrophic subaortic stenosis. **Adverse reactions:** Hypotension if hypovolemic, arrhythmias, tachycardia (with high doses), cutaneous vasodilation, increased blood pressure and dyspnea. **Monitoring:** Continuous heart rate and arterial blood pressure.

DOPAMINE

Classification: Sympathomimetic, adrenergic agonist agent. **Indications:** Treatment of hypotension. **Dosage/administration:** 2.5 to 25 µg/kg/min via continuous intravenous infusion on intravenous pump. Once 20 to 25 µg/kg/min is reached, consideration should be given to adding a second pressor. Clinical benefits have been noted at doses of up to 40 µg/kg/min. Begin at a low dose and titrate to obtain desired mean arterial pressure. Central *venous* access preferred. ***Do not administer via* umbilical arterial catheter (UAC).** Maximum concentration is 90 mg/100 mL = 900 µg/mL mixed in normal saline (NS) or dextrose. **Precautions:** Hypovolemia should be corrected before use. Extravasation may cause tissue necrosis. Treat dopamine extravasation with phentolamine. **Contraindications:** Pheochromocytoma, tachyarrhythmias, or hypovolemia may increase pulmonary artery pressure. Use with caution in neonates with pulmonary hypertension. **Adverse reactions:** Arrhythmias, tachycardia, vasoconstriction, hypotension, widened QRS complex, bradycardia, hypertension, excessive diuresis and azotemia, reversible suppression of prolactin and thyrotropin secretion. **Monitoring parameters:** Continuous heart rate and arterial blood pressure, urine output, peripheral perfusion.

ENALAPRILAT

Classification: Angiotensin-converting enzyme inhibitor, antihypertensive. **Indications:** Hypertension, congestive heart failure. **Dosage/administration:** *Neonatal hypertension:* Enalaprilat: 5 to 10 µg/kg/dose (0.005–0.01 mg/kg/dose), intravenously every 8 to 24 hours. *Congestive heart failure:* Enalapril maleate: Initial dose: 0.1 mg/kg/day orally every 24 hours; may be given without regard to feeding times; increased according to response, every 3 to 4 days, to a maximum of 0.43 mg/kg/day. Oral suspension prepared by dissolving a crushed 2.5-mg tablet in 12.5 mL of sterile water, yielding final concentration of 0.2 mg/mL (200 µg/mL). Use immediately, discard remaining portion. **Precautions:** Impaired renal function. **Monitoring:** Blood pressure, renal function, serum electrolytes. Hold for mean arterial pressure less than 30 and heart rate less than 100. **Adverse reactions:** Transient or prolonged episodes of hypotension, oliguria, mild nonoliguric renal failure, hypotension in volume-depleted neonates, and hyperkalemia in neonates receiving potassium supplements and/or potassium-sparing diuretics.

ENOXAPARIN

Classification: Low-molecular-weight heparin, anticoagulant. **Indication:** Prophylaxis and treatment of thromboembolic disorders. **Dosage/administration:** Prophylaxis: 0.75 mg/kg/dose subcutaneously every 12 hours. Treatment: 1.5 mg/kg/dose subcutaneously every 12 hours. **Clinical considerations:** Adjust dose to maintain anti–factor Xa level between 0.5 and 1.0 U/mL. Peak anti–factor Xa activity is obtained 4 hours after dose. For subcutaneous administration only. To minimize bruising, do not administer intramuscularly or intravenously; do not rub injection site. **Precautions:** Reduce dose by 30% in severe renal impairment. **Contraindications:** Avoid in infants who require spinal puncture to minimize risk of epidural/spinal hematoma. **Adverse effects:** Fever, edema, hemorrhage, thrombocytopenia, pain/erythema at injection site.

EPINEPHRINE

Classification: Adrenergic agent. **Indications:** Cardiac arrest, refractory hypotension, bronchospasm.
Dosage/administration:

TABLE A.11

Indication	Dose	Comments
Severe bradycardia and hypotension	IV push: 0.1 to 0.3 mL/kg of **1:10,000** concentration (equal to 0.01–0.03 mg/kg or 10–30 µg/kg) Endotracheal tube (ETT): 0.1 to 0.3 mL/kg of **1:10,000** concentration (equal to 0.01–0.03 mg/kg or 10–30 µg/kg)	May repeat 2 to 3 times Q3–5 min.
Continuous IV	Start at 0.1 µg/kg/min. Adjust dose to desired response, to a max of 1 µg/kg/min	Use the **1:1,000** formulation for mixing continuous IV preparations. Max IV concentration = 1 mg/50 mL

IV = intravenous; Q3–5 min = every 3 to 5 minutes.

Monitoring: Continuous heart rate and blood pressure monitoring. **Drug interactions:** Incompatible with alkaline solutions (sodium bicarbonate). **Precautions:** Note the differences in concentration for emergency administration and continuous intravenous epinephrine doses. High doses of preservative-containing epinephrine will necessitate caution in selection of epinephrine preparations. Always use a 1:10,000 concentration (0.1 mg/mL) for individual doses, endotracheal tube doses, and for emergency administration (IV and endotracheal). Use the 1:1000 concentration for preparation of continuous infusions. Correction of acidosis before administration of catecholamines enhances their effectiveness. **Contraindications:** Hyperthyroidism, hypertension, and diabetes. **Adverse reactions:** Ventricular arrhythmias, tachycardia, pallor and tremor, severe hypertension with possible intraventricular hemorrhage, myocardial ischemia, hypokalemia, and decreased renal and splanchnic blood flow. Intravenous infiltration may cause tissue ischemia and necrosis (consider treatment with phentolamine).

EPINEPHRINE RACEMIC

Classification: Adrenergic agonist. **Indications:** Treatment of postextubation stridor. **Dosage/administration:** 0.25 to 0.5 mL of 2.25% *racemic epinephrine* solution diluted in 3 mL normal saline (NS). Given by nebulizer every 2 hours as needed. **Clinical considerations:** Observe closely for rebound airway edema. Closely monitor heart rate (hold for heart rate greater than 180 beats per minute) and blood pressure during administration. **Adverse reactions:** Tachyarrhythmias, hypokalemia.

ERYTHROMYCIN

Classification: Macrolide antibiotic. **Indications:** Treatment of infections caused by chlamydia, mycoplasma, and ureaplasma; treatment and prophylaxis of *Bordetella pertussis* and ophthalmia neonatorum; also used as a prokinetic agent.
Dosage/administration:

TABLE A.12

Indication	Dosage	Comment
Systemic infections	E. Estolate (Ilosone): 10 mg/kg/dose PO Q8h. E. Ethylsuccinate (ESS, EryPed): 10 mg/kg/dose PO Q6h.	Administer with feeding to enhance absorption of E. Ethylsuccinate and to reduce possible GI upset
Severe systemic infections or PO route unavailable	5–10 mg/kg/dose, IV Q6h. (Dilute to 1–5 mg/mL and infuse over 1 h)	Use only preservative-free IV erythromycin formulations
Ophthalmia neonatorum	Prophylaxis: 0.5–1 cm ribbon of 0.5% ointment into each conjunctival sac × 1	Administered at birth
Chlamydia conjunctivitis	0.5–1 cm ribbon of 0.5% ointment into each conjunctival sac Q6h × 7 days	PO therapy is preferable to topical therapy for eradication of nasopharyngeal carrier state. Treat mother and her sexual partner
Prokinetic agent	Initial: 3 mg/kg/ IV over 60 minutes, followed by 20 mg/kg/day PO in 3–4 divided doses 30 minutes before meals	
Ureaplasma urealyticum	5–10 mg/kg/dose PO or IV Q6h and treat for 10–14 days	

GI = gastrointestinal; IV = intravenously; PO = orally; Q6h = every 6 hours; Q8h = every 8 hours.

Precautions: Do not administer intramuscularly (causes pain and necrosis). Cholestatic jaundice occurs with estolate. Hepatotoxicity can occur with preexisting liver impairment. **Contraindications:** Preexisting hepatic dysfunction. **Drug interactions:** Increased blood levels of carbamazepine, digoxin, cyclosporine, warfarin, methylprednisolone, and theophylline. **Test interactions:** False-positive urine catecholamines. **Monitoring:** Liver function tests (LFTs), complete blood count (eosinophilia). **Adverse reactions:** Anaphylaxis, rash, stomatitis, candidiasis, hepatotoxicity, ototoxicity (high-dose erythromycin), intrahepatic cholestasis, and vomiting.

FENTANYL CITRATE

Classification: Narcotic analgesic. **Indication:** Analgesia, sedation, anesthesia. **Dosage/administration:** *Sedation/analgesia:* Intravenous: 1 to 5 µg/kg/dose every 2 to 4 hours over 10 minutes on syringe pump. Maximum concentration for continuous intravenous infusion is 10 µg/mL in NS or dextrose. *Bolus:* 1 to 2 µg/kg; then 1 to 5 µg/kg/hr titrate as needed. *Intravenous bolus:* Mix 1 cc of 100 µg/2 cc fentanyl in 9 cc NS<, mixture = 10 µg/cc of fentanyl. *Anesthesia:* 5 to 50 µg/kg per dose. **Precautions:** Give intravenous bolus dose over 10 minutes on syringe pump to avoid apnea and fentanyl-induced decreased total lung and chest wall compliance. **Contraindications:** Increased intracranial pressure, severe respiratory depression, severe liver or renal insufficiency. **Adverse reactions:** Central nervous system and respiratory depression, skeletal/thoracic muscle rigidity, vomiting, constipation, peripheral vasodilation, miosis, biliary or urinary tract spasms and antidiuretic hormone release; tolerance develops in association with continuous intravenous infusions for more than 5 days. **Monitoring:** Respiration rate (RR), heart rate, blood pressure, abdominal status, muscle rigidity. Adherence to extracorporeal membrane oxygenation (ECMO) membranes may necessitate increased dose.

FERROUS SULFATE

Classification: Oral mineral supplement. **Indication:** Prophylaxis for prevention of iron-deficiency anemia in preterm newborns. **Dosage/administration:** 2 to 4 mg of elemental iron/kg/day orally every day. Ferrous sulfate drops contain 25 mg elemental iron/mL. Iron supplements are available in different concentrations. When ordering, specify exact amount in mg to avoid over- or underdosing. Iron supplementation may increase hemolysis if adequate vitamin E therapy is not supplied. Start iron therapy no later than 2 months of age. **Clinical considerations:** Absorption is variable. **Contraindications:** Peptic ulcer disease, ulcerative colitis, enteritis, hemochromatosis, and hemolytic anemia. **Drug interactions:** Decreased absorption of both iron and tetracycline when given together. Antacids and chloramphenicol decrease iron absorption. **Monitoring:** Hemoglobin and reticulocyte counts during therapy. Observe stools (may color the stool black and cause false-positive guaiac test for blood), and monitor for constipation. **Adverse reactions:** Constipation, diarrhea, and gastrointestinal irritation. **Overdose:** Serum iron level greater than 300 mcg/dL usually requires treatment because of severe toxicity; acute gastrointestinal irritation, erosion of gastrointestinal mucosa, hematemesis, lethargy, acidosis, hepatic and renal dysfunction, circulatory collapse, coma, and death. Antidote is deferoxamine chelation therapy. Gastric lavage with 1 to 5% sodium bicarbonate or sodium phosphate solution prevents additional absorption of iron.

FLUCONAZOLE

Classification: Systemic antifungal agent. **Indications:** Treatment of systemic fungal infections, meningitis, and severe superficial mycoses. Alternative to amphotericin-B in patients with preexisting renal impairment or when concomitant therapy with other potentially nephrotoxic drugs is required. **Dosage/administration:** *Systemic infection, meningitis:* Loading 12 mg/kg intravenously/orally followed 24 hours later by 6 mg/kg intravenously/orally every day. *Oropharyngeal/esophageal candidiasis:* 6 mg/kg intravenously/orally on day 1, then 3 mg/kg intravenously/orally daily. Administer intravenous dose on syringe pump for 30 minutes. **Clinical considerations:** Well-absorbed orally. Good cerebrospinal fluid penetration by both intravenous and oral routes. **Precautions:** Adjust dosage for impaired renal function. **Drug interactions:** Warfarin, phenytoin, rifampin. Possible interference with metabolism of caffeine and theophylline. **Monitoring:** Renal and liver function tests (LFTs). **Adverse reactions:** Vomiting, diarrhea, exfoliative skin disorders, and reversible increased aspartate aminotransferase, alanine aminotransferase, alkaline phosphatase.

FOLIC ACID

Classification: Vitamin, mineral, nutritional supplement. **Indication:** Treatment of megaloblastic and macrocytic anemias as a result of folate deficiency. **Dosage/administration:** 15 µg/kg/dose or up to maximum of 50 µg/day. May be given orally/intramuscularly/intravenously/subcutaneously. The parenteral form may be diluted to a concentration of 0.1 mg/mL (100 µg/mL) and administered orally. Administer deeply if intramuscular route is used. The oral form may be given without regard to feeds. **Clinical considerations:** May mask hematologic defects of vitamin B_{12} deficiency, but will not prevent progression of irreversible neurologic abnormalities, despite the absence of anemia. **Precautions:** The injection contains benzyl alcohol (1.5%) as a preservative; avoid using in preterm infants. **Contraindications:** Pernicious, aplastic, and normocytic anemias. **Drug interactions:** May decrease phenytoin serum concentrations. **Monitoring parameters:** Hematocrit, hemoglobin, reticulocyte. **Adverse effects:** Gastrointestinal upset, slight flushing but generally well tolerated.

FOSPHENYTOIN

Classification: Anticonvulsant. **Indications:** Management of generalized convulsive status epilepticus refractory to phenobarbital. For short term (< 5 days) parenteral (intravenous or intramuscular) administration when other means of phenytoin administration are unavailable, inappropriate, or less advantageous. **Dosage/ administration:** PE: phenytoin equivalent. Fosphenytoin 1 mg PE = Phenytoin 1 mg = Fosphenytoin 1.5 mg. *Loading dose:* 15 to 20 mg PE/kg intramuscularly or intravenously. Infuse loading dose over 10 minutes on syringe pump. *Maintenance dose:* 4 to 8 mg PE/kg intramuscularly or intravenously, slow push every 24 hours. Begin maintenance dose 24 hours after the loading dose. Modify dose in infants with hepatic or renal impairment. Maximum concentration for intravenous or intramuscular administration is 25 mg/mL. Flush intravenous line with normal saline (NS) before/after administration. **Precautions:** To avoid medication errors, always prescribe and dispense fosphenytoin in mg of PE. Consider the amount of phosphate delivered by fosphenytoin in infants who require phosphate restriction. Each 1 mg PE fosphenytoin delivers 0.0037 mmol of phosphate. Use with caution in infants with hyperbilirubinemia. Fosphenytoin and bilirubin compete with phenytoin and displace phenytoin from plasma protein-binding sites. This results in an increased serum concentration of free phenytoin. Use with caution in hypotension and myocardial insufficiency. **Contraindications:** Heart block, sinus bradycardia. **Adverse reactions:** Hypotension, vasodilation, tachycardia, bradycardia, fever, hyperglycemia, neutropenia, thrombocytopenia, megaloblastic anemia, osteomalacia. **Monitoring considerations:** Monitor blood pressure, electrocardiogram during intravenous loading doses. **Monitoring parameters:** Therapeutic levels: 10 to 20 mg/L total phenytoin *or* 1 to 2 mg/L unbound phenytoin only. **Guidelines for obtaining levels:** Obtain phenytoin levels 2 hours after end of intravenous infusion or 4 hours after intramuscular dose. Obtain the first level 48 hours after the loading dose.

FUROSEMIDE

Classification: Loop diuretic. **Indications:** Management of pulmonary edema. To provide diuresis and improve lung function when a greater diuretic effect than produced by chlorothiazide (DIURIL) is needed. **Dosage/administration:** Intravenous =

1 mg/kg/dose. Oral = 2 mg/kg/dose. For long-term use, consider alternate day therapy or longer (every 48–72 hours) in order to prevent toxicities. Give with feeds to reduce gastrointestinal irritation. Give the alcohol and sugar-free product to neonates. Intravenous form may be used orally. **Monitoring:** Follow daily weight changes, urine output, serum phosphate, and serum electrolytes. Closely monitor potassium levels in neonates receiving digoxin. **Precautions:** Use with caution in hepatic and renal disease. **Adverse reactions:** Fluid and electrolyte imbalance, hypokalemia, hypocalcemia/hypercalciuria, hypochloremic alkalosis, nephrocalcinosis (associated with long-term therapy), potential ototoxicity (especially if receiving aminoglycosides), prerenal azotemia, hyperuricemia, agranulocytosis, anemia, thrombocytopenia, interstitial nephritis, pancreatitis, and cholelithiasis [in bronchopulmonary dysplasia (BPD) or congestive heart failure and long-term total parenteral nutrition and furosemide therapy].

GAMMA GLOBULIN

Classification: Immune globulin. **Indications:** Alloimmune thrombocytopenia. **Dosage/administration:** 0.8 to 1.0 g/kg intravenously for 1 to 2 doses given over 2 to 3 hours. Usual concentration for intravenous administration is 5 to 10% (50–100 mg/mL). Maximum concentration for infusion is 12% (12% concentration should be given via central line). **Precautions:** Delay immunizations with live virus vaccines until 3 to 11 months after intravenous immunoglobulin administration. **Monitoring:** Continuous heart rate and blood pressure monitoring during administration. **Adverse reactions:** Transient hypoglycemia, tachycardia, and hypotension (resolved with cessation of infusion). Tenderness, erythema, and induration at injection site and allergic manifestations. Rare hypersensitivity reactions reported with rapid intravenous administration.

GANCICLOVIR

Classification: Antiviral agent. **Indications:** Treatment or prophylaxis of cytomegalovirus (CMV) infections. **Dosages/administration:** For congenital CMV infection, 10 to 15 mg/kg/day divided every 12 hours for 3 to 6 weeks; infuse over 1 hour on syringe pump. Maximum concentration for infusion must not exceed 10 mg/mL in dextrose or normal saline (NS). *Administer via central line to minimize risk of phlebitis.* If central line is not available, it may be administered peripherally at a concentration no greater than 2 mg/mL. Do not administer intramuscularly or subcutaneously to avoid severe tissue irritation that is due to its high pH. **Precautions:** Treat ganciclovir as *cytotoxic* drug. *Avoid all contact* with skin and mucous membranes. Wear impervious protective gown, nonlatex procedure gloves, and mask. Priming of intravenous set should not allow any drug to be released into the environment. **Contraindications:** For infants with neutropenia with an absolute neutrophil count less than 500 or thrombocytopenia with a platelet count less than 25,000. Consider treatment with G-CSF (Neupogen) in patients with neutropenia. Adjust dose in renal impairment. Avoid dehydration during therapy. **Adverse reactions:** Neutropenia, thrombocytopenia, anemia. Thrombocytopenia is usually reversible and responds to a decreased dose. Inflammation at intravenous site. Increased liver function tests (LFTs), increased blood urea nitrogen/serum creatinine, decrease dosage if renal function worsens. **Monitoring considerations:** Obtain daily complete blood count with differential and platelet count. Obtain weekly blood urea nitrogen, serum creatinine. At the first sign of significant renal dysfunction, the dose of ganciclovir should be adjusted by either reducing the number of mg/dose or by prolonging the dosing interval.

GENTAMICIN SULFATE

Classification: Aminoglycoside, antibiotic. **Indications:** Active against gram-negative aerobic bacteria, some activity against coagulase-positive staphylococci, ineffective against anaerobes, streptococci.

Dosage/administration:

TABLE A.13

Age	IV Dosage
< 35 weeks corrected gestational age	3 mg/kg/dose Q24h
≥ 35 weeks corrected gestational age	4 mg/kg/dose Q24h

IV = intravenous; Q24h = every 24 hours.

Administer intravenous infusion on syringe pump over 30 minutes. Intravenous route preferred because intramuscular absorption is variable. **Precautions:** Modify dosage in patients with renal impairment. **Drug interactions:** Indomethacin decreases gentamicin clearance and prolongs its half-life. Increased neuromuscular blockade is observed when aminoglycosides are used with neuromuscular blocking agents (e.g., pancuronium). The risk of aminoglycoside-induced ototoxicity and/or nephrotoxicity is increased when used concurrently with loop diuretics (e.g., furosemide, bumetanide) or vancomycin. Penicillins, cephalosporins, amphotericin B, blunt gentamicin serum peak concentration if administered less than 1 hour before/after these agents. Neuromuscular weakness or respiratory failure may occur in infants with hypermagnesemia. **Adverse reactions:** Vestibular and auditory ototoxicity (associated with high peak and trough levels) and renal toxicity (occurs in the proximal tubule, associated with high trough levels, usually reversible). Treat extravasation with hyaluronidase around periphery of affected area. **Monitoring considerations:** Assess renal function. **Guidelines for obtaining levels:** Draw trough levels within 30 minutes before the next dose. Draw peak levels at 30 minutes after the end of a 30-minute infusion or 1 hour after an intramuscular injection. **Monitoring parameters:** For all infants, *obtain blood levels pre– and post–third dose. Trough:* Less than 1.5 µg/mL. *Peak:* 6 to 15 µg/mL. *Dose adjustment:* For trough levels between 1.5 and 2.0 µg/mL, obtain another trough with next dose. For trough greater than 2.0 µg/mL, increase interval by 12 hours. For peak less than 6 µg/mL, increase dose by 20 to 25% to achieve peak of 6 to 15. For peak greater than 15 µg/mL, decrease dose by 20 to 25% to achieve peak of 6 to 15.

GLUCAGON

Classification: Antihypoglycemic agent. **Indications:** Treatment of hypoglycemia in cases of documented glucagon deficiency. **Dosage/administration:** 25 to 300 µg/kg/dose (0.025–0.3 mg/kg/dose) intravenous push/intramuscular/subcutaneous every 20 minutes as needed. *Maximum dose:* 1 mg. *Continuous intravenous:* Administer in dextrose 10% water (DW10) solution, starting at 0.5 mg/kg/day. Add hydrocortisone if no response within 4 hours. Further dosage increases greater than 2 mg/day unlikely to be effective. After effect seen, slowly taper over at least 24 hours. Compatible with dextrose solutions. **Contraindications:** Should not be used in small-for-gestational-age (SGA) infants. **Precautions:** Do not delay starting glucose infusion while awaiting effect of glucagon. Use caution in infants with history of insulinoma or pheochromocytoma. Incompatible with electrolyte-containing solutions. **Monitoring:** Serum glucose. **Adverse reactions:** Vomiting, tachycardia, hypertension, and gastrointestinal upset.

HEPARIN SODIUM

Classification: Anticoagulant. **Indications:** Line flushing for heparin locks and to maintain patency of single- and double-lumen central catheters.

Dosage/administration:

TABLE A.14

Indication	Dosage	Comment
Heparin lock for peripheral IV, central lines	1–2 mL of 10 U/mL solution Q4–6h and prn	To keep line open
Continuous infusion for central venous and/or arterial line	Add heparin to make a final concentration of 0.5–1 U/mL	To keep line open

IV = intravenous; prn = as needed; Q4–6h = every 4 to 6 hours.

Contraindications: Platelet count less than 50,000/mm^3, suspected intracranial hemorrhage, gastrointestinal bleeding, shock, severe hypotension, and uncontrolled bleeding. **Precautions:** Risk factors for hemorrhage include intramuscular injections, venous and arterial blood sampling, and peptic ulcer disease. Use preservative-free heparin in neonates. To avoid systemic heparinization in small neonates, use more dilute (0.5 U/mL) heparin flush concentrations. **Monitoring:** Follow platelet counts every 2 to 3 days. Assess for signs of bleeding and thrombosis. **Drug interactions:** Thrombolytic agents and intravenous nitroglycerin. **Adverse reactions:** Heparin-induced thrombocytopenia reported in some heparin-exposed newborns. Other adverse reactions include hemorrhage, fever, urticaria, vomiting, increased liver function tests (LFTs), osteoporosis, and alopecia. **Antidote:** Protamine sulfate (1 mg/100 U of heparin given in the previous 4 hours).

HYALURONIDASE

Classification: Antidote, extravasation. **Indications:** Prevention of tissue injury caused by intravenous extravasation of hyperosmolar or extremely alkaline solutions. **Dosage/administration:** Subcutaneous or intradermal: Dilute to 150 U/mL in normal saline (NS). Inject 5 separate 0.2-mL injections into the leading edge of the infiltrate. Use a 25- or 27-gauge needle, and change after each injection. Elevate the extremity. Do not apply heat and do not administer intravenously. Best results are obtained when used within 1 hour of extravasation. May repeat if necessary. **Clinical considerations:** Some agents for which hyaluronidase is effective include aminophylline, amphotericin, calcium, diazepam, erythromycin, gentamicin, methicillin, nafcillin, oxacillin, phenytoin, potassium chloride, sodium bicarbonate, tromethamine, vancomycin, total parenteral nutrition, and concentrated intravenous solutions. **Warnings:** Hyaluronidase is neither effective nor indicated for treatment of extravasations of vasoconstrictive agents (phentolamine is the preferred agent for treatment of extravasation with vasoconstrictive agents).

HYDRALAZINE

Classification: Antihypertensive, vasodilator. **Indication:** Blood pressure reduction in neonatal hypertension. After load reduction in congestive heart failure. **Dosage/administration:** *Initial dose:* 0.1 to 0.5 mg/kg/dose intravenously every 6 to 8 hours. Increase gradually to a maximum of 2 mg/kg/dose intravenously every 6 hours as required for blood pressure control. Usual concentration for intravenous administration is 1 mg/mL. Maximum concentration for intravenous administration is 20 mg/mL. *Oral dose:* 0.25 to 1 mg/kg/dose orally every 6 to 8 hours. Administer with food to enhance absorption. *Maximum dose:* 7 mg/kg/day. Double the dose when changing from intravenous to oral because hydralazine is only about 50% absorbed.

Precautions: Use with caution in severe renal and cardiac disease. **Clinical considerations:** May cause reflex tachycardia. Concurrent beta-blocker therapy recommended to reduce the magnitude of reflex tachycardia and to enhance antihypertensive effect. Maximum effect occurs in 3 to 4 days. Tachyphylaxis reported with chronic therapy. **Drug interactions:** Concurrent use with other antihypertensives allows reduced dosage requirements of hydralazine to less than 0.15 mg/kg/dose. **Monitoring:** Daily monitoring of heart rate, blood pressure, urine output, and weight. Guaiac all stools, and obtain complete blood count at least twice weekly. **Adverse reactions:** Tachycardia, vomiting, diarrhea, orthostatic hypotension, edema, gastrointestinal irritation and bleeding, anemia, and agranulocytosis.

HYDROCORTISONE

Classification: Adrenal corticosteroid. **Indication:** Blood pressure support for $\leq$ 28 weeks and $\leq$ 1000 g and/or inadequate response to volume or pressors adjunct therapy for persistent hypoglycemia; treatment of cortisol insufficiency. **Dosage/administration:** Give 1 mg/kg/dose intravenously initial dose; may only need 1 dose or may repeat in 8 hours. Give the first dose as a slow push over 3 to 5 minutes. Administer subsequent doses over 30 minutes on syringe pump. If response: 1 mg/kg intravenously Q12 $\times$ 1 then 0.5 mg/kg intravenously Q12 $\times$ 2 then discontinue (D/C). May repeat sequence. Final concentration for infusion is 1 mg/mL in dextrose or saline. Maximum infusion concentration is 10 mg/mL. Use preservative-free hydrocortisone sodium succinate formulation for intravenous dosing. **Precautions:** Acute adrenal insufficiency may occur with abrupt withdrawal following long-term therapy or during periods of stress. **Adverse reactions:** Hypertension, edema, cataracts, peptic ulcer, immunosuppression, hypokalemia, hyperglycemia, dermatitis, Cushing's syndrome, and skin atrophy.

INDOMETHACIN

Classification: Cardiovascular agent. **Indications:** Pharmacologic alternative to surgical closure of patent ductus arteriosus (PDA).
Dosage/administration:

TABLE A.15

Age at First Dose	First Dose (mg/kg/dose IV)	Second Dose (mg/kg/dose IV)	Third Dose (mg/kg/dose IV)
< 48 h	0.2	0.1	0.1
2–7 days	0.2	0.2	0.2
> 7 days	0.2	0.25	0.25

IV = intravenous.

Intravenous dosing only—oral dosing not recommended. Give by intravenous syringe pump over 30 minutes, 3 doses per course with a usual maximum of 2 courses, given at 12- to 24-hour intervals. Some infants require a longer treatment course (0.2 mg/kg every 24 hours for 5 to 7 days). **Clinical considerations**: Hold enteral feeds until 12 hours after last indomethacin dose. **Contraindications:** Impaired renal function (blood urea nitrogen greater than 30 mg/dL, urine output less than 0.6 mLkg/h for preceding 8 hours, and creatinine greater than 0.8 mg/dL), active bleeding, ulcer disease, necrotizing enterocolitis (NEC) or stool hema test greater than 3+, platelet count less than 60,000/mm³, and coagulation defects. **Precautions:** Use with caution in neonates with cardiac dysfunction and hypertension. Because indomethacin causes a decrease in renal and gastrointestinal blood flow, withhold enteral feedings during therapy. Reduction in cerebral flow reported with intravenous infusions of less than 5 minutes' duration. **Monitoring:** Urine output (keep >0.6 mL/kg/hour), serum electrolytes, serum blood urea nitrogen and creatinine, platelet count. Closely assess pulse pressure, cardiopulmonary status, and patent ductus arteriosus murmur for evidence of success/failure of therapy. Guaiac all stools and test gastric aspirates to detect gastrointestinal bleeding. Observe for prolonged bleeding from puncture sites. **Drug interactions:** Concurrent administration with digoxin and/or with aminoglycosides results in increased plasma concentrations of these respective agents. **Adverse reactions:** Decreased platelet aggregation, ulcer, gastrointestinal intolerance, hemolytic anemia, bone marrow suppression, agranulocytosis, thrombocytopenia, ileal perforation, transient oliguria, electrolyte imbalance, hypertension, hypoglycemia, indirect hyperbilirubinemia, and hepatitis.

INSULIN, REGULAR

Classification: Pancreatic hormone, hypoglycemic agent. **Indication:** Hyperglycemia, hyperkalemia. **Dosage/administration:** For intravenous bolus and intravenous infusion, use regular human insulin. Mix 15 units regular insulin in 150-mL intravenous bag normal saline (NS) or dextrose 5% water (D5W) = 10 U/100 mL or 0.1 U/mL. Maximum recommended concentration is 1 U/mL.

TABLE A.16

Indication	Dosage	Administration	Comment
Bolus	0.05–0.1 U/kg Q4–6h prn	Infuse over 15–20 minutes via syringe pump	Monitor glucose every 30 minutes to 1 hour
Continuous IV infusion	0.05–0.2 U/kg/h	If BG remains > 180 mg/dL, titrate in increments of 0.01 U/kg/hr. If hypoglycemia occurs, D/C insulin infusion and give D10W at 2 mL/kg (0.2 g/kg)	Before start of infusion, purge IV tubing with minimum of 25 mL of the infusion solution to saturate plastic binding sites. Titrate to maintain euglycemia
Hyperkalemia	First administer calcium gluconate 50 mg/kg/dose IV, then sodium bicarbonate 1 mEq/kg/dose IV. Calcium gluconate is *not* compatible with NaHCO$_3$. Flush IV lines between infusions	Follow with dextrose 300–600 mg/kg/dose + regular insulin 0.2 U/kg/dose IV	May repeat dose in 30 to 60 minutes or begin dextrose infusion at 0.25–0.5 g/kg/h with regular insulin 0.1 U/kg/h

BG = blood glucose; D/C = discontinue; IV = intravenously; prn = as needed; Q4–6h = every 4 to 6 hours.

Monitoring: Follow blood glucose concentration every 30 minutes to 1 hour after starting infusion and after changes in infusion rate. Follow these parameters every 2 to 4 hours after achieving a stable euglycemic state. **Clinical considerations:** Reduce loss of insulin that is due to adsorption to the plastic tubing by flushing tubing with minimum of 25 mL of insulin solution before beginning the infusion. **Precaution:** Only regular insulin may be administered intravenously. **Adverse reactions:** Hyperglycemic rebound, urticaria, anaphylaxis; may rapidly induce hypoglycemia. Insulin resistance may develop with prolonged use and necessitate an increased dose.

LEVOTHYROXINE SODIUM

Classification: Thyroid hormone. **Indications:** Replacement or supplementary therapy for hypothyroidism. **Dosage/administration:** *To avoid differences in bioavailability, use the same brand of thyroid hormone (100 mg levothyroxine = 65 mg thyroid USP).* *Initial oral dose:* 10 to 15 µg/kg/day every 24 hours; adjust in 12.5-µg increments every 2 weeks until T_4 is 10 to 15 µg/dL and thyroid-stimulating hormone (TSH) is less than 15 mU/L. *Maintenance dose:* Term infant 37.5 to 50 µg/day. Administer oral dose on an empty stomach. *Initial intravenous dose:* 5 to 10 µg/kg/day, every 24 hours, increase every 2 weeks by 5 to 10 µg. When switching from oral to intravenous, intravenous dose should be 80 % of the oral dose per day. Use only normal saline (NS) to reconstitute intravenous preparations. Use immediately after mixing. Do not add to any other solution. Usual concentration for infusion is 20 to 40 µg/mL. Maximum concentration for infusion is 100 µg/mL. Administer as a slow push. May also be given intramuscularly. **Clinical considerations:** Oral route preferred: use intravenous when oral route unavailable or with myxedema stupor/coma. **Contraindications:** Thyrotoxicosis and uncorrected adrenal insufficiency. **Precautions:** Use with caution in infants receiving anticoagulants. In infants with cardiac disease, begin with one-fourth of usual maintenance dose and increase weekly. Do not use the intravenous form orally because it crystallizes when exposed to acid. **Monitoring:** Adjust dosage based on clinical status and serum T_4 and TSH. Serum T_4 and TSH levels should be measured every 1 to 2 months or 2 to 3 weeks after any change in dose. Obtain serum T_4, free T_4 index, and TSH levels. Adequate therapy should suppress TSH values to less than 15 mU/L within 3 to 4 months of starting therapy. Assess for signs of hypothyroidism: lethargy, poor feeding, constipation, intermittent cyanosis, and prolonged neonatal jaundice. Also closely assess for signs of thyrotoxicosis: hyperreactivity, tachycardia, tachypnea, fever, exophthalmos, and goiter. Periodically assess growth and bone-age development. **Adverse reactions:** Hyperthyroidism, rash, weight loss, diarrhea, tachycardia, cardiac arrhythmias, tremors, fever, and hair loss. Prolonged overtreatment can produce premature craniosynostosis and acceleration of bone age.

LORAZEPAM

Classification: Benzodiazepine, anticonvulsant, sedative hypnotic. **Indication:** Status epilepticus refractory to conventional therapy. **Dosage/administration:** *Initial dose:* 0.05 to 0.1 mg/kg/dose, intravenously over 5 minutes; repeat in 10 to 15 minutes if necessary. *Maximum dose:* 4 mg/dose. *Maintenance dose:* 0.05 mg/kg/dose intravenously/intramuscularly/orally/rectally, every 6 to 24 hours, depending on response. Reduce dosage in hepatic or renal impairment. The intravenous formulation may be given orally. May administer with feeds to decrease gastrointestinal distress. **Contraindications:** Preexisting central nervous system (CNS) depression or severe hypotension. **Warning:** Stereotypic movements have been observed in preterm infants. **Precautions:** Some preparations contain 2% benzyl alcohol and may be hazardous to neonates in high doses. Dilute before intravenous use with equal volume of normal saline (NS) or sterile water (to minimize benzyl alcohol content). Use with caution in infants with renal or hepatic impairment or myasthenia gravis. **Monitoring:** Respiratory status during and after administration. **Adverse reactions:** CNS depression, bradycardia, circulatory collapse, respiratory depression, blood pressure instability, and gastrointestinal symptoms. Discontinue therapy if syncope and paradoxic CNS stimulation occur.

METHADONE

Classification: Narcotic, analgesic. **Indications:** Treatment of neonatal opiate withdrawal. **Dosage/administration:** *Initial dose:* 0.05 to 0.2 mg/kg/dose, oral or slow intravenous push, every 12 to 24 hours. Titrate dose based on neonatal abstinence score (NAS). Wean dose by 10 to 20% per week over a 4 to 6 week period. **Clinical considerations:** Tapering is difficult because of its long elimination half-life. Consider alternative agents. Reserve for use in infants born to methadone-treated mothers only. **Monitoring:**

Respiratory and cardiac status. **Drug interactions:** Methadone metabolism accelerated by rifampin and phenytoin; this may precipitate withdrawal symptoms. **Adverse reactions:** Respiratory depression, ileus, delayed gastric emptying.

METOCLOPRAMIDE

Classification: Antiemetic, prokinetic agent. **Indications:** Improve gastric emptying and gastrointestinal motility. **Dosage/administration:** Gastrointestinal dysmotility: 0.4 to 0.8 mg/kg/day divided every 6 hours intravenously/orally; orally administer 30 minutes before feeds. Orally available as 0.1 mg/mL and 1 mg/mL. Administer intravenous over 30 minutes on syringe pump. Maximum concentration for intravenous infusion is 5 mg/mL (usual concentration: 1 mg/mL) in normal saline (NS) or dextrose. Intravenous form may be given orally. **Contraindications:** Gastrointestinal obstruction, pheochromocytoma, history of seizure disorder. **Monitoring:** Measure gastric residuals. **Adverse reactions:** Drowsiness, restlessness, agitation, diarrhea, methemoglobinemia, and extrapyramidal symptoms (usually occur following intravenous administration of large doses and within 24 to 48 hours of starting therapy; responds rapidly to Benadryl and subsides within 24 hours after stopping metoclopramide). **Overdose:** Associated with doses greater than 1 mg/kg/day, characterized by drowsiness, ataxia, extrapyramidal reactions, seizures, and methemoglobinemia (treat with methylene blue).

MIDAZOLAM

Classification: Benzodiazepine, sedative hypnotic, anticonvulsant. **Indications:** Sedation. **Dosage/administration:** 0.05 to 0.15 mg/kg/dose every 2 to 4 hours as needed. Infuse over 15 minutes on syringe pump. Final infusion concentration is 0.5 mg/mL in normal saline (NS) or dextrose. **Contraindications:** Preexisting central nervous system (CNS) depression or shock. **Precautions:** Congestive heart failure and renal impairment. Contains 1% benzyl alcohol (minimize neonate exposure by diluting the 5 mg/mL concentration to 0.5 mg/mL). **Monitoring:** Respiration rate (RR), heart rate, blood pressure. **Drug interactions:** CNS depressants, anesthetic agents, cimetidine, and theophylline. Decrease midazolam dose by 25% during prolonged concurrent narcotic administration. **Adverse reactions:** Sedation, respiratory depression, apnea, cardiac arrest, hypotension, bradycardia, and seizures (following rapid bolus administration and in neonates with underlying CNS disorders). Encephalopathy reported in several infants sedated for 4 to 11 days with midazolam and fentanyl.

MILRINONE

Classification: Phosphodiesterase inhibitor. **Indications:** Effective inotropic agent indicated for the short-term intravenous treatment of congestive heart failure. In infants with decreased myocardial function, milrinone increases cardiac output, decreases pulmonary capillary wedge pressure, and decreases vascular resistance. It increases myocardial contractility and improves diastolic function by improving left ventricular diastolic relaxation. **Dosage/administration:** Milrinone is administered with a loading dose followed by a continuous infusion. *Loading dose:* 50 µg/kg administered via syringe pump over 20 minutes. *Maintenance dose:* 0.25 to 0.5 µg/kg/min. *Maximum infusion rate:* 1 µg/kg/min. Usual concentration for infusion is 100 µg/mL. Maximum is 250 µg/mL in normal saline (NS) or dextrose. Central line preferred. *Do not administer via* umbilical arterial catheter (UAC). Monitoring parameters: Electrocardiogram, blood pressure, complete blood count, electrolytes. Volume expanders may be needed to counteract the vasodilatory effect and potential decrease in filling pressures. **Adverse effects:** Thrombocytopenia, arrhythmias, hypotension.

MORPHINE SULFATE

Classification: Opiate, narcotic analgesic. **Indication:** Analgesia, sedation, treatment of opiate withdrawal. **Dosage/administration:** *Analgesia / sedation:* 0.05 mg/kg/dose intravenously/intramuscularly/subcutaneously every 4 to 8 hours as needed for pain. Administer bolus over 5 minutes on syringe pump. *Continuous intravenous infusion:* 0.01 to 0.02 mg/kg/h. Use only preservative-free formulation. *Concentration for administration:* 0.1 –to 1 mg/mL in normal saline (NS) or dextrose. **Treatment of opiate withdrawal** *(Use only 0.4 mg/mL preservative-free morphine concentration):*

TABLE A.17

For NAS Score	Initial Oral Dose
8–10	0.32 mg (0.8 mL)/kg/day divided Q4h
11–13	0.48 mg (1.2 mL)/kg/day divided Q4h
14–16	0.64 mg (1.6 mL)/kg/day divided Q4h
> 17	0.8 mg (2.0 mL)/kg/day divided Q4h

NAS = neonatal abstinence score; Q4h = every 4 hours.

TABLE A.18

For NAS Score	Maintenance Oral Dose
> 8 × 3 successive scores	↑ dose by 0.16 mg (0.4 mL)/kg/day divided Q4h to max dose.
< 8 × 3 successive scores	Wean by 10% of the max daily dose. If infant has been weaned too quickly, go back to last effective dose.

NAS = neonatal abstinence score; Q4h = every 4 hours.

If neonatal abstinence scores are too low, make sure that the infant is not obtunded because of overdosage. Discontinue when dose is less than 25% of maximum dose. Administration of oral morphine solution with food may increase bioavailability. **Precautions:** Fentanyl is preferred over morphine in neonates with cardiovascular and hemodynamic instability. Morphine causes histamine release leading to increased venous capacitance and suppression of adrenergic tone. Hypotension and chest wall rigidity may occur with rapid intravenous administration. Tolerance may develop following prolonged use (> 96 hours). **Contraindications:** Increased intracranial pressure. Use with caution in severe hepatic, renal impairment, necrotizing enterocolitis (NEC). **Adverse reactions:** Hypotension, respiratory depression, constipation, and urinary retention. Naloxone should be available to reverse adverse effects. **Monitoring:** Monitor respiration rate (RR), heart rate, and blood pressure closely; observe for abdominal distention and loss of bowel sounds; monitor input and output to evaluate urinary retention.

NAFCILLIN

Classification: Semisynthetic penicillinase-resistant antistaphylococcal penicillin. **Indications:** Primarily active against staphylococci. Reserve for penicillin-resistant *S. aureus* infections. **Dosage/administration:** *Intravenous:* Final concentration of 25 mg/mL infused over 30 minutes on syringe pump (see Table A.19).
Precautions: Dosing interval increased with hepatic dysfunction. Oral route not recommended because of poor absorption. Avoid intramuscular administration if possible. **Monitoring:** Complete blood count, blood urea nitrogen, creatinine, and liver function tests (LFTs). Observe for hematuria and proteinuria. **Clinical considerations:** Better cerebrospinal fluid penetration than methicillin. Decrease dose by 33 to 50% in infants with combined renal/hepatic impairment. **Drug interactions:** Blunting of peak aminoglycoside concentration when administered simultaneously with nafcillin. **Adverse reactions:** Agranulocytosis hypersensitivity, granulocytopenia, and nephro-

TABLE A.19

Age	Weight	IV Dosage
≤ 7 days	< 2 kg	25 mg/kg/dose Q12h
≤ 7 days	≥ 2 kg	25 mg/kg/dose Q8h
> 7 days	< 1200 g	25 mg/kg/dose Q12h
> 7 days	1200–2000 g	25 mg/kg/dose Q8h
> 7 days	> 2000 g	25 mg/kg/dose Q6h

IV = intravenous; Q6h = every 6 hours; Q8h = every 8 hours; Q12h = every 12 hours.

toxicity (eosinophilia may precede renal damage). Treat extravasation with hyaluronidase.

NALOXONE

Classification: Narcotic antagonist. **Indications:** Used concurrently during neonatal resuscitation for narcotic-induced central nervous system depression. **Dosage/ administration:** 0.1 mg/kg bolus intravenously/endotracheally/intramuscularly/ subcutaneously. May repeat every 3 to 5 minutes if no response. Multiple doses may be necessary because of its short duration of action. Intravenous or endotracheal tube route preferred, intramuscular or subcutaneous route may lead to delayed onset of action. **Contraindications:** Use with caution in infants with chronic cardiac disease, pulmonary disease, or coronary disease. Do not administer to newborns of narcotic dependent mothers, as it may precipitate seizures. **Adverse reactions:** Will produce narcotic withdrawal syndrome in newborns with chronic dependence. Abrupt reversal may result in vomiting, diaphoresis, tachycardia, hypertension, and tremors. **Monitoring:** Heart rate, respiratory rate, blood pressure.

NYSTATIN

Classification: Nonabsorbed antifungal agent. **Indications:** Treatment of susceptible cutaneous, mucocutaneous, and oropharyngeal fungal infections caused by Candida species. **Dosage/administration:** *Oral:* Preterm infant: 0.5 mL (50,000 U) every 6 hours. Term infant: 1 mL (100,000 U) every 6 hours. Apply suspension with swab to each side of mouth every 6 hours after feedings. *Topical therapy:* Apply ointment or cream to affected area every 6 hours. Continue oral therapy and topical application for 3 days beyond resolution of fungal infection. Breastfeeding mothers should be concurrently treated topically. **Clinical considerations:** Combination therapy for candidal perineal infections with oral and topical nystatin is possible because of nystatin's poor absorption in the gastrointestinal tract and because the gastrointestinal tract serves as the reservoir for fungi causing perineal infection. Eliminate factors contributing to fungal growth (wet, occlusive diapers and the use of contaminated nipples). **Adverse reactions:** Irritation, contact dermatitis, diarrhea, and vomiting.

OMEPRAZOLE

Classification: Gastric acid secretion inhibitor, gastrointestinal agent, gastric or duodenal ulcer treatment. **Indications:** Short-term (< 8 weeks) treatment of documented reflux esophagitis or duodenal ulcer refractory to conventional therapy. **Dosage/administration:** 0.5 to 1.5 mg/kg per dose orally, via nasogastric tube, or jejunostomy tube daily for 4 to 8 weeks. **Precautions:** Mild transaminase elevations have been reported in children who received omeprazole for extended periods of time. **Contraindications:** Hypersensitivity to omeprazole or any component. **Adverse reactions:** Tachycardia, bradycardia, palpitations, altered sleeping patterns, hemifacial dysesthesia, fever, irritability, dry skin, rash, hypoglycemia, diarrhea, vomiting, constipation, discoloration of feces, feeding intolerance because of anorexia, irritable colon, urinary frequency, agranulocytosis, pancytopenia, thrombocytopenia, anorexia, leukocytosis, hepatitis, increased liver function tests (LFTs), jaundice, hematuria, pyuria, proteinuria, glycosuria, cough, and epistaxis. **Monitoring:** Observe for symptomatic improvement within 3 days. Consider esophageal pH monitoring to assess for efficacy (pH > 4.0). Aspartate aminotransferase/alanine aminotransferase if duration of therapy is greater than 8 weeks.

PALIVIZUMAB

Classification: A humanized monoclonal antibody to respiratory syncytial virus (RSV). **Indications:** Prophylaxis for the prevention of RSV in high-risk infants; infants less than 6 months of age with a history of prematurity (< 32 weeks' gestational age) or less than 24 months of age with chronic lung disease. **Dosage/administration:** 15 mg/kg/dose intramuscularly, given every 30 days for up to 5 doses during the RSV season (i.e., October/November through March/April). **Precautions:** History of hypersensitivity related to the use of other immunoglobulin preparations, blood products, or other medications. Efficacy has not been demonstrated in the treatment of established RSV infection. Give with caution to patients with thrombocytopenia or any coagulation disorder. Not recommended for children with cyanotic congenital heart disease. **Adverse effects:** Vomiting, diarrhea, rash, rhinitis, and erythema and moderate induration at the injection site.

PANCURONIUM BROMIDE

Classification: Nondepolarizing neuromuscular blocking agent. **Indications:** Skeletal muscle relaxation, increased pulmonary compliance during mechanical ventilation, facilitate endotracheal intubation. **Dosage/administration:** 0.05 to 0.1 mg/kg/dose intravenously (may be administered undiluted by slow intravenous push) every 1 to 4 hours as needed. **Precautions:** Preexisting pulmonary, hepatic, or renal impairment. In neonates with myasthenia gravis, small doses of pancuronium may have profound effects (may need to decrease dosage). **Monitoring:** Continuous cardiac, blood pressure monitoring, assisted ventilation status. Because sensation remains intact, administer concurrent sedation and analgesia as needed. Apply ophthalmic lubricant.

Factors influencing duration of neuromuscular blockade:

TABLE A.20

Potentiation	Antagonism
Acidosis, hypothermia, neuromuscular disease, hepatic disease, renal failure, cardiovascular disease, aminoglycosides, succinylcholine, hypermagnesemia, and hypokalemia- or potassium-depleting drugs (e.g., amphotericin-B, corticosteroids, diuretics), clindamycin	Pyridostigmine, neostigmine, or edrophonium in conjunction with atropine, alkalosis, epinephrine, theophylline, hyperkalemia

Adverse reactions: Tachycardia, hypertension, hypotension, excessive salivation, rashes, bronchospasm. **Antidote:** Neostigmine 0.025 mg/kg intravenously (with atropine 0.02 mg/kg).

PENICILLIN G PREPARATIONS

Classification: Antibiotic. **Indications:** Treatment of neonatal meningitis and bacteremia, group B streptococcal infections, and congenital syphilis. **Dosage/adminis-

tration: Intramuscularly, intravenously (intravenous route is preferred to avoid muscle fibrosis and atrophy). Only aqueous penicillin G should be used intravenously. Final concentration for intravenous infusion is 50,000 U/mL infused over 30 minutes on syringe pump. When treating bacteremia, use the meningitis dose until meningitis is ruled out. **Group B streptococcal infections:** *Bacteremia:* 200,000 U/kg/day in divided doses every 6 hours. *Meningitis:* 400,000 U/kg/day in divided doses every 6 hours.
Infections due to other organisms:

TABLE A.21

Dosages: Bacteremia: 50,000 U/kg/dose; Meningitis: 100,000 U/kg/dose

Postconceptional Age	Postnatal Age	Frequency
≤ 29 weeks	0–4 weeks	Q12h
≤ 29 weeks	> 4 weeks	Q8h
30–36 weeks	0–2 weeks	Q12h
30–36 weeks	> 2 weeks	Q8h
37–44 weeks	0–1 week	Q8h
> 45 weeks	All	Q6h

Q6h = every 6 hours; Q8h = every 8 hours; Q12h = every 12 hours.

Monitoring: Serum potassium and sodium for renal failure and high-dose therapy. Weekly complete blood count, blood urea nitrogen, creatinine. **Precautions:** Dosage adjustment for renal failure. Use only aqueous penicillin G for intravenous administration. **Drug interactions:** Blunting of peak aminoglycoside serum concentration if administered simultaneously with penicillin G preparations. **Test interactions:** Positive direct Coombs' test. **Adverse reactions:** Bone marrow suppression, granulocytopenia, anaphylaxis, hemolytic anemia, interstitial nephritis, Jarisch-Herxheimer reaction, change in bowel flora (Candida superinfection, diarrhea), central nervous system toxicity.

PHENOBARBITAL

Classification: Anticonvulsant, sedative, hypnotic. **Indications:** Drug of choice to control neonatal seizures. Management of withdrawal, direct hyperbilirubinemia, cholestasis. **Dosage/administration:** *Seizures:* Loading dose: 20 mg/kg/dose, administer intravenous loading dose over 15 minutes (<1 mg/kg/min) on syringe pump. Administer additional doses of 5 mg/kg every 5 minutes until cessation of seizures or a total dose of 40 mg/kg is administered. Use the intravenous route if possible because of unreliable intramuscular absorption. Maintenance therapy: 3 to 5 mg/kg/day intravenously/ intramuscularly/ orally daily. Begin maintenance therapy 24 hours after loading dose. Parenteral dose preferred for seriously ill neonate. *Cholestasis:* 4 to 5 mg/kg/day, intravenously/intramuscularly/ orally for 4 to 5 days. *Neonatal withdrawal syndrome:* Administer loading dose, then titrate based on neonatal abstinence score. Loading dose: 15 to 20 mg/kg/dose. Closely follow blood levels after stabilization of abstinence symptoms for 24 to 48 hours, decrease the daily dose by 10 to 20% per day. See Table A.22. **Clinical considerations:** *Direct hyperbilirubinemia:* More effective in full-term infants. *Neonatal withdrawal syndrome:* Avoid using in infants with gastrointestinal symptoms. **Warnings:** Abrupt discontinuation in infants with seizures may precipitate status seizures. **Precautions:** Hepatic or renal impairment. **Monitoring:** *Therapeutic serum concentration:* 15 to 40 μg/mL. Obtain trough levels just before the next dose. Monitor respiratory status. **Drug interactions:** Benzodiazepines, primidone,

TABLE A.22

Neonatal Abstinence Score	Dosage
8–10	6 mg/kg/day divided Q8h
11–13	8 mg/kg/day divided Q8h
14–16	10 mg/kg/day divided Q8h
> 17	12 mg/kg/day divided Q8h

Q8h = every 8 hours.

warfarin, corticosteroids, and doxycycline. Increased serum concentrations with concurrent phenytoin or valproate. **Adverse reactions:** Respiratory depression (with serum concentrations > 60 µg/mL), hypotension, circulatory collapse, paradoxical excitement, megaloblastic anemia, hepatitis, and exfoliative dermatitis. Sedation reported at serum concentrations greater than 40 µg/mL.

PHENTOLAMINE MESYLATE

Classification: Extravasation antidote, vasodilator, alpha-adrenergic blocking agent. **Indication:** Local treatment of dermal necrosis caused by extravasation of vasoconstrictive agents (e.g., dopamine, dobutamine, epinephrine, norepinephrine, and phenylephrine). **Dosage/administration:** Phentolamine, 5 mg, diluted in 4 mL normal saline (NS) to concentration of 1 mg/mL. Use immediately after reconstitution. Using a 25- to 30-gauge needle, inject 0.2 mL subcutaneously at 5 separate sites around edge of infiltration; change needle between each skin entry. Repeat if necessary. Best results if used within 12 hours after extravasation occurrence. **Clinical considerations:** Topical 2% nitroglycerin ointment may be used for significantly swollen extremity. **Contraindications:** Renal impairment. **Precautions:** Gastritis or peptic ulcer. **Monitoring:** Assess affected area for reversal of ischemia. Closely monitor blood pressure, heart rate/rhythm. **Adverse reactions:** Hypotension, tachycardia, arrhythmias, nasal congestion, vomiting, diarrhea, exacerbation of peptic ulcer.

PHENYTOIN

Classification: Anticonvulsant. **Indication:** Treatment of seizures that are refractory to phenobarbital. **Dosage/administration:** *Loading dose:* 15 to 20 mg/kg/ intravenous infusion on syringe pump over 30 minutes. Dilute to 5 mg/mL with normal saline (NS). Use a 0.22-µm in-line filter. Start infusion immediately after preparation. Observe for precipitates. *Avoid using in central lines because of the risk of precipitation. If must use a central line, then flush catheter with 1 to 3 mL NS before and after administration because of heparin incompatibility.* *Maintenance dose:* 4 to 8 mg/kg every 24 hours intravenous infusion on syringe pump over 30 minutes. Maintenance doses usually start 12 hours after loading dose. Avoid intramuscular route because of erratic absorption, pain on injection, and precipitation of drug at injection site. **Precautions:** Rapid intravenous administration has resulted in hypotension, cardiovascular collapse, and central nervous system depression. May cause local irritation, inflammation, necrosis, and sloughing with or without signs of infiltration. **Contraindications:** Heart block, sinus bradycardia. **Adverse reactions:** Hypersensitivity reaction, arrhythmias, hypotension, hyperglycemia, cardiovascular collapse, liver damage, blood dyscrasias; extravasation may cause tissue necrosis. Treat with hyaluronidase around the periphery of affected site. **Monitoring:** Heart rate, rhythm, hypotension during infusion. **Monitoring parameters:** Obtain trough level 48 hours after intravenous loading dose. Therapeutic serum concentration: 8 to 15 µg/mL.

RANITIDINE

Classification: Histamine-2 antagonist. **Indications:** Duodenal and gastric ulcers, gastroesophageal reflux, and hypersecretory conditions. **Dosage/administration:** *Oral dose:* 6 mg/kg/day orally divided in 3 to 4 doses. *Intravenous dose:* 0.5 mg/kg/ dose intravenously every 6 hours infused over 30 minutes on syringe pump. Usual concentration for infusion is 1 mg/mL mixed with dextrose or normal saline (NS). Maximum concentration for intravenous infusion is 2.5 mg/mL. *Continuous intravenous dose:* 0.0625 mg/kg/h. Titrate dose to maintain a gastric pH greater than 4. **Clinical considerations:** Because of the absence of possible endocrine toxicity and drug interactions, ranitidine is preferred over cimetidine. Ranitidine effectively increases gastric pH. Increased gastric pH may promote the development of gastric colonization with pathogenic bacteria or yeast. **Precautions:** Use with caution in infants with liver and renal impairment. Intravenous formulation contains 0.5% phenol; no short-term toxicity has been reported. Manufacturer's oral solution contains 7.5% alcohol. **Drug interactions:** May increase serum levels of theophylline, warfarin, and procainamide. **Monitoring:** Monitor gastric pH to assess ranitidine efficacy. **Adverse reactions:** Gastrointestinal disturbance, sedation, thrombocytopenia, hepatotoxicity, vomiting, bradycardia or tachycardia.

SODIUM BICARBONATE

Classification: Alkalinizing agent. **Indications:** Treatment of documented or assumed metabolic acidosis during prolonged resuscitation after establishment of effective ventilation. Treatment of bicarbonate deficit caused by renal or gastrointestinal losses. Adjunctive treatment of hyperkalemia. **Dose/administration:** *Replacement:* Infuse over 20 to 30 minutes on syringe pump. *Resuscitation:* 1 to 2 mEq/kg intravenous slow push over at least 2 minutes. *Correction of metabolic acidosis:* HCO_3 needed (mEq) = HCO_3 deficit (mEq/L) × (0.3 × body wt [kg]). Administer half of calculated dose, then assess need for remainder. Usual concentration for infusion is 0.5 mEq/mL; maximum concentration is 1 mEq/mL. *For continuous intravenous infusion:* Use 50 mEq sodium bicarbonate (8.4% concentration) and add to 50 cc of appropriate diluent (e.g, dextrose, maximum 10%; normal saline (NS); or sterile water). Concentration is 0.5 mEq/mL. Maximum infusion rate for continuous intravenous administration is 1 mEq/kg/h. **Precautions:** Rapid injection of hypertonic sodium bicarbonate (1 mEq/mL) solution has been linked to cerebral hemorrhage. **Adverse effects:** Pulmonary edema, respiratory acidosis, local tissue necrosis, hypocalcemia, hypernatremia, metabolic alkalosis. **Monitoring:** Follow acid–base status; arterial blood gases; serum electrolytes, including calcium; and urinary pH. Use hyaluronidase to treat intravenous extravasation.

SPIRONOLACTONE

Classification: Potassium-sparing diuretic. **Indications:** Mild diuretic with potassium-sparing effects. Used in conjunction with thiazide diuretics in the treatment of congestive heart failure, hypertension, edema, and bronchopulmonary dysplasia (BPD) when prolonged diuresis is desirable. **Dosage/administration:** 1 to 3 mg/kg/day orally divided every 12 hours. *BPD therapy:* Chlorothiazide, 20 mg/kg/dose orally every 12 hours for 8 weeks, plus spironolactone 1.5 mg/kg/dose orally every 12 hours for 8 weeks. **Clinical considerations:** Offers no additional benefit when included as part of the regimen to treat BPD. **Contraindications:** Renal failure, anuria, hyperkalemia. **Monitoring:** Serum and urine potassium. **Drug interactions:** May potentiate ganglionic blocking agents and other antihypertensive agents. **Adverse reactions:** Hyperkalemia, vomiting, diarrhea, hyperchloremic metabolic acidosis, dehydration, hyponatremia.

SURFACTANTS

Classification: Natural, animal-derived exogenous surfactant agent. **Indications:** *Prophylaxis:* Infants with high risk for respiratory distress syndrome (RDS), defined in clinical trials as a birth weight less than 1250 g, and larger infants with evidence of pulmonary immaturity. *Rescue therapy*: Infants with moderate to severe RDS, defined in clinical trials as requirement for mechanical ventilation and fractional concentraton of inspired oxygen (FiO_2) higher than 40%. Treatment of full-term infants with respiratory failure that is due to meconium aspiration, pneumonia, or persistent pulmonary hypertension.

Dosage/administration:

TABLE A.23

Surfactant	Doses	Comments
Beractant (Survanta)	4 mL/kg/dose	Divided into 4 aliquots, with up to 3 additional doses (4 total), administered Q6h if needed
Calfactant (Infasurf)	3 mL/kg/dose	Divided into 2 aliquots, with up to 3 additional doses, administered Q12h, if needed
Poractant alfa (Curosurf)	Initial dose = 2.5 mL/kg/dose. Subsequent doses = 1.25 mL/kg/dose	Divided into 2 aliquots, followed by up to 2 additional doses of 1.25 mL/kg/dose, administered Q12h if needed

Q6h = every 6 hours; Q12h = every 12 hours.

Administered intratracheally by instillation into a 5 French end-hole catheter inserted into the infant's endotracheal tube with the tip of the catheter protruding just beyond the end of the endotracheal tube and above the infant's carina. *Prophylactic therapy*: Intratracheally as soon as possible after birth. *Rescue therapy*: Intratracheally immediately following the diagnosis of RDS. **Clinical considerations:** Suction endotracheal tube before administration. Delay suctioning postadministration as long as possible (minimum of 1 hour). **Monitoring:** Assess endotracheal tube patency and correct anatomic location before administration of surfactant. Monitor oxygen saturation and heart rate continuously during administration of doses. After administration of each dose, monitor arterial blood gases frequently to detect and correct postdose abnormalities of ventilation and oxygenation. **Precautions:** A videotape demonstrating surfactant administration procedure is available from Ross Laboratories and Forest Laboratories and should be viewed before use of their products. **Adverse reactions:** Transient bradycardia, hypoxemia, pallor, vasoconstriction, hypotension, endotracheal tube blockage, hypercapnia, apnea, and hypertension may occur during the administration process.

THEOPHYLLINE

Classification: Bronchodilator, respiratory stimulant. **Indications:** Apnea. **Dosage/administration:** *Loading dose:* 5 mg/kg/dose orally. *Maintenance dose:* 6 mg/kg/day orally, divided every 6 to 8 hours. Start 6 to 8 hours after loading dose. For intravenous use, see Aminophylline. **Contraindications:** Uncontrolled arrhythmias, hyperthyroidism. **Clinical considerations:** Consider caffeine as first-line agent for apnea of prematurity. **Precautions:** Peptic ulcer, hypertension, and compromised cardiac function. Some elixir preparations may contain alcohol. **Drug interactions:** Increased theophylline elimination: carbamazepine, isoproterenol, phenytoin, phenobarbital, and rifampin. Decreased theophylline elimination: erythromycin, quinolones, calcium channel blockers, nonselective beta-blockers, and cimetidine. **Monitoring:** Heart rate, blood glucose during loading dose, agitation, feeding intolerance. Hold dose if heart rate is greater than 180 beats per minute. **Therapeutic ranges:** Check levels at fifth dose (or before fifth dose if increased number/severity of apnea spells), then every week, or as needed for increased number/severity of apnea spells. Desired serum level in apnea of prematurity is 5 to 15 µg/mL. 1 mg/kg is given for each desired 2 µg/mL increase in serum theophylline level. **Adverse reactions:** Vomiting, sinus tachycardia, hyperglycemia, diuresis, dehydration, feeding intolerance, central nervous system irritability, gastroesophageal reflux, seizures. **Overdosage:** Tachycardia, vomiting, seizures, circulatory failure, failure to gain weight, hyperreflexia, encephalopathy. **Theophylline toxicity treatment:** Activated charcoal, 1 g/kg slurry via gavage tube every 2 to 4 hours. Sorbitol-containing preparations used for toxicity treatment may cause osmotic diarrhea and should be avoided.

URSODIOL

Classification: Gallstone dissolution agent. **Indications:** Facilitates bile excretion in infants with biliary atresia, improves hepatic metabolism of essential fatty acids in infants with cystic fibrosis. **Dosages/administration:** *Biliary atresia:* 10 mg/kg/dose orally every 12 hours. *Cystic fibrosis:* 15 mg/kg/dose orally every 12 hours. Administer with food. Must be refrigerated. Available as a pharmaceutical extemporaneous preparation in concentration of 10 mg/mL or 20 mg/mL oral suspension. **Precautions:** Obtain baseline alanine aminotransferase, aspartate aminotransferase, alkaline phosphate, bilirubin. **Contraindications:** Use with caution in infants with chronic liver disease. **Adverse reactions:** Hepatotoxicity.

VANCOMYCIN HYDROCHLORIDE

Classification: Antibiotic. **Indications:** Drug of choice for serious infections caused by methicillin-resistant staphylococci, penicillin-resistant pneumococci, and coagulase-negative staphylococcus. The oral route is used for the treatment of *Clostridium difficile.*
Dosage/administration:

TABLE A.24

Postnatal Age	Weight (kg)	Dose (mg/kg/dose)
≤ 7 days	< 1.2 kg	15 mg/kg IV Q24h
≤ 7 days	1.2–2 kg	10 mg/kg IV Q12h
≤ 7 days	> 2 kg	15 mg/kg IV Q12h
> 7 days	< 1.2 kg	15 mg/kg IV Q24h
> 7 days	1.2–2 kg	15 mg/kg IV Q12h
> 7 days	> 2 kg	10 mg/kg IV Q8h

IV = intravenously; Q12h = every 12 hours; Q24h = every 24 hours; Q8h = every 8 hours.

Intravenous infusion over 60 minutes on syringe pump. Final concentration for infusion is 5 mg/mL. Concentrations greater than 5 mg/mL up to a maximum of 10 mg/mL should be administered centrally. Mix in normal saline (NS) or dextrose. **Precautions:** Use with caution in patients with renal impairment or those receiving other nephrotoxic or ototoxic drugs; dosage modification required in patients with impaired renal function. **Adverse reactions:** Red neck or red man syndrome (erythema multiforme-like reaction with intense pruritus; tachycardia; hypotension; rash involving face, neck, upper trunk, back, and upper arms) usually develops during a rapid infusion of vancomycin or with doses greater than 15 to 20 mg/kg/h and usually dissipates in 30 to 60 minutes. Lengthening infusion time usually eliminates risk for subsequent doses. Cardiac arrest, fever, chills, eosinophilia, and neutropenia reported after prolonged administration (> 3 weeks); phlebitis may be minimized by slow infusion and more dilution of the drug. If extravasation occurs, consider using hyaluronidase around periphery of affected area. Also reported are ototoxicity, enhanced by aminoglycoside therapy and associated with prolonged serum concentration greater than 40 µg/mL, and nephrotoxicity (higher incidence with trough concentrations > 10 µg/mL). **Monitoring:** Assess renal function. Therapeutic serum concentrations: Trough 5 to 15 µg/ mL. Sample drawn 30 minutes to just before next dose. Peak levels are not clinically significant.

VITAMIN A INJECTION

Classification: Nutritional supplement, fat soluble vitamin. **Indication:** To minimize incidence of chronic lung disease in high-risk, preterm newborns. **Dosage/administration:** 5000 IU, intramuscularly 3 times per week for 12 doses total. Start within 72 hours of birth in infants with birth weights less than 1000 g. Administer with a 25- to 27-gauge needle. **Caution:** Do not use concurrently with dexamethasone. **Contraindications:** Do not administer intravenously. **Adverse effects:** Full fontanel, hepatomegaly, edema, mucocutaneous lesions, bony tenderness.

VITAMIN B₁

Classification: Water-soluble vitamin supplement. **Indications:** Treatment of thiamine deficiency.

TABLE A.25

Indications	Dosage/administration (for preterm and term infants)
Thiamine RDA	300 µg/day
Thiamine deficiency	Preventive dose 0.5–1.0 mg/day PO
Thiamine deficiency	Therapeutic dose 5–10 mg/day, divided Q6–8h

PO = orally; Q6–8h = every 6 to 8 hours; RDA = recommended daily allowance.

Thiamine sources: 1 mL of PolyViSol or ViDaylin supplies 500 µg. Human milk supplies 56 µg/day. **Drug interactions:** Thiamine requirements increased with high-carbohydrate diets or high-concentration intravenous dextrose solutions. **Test interactions:** Large doses may interfere with spectrophotometric determination of serum theophylline. **Adverse reactions:** Allergic reaction, angioedema, and cardiovascular collapse. Severity and frequency of adverse reactions increases with parenteral route of administration.

VITAMIN B₆

Classification: Water-soluble vitamin supplement. **Indications:** Prevention and treatment of pyridoxine-dependent seizures. **Dosage/administration:** 50 to 100 mg intravenously over 1 minute, or intramuscularly as a single test dose; followed by 30-minute observation period. Intravenous route is preferred. If response seen, begin maintenance dose of 50 to 100 mg orally every day. The injectable form may be given orally. Mix with feeds if desired. **Monitoring:** Electroencephalogram monitoring recommended during initial therapy for pyridoxine-dependent seizures, respiration rate (RR), heart rate, blood pressure. **Precautions:** Risk of profound sedation and respiratory depression; ventilatory support may be required. **Adverse reactions:** Sedation, increased aspartate aminotransferase, decreased serum folic acid level, allergic reaction. Seizures reported following intravenous administration of very large doses.

VITAMIN D₂

Classification: Fat-soluble vitamin. **Indications:** Refractory rickets, hypophosphatemia, hypoparathyroidism. **Dosage/administration:** *Less than 37 weeks*: 10 to

20 µg/day (400–800 IU/day). *37 weeks or more:* 10 µg/day (400 IU/day) orally. Administer intramuscularly for fat malabsorption. Ergocalciferol 1.25 mg provides 50,000 IU of vitamin D activity. **Contraindications:** Hypercalcemia, evidence of vitamin D toxicity. **Monitoring:** Serum calcium, phosphorus, alkaline phosphatase levels. Excessive doses may lead to hypervitaminosis D manifested by hypercalcemia, azotemia, increased serum creatinine, mild hypokalemia, diarrhea, polyuria, metastatic calcification, nephrocalcinosis. **Adverse reactions:** Acidosis, polyuria, nephrocalcinosis, hypertension, arrhythmias.

VITAMIN E

Classification: Fat-soluble vitamin. **Indications:** Prevention and treatment of vitamin E deficiency. **Dosage/administration:** *Usual dose:* 5 IU orally every day. *Range:* 5 to 25 IU orally every day. **Precautions:** Aquasol E is very hyperosmolar (3000 µOsm); a 1:4 dilution with sterile water is required. Poorly absorbed in malabsorption disorders; use water-soluble forms. **Monitoring:** Physiologic serum levels for preterm infants are 1 to 2 mg/dL and should be monitored during administration of pharmacologic doses of vitamin E. **Clinical considerations:** Requirements for vitamin E increase as the intake of polyunsaturated fatty acids increases. **Adverse reactions:** Feeding intolerance, necrotizing enterocolitis (NEC), increased incidence of sepsis.

VITAMIN K$_1$

Classification: Fat-soluble vitamin. **Indications:** Prevention and treatment of hemorrhagic disease of the newborn, hypoprothrombinemia caused by drug-induced or anticoagulant-induced vitamin K deficiency. **Dosage/administration:** Prophylaxis (administered at birth). *Less than 1.5 kg:* 0.5 mg intramuscularly/subcutaneously *1.5 kg or more:* 1 mg intramuscularly/subcutaneously. **Warnings:** Ineffective in hereditary hypoprothrombinemia or hypoprothrombinemia caused by severe liver disease. Severe hemolytic anemia or hyperbilirubinemia reported in neonates following administration of doses greater than 20 mg. Intramuscular administration not associated with an increased risk of childhood cancer. **Precautions:** Despite proper dilution and rate of administration, severe anaphylactoid or hypersensitivitylike reactions (including shock and cardiac/respiratory arrest) have been reported to occur during or immediately after intravenous administration. Intravenous administration is restricted to emergency use, should not exceed 1 mg/minute, and should occur with a physician in attendance. Use with caution in neonates with severe hepatic disease. **Drug interactions:** Antagonizes action of warfarin. **Monitoring:** Prothrombin time/partial thromboplastin time (PT/PTT) if giving maintenance therapy. Allow a minimum of 2 to 4 hours to detect measurable improvement in these parameters.

ZIDOVUDINE

Classification: Antiretroviral agent, nucleoside analog reverse transcriptase inhibitor. **Indications:** Treatment of neonates born to human immunodeficiency virus (HIV)-infected women. **Dosage/administration:** *Term infants:* 2 mg/kg/dose every 6 hours orally. *Preterm infants 2 weeks of age or younger:* 1.5 mg/kg/dose orally every 12 hours. *Preterm infants older than 2 weeks of age:* 2 mg/kg/dose orally every 8 hours. May be administered with feeds but manufacturer recommends administration 30 minutes before or 1 hour after feeds. Initiate therapy within 12 hours of birth and continue for 6 weeks, with subsequent treatment contingent on clinical status and results of HIV studies. *Intravenous:* 1.5 mg/kg/dose every 6 hours given on infusion pump over 1 hour. *Final concentration for intravenous administration:* 4 mg/mL. Do not administer intramuscularly. **Clinical considerations:** Intravenous dose is two-thirds of oral dose. **Precautions:** Use with caution in patients with bone marrow compromise or renal or hepatic impairment. **Adverse reactions:** Anemia and neutropenia. **Drug interactions:** Acetaminophen, acyclovir (increased toxicity), ganciclovir (increased hematological toxicity), cimetidine, indomethacin, and lorazepam. Coadministration with other drugs metabolized by glucuronidation increases toxicity of either drug and increases granulocytopenia. **Monitoring consideration:** Weekly complete blood count, renal, liver function tests (LFTs), CD4 cell count, HIV RNA plasma levels.

ZINC ACETATE ORAL SOLUTION

Classification: Mineral supplement. **Indication:** Prevention and treatment of zinc deficiency states. **Dosage/administration:** 0.5 to 1 mg of elemental Zn/kg/day orally every day. **Clinical considerations:** May administer with food if gastrointestinal upset occurs. **Drug interactions:** Iron and agents that increase gastric pH (e.g., H-2 blockers, proton pump inhibitors) may decrease zinc absorption. **Monitoring:** Periodic serum copper, zinc levels. **Adverse effects:** Nausea, vomiting, leukopenia, diaphoresis, gastrointestinal disturbances. At excessive doses, hypotension, tachycardia, and gastric ulcers.

Intravenous Compatibility chart

BWH
NICU IV COMPATIBILITY CHART

	Ampicillin 100mg/ml	Caffeine citrate 20mg/ml	Clindamycin 6mg/ml	Dobutamine 90mg/100ml	Dopamine 90mg/100ml	Epinephrine 1mg/50ml	Fentanyl 500micg/50ml	Gentamicin 10mg/ml	Heparin 0.5u/ml	Indomethacin 0.5mg/ml	Insulin 15u/100ml	Lipids 20%	Milrinone 20mg/100ml	Morphine sulfate 1mg/ml	Na bicarb 1meq/ml	Vancomycin 10mg/ml	TPN
Ampicillin 100mg/ml		I	Y	I	Y	Y	Y	I	Y	I	Y	Y	I	Y	I	Y	Y
Caffeine citrate 20mg/ml	I		Y	Y	Y	Y	Y	Y	Y	I	Y	Y	Y	Y	Y	Y	Y
Clindamycin 6mg/ml	Y	Y		I	I	I	I	Y	Y	I	I	Y	I	Y	Y	I	Y
Dobutamine 90mg/100ml	I	Y	I		Y	Y	Y	I	Y	I	Y	Y	Y	Y	I	I	Y
Dopamine 90mg/100ml	Y	Y	I	Y		Y	Y	Y	A,Y	I	Y	Y	Y	Y	I	I	Y
Epinephrine 1mg/50ml	Y	Y	I	Y			Y	Y	I	Y	I	I	Y	Y	I	I	Y
Fentanyl 500mcg/50ml	Y	Y	I	Y	Y	Y		I	Y	I	I	Y	Y	Y	I	I	Y
Gentamicin 10mg/ml	I	Y	Y	I	Y	I	I		Y	I	Y	Y	I	Y	I	I	Y
Heparin 0.5u/ml	Y	Y	Y	Y	A,Y	Y	Y	Y		I	Y	A,Y	Y	A,Y	Y	Y	A,Y
Indomethacin 0.5mg/ml	I	I	I	I	I	I	I	I	I		Y	I	I	I	Y	I	I
Insulin 15 u/100ml	Y	Y	I	Y	Y	I	I	Y	Y	Y		A,Y	Y	Y	Y	Y	A,Y
Lipids 20%	Y	Y	Y	Y	Y	Y	Y	Y	A,Y	I	A,Y		I	Y	I	I	A,Y
Milrinone 20mg/100ml	I	Y	I	Y	Y	Y	Y	I	Y	I	Y	I		Y	I	I	Y
Morphine sulfate 1mg/ml	Y	Y	Y	Y	Y	Y	Y	Y	A,Y	I	Y	Y	Y		I	Y	Y
Na bicarb 1meq/ml	I	Y	Y	I	I	I	I	I	Y	Y	Y	I	I	I		I	I
Vancomycin 10mg/ml	Y	Y	I	I	I	I	I	I	Y	I	Y	I	I	Y	I		Y
TPN	Y	Y	Y	Y	Y	Y	Y	Y	A,Y	I	A,Y	A,Y	Y	Y	I	Y	

KEY: A= ADDITIVE; Y= Y-SITE; I= INCOMPATIBLE
Concentrations shown are the MAXIMUM concentrations for compatibilty in neonates.

FIG. APP.01. Intravenous Compatibility chart

Suggested Readings

American Academy of Pediatrics. *2001 Red Book: Report of the Committee on Infectious Diseases,* 25th ed. 2001. Elk Grove Village, Ill.: American Academy of Pediatrics.

American Heart Association and American Academy of Pediatrics. *Handbook for Neonatal Resuscitation Textbook,* 4th ed. 2000. Washington, DC: AHA/AAP.

Gunn V.L. *The Harriet Lane Handbook,* 16th ed. 2002. Philadelphia: Mosby-Year Book, Inc.

Nelson J.D. *Nelson's 2000–2001 Pocket Book of Pediatric Antimicrobial Therapy,* 14th ed. 2000. Baltimore: Williams & Wilkins.

Taketomo C.K., et al. *Pediatric Dosage Handbook,* 9th ed. 2002. Cleveland, Ohio: American Pharmaceutical Association.

Trissel L. *Handbook of Injectable Drugs,* 11th ed. Bethesda, MD: Board of the American Society of Health-System Pharmacists, 2001.

Young T.E., Mangum B. *Neofax,* 15th ed. 2002. Raleigh, N.C.: Acorn Publishing.

APPENDIX B. EFFECTS OF MATERNAL DRUGS ON THE FETUS

Camilia R. Martin

I. Introduction

A. In most instances, the **risk** of adverse fetal effects from drugs taken by the mother is not known. Properly designed scientific studies cannot be performed ethically, because they would require that women take drugs when they did not need them in order to eliminate the confounding effect of maternal disease or disorder. The current investigational methods (retrospective analysis, cohort studies, and case reports) often cannot differentiate the cause of the malformation or other adverse outcome. When a problem occurs in association with a history of maternal drug ingestion, any of the following can be the cause:

1. **The drug itself.**
2. **The maternal disease state** (e.g., diabetes, maternal infection, or environmental toxicity).
3. **Preexistent physical disorders** (e.g., amniotic bands), producing deformation and disruption.
4. **Unrecognized illness** (e.g., unrecognized viral illness).
5. An **already anomalous pregnancy** may have produced symptoms that led to drug ingestion.
6. **Genetic aberration.**
7. A **spontaneous malformation** rate of 2 to 3%, a **stillbirth risk** of 1%, and a **spontaneous abortion rate** of 10%.
8. **Other or unknown cause.** In addition, maternal drug histories are extremely unreliable, and findings often depend on how the interview was conducted.

B. Teratogenic effects. Because of tremendous variability in maternal elimination and drug disposition characteristics, very little predictability comes from knowing the maternal dose. Timing of drug exposure is important. Drugs taken when the embryo is extremely undifferentiated are unlikely to produce physical malformation unless the drug persists in the body or alters the gamete. The most critical period for the induction of physical defects is believed to be 15 to 60 days after conception. Because the timing of this event is rarely known with certainty, however, one cannot exclude the possibility of malformation in any clinical situation. Drugs taken after organogenesis can affect the growth and development of the fetus. The brain, in particular, continues to grow and develop in the latter trimesters and beyond. A drug taken during gestation also can act as a transplacental carcinogen. In short, there is no "guaranteed safe" time for a pregnant woman to take a drug.

C. Even when a drug is associated with a statistically significant increase in the risk of a birth defect, the actual risk may remain low. For example, a birth defect that naturally occurs once in 1 million births may be made 1000 times more likely by drug exposure and still would be seen in only 0.1% of the drug exposures. A real example of this is with phenytoin exposure. This drug produces a 200 to 400% increase in the risk of common birth defects (cleft lip, heart defects); however, 85% of children born to women who take phenytoin are normal or have minor effects of exposure. Numerical risks cannot be stated with certainty for most drugs because the data have been collected retrospectively. Where a risk is stated, the value should be interpreted with caution. For a given pregnancy, studied risk may not accurately reflect the risk to the fetus; genetic factors may have a strong influence on susceptibility to certain teratogens.

D. Manufacturer's recommendations and package inserts should be checked before the fetus is exposed to these agents.

II. Effects of common maternal drugs on the fetus (Table B.1)

TABLE B.1. EFFECTS OF COMMON MATERNAL DRUGS ON THE FETUS

Class	Drug	Risk category*	Pharmacokinetics/reported effects on fetus
Analgesics/anti-pyretics and NSAIDs	Acetaminophen	B	Crosses placenta Not implicated as a teratogen When used within dosing recommendations and for short-term use, acetaminophen considered safe Continuous use or high-toxic dosages have been associated with maternal anemia, maternal hepatorenal failure, maternal death, fetal hepatorenal failure, fetal death
	Acetylsalicylic acid (aspirin)	C D—full dose aspirin in 3rd trimester	Crosses placenta Not implicated as an important teratogen No fetal or newborn effects have been shown with *low-dose aspirin therapy* *Full-dose* aspirin associated with delayed onset and prolonged duration of labor (inhibition of prostaglandin synthesis) *Full-dose* ingestion within 5 days of delivery is associated with an increase risk of bleeding in both mother and baby Platelet dysfunction has been described (see Chap. 26) Association between *full-dose* maternal aspirin near-term and premature closure of the ductus arteriosus (inhibition of prostaglandin synthesis) and the syndrome of pulmonary hypertension in the newborn (see Chap. 24)
	Ibuprofen	B D—full dose aspirin in 3rd trimester	Not implicated as a teratogen When used as a tocolytic agent, use associated with reduced amniotic fluid volume Like aspirin, another prostaglandin synthesis inhibitor, use associated with delayed onset and prolonged duration of labor, premature closure of the ductus arteriosus, and pulmonary hypertension in the newborn
Anesthetic agents used during labor and delivery	Analgesics/narcotic agents		See Chap. 19

*Risk Categories are defined at the end of this appendix.

Atropine (anesthetic premedication)	C	Parasympatholytic/anticholinergic Rapidly crosses the placenta with fetal uptake May directly affect fetal heart rate When used for premedication at 0.01 mg/kg, no fetal effects on heart rate or variability, and no effects on uterine activity were reported
Benzodiazepines	D	See Psychotherapeutic agents, antipsychotics, below
Induction agents		
Ketamine	B	Rapid-acting IV general anesthetic agent Not implicated as a teratogen Rapidly crosses the placenta When used in high doses (1.5–2.2 mg/kg), ketamine associated with an increase in maternal blood pressure, increased uterine tone and contractions, newborn depression, and increased muscle tone in the infant These maternal/newborn effects were rarely observed with lower doses (0.2–0.5 mg/kg), which are commonly used today
Propofol	B	Hypnotic agent Not implicated as a teratogen Rapidly crosses the placenta Associated with decreased Apgar scores and decreased neurobehavioral scores compared with infants born by spontaneous vaginal delivery
Thiopental	C	Rapid and ultrashort-acting IV general anesthetic agent Not implicated as a teratogen Rapidly crosses the placenta Associated with decreased Apgar scores and decreased neurobehavioral scores compared with infants born by spontaneous vaginal delivery

(continues)

*Risk Categories are defined at the end of this appendix.

TABLE B.1. *(Continued)*

Class	Drug	Risk category*	Pharmacokinetics/reported effects on fetus
Inhalation agents	Enflurane	B	Rapid fetal uptake No adverse effects on Apgar scores or neurobehavioral status in the newborn
	Halothane	C	Associated with uterine muscle relaxation and increased blood loss; however, low-dose halothane (0.5%) not shown to have adverse maternal or newborn effects
	Isoflurane	C	Preferred agent in patients receiving beta-adrenergic therapy because of a reduced incidence of arrhythmias
	Nitrous oxide	?	Short-term use as an obstetric anesthetic considered safe
Local anesthetics	Bupivacaine	C	Long-acting local anesthetic Reports of associated neonatal depression, hypoxia, fetal acidosis, and bradycardia High concentrations may increase forceps delivery rate
	Chloroprocaine	C	
	Lidocaine	C_B, B_M	Not implicated as a teratogen when used early in pregnancy Injection into paracervical tissues or uterine cavity results in fetal heart rate decelerations Epidural use associated with maternal hypotension
	Ropivacaine	B	Rapidly crosses the placenta Use as an obstetric anesthetic is considered safe
Scopolamine		C	Parasympatholytic/anticholinergic Used to prevent nausea and vomiting associated with anesthesia and surgery Readily crosses the placenta

*Risk Categories are defined at the end of this appendix.

Drug	Risk Category*	Effects
Scopolamine (cont.)		Fetal effects may include tachycardia and decreased heart rate variability Report of newborn toxicity with fever, tachycardia, and lethargy; symptoms reversed with physostigmine
Skeletal muscle relaxants Pancuronium Vecuronium	C	Crosses the placenta in small amounts near term, placenta transfer early in pregnancy has not been reported Short-term use has shown no demonstrable adverse effects on the fetus Repetitive or large doses have been associated with neonatal depression and transient fetal heart rate changes, which do not seem to correlate or indicate fetal compromise
Anticoagulants		
Heparin	C	Does not cross the placenta Not considered a teratogen Maternal complications include bleeding
Warfarin and other coumarin derivatives	D_B, X_M	Oral anticoagulants Crosses the placenta Considered a teratogen Fetal effects include: Embryopathy (fetal warfarin syndrome)—growth restriction, blindness, optic atrophy, microphthalmia, nasal hypoplasia, hypoplasia of the extremities, stippled epiphyses, mental deficiency, seizures, hearing loss, congenital heart disease, scoliosis, death Central nervous system defects Spontaneous abortion Stillbirth Prematurity Hemorrhage
Anticonvulsants		
Carbamazepine	D	Crosses the placenta Considered a teratogen Associated with spina bifida, craniofacial defects, fingernail hypoplasia, and developmental delay
Ethosuximide (Zarontin)	C	Used for the treatment of petit mal epilepsy Not well studied, making conclusions regarding teratogenicity difficult

(continues)

*Risk Categories are defined at the end of this appendix.

TABLE B.1. *(Continued)*

Class	Drug	Risk category*	Pharmacokinetics/reported effects on fetus
	Ethosuximide (Zarontin) (cont.)		Some reported newborn associations in a limited number of exposures include patent ductus arteriosus, cleft lip/palate, mongoloid facies, altered palmar crease, accessory nipple, hydrocephalus Spontaneous hemorrhage in the newborn has been reported
	Phenobarbital	D	Crosses the placenta Considered a teratogen No specific phenotype (in contrast to phenytoin) Associated findings: cardiovascular defects, cleft lip/palate, early hemorrhagic disease of the newborn (induction of fetal liver microsomal enzymes depleting vitamin K and suppressing vitamin K–dependent coagulation factors) (See Chap. 26), barbiturate withdrawal, impaired cognitive development
	Phenytoin (Dilantin)	D	Crosses the placenta Considered a teratogen; some suggestion that this is dose-related Recognizable pattern of malformations known as fetal hydantoin syndrome. Features include broad nasal bridge, wide fontanelle, low-set hairline, broad alveolar ridge, metopic ridging, short neck, ocular hypertelorism, microcephaly, cleft lip/palate, abnormal or low-set ears, epicanthal folds, ptosis of eyelids, coloboma, coarse scalp hair, small or absent nails, hypoplasia of distal phalanges, altered palmar crease, digital thumb, dislocated hip, impaired growth, congenital heart defects, central nervous system malformations, mental deficiency May cause early hemorrhagic disease of the newborn (induction of fetal liver microsomal enzymes depleting vitamin K and suppressing vitamin K–dependent coagulation factors) (see Chap. 26)
	Primidone (Mysoline)	D	Structural analog of phenobarbital Considered a teratogen Also may be associated with hemorrhagic disease of the newborn

*Risk Categories are defined at the end of this appendix.

		Risk Category*	
Antiinfectives	**Valproic acid (Depakene)**	D	Readily crosses the placenta Associated fetal/newborn complications, including: congenital abnormalities: Valproic acid syndrome: neural tube defects, craniofacial, microcephaly, abnormal digits, hypospadias, congenital heart disease, delayed psychomotor development, growth restriction Other: hyperbilirubinemia, hepatotoxicity, transient hyperglycemia, withdrawal
	Amebicides Metronidazole	B	Crosses the placenta Although mutagenic and carcinogenic in bacteria and rats, no clear association of these properties in humans Majority of evidence suggests that there is no significant risk to the fetus
	Aminoglycosides Amikacin	C_B, D_M	Rapidly crosses the placenta Not considered a teratogen Theoretical risk of ototoxicity
	Gentamicin Neomycin Tobramycin Streptomycin	C	Rapidly crosses the placenta Not considered a teratogen Theoretical risk of ototoxicity Neonatal potentiation of $MgSO_4$-induced (magnesium sulfate) neuromuscular weakness has been reported, ototoxicity
	Antibiotics—general Chloramphenicol	C	Crosses the placenta at term Not considered a teratogen One report associating cardiovascular collapse (gray baby syndrome) in infants born to mothers receiving chloramphenicol during the latter stage of pregnancy
	Clindamycin	B	Crosses the placenta Not considered a teratogen

(continues)

Risk Categories are defined at the end of this appendix.

TABLE B.1. *(Continued)*

Class	Drug	Risk category*	Pharmacokinetics/reported effects on fetus
	Erythromycin	B	Crosses the placenta, but in very low concentrations Not considered a teratogen
	Pentamidine	C	Antiprotozoal agent
	Trimethoprim	C	Folate antagonist May be used alone or in combination with sulfonamides Crosses the placenta Some suggestion that use in the first trimester may cause structural defects: cardiovascular defects, neural tube defects
Antifungal Amphotericin B		B	Crosses the placenta Not considered a teratogen
Miconazole		C	Topical antifungal agent No reports documenting associated congenital malformations
Antiviral Acyclovir		B	Crosses the placenta No documented reports of adverse effects to the fetus or newborn
Cephalosporins Moxalactam		B C	Cephalosporins as a class of drug are generally considered safe to use during pregnancy Many have been shown to cross the placenta Some reports of possible cardiovascular malformations and oral cleft defects with cefaclor, ceftriaxone, cephalexin, and cephradrine
Povidone-iodine (Betadine)		D	Readily crosses the placenta May cause transient hypothyroidism
Penicillins		B	Many penicillin derivatives have been shown to readily cross the placenta As a class of drug, penicillins not considered teratogenic

*Risk Categories are defined at the end of this appendix.

756

Quinolones e.g., Ciprofloxacin Norfloxacin	C	Unknown for many quinolone derivatives whether transplacental passage occurs, although the molecule is small enough for this theoretically to be possible Norfloxacin and ofloxacin have been documented to cross the placenta Animal evidence suggests association with cartilage damage and arthropathy, although this has never been shown in human studies No strong or convincing evidence that quinolone use is associated with congenital abnormalities Some small reports of possible associated birth defects, although a consistent pattern has not been identified Most recommend not to use quinolones during pregnancy as safer alternatives exist
Sulfonamides	C D—if administered near term	Readily cross the placenta When close to term, documented associated toxicities include jaundice (competes with bilirubin for albumin-binding sites) and hemolytic anemia No strong evidence to suggest an association with congenital abnormalities
Tetracyclines e.g., Doxycycline Tetracycline	D	Crosses the placenta Associated with maternal hepatotoxicity Associated with disruption of fetal mineralized structures such as teeth (intense yellow staining) and bones Possible risk for minor fetal anomalies
Urinary germicides Nitrofurantoin	B	Not considered a teratogen Caution with use close to term secondary to reports of newborn hemolytic anemia in *G6PD* deficient infants
Antimalarials		
Chloroquine	C	Crosses the placenta Not considered a major teratogen, although a small association to birth defects could not be excluded
Hydroxychloroquine (Plaquenil)	C	Crosses the placenta Generally considered safe to use during pregnancy; however, studies and the number of exposures limited

(continues)

*Risk Categories are defined at the end of this appendix.

TABLE B.1. (Continued)

Class	Drug	Risk category*	Pharmacokinetics/reported effects on fetus
	Quinine	D_B, X_M	Considered a teratogen Reported associated congenital anomalies including CNS anomalies, limb defects, facial defects, heart defects, digestive organ anomalies, urogenital anomalies, hernias, and vertebral anomalies Reports of maternal and neonatal thrombocytopenia purpura Reports of neonatal hemolysis in *G6PD* deficient newborns
Antiparasitics	**Crotamiton 10%** (Eurax)	B	No toxicity reported in use in pregnancy and infants
	Lindane (gamma benzene hydrochloride, Kwell)	B	Possible association with hypospadias Theoretical concern for neurotoxicity, convulsions, and aplastic anemia, CNS toxicity has been reported in infants
	Mebendazole (Vermox)	C	No strong evidence to suggest association with congenital malformations
	Paromomycin	C	No linkage to congenital malformations
	Pyrethins piperonyl butoxide (A-200, RID, RTC)	C	Little data to assess safety Poorly absorbed, so should have minimal potential toxicity
	Thiabendazole	C	No reports of human teratogenicity
Antituberculars (see Chap. 23)	**Ethambutol**	B	Crosses the placenta No reports of associate congenital defects
	Ethionamide	C	One report of increased congenital anomalies
	Isoniazid	C	Crosses the placenta No strong association to congenital anomalies Two case reports of association with hemorrhagic disease of the newborn
	Rifampin	C	Crosses the placenta No strong association to congenital anomalies Association with hemorrhagic disease of the newborn

*Risk Categories are defined at the end of this appendix.

		D/X	
Cardiovascular	**Streptomycin**		Ototoxicity—other drugs available
	ACE inhibitors e.g., Captopril Enalapril	C D—if used in 2nd and 3rd trimesters	No apparent increased human fetal risk when used in first trimester 2nd- and 3rd-trimester use associated with fetal teratogenicity secondary to fetal hypotension and reduced renal blood flow resulting in anuria, renal dysgenesis, and renal failure. Anuria-associated oligohydramnios may result in fetal growth restriction, pulmonary hypoplasia, limb contractures, craniofacial deformation, and neonatal death
	Antiarrhythmic agents Lidocaine	B	Rapidly crosses the placenta Limited data with use as an antiarrhythmic during pregnancy; the few reports available do not suggest a significant risk to the fetus
	Procainamide	C	Has not been linked to congenital anomalies or adverse fetal or newborn effects
	Quinidine	C	Crosses the placenta Has not been linked to congenital anomalies Report of neonatal thrombocytopenia after maternal use
	Beta blockers Propranolol	C D—if used in 2nd or 3rd trimesters	Crosses the placenta Oxytocic effects Multiple reported fetal and neonatal effects: most commonly intrauterine growth restriction, hypoglycemia, and bradycardia
	Calcium channel blockers Diltiazem	C	Suggestion of increased risk for cardiovascular effects
	Verapamil	C	Crosses the placenta Has not been linked to congenital anomalies
	Digoxin	C	Transplacental passage and uptake by the fetus increasing with advancing gestational age No linkage to congenital anomalies Neonatal death has been reported after maternal overdose

(continues)

*Risk Categories are defined at the end of this appendix.

TABLE B.1. (Continued)

Class	Drug	Risk category*	Pharmacokinetics/reported effects on fetus
Diuretics	Acetazolamide	C	Carbonic anhydrase inhibitor No linkage to congenital anomalies in humans One report of neonatal sacrococcygeal teratoma; this possible association has not been supported by other reports
	Thiazidie diuretics	C D if used in PIH	Chlorothiazide, chlorthalidone, hydrochlorothiazide Readily crosses the placenta May decrease placental perfusion (use not recommended in pregnancy-induced hypertension due to baseline hypovolemic status) Can induce maternal hyperglycemia (infant should be observed for hypoglycemia secondary to hyperinsulinemic response to maternal hyperglycemia) Conflicting reports exist regarding association with congenital abnormalities; possible linkage to congenital heart defects with chlorthalidone with first-trimester use Neonatal thrombocytopenia, hemolytic anemia, and electrolyte imbalances have been reported
	Furosemide	C D if used in PIH	Crosses the placenta May decrease placental perfusion (use not recommended in pregnancy-induced hypertension due to baseline hypovolemic status) Associated with increased fetal urine production No strong association to major congenital anomalies; possibly associated with an increased risk for hypospadias
	Spironolactone	C D if used in PIH	Potassium-conserving diuretic Aldosterone antagonist in the distal convoluted renal tubule May decrease placental perfusion (use not recommended in pregnancy-induced hypertension due to baseline hypovolemic status) No strong association to major congenital anomalies; however, concern that the antiandrogenic effect caused feminization in male rat fetuses

*Risk Categories are defined at the end of this appendix.

Drug	Risk Category*	Comments
Other antihypertensives		
Diazoxide	C	Crosses the placenta May cause a rapid decrease in maternal blood pressure, decrease placental perfusion and fetal bradycardia; fewer effects seen with small doses at frequent intervals Uterine relaxant and therefore may inhibit uterine contractions Use associated with neonatal hyperglycemia
Methyldopa	B	Central-acting, antiadrenergic agent Crosses the placenta No association to congenital abnormalities Reports of neonatal decreased intracranial volume and reduced systolic blood pressure; neither considered clinically significant
Nitroprusside	C	Crosses the placenta No association to congenital abnormalities May see transient fetal bradycardia Standard maternal dosing does not appear to increase the risk for excessive cyanide accumulation in the fetus
Prazosin	C	Alpha 1-adrenergic blocking agent Crosses the placenta No association to congenital abnormalities
Vasodilators		
Dipyridamole	C	No association to congenital abnormalities Increases placental perfusion Clinical intervention trial suggests benefits of this therapy, including reduced incidence of stillbirth, placental infarction, and intrauterine growth restriction
Disopyramide	C	Crosses the placenta No association to congenital abnormalities Reports of oxytocic effect

(continues)

*Risk Categories are defined at the end of this appendix.

761

TABLE B.1. *(Continued)*

Class	Drug	Risk category*	Pharmacokinetics/reported effects on fetus
	Hydralazine	C	Crosses the placenta No association to congenital abnormalities Reports of fetal arrhythmia Neonatal reports of thrombocytopenia and bleeding; however, this may be related to severe maternal hypertension rather than the drug exposure One report of lupuslike syndrome developing in mother and baby after exposure resulting in a neonatal death
	Nitroglycerin	B_B, C_M	Rapid onset, short acting Reports, although limited in number, suggest no significant harm to the fetus Some reports of fetal bradycardia and loss of beat-to-beat variability in response to a reduction in maternal blood pressure; these fetal cardiac effects are apparently of no lasting clinical significance
Chemotherapy agents			Use of antineoplastic agents associated with low birth weight Limited exposures with often multiple agents used at once makes final interpretation of observations difficult Congenital anomalies of virtually all organ systems have been described
Alkylating agents			
	Cytarabine	D	Early use in the 1st and 2nd trimester is associated with chromosomal and congenital abnormalities Pancytopenia in the newborn has been reported with use during the third trimester
	Dactinomycin	C	Limited reports of use during pregnancy One report of six exposed pregnancies did not reveal an association with congenital anomalies
	Daunorubicin	D	In one series of 29 exposed pregnancies, newborn complications included anemia, hypoglycemia, electrolyte disturbances, and transient neutropenia
	Doxorubicin	D	Safe use in pregnancy not established Embryotoxic and teratogenic in rats

*Risk Categories are defined at the end of this appendix.

Drug	Risk Category*	Comments
Doxorubicin (cont.)		Embryotoxic and abortifacient in rabbits
5-Fluorouracil	D_B, X_M	Reported association with spontaneous abortions, cleft lip/palate, and ventricular septal defect (VSD)
6-Mercaptopurine	D	Neonatal pancytopenia and hemolytic anemia
Methotrexate	X	Folic acid antagonist Crosses the placenta Considered a teratogen Associated with severe newborn myelosuppression
Procarbazine	D	Associated with congenital abnormalities May produce gonadal dysfunction
Thioguanine	D	Purine analog interrupting nucleic acid biosynthesis Use associated with chromosomal abnormalities, missing digits
Vinca alkaloids	D	Antimitotic May produce gonadal dysfunction Associated with chromosomal abnormalities
Drugs of habit or abuse		
Caffeine	B	Crosses the placenta No association with congenital anomalies Moderate to heavy consumption associated with increased risk of late 1st- and 2nd-trimester spontaneous abortion In mothers who have experienced a prior loss, even light use has been shown to increase the risk of fetal loss Demonstration of increased fetal breathing and decreased heart rate after caffeine consumption Fetuses of mothers with high caffeine consumption have been shown to have less time in active sleep, and a greater time in arousal High caffeine consumption with cigarette smoking increases the risk for low birth weight more than with cigarette smoking alone Newborn cardiac arrhythmias have been described possibly related to caffeine withdrawal

(continues)

*Risk Categories are defined at the end of this appendix.

TABLE B.1. *(Continued)*

Class	Drug	Risk category*	Pharmacokinetics/reported effects on fetus
	Cocaine	C X if nonmedicinal	See Chap. 19
	Ethanol	D X if excessive or prolonged use	See Chap. 19
	Marijuana	C	See Chap. 19
	Tobacco	C	See Chap. 19
Gastrointestinal	**Anti-inflammatory** Sulfasalazine	B D—if used near term	Crosses the placenta No strong linkage to congenital abnormalities; however, reports of potential associations including cleft lip/palate, hydrocephalus, VSD, coarctation of the aorta, genitourinary abnormalities Caution near term due to the association between sulfonamides and newborn jaundice
	Antilipemic Cholestyramine	B	Resin that binds bile acids No linkage to congenital malformations One report of fetal subdural hematomas thought to be secondary to vitamin K deficiency caused by the drug or mother's underlying cholestasis
	Antisecretory Cimetidine	B	H_2-receptor antagonist inhibiting gastric acid secretion Crosses the placenta Antiadrenergic activity in animals, though not shown in humans No increased risk of congenital malformations
	Ranitidine	B	Like cimetidine; however, ranitidine does not shown antiadrenergic activity in animal or human studies

*Risk Categories are defined at the end of this appendix.

		Risk Category*	Comments
	Laxative		
	Docusate	C	No linkage to fetal toxicity or congenital malformations One report of maternal and neonatal hypomagnesemia thought to be secondary to docusate sodium
	Metoclopramide	B	Used in pregnancy for antiemetic effect and to decrease gastric emptying time Crosses the placenta at term No linkage to fetal toxicity or congenital malformations
Narcotics	**Butorphanol**	C	See Chap. 19
	Meperidine	B	
	Pentazocine	C	
	Propoxyphene	C for all, D if excessive or prolonged use at term	
Psychotherapeutic Agents	**Antipsychotics/ tranquilizers** *For schizophrenia:*		*General comments:* For drugs in this class that are used for schizophrenia, reports of newborn toxicity when used close to term. Two clinical syndromes described: 1. Syndrome more commonly seen with low-potency agents (e.g., chlorpromazine, prochlorperazine, thioridazine)—neonatal depression, lethargy, gastrointestinal dysfunction, and hypotension. These symptoms may last a few days. 2. Syndrome more commonly seen with high-potency agents (e.g., haloperidol)—extrapyramidal signs including tremors, increased tone, spasticity, posturing, arching of the back, hyperactive deep tendon reflexes, and shrill crying. These symptoms may last for several months. *(continues)*

*Risk Categories are defined at the end of this appendix.

TABLE B.1. *(Continued)*

Class	Drug	Risk category	Pharmacokinetics/reported effects on fetus
	Chlorpromazine	C	Crosses the placenta Considered safe when used in smaller, antiemetic dosages When used for analgesia during labor, marked drop in maternal blood pressures have been noted Most studies report no linkage to congenital anomalies
	Haloperidol	C	Conflicting reports regarding an association with limb reduction defects Possible association with cardiovascular defects Use during labor at suggested dosages has not been linked with neonatal effects
	Prochlorperazine, thioridazine	C	Crosses the placenta Use for nausea and vomiting considered safe Although conflicting results, most suggest that phenothiazines are safe when used in low doses
For bipolar disease:			
	Lithium	D	Crosses the placenta Serum half-life in newborns longer compared with adult values Strong association with congenital anomalies, especially cardiovascular defects (Ebstein's anomaly) Reported fetal and newborn toxicities, including cyanosis, hypotonia, bradycardia, thyroid depression and goiter, cardiomegaly, and diabetes insipidus Most neonatal toxic effects are self-limited
Benzodiazepines			
	Alprazolam	D	Most documented to readily cross the placenta with fetal accumulation of levels No linkage to congenital anomalies with alprazolam; however, reported associations with other drugs in this class:

*Risk Categories are defined at the end of this appendix.

Clonazepam	D	Clonazepam—congenital heart defects
Diazepam	D	Diazepam—cleft lip/palate (controversial, no linkage with more recent large cohort and case-control studies), inguinal hernia, dysmorphic features, fetal growth restriction, CNS defect
Lorazepam	D	Lorazepam—anal atresia
		Risk of newborn toxicity and withdrawal especially with increased dosages or prolonged use; described clinical presentation of toxicity and withdrawal include:
		1. "Floppy infant syndrome"—hypothermia, hypotonia, lethargy, sucking difficulties, apnea, cyanosis
		2. "Withdrawal syndrome"—tremors, irritability, inconsolable crying, restlessness, abnormal sleep pattern, hypertonicity, hyperreflexia, seizures, diarrhea, vomiting, vigorous sucking. These symptoms may present up to 3 weeks after delivery and last for several months.
		Long-term neurobehavioral consequences controversial and inadequately studied
Tricyclic antidepressants		
Amitriptyline	C	Crosses the placenta
Imipramine	D	Conflicting reports regarding association with limb reduction defects
Nortriptyline	D	Although small number of exposures, possible association with cardiovascular defects with imipramine and nortriptyline
		The following newborn effects have been described with imipramine and nortriptyline use: periodic apnea, cyanosis, tachypnea, respiratory distress, irritability, seizures, feeding difficulties, heart failure, tachycardia, myoclonus, and urinary retention
		Long-term neurodevelopmental studies lacking, one report of no lasting neurodevelopmental effect
Selective serotonin reuptake inhibitors		
Fluoxetine	C	No apparent linkage to congenital anomalies
Fluvoxamine	C	A neonatal withdrawal syndrome has been described. Onset may occur up to a few days after delivery and last for several months. Symptoms similar to those described for benzodiazepines

(continues)

*Risk Categories are defined at the end of this appendix.

TABLE B.1. *(Continued)*

Class	Drug	Risk category*	Pharmacokinetics/reported effects on fetus
	Selective serotonin reuptake inhibitors (cont.)		Long-term neurobehavioral data for exposed infants is lacking, one report of no lasting neurodevelopmental effect with fluoxetine use (Nulman)
	Paroxetine	C	
	Sertraline	B	
	Venlafaxine	C	
Thyroid medications	**Thyroid supplementation**		
	Levothyroxine	A	See Chap. 2
	Antithyroid		
	Methimazole	D	See Chap. 2
	Propylthiouracil	D	

ACE = angiotensin converting enzyme; CNS = central nervous system; IV = intravenous; NSAIDs = nonsteroidal anti-inflammatory drugs; PIH = pregnancy-induced hypertension; VSD = ventricular septal defect.

*Risk Categories are defined at the end of this appendix.

A. References used to create the summary table are stated at the end of this appendix.

B. **Pregnancy risk category**

   1. **The Food and Drug Administration** has offered a classification system to assign the risk of a particular drug to the fetus during pregnancy (*Federal Register* 1980;44:37434–37467). The classification system is as follows:

   a. **Category A.** Controlled studies show no risk. Adequate, well-controlled studies in pregnant women have not demonstrated a risk to the fetus in the first trimester of pregnancy, and there is no evidence of risk in later trimesters.

   b. **Category B.** No evidence of risk in humans. Animal studies have not demonstrated a risk to the fetus, but there are no adequate studies in pregnant women; or animal studies have shown an adverse effect, but adequate studies in pregnant women have not demonstrated a risk to the fetus during the first trimester of pregnancy, and there is no evidence of risk in later trimesters.

   c. **Category C.** Risk cannot be ruled out. Animal studies have shown an adverse effect on the fetus, but there are no adequate studies in humans, or there are no animal reproduction studies and no adequate studies in humans.

   d. **Category D.** There is evidence of human fetal risk, but the potential benefits from the use of the drug in pregnant women may be acceptable despite its potential risks.

   e. **Category X.** Contraindicated in pregnancy. Studies in animals or humans demonstrate fetal abnormalities or adverse reaction; reports indicate evidence of fetal risk. The risk of use in pregnant women clearly outweighs any possible benefit to the patient.

   2. **All medications have a risk/benefit ratio.** The clinician must get the best information available, inadequate as it may be, and decide if the mother's condition is such that use of a certain medication is required.

   3. The **risk category was assigned** by referencing the textbook by Briggs et al. (Briggs G.G., Freeman R.K., Yaffe S.J. *Drugs in Pregnancy and Lactation: A Reference Guide to Fetal and Neonatal Risk*, 6th ed. 2002; Philadelphia: Lippincott Williams & Wilkins) or by using the manufacturer's ratings. If Briggs et al. and the manufacturer's ratings differed from one another, both categories were listed (Briggs = subscript B; Manufacturer = subscript M).

   4. Briggs et. al. provided additional information beyond that provided by the manufacturer, which is helpful to the reader.

   5. Manufacturer's recommendations and package inserts should be checked before the fetus is exposed to these agents for the most current information.

   6. Additional information can be found at the Pregnancy Environmental Hotline (800-322-5014 or 617-466-8471, fax 617-487-2361), sponsored by the National Birth Defects Center and the Genesis Fund.

Suggested Readings

American Academy of Pediatrics, Committee on Drugs. Use of psychoactive medication during pregnancy and possible effects on the fetus and newborn. *Pediatrics* 2000;105:880–887.

Berkovitch M. Fetal effects of metoclopramide therapy for nausea and vomiting of pregnancy. *N Engl J Med* 2000;343:445–446.

Berlin C.M., Jr. Effects of drugs on the fetus. *Pediatr Rev* 1991;12:282–287.

Bodendorfer T.W. Obtaining drug exposure histories during pregnancy. *Am J Obstet Gynecol* 1979;135:490–494.

Boyle R.J. Effects of certain prenatal drugs on the fetus and newborn. *Pediatr Rev* 2000;23:17–24.

Briggs G.G. *Drugs in Pregnancy and Lactation.* 2002; Philadelphia: Lippincott Williams & Wilkins.

Briggs G.G., Freeman R.K., Yaffe S.G. *Drugs in Pregnancy and Lactation: A Reference Guide to Fetal and Neonatal Risk,* 6th ed., 2002; Philadelphia: Lippincott Williams & Wilkins.

Dean J.C. Long-term health and neurodevelopment in children exposed to antiepileptic drugs before birth. *J Med Genet* 2002;39:251–259.

Holmes L.B. The teratogenicity of anticonvulsant drugs. *N Engl J Med* 2001; 344:1132–1138.

Kalter H. Medical progress: Congenital malformations: Etiologic factors and their role in prevention (first of two parts). *N Engl J Med* 1983;308:424–431.

Kalter H. Medical progress: Congenital malformations: (second of two parts). *N Engl J Med* 1983;308:491–497.

Koren G. Drugs in pregnancy. *N Engl J Med* 1998;338:1128–1137.

Levy G. Pharmacokinetics of fetal and neonatal exposure to drugs. *Obstet Gynecol* 1981;58:9S–16S.

Murray L. Drug therapy during pregnancy and lactation. *Emerg Med Clin North Am* 1994;12:129–149.

Neubert D. Principles and problems in assessing prenatal toxicity. *Arch Toxicol* 1987;60:238–245.

Nordeng H. Neonatal withdrawal syndrome after in utero exposure to selective serotonin reuptake inhibitors. *Acta Paediatr* 2001;90:288–291.

Nulman I. Neurodevelopment of children exposed in utero to antidepressant drugs. *N Engl J Med* 1997;336:258–262.

Szeto H.H. Maternal-fetal pharmacokinetics and fetal dose-response relationships. *Ann NY Acad Sci* 1989;562:42–55.

Szeto H.H. Kinetics of drug transfer to the fetus. *Clin Obstet Gynecol* 1993; 36:246–254.

Szeto H.H. Maternal-fetal pharmacokinetics: Summary and future directions. *NIDA Res Monogr* 1995;154:203–217.

Ward R.M. Maternal-placental-fetal unit: Unique problems of pharmacologic study. *Pediatr Clin North Am* 1989;36:1075–1088.

Ward R.M. Drug therapy of the fetus. *J Clin Pharmacol* 1993;33:780–789.

APPENDIX C. MATERNAL MEDICATIONS AND BREASTFEEDING

Karen M. Puopolo

I. **Background.** Questions commonly arise regarding the safety of maternal medication use during breastfeeding. A combination of the biological and chemical properties of the drug and the physiology of the mother and infant determine the safety of any individual medication. Consideration is given to the amount of drug that is found in breast milk, the half-life of the drug in the infant, and the biological effect of the drug on the infant.

   A. **Drug properties that affect entry into breast milk.** Molecular size, pH, pKa, lipid solubility, and protein-binding properties of the drug all affect the **M/P ratio,** which is defined as the relative concentration of the protein-free fraction of the drug in milk and maternal plasma. Small molecular size, slightly alkaline pH, nonionization, high lipid solubility, and lack of binding to serum proteins all favor entry of a drug into breast milk. The half-life of the medication and frequency of drug administration are also important; the longer the cumulative time the drug is present in the maternal circulation, the greater the opportunity for it to appear in breast milk.

   B. **Maternal factors.** The total maternal dose and mode of administration (intravenous versus oral) as well as maternal illness (particularly renal or liver impairment) can affect the persistence of the drug in the maternal circulation. Medications taken in the first few days postpartum are more likely to enter breast milk as the mammary alveolar epithelium does not fully mature until the end of the first postpartum week.

   C. **Infant factors.** The maturity of the infant is the primary factor determining the persistence of a drug in the infant's system. Preterm infants and term infants in the first month after birth metabolize drugs more slowly because of renal and hepatic immaturity. The total dose of drug that the infant is exposed to is determined by the volume of milk ingested (per kg of body weight) as well as the frequency of feeding (or frequency of milk expression in the case of preterm infants).

II. **Determination of drug safety during breastfeeding.** A number of available resources evaluate the risk of individual medications to the breastfed infant. Ideally, direct measurements of the entry of a drug into breast milk, and the level and persistence of the drug in the breastfed infant, as well as experience with exposure of infants to the drug, are all used to make a judgment regarding drug safety. Unfortunately, this type of information is available for relatively few medications. In the absence of specific data, a judgment is made on the basis of both the known pharmacologic properties of the drug and the known or predicted affects of the drug on the developing infant. Clinicians providing advice to the nursing mother about the safety of a particular medication should be aware of the following points.

   A. **Resources may differ in their judgment of a particular drug.** Information about some medications (especially newer ones) is in flux, and safety judgments may change over a relatively short period of time. Different resources approach the question of medication use in breastfeeding with different perspectives. For example, *The Physicians Desk Reference* is a compendium of commercially supplied drug information. In the absence of specific data regarding the entry of a drug into breast milk, drug manufacturers generally do not make a definitive statement about the safety of drugs in breastfeeding. Other resources, such as *Medications in Mother's Milk,* take the available data and make a judgment about relative safety of the drug.

   B. **The safety of a drug in pregnancy is often not the same as the safety of the drug during breastfeeding.** Occasionally a medication that is contraindicated in pregnancy (for example, warfarin or ibuprofen) is safe to use while breastfeeding.

C. **Definitive data are not available for most medications or for specific clinical situations.** There is a need for individualized clinical judgment in many cases, taking into account the available information, the need of the mother for the medication, and the risk to the infant of both exposure to the drug and of exposure to breast-milk substitutes. Consultation with the **Breastfeeding and Human Lactation Study Center** at the University of Rochester can aid the clinician in making specific clinical judgments.

III. **Resources.** Resources listed as items III.A, III.B, III.C, III.D, and III.E served as source material for this appendix. Resources III.A–E are used to guide clinical decision making regarding breastfeeding at our institution.

A. **American Academy of Pediatrics, Committee on Drugs. Transfer of drugs and other chemicals into human milk.** *Pediatrics* 108(3): 2001;776–789. This AAP Pediatrics Policy Statement on medication use and breastfeeding is available via the Internet at http://www.aap.org/policy/0063.html. This statement sites nearly 400 primary references to place more than 150 substances in six different categories:

1. **Cytotoxic drugs** that may interfere with cellular metabolism of the nursing infant and are contraindicated during breastfeeding.
2. **Drugs of abuse** for which adverse effects on the infant during breastfeeding have been reported and are contraindicated during breastfeeding.
3. **Radioactive compounds** that require temporary cessation of breastfeeding.
4. **Drugs for which the effect on nursing infants is unknown** but may be of concern.
5. **Drugs that have been associated with significant effects** on some nursing infants and should be given to nursing mothers with caution.
6. **Maternal medication** usually compatible with breastfeeding.
7. **Food and environmental agent** effects on breastfeeding are also included in a separate evaluation.

B. Briggs G.G., et al. (Eds.) *Drugs in Pregnancy and Lactation,* 6th ed. 2001; Baltimore: Williams and Wilkins. This book lists primary references and reviews data on hundreds of medications with respect to the risk to the developing fetus and the risk in breastfeeding. The book lists the Food and Drug Administration's Pregnancy Risk Category and the American Academy of Pediatrics rating (when available) for each medication.

C. Hale T. *Medications and Mother's Milk,* 10th ed. 2002; Amarillo, Tex.: Pharmasoft Medical Publishing. This book is a comprehensive listing of hundreds of medications, with primary references sited for most. The Food and Drug Administration–assigned Pregnancy Risk Category and American Academy of Pediatrics evaluation are provided for each drug. The author's own evaluation category is as follows:

1. L1: Safest.
2. L2: Safer.
3. L3: Moderately safe. Many drugs fall into this category, which is defined as follows: "There are no controlled studies in breastfeeding women, however, the risk of untoward effects to a breastfed infant is possible, or controlled studies show only minimal, unthreatening effects. Drugs should be given only if the potential benefit justifies the risk to the infant."
4. L4: Possibly hazardous.
5. L5: Contraindicated.
6. Specific drug updates and supplemental information for this reference are available on the Internet at http://neonatal.ttuhsc.edu.

D. Lawrence R. *Breastfeeding: A Guide for the Medical Professional,* 5th ed. 1999; St. Louis: CV Mosby Co. This book includes an extended discussion of the pharmacology of drug entry into breast milk. An appendix contains a listing of more than 500 drugs listed by drug category (analgesics, antibiotics, etc.) with the American Academy of Pediatrics safety rating, if available. The appendix also contains extensive pharmacokinetic data for each drug, including values for the M/P ratio and maximum amount (mg/mL) of drug found in breast milk.

E. Riordan J., Auerbach K.G. *Breastfeeding and Human Lactation,* 2nd ed. 1998; Sudbury, Mass.: Jones and Bartlett Publishers. This book discusses the pharmacology of drugs and breast milk, the effect of drugs on milk volume, and the safety of broad categories of drugs in breastfeeding. An appendix contains the American Academy of Pediatrics Policy Statement on the Transfer of Drugs and Other Chemicals into Human Milk and a listing of generic and trade names of common medications.

F. **The Breastfeeding and Human Lactation Study Center.** The Study Center maintains a drug data bank that is updated monthly. Health professionals may call the phone number listed below to talk to staff members regarding the safety of a particular drug in breastfeeding. The Study Center will provide information immediately by telephone or will supply information by E-mail, return mail, or fax. The Study Center will only take calls from healthcare professionals (not parents). General information about this program can be found at www.cdc.gov/breastfeeding/compend-bhlsc.htm. Contact information: The Breastfeeding and Human Lactation Study Center, University of Rochester School of Medicine and Dentistry, Department of Pediatrics, Box 777, 601 Elmwood Avenue, Rochester, NY 14642; Telephone: (585) 275–0088, Fax: (585) 461–3614.

G. **The Food and Drug Administration's Pregnancy Risk Categories** for drugs are detailed at http://www.fda.gov/fdac/features/2001/301_preg.html#categories. A brief summary is as follows:

1. **Category A.** Controlled studies in women fail to demonstrate a risk to the fetus.

2. **Category B.** Either animal-reproduction studies have not demonstrated a fetal risk or, if such a risk was found, it was not confirmed in later controlled studies in women.

3. **Category C.** Either studies in animals have revealed adverse effects on the fetus and there are no controlled studies in women, or studies in women and animals are not available. Drugs should be given only if the potential benefit justifies the potential risk to the fetus.

4. **Category D.** There is positive evidence of human fetal risk, but the benefits from use in pregnant women may be acceptable despite the risk (e.g., in a life-threatening situation or for a serious disease).

5. **Category X.** Studies in animals or human beings have demonstrated fetal abnormalities, and the risk of the use of the drug in pregnant women clearly outweighs any possible benefit.

IV. **Information on common medications.** Following are tables of medications commonly prescribed to breastfeeding women. They are organized by category and are listed alphabetically within each category, with the Food and Drug Administration Pregnancy Risk Category (PRA), A–D and X; American Academy of Pediatrics (AAP) rating (1–6, or NR = not reviewed), the *Medications in Mother's Milk* (MMM) rating (L1–L5).

TABLE C.1. ANTIBIOTICS

Medication	PRC	AAP	MMM
Acyclovir	C	6	L2
Amikacin	C	NR	L2
Amoxicillin	B	6	L1
Amphotericin B	B	NR	L3
Ampicillin/Unasyn	B	NR	L1
Augmentin	B	NR	L1
Azithromycin	B	NR	L2
Aztreonam	B	6	L2
Carbenicillin	B	NR	L1
Cefprozil	C	6	L1

Cephalosporins:
  *List 1:
  †List 2:
	
	B
	B
		
		6 or NR
		6 or NR
			
			L1
			L2

Ciprofloxacin	C	6	L4
Clarithromycin	C	NR	L2
Clindamycin	B	6	L3
Doxycycline	D	NR	L3 (acute), L4 (chronic)
Erythromycin	B	6	L1
Famciclovir	B	NR	L2
Floxacillin	B1	NR	L1
Fluconazole	C	6	L2
Gentamicin	C	NR	L2
Griseofulvin	C	NR	L2
Imipenem-cilastatin	C	NR	L2
Isoniazid	C	6	L3
Itraconazole	C	NR	L2
Kanamycin	D	6	L2
Ketoconazole	C	6	L2
Loracarbef	B	NR	L2
Methicillin	B	NR	L3
Metronidazole	B	4	L2
Minocycline	D	NR	L2 (acute), L4 (chronic)
Mupirocin	B	NR	L1
Nafcillin	B	NR	L1
Nitrofurantoin	B	6	L2

(continues)

TABLE C.1. *Continued*

Medication	PRC	AAP	MMM
Norfloxacin	C	NR	L3
Ofloxacin	C	6	L3
Penicillin G	B	6	L1
Piperacillin/Zosyn	B	NR	L2
Sulfamethoxazole	C	NR	L3
Trimethoprim	C	6	L3

AAP = American Academy of Pediatrics; MMM = *Medications in Mother's Milk;* NR= not reviewed; PRC = pregnancy risk category.
*List 1: cefadroxil, cefazolin, cefoxitin, ceftazidime, cephalexin, cephapirin, cephradine.
†List 2: cefaclor, cefdinir, ceftibulen, cefepime, cefixime, cefoperazone, cefotaxime, cefotetan, cefpodoxime, ceftriaxone, cefuroxime, cephalothin.

TABLE C.2. ANALGESICS

Medication	PRC	AAP	MMM
Acetaminophen	B	6	L1
Aspirin	C/D	5	L3
Butorphanol	B/D	6	L3
Codeine	C	6	L3
Fentanyl	B	6	L2
Hydrocodone	B	NR	L3
Hydromorphone	C	NR	L3
Ibuprofen	B/D	6	L1
Indomethacin	B/D	6	L3
Ketorolac	B/D	6	L2
Meperidine	B	6	L2/L3 (early postpartum)
Methadone	B	6	L3
Morphine	B	6	L3
Nubain	B	NR	L3
Naproxen	B	6	L3/L4 (chronic use)
Oxycodone	B	NR	L3

AAP = American Academy of Pediatrics; MMM = *Medications in Mother's Milk;* NR = not reviewed; PRC = pregnancy risk category.

TABLE C.3. **ANTIHYPERTENSIVE AND CARDIAC MEDICATIONS**

Medication	PRC	AAP	MMM
Amiodarone	C	4	L5
Atenolol	C	5	L3
Captopril	D	6	L4 (L3 after 30 days of age)
Clonidine	C	NR	L3
Digoxin	C	6	L2
Diltiazem	C	6	L3
Dopamine/dobutamine	C	NR	L2
Enalapril	C/D	6	L4 (early postpartum)/L2
Epinephrine	C	NR	L1
Flecainide	C	6	L4
Hydralazine	C	6	L2
Labetalol	C	6	L2
Magnesium sulfate	B	6	L1
Methyldopa	C	6	L2
Nifedipine	C	6	L2
Nimodipine	C	NR	L2
Procainamide	C	6	L2
Propanolol	C	6	L3

AAP = American Academy of Pediatrics; MMM = *Medications in Mother's Milk*; NR = not reviewed; PRC = pregnancy risk category.

TABLE C.4. ALLERGY AND RESPIRATORY MEDICATIONS

Medication	PRC	AAP	MMM
Albuterol	C	NR	L1
Beclomethasone	C	NR	L2
Betamethasone	C	NR	L3
Budesonide	C	NR	L3
Cetirizine (Zyrtec)	B	NR	L2
Clemastine (Tavist)	C	5	L4
Cromolyn sodium	B	NR	L1
Dexamethasone	C	NR	L3
Dextromethorphan	C	NR	L1
Diphenhydramine	C	NR	L2
Fexofenadine (Allegra)	C	6	L3
Flunisolide	C	NR	L3
Hydrocortisone (topical)	C	NR	L2
Loratadine (Claritin)	B	6	L2
Methylprednisolone	C	6	L2
Montelukast (Singulair)	B	NR	L3
Phenylephrine	C	NR	L3
Prednisone	B	6	L2/L4 (chronic high dose)
Pseudoephedrine*	C	6	L3/L4
Theophylline	C	6	L3

AAP = American Academy of Pediatrics; MMM = *Medications in Mother's Milk*; NR = not reviewed; PRC = pregnancy risk category.
*Pseudoephedrine and most antihistamines can decrease milk production.

TABLE C.5. PSYCHOACTIVE MEDICATIONS

Medication	PRC	AAP	MMM
Alprazolam	D	4	L3
Amitryptyline	D	4	L2
Bupropion	B	4	L3
Caffeine	B	6	L2
Carbamazepine	C	6	L2
Chloral hydrate	C	6	L3
Chlordiazepoxide	D	NR	L3
Chlorpromazine	C	4	L3
Citalopram (Celexa)	C	NR	L3
Clomipramine	C	4	L2
Clonazepam	C	NR	L3
Clozapine	C	4	L3
Desipramine	C	4	L2
Diazepam	D	4	L3/L4 (chronic use)
Domperidone	NR	6	L2
Fluoxetine (Prozac)	B	4	L3 (neonatal), L2 (older infant)
Gabapentin	C	NR	L3
Haloperidol	C	4	L2
Lithium	D	5	L4
Lorazepam	D	4	L3
Methylphenidate (Ritalin)	C	NR	L4
Midazolam	D	4	L3
Oxazepam	D	NR	L3
Paroxetine (Paxil)	B	4	L2
Pentobarbital	D	NR	L3
Phenobarbital	D	5	L3
Phenytoin	D	6	L2
Prochlorperazine	C	NR	L3
Sertraline (Zoloft)	B	4	L2
Valproic acid	D	6	L2

AAP = American Academy of Pediatrics; MMM = *Medications in Mother's Milk*; NR = not reviewed; PRC = pregnancy risk category.

TABLE C.6. GASTROINTESTINAL MEDICATIONS

Medication	PRC	AAP	MMM
Bismuth subsalicylate	C/D	4	L3
Cimetidine	B	6	L2
Docusate	C	NR	L2
Kaolin-pectin	C	NR	L2
Loperamide	B	6	L2
Metoclopramide	B	4	L2
Nizatidine	C	NR	L2
Omeprazole	C	NR	L2
Ondansetron	B	NR	L2
Ranitidine	B	NR	L2

AAP = American Academy of Pediatrics; MMM = *Medications in Mother's Milk*; NR = not reviewed; PRC = pregnancy risk category.

TABLE C.7. MEDICATIONS CONTRAINDICATED IN BREASTFEEDING

Amiodarone

Antineoplastic agents

Bromocriptine

Chloramphenicol

Drugs of abuse

Diethylstilbestrol

Disulfiram

Lithium*

Radioisotopes—usually require only temporary cessation of breastfeeding

Tamoxifen

Note on oral contraceptives: Estrogen-containing preparations can reduce milk supply. Progestin-only oral contraceptives are safer with respect to milk production.
*Note on Lithium: Listed as PRC=D, AAP=5, MMM=L4. Infant serum lithium levels 30–40% of mother's level. Infant must be closely monitored by a pediatrician if used during breastfeeding. Drug has potential effects on infant neurodevelopment, cardiac rhythm, and thyroid function.

APPENDIX D. SELECTED CHEMISTRY NORMAL VALUES

Ann R. Stark

Test	Age	Normal Range	Units
Alanine aminotransferase (ALT)		3–54	U/L
Albumin		2.5–4.0	g/dL
Alkaline phosphatase		110–400	U/L
Ammonia		20–80	μg/dL
Aspartate aminotransferase (AST)		10–65	U/L
Bicarbonate		19–25	mEq/L
Bilirubin, direct		<0.6	mg/dL
Bilirubin, total (TSB)	cord	<2.8	mg/dL
	24 h[†]	<8.0	mg/dL
	48 h[†]	<13.0	mg/dL
	72 h[†]	<16.0	mg/dL
	3–7 d	<12.0	mg/dL
	7–30 d	<7.0	mg/dL
Blood urea nitrogen (BUN)		3–25	mg/dL
Calcium	term, <1 wk	7.0–12.0	mg/dL
	preterm, <1 wk	6.0–10.0	mg/dL
Chloride		88–111	mEq/L
Creatinine	1–4 d	0.3–1.0	mg/dL
	5 d–2 yr	0.2–0.4	mg/dL
Glucose		40–100	mg/dL
Magnesium		1.6–2.2	mg/dL
Phosphorus		4.5–9.0	mg/dL
Potassium		3.5–5.5	mEq/dL
Sodium		135–148	mEq/L
Total protein		4.2–6.6	g/dL
Uric acid		2.0–5.5	mg/dL

*Values for term newborns, unless indicated.
†Values represent 95th percentile for TSB at the indicated hour (see Chap. 18 and Bhutani V.K., et al. Predictive ability of a predischarge hour-specific serum bilirubin for subsequent significant hyperbilirubinemia in healthy term and near-term newborns. *Pediatrics* 1999;103:6.
Source: Chemistry Normal Values, Children's Hospital Boston.

SUBJECT INDEX

Page numbers followed by *f* indicate figures; page numbers followed by *t* indicate tables.

A

AAP. *See* American Academy of
Pediatrics (AAP)
Abandonment, 170
Abdomen
distention of, 652–653, 666
examination of, 38, 42
masses of, 624*t*, 664
paracentesis, 701
x-rays of
for necrotizing enterocolitis, 645
in surgical emergencies, 665
ABG, 362
with pneumothorax, 372
transient tachypnea, 384
Abnormal urine odors
associated with inborn errors of
metabolism, 593, 595*t*
ABO hemolytic disease, 218–219
Abused drugs
contraindicating breastfeeding, 140
Acardia, 91
Acetaminophen, 709*t*
fetal effects of, 750*t*
Acetazolamide, 717
fetal effects of, 760*t*
for germinal matrix hemorrhage/
intraventricular hemorrhage,
533
Acetylsalicylic acid (aspirin)
fetal effects of, 750*t*
Acid
handling, 622–623
Acid-base
normal physiology, 107–108
Acid-base balance
complicating exchange transfusion,
212
Acid-base disorders
with inborn errors of metabolism,
592–593
Acquired heart disease, 449
Acquired immunodeficiency syndrome
(AIDS), 267
Acquired mechanical obstruction, 658
Acquired thrombophilia, 494
Acute hemolytic transfusion reactions,
490–491
Acute lung injury, 393
Acute renal failure, 630–631
Acute transfusion reactions, 490–491
Acyclovir, 717
fetal effects of, 756*t*

for herpes simplex virus (HSV),
262–263
Adenosine, 458–459
Adhesives
avoidance of, 669
Adjunctive immunotherapy
for bacterial meningitis and sepsis,
289
Adrenal glands
injuries of, 245
AFP, 95
African Americans
prematurity among, 45–46
Afterload reducing agents, 450–451
AIDS, 267
Air leak, 360
during delivery, 67
with meconium aspiration syndrome
(MAS), 405
pulmonary, 371–377
with respiratory distress syndrome
(RDS), 347
Air transports, 157
Air travel
by very low birth weight (VLBW),
163
Alagille syndrome, 415*t*
Albinism, 674
Albright syndrome, 673
Albumin, 185
drugs causing displacement of from
bilirubin, 186*f*
Alcohol
and breastfeeding, 140
Allergic transfusion reactions,
491
Allergy medications
breastfeeding, 777*t*
Alloimmune thrombocytopenia,
482–484
Alpha-fetoprotein (AFP), 95
Alprazolam
fetal effects of, 766*t*
Alprostadil, 717–718
Ambiguous genitalia, 607–618
causes of, 614*t*–615*t*
evaluation of, 617*f*
nursery evaluation of, 609–611
American Academy of Pediatrics (AAP)
breastfeeding
medications, 772
pain
management of, 704

WEIGHT (MASS) (POUNDS [LB] AND OUNCES [OZ] TO GRAMS [G])

Example: To obtain g equivalent to 6 lb, 8 oz, read 6 on top scale, 8 on side scale; equivalent is 2948 g.

Ounces (oz)	Pounds (lb)										
	0	1	2	3	4	5	6	7	8	9	10
0	0	454	907	1361	1814	2268	2722	3175	3629	4082	4536
1	28	482	936	1389	1843	2296	2750	3203	3657	4111	4564
2	57	510	964	1417	1871	2325	2778	3232	3685	4139	4593
3	85	539	992	1446	1899	2353	2807	3260	3714	4167	4621
4	113	567	1021	1474	1928	2381	2835	3289	3742	4196	4649
5	142	595	1049	1503	1956	2410	2863	3317	3770	4224	4678
6	170	624	1077	1531	1984	2438	2892	3345	3799	4252	4706
7	198	652	1106	1559	2013	2466	2920	3374	3827	4281	4734
8	227	680	1134	1588	2041	2495	2948	3402	3856	4309	4763
9	255	709	1162	1616	2070	2523	2977	3430	3884	4337	4791
10	283	737	1191	1644	2098	2551	3005	3459	3912	4366	4819
11	312	765	1219	1673	2126	2580	3033	3487	3941	4394	4848
12	340	794	1247	1701	2155	2608	3062	3515	3969	4423	4876
13	369	822	1276	1729	2183	2637	3090	3544	3997	4451	4904
14	397	850	1304	1758	2211	2665	3118	3572	4026	4479	4933
15	425	879	1332	1786	2240	2693	3147	3600	4054	4508	4961

Note: 1 lb = 453.59237 g; 1 oz = 28.349523 g; 1000 g = 1 kg. Gram equivalents have been rounded to whole numbers by adding 1 when the first decimal place is 5 or greater.

LENGTH (INCHES [IN.] TO CENTIMETERS [CM])

1-in. increments
Example: To obtain cm equivalent to 22 in., read *20* on top scale, *2* on side scale; equivalent is 55.9 cm.

In.	0	10	20	30
0	0	25.4	50.8	76.2
1	2.5	27.9	53.3	78.7
2	5.1	30.5	55.9	81.3
3	7.6	33.0	58.4	83.8
4	10.2	35.6	61.0	86.4
5	12.7	38.1	63.5	88.9
6	15.2	40.6	66.0	91.4
7	17.8	43.2	68.6	94.0
8	20.3	45.7	71.1	96.5
9	22.9	48.3	73.7	99.1

One-quarter (¼)-in. increments
Example: To obtain cm equivalent to 14¾ in., read *14* on top scale, ¾ on side scale; equivalent is 37.5 cm.

10–15 in.	10	11	12	13	14	15
0	25.4	27.9	30.5	33.0	35.6	38.1
¼	26.0	28.6	31.1	33.7	36.2	38.7
½	26.7	29.2	31.8	34.3	36.8	39.4
¾	27.3	29.8	32.4	34.9	37.5	40.0

16–21 in.	16	17	18	19	20	21
0	40.6	43.2	45.7	48.3	50.8	53.3
¼	41.3	43.8	46.4	48.9	51.4	54.0
½	41.9	44.5	47.0	49.5	52.1	54.6
¾	42.5	45.1	47.6	50.2	52.7	55.2

Note: 1 in. = 2.540 cm. Centimeter equivalents rounded one decimal place by adding 0.1 when second decimal place is 5 or greater; for example, 33.48 becomes 33.5.

TEMPERATURE (FAHRENHEIT [F] TO CENTIGRADE [C])

°F	°C	°F	°C	°F	°C	°F	°C
95.0	35.0	98.0	36.7	101.0	38.3	104.0	40.0
95.2	35.1	98.2	36.8	101.2	38.4	104.2	40.1
95.4	35.2	98.4	36.9	101.4	38.6	104.4	40.2
95.6	35.3	98.6	37.0	101.6	38.7	104.6	40.3
95.8	35.4	98.8	37.1	101.8	38.8	104.8	40.4
96.0	35.6	99.0	37.2	102.0	38.9		
96.2	35.7	99.2	37.3	102.2	39.0		
96.4	35.8	99.4	37.4	102.4	39.1		
96.6	35.9	99.6	37.6	102.6	39.2		
96.8	36.0	99.8	37.7	102.8	39.3		
97.0	36.1	100.0	37.8	103.0	39.4		
97.2	36.2	100.2	37.9	103.2	39.6		
97.4	36.3	100.4	38.0	103.4	39.7		
97.6	36.4	100.6	38.1	103.6	39.8		
97.8	36.6	100.8	38.2	103.8	39.9		

Note: °C = (F − 32) × ⅝. Centigrade temperature equivalents rounded to one decimal place by adding 0.1 when second decimal place is 5 or greater.
The metric system replaces the term *centigrade* with *Celsius* (the inventor of the scale).